MAJOR DRUG CLASSES AND THEIR PROTOTYPES

DIURETICS

High-Ceiling (Loop) Diuretics
    Furosemide
Thiazide Diuretics
    Hydrochlorothiazide
Potassium-Sparing Diuretics
    Spironolactone
    Triamterene

CARDIOVASCULAR DRUGS

Angiotensin-Converting Enzyme (ACE) Inhibitors
    Captopril
Calcium Channel Blockers
    Agents That Affect the Heart and Blood Vessels
        Verapamil
    Agents That Affect Blood Vessels Primarily
        Nifedipine
Drugs for Hypertension
    Diuretics
        Hydrochlorothiazide
        Furosemide
        Spironolactone
    Beta-Adrenergic Blockers
        Propranolol
        Metoprolol
    Alpha-Adrenergic Blockers
        Prazosin
    Combined Alpha / Beta Blocker
        Labetalol
    Centrally Acting Antiadrenergics
        Clonidine
        Methyldopa
    ACE Inhibitors
        Captopril
        Enalapril
    Calcium Channel Blockers
        Verapamil
        Nifedipine
Drugs for Angina Pectoris
    Organic Nitrates
        Nitroglycerin
    Beta Blockers
        Propranolol
        Metoprolol
    Calcium Channel Blockers
        Verapamil
        Nifedipine
Drugs for Congestive Heart Failure
    Diuretics
        Hydrochlorothiazide
        Furosemide
        Spironolactone
    Vasodilators
        Captopril (ACE inhibitor)

Inotropic Agents
    Digoxin (a cardiac glycoside)
    Dopamine (a sympathomimetic)
Antidysrhythmic Drugs
    Class I: Sodium Channel Blockers
        Quinidine (Class IA)
        Lidocaine (Class IB)
    Class II: Beta Blockers
        Propranolol
    Class III: Drugs That Delay Repolarization
        Bretylium
    Class IV: Calcium Channel Blockers
        Verapamil
    Others
        Adenosine
        Digoxin
Drugs Used to Lower Blood Cholesterol
    Bile Acid–Binding Resins
        Cholestyramine
    HMG-CoA Reductase Inhibitors
        Lovastatin
    Others
        Nicotinic acid
        Gemfibrozil
Anticoagulant, Antiplatelet, and Thrombolytic Drugs
    Anticoagulants
        Heparin (parenteral)
        Warfarin (oral)
    Antiplatelet Drugs
        Aspirin
    Thrombolytic Drugs
        Streptokinase
        Alteplase (tPA)

ENDOCRINE DRUGS

Drugs for Diabetes
    Insulin Preparations
        Regular insulin (insulin injection)
        Lente insulins
    Sulfonylureas (Oral Hypoglycemics)
        Tolbutamide
Drugs for Thyroid Disorders
    Drugs for Hypothyroidism
        Levothyroxine (T_4)
    Drugs for Hyperthyroidism
        Propylthiouracil
Contraceptive Agents
    Combination Oral Contraceptives
        Ethinyl estradiol plus norethindrone
    Progestin-Only Oral Contraceptives
        Norethindrone
    Long-Acting Contraceptives
        Subdermal progestin implant [Norplant]
        Depot medroxyprogesterone acetate
    Emergency Postcoital Contraceptives
        Ethinyl estradiol plus norgestrel
        Mifepristone (RU 486)

Pharmacology for Nursing Care

$

Tuc

Pharmacology for Nursing Care

Second Edition

Richard A. Lehne, PhD

Formerly:
Lecturer, University of Arizona College of Nursing
Lecturer, University of Virginia College of Nursing
Research Assistant Professor, Department of Pharmacology
University of Virginia School of Medicine

in consultation with

Linda A. Moore, EdD, RN
Associate Professor of Nursing
University of North Carolina at
Charlotte
Charlotte, North Carolina

Diane B. Hamilton, PhD, RN
Assistant Professor of Nursing
University of Rochester
College of Nursing
Rochester, New York

Leanna J. Crosby, DNSc, RN
Assistant Professor
Director of Research Laboratories
College of Nursing
University of Arizona
Tucson, Arizona

W.B. SAUNDERS COMPANY
A Division of Harcourt Brace & Company
Philadelphia   London   Toronto   Montreal   Sydney   Tokyo

W. B. SAUNDERS COMPANY
A Division of
Harcourt Brace & Company

The Curtis Center
Independence Square West
Philadelphia, Pennsylvania 19106

Library of Congress Cataloging-in-Publication Data

Lehne, Richard A.

Pharmacology for nursing care / Richard A. Lehne, in consultation
with Linda A. Moore, Leanna J. Crosby, Diane B. Hamilton.—2nd
ed.
p. cm.
Includes bibliographical references and index.

ISBN 0–7216–5166–6

1. Pharmacology.   2. Nursing.   I. Title.   [DNLM
  1. Drug Therapy—nurses' instruction.   2. Pharmacology—
nurses' instruction.   QV 4 L523p 1994]

RM301.P457   1994

615.1—dc20

DNLM/DLC   93-26136

Notice

In preparing this text, the author and publisher have exerted every effort to ensure that the drug dosages and usages presented herein are accurate and in accord with standards set by the United States Food and Drug Administration or considered appropriate by the general medical community. However, because standards for drug therapy are continually evolving, the reader is advised, before administering any drug, to consult the manufacturer's package insert for any changes in recommended dosages or indications, and for any additional warnings and precautions. This is especially important when administering newer drugs or those that are infrequently used. Any discrepancies or errors should be brought to the attention of the publisher.

PHARMACOLOGY FOR NURSING CARE, 2nd edition   ISBN 0–7216–5166–6

Printed in the United States of America.

Last digit is the print number: 9   8   7   6   5   4   3   2

Dedicated to the memory of
Betsey Abell
my dear friend

Somphet Manivong

Biographic Information

Richard A. Lehne, PhD, received his BA from Drew University and his doctorate in pharmacology from George Washington University. Over the past fourteen years, he has taught pharmacology to undergraduate and graduate nursing students at the University of Arizona College of Nursing and the University of Virginia School of Nursing, and has been voted best teacher by his students. Dr. Lehne now lives in Charlottesville, VA, where he is occupied with writing, guest lecturing and learning to dance.

Linda A. Moore, EdD, RN, is an Associate Professor at the University of North Carolina at Charlotte. She received her BSN from Duke University and her MSN and EdD from the University of Virginia. She is currently Academic Coordinator of the Nurse Anesthesia program at UNC Charlotte/ Carolinas Medical Center. In addition, she is Director of Continuing Education in the College of Nursing. Her major clinical and research interest is cardiovascular nursing, both cardiac risk prevention and care of the critically ill cardiac client. Dr. Moore is a member of the North Carolina Nurses' Association, Sigma Theta Tau, and the American Association of Critical Care Nurses.

Leanna J. Crosby, DNSc, RN, received her diploma in nursing from St. Luke's Hospital School of Nursing, her baccalaureate and master's degrees in nursing from the University of Virginia, and her doctorate in nursing science from Catholic University of America. She is now an Assistant Professor and Director of Research Laboratories at the University of Arizona College of Nursing. Her primary teaching responsibilities are graduate physiology and undergraduate pathophysiology. Her area of research is chronic rheumatoid disease, and she is a member of the University of Arizona Health Science Arthritis Center. In addition, Dr. Crosby is a member of the Arthritis Health Professions Association, Sigma Xi Scientific Research Society, and Sigma Theta Tau and other nursing organizations.

Diane B. Hamilton, PhD, RN, received her BA from Northwestern University, her BSN from West Texas State University, her MA in Community Mental Health and Gerontologic Nursing from the University of Iowa, and her PhD in Psychosocial Nursing and Nursing History from the University of Virginia. She has extensive experience in psychiatric nursing, including serving as attending nurse at the Institute of Psychiatry of the Medical University of South Carolina. She has taught psychiatry and behavioral science to medical students, and gerontology, community health, psychiatric nursing, and nursing history to nursing students. Currently, she is an Assistant Professor at the University of Rochester College of Nursing, where she teaches psychiatric nursing and nursing history and does nursing history research.

Dr. Hamilton is a member of the American Nurses Association, the American Association of the History of Nursing, the American Association for the History of Medicine, the American Association of University Women, and Sigma Theta Tau; she is also an Associate of the Susan B. Anthony Center. Dr. Hamilton is a recipient of the Best of *Image* Award in nursing history, the Lavinia Dock Award for historical scholarship, the Best Investigator Award from the University of Rochester, and the Golden Apple Teaching Award from the Medical University of South Carolina.

Preface to the Second Edition

OVERVIEW OF THE BOOK

Welcome to the second edition of *Pharmacology for Nursing Care,* the pharmacology text nursing students *like* to read. This edition, like the first, was written to be a true *text*book—that is, a book that focuses on essentials and downplays secondary details. To give the book its focus, three principal techniques are employed: (1) teaching through prototypes, (2) using large print for essential information and small print for secondary information, and (3) limiting discussion of adverse effects and drug interactions to ones that are of particular clinical significance. To reinforce the relationship of pharmacologic knowledge to nursing practice, nursing implications are integrated into the body of each chapter. In addition, to provide rapid access to nursing information, nursing implications are summarized at the end of most chapters. Like the first edition, the second emphasizes conceptual material, thereby reducing rote memorization and increasing reader friendliness. A detailed description of the book's distinguishing features is given in the preface to the first edition, which is reprinted herein.

NEW IN THIS EDITION

Incorporation of Nursing Process. The objective of drug therapy is to produce maximum benefits with minimum harm. To accomplish this objective, we must individualize treatment. The nursing process is well suited to help us do this. To demonstrate the applications of nursing process in drug therapy, we have (1) added a new chapter discussing the relationship of nursing process to drug therapy, and (2) restructured the summaries of nursing implications employing a modified nursing process format.

New Chapters. In response to developments in pharmacology and to suggestions from students and teachers, we have added nine new chapters:

- Pharmacology and the Nursing Process
- Drug Therapy in Pediatric and Geriatric Patients
- Drugs for Headache
- Angiotensin-Converting Enzyme Inhibitors
- Management of Myocardial Infarction
- Hematopoietic Growth Factors
- Drug Therapy of Urinary Tract Infections
- Drugs for Sexually Transmitted Diseases
- Immunosuppressive Drugs

Updates of Existing Chapters. All chapters have been extensively revised. Revisions include updated guidelines for managing common disorders (e.g., myocardial infarction, hypertension, high blood cholesterol, asthma, diabetes mellitus, peptic ulcer disease). More than 120 new drugs have been added.

TEACHING AIDS FOR INSTRUCTORS

An *Instructor's Manual* and *Transparency Set* are available at no charge to teachers using this text. The Transparency Set contains 100 color transparencies of figures (and a few tables) from the text. The Instructor's Manual contains (1) suggestions for setting up a pharmacology course, (2) over 70 case studies, including more than 350 short answer questions with answers and rationales, and (3) an exam bank with over 700 questions, most in NCLEX format. To obtain your Instructor's Manual and Transparency Set, contact your W. B. Saunders educational sales representative. (If you do not know who your sales representative is, you can find out from your school bookstore, or by calling W. B. Saunders sales support at 1-215-238-8406.)

RICHARD A. LEHNE

Preface to the First Edition

Pharmacology pervades all phases of nursing practice and relates directly to patient care and patient education. Despite its pervasiveness and importance, pharmacology remains an area in which students, practitioners, and teachers are often uneasy. Much of this uneasiness stems from traditional approaches to the subject, in which memorization of details takes precedence over understanding. In this text, the opposite approach is taken. Here, the guiding principle is to establish a basic understanding of drugs, after which secondary details can be learned as needed.

This text was written with two major objectives. The first is to help nursing students establish a knowledge base in the basic science of drugs. The second is to demonstrate how that knowledge can be directly applied in providing patient care and patient education. To achieve these goals, several innovative techniques are employed. These are described below.

Laying Foundations in Basic Principles. Understanding drugs requires a strong foundation in basic pharmacologic principles. To establish this foundation, major chapters are dedicated to the following topics: basic principles that apply to all drugs (Chapters 5 through 10), basic principles of neuropharmacology (Chapter 11), basic principles of antimicrobial chemotherapy (Chapter 73), and basic principles of cancer chemotherapy (Chapter 90).

Reviewing Physiology and Pathophysiology. To understand the actions of a drug, we must first understand the biologic systems that the drug influences. For all major drug families, relevant physiology and pathophysiology are reviewed. Reviews are presented at the beginning of each chapter, rather than in a systems review at the beginning of a unit. For example, in the unit on cardiovascular drugs, which includes separate chapters on hypertension, angina pectoris, congestive heart failure, myocardial infarction, and dysrhythmias, reviews of relevant physiology and pathophysiology begin *each chapter*. This juxtaposition of pharmacology, physiology, and pathophysiology is designed to facilitate understanding of the inter-relationships among these subjects.

Teaching Through Prototypes. Within each drug family, we can usually identify one agent that embodies the features that characterize all members of the group. Such a drug can be viewed as a prototype. Since other family members are generally very similar to the prototype, to know the prototype is to know the basic properties of all group members.

The benefits of teaching through prototypes can best be appreciated with an example. Let's consider the nonsteroidal anti-inflammatory drugs (NSAIDs), a family that includes aspirin, ibuprofen [Motrin, others], naproxen [Naprosyn, Anaprox], indomethacin [Indocin], and more than twenty other drugs. Traditionally, information on these drugs is presented in a series of paragraphs describing each drug in turn. When attempting to study from such a list, students are likely to learn many drug names and little else; the important concept of similarity among family members is easily lost. In this text, the family prototype—aspirin—is discussed first and in depth. After this, instruction is completed by pointing out the relatively minor ways in which individual NSAIDs differ from aspirin. Not only is this approach more efficient than the traditional approach, it is also more effective in that similarities among family members are emphasized.

Large Print and Small Print: A Way to Focus on Essentials. Pharmacology is exceptionally rich in detail. There are many drug families, each with multiple members and each member with its own catalogue of indications, contraindications, adverse effects, and drug interactions. This abundance of detail confronts the teacher with the difficult question of what to teach and confronts the student with the equally difficult question of what to study. Attempts to answer these questions can frustrate teacher and student alike. Even worse, in the presence of myriad details, basic concepts can become obscured.

To help establish a focus on essentials, this text employs two type sizes. Large print is intended to say, "On your first exposure to this topic, this is the core of information that you should learn." Small print is intended to say, "Here is additional information that you may want to learn after mastering the material in large print." As a rule, large print is reserved for prototypes, basic principles of pharmacology, and reviews of physiology and pathophysiology. Small print is used for secondary information about the prototypes and for discussion of drugs that are not prototypes. By employing this technique, we have been able to incorporate a large body of detail into this book without having that detail cloud the big picture. Furthermore, because the technique highlights essentials, it minimizes questions about what to teach and what to study.

The use of large and small print is especially valuable for discussing adverse effects and drug interactions. Most drugs are associated with many adverse effects and interactions. As a rule, however, only a few of these are noteworthy. In traditional texts, practically all adverse effects and interactions are presented, creating long and tedious lists. In this text, those few adverse effects and interactions that are especially characteristic are highlighted through presentation in large print; the remainder are noted briefly in small print. As a result, rather than overwhelming students with a long and forbidding list, which can impede comprehension, the approach employed here, by delineating a moderate body of important information, serves to promote comprehension.

Nursing Implications: Demonstrating the Application of Pharmacology to Nursing Practice. The principal reason for asking a nursing student to learn pharmacology is to enhance his or her ability to care for and educate patients. To show students how they can apply pharmacologic knowledge to nursing practice, nursing implications are *integrated into the body of each chapter.* That is, as specific drugs and drug families are discussed, the nursing implications inherent in the pharmacologic information are discussed side-by-side with the basic science. To facilitate access to nursing information, nursing implications are also *summarized at the end of most chapters.* These

summaries should serve to reinforce the information presented in the main text.

In chapters that are especially brief or that address drugs that are infrequently used, summaries of nursing implications have been omitted. However, even in these chapters, nursing implications are incorporated into the chapter body.

A Note About Drug Therapy. Throughout this text, as we discuss specific drug families (e.g., beta-adrenergic blockers), we discuss the clinical applications of those drugs. Similarly, in chapters that focus on specific diseases (e.g., Parkinson's disease, hypertension), we indicate which drugs are generally considered most appropriate for treatment. However, it is important to note that clinical applications of individual drugs may change over time: a drug may acquire new indications that are not discussed here, or it may cease to be used for indications that *are* discussed here. Likewise, drug therapy of specific diseases is continually evolving: as superior drugs are developed, they tend to replace older, less desirable agents. Accordingly, although the drug therapies presented in this text reflect a general consensus on what is considered best *today*, these therapies may not be considered best a few years from now—and, in therapeutic areas where there is controversy or where change is especially rapid, the treatments discussed here may be considered inappropriate by some clinicians right now.

About Dosage Calculations. Unlike many nursing pharmacology texts, this one has no section on dosage calculation. The reasons for this departure from tradition are twofold. First, adequate presentation of this important subject simply isn't feasible in a text dedicated to the basic science of drugs; the amount of space that can be allotted is too small. Second, thanks to the availability of several excellent publications on the subject (e.g., *Math for Nurses,* W. B. Saunders Company), the need to include this information in pharmacology texts has been obviated.

Ways to Use This Textbook. Because of its focus on essentials, this text is especially well suited to serve as the primary text for courses dedicated specifically to pharmacology. In addition, the book's focused approach makes it a valuable resource for pharmacologic instruction within integrated curriculums and for self-directed learning by students and practitioners.

RICHARD A. LEHNE

Acknowledgments

In writing this edition, as in the first, I have enjoyed the wise counsel, warm friendship, and good humor of Drs. Linda A. Moore, Diane B. Hamilton, and Leanna J. Crosby. Special appreciation is due Dr. Moore for creating and coordinating the greatly expanded Instructor's Manual that accompanies this edition.

I want to thank Dr. Alfred J. Rémillard for revising and updating the section on Canadian Drug information, which he wrote originally for the first edition of this book.

I am grateful to a small army of extraordinary people at W. B. Saunders Company. Daniel T. Ruth, nursing editor, has given this project unfailing support; applied his considerable diplomatic skills to keep volatile situations from going ballistic (usually); coaxed a reluctant author into making changes that, in retrospect, really *are* improvements; and extended genuine friendship, which can be rare in our professional world. Special acclaim is due Arlene Friday, copy editor, for giving this text its final form, and for making an arduous and potentially contentious process go as smoothly and painlessly as this author could hope for. I am grateful also to Melissa Walter for creating the new artwork for this edition, to Sharon Iwanczuk for creating the artwork transported from the first edition, and to Joan Wendt for giving this edition its elegant design. Of course, I want to thank Susan Bielitsky, editorial assistant, who was always upbeat, sympathetic, and helpful, despite my frequent calls for aid. Finally, I want to thank Peter Faber, production manager, along with the entire production staff, for transmuting this book into tangible form.

I am grateful to the reviewers who have enhanced this book with their comments and corrections. Ruth Kingdon, MSN, RN, and Robert J. Kizior, BS, RPh, did the Herculean task of critiquing the entire manuscript. The contributors to the Instructor's Manual—Rebecca Kent Bevilacqua, RN,C, SNP; Diane Blanchfield, CRNA, MS; Judy Gias, BSN, RN, CCRN; Sonya Hardin, PhD, RN, CCRN, CS; Frances Rhyne King, MEd, MN, RN; Judith C. Mann, MSN, RN: Rosemary Martines, RN; Ann Mabe Newman, DSN, RN,C; Elaine Nishioka, MSN, RN, PNP; Carol O'Neil, PhD, RN: Sherry Walter, MSN, RN: and Willie Wachoviak, RN,C, FNP—provided insightful feedback within their areas of expertise; thank you all.

I want to thank my friends and colleagues at the University of Arizona College of Pharmacy, Tucson, AZ, who will recognize their influence throughout this book. It was my great pleasure to work with the faculty of the Department of Pharmacology and Toxicology teaching basic pharmacology to BSN students at the College of Nursing, and with Drs. Martin D. Higbee and Marie E. Gardner of the Department of Pharmacy Practice, who shared their considerable expertise in gerontology as we taught pharmacology and therapeutics to graduate students in the Gerontologic Nurse Practitioner program.

Lastly, I want to thank the friends and associates who have provided comfort and encouragement over the past year and a half as this revision took form. Four of you deserve special recognition: Jean Gratz, a steadfast friend with a talent for calling just when she's needed most; Bill Curtis, a longtime friend, who, despite the demands of maintaining the formularies at both the C.S.T. and his new dispensary, somehow found time for our frequent and lengthy commiserations; Sam Adams, always on tap, and never failing to provide solace during the occasional crisis; and, of course, the Muse of Pharmacology—my aging companion, Cat.

RAL

Contents

UNIT XIII

Ophthalmic Drugs

UNIT XIV

Dermatologic Drugs

UNIT XV

Nutrients

UNIT XVI

Chemotherapy of Infectious Diseases

UNIT XVII

Chemotherapy of Parasitic Diseases

Detailed Contents

UNIT XIII

Ophthalmic Drugs

UNIT XIV

Dermatologic Drugs

UNIT XV

Nutrients

UNIT XVI

Chemotherapy of Infectious Diseases

UNIT XVII

Chemotherapy of Parasitic Diseases

UNIT XVIII

Cancer Chemotherapy

UNIT XIX

Immunosuppressive Drugs

UNIT XX

Toxicology

APPENDICES

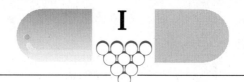

Introduction

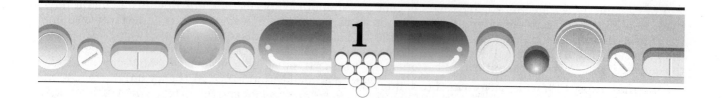

Orientation to Pharmacology

FOUR BASIC TERMS

PROPERTIES OF AN IDEAL DRUG
    The Big Three: Effectiveness, Safety, and
    Selectivity
    Additional Properties of an Ideal Drug

THE THERAPEUTIC OBJECTIVE

**FACTORS THAT DETERMINE THE
INTENSITY OF DRUG RESPONSES**
    Administration
    Pharmacokinetics
    Pharmacodynamics
    Sources of Individual Variation

If you are typical of the students for whom this book was written, by this time in your life you have spent 15 or more years in school and have probably asked yourself, "What's the purpose of all this education?" In the past your question may have lacked a satisfying answer. Happily, now you have one: You have undergone all that education to prepare yourself to study pharmacology!

There is good reason why you haven't approached pharmacology before now. Pharmacology is a science that draws upon information from a number of disciplines, including anatomy, physiology, psychology, chemistry, and microbiology. Consequently, before you could begin to study pharmacology, you first had to become familiar with these other sciences. Now that you've established the requisite knowledge base, you're finally ready to learn about drugs.

FOUR BASIC TERMS

At this point it will be helpful to define four basic terms: *drug, pharmacology, clinical pharmacology,* and *therapeutics.* As we go through these definitions, we will also discuss what the focus of this text will be.

Drug. A drug is defined as *any chemical that can affect living processes.* By this definition, virtually all chemicals can be considered drugs, since, when given in large enough amounts, all chemicals

will have some effect on life. Clearly, it is beyond the scope of this text to consider all compounds that fit the definition of a drug. Accordingly, rather than studying all drugs, we will limit discussion to those drugs that have therapeutic applications.

Pharmacology. Pharmacology can be defined as *the study of drugs and their interactions with living systems.* Given this definition, the science of pharmacology can claim a large body of knowledge as its own. Under our definition, pharmacology encompasses the study of the biochemical and physiologic effects of drugs as well as the study of drug absorption, distribution, metabolism, and excretion. In addition, pharmacology includes knowledge of the history, sources, physical and chemical properties, and therapeutic and other uses of drugs. Since pharmacology encompasses such a broad spectrum of information, it would be inappropriate (not to mention impossible) to address the entire scope of pharmacology in this text. Consequently, we will restrict consideration to information relevant to the clinical setting.

Clinical Pharmacology. Clinical pharmacology is defined as *the study of drugs in humans.* This discipline includes the study of drugs in *patients* as well as in *healthy volunteers* (during new drug development). Since clinical pharmacology encompasses all aspects of the interaction between drugs and people, and since our primary interest is the use of drugs to treat patients, clinical pharmacology includes some information that will be outside the scope of this text.

Therapeutics. Therapeutics, also known as *pharmacotherapeutics,* is defined as *the use of drugs to diagnose, prevent, or treat disease or to prevent pregnancy.* Alternatively, therapeutics can be defined simply as the medical use of drugs.

Therapeutics will provide the focus of this book. That is, discussions will focus on the basic science information needed to understand the use of drugs as therapeutic agents. The information provided here should help you understand how drugs produce their effects—both therapeutic and adverse; the reasons for giving a particular drug to a particular patient; and the rationale underlying selection of dosage, route, and schedule of administration. In addition, knowledge of pharmacology will help you understand the strategies employed to promote beneficial drug effects and to minimize undesired reactions. It is hoped that application of this knowledge will result in improved patient care and education. It is also hoped that your knowledge of pharmacology will render working with medications a more gratifying activity.

PROPERTIES OF AN IDEAL DRUG

If we were developing a new drug, we would want that drug to be as good as possible. In order

to approach perfection, our new drug should have certain properties, such as effectiveness and safety. In the discussion below, we will consider the characteristics that an ideal drug might possess. It must be emphasized, however, that the ideal medication exists in theory only—*there is no such thing as a perfect drug.* The truth of this statement will become apparent as we consider the properties that an ideal drug should have.

THE BIG THREE: EFFECTIVENESS, SAFETY, AND SELECTIVITY

The three most important characteristics that any drug can have are effectiveness, safety, and selectivity.

Effectiveness. An effective drug is one that elicits the responses for which it has been administered. *Effectiveness is the most important property that a drug can have.* Regardless of its other virtues, if a drug is not effective, that is, if it doesn't do anything useful, there is little justification for giving it. Current law requires that all new drugs be proved effective prior to release for marketing in the United States.

Safety. A safe drug is defined as one that cannot produce harmful effects—even if administered in very high doses and for a very long time. *There is no such thing as a safe drug.* All drugs have the ability to cause injury. The chances of producing adverse effects can be reduced by proper drug selection and proper administration. However, the risk of adverse effects can never be eliminated. Certain anticancer drugs, for example, are always associated with an increased risk of serious infection. With other drugs (e.g., barbiturates), excessive dosage always carries a risk of fatal respiratory depression. Clearly, drugs are not safe. The fact that drugs are dangerous may explain why the Greeks chose the word *pharmakon,* which can be translated as *poison,* as a name for these compounds.

Selectivity. A selective drug is defined as one that elicits only those responses for which it is given. A selective drug would not produce side effects. *There is no such thing as a selective drug: all medications cause side effects.* Common examples of side effects include the drowsiness that can be caused by antihistamines; the morning sickness, cramps, and depression that can be caused by oral contraceptives; and the constipation, urinary hesitancy, and respiratory depression that can be caused by morphine.

ADDITIONAL PROPERTIES OF AN IDEAL DRUG

Reversible Action. For most drugs, it is important that effects be reversible. That is, in most

cases, we want drug actions to subside within some appropriate period of time. General anesthetics, for example, would be useless if patients never woke up. Likewise, it is unlikely that oral contraceptives would find widespread acceptance if their use resulted in permanent sterility. For a few drugs, most notably antibiotics and anticancer agents, reversibility is not a desirable attribute. When using these compounds, we want toxicity to target cells to endure.

Predictability. It would be very helpful if, prior to drug administration, we could know with certainty just how a given patient will respond. Unfortunately, since each patient is unique, the accuracy of predictions cannot be guaranteed. Accordingly, in order to maximize the chances of eliciting desired responses, we must tailor therapy to the individual.

Ease of Administration. An ideal drug should be simple to administer: the route should be convenient, and the number of doses per day should be low. The diabetic patient who faces a lifetime of multiple daily injections is not likely to judge insulin ideal. Likewise, drugs that require intravenous infusion are rarely considered ideal by the nurse who must set up the infusion apparatus and monitor its function.

In addition to convenience, ease of administration has two additional benefits: (1) it can enhance patient compliance, and (2) it can decrease errors in drug administration. Patients are more likely to comply with a dosing schedule that consists of once-a-day administration than with one that requires multiple daily doses. Similarly, hospital personnel are less likely to commit medication errors when administering oral drugs than when preparing and administering intravenous formulations.

Freedom from Drug Interactions. When a patient is taking two or more drugs, those drugs can interact with one another. Such interactions may either augment or reduce drug responses. For example, the degree of respiratory depression caused by diazepam [Valium], which is normally minimal, can be greatly *intensified* in the presence of alcohol. On the other hand, the antibacterial effects of tetracycline can be substantially *reduced* if this drug is taken concurrently with an iron or calcium supplement. Because of the potential for interactions between drugs, when a patient is taking more than one agent, the possible impact of drug interactions must be considered. An ideal drug would not interact with other agents. Unfortunately, few medicines are devoid of significant interactions.

Low Cost. An ideal drug would be readily affordable. The cost of some drugs can be a substantial financial burden. As an extreme example, 1 year of therapy with human growth hormone (so-matrem) can cost between $10,000 and $20,000. More commonly, expense becomes a significant factor for patients who must take drugs chronically. People with diseases such as hypertension, arthritis, and diabetes, for example, require drug therapy for life. The cumulative expense of such treatment can be huge—even for drugs of moderate price.

Chemical Stability. Some drugs lose effectiveness during storage. Others, which may be stable on the shelf, can rapidly lose effectiveness when put into solution (e.g., in preparation for injection). These losses in efficacy result from chemical instability. Because of chemical instability, stocks of certain drugs must be periodically discarded and replaced with fresh supplies. An ideal drug would retain its activity indefinitely, both on the shelf and in solution.

Possession of a Simple Generic Name. Generic names of drugs are often complex and, therefore, difficult to remember and pronounce. As a rule, the trade name for a drug is simpler than its generic name. Examples of drugs that have simple trade names and complex generic names include chlordiazepoxide [Librium], acetaminophen [Tylenol], and cephalexin [Keflex]. Since generic names are preferable to trade names (for reasons discussed in Chapter 3), an ideal drug should have a generic name that is easy to recall and pronounce.

SUMMARY OF PROPERTIES OF AN IDEAL DRUG

From the preceding discussion, it should be obvious that currently available medications are far from ideal. No drug has all of the properties discussed above: no drug is safe; all drugs produce side effects; responses may be difficult to predict and may be altered by drug interactions; and drugs may be expensive, unstable, and difficult to administer. Because medications are not ideal, care must be exercised by all members of the health care team to promote therapeutic effects while minimizing the potential for drug-induced injury.

THE THERAPEUTIC OBJECTIVE

The objective of drug therapy is to provide the maximum benefit with minimum harm. If drugs were ideal, this objective could be achieved with relative ease. However, since drugs are less than perfect, skill and care must be exercised if treatment is to result in more good than harm.

As detailed in Chapter 2, the nurse has a critical

responsibility in achieving the therapeutic objective. In order to meet this responsibility, you must understand drugs. The primary purpose of this text is to help you establish that understanding.

FACTORS THAT DETERMINE THE INTENSITY OF DRUG RESPONSES

Multiple factors determine how an individual will respond to a prescribed dose of a particular drug (Fig. 1–1). Knowledge of these factors is needed if we want to think rationally about how a drug interacts with the patient to produce its effects. Furthermore, knowledge of drug-patient interactions is needed if the nurse is to contribute maximally to efforts at achieving the therapeutic objective.

Our ultimate concern when administering a drug is the intensity of the responses that the drug will elicit. Working our way up from the bottom of Figure 1–1, we can see that the intensity of the response is determined ultimately by the concentration of a drug at its sites of action. As the figure suggests, the prime determinant of this concentration is the administered dose. When administration is performed correctly, the dose that was given will bear a close relationship to the dose that was prescribed. The steps leading from prescribed dose to intensity of drug response are considered below.

ADMINISTRATION

Dosage size and the route and timing of administration are important determinants of drug responses. Accordingly, the prescribing physician will consider these variables with care. Unfortunately, drugs are not always administered as pre-

scribed: poor patient compliance and medication errors by hospital staff can result in major discrepancies between the dose that was prescribed and the dose that is actually administered. Such discrepancies can significantly alter the outcome of treatment. To help minimize errors caused by poor compliance, patients should be fully informed about the nature of their medications and the proper methods of administration.

Medication errors made by hospital staff may result in drug administration via the wrong route, in the wrong dose, or at the wrong time. The patient may even be given the wrong drug. These errors can be made by pharmacists, physicians, and nurses. Any of these errors will detract from achieving the therapeutic objective.

PHARMACOKINETICS

Pharmacokinetic processes determine how much of an administered dose will reach its sites of action. There are four major pharmacokinetic processes: (1) drug absorption, (2) drug distribution, (3) drug metabolism, and (4) drug excretion. Collectively, these processes can be thought of as *the impact of the body on the drug*. The pharmacokinetic processes are discussed at length in Chapter 5.

PHARMACODYNAMICS

Once a drug has reached its site of action, pharmacodynamic processes determine the nature and intensity of the response. Pharmacodynamics can be thought of as *the impact of drugs on the body*. In most cases, the initial step leading to a response is the binding of a drug to its *receptor*. This drug-receptor interaction is followed by a sequence of

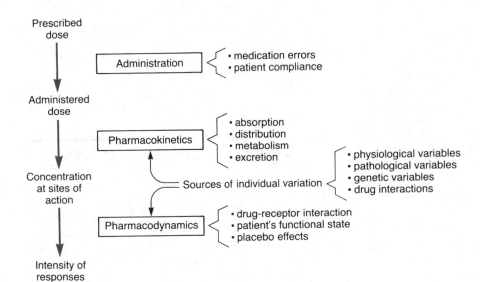

Figure 1–1. Factors that determine the intensity of drug responses. (Adapted from Koch-Weser, J. Drug therapy. Serum drug concentrations as therapeutic guides. N. Engl. J. Med. 287:227, 1972.)

events that ultimately results in a response. As indicated in Figure 1–1, the patient's "functional state" can influence pharmacodynamic processes. For example, individuals who have developed tolerance to morphine will respond less to a particular dose than will patients who lack tolerance. Placebo (psychologic) effects also help determine the responses that a drug will elicit. The topic of pharmacodynamics is discussed at length in Chapter 6.

SOURCES OF INDIVIDUAL VARIATION

Characteristics unique to each patient can influence pharmacokinetic and pharmacodynamic processes and, by doing so, can help determine a patient's responses to drugs. As indicated in Figure 1–1, sources of individual variation include drug interactions; physiologic variables (e.g., age, sex, weight); pathophysiologic variables (especially diminished function of the kidneys and liver, the major organs of drug elimination); and genetic variables. Genetic factors can alter the metabolism of drugs and can predispose the patient to unique drug reactions. Because individuals differ from one another, no two patients will respond identically to the same drug regimen. Accordingly, if the therapeutic objective is to be achieved, it is essential that drug therapy be matched to the individual. The subject of individual variation in drug responses is discussed at length in Chapter 9.

SUMMARY

Whenever medicines are used, our goal is to promote desired effects and minimize adverse effects. In order to achieve this objective, we need to understand pharmacokinetics and pharmacodynamics, the principal determinants of drug responses. In addition, it is essential that we account for potential sources of individual variation in drug responses. When all these considerations are made, the resulting regimen will be tailored to the individual and, therefore, should produce maximum benefit with minimum harm.

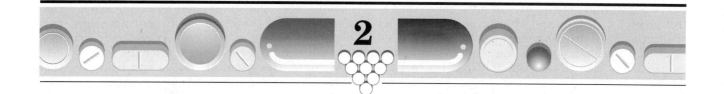

Application of Pharmacology in Nursing

O ur objective in this chapter is to answer the following question, "Why should a nursing student learn pharmacology?" To answer this question, we will examine the ways in which a nurse can put knowledge of pharmacology to practical use. Hopefully, you will complete this chapter being convinced that an understanding of drugs is necessary for the practice of nursing and, therefore, that putting time and energy into learning about drugs will constitute a worthwhile investment.

EVOLUTION OF NURSING RESPONSIBILITIES IN REGARD TO DRUGS

At one time, the nurse's responsibility regarding medications was limited to the *Five Rights of Drug Administration*, namely, give the *right drug* to the *right patient* in the *right dose* by the *right route* at the *right time*. Clearly, the Five Rights are important. However, although these basics are essential, much more is required if the therapeutic objective is to be achieved. The Five Rights guarantee only that a drug will be administered as prescribed. Correct administration, without additional interventions, cannot insure that treatment will result in maximum benefit and minimum harm.

The limitations of the Five Rights can be illustrated with this analogy: The nurse who sees his or her responsibility as being over as soon as he or she has administered a patient's medicine would be like a baseball pitcher who felt that his responsibility was over once he had thrown the ball toward the batter. As the pitcher must be ready to respond to the consequences of the interaction between ball and bat, the nurse must be ready to respond to the consequences of the interaction between drug and patient. Put another way, although both the nurse and the pitcher have a clear obligation to deliver their respective "pills" in the most appropriate fashion, proper delivery is only the beginning of their responsibilities: *important events will take place after the "pill" is delivered, and these must be responded to.* Like the pitcher, the nurse can respond rapidly and effectively only by *anticipating* (knowing in advance) what the possible reactions to the pill might be. In order to anticipate possible reactions, both the nurse and the pitcher require certain kinds of knowledge. Just as the pitcher must understand the abilities of the opposing batter, the nurse must understand the patient and the disorder for which he or she is being treated. As the pitcher must know the most appropriate pitch (e.g., fast ball, curve) to deliver in specific circumstances, the nurse must know what medications are appropriate for the patient and must check to insure that the medication ordered is among them. Conversely, as the pitcher must know what pitches *not* to throw at a particular batter, the nurse must know what drugs are *contraindicated* for the patient. As the pitcher must know the most likely outcome after the ball and bat interact, the nurse must know the probable consequences of the interaction between drug and patient. Although this analogy is not perfect (the nurse and patient are on the same team, whereas the pitcher and batter are not), it does help us appreciate that the nurse's responsibility extends well beyond the Five Rights. Consequently, in addition to the limited information needed to administer drugs in accordance with the Five Rights, you need to acquire a broad base of pharmacologic knowledge so as to contribute fully to achieving the therapeutic objective.

In drug therapy today, nurses, together with physicians and pharmacists, participate in a system of checks and balances designed to promote beneficial effects and minimize harm. Nurses are especially important within this system because it is the nurse—not the physician—who follows patients' status most closely. As a result, you are likely to be the first member of the health care team to observe and evaluate drug responses, and to intervene if required. In order to observe and evaluate drug responses, and in order to intervene rapidly and appropriately, you must know *in advance* the responses that a medication is likely to elicit. Put another way, in order to provide professional care, you must understand drugs; the stronger your knowledge of pharmacology, the more you will be able to *anticipate* drug responses and not simply *react* to them after the fact.

Within our system of checks and balances, the nurse has an important role as *patient advocate*. It is your responsibility to detect errors made by pharmacists and physicians—and mistakes *will* be made. For example, the physician may overlook potential drug interactions; or may be unaware of alterations in the patient's status that would preclude use of a particular drug; or may select the correct drug, but may order an inappropriate dosage or route of administration. Since it is the nurse who actually administers drugs, the nurse is the last person to check medications prior to administration. Consequently, *you are the patient's last line of defense against errors.* It is ethically and legally unacceptable for you to administer a drug that is harmful to the patient—even though the medication has been prescribed by a licensed physician and dispensed by a licensed pharmacist: in your role as patient advocate, you must protect the patient against medication errors made by other members of the health care team. In serving as patient advocate, it is impossible for you to know too much about drugs.

APPLICATION OF PHARMACOLOGY IN PATIENT CARE

The two major areas in which you can apply pharmacolgic knowledge are patient care and patient education. Patient care is considered in this section. Patient education is considered in the next section. In discussing the applications of pharmacology in patient care, we will focus on seven aspects of drug therapy: (1) preadministration assessment, (2) dosage and administration, (3) evaluating and promoting therapeutic effects, (4) minimizing adverse effects, (5) minimizing adverse interactions, (6) making PRN decisions, and (7) managing toxicity.

PREADMINISTRATION ASSESSMENT

All drug therapy begins with assessment of the patient. Assessment has three basic goals: (1) collecting baseline data needed to evaluate therapeutic and adverse responses, (2) identifying high-risk patients, and (3) assessing the patient's capacity for self care. The first two goals are highly specific for each drug. Accordingly, we cannot achieve these goals without understanding pharmacology. The third goal applies generally to all drugs; hence, it does not usually require specific knowledge of the drug to be used. Preadministration assessment is discussed further in Chapter 3 (Pharmacology and the Nursing Process).

Collecting Baseline Data. Baseline data are needed to evaluate drug responses, both therapeutic and adverse. For example, if we plan to give a drug to lower blood pressure, we must know the patient's blood pressure prior to treatment. Without this baseline data, we would have no way of determining the effectiveness of our drug. Similarly, if we are planning to give a drug that can decrease blood cell counts, we need to know baseline counts in order to evaluate the adverse effects of treatment. Obviously, in order to collect appropriate baseline data, we must first know the effects that our drug is likely to produce.

Identifying High-Risk Patients. Multiple factors can predispose an individual patient to adverse reactions from specific drugs. Important predisposing factors are pathophysiology (especially liver and kidney dysfunction), genetic factors, drug allergies, pregnancy, old age, and extreme youth.

Patients with penicillin allergy provide a dramatic example of those at risk: giving penicillin to these people can kill them. Accordingly, whenever treatment with penicillin is under consideration, we must determine if the patient has had an allergic reaction to this drug in the past. If the patient has a history of penicillin allergy, an alternative antibiotic should be employed. If there is no effective alternative, facilities for managing a severe reaction should be in place before the drug is given.

From the preceding example, we can see that when drug therapy is being planned, patients at high risk of reacting adversely must be identified. The tools for identification are the patient history, physical examination, and laboratory tests. Of course, if identification is to be successful, you must know what to look for (i.e., you must know the factors that can increase the risk of severe reactions to the drug in question). Once the high-risk patient has been identified, we can take steps to reduce the risk. We might select an alternative drug, or, if no alternative is available, we can at least prepare in advance to manage a possible reaction.

DOSAGE AND ADMINISTRATION

Earlier, we noted the Five Rights of Drug Administration and agreed on their importance. Although you can implement the Five Rights without a detailed knowledge of pharmacology, having such knowledge can help reduce your contribution to medication errors. Some examples will illustrate this point:

1. Certain drugs have more than one applica-

tion, and dosage may vary depending upon the reason for drug use. Aspirin, for example, is given in low doses to relieve pain and in higher doses to suppress inflammation (e.g., in patients with arthritis). If you didn't know about these differences, you might administer too much aspirin to the patient with pain or too little to the patient with inflammation.

2. Many drugs can be administered by more than one route, and dosage may vary depending upon the route selected. Morphine, for example, may be administered by mouth or by injection (subcutaneous, intramuscular, intravenous). Oral doses are generally *much larger* than injected doses. Accordingly, if a large dose intended for oral use were to be mistakenly administered by injection, the result could prove fatal. The nurse who understands the pharmacology of morphine is unlikely to make this medication error.

3. Certain intravenous agents can cause severe local injury if the line through which they are being administered becomes extravasated. Accordingly, when such drugs are given, special care must be taken to prevent extravasation. The infusion must be monitored closely, and, if extravasation occurs, corrective steps must be taken immediately to minimize harm. The nurse who doesn't understand these drugs will be unprepared to administer them safely.

The following basic guidelines can help insure correct administration:

1. Read the medication order carefully. If the order is unclear, verify it with the prescribing physician.
2. Verify the identity of the patient by comparing the name on the wristband with the name on the drug order or administration record.
3. Read the medication label carefully. Verify the identity of the drug, the amount of drug (per tablet, volume of liquid, etc.), and its suitability for administration by the intended route.
4. Verify dosage calculations.
5. Implement any special handling that the drug may require.
6. Do not administer any drug if you do not understand the reason for its use.

EVALUATING AND PROMOTING THERAPEUTIC EFFECTS

Evaluating Therapeutic Responses. Evaluation is one of the most important aspects of drug therapy. After all, this is the process that tells us whether or not our drug is doing anything useful. Because the nurse follows the patient's status most closely, the nurse is in the best position to evaluate therapeutic responses.

In order to make an evaluation, you must know the rationale for treatment and the nature and time course of the desired response. If you lack this knowledge, you will be unable to evaluate the patient's progress. When beneficial responses develop as hoped for, ignorance of expected effects might not be so bad. However, when desired responses do not occur, it may be essential to identify this failure quickly, since timely implementation of alternative therapy may be needed.

When evaluating responses to a drug that has more than one application, you can do so only if you know the specific indication for which the medication is being used. Nifedipine, for example, is given for two cardiovascular disorders: hypertension and angina pectoris. When the drug is used to treat hypertension, you should monitor for a reduction in blood pressure. In contrast, when this drug is used to treat angina, you should monitor for a reduction in chest pain. Clearly, if you are to make the proper evaluation, you must understand the reason for drug use.

Promoting Compliance. Drugs can be of great value to patients, but only if they are taken correctly. Drugs that are self-administered in the wrong dose, by the wrong route, or at the wrong time cannot produce maximum benefit—and may even prove harmful. Obviously, successful therapy requires active and informed participation by the patient. By educating patients about the drugs they are taking, you can help elicit the required level of participation.

Implementing Nondrug Measures. The benefits of drug therapy can often be enhanced by nonpharmacologic measures. Examples include (1) enhancing drug therapy of asthma through breathing exercises, biofeedback, and emotional support; (2) enhancing drug therapy of arthritis through exercise, physical therapy, and rest; and (3) enhancing drug therapy of hypertension through weight reduction, smoking cessation, and sodium restriction. As a nurse, you may provide these supportive measures directly, through patient education, or by coordinating the activities of other health care providers.

MINIMIZING ADVERSE EFFECTS

All drugs have the potential to produce undesired effects. Common examples include gastric erosion caused by aspirin, sedation caused by antihistamines, hypoglycemia caused by insulin, and excessive fluid loss caused by diuretics. When drugs are employed properly, the incidence and severity of such effects can be reduced. Measures to reduce adverse effects include identifying high-risk patients through the patient history, insuring proper administration through patient education,

and forewarning patients about activities that might precipitate an adverse reaction.

When untoward effects cannot be avoided, discomfort and injury can often be minimized by appropriate intervention. For example, timely administration of glucose will prevent brain damage from insulin-induced hypoglycemia. In order to help reduce adverse effects, you must know the following about the drugs you are working with: (1) the major adverse effects that the drug can produce, (2) the time when these reactions are likely to occur, (3) early signs that an adverse reaction is developing, and (4) the interventions that can minimize discomfort and harm.

MINIMIZING ADVERSE INTERACTIONS

When a patient is taking two or more drugs, those drugs may interact with one another to diminish therapeutic effects or intensify adverse effects. For example, the ability of oral contraceptives to protect against pregnancy can be reduced by concurrent therapy with phenobarbital (an antiseizure drug), and the risk of thromboembolism from oral contraceptives can be increased by smoking cigarettes.

As a nurse, you can help reduce the incidence and intensity of adverse interactions in several ways. These include taking a thorough drug history, advising the patient to avoid over-the-counter drugs that can interact with the prescribed medication, monitoring the patient for adverse interactions *known* to occur between the drugs the patient is taking, and being alert for as yet *unknown* interactions.

MAKING PRN DECISIONS

A PRN medication order is one in which the nurse has discretion regarding how much drug to give and when to give it. (PRN is an acronym that stands for *pro re nata*, a Latin phrase meaning *as needed* or *as the occasion arises*.) PRN orders are common for hypnotics (sleeping pills) and for analgesics (pain medications). In order to implement a PRN order rationally, you must know the reason for drug use and be able to assess the patient's medication needs. Clearly, the better your knowledge of pharmacology, the better your PRN decisions are likely to be.

MANAGING TOXICITY

Some adverse drug reactions are extremely dangerous. If toxicity is not diagnosed early and responded to quickly, irreversible injury or death can result. In order to minimize harm, you must know the early signs of toxicity and the procedure for toxicity management.

APPLICATION OF PHARMACOLOGY IN PATIENT EDUCATION

In most cases, it is the responsibility of the nurse to educate patients about medications. In your role as educator, you must provide the patient with the following information:

1. Drug name and therapeutic category (e.g., penicillin: antibiotic)
2. Dosage size and schedule
3. Route and technique of administration
4. Expected therapeutic response and when it should develop
5. Nondrug measures to enhance therapeutic responses
6. Duration of treatment
7. Method of drug storage
8. Symptoms of major adverse effects, and measures to minimize discomfort and harm
9. Major adverse drug-drug and drug-food interactions
10. Who to contact in the event of therapeutic failure, severe adverse reactions, or severe adverse interactions

In order to communicate this information effectively and accurately, you must first understand it. That is, to be a good educator, you must know pharmacology.

In the discussion below, we will consider the relationship between patient education and the following aspects of drug therapy: dosage and administration, promoting therapeutic effects, minimizing adverse effects, and minimizing adverse interactions.

DOSAGE AND ADMINISTRATION

Drug Name. The patient should know the name of the medication he or she is taking. If the drug has been prescribed by a trade name, the patient should be given the drug's generic name in addition to the trade name. This information will reduce the risk of overdosage that can result when a patient fails to realize that two prescriptions that bear different names actually contain the same medication.

Dosage Size and Schedule of Administration. Patients must be told how much drug to take and when to take it. For some medications, dosage must be adjusted by the patient. Insulin provides a good example. For insulin therapy to be successful, the patient must adjust the dosage to accommodate alterations in caloric intake. How to make this adjustment is taught by the nurse.

With PRN medications, the schedule of administration is not fixed. Rather, these drugs are taken as conditions require. For example, some people with asthma experience exercise-related respiratory distress. To minimize such attacks, these individuals can take supplementary medication prior to anticipated exertion. It is the responsibility of the nurse to teach patients when PRN drugs should be taken.

The patient should know what to do if a dose is missed. With oral contraceptives, for example, if one dose is missed, the omitted dose should be taken together with the next scheduled dose. However, if three or more doses are missed, a new cycle of administration must be initiated.

Some patients have difficulty remembering whether or not they have taken their medication. Possible causes include mental illness, advanced age, and complex regimens. To facilitate accurate dosing, you can provide the patient with a pill box that has separate compartments for each day of the week, and then teach him or her to load the compartments weekly. To determine if they have taken their medicine, patients can simply examine the box.

Technique of Administration. Patients must be taught how to administer drugs. This is especially important for routes that may be unfamiliar (e.g., sublingual for nitroglycerin) and for techniques that are difficult (e.g., subcutaneous injection of insulin). Patients taking oral medications may require special instructions. For example, some oral preparations must not be chewed or crushed; some should be taken with fluids; and some should be taken with meals, whereas others should not. Careful attention must be paid to the patient who, because of disability (e.g., visual or intellectual impairment, limited manual dexterity), may find self-medication difficult.

Duration of Drug Use. Just as patients must know when to take their medicine, they must know when to stop. In some cases (e.g., treatment of acute pain), patients should discontinue drug use as soon as symptoms subside. In other cases (e.g., treatment of hypertension), patients should know that therapy will probably continue lifelong. For other conditions (e.g., gastric ulcers), medication may be prescribed for a specific time interval, after which the patient should return for re-evaluation.

Drug Storage. Certain medications are chemically unstable and deteriorate rapidly if stored improperly. Patients who are using unstable drugs must be taught how to store them correctly (e.g., under refrigeration, in light-proof containers). All drugs should be stored where children can't reach them.

PROMOTING THERAPEUTIC EFFECTS

In order to participate fully in achieving the therapeutic objective, patients must know the nature and time course of expected beneficial effects. With this knowledge, patients can help evaluate the success or failure of treatment. By recognizing treatment failure, the informed patient will be able to seek timely implementation of alternative therapy.

With some drugs, such as those used to treat depression and schizophrenia, beneficial effects are delayed, taking weeks or months to develop. Awareness that treatment may not produce immediate results will allow the patient to have realistic expectations, and will help reduce anxiety about therapeutic failure.

As noted above, nondrug measures can complement drug therapy. For example, although drugs are useful in managing adult-onset diabetes, exercise and caloric restriction are at least as important. Teaching the patient about nondrug measures can greatly increase the chances of success.

MINIMIZING ADVERSE EFFECTS

Knowledge of adverse drug effects will enable the patient to avoid some adverse effects and reduce others through early detection. The following examples should underscore the value of educating patients about the undesired effects of drugs:

1. Insulin overdosage can cause blood glucose levels to drop precipitously. Early signs of hypoglycemia include sweating and increased heart rate. The patient who has been taught to recognize these early signs can respond by ingesting glucose-rich foods, thereby restoring blood sugar to a safe level. In contrast, the patient who fails to recognize evolving hypoglycemia and does not ingest glucose may become comatose, and may even die.

2. Many anticancer drugs predispose patients to acquiring serious infections. The patient who is aware of this possibility can take steps to avoid contagion (e.g., avoiding contact with people who have an infection; avoiding foods likely to contain pathogens). In addition, the informed patient is in a position to notify the physician at the first sign that an infection is developing, thereby allowing rapid treatment. In contrast, the patient who has not received adequate education is at increased risk of death from infectious disease.

3. Some side effects, although benign, can be disturbing if they occur without warning. For example, rifampin (a drug for tuberculosis) imparts a harmless red-orange color to urine, sweat, saliva, and tears. Patients will appreciate knowing about this effect *before* it occurs.

MINIMIZING ADVERSE INTERACTIONS

Patient education can help avoid hazardous drug-drug and drug-food interactions. For example, phenelzine (an antidepressant) can cause dangerous elevations in blood pressure if taken in combination with certain drugs (e.g., amphetamines) or certain foods (e.g., most cheeses, figs, avocados). Accordingly, it is essential that patients taking phenelzine be given explicit and emphatic instruction regarding the drugs and foods they must avoid.

SUMMARY

We began this chapter by asking, "Why should a nursing student learn pharmacology?" To answer the question, we explored the applications of pharmacology in nursing practice. We observed that nursing responsibilities regarding drugs go far beyond the Five Rights of Drug Administration. We observed also that the nurse has a critical role as patient advocate, serving as the patient's last line of defense against medication errors. We then discussed the many ways in which pharmacologic knowledge can be put to practical use in patient care and patient education. We saw that by applying knowledge of pharmacology, you can have a positive influence on virtually all aspects of drug therapy, thereby helping to maximize benefits and minimize harm. Hopefully, your appreciation of the importance of pharmacology in nursing practice, coupled with your desire to provide the best patient care, will provide the motivation you will need to develop an in-depth understanding of drugs.

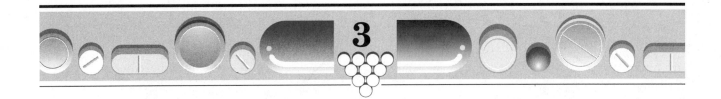

Pharmacology and the Nursing Process

The nursing process is a conceptual framework that nurses employ to guide health care delivery. In this chapter we will consider how the nursing process can be applied in drug therapy.

REVIEW OF THE NURSING PROCESS

Before discussing the nursing process as it applies to drug therapy, we need to review the process itself. Since you are probably familiar with the process already, our review will be brief.

In its simplest form, the nursing process can be viewed as a cyclic procedure that has five basic steps: (1) assessment, (2) analysis (including nursing diagnoses), (3) planning, (4) implementation, and (5) evaluation. These steps are shown schematically in Figure 3–1.

Assessment. Assessment consists of collecting data about the patient. These data are used to identify actual and potential health problems. The data base established during assessment provides a foundation for subsequent steps in the process. Important methods of data collection are the patient interview, medical and drug-use histories, the physical examination, observation of the patient, and laboratory tests.

Analysis: Nursing Diagnoses. In this step, the nurse analyzes the data base to determine actual and potential health problems. These problems

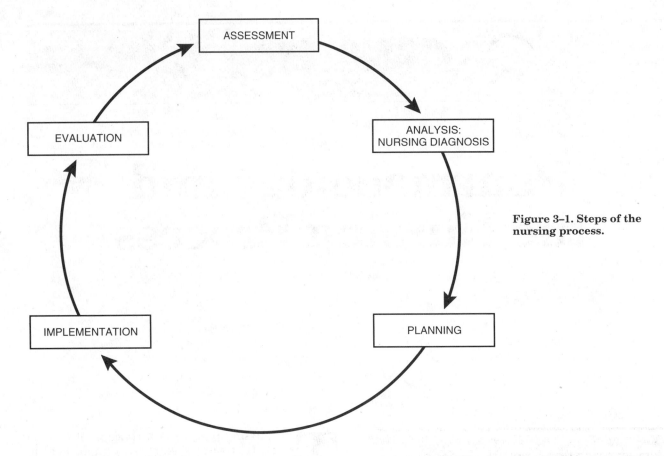

Figure 3–1. Steps of the nursing process.

may be physiologic, psychologic, or sociologic. Each problem is stated in the form of a *nursing diagnosis*, which can be defined as an actual or potential health problem that nurses are qualified and licensed to treat. Nursing diagnoses approved by the North American Nursing Diagnosis Association (NANDA) are listed in Table 3–1.

A complete nursing diagnosis consists of two statements: (1) a statement of the patient's actual or potential health problem, followed by (2) a statement of the problem's probable cause or risk factors. Typically, the statements are separated by the phrase *related to*, as in this example of a drug-associated nursing diagnosis: noncompliance with the prescribed regimen [the problem] related to inability to self-administer medication [the cause].

Planning. In the planning step, the nurse delineates specific interventions directed at solving or preventing the problems identified in analysis. The plan must be individualized for each patient. When creating a care plan, the nurse must define goals, set priorities, identify nursing interventions, and establish criteria for evaluating success. In addition to nursing interventions, the plan should include interventions performed by other health care providers. Planning is an ongoing process that must be modified as new data are gathered.

Implementation (Intervention). Implementation begins with carrying out the interventions identified during planning. Some interventions are collaborative and others are independent. Collaborative interventions require a physician's order, whereas independent nursing interventions do not. In addition to carrying out interventions, implementation involves coordinating actions of other members of the health care team. Implementation is completed by observing and recording the outcomes of treatment. Records should be thorough and precise.

Evaluation. This step is performed to determine the degree to which treatment has been successful. Evaluation is accomplished by analyzing the data collected during implementation. Evaluation should identify those interventions that should be continued, those that should be discontinued, and potential new interventions that should be implemented. Evaluation completes the initial cycle of the nursing process and provides the basis for beginning the cycle anew.

APPLICATION OF THE NURSING PROCESS IN DRUG THERAPY

Having reviewed the nursing process itself, we can now discuss the process as it pertains to drug therapy. As you will recall from Chapter 1, the overall objective in drug therapy is to produce maximum benefit with minimum harm. To accom-

Table 3–1. NANDA-Approved Nursing Diagnoses

Pattern 1: Exchanging
　Altered Nutrition: More than body requirements
　Altered Nutrition: Less than body requirements
　Altered Nutrition: Potential for more than body
　　requirements
　High Risk for Infection
　High Risk for Altered Body Temperature
　Hypothermia
　Hyperthermia
　Ineffective Thermoregulation
　Dysreflexia
　*Constipation
　Perceived Constipation
　Colonic Constipation
　*Diarrhea
　*Bowel Incontinence
　Altered Urinary Elimination
　Stress Incontinence
　Reflex Incontinence
　Urge Incontinence
　Functional Incontinence
　Total Incontinence
　Urinary Retention
　*Altered (specify type) Tissue Perfusion (renal, cerebral,
　　cardiopulmonary, gastrointestinal, peripheral)
　Fluid Volume Excess
　Fluid Volume Deficit
　High Risk for Fluid Volume Deficit
　*Decreased Cardiac Output
　Impaired Gas Exchange
　Ineffective Airway Clearance
　Ineffective Breathing Pattern
　†Inability to Sustain Spontaneous Ventilation
　†Dysfunctional Ventilatory Weaning Response (DVWR)
　High Risk for Injury
　High Risk for Suffocation
　High Risk for Poisoning
　High Risk for Trauma
　High Risk for Aspiration
　High Risk for Disuse Syndrome
　Altered Protection
　Impaired Tissue Integrity
　*Altered Oral Mucous Membrane
　Impaired Skin Integrity
　High Risk for Impaired Skin Integrity

Pattern 2: Communicating
　Impaired Verbal Communication

Pattern 3: Relating
　Impaired Social Interaction
　Social Isolation
　*Altered Role Performance
　Altered Parenting
　High Risk for Altered Parenting
　Sexual Dysfunction
　Altered Family Processes
　†Caregiver Role Strain
　†High Risk for Caregiver Role Strain
　Parental Role Conflict
　Altered Sexuality Patterns

Pattern 4: Valuing
　Spiritual Distress (distress of the human spirit)

Pattern 5: Choosing
　Ineffective Individual Coping
　Impaired Adjustment
　Defensive Coping
　Ineffective Denial
　Ineffective Family Coping: Disabling
　Ineffective Family Coping: Compromised
　Family Coping: Potential for Growth
　†Ineffective Management of Therapeutic Regimen
　　(individuals)
　Noncompliance (specify)
　Decisional Conflict (specify)
　Health Seeking Behaviors (specify)

Pattern 6: Moving
　Impaired Physical Mobility
　†High Risk for Peripheral Neurovascular Dysfunction
　Activity Intolerance
　Fatigue
　High Risk for Activity Intolerance
　Sleep Pattern Disturbance
　Diversional Activity Deficit
　Impaired Home Maintenance Management
　Altered Health Maintenance
　*Feeding Self-Care Deficit
　Impaired Swallowing
　Ineffective Breast-feeding
　†Interrupted Breast-feeding
　Effective Breast-feeding
　†Ineffective Infant Feeding Pattern
　*Bathing/Hygiene Self-Care Deficit
　*Dressing/Grooming Self-Care Deficit
　*Toileting Self-Care Deficit
　Altered Growth and Development
　†Relocation Stress Syndrome

Pattern 7: Perceiving
　*Body Image Disturbance
　*Self Esteem Disturbance
　Chronic Low Self-Esteem
　Situational Low Self-Esteem
　*Personal Identity Disturbance
　Sensory/Perceptual Alterations (specify) (visual, auditory,
　　kinesthetic, gustatory, tactile, olfactory)
　Unilateral Neglect
　Hopelessness
　Powerlessness

Pattern 8: Knowing
　Knowledge Deficit (specify)
　Altered Thought Processes

Pattern 9: Feeling
　*Pain
　Chronic Pain
　Dysfunctional Grieving
　Anticipatory Grieving
　High Risk for Violence: Self-directed or directed at others
　†High Risk for Self-Mutilation
　Post-Trauma Response
　Rape-Trauma Syndrome
　Rape-Trauma Syndrome: Compound Reaction
　Rape-Trauma Syndrome: Silent Reaction
　Anxiety
　Fear

*Categories with modified label terminology.
†New diagnostic categories approved 1992.

plish this objective, we must take into account the unique characteristics of each patient. That is, we must individualize therapy. The nursing process is well suited to help us do this. As the discussion below indicates, in order to apply the nursing process in drug therapy, you must first have a solid knowledge base in pharmacology. You will also see from the discussion that applying the nursing process to drug therapy is, in large part, an exercise in common sense.

PREADMINISTRATION ASSESSMENT

Preadministration assessment establishes the baseline data needed to tailor drug therapy to the individual. By identifying the variables that can affect an individual's responses to drugs, we can adapt treatment so as to maximize benefits and minimize harm. Preadministration assessment has four basic goals:

1. Collection of baseline data needed to evaluate therapeutic responses.
2. Collection of baseline data needed to evaluate adverse effects.
3. Identification of high-risk patients.
4. Assessment of the patient's capacity for self-care.

The first three goals are specific to the particular drug being used. Accordingly, in order to achieve these goals, you must know the pharmacology of the drug under consideration. The fourth goal applies more or less equally to all drugs—although this goal may be more critical for some drugs than others.

Important methods of data collection include interviews with the patient and family, observation of the patient, physical examination, laboratory tests, the patient's medical history, and the patient's drug history. The drug history should include prescription drugs, over-the-counter drugs, and drugs taken for nonmedical purposes (alcohol, nicotine, caffeine, illicit drugs). Prior adverse drug reactions should be noted, including drug allergies and idiosyncratic reactions.

Baseline Data Needed to Evaluate Therapeutic Effects. Drugs are administered to achieve a desired response. In order to know if we have produced that response, we need to establish baseline measurements of the parameter that therapy is directed at changing. For example, if we are giving a drug to lower blood pressure, we need to know what the pressure was prior to treatment. Without this information, we have no basis for determining the effect of our drug. And if we can't determine whether or not a drug is working, there's little justification for giving it. In order to know what baseline measurements to make, you must know the reason for drug use. This knowl-

edge comes in large part from studying pharmacology.

Baseline Data Needed to Evaluate Adverse Effects. All drugs have the ability to produce undesired effects. In practically all cases, the adverse effects that a particular drug can produce are known. In many cases, development of an adverse effect will be completely obvious in the absence of any baseline data. For example, we don't need special baseline data to know that hair loss following cancer chemotherapy was caused by the drug. However, in other cases, baseline data *are* needed to determine whether or not an adverse effect has occurred. For example, some drugs can impair liver function. In order to know if a drug has disrupted liver function, we need to know the state of liver function prior to drug use. Without this information, we can't tell from later measurements whether apparent liver dysfunction was pre-existing or caused by the drug. Clearly, in cases like this, baseline data are needed. As noted earlier, knowing what data to collect comes directly from your knowledge of the drug under consideration.

Identification of High-Risk Patients. Because of individual characteristics, a particular patient may be at high risk of experiencing adverse responses to a particular drug. Just which individual characteristics will predispose a patient to adverse reactions depends on the drug under consideration. For example, if a drug is eliminated from the body primarily by renal excretion, an individual with impaired kidney function will be at risk of having this drug accumulate to toxic levels. Similarly, if a drug is eliminated by the liver, an individual with impaired liver function will be at risk of having that drug accumulate to toxic levels. The message here is that in order to identify the patient at risk, you must know the pharmacology of the drug to be administered.

Multiple factors can increase the patient's risk of adverse reactions to a particular drug. Impaired liver and kidney function were just mentioned. Other characteristics that can predispose the patient to adverse responses include age, body composition, pregnancy, diet, genetic heritage, other drugs being used concurrently, and practically any pathophysiologic condition. These factors are discussed at length in Chapter 7 (Drug Interactions), Chapter 8 (Adverse Drug Reactions), Chapter 9 (Sources of Individual Variation in Drug Responses), and Chapter 10 (Drug Therapy in Pediatric and Geriatric Patients).

When identifying factors that put the patient at risk, you should distinguish between factors that put the patient at extremely high risk versus factors that put the patient at moderate or low risk. The terms *contraindication* and *precaution* can be used for this distinction. A *contraindication* is defined as a pre-existing condition that precludes use of a particular drug under all but the most desperate circumstances. For example, a previous *severe* allergic reaction to penicillin (which can be life threatening) would be a contraindication to using penicillin again—unless the patient had a life-threatening infection that could not be controlled with other antibiotics. A *precaution*, by contrast, can be defined as a pre-existing condition that significantly increases the risk of an adverse reaction to a particular drug, but not to a degree that is life threatening. For example, a previous *mild* allergic reaction to penicillin would constitute a precaution to using this drug again. That is, the drug may be used, but greater than normal caution must be exercised. Preferably, an alternative drug would be selected.

Assessment of the Patient's Capacity for Self-Care. If drug therapy is to succeed, the outpatient must be willing and able to self-administer medication as prescribed. Accordingly, his or her capacity for self-care must be assessed. If assessment reveals that the patient is incapable of self-medication, alternative care must be arranged.

Multiple factors can affect the capacity for self-care and the probability of adhering to the prescribed regimen. The patient with reduced visual acuity or limited manual dexterity may be unable to self-medicate, especially if the technique of administration is complex. The patient with limited intellectual ability may be incapable of understanding or remembering what he or she is supposed to do. The patient with severe mental illness (e.g., depression, schizophrenia) may lack the understanding or motivation needed to self-medicate. Some patients may lack the money to pay for drugs. Others may fail to take medications as prescribed because of individual or cultural attitudes toward drugs. Among geriatric patients, the most common cause for failed self-medication is a conviction that the drug was simply not needed in the dosage prescribed. A thorough assessment will identify all of these factors, thereby enabling you to account for them when formulating nursing diagnoses and the patient care plan.

ANALYSIS AND NURSING DIAGNOSES

With respect to drug therapy, the analysis phase of the nursing process has three objectives. First, you must judge the appropriateness of the prescribed regimen. Second, you must identify potential health problems that the drug might cause. Third, you must determine the patient's capacity for self-care.

As the last link in the patient's chain of defense against inappropriate drug therapy, the nurse must analyze the data collected during assessment to determine if the proposed treatment has a reasonable likelihood of being effective and safe. This

judgment is made by considering the medical diagnosis, the known actions of the prescribed drug, the patient's prior responses to the drug, and the presence of contraindications to the drug. You should question the drug's appropriateness if (1) the drug has no actions that are known to benefit individuals with the patient's medical diagnosis, (2) the patient failed to respond to the drug in the past, (3) the patient had a serious adverse reaction to the drug in the past, or (4) the patient has a condition or is using a drug that contraindicates the prescribed drug. If any of these conditions apply, you should consult with the prescribing physician to determine if the drug should be given.

Analysis must identify potential adverse effects and drug interactions. This is accomplished by synthesizing knowledge of the drug under consideration and the data collected during assessment. Knowledge of the drug itself will indicate adverse effects that practically all patients are likely to experience. Data on the individual patient will indicate *additional* adverse effects and interactions to which the particular patient is predisposed. Once potential adverse effects and interactions have been identified, pertinent nursing diagnoses can be easily formulated. For example, if treatment is likely to cause respiratory depression, an appropriate nursing diagnosis would be: impaired gas exchange related to drug therapy. Table 3–2 presents additional examples of nursing diagnoses that can be readily derived from knowledge of the adverse effects and interactions that treatment may cause.

Analysis must characterize the patient's capacity for self-care. The analysis should indicate potential impediments to self-care (e.g., visual impairment, reduced manual dexterity, impaired cognitive function, insufficient understanding of the prescribed regimen) so that these factors can be addressed in the care plan. To varying degrees, nearly all patients will be unfamiliar with self-medication and the drug regimen. Accordingly, a nursing diagnosis applicable to almost every patient is: knowledge deficit related to the drug regimen.

PLANNING

Planning consists of defining goals, establishing priorities, identifying specific interventions, and establishing criteria for evaluating success. Good planning will allow you to promote beneficial drug effects. Of equal or greater importance, good planning will allow you to *anticipate* adverse effects—rather than react to them after the fact.

Defining Goals. In all cases, the goal of drug therapy is to produce maximum benefits with minimum harm. That is, we want to employ drugs in such a way as to maximize therapeutic responses

	Table 3–2. Examples of Nursing Diagnoses That Can be Derived from Knowledge of Adverse Drug Effects	
Drug	**Adverse Effect**	**Related Nursing Diagnosis**
Amphetamine	CNS stimulation	Altered sleep pattern related to drug-induced CNS excitation
Aspirin	Gastric erosion	Pain related to aspirin-induced gastric erosion
Atropine	Urinary retention	Urinary retention related to drug therapy
Bethanechol	Stimulation of GI smooth muscle	Bowel incontinence related to drug-induced increase in bowel motility
Clonidine	Impotence	Sexual dysfunction related to drug-induced impotence
Cyclophosphamide	Reduction in white blood cell counts	Potential for infection related to drug-induced neutropenia
Digoxin	Dysrhythmias	Reduced tissue perfusion related to drug-induced cardiac dysrhythmias
Furosemide	Excessive urine production	Fluid volume deficit related to drug-induced diuresis
Gentamicin	Damage to the eighth cranial nerve	Perceptual/sensory alteration: hearing impairment related to drug therapy
Glucocorticoids	Thinning of the skin	Impaired skin integrity related to drug therapy
Haloperidol	Involuntary movements	Disturbance in self-esteem related to drug-induced involuntary movements
Nitroglycerin	Hypotension	Potential for injury related to dizziness caused by drug-induced hypotension
Propranolol	Bradycardia	Decreased cardiac output related to drug-induced bradycardia
Warfarin	Spontaneous bleeding	Potential for injury related to drug-induced bleeding

CNS = central nervous system, GI = gastrointestinal.

while preventing or minimizing adverse reactions and interactions. The objective of planning is to formulate ways to achieve this goal.

Setting Priorities. This requires knowledge of the drug under consideration and the patient's unique characteristics—and even then, setting priorities can be difficult. Highest priority is given to life-threatening conditions (e.g., anaphylactic shock, ventricular fibrillation). These may be drug induced or the result of disease. High priority is also given to reactions that cause severe, acute discomfort and to reactions that can result in long-term harm. Since we cannot manage all problems simultaneously, less severe problems must wait until the patient and care provider have the time and resources to address them.

Identifying Interventions. The heart of planning is identification of nursing interventions. These interventions can be divided into four major groups: (1) drug administration, (2) interventions to enhance therapeutic effects, (3) interventions to minimize adverse effects and interactions, and (4) patient education (which encompasses information in the first three groups).

When planning drug administration, you must consider dosage size, route of administration, and less obvious factors, including timing of administration with respect to meals and to other drugs. Timing with respect to side effects is also important. For example, if a drug causes sedation, it may be desirable to give the drug at bedtime, rather than in the morning or during the day.

Nondrug measures can help promote therapeutic effects and should be included in the plan. For example, drug therapy of hypertension can be com-bined with weight loss (in obese patients), salt restriction, and cessation of smoking.

Interventions to prevent or minimize adverse effects are of obvious importance. When planning these interventions, you should distinguish between reactions that develop quickly and those that are delayed. A few drugs can cause severe adverse reactions (e.g., anaphylactic shock) shortly after administration. When planning to administer such a drug, you should insure that facilities for managing possible reactions are immediately available. Delayed reactions can often be minimized, if not avoided entirely. The plan should include interventions to do so.

Well-planned patient education is central to success. The plan should account for the patient's capacity to learn, and it should address the following: technique of administration, dosage size and timing, duration of treatment, method of drug storage, measures to promote therapeutic effects, and measures to minimize adverse effects. Patient education is discussed at length in Chapter 2.

Establishing Criteria for Evaluation. The need for objective criteria by which to measure desired drug responses is obvious: without such criteria we could not determine if our drug was doing anything useful. As a result, we would have no rational basis for making dosage adjustments and for deciding how long treatment should continue. If the drug is to be used on an outpatient basis, follow-up visits for evaluation should be planned.

IMPLEMENTATION

Implementation of the care plan in drug therapy has four major components: (1) drug administration, (2) patient education, (3) interventions to promote therapeutic effects, and (4) interventions to minimize adverse effects. These critical nursing activities are discussed at length in Chapter 2.

EVALUATION

Over the course of drug therapy, the patient must be evaluated for (1) therapeutic responses, (2) adverse drug reactions and interactions, (3) compliance (adherence to the prescribed regimen), and (4) satisfaction with treatment. How frequently evaluations are performed depends on the expected time course of therapeutic and adverse effects. Like assessment, evaluation is based on laboratory tests, observation of the patient, physical examination, and patient interviews. The conclusions drawn during evaluation provide the basis for modifying nursing interventions and the drug regimen.

Therapeutic responses are evaluated by comparing the patient's current health status with the baseline data. In order to evaluate treatment, you must know the reason for drug use, the criteria for success (as defined during planning), and the expected time course of responses (some drugs act within minutes, whereas others may take weeks or even months to produce beneficial effects).

The need to anticipate and evaluate adverse effects is self-evident. To make these evaluations, you must know which adverse effects are likely to occur, how they are manifested, and their probable time course. The method of monitoring is determined by the expected effect. For example, if hypotension is expected, blood pressure is monitored; if constipation is expected, bowel function is monitored; and so on. Since some adverse effects can be fatal in the absence of timely detection, it is impossible to overemphasize the importance of monitoring and preparedness for rapid intervention.

Evaluation of compliance is desirable in all patients—and is especially valuable when therapeutic failure occurs or when adverse effects are unexpectedly severe. Methods of evaluating compliance include measurement of plasma drug levels, interviewing the patient, and counting pills. The evaluation should determine if the patient understands when to take medication, what dosage to take, and the technique of administration.

Patient satisfaction with drug therapy increases quality of life and promotes compliance. If the patient is dissatisfied, an otherwise effective regimen may not be taken as prescribed. Factors that can cause dissatisfaction include unacceptable side effects, an inconvenient dosing schedule, difficulty of administration, and high cost. When evaluation reveals dissatisfaction, an attempt should be made to alter the drug regimen to make it more acceptable.

USE OF A MODIFIED NURSING PROCESS FORMAT TO SUMMARIZE NURSING IMPLICATIONS IN THIS TEXT

Throughout this text, nursing implications are integrated into the body of each chapter. The reason for integrating nursing information with basic science information is to reinforce the relationship between pharmacologic knowledge and nursing practice. In addition to being integrated, nursing implications are *summarized* at the end of most chapters. The purpose of the summaries is to provide a concise and readily accessible reference on patient care and patient education related to specific drugs and drug families.

The format employed for the summaries of nursing implications reflects the nursing process (Table 3–3). However, as you can see, we have modified the headings somewhat. This was done to accommodate the needs of pharmacology instruction and to keep the summaries concise. The components of the format are discussed below.

Preadministration Assessment. This section summarizes the information you should have before giving a drug. The section begins by stating the reason for drug use. This is followed by a summary of the baseline data needed to evaluate therapeutic and adverse effects. After this, contraindications and precautions are summarized under the heading *Identifying High-Risk Patients*.

Implementation: Administration. This section summarizes routes of administration, guidelines for dosage adjustment, and special considerations in administration, such as timing with respect to meals, preparation of intravenous solutions, and unusual techniques of administration.

Implementation: Measures to Enhance Therapeutic Effects. This section addresses issues such as diet modification, measures to in-

Table 3–3. Modified Nursing Process Format for Summaries of Nursing Implications
Preadministration Assessment
Therapeutic Goal
Baseline Data
Identifying High-Risk Patients
Implementation: Administration
Routes
Administration
Implementation: Measures to Enhance Therapeutic Effects
Ongoing Evaluation and Interventions
Summary of Monitoring
Evaluating Therapeutic Effects
Minimizing Adverse Effects
Minimizing Adverse Interactions

crease comfort, and ways to promote adherence with the prescribed regimen.

Ongoing Evaluation and Interventions. This section summarizes nursing implications that relate to drug responses, both therapeutic and undesired. As indicated in Table 3–3, the section has four subsections: (1) summary of monitoring, (2) evaluating therapeutic effects, (3) minimizing adverse effects, and (4) minimizing adverse interactions. The monitoring section summarizes the physiologic and psychologic parameters that must be monitored in order to evaluate therapeutic and adverse responses. The section on therapeutic effects summarizes criteria and procedures for evaluating therapeutic responses. The section on adverse effects summarizes the major adverse reactions that should be monitored for and presents interventions to minimize them. The section on adverse interactions summarizes the major interactions to be alert for and gives interventions to minimize them.

Patient Education. This topic does not have a section of its own. Rather, patient education is integrated into the other sections. That is, as we summarize the nursing implications that relate to a particular topic, such as drug administration or a specific adverse effect, patient education related to that topic is discussed concurrently. This integration is done to promote clarity and efficiency of communication. In order to make this important information stand out, it appears in color.

What About Diagnosis and Planning? These headings are not used in the summaries. There are several reasons for the omission, the dominant one being efficiency of communication.

Nursing diagnoses have been left out because they are extremely numerous and largely self-evident. Yes, we could have included a list of diagnoses for each drug. However, since nursing diagnoses derive from drug effects, and since all drugs cause many effects (primarily adverse), the list of diagnoses for each drug would be very long. Accordingly, since nursing diagnoses can be readily formulated from one's knowledge of pharmacology, and since a long list of diagnoses would dilute the impact of other important information, we decided to omit nursing diagnoses from the summaries.

Planning has not been used as a heading for three reasons. First, planning applies primarily to the overall management of the disorder for which a particular drug is being used—and much less to the drug itself. Second, planning is discussed at length and more appropriately in nonpharmacology nursing texts, such as those on medical-surgical nursing. There is no need to repeat this information here. Third, most planning is done with the aid of standardized nursing care plans—either computerized or in print format. These standardized plans are sufficient for most drug-related planning. Please note, however, that although we don't have a separate heading for planning, critical issues in planning *are* included nonetheless.

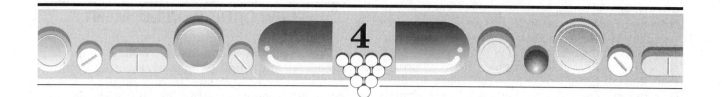

Drug Legislation, Development, Names, and Information

In this chapter we will complete our introduction to pharmacology by considering four diverse but important topics. These are (1) drug legislation, (2) new drug development, (3) the annoying problem of drug names, and (4) sources of drug information.

LANDMARK DRUG LEGISLATION

The history of drug legislation in the United States reflects an evolution in our national posture toward regulating the pharmaceutical industry. That posture has changed from one of minimal control to one of extensive control. For the most part, increased regulation has been beneficial, resulting in safer and more effective drugs.

The first American law to regulate drugs was the *Federal Pure Food and Drug Act of 1906*. This law was very weak: its only requirement was that drugs be *free of adulterants*. The law said nothing about drug safety and effectiveness.

The Food, Drug and Cosmetic Act, passed in 1938, was much stronger than the Pure Food and Drug Act and was the first legislation to regulate drug *safety*. The motivation for the 1938 law was a tragedy in which more than 100 people died following use of a new medication. The lethal preparation contained an antibiotic (sulfanilamide) plus a solubilizing agent (diethylene glycol). Tests revealed that the solvent was the cause of death. (Diethylene glycol is commonly used as automotive antifreeze.) To reduce the chances that such a tragedy might recur, Congress required that all new drugs undergo testing for toxicity. The results of these tests were to be reviewed by the *Food and Drug Administration* (FDA), and only those drugs judged to be safe would receive FDA approval for marketing.

The next major development in drug regulation was the *Kefauver-Harris Act of 1962*. This law was created in response to the thalidomide tragedy, which occurred in Europe in the early 1960's. Thalidomide is a sedative now known to cause birth defects. Because the drug was used widely by pregnant women, many infants were born with phocomelia, a rare birth defect characterized by the gross malformation or complete absence of arms or legs. This tragedy was especially poignant in that it resulted from nonessential drug use: the women who took thalidomide could have done very well without it. Thalidomide was not a problem in the United States because the drug had been withheld by the FDA.

Because of the European experience with thalidomide, the Kefauver-Harris Act sought to strengthen all aspects of drug regulation. One of the bill's major provisions was to require proof of *effectiveness* before a new drug could be marketed. Remarkably, this was the first law to demand that drugs actually be of some benefit. The new act also required that all old drugs that had been introduced between 1932 and 1962 undergo testing for effectiveness; those drugs that could not be proved useful would be withdrawn. Lastly, the Kefauver-Harris Act established rigorous procedures for testing new drugs. These procedures are discussed later under *New Drug Development*.

In 1970, Congress passed the *Controlled Substances Act* (Title II of the Comprehensive Drug Abuse Prevention and Control Act). This legislation set rules for the manufacture and distribution of drugs considered to have the potential for abuse. One provision of the law defines categories into which controlled substances are placed. These categories are labeled Schedules I, II, III, IV, and V. Drugs in Schedule I have no accepted medical use in the United States and are deemed to have a high potential for abuse. Examples include heroin, mescaline, and lysergic acid diethylamide (LSD). Drugs in Schedules II through V have accepted medical applications but also have the potential for abuse. The abuse potential of these agents becomes progressively less as we proceed from Schedule II to Schedule V. The Controlled Substances Act is discussed further in Chapter 34 (Drugs of Abuse).

NEW DRUG DEVELOPMENT

The development and testing of new drugs is an expensive and lengthy process, requiring from 6 to 12 years for completion. It is estimated that for every 5000 compounds that enter testing, only one emerges as a new product.

Rigorous testing procedures have been established so that newly released drugs might be both safe and effective. Unfortunately, although testing can determine effectiveness, testing cannot guarantee that a new drug will be safe: significant adverse effects may evade detection during testing only to become apparent once a new drug has been released for general use.

STAGES OF NEW DRUG DEVELOPMENT

The testing of new drugs has two principal steps: *preclinical testing* and *clinical testing*. Preclinical tests are performed in animals. Clinical testing is done in humans. The steps in drug development are outlined in Table 4–1.

Preclinical Testing

Preclinical testing is required before a new drug may be tested in humans. During preclinical testing, drugs are evaluated for *toxicities, pharmacokinetic properties,* and *potentially useful biologic effects*. Preclinical tests may take 1 to 3 years. When sufficient preclinical data have been gath-

---

Table 4–1. Steps in New Drug Development

Preclinical Testing (in animals)
  Toxicity
  Pharmacokinetics
  Possible Useful Effects
    ↓
  Investigational New Drug (IND) Status
    ↓
Clinical Testing (in humans)

  Phase I
    Subjects: normal volunteers
    Tests: metabolism and biologic effects
  Phase II
    Subjects: patients
    Tests: therapeutic utility and dosage range
  Phase III
    Subjects: patients
    Tests: safety and effectiveness
  Conditional Approval of New Drug Application (NDA)
    ↓
  Phase IV
      Early: limited, closely monitored marketing
      Late: Unlimited marketing with postmarketing
        surveillance

ered, the drug developer may apply to the FDA for permission to begin testing in humans. If the application is approved, the drug is awarded *Investigational New Drug* status, and clinical trials may commence.

Clinical Testing

Clinical trials occur in four phases and may take 5 to 9 years for completion. The first three phases are done before a new drug is marketed. The fourth phase is performed after marketing has begun.

Phases I, II, and III. Phase I trials are conducted in *normal volunteers.* The goal of these tests is twofold: evaluation of drug *metabolism* and determination of *effects in humans.* In phases II and III, drugs are tested in *patients.* The purpose of these tests is to establish *therapeutic effects, dosage range,* and *safety.* Upon completing phase III, a drug company applies to the FDA for conditional approval of a *New Drug Application.* If conditional approval is granted, phase IV trials may begin.

Phase IV: Postmarketing Surveillance. Phase IV testing has two stages, referred to as *early* and *late.* During the early phase, a new drug is released for marketing but on a limited basis; *all* patients are monitored. The value of early phase IV testing is that it permits observation of drug effects in a population much larger than the populations that participated in phase II and phase III. In the late stage of phase IV, the new drug is released for general marketing. During this phase, voluntary reporting by prescribing physicians expands our knowledge of what the new drug can do.

LIMITATIONS OF THE TESTING PROCEDURE

It is important for nurses and other health care professionals to appreciate the limitations of the drug development process. Two problems are of particular concern. First, information on beneficial and adverse effects in women is very limited. Second, new drugs are likely to have adverse effects that were not detected during clinical trials.

Limited Information in Women

Very little drug testing is done in women. In practically all cases, women of child-bearing potential are excluded from early clinical trials. The rationale for this exclusion is concern for fetal safety. Unfortunately, FDA policy has taken this concern to an extreme, effectively barring all women of child-bearing age from phase I and phase II trials—whether or not they are actually pregnant or using adequate contraception. At this time, the only women allowed to participate in early clinical trials are those who have life-threatening illnesses that might respond to the drugs under study.

Because of limited drug testing in women, we don't know with precision how women will respond to drugs. We don't know if beneficial effects in women will be equivalent to those seen in men. Nor do we know if adverse effects will be equivalent to those in men. We don't know how timing of drug administration with respect to the menstrual cycle will affect beneficial and adverse responses. We don't know if drug disposition (absorption, distribution, metabolism, excretion) will be the same in women as in men. Furthermore, of the various drugs that might be used to treat a particular illness, we don't know if the ones that are most effective in men will also be most effective in women. Lastly, we don't know about the safety of drug use during pregnancy.

Very recently, the FDA indicated that it will revise its guidelines to remove some of the restrictions that now bar women of child-bearing age from early trials. However, even if this is done, it will take a long time to close the gender gap in our knowledge of drugs.

Failure to Detect All Adverse Effects

The testing procedure cannot detect all adverse effects before a new drug is released. There are three reasons for this problem: (1) during clinical trials a relatively small number of patients are given the drug; (2) because these patients are carefully selected, they do not represent the variety of individuals who will eventually take the drug; and (3) patients in trials take the drug for a relatively short time. Because of these unavoidable limitations in the testing process, effects that occur infrequently and effects that take a long time to develop may go undetected. Hence, despite our best efforts, when a new drug is released, it may well have adverse effects of which we are as yet unaware.

Consequently, when working with a new drug, you should be especially watchful for previously unreported drug reactions. If a patient taking a new drug begins to show unusual symptoms, it is prudent to suspect that the new drug may be the cause—even though the symptoms are not yet mentioned in the literature.

EXERCISING DISCRETION REGARDING NEW DRUGS

When thinking about prescribing a new drug, the clinician would do well to follow this guideline: *Be neither the first to adopt the new nor the last to abandon the old.* Recall that the therapeutic objective is to produce maximum benefit with minimum harm. To achieve this objective, we must balance the inherent risks in giving a drug against the potential benefits. As a rule, new drugs have actions very similar to those of older agents: it is rare for a new drug to be able to do something that an older drug can't do already. Consequently, the need to treat a particular disorder seldom constitutes a compelling reason to select a new drug over an agent that has been available for years. Furthermore, new drugs generally present greater risks than the old ones. As noted above, at the time of its introduction, a new drug is likely to have adverse effects that have not yet been reported, and these effects may prove very bad for some patients. In contrast, older, more familiar drugs are less likely to cause unpleasant surprises. Consequently, when we weigh the benefits of a new drug against the risks, it is likely that the benefits will be insufficient to justify the risks—especially when an older drug whose properties are well known would probably provide adequate treatment. Accordingly, when it comes to the use of new drugs, it is usually better to adopt a wait-and-see policy, letting more adventurous clinicians discover the hidden dangers that a new drug may present.

DRUG NAMES

The topic of drug names is important and can be confusing. The topic is important because the names we employ affect our ability to communicate about medicines. The subject is confusing because we have evolved a system in which any drug can have a large number of names.

In approaching the discussion of drug names, we will begin by defining the types of names that drugs have. We will then consider (1) the complications that arise from assigning multiple names to a drug, and (2) the benefits of using just one name: the generic name.

THE THREE TYPES OF DRUG NAMES

Drugs have three types of names: (1) a chemical name, (2) a generic or nonproprietary name, and (3) a trade or proprietary name. Examples of these appear in Table 4–2. All of the names in the table are for the same drug, a compound most familiar to us under the trade name Tylenol.

Chemical Name. The chemical name constitutes a description of a drug using the nomenclature of chemistry. As you can see from the example in Table 4–2, a drug's chemical name can be long and complex. Because of their complexity, chemical names are inappropriate for everyday use. For example, few people would communicate using the chemical term *N-acetyl-para-aminophenol* when a

Table 4–2. The Three Types of Drug Names	

$$H_3C - \overset{\overset{\textstyle O}{\|}}{C} - \overset{\overset{\textstyle H}{|}}{N} - \!- OH$$

Type of Drug Name	Examples
Chemical Name	*N*-Acetyl-para-aminophenol
Generic Name (nonproprietary name)	Acetaminophen
Trade Name (proprietary name)	Acephen, Aceta, Anacin-3, Apacet, Arthritis Pain Formula Aspirin Free, Aspirin Free Pain Relief, Banesin, Bromo Seltzer, Dapa, Datril, Dolanex, Dorcol Children's Fever and Pain Reducer, Feverall, Genapap, Genebs, Halenol, Liquiprin Elixir, Meda Tab, Myapap, Neopap, Oraphen-PD, Panadol, Panex, Panex 500, Phenaphen Caplets, Snaplets-FR Granules, St. Joseph Aspirin-Free for Children, Suppap-325, Tapanol Extra Strength, Tempra, Tylenol

The chemical, generic, and trade names listed are all names for the drug whose structure is pictured in this table. This drug is most familiar to us under its trade name of Tylenol.

more simple generic name (acetaminophen) or trade name (e.g., Tylenol) could be used instead.

Generic Name. The generic name of a drug is assigned by the United States Adopted Names Council. Each drug has only one generic name. The generic name is also known as the *nonproprietary name*. Generic names are less complex than chemical names but usually more complex than trade names. For the reasons presented below, generic names are preferable to trade names for general usage.

Trade Name. Trade names, also known as *proprietary* or *brand* names, are the names under which a drug is marketed. Trade names are created by drug companies with the intention that the name be easy for nurses, physicians, and consumers to recall and pronounce. Since any drug can be marketed in different formulations and by multiple companies, the number of trade names that a drug can have is large. By way of illustration, Table 4–2 gives the 31 trade names, including Tylenol, that exist for the drug whose generic name is *acetaminophen*.

WHICH NAME TO USE, GENERIC OR TRADE?

We employ drug names in two ways: (1) for written and verbal communication about medicines, and (2) to put on labels to identify medications in containers. In both cases, accurate communication is imperative. For communication to be accurate, when we read or hear a drug name, we must know what compound that name is referring to. We can't know what's in a bottle if we don't know what the name on the bottle means. Likewise, we can't communicate verbally about drugs if the names we employ go unrecognized. Clearly, if we are to communicate accurately, name recognition is essential. As discussed below, name recognition would be enhanced through universal use of generic names.

The Little Problem with Generic Names

In almost all cases, the generic name for a drug is longer and more complicated than the trade name. This fact is illustrated in Table 4–3, which compares the generic and trade names for six common drugs. A simple analysis reveals that the average generic name in the table has 4.8 syllables. In contrast, the average trade name has only 2.5 syllables. That is, the generic names are nearly twice as long as the trade names.

Because generic names are more complex than trade names, generic names can be more difficult to remember and pronounce. As an exercise, try pronouncing the names in Table 4–3. While trade names like Motrin and Elavil roll off the tongue with ease, their generic counterparts—ibuprofen and amitriptyline—tend to tie the tongue in knots.

Why is it that generic names are more complicated than trade names? One reason is that the pharmaceutical industry has an important role in establishing generic names. When a pharmaceutical company has developed a new drug, that company submits a suggested generic name to the United States Adopted Names Council, the body responsible for assigning a drug its generic name. As a rule, the Council adopts the name the company suggests. Since, from a marketing perspective, it's to the company's advantage to have a product whose trade name is more easily recognized than its generic name, it seems unlikely that a company will suggest a simple, euphonious ge-

neric name. Also contributing to the complexity of generic names are the guidelines established by the Council for naming drugs.

The Big Problems with Trade Names

The Problem of Multiple Names for the Same Medication. The principal objection to trade names is their vast number. Although a drug can have only one generic name, the number of trade names it can have is unlimited. As the number of trade names for a single drug increases, the problem of name recognition becomes progressively larger. By way of illustration, the drug whose generic name is *acetaminophen* has trade names that number in excess of 30 (see Table 4–2). Although most clinicians will recognize this drug's generic name, few are familiar with all of the trade names. As we can see, even though a generic name may be complex, to recall a single generic name for a particular drug remains an easier task than to recall a multitude of trade names for that same drug. Accordingly, if generic names were to be employed universally, accurate communication would be facilitated. Conversely, the use of multiple trade names can do nothing but create confusion.

By clouding communication about drugs, use of trade names can result in "double medication," with potentially disastrous results. Because a patient frequently sees more than one physician, it is possible for a patient to be given prescriptions for the same drug by two different doctors. If those prescriptions are written for different brand names, then the two bottles the patient receives will be labeled with different names. Consequently, although both bottles contain the same drug, the patient may be unaware of this fact. If both medications are taken as prescribed, excessive dosing will result. However, if generic names had been used, both labels would bear the same name, thereby informing the patient that both bottles contain the same drug. Given this information, the patient is likely to consult with the prescribing physicians to determine if both prescriptions should be honored.

The Problem of Using Trade Names for Combination Products. Many pharmaceutical preparations are composed of more than one drug. When such combination products are referred to by trade name, the name is unlikely to indicate either the number of drugs present or their identity. Referring to Table 4–4, there is nothing about the trade name *Excedrin Tablets* to suggest that the product bearing this name consists of three different drugs: aspirin, acetaminophen, and caffeine. By discarding the trade name and labeling this product *aspirin plus acetaminophen plus caffeine,* we could eliminate confusion about its composition.

Table 4–3. Generic Names and Trade Names of Some Commonly Used Drugs	
Generic Name	**Trade Name**
Chlordiazepoxide	Librium
Ibuprofen	Motrin
Furosemide	Lasix
Amitriptyline	Elavil
Acetaminophen	Tyyenol
Cephalexin	Keflex

Table 4–4. Composition of Some Common Preparations That Contain a Combination of Drugs	
Product Name	**Drugs in the Preparation**
Excedrin Tablets	Acetaminophen + aspirin + caffeine
Excedrin P.M.	Acetaminophen + diphenhydramine
4-Way Long-Acting Nasal Spray	Oxymetazoline
4-Way Fast-Acting Nasal Spray	Phenylephrine + naphazoline + pyrilamine
4-Way Cold Tabs	Acetaminophen + phenylpropanolamine + chlorpheniramine

The group of *4-Way* products listed in Table 4–4 illustrates the potential for trade names to be misleading, with a resultant impairment of accurate communication. If nothing else, the name *4-Way* suggests that the product contains more than one drug. In fact, the name seems to imply the presence of *four* drugs. However, as can be seen from the table, this implication is not correct: none of the 4-Way preparations is composed of four drugs. One preparation—4-Way Long-Acting Nasal Spray—contains only one drug. Each of the other preparations contains three drugs. Furthermore, it should be noted that all three of these similarly named products are, in fact, completely different from one another—none has ingredients in common with the others. Hence, in the case of these 4-Way products, we can see that the trade name cannot be taken to mean either (1) the presence of four different drugs, or (2) that these preparations that bear similar names have the same composition. Had generic names been employed to label these products, there could be no confusion about their makeup.

What If Peas Were Marketed Like Drugs?

Given the problems that trade names create, why do we use trade names at all? We use trade names because the pharmaceutical industry wants them. Why? Because trade names give this industry a unique and powerful tool with which to market its products. As we shall see, the extent to which trade names are exploited to promote drug sales is without parallel in the marketing of any other product.

To understand the immense marketing value that trade names have for the drug companies, it will be helpful to consider the marketing of a product that is not a drug. Take peas, for example. All companies that sell peas use the same name—peas—to identify their product. When we buy peas, no matter whose, all pea packages say PEAS in big letters on the label. Pea packages even have a picture of peas to help us properly identify what's inside. Consequently, when we choose a package of peas, we know with certainty what we are buying.

When we want to compare different brands of peas, the task is easy. Company A's peas are easily distinguished from those of company B or company C by the presence of a company name on the label. Consequently, thanks to the way peas are marketed, we have no trouble understanding (1) just what we are buying, and (2) who made it. As a result, we can easily select the product we want from the manufacturer we like best.

Now let's consider what we could expect if peas were marketed like drugs. Under the new system, pea packages would have no pictures of peas on them. Nor would pea packages proclaim PEAS in big letters to help us identify their contents. Instead, pea packages would be emblazoned with trade names—names like *Vegi-P* or *Producin* or *NuPod-500's*. If peas were marketed using trade names, when we went shopping for peas we'd be obliged to read a lot of fine print to find the product we wanted. And once we finally did turn up a package with peas in it, for example the one labeled *NuPod-500's*, we'd probably buy *NuPod-500's* for life—it being too much trouble to figure out which of the other packages with meaningless names on them also contain peas. From the point of view of the people who sell *NuPod-500's*, this technique of marketing by trade names is a terrific arrangement. Consumers will be loyal to their product not because that product is better or cheaper than someone else's, but because product labeling with trade names makes it very difficult to identify the competition so that comparisons can be made. Fortunately, we don't allow this kind of marketing for peas. When we shop for peas, we demand that all pea packages bear the word PEAS—not *Vegi-P* or *NuPod-500's* or any other trade name. Why we permit medicines to be marketed in any less informative a manner is a disturbing question.

When we consider that drugs, unlike peas, cannot be identified by simple observation, the use of trade names for marketing becomes especially unsettling. With peas, once we open the package, we no longer need the label to identify the contents. We know what peas look like. Hence, even if peas were marketed like drugs, we would not be completely dependent upon labeling to identify the product. With drugs we have no options: since we cannot identify a drug by looking at it, we cannot escape reliance on package labeling to inform us about the medicine inside. It is ironic that a product whose label is so essential for identification can be marketed under a system that employs multiple trade names, thereby making product identification needlessly and dangerously difficult.

Generic Products versus Brand Name Products

To complete our discussion of drug names, we need to address two questions: (1) Do significant differences exist between different brands of the same drug? and (2) If such differences do exist, do they justify the use of trade names?

The answer to our first question is a qualified *Yes.* Yes, examples can be found in which different brands of the same drug are not therapeutically equivalent. However, these examples are rare. In most cases, there is no significant difference among preparations of a drug made by company A, company B, and company Z. Furthermore, it should be noted that drugs marketed under generic names are chemically identical to those marketed under trade names. For example, the medication present in tablets available generically as *diazepam* is identical to that in tablets marketed under the trade name *Valium.*

In those cases in which drug preparations *do* differ from one another, the differences are not in the chemical composition of the drugs themselves. Rather, differences concern either the rate or extent of drug absorption. Differences in absorption can occur because of differences in the way that drug formulations (e.g., tablets, capsules, sustained-release preparations) are manufactured. Hence, even though brand A and brand B contain the same amount of the same drug, these preparations may be absorbed differently and, as a result, may produce quantitatively different effects. Occasionally, such differences are large enough to be of therapeutic significance.

Since, in some cases, variations in absorption between different brands of the same drug can be large enough to affect the outcome of therapy, do such variations justify the use of trade names in order to identify a preferred product? The answer to this question is a resounding NO! If physicians want to prescribe a drug made by a particular company, they needn't resort to trade names to do so; their preference can be indicated simply by including the manufacturer's name on the prescription. As with peas, if we prefer a particular brand (e.g., Bird's Eye), that's what we ask for. We haven't found it necessary to create a complicated system of alternative names for peas in order to distinguish one brand from another. On the contrary, common sense tells us that such a system of trade names would make it more difficult, not easier, for us to clearly communicate our needs. Perhaps some day we will market medicines with as much common sense as we use to market vegetables.

Conclusion Regarding Generic Names and Trade Names

In the preceding discussion we considered the advantages and disadvantages associated with trade names and generic names. We noted that although generic names may be long, this disadvantage is more than offset by the fact that each drug has only one generic name. In contrast, the sole virtue of trade names—ease of recall and pronunciation—is far outweighed by the problems that stem from the existence of multiple trade names for a single drug. Multiple trade names can impede name recognition and can thereby promote medication errors and miscommunication about drugs. With generic names, the opposite is achieved: facilitation of communication and promotion of safe and effective drug use. Clearly, generic names are preferable to trade names. Accordingly, until such time as trade names are outlawed, the least we can do is actively discourage their use. In this text, generic names are employed for routine discussion. Although trade names are presented, they are not emphasized. We may eventually see the day when trade names are abandoned and generic names are employed universally. On that day, efforts to achieve the therapeutic objective will receive a significant boost.

SOURCES OF DRUG INFORMATION

There is much more to pharmacology than we can address in this text. When you need additional information, the sources discussed below should be helpful.

PEOPLE

Clinicians and Pharmacists. Nurses and other clinicians can be invaluable sources of information about medicines. Pharmacists know a great deal about drugs and are usually eager to share their expertise.

Poison Control Centers. Poison control centers are present throughout the country. These centers are accessible by telephone, permitting rapid access to information about medicines and toxic compounds. Appendix E lists the names, addresses, and telephone numbers of the certified regional poison centers in the United States.

Pharmaceutical Sales Representatives. Pharmaceutical sales representatives (drug representatives) can be useful sources of drug information. These people know their own products very well, and they can provide detailed, authoritative information about them. Keep in mind, however, that the ultimate job of the drug representative is *sales—not education.* Because the objective is sales, drug representatives may fail to volunteer negative information about their product. Likewise, they are unlikely to point out superior qualities in a competing drug. (Is a Chevrolet salesperson going to extol the virtues of a Ford?) Such a lack of complete candor does not mean that drug representatives are unethical, they are simply doing their job. However, since full disclosure may be inconsistent with success, the drug representative may not be your best source of information—especially if you are trying to establish an unbiased comparison between the representative's product and a drug from a competing manufacturer.

PUBLISHED INFORMATION

The publications described below are general references. These works cover a broad range of topics but in limited depth. Accordingly, these references are most useful as initial sources of information. If more detail is needed, specialty publications should be consulted. Some important drug references, including the ones described below, are listed in Table 4–5.

Text-like Books

Goodman and Gilman's The Pharmacological Basis of Therapeutics is the classic text/reference on pharmacology used by medical students and practicing physicians. As its name implies, this book focuses on the basic science information that underlies drug use—and not on therapeutics per se. New editions are released about every 5 years.

Drug Evaluations, a comprehensive reference prepared by the American Medical Association, discusses drugs from the perspective of therapeutics. Hence, in contrast to the text originated by Goodman and Gilman, this book emphasizes clinical aspects of pharmacology rather than basic science. Since the organizing principle for most chapters is drugs used to treat a particular disease, the book is especially helpful for obtaining *comparative* information on the various agents that might be employed to manage a specific disorder. The book is updated annually.

Pharmacotherapy: A Pathophysiologic Approach is a comprehensive text on drug therapy. As in *Drug Evaluations*, each chapter focuses on the treatment of a specific disorder. To facilitate understanding of drug therapy, the book presents thorough reviews of pathophysiology.

Newsletter

The Medical Letter is a bimonthly publication that gives very current information on drugs. A typical issue discusses two or three agents. Discussions consist of a summary of data from clinical

---

Table 4–5. Some Important Drug References

General Information on Drug Actions, Pharmacokinetics, Therapeutics, Adverse Effects, and Drug Interactions

Drug Evaluations. American Medical Association, Chicago (updated annually)

Goodman and Gilman's The Pharmacological Basis of Therapeutics, 8th ed. Gilman, A.G., Rall, T.W., Nies, A.S., Taylor, P. (eds.). McGraw-Hill, New York, 1990

Pharmacotherapy: A Pathophysiologic Approach, 2nd ed. DiPiro, J.T., et al (eds.). Elsevier Science Publishing, New York, 1992

Principles of Drug Action: The Basis of Pharmacology, 3rd ed. Pratt, W.P., Taylor, P., Churchill Livingstone, New York, 1990

Detailed Information on Specific Drugs and Drug Families

AHFS Drug Information, 1992. McEvoy, G.K. (ed.). American Society of Hospital Pharmacists, Bethesda, MD (updated annually)

Drug Facts and Comparisons, Loose-leaf ed. Facts and Comparisons, St. Louis (updated monthly)

Physicians' Desk Reference. Medical Economics Data, Montvale, NJ (updated annually)

United States Pharmacopeia Drug Information (USP DI): Drug Information for the Health Care Professional. The United States Pharmacopeial Convention, Inc., Rockville, MD (updated bimonthly)

Very Current Information

The Medical Letter. The Medical Letter, Inc., New Rochelle, NY (published biweekly)

International Drug Information

British Pharmacopoeia. Office of the British Pharmacopoeia Commission, Pharmaceutical Press, London, 1988

Compendium of Pharmaceuticals and Specialties. Canadian Pharmaceutical Association, Ottawa, Ontario, Canada (updated annually)

Drugs Available Abroad. Gale Research, Inc., Detroit, MI, 1991

Index Nominum: International Drug Directory. edited by Swiss Pharmaceutical Society. Medpharm Scientific Publishers, Stuttgart, Germany (updated annually)

---

trials plus a conclusion regarding the drug's therapeutic utility. The conclusions can be a valuable guide for the clinician who is considering using a new drug.

Reference Books

The *Physicians' Desk Reference*, also known as the PDR, is a reference work financed by the pharmaceutical industry. For each drug discussed, the information presented is identical to that on the package insert for that drug. In addition to its textual content, the PDR contains a pictorial section for product identification. The PDR is updated annually.

Drug Facts and Comparisons is a comprehensive reference that contains monographs on virtually every drug marketed in the United States. Information is provided on drug actions, indications, warnings, precautions, adverse reactions, dosage, and administration. In addition to describing the properties of single medications, the book lists the contents of all combination products sold in this country. Indexing is by generic name and by trade name. Revised editions are published annually.

A number of drug references have been compiled expressly for nurses. All of these address topics of special interest to the nurse, including information on administration, assessment, evaluation, and patient education. Representative nursing drug references include *Drugs and Nursing Implications, The Nurse's Drug Handbook,* and *Nurses' Drug Reference.*

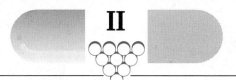

Basic Principles of Pharmacology

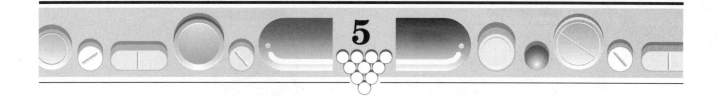

Pharmacokinetics

The term *pharmacokinetics* is derived from two Greek words: *pharmakon* (drug or poison) and *kinesis* (motion). As this derivation implies, pharmacokinetics is the study of drug movement throughout the body. Pharmacokinetics also includes the study of drug metabolism and excretion.

There are four basic pharmacokinetic processes: *absorption, distribution, metabolism,* and *excretion* (Fig. 5–1). *Absorption* is defined as the movement of drugs from their site of administration into the blood. *Distribution* is defined as drug movement from the blood to the interstitial space of tissues and from there into cells. *Metabolism* (biotransformation) is defined as enzymatically mediated alteration of drug structure. *Excretion* is the movement of drugs and their metabolites out of the body. (The combination of drug metabolism plus excretion is called *elimination.*) The four pharmacokinetic processes, acting in concert, determine the concentration of a drug at its sites of action.

APPLICATION OF PHARMACOKINETICS IN THERAPEUTICS

By applying knowledge of pharmacokinetics to drug therapy, we can help maximize desirable effects and minimize harm. Recall that the intensity of drug responses is directly related to the concentration of a drug at its sites of action. To maximize beneficial effects, we must achieve concentrations that are high enough to elicit desired responses. To minimize harm, we must avoid unnecessarily high concentrations. This balance is achieved by selecting the most appropriate route, dosage, and schedule of drug administration. The only means by which we can rationally choose the most effec-

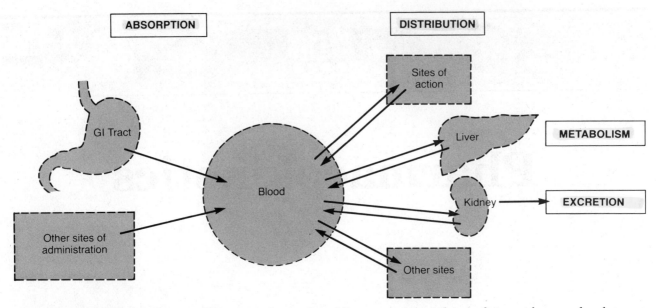

Figure 5-1. The four basic pharmacokinetic processes. Dotted lines represent membranes that must be crossed as drugs move throughout the body.

tive route, dosage, and schedule is through careful consideration of pharmacokinetic factors.

As a nurse, you will have ample opportunity to apply knowledge of pharmacokinetics in clinical practice. For example, by understanding the reasons behind selection of route, dosage, and timing of drug administration, you will be less likely to commit medication errors than will the nurse who, through lack of this knowledge, administers medications by blindly following physicians' orders. Also, as noted in Chapter 2, physicians do make mistakes. Accordingly, you will have occasion to question or even challenge physicians regarding their selection of dosage, route, or schedule of drug administration. In order to alter a physician's decision, you will need a rational argument to support your position. To present such an argument, you will need knowledge of pharmacokinetics.

Knowledge of pharmacokinetics can increase job satisfaction. Working with medications can be a significant component of nursing practice. For the nurse who lacks knowledge of pharmacokinetics, drugs will always be somewhat mysterious and, as a result, will be a potential source of ill ease. By helping to demystify drug therapy, pharmacokinetic knowledge can decrease some of the stress of nursing practice and can increase intellectual and professional satisfaction.

A NOTE TO CHEMOPHOBES

Before we proceed to the heart of this chapter, some advance notice and encouragement are in order for the chemophobes (those who fear chemistry) who may be reading this text. Since drugs are

chemicals, we cannot discuss pharmacology meaningfully without occasionally talking about chemistry. This chapter has some chemistry in it. In fact, the chemistry presented here is the most difficult in the book. Accordingly, once we've worked our way through this chapter, the chapters that follow will be a relative breeze. Since the concepts addressed here are fundamental, and since these concepts reappear frequently, all students, including chemophobes, are encouraged to learn this material now—regardless of the effort required.

PASSAGE OF DRUGS ACROSS MEMBRANES

All four phases of pharmacokinetics—absorption, distribution, metabolism, and excretion—involve drug movement. To move throughout the body, drugs must cross membranes. Drugs must cross membranes to enter the blood from their site of administration. Once in the blood, drugs must cross membranes to reach their sites of action. In addition, drugs must cross membranes to undergo metabolism and excretion. Accordingly, the factors that determine the passage of drugs across biologic membranes have a profound influence on all aspects of pharmacokinetics.

MEMBRANE STRUCTURE

Biologic membranes are composed of layers of individual cells. The cells composing most membranes are very close to one another—so close, in fact, that drugs must usually pass *through* cells, rather than between them, in order to cross the membrane. Hence, the ability of a drug to cross a biologic membrane is determined primarily by the ability of the drug to pass through single cells. The major barrier to passage through a cell is the cytoplasmic membrane (the membrane that surrounds every cell).

The basic structure of the cell membrane is depicted in Figure 5–2. As indicated, the basic membrane structure consists of a double layer of molecules known as *phospholipids*. Phospholipids are simply lipids (fats) that contain an atom of phosphate.

In Figure 5–2, the phospholipid molecules are depicted as having a round head (the phosphate-containing component) and two tails (long-chain hydrocarbons). The large objects embedded in the membrane represent protein molecules. These proteins serve a variety of functions.

THREE WAYS TO CROSS A CELL MEMBRANE

The three most important ways by which drugs cross cell membranes are (1) passage through channels or pores, (2) passage with the aid of a transport system, and (3) direct penetration of the membrane itself. Of these three, direct penetration of the membrane is most common.

Channels and Pores

Very few drugs cross membranes via channels or pores. The channels in membranes are extremely small (approximately 4 angstroms). Consequently, only the smallest of compounds (molecular weight less than 200) can use these holes as a route of transit. Agents with the ability to cross membranes via channels include small ions, such as potassium and sodium.

Transport Systems

Transport systems are carriers that can move drugs from one side of the cell membrane to the other. Some transport systems require the expenditure of energy, whereas others do not. All transport systems are selective; they will not carry just any drug. Whether or not a transporter will carry a particular drug depends upon that drug's structure.

Transport systems are an important means of drug transit. For example, certain orally administered drugs could not be absorbed unless there were transport systems to move them across the membranes that separate the lumen of the intestine from the blood. A number of drugs could not reach intracellular sites of action without a transport system to move them across the cell membrane. Renal excretion of many drugs would be extremely slow were it not for transport systems

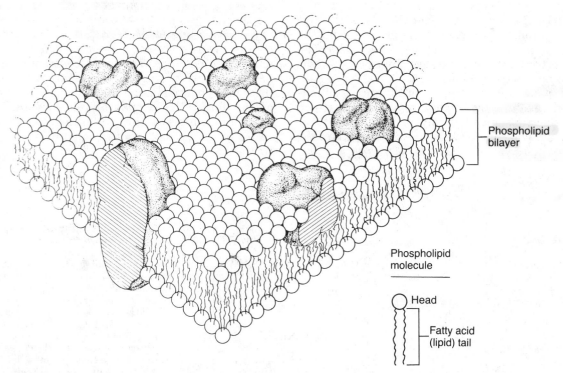

Figure 5–2. Structure of the cell membrane. The cell membrane consists primarily of a double layer of phospholipid molecules. The large globular structures represent protein molecules imbedded in the lipid bilayer. (Modified from Singer, S.J. and Nicolson, G.L. The fluid mosaic model of the structure of cell membranes. Science 175:720, 1972. Copyright 1972 by AAAS.)

in the kidney that can pump drugs from the blood into the renal tubules.

Direct Penetration of the Membrane

For most drugs, movement throughout the body is dependent on an ability to penetrate membranes directly. This is because most drugs are too large to pass through channels or pores and because, for most drugs, there are no transport systems to help them cross all the membranes that separate them from sites of action, metabolism, and excretion.

In order to directly penetrate membranes, a drug must be *lipid soluble* (lipophilic). Recall that membranes are composed primarily of lipids. Consequently, if a drug is to penetrate membranes, it must have the ability to dissolve into the lipids of which membranes are composed.

Certain kinds of molecules are *not* lipid soluble and, therefore, cannot penetrate membranes. Compounds in this category are *polar molecules* and *ions (molecules that carry an electrical charge)*.

POLAR MOLECULES

Polar molecules are molecules with uneven distribution of electrical charge. That is, positive and negative charges within the molecule tend to congregate separately from one another. Water is the classic example of a polar molecule. As depicted in Figure 5–3A, the electrons (negative charges) in the water molecule spend more time in the vicinity of the oxygen atom than in the vicinity of the two hydrogen atoms. As a result, the area around the oxygen atom tends to be negatively charged, whereas the area around the hydrogen atoms tends to be positively charged.

Kanamycin (Fig. 5–3B), an antibiotic, is an example of a polar drug. The hydroxyl groups, which attract electrons, give kanamycin its polar nature.

Although polar molecules have an uneven *distribution* of charge, they have no *net charge*. Polar

molecules have an equal number of protons (which bear a single positive charge) and electrons (which bear a single negative charge). As a result, the positive and negative charges balance each other exactly, and the molecule as a whole has neither a net positive nor a net negative charge. (Molecules that *do* bear a net charge are called *ions*. These are discussed below.)

There is a general rule in chemistry that states: "like dissolves like." In accord with this rule, *polar* molecules will dissolve in *polar* solvents (such as water) but will not dissolve in *nonpolar* solvents (such as oil). Table sugar provides a common example of the rule. Most of us have noted that sugar (a polar compound) readily dissolves in water but does not dissolve in lipids (e.g., salad oil, butter), which are nonpolar compounds. Just as sugar is unable to dissolve in lipids, polar drugs are unable to dissolve in the lipid bilayer of the cell membrane.

IONS

Ions are defined as molecules that have a *net electrical charge* (either positive or negative). With rare exceptions, *ions are unable to cross membranes*.

Quaternary Ammonium Compounds

Quaternary ammonium compounds are molecules that contain at least one atom of nitrogen and *carry a positive charge at all times*. The constant charge on these compounds results from atypical bonding to the nitrogen. In most nitrogen-containing compounds, the nitrogen atom bears only three chemical bonds. In contrast, the nitrogen atoms of quaternary ammonium compounds have four chemical bonds (Fig. 5–4A). It is because of the fourth bond that quaternary ammonium compounds always carry a positive charge. Because of the charge, these compounds are unable to cross most membranes.

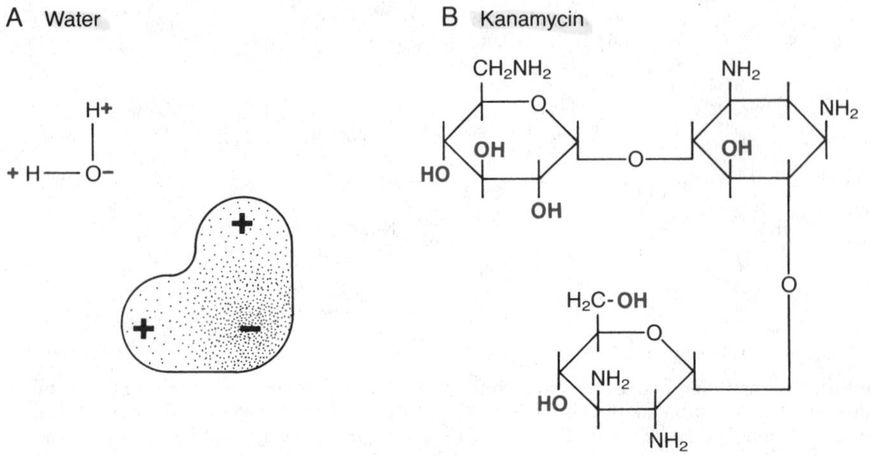

A   Water

B   Kanamycin

Figure 5–3. Polar molecules. *A,* Stippling shows the distribution of electrons within the water molecule. As indicated, water's electrons spend more time near the oxygen atom than hydrogen atoms, making the area near the oxygen atom somewhat negative and the area near the hydrogen atoms more positive. *B,* Kanamycin is a polar drug. The—OH groups of kanamycin attract electrons, thereby causing the area around these groups to be more negative than the rest of the molecule.

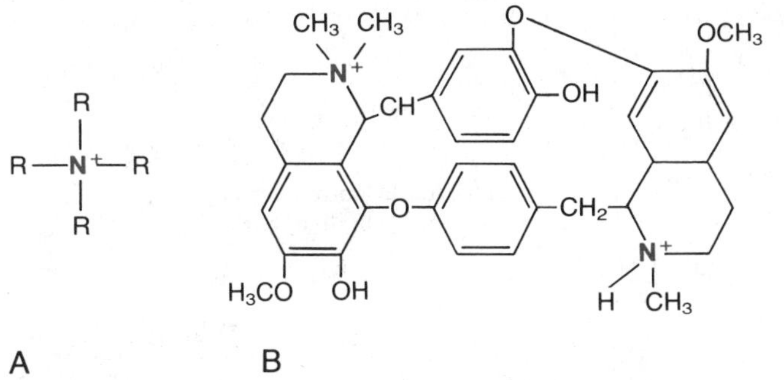

Figure 5–4. Quaternary ammonium compounds. *A,* The basic structure of quaternary ammonium compounds. Because the nitrogen atom is bonded to four organic radicals, the quaternary ammonium compound always carries a positive charge. Because of this charge, quaternary ammonium compounds are not lipid soluble and are unable to cross most membranes. *B,* Tubocurarine is a representative quaternary ammonium compound. Note that this agent contains two "quaternized" nitrogen atoms.

Tubocurarine (Fig. 5–4B) is representative of the quaternary ammonium compounds. In purified form, tubocurarine is employed as a muscle relaxant during surgery and other procedures. A crude preparation—curare—is used by South American Indians as an arrow poison. When employed for hunting, tubocurarine (curare) produces paralysis of the diaphragm and other skeletal muscles, causing death by asphyxiation. Interestingly, even though meat from animals killed with curare is laden with poison, it can be eaten without ill effect. The reason that this poison can be ingested safely is that tubocurarine, being a quaternary ammonium compound, cannot cross membranes and, therefore, cannot be absorbed from the intestine; as long as the drug remains in the intestine it can do no harm. As you might gather, when tubocurarine is used clinically, it cannot be administered by mouth. Instead, the drug must be given by injection. Once in the bloodstream, tubocurarine has ready access to its sites of action on muscles.

pH-Dependent Ionization

Unlike the quaternary ammonium compounds, which always carry a charge, certain drugs can exist in either a charged or an uncharged form. Many drugs are either weak organic acids or weak organic bases. Weak acids and bases can exist in charged and uncharged forms. Whether a weak acid or base will carry a charge is determined by the pH of the surrounding medium.

A review of acid-base chemistry will be helpful. An acid is defined as a compound that can give up a hydrogen ion (proton). Put another way, *an acid is a proton donor.* A base is defined as a compound that can take on a hydrogen ion. That is, *a base is a proton acceptor.* When an acid gives up its proton, which is positively charged, the acid itself becomes negatively charged. Conversely, when a

base accepts a proton, the base becomes positively charged. These reactions are depicted in Figure 5–5, using aspirin as an example of an acid and amphetamine as an example of a base. Because the process of an acid giving up a proton or a base accepting a proton converts the acid or base into a charged particle (ion), the process for either an acid or a base is termed *ionization.*

The extent to which a weak acid or weak base becomes ionized is determined by the pH of its environment. The following rules apply:

1. *Acids* tend to ionize in *basic* (alkaline) media.
2. *Bases* tend to ionize in *acidic* media.

An example of the pH-dependent ionization of drugs will illustrate the significance of this phenomenon. We will use aspirin for our example. Being an acid, aspirin tends to give up its proton (become ionized) in basic media. Conversely, aspirin will keep its proton and remain nonionized in acidic media. Hence, when aspirin is in the stomach (an acidic medium) most of the aspirin molecules will remain nonionized. Because aspirin molecules are nonionized in the stomach, they are able to be absorbed across the membranes that separate the stomach from the bloodstream. When aspirin molecules pass from the stomach to the small intestine, where the environment is relatively alkaline, they will change to their ionized form. As a result, absorption of aspirin from the intestine is impeded.

Ion Trapping (pH Partitioning)

Because the ionization of drugs is pH-dependent, when the pH of the fluid on one side of a membrane differs from the pH of the fluid on the other side, drug molecules will tend to accumulate on the side where the pH most favors their ionization. Accordingly, since acidic drugs tend to ionize in basic media, and since basic drugs tend to ionize in acidic media, *when there is a pH gradient between two sides of a membrane*

1. *Acidic* drugs will accumulate on the *alkaline* side.
2. *Basic* drugs will accumulate on the *acidic* side.

The process whereby a drug accumulates on the side of a membrane where the pH most favors its ionization is referred to as *ion trapping* or *pH partitioning.* Figure 5–6 shows the steps of ion trapping using aspirin as an example.

Since ion trapping can influence the movement of drugs throughout the body, the process is not simply of academic interest. Rather, ion trapping has practical clinical implications. Knowledge of ion trapping helps us to understand drug absorption as well as the movement of drugs to sites of action, metabolism, and excretion. An understanding of ion trapping can be put to practical use on

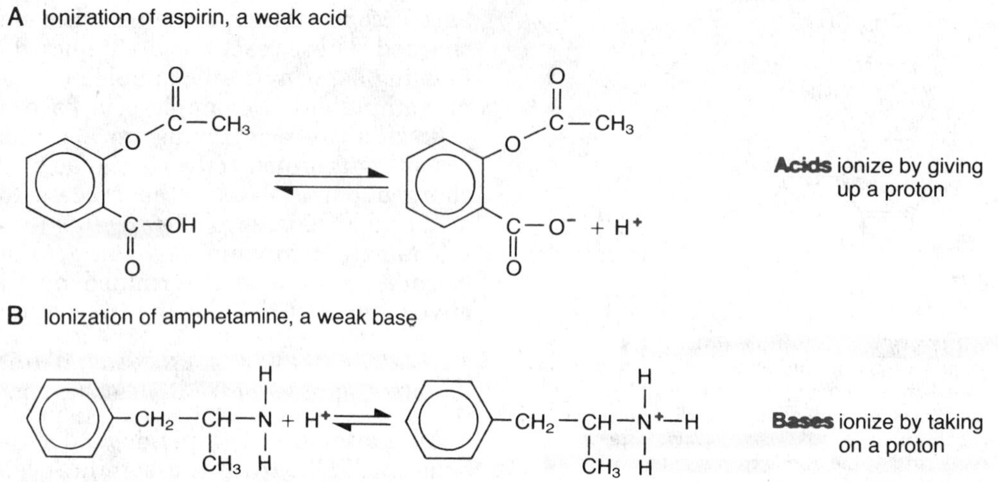

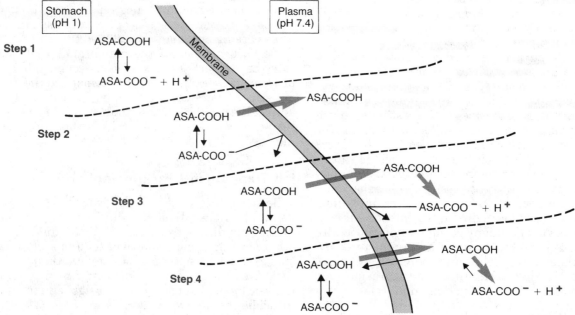

A Ionization of aspirin, a weak acid

Acids ionize by giving up a proton

B Ionization of amphetamine, a weak base

Bases ionize by taking on a proton

Figure 5–5. Ionization of weak acids and weak bases. The extent of ionization of weak acids (A) and weak bases (B) depends upon the pH of their surroundings The ionized (charged) forms of acids and bases are not lipid soluble and do not readily cross membranes.

Figure 5–6. Ion trapping of drugs. This figure demonstrates ion trapping using aspirin as an example. Because it is an acidic drug, aspirin will be nonionized in acid media and ionized in alkaline media. This figure demonstrates how the process of ion trapping will cause molecules of orally administered aspirin to move from the acidic (pH 1) environment of the stomach to the more alkaline (pH 7.4) environment of the plasma, thereby causing aspirin to accumulate in the blood. In the figure, aspirin (acetylsalicylic acid) is depicted as ASA with its COOH (carboxylic acid) group attached. **Step 1,** Once ingested, ASA dissolves in the stomach contents. After dissolving, some of the ASA molecules will give up a proton and become ionized. However, most of the ASA in the stomach will remain nonionized. (Most of the aspirin molecules in the stomach will be nonionized because the stomach is acidic and acidic drugs don't ionize in acidic media.) **Step 2,** Since most of the ASA molecules in the stomach are nonionized (and therefore lipid soluble), most ASA molecules in the stomach can readily cross the membranes that separate the stomach lumen from the plasma. Because of the concentration gradient that exists between the stomach and plasma, nonionized ASA molecules will begin moving into the plasma. (Note that because of their charge, ionized ASA molecules cannot leave the stomach.) **Step 3,** As the nonionized ASA molecules enter the relatively alkaline environment of the plasma, most of these molecules will give up an H+ and become negatively charged ions. Those ASA molecules that become ionized in the plasma cannot diffuse back into the stomach. **Step 4,** As the nonionized ASA molecules in the plasma become ionized, more nonionized molecules will pass from the stomach to the plasma to replace them. This passage will occur because the laws of diffusion demand equal concentrations of diffusible substances on both sides of the membrane. Since only the nonionized form of the ASA is able to diffuse across the membrane, it is this form that the laws of diffusion will attempt to equilibrate. Nonionized ASA will continue to move from the stomach to the plasma until the amount of ionized ASA in plasma has become large enough to prevent conversion of newly arrived nonionized molecules to the ionized form. Equilibrium will then be established between the plasma and the stomach. At equilibrium, there will be *equal* amounts of *non*ionized ASA in stomach and plasma. However, on the plasma side, the amount of ionized ASA will be much larger than on the stomach side. Since there are equal amounts of nonionized ASA on both sides of the membrane but much more ionized ASA in the plasma, the *total* amount of ASA in plasma will be much higher than in the stomach.

those occasions when it is necessary to actively influence drug movements. Management of poisoning is such an occasion: by manipulating urinary pH, we can employ ion trapping to draw toxic substances from the blood into the urine, thereby accelerating their removal from the body.

ABSORPTION

Absorption is defined as the *movement of a drug from its site of administration into the blood.* The *rate* of absorption determines *how soon* effects will begin. The *amount* of absorption helps determine *how intense* the effects will be.

FACTORS AFFECTING DRUG ABSORPTION

The rate at which a drug is absorbed is influenced by the physical and chemical properties of the drug itself and by physiologic and anatomic factors at the site of absorption.

Rate of Dissolution. Before a drug can be absorbed it must first dissolve. Hence, the rate of dissolution helps determine the rate of absorption. Drugs present in formulations that allow rapid dissolution will have a faster onset than will drugs formulated in such a way that their dissolution is delayed.

Surface Area. The surface area available for drug absorption is a major determinant of the rate and extent of absorption. The larger the surface area, the faster absorption will be. For this reason, orally administered drugs are usually absorbed from the small intestine rather than from the stomach. (Recall that the small intestine, because of its lining of microvilli, has an extremely large surface area, whereas the surface area of the stomach is relatively small.)

Blood Flow. Drugs are absorbed most rapidly from sites where blood flow is high. This is because blood containing newly absorbed drug will be replaced rapidly by drug-free blood, thereby maintaining a large gradient between the concentration of drug outside the blood and the concentration of drug in the blood. The greater this concentration gradient, the more rapid absorption will be.

Lipid Solubility. As a rule, highly lipid-soluble drugs are absorbed more rapidly than drugs whose lipid solubility is low. This is because lipid-soluble drugs can readily cross the membranes that separate them from the blood, whereas drugs of low lipid solubility cannot.

pH Partitioning. pH partitioning can influence drug absorption. Absorption will be enhanced when the difference between the pH of plasma and the pH at the site of administration is such that drug molecules will have a greater tendency to be ionized in the plasma.

CHARACTERISTICS OF COMMONLY USED ROUTES OF ADMINISTRATION

The routes of administration that are used most commonly fall into two major groups: *enteral* (via the gastrointestinal tract) and *parenteral*. The literal definition of *parenteral* is *outside the gastrointestinal tract.* However, in common parlance, the term parenteral is used to mean *by injection.* The principal parenteral routes are *intravenous, subcutaneous,* and *intramuscular.*

For each of the major routes of administration—oral, intravenous (IV), intramuscular (IM), and subcutaneous (SC)—the pattern of drug absorption (the rate and extent of absorption) is unique. Consequently, the route by which a drug is administered will significantly affect both the time of onset and the intensity of its effects. Why do patterns of absorption differ between routes? Because the barriers to absorption associated with each route are different. In the discussion below, we will examine these barriers and their influence on absorption pattern. In addition, as we discuss each major route, we will consider its clinical advantages and disadvantages.

Intravenous

Barriers to Absorption. When a drug is administered intravenously, there are *no barriers* to absorption. Recall that absorption is defined as the movement of a drug from its site of administration into the blood. Since IV administration puts a drug directly into the blood, this technique bypasses all barriers to absorption.

Absorption Pattern. Intravenous administration results in "absorption" that is both *instantaneous* and *complete.* Intravenous "absorption" is instantaneous in that drug enters the blood directly. "Absorption" is complete in that virtually all of the administered dose reaches the blood.

Advantages. *Rapid Onset.* Intravenous administration results in rapid onset of drug action. Although rapid onset is not always important, it is clearly beneficial in emergencies.

Control. Since the entire dose is administered directly into the blood, we have precise control over levels of drug in the blood. As discussed below, this contrasts with the other major routes of administration, and especially with oral administration.

Use of Large Fluid Volumes. The intravenous route is the only parenteral route that permits the use of large volumes of fluid. Some drugs that require parenteral administration are poorly soluble in water and, therefore, must be dissolved in a large volume. Because of the physical limitations presented by soft tissues (e.g., muscle, subcutaneous tissue), injection of large volumes at these sites is not possible. In contrast, the amount of fluid that can be infused into a vein, although limited, is still relatively large.

Use of Irritant Drugs. Certain drugs, because of their irritant properties, can be administered only by the intravenous route. A number of anticancer drugs, for example, are very chemically reactive. If present in high concentrations, these agents can cause severe local injury. However, when administered through a freely flowing IV line, these drugs are rapidly diluted in the blood, thereby minimizing the risk of harm.

Disadvantages. ***High Cost, Difficulty, and Inconvenience.*** Intravenous administration is expensive, difficult, and inconvenient. The cost of IV administration sets and their set-up charges can be substantial. Setting up an IV line takes time and special training. Because of the difficulty involved, most patients are unable to self-administer IV drugs and, therefore, must depend on a health care professional. Because patients are tethered to lines and bottles, their mobility is limited. In sharp contrast to this picture, oral administration is easy, convenient, and cheap.

Irreversibility. More important than cost or convenience, IV administration can be dangerous. Once a drug has been injected, there is no turning back—the drug is in the body and cannot be retrieved. Hence, if dosage is excessive, avoiding toxicity may be impossible.

To minimize risk, intravenous drugs should be injected slowly (over 1 minute or more). Since all of the blood in the body is circulated about once every minute, by injecting a drug over a 1-minute interval, we can cause that drug to be diluted in the largest volume of blood possible. By doing so, we can avoid drug concentrations that are unnecessarily—or even dangerously—high.

Performing IV injections slowly has the additional advantage of reducing the risk of toxicity to the central nervous system (CNS). When a drug is injected into the antecubital vein of the arm, about 15 seconds is required for the drug to reach the brain. Consequently, if the dosage is sufficient to cause CNS toxicity, signs of toxicity may become apparent 15 seconds after starting the injection. If the injection is being done slowly (e.g., over a 1-minute interval), only 25% of the total dose will have been administered when signs of toxicity appear. If administration is discontinued immediately, adverse effects will be much less than they would have been had the entire dose been injected.

Fluid Overload. When drugs are administered in a large volume, fluid overload can occur. This can be a significant problem for patients with hypertension, kidney disease, or congestive heart failure.

Infection. Infection can occur from injecting a contaminated drug. Fortunately, the risk of infection is much lower today than it was before we developed modern techniques for sterilizing drugs intended for IV use.

Embolism. Intravenous administration carries a risk of embolism (blood vessel blockage at a site distant from the point of administration). Embolism can be caused in several ways. First, insertion of an IV needle can injure the venous wall, leading to formation of a thrombus (clot); embolism can result if the clot breaks loose and becomes lodged in another vessel. Second, injection of hypotonic or hypertonic fluids can destroy red blood cells; the debris from these cells can produce embolism.

Lastly, injection of drugs that are not fully dissolved can lead to embolism. Particles of undissolved drug are like small grains of sand. These can become embedded in blood vessels to produce blockage. Because of the risk of embolism, it is important to check intravenous solutions prior to administration to insure that drugs are completely dissolved. If the fluid is cloudy or contains particulate matter, the drug is not dissolved and the fluid must not be administered.

The Importance of Reading Labels. Not all formulations of the same drug are appropriate for IV administration. Accordingly, it is essential to read the label before giving a drug intravenously. Two examples will illustrate the importance of this admonition. Our first example is insulin. Only one preparation of insulin can be administered safely IV. That preparation, which is usually labeled *insulin injection*, consists of insulin in *solution*. In all other preparations, insulin is present as a *particulate suspension*. These preparations are intended for subcutaneous administration only. Because of their particulate nature, these preparations could prove fatal if administered IV. By checking the label, inadvertent intravenous administration of particulate insulin can be avoided.

Epinephrine provides our second example of the importance of reading the label before giving a drug intravenously. Epinephrine, a drug that stimulates the cardiovascular system, can be injected by several routes (intramuscular, intravenous, subcutaneous, intracardiac, intraspinal). It must be noted, however, that solutions prepared for use by one route will differ in concentration from solutions prepared for use by other routes. For example, whereas solutions intended for *subcutaneous* administration are quite *concentrated*, solutions intended for *intravenous* use are *dilute*. If a solution prepared for subcutaneous use were to be inadvertently administered intravenously, the result could prove *fatal*. (Intravenous administration of concentrated epinephrine could overstimulate the heart and blood vessels, causing severe hypertension, cerebral hemorrhage, stroke, and death.) The message here is that it is not sufficient to simply administer the *right drug*; the preparation and concentration must also be *appropriate for the intended route.*

Intramuscular

Barriers to Absorption. When drugs are injected intramuscularly, the only barrier to absorption is the *capillary wall.* In the capillary beds that serve muscles and most other tissues, there are "large" spaces between the cells that compose the capillary wall (Fig. 5–7). Drugs can pass through these spaces with ease. No cell membranes need to be crossed in order to enter the bloodstream. Hence, like intravenous administration, intramuscular administration presents no significant barriers to absorption.

Absorption Pattern. Drugs administered intramuscularly may be absorbed rapidly or slowly. The rate of absorption is determined largely by two factors: (1) water solubility of the drug, and (2) blood flow to the site of injection. Drugs that are highly water soluble will be absorbed rapidly (within 10 to 30 minutes). Drugs that are poorly soluble in water will be absorbed more slowly. Drugs injected into sites with a high blood flow will be absorbed more rapidly than drugs injected into sites whose blood flow is low.

Advantages. The intramuscular route can be used for parenteral administration of *poorly soluble drugs.* Recall that drugs must be dissolved if they are to be administered intravenously. Consequently, the IV route cannot be used for poorly soluble compounds. In contrast, since little harm will come from depositing a suspension of undissolved drug in the interstitial space of muscle tissue, the IM route is acceptable for drugs whose water solubility is poor.

A second advantage of the IM route is that it allows administration of drugs as *depot preparations* (preparations from which the drug is absorbed gradually over an extended time). The effects of a single depot preparation may last for weeks or even months. For example, *benzathine penicillin G,* a depot preparation of penicillin, can release therapeutically effective amounts of penicillin for a month or more following a single IM injection. In contrast, a single IM injection of penicillin G itself would be absorbed and excreted in less than 1 day. The obvious advantage of depot preparations is that they can greatly reduce the number of injections required during long-term therapy.

Disadvantages. The major drawbacks of IM administration are *discomfort* and *inconvenience.* Intramuscular injection of some preparations can be painful. Also, IM injections can cause local tissue injury and possibly nerve damage (if the injection is done improperly). Like all other forms of parenteral administration, IM injections are less convenient than oral administration.

Subcutaneous

From a pharmacokinetic perspective, SC administration is nearly identical to IM administration. As with IM administration, there are no significant barriers to the absorption of drugs administered subcutaneously: drugs simply enter the bloodstream through the spaces between cells of the capillary wall. As with IM administration, blood flow and drug solubility are the major determinants of the rate at which subcutaneous drugs are absorbed. Because of the above similarities between SC and IM administration, these routes have similar advantages (can be used for poorly soluble drugs, potential for prolonged action) and drawbacks (discomfort, inconvenience, potential for injury).

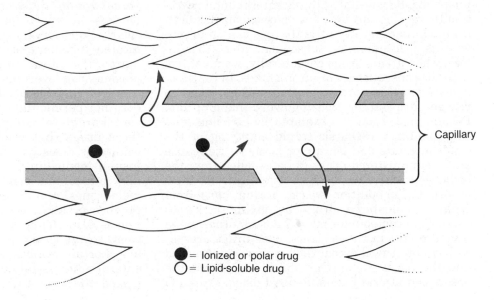

Figure 5–7. Drug movement at typical capillary beds. In most capillary beds, "large" gaps exist between the cells that compose the capillary wall. Drugs and other molecules can pass freely into and out of the bloodstream through these gaps. (Lipid-soluble compounds can also pass directly through the cells of the capillary wall.)

Capillary

● = Ionized or polar drug
○ = Lipid-soluble drug

Oral

In the discussion below, the abbreviation PO is used in reference to oral administration. This abbreviation stands for *per os*, a Latin phrase meaning *by way of the mouth*.

Barriers to Absorption. Following oral administration, drugs may be absorbed from the stomach or from the intestine. In either case, there are two barriers to cross: (1) the layer of *epithelial cells* that lines the gastrointestinal (GI) tract, and (2) the *capillary wall*. Since the walls of the capillaries that serve the GI tract offer no significant resistance to absorption, the major barrier to absorption is the gastrointestinal epithelium. To cross this layer of tightly packed cells, drugs must pass through the cells rather than between them.

Absorption Pattern. Because of multiple factors, the rate and extent of drug absorption following oral administration can be *highly variable*. Factors that can influence absorption include (1) solubility and stability of the drug, (2) gastric and intestinal pH, (3) gastric emptying time, (4) food in the gut, (5) coadministration of other drugs, and (6) special coatings on the drug preparation.

Advantages. Oral administration is easy, convenient, and inexpensive. (By inexpensive, we don't mean that oral drugs themselves are inexpensive, but rather that there is no cost for the process of administration.) Because of its relative ease, oral administration is the preferred route for self-medication.

Although absorption of orally administered drugs can be highly variable, this route is still *safer than parenteral injection*. With oral administration, there is no risk of fluid overload, infection, or embolism. Furthermore, since oral administration is potentially reversible, whereas injections are not, oral administration is much safer than injections. Recall that with parenteral administration there is no turning back: once a drug has been injected, there is very little that we can do to prevent its absorption and subsequent effects. Therefore, when giving drugs parenterally, we must live with the consequences of our mistakes. In contrast, if need be, there are steps that can be taken to prevent drug absorption following inappropriate PO administration. For example, by inducing emesis (vomiting), catharsis (rapid emptying of the small intestine and bowel), or both, we can cause orally administered drugs to be expelled from the body before there has been sufficient time for their absorption. In addition, we can prevent harm from orally administered drugs by giving activated charcoal, a compound that will adsorb drugs while they are still in the GI tract; once drugs are adsorbed onto the charcoal they cannot be absorbed into the bloodstream. Our ability to prevent the absorption of orally administered drugs gives PO

medications a safety factor that is unavailable with drugs injected parenterally.

Disadvantages. *Variability.* The major disadvantage of PO drug use is that absorption can be highly variable: a drug administered to patient A may be absorbed rapidly and completely, whereas administration of the same preparation to patient B may result in absorption that is delayed and incomplete. This variability makes it difficult to control the concentration of a drug at its sites of action and, therefore, makes it difficult to control the onset, intensity, and duration of responses.

Inactivation. Oral administration can lead to inactivation of certain drugs. Penicillin G, for example, cannot be taken orally because it would be destroyed by acid in the stomach. Insulin cannot be taken orally because it would be destroyed by digestive enzymes.

Some drugs cannot be taken orally because they would undergo rapid inactivation by hepatic enzymes as they pass through the liver on their way from the GI tract to the general circulation. This phenomenon, known as the "first-pass effect," is discussed later in the chapter.

Patient Requirements. Oral drug administration requires a conscious, cooperative patient. Drugs cannot be administered PO to comatose individuals or to individuals who, for whatever reason (e.g., psychosis, seizure, obstinacy, nausea), are unable or unwilling to swallow oral medications.

Local Irritation. Some oral preparations cause local irritation of the GI tract, which can result in discomfort, nausea, and vomiting.

Comparing Oral Administration with Parenteral Administration

Because of ease, convenience, and relative safety, *oral administration is generally preferred to parenteral administration.* However, there are situations in which parenteral administration is clearly superior. Parenteral administration is indicated in emergencies when rapid onset is required. Parenteral administration is needed when plasma drug levels must be tightly controlled. (Because of variable absorption, oral administration does not permit tight control of plasma drug levels.) Parenteral administration is preferred for those drugs that would be destroyed by gastric acidity or digestive enzymes if given orally (e.g., insulin, penicillin G). Drugs such as the quaternary ammonium compounds, which cannot cross membranes, require parenteral administration to produce systemic effects. Parenteral administration is also required for those drugs that would cause severe local injury if administered by mouth (e.g., certain anticancer agents). In addition, parenteral administration is indicated when the prolonged effects of a depot preparation are desired.

Lastly, parenteral therapy is superior to oral therapy for those patients who cannot or will not take drugs orally.

PHARMACEUTICAL PREPARATIONS FOR ORAL ADMINISTRATION

There are several kinds of "packages" (formulations) into which a drug can be put for oral administration. Three such formulations—*tablets, enteric coatings,* and *sustained-release preparations*—are discussed below.

Before we discuss drug formulations, it will be helpful to define two terms: *chemical equivalence* and *bioavailability*. Two drug preparations would be considered *chemically equivalent* if they contained the same amount of the identical chemical compound (drug). Two preparations would be considered equal in *bioavailability* if the drug they contained were absorbed at the same rate and to the same extent from both preparations. Please note that it is possible for two formulations of the same drug to be chemically equivalent while differing in bioavailability.

Tablets. A tablet is a mixture of a drug plus binders and fillers, all of which have been compressed together. Tablets made by different manufacturers can differ in their rates of disintegration and dissolution, causing differences in their bioavailability. As a result, two tablets that contain the same amount of the same drug can have quantitative differences in their therapeutic effects.

Enteric-Coated Preparations. Enteric-coated preparations are drugs that have been covered with a material designed to dissolve in the intestine but not in the stomach. Materials used for enteric coatings include fatty acids, waxes, and shellac. Since enteric-coated preparations release their contents into the intestine and not into the stomach, these preparations are employed for two general purposes: (1) to protect drugs from acid and pepsin in the stomach, and (2) to protect the stomach from drugs that can cause gastric discomfort.

The primary disadvantage of enteric-coated preparations is that they can be even more variable in their absorption than tablets. Since gastric emptying time can vary from minutes up to 12 hours, and since enteric-coated preparations cannot be absorbed until they leave the stomach, variations in gastric emptying time can alter the time of onset of these drugs. Furthermore, there are occasions when enteric coatings fail to dissolve, thereby allowing medication to pass through the GI tract without being absorbed at all.

Sustained-Release Preparations. Sustained-release formulations are capsules filled with tiny spheres that contain the actual drug; the spheres have coatings that are designed to dissolve at variable rates. Since some spheres dissolve more slowly than others, drug is released steadily throughout the day. The primary advantage of sustained-release preparations is that they permit a reduction in the number of daily doses. These formulations have the additional advantage of producing relatively steady drug levels for an extended time (much like giving a drug by infusion). The major disadvantages of sustained-release formulations are high cost and the potential for variable absorption.

ADDITIONAL ROUTES OF ADMINISTRATION

Drugs can be administered by a number of routes in addition to those discussed above. Drugs can be applied *topically* for local therapy of the skin, eyes, ears, nose, mouth, and vagina. In a few cases, topical agents (e.g., nitroglycerin, nicotine) are formulated for *transdermal* absorption into the systemic circulation. Some drugs are *inhaled* to elicit local effects in the lung, especially in the treatment of asthma. Other inhalational agents (e.g., volatile anesthetics, oxygen) are used for their systemic effects. *Rectal suppositories* may be employed to elicit effects locally or throughout the body. *Vaginal suppositories* may be employed to treat local disorders. For management of some conditions, drugs must be injected directly into a specific tissue or organ (e.g., heart, joints, nerves, central nervous system). The unique characteristics of these routes will be addressed as we discuss specific drugs that are given by these routes.

DISTRIBUTION

Distribution is defined as *the movement of drugs throughout the body*. Drug distribution is determined by three major factors: (1) blood flow to tissues, (2) the ability of a drug to exit the vascular system, and (3) the ability of a drug to enter cells.

BLOOD FLOW TO TISSUES

In the first phase of distribution, drugs are carried in the blood to the tissues and organs of the body. The rate at which drugs are delivered to a particular tissue is determined by the blood flow to that tissue. Since most tissues are well perfused, regional blood flow is rarely a limiting factor in drug distribution.

There are two pathologic conditions—abscesses and tumors—in which low regional blood flow can affect drug therapy. An abscess is a pus-filled pocket of infection that is devoid of internal blood vessels. Because abscesses lack a blood supply, antibiotics cannot reach the bacteria within. Accordingly, if drug therapy of an abscess is to be effective, the abscess must first be surgically drained.

Solid tumors have a restricted blood supply. Although blood flow to the outer regions of tumors is relatively high, blood flow becomes progressively lower toward the core. As a result, we cannot achieve high drug levels deep within solid tumors. This limited blood flow is a major reason why solid tumors are resistant to drug therapy.

EXITING THE VASCULAR SYSTEM

Once a drug has been delivered to an organ or a tissue via the blood, the next phase of distribution is to exit the vasculature. Leaving the blood occurs at capillary beds. Since most drugs do not produce their effects within the blood, the ability to leave the vascular system is an important determinant of a drug's actions. Exiting the vascular system is also necessary for drugs to undergo metabolism and excretion.

Typical Capillary Beds

Most capillary beds offer no resistance to the departure of drugs. In most tissues, drugs can leave the vasculature by passing through pores in the capillary wall. Since drugs pass *between* capillary cells rather than *through* them, movement into the interstitial space is not impeded. The exit of drugs from a typical capillary bed is illustrated in Figure 5–7.

The Blood-Brain Barrier

The term *blood-brain barrier* refers to the unique anatomy of the capillaries that serve the CNS. As shown in Figure 5–8, there are *tight junctions* between the cells that compose the walls of most capillaries in the CNS. These junctions are so tight that they prevent the passage of drugs. Consequently, in order to leave the blood and reach sites of action within the brain, a drug must have the ability to pass *through* cells of the capillary wall. Only drugs that are *lipid soluble* or have a *transport system* are able to cross the blood-brain barrier to a significant degree.

The presence of the blood-brain barrier is a mixed blessing. The good news is that the barrier protects the brain from injury by potentially toxic substances. The bad news is that the barrier can be a significant obstacle to drug therapy of CNS disorders. The barrier can, for example, impede access of antibiotics to CNS infections.

The blood-brain barrier is not fully developed at birth. As a result, newborns are much more sensitive than older children and adults to medicines that act on the brain. Likewise, neonates are especially vulnerable to CNS poisons.

Placental Drug Transfer

The membranes of the placenta separate the maternal circulation from the fetal circulation (Fig. 5–9). *The membranes of the placenta do NOT constitute an absolute barrier to the passage of drugs.* The same factors that determine the movement of drugs across other membranes determine the movement of drugs across the placenta. Accordingly, lipid-soluble, nonionized compounds will readily pass from the maternal bloodstream into the blood of the fetus. In contrast, compounds that are ionized, highly polar, or protein bound (see below) will be excluded.

Drugs that have the ability to cross the placenta can cause serious harm. Many compounds can cause birth defects, ranging from low birth weight to mental retardation to gross malformations. (Recall the thalidomide experience.) If a pregnant woman is a habitual user of opioids (e.g., heroin), her child will be born drug dependent, requiring treatment with a heroin substitute to suppress symptoms of withdrawal. The use of respiratory depressants (anesthetics and analgesics) during delivery can suppress respiration in the neonate. Hence, infants exposed to respiratory depressants during delivery must be monitored closely until breathing has normalized.

Protein Binding

Drugs can form reversible bonds with various proteins in the body. Of all the proteins to which drugs can bind, *plasma albumin* is the most important.

Albumin is the most abundant protein in plasma. Like other proteins, albumin is a large molecule (molecular weight = 69,000 daltons). Because of its size, *albumin always remains within the bloodstream*; albumin is too large to squeeze through pores in the capillary wall, and no transport system exists by which albumin might exit the vascular system.

Figure 5–10A depicts the binding of drug molecules to albumin. Note that the drug molecules are much smaller than albumin. (The molecular weight of the average drug is about 300 to 500 daltons compared with 69,000 daltons for albumin.) As indicated by the two-way arrows, binding between albumin and drugs is *reversible*. As a result, a drug may exist in either a *bound* or an *unbound* (free) state.

For those drugs with the ability to bind albumin, only some of the molecules present in plasma will be bound at any particular moment. The percentage of drug molecules that will be bound is determined by the strength of the attraction between the albumin and the drug. For example, the attrac-

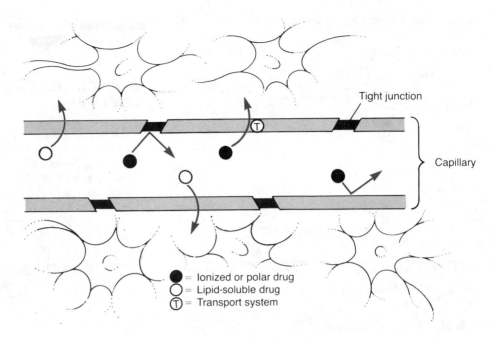

Figure 5–8. Drug movement across the blood-brain barrier. Tight junctions between the cells that compose the walls of the capillaries that serve the central nervous system prevent drugs from passing between cells to exit the vascular system. Consequently, in order to reach sites of action within the brain, a drug must pass directly through the cells of the capillary wall. To do this, a drug must be lipid soluble or able to use an existing transport system.

tion between albumin and warfarin (an anticoagulant) is relatively strong, causing nearly all (99%) of the warfarin molecules in plasma to be bound, leaving only 1% free. For gentamicin (an antibiotic), the ratio of bound to free is quite different. Since the attraction between gentamicin and albumin is relatively weak, less than 10% of the gentamicin molecules present in plasma will be bound, leaving more than 90% free.

An important consequence of protein binding is the restriction of drug distribution. Because albumin is too large to leave the bloodstream, drug molecules bound to albumin cannot leave the bloodstream either (Fig. 5–10B). Only those drug molecules that are free (not protein bound) can exit capillaries and become distributed to spaces outside the vasculature. Drug molecules that are protein bound cannot leave the bloodstream to reach sites of action, metabolism, or excretion.

In addition to restricting the distribution of drugs, protein binding can be a source of drug interactions. As suggested by Figure 5–10A, each molecule of albumin has only a few sites to which drug molecules can bind. Because the number of

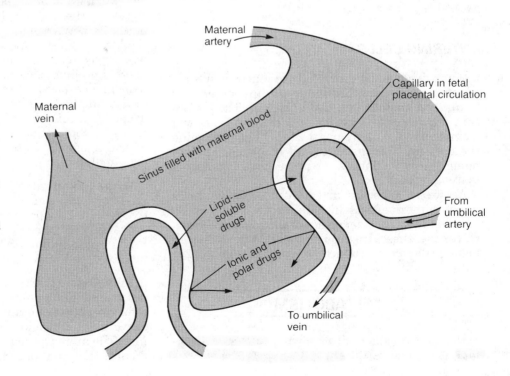

Figure 5–9. Placental drug transfer. Membranes of the maternal and fetal vascular systems must be crossed for drugs to enter the fetal circulation. Lipid-soluble drugs can readily cross these membranes and enter the fetal circulation. In contrast, ions and polar molecules are retained in the maternal blood.

A Reversible Binding of a Drug to Albumin

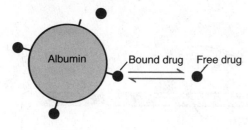

B Retention of Protein-Bound Drug Within the Vasculature

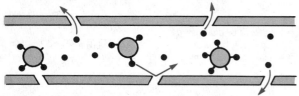

Figure 5–10. Protein binding of drugs. *A,* Albumin is the most prevalent protein in plasma and the most important of the proteins to which drugs can become bound. *B,* Only unbound (free) drugs can leave the vascular system. Bound drugs are too large to fit through the gaps between cells in the capillary wall.

binding sites is limited, drugs that bind to albumin will compete with one another for those sites. As a result, one drug can displace another from albumin, causing the free concentration of the displaced drug to rise. By increasing levels of free drug, competition for binding can increase the intensity of drug responses. If the intensity increases excessively, toxicity can result.

ENTERING CELLS

Some drugs must enter cells to reach their sites of action, and practically all drugs must enter cells to undergo metabolism and excretion. The factors that determine the ability of a drug to cross cell membranes are the same factors that determine the passage of drugs across all other membranes, namely, lipid solubility, the presence of a transport system, or both.

As we will discuss in Chapter 6, many drugs produce their effects by binding to receptors located on the external surface of the cell membrane. Obviously, these drugs do not need to cross the cell membrane in order to act.

METABOLISM

Drug metabolism, also known as *biotransformation*, is defined as the *enzymatic alteration of drug structure*. Practically all drug metabolism takes place in the *liver*.

HEPATIC DRUG-METABOLIZING ENZYMES

Much of the drug metabolism that takes place in the liver is performed by the *hepatic microsomal enzyme system*, also known as the *P-450 system*. (The name P-450 refers to cytochrome P-450, a key component of this enzyme system.)

Hepatic microsomal enzymes are capable of catalyzing a wide variety of reactions that employ drugs as substrates. Some of these reactions are illustrated in Figure 5–11. As these examples indicate, drug metabolism doesn't always result in the breakdown of drugs into smaller molecules; drug metabolism can also result in the synthesis of a molecule that is larger than the parent drug.

THERAPEUTIC CONSEQUENCES OF DRUG METABOLISM

Drug metabolism has five possible consequences of therapeutic significance: (1) accelerated renal excretion of drugs, (2) inactivation of drugs, (3) increased therapeutic action, (4) activation of prodrugs, and (5) increased or decreased toxicity. Figure 5–11 depicts reactions that illustrate these consequences of drug metabolism.

Accelerated Renal Drug Excretion. The most important consequence of drug metabolism is the promotion of renal drug excretion. As discussed in the next section of this chapter, the kidney, which is the major organ of drug excretion, is unable to excrete drugs that are highly lipid soluble. By converting lipid-soluble drugs into *more polar* (less lipid-soluble) compounds, drug metabolism makes possible the renal excretion of many drugs. In the case of certain highly lipid-soluble drugs (e.g., thiopental), renal excretion would take years for completion were it not for the conversion of these agents into more polar compounds by drug-metabolizing enzymes.

Drug Inactivation. Drug metabolism can convert pharmacologically active compounds to inactive forms. This phenomenon is illustrated by the conversion of procaine (a local anesthetic) into PABA (para-aminobenzoic acid), an inactive metabolite (see Fig. 5–11).

Increased Therapeutic Action. Metabolism can increase the effectiveness of some drugs. This consequence of metabolism is illustrated by the conversion of codeine into morphine (see Fig. 5–11). (The analgesic activity of morphine is so much greater than that of codeine that formation of mor-

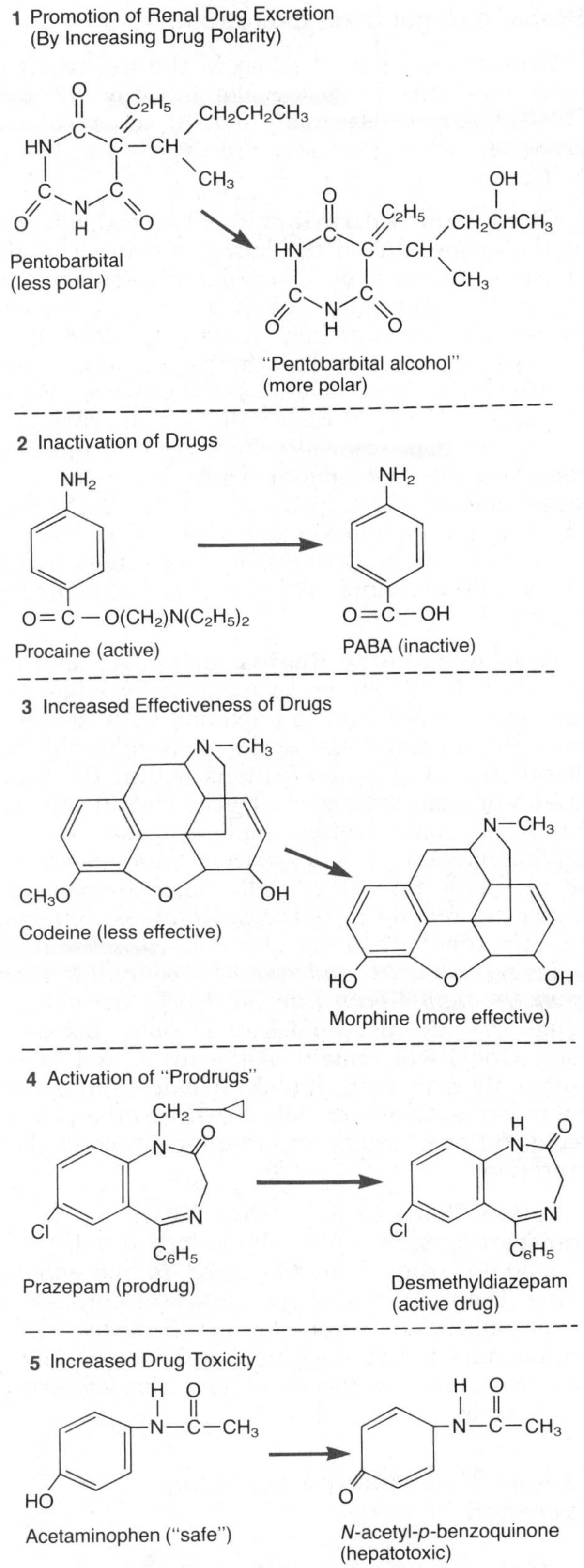

1 Promotion of Renal Drug Excretion
(By Increasing Drug Polarity)

Pentobarbital
(less polar)

"Pentobarbital alcohol"
(more polar)

- -

2 Inactivation of Drugs

Procaine (active)

PABA (inactive)

- -

3 Increased Effectiveness of Drugs

Codeine (less effective)

Morphine (more effective)

- -

4 Activation of "Prodrugs"

Prazepam (prodrug)

Desmethyldiazepam
(active drug)

- -

5 Increased Drug Toxicity

Acetaminophen ("safe")

N-acetyl-*p*-benzoquinone
(hepatotoxic)

Figure 5–11. Therapeutic consequences of drug metabolism.

phine may account for virtually all the pain relief that occurs following codeine administration.)

Activation of Prodrugs. A prodrug is a compound that is pharmacologically inactive as administered and then undergoes conversion to its active form within the body. Activation of a prodrug is illustrated by the metabolic conversion of prazepam into desmethyldiazepam (see Fig. 5–11). (Prazepam is a close relative of diazepam, a drug familiar to us under the trade name Valium.)

Increased or Decreased Toxicity. By converting drugs into inactive forms, metabolism can decrease toxicity. Conversely, metabolism can increase the potential for harm by converting relatively safe compounds into forms that are toxic. Increased toxicity is illustrated by the conversion of acetaminophen into a hepatotoxic metabolite (see Fig. 5–11). It is this product of metabolism, and not acetaminophen itself, that causes injury when acetaminophen is taken in excessive dosage.

SPECIAL CONSIDERATIONS IN DRUG METABOLISM

Several factors can influence the rate at which drugs are metabolized. These factors must be accounted for in drug therapy.

Age. The drug-metabolizing capacity of infants is *limited*. The liver does not develop its full capacity to metabolize drugs until about 1 year after birth. *During the time prior to hepatic maturation, infants are especially sensitive to drugs, and care must be taken to avoid injury.*

Induction of Drug-Metabolizing Enzymes. Some drugs act on the liver to increase rates of drug metabolism. For example, when phenobarbital is administered for a few days, it can cause the drug-metabolizing capacity of the liver to double. Phenobarbital increases metabolism by causing the liver to synthesize drug-metabolizing enzymes. This process of stimulating enzyme synthesis is referred to as *induction*.

Induction of drug-metabolizing enzymes can have two therapeutic consequences. First, by stimulating the liver to produce more drug-metabolizing enzymes, a drug can increase the rate of its own metabolism, thereby necessitating an increase in its dosage to maintain therapeutic effects. Second, induction of drug-metabolizing enzymes can accelerate the metabolism of other drugs used concurrently, necessitating an increase in *their* dosage.

First-Pass Effect. The term *first-pass effect* refers to the rapid hepatic inactivation of certain oral drugs. When drugs are administered orally, they are absorbed from the GI tract and carried directly to the liver by way of the hepatic portal circulation. If the capacity of the liver to metabolize a drug is extremely high, that drug will be completely inactivated on its first pass through the liver; hence, no therapeutic effects will occur. To circumvent the first-pass effect, drugs that undergo rapid hepatic metabolism are often administered parenterally. This permits the drug to temporarily bypass the liver, thereby allowing it to reach therapeutic levels in the systemic blood.

Nitroglycerin is the classic example of a drug that undergoes such rapid hepatic metabolism that it is without effect following oral administration. However, when administered sublingually (under the tongue), nitroglycerin is very active. Sublingual administration is effective because it permits nitroglycerin to be absorbed through the oral mucosa directly into the systemic circulation. Once in systemic circulation, the drug is carried to its sites of action prior to passage through the liver. Hence, therapeutic action can be exerted before the drug is exposed to hepatic enzymes.

Nutritional Status. Hepatic drug-metabolizing enzymes require a number of co-factors to function. In the malnourished patient, these co-factors may be deficient, causing drug metabolism to be compromised.

Competition Between Drugs. When two drugs are metabolized by the same metabolic pathway, they may compete with each other for metabolism. This competition can decrease the rate at which one or both agents is metabolized. However, in actual practice, competition for metabolism is rarely significant.

EXCRETION

Drug excretion is defined as the *removal of drugs from the body*. Drugs and their metabolites can exit the body in urine, bile, sweat, saliva, breast milk, and expired air. The most important organ for drug excretion is the kidney.

RENAL DRUG EXCRETION

The kidneys account for the majority of drug excretion. When the kidneys are healthy, they serve to limit the duration of action of many drugs. Conversely, if renal failure occurs, both the duration and intensity of drug responses may be increased.

Steps in Renal Drug Excretion

Urinary excretion of drugs is the net result of three processes: (1) glomerular filtration, (2) passive tubular reabsorption, and (3) active tubular secretion. These processes are depicted in Figure 5–12.

Glomerular Filtration. Renal excretion begins at the glomerulus of the kidney tubule. The glomerulus consists of a capillary network surrounded by Bowman's capsule; small pores are present in the capillary walls. As blood flows through the glomerular capillaries, fluids and small molecules—including drugs—are forced through the pores of the capillary wall. This process, called glomerular filtration, moves drugs from the blood into the tubular urine. Blood cells and large molecules (e.g., proteins) are too big to pass through the capillary pores and, hence, do not undergo filtration. Because large molecules are not filtered, drugs bound to albumin remain behind in the blood.

Passive Tubular Reabsorption. As depicted in Figure 5–12, the vessels that deliver blood to the glomerulus return to proximity with the renal tubule at a point distal to the glomerulus. At this distal site, drug concentrations within the blood are lower than drug concentrations within the tubule. This concentration gradient can serve as a driving force to move drugs from the lumen of the tubule back into the blood. Since lipid-soluble drugs can readily cross the membranes that compose the tubular and vascular walls, *drugs that are lipid soluble will undergo passive reabsorption from the tubule back into the blood*. In contrast, drugs that are not lipid soluble (ions and polar compounds) will remain in the urine and be excreted. By converting lipid-soluble drugs into more polar forms, drug metabolism reduces the passive reabsorption of drugs, and thereby promotes their excretion.

Active Tubular Secretion. There are active transport systems within the kidney tubules that can pump drugs from the blood to the tubular urine. The tubules have two classes of pumps, one for organic acids and one for organic bases. These pumps have a relatively high capacity and play a significant role in the renal excretion of certain compounds.

Factors That Modify Renal Drug Excretion

pH-Dependent Ionization. The phenomenon of pH-dependent ionization can be used to accelerate renal excretion of drugs. Recall that passive tubular reabsorption is limited to lipid-soluble compounds. Since ions are not lipid soluble, drugs that are ionized at the pH of tubular urine will

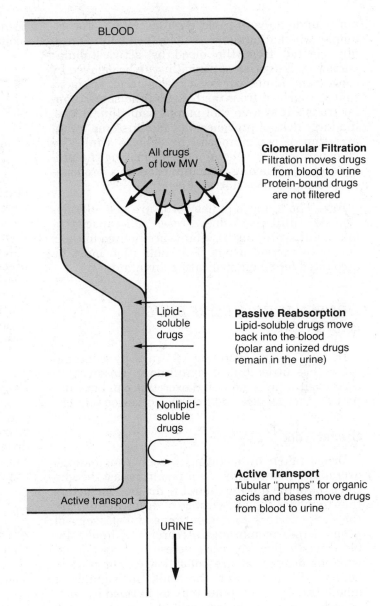

BLOOD

All drugs
of low MW

Glomerular Filtration
Filtration moves drugs
from blood to urine
Protein-bound drugs
are not filtered

Lipid-
soluble
drugs

Passive Reabsorption
Lipid-soluble drugs move
back into the blood
(polar and ionized drugs
remain in the urine)

Nonlipid-
soluble
drugs

Active transport

Active Transport
Tubular "pumps" for organic
acids and bases move drugs
from blood to urine

URINE

Figure 5–12. Renal drug excretion. (Redrawn from Binns, T.B. [ed.]. Absorption and Distribution of Drugs. Edinburgh, Churchill Livingstone, 1964.)

remain in the tubule and be excreted. Consequently, by manipulating urinary pH in such a way as to promote the ionization of a drug, we can decrease the passive reabsorption of that drug and thereby hasten its excretion. This principle has been employed to promote the excretion of ingested poisons and medications that have been taken in toxic doses.

The treatment of aspirin poisoning provides an example of how manipulation of urinary pH can be put to therapeutic advantage. When children have been exposed to toxic doses of aspirin, they can be treated, in part, by giving an agent that will elevate urinary pH (i.e., makes the urine more basic). Since aspirin is an acidic drug, and since acids tend to ionize in basic media, elevation of urinary pH will cause more of the aspirin molecules present in urine to become ionized. As a result, less

drug will be passively reabsorbed and, therefore, more will be excreted.

Competition for Active Tubular Transport. Competition between drugs for active tubular transport can delay their renal excretion, thereby prolonging their effects. The active transport systems of the renal tubules can be envisioned as motor-driven revolving doors that carry drugs from the plasma into the renal tubules. These "revolving doors" can carry only a limited number of drug molecules per unit time. Accordingly, if there are too many molecules present, some must wait their turn. Because of competition, if we administer two drugs at the same time, and if both drugs use the same system of transport, the excretion of each will be delayed by the presence of the other.

Competition for transport has been employed clinically to prolong the effects of drugs that normally undergo very rapid renal excretion. For example, when administered alone, penicillin is rapidly cleared from the blood by active tubular transport. Excretion of penicillin can be delayed by concurrent administration of probenecid, an agent that is removed from the blood by the same tubular transport system that pumps penicillin. Hence, if a large dose of probenecid is administered, renal excretion of penicillin will be delayed while the transport system is occupied with moving the probenecid. By delaying penicillin excretion, probenecid prolongs antibacterial effects.

Age. The kidneys of newborns are not fully developed. Until the kidneys reach full capacity (a few months after birth), infants are limited in their ability to excrete drugs. This limitation must be accounted for when medicating an infant.

NONRENAL ROUTES OF DRUG EXCRETION

In most cases, excretion of drugs by nonrenal routes has little clinical significance. However, in certain situations, nonrenal excretion can have important therapeutic and toxicologic consequences.

Breast Milk

Drugs taken by lactating women can undergo excretion into the milk. As a result, breast-feeding can expose the nursing infant to drugs. The factors that influence the appearance of drugs in milk are the same factors that determine the passage of drugs across membranes. Accordingly, lipid-soluble drugs will have ready access to breast milk, whereas drugs that are polar, ionized, or protein bound will not enter the milk in significant amounts. Because infants may be harmed by compounds excreted in breast milk, it is recommended that nursing mothers avoid all drugs. If a woman *must* take medication, she should consult with her physician to insure that the medication will not appear in her milk in concentrations high enough to harm her baby. If toxic amounts *will* be excreted in milk, breast-feeding must cease.

Other Nonrenal Routes of Excretion

The *bile* is an important route of excretion for certain drugs. Recall that bile is secreted into the intestine, and then leaves the body in the feces. In some cases, drugs entering the intestine in bile may undergo reabsorption back into the portal blood. This reabsorption, referred to as *enterohepatic recirculation*, can substantially prolong a drug's sojourn in the body.

The *lungs* are the major route by which volatile anesthetics are excreted.

Small amounts of drugs can appear in *sweat* and *saliva*. These routes have little therapeutic or toxicologic significance.

TIME COURSE OF DRUG RESPONSES

To achieve the therapeutic objective, we must control the time course of drug responses. We need to regulate the time at which drug responses will start, the time they will be most intense, and the time they will cease. Since the four pharmacokinetic processes—absorption, distribution, metabolism, and excretion—determine how much drug will be at its sites of action at any given time, these processes are the major determinants of the time course over which drug responses will take place. Having discussed the individual processes that contribute to determining the time course of drug action, we are now prepared to discuss the time course itself.

PLASMA DRUG LEVELS

In most cases, the time course of drug action bears a direct relationship to the concentration of drug in the blood. Before discussing the time course per se, it will be helpful to review several important concepts related to plasma drug levels.

Clinical Significance of Plasma Drug Levels

Clinicians frequently monitor plasma drug levels in efforts to regulate drug responses. When measurements indicate that drug levels are inappropriate, these levels can be adjusted up or down by changing the dosage or the timing of drug administration.

The practice of regulating plasma drug levels in order to control drug responses should seem a bit odd given that (1) drug responses are related to drug concentrations at *sites of action* and that (2) the site of action of most drugs is not in the plasma. The question arises, "Why adjust plasma levels of a drug when what really matters is the concentration of that drug at its sites of action?" The answer to this question begins with the following observation: more often than not, it is a practical impossibility to measure drug concentrations at sites of action. For example, when a patient with epilepsy takes phenytoin (an anticonvulsant), we cannot routinely draw samples from inside the skull to see if brain levels of the medication are adequate for seizure control. Fortunately, in the case of phenytoin and most other drugs, it is not necessary to measure drug concentrations at actual sites of action in order to have an objective basis for adjusting dosage. Experience has shown that for most drugs *there is a direct correlation between therapeutic and toxic responses and the amount of drug present in plasma.* Therefore, although we can't usually measure drug concentrations at sites of action, we *can* determine plasma drug concentrations that, in turn, are highly predictive of therapeutic and toxic responses. Accordingly, the dosing objective is commonly spoken of in terms of achieving a specific plasma level of a drug.

Two Plasma Drug Levels Defined

Two plasma drug levels are of special importance: (1) the minimum effective concentration, and (2) the toxic concentration. These levels are depicted in Figure 5–13 and defined below.

Minimum Effective Concentration. The minimum effective concentration (MEC) is defined as *the plasma drug level below which therapeutic effects will not occur.* Hence, to be of benefit, a drug must be present in concentrations at or above the MEC.

Toxic Concentration. Toxicity occurs when plasma drug levels climb too high. The plasma level at which toxic effects begin to appear is termed the toxic concentration. Doses must be kept small enough so that the toxic concentration is not exceeded.

Therapeutic Range

As indicated in Figure 5–13, there is a range of plasma drug levels, falling between the MEC and the toxic concentration, that is termed the *therapeutic range.* When plasma levels are within the therapeutic range, there is enough drug present to produce therapeutic responses, but not so much drug that toxicity results. *The objective of drug dosing is to maintain plasma drug levels within the therapeutic range.*

The width of the therapeutic range is a major determinant of the ease with which a drug can be used safely. Drugs that have a narrow therapeutic range are difficult to administer safely. Conversely, drugs that have a wide therapeutic range can be administered safely with relative ease. Acetaminophen, for example, has a relatively wide therapeutic range—the toxic concentration is about 30 times greater than the MEC. Because of this wide therapeutic range, the dosage need not be highly precise: a broad range of doses can be employed to produce plasma levels that will be above the MEC but that will not exceed the toxic concentration. In contrast, lithium (used for manic-depressive illness) has a very narrow therapeutic range—the toxic concentration is only three times greater than the MEC. Since toxicity can result from lithium levels that are not much greater than those needed to produce therapeutic effects, lithium dosing must be done carefully if therapeutic effects are to be achieved without causing toxicity. If lithium had a wider therapeutic range, the drug would be much easier to use.

Understanding the concept of therapeutic range can facilitate patient care. Because drugs with a narrow therapeutic range are more dangerous than drugs with a wide therapeutic range, patients taking drugs with a narrow therapeutic range are the patients who are most likely to require nursing intervention for drug-related complications. The nurse who is aware of this fact can focus attention on these patients. In contrast, the nurse who has no basis for predicting which drugs are most likely to produce toxicity has no basis for allocating attention and, therefore, is obliged to monitor all patients with equal diligence—a process that is both stressful and inefficient.

However, lest you get the wrong impression, the above advice should not be construed as an invitation to be lax about patients taking drugs that have a wide therapeutic range. Even these drugs can cause harm. Hence, although patients receiving drugs with a narrow therapeutic range should be monitored most closely, common sense dictates that patients receiving safer drugs must not be neglected.

SINGLE-DOSE TIME COURSE

Figure 5–13 shows how plasma drug levels change over time following administration of a single dose of an oral medication. The rise in drug levels occurs as the medicine undergoes absorption. Drug levels then decline as metabolism and excretion eliminate the drug from the body.

Because responses cannot occur until plasma drug levels have reached the MEC, there is a period of latency between the time of administration and the onset of effects. The extent of this delay is determined by the rate of absorption.

The duration of drug effects is determined

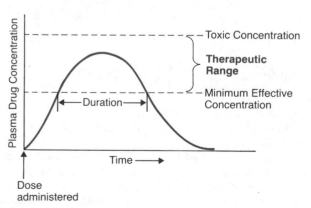

Figure 5–13. Single-dose time course.

largely by the combination of metabolism and excretion. As long as plasma levels remain above the MEC, therapeutic responses will be maintained; when plasma levels fall below the MEC, responses will cease. Since metabolism and excretion are the processes most responsible for causing plasma drug levels to fall, these processes are the primary determinants of how long drug effects will persist.

DRUG HALF-LIFE

Before proceeding to the topic of multiple dosing, we need to discuss the concept of drug half-life. When a patient ceases drug use, the combination of metabolism and excretion will cause the amount of drug in the body to decline. The half-life of a drug is an index of just how rapidly that decline will occur.

Drug half-life is defined as *the time required for the amount of drug in the body to decrease by 50%*. A few drugs have half-lives that are extremely short—in the order of minutes. In contrast, the half-lives of some drugs may exceed 1 week. Drugs with short half-lives leave the body quickly. Drugs with long half-lives leave slowly.

Note that in our definition of half-life, a *percentage*—not a specific *amount*—of drug is lost during one half-life. That is, the half-life does not specify, for example, that 2 gm or 18 mg will leave the body in a given time. Rather, the half-life tells us that no matter what the amount of drug in the body may be, half (50%) will leave during a specified period of time (the half-life). The actual *amount* of drug that is lost during one half-life will depend upon just how much drug is present—the more drug that is in the body, the larger the amount that will be lost during one half-life.

The concept of half-life is best understood through an example. Morphine provides a good illustration. The half-life of morphine is approximately 3 hours. By definition, this means that body stores of morphine will decrease by 50% every 3 hours—regardless of how much morphine is in the body. If there is 50 mg of morphine in the body, 50% (25 mg) will be lost in 3 hours; if there is only 2 mg of morphine in the body, only 1 mg (50% of 2 mg) will be lost in 3 hours. Note that in both cases, morphine levels drop by 50% during an interval of one half-life. However, the actual *amount* lost is larger when total body stores of the drug are higher.

When drug administration is discontinued, most of the drug in the body will be eliminated over an interval equal to four half-lives. This statement can be validated with simple arithmetic. Let's consider a patient who has been taking morphine. In addition, let's assume that, at the time dosing ceased, total body content of morphine was 40 mg. Within one half-life after drug withdrawal, morphine stores will decline by 50%—down to 20 mg. During the second half-life, stores will again decline by 50%, dropping from 20 mg to 10 mg. During the third half-life, the level will decline once more by 50%—from 10 mg down to 5 mg. During the fourth half-life, the level will again decline by 50%—from 5 mg down to 2.5 mg. Hence, over a period of four half-lives, total body stores of morphine will drop from an initial level of 40 mg down to 2.5 mg, an overall decline of 94%. Most of the drug in the body will be cleared within four half-lives.

The time required for drugs to leave the body is more important toxicologically than therapeutically. Let's consider the elimination of digitoxin (a drug used to treat heart failure) as an example. Digitoxin, true to its name, is a potentially dangerous drug with a narrow therapeutic range. In addition, the half-life of digitoxin is very long—about 7 days. What will be the consequence of digitoxin overdosage? Toxic levels of the drug will remain in the body for a long time: since digitoxin has a half-life of 7 days, and since four half-lives are required for most of the drug to be cleared from the body, it could take weeks for digitoxin stores to fall to a safe level. During the time that excess drug remains in the body, significant effort will be required to keep the patient alive. If digitoxin had a shorter half-life, body stores would decline more rapidly, thereby making management of overdosage less difficult.

It is important to note that the concept of half-life does not apply to the elimination of all drugs. A few agents, most notably ethanol (alcohol), leave the body at a *constant rate*, regardless of how much is present. The implications of this kind of decline for ethanol are discussed in Chapter 33.

DRUG LEVELS PRODUCED WITH REPEATED DOSES

Multiple dosing leads to drug accumulation. When a patient takes a single dose of a drug, plasma levels simply go up and then come back down. In contrast, when a patient takes repeated doses of a drug, the process is more complex and results in drug accumulation. The factors that determine the rate and extent of accumulation are considered below.

The Process by Which Plateau Drug Levels are Achieved

Administering repeated doses of a drug will cause that drug to build up in the body until a *plateau* (steady level) has been achieved. What causes drug levels to reach a plateau? To begin with, common sense tells us that if a second dose of a drug is administered before all of the prior dose has been eliminated, total body stores of that drug will be higher after the second dose than after the initial dose. As succeeding doses are administered, drug levels will climb even higher. The drug will continue to accumulate until a state has been achieved in which the amount of drug eliminated between doses equals the amount administered. *When the amount of drug eliminated between doses equals the dose administered, average drug levels will remain constant and a plateau will have been reached.*

The process by which multiple dosing produces a plateau is illustrated in Figure 5–14. The drug in this figure is a hypothetical agent with a half-life of exactly 1 day. The regimen consists of a 2-gm dose administered once daily. For purposes of illustration, we will assume that absorption takes place instantaneously. Upon administration of the first 2-gm dose (day 1 in the figure), total body stores go from zero to 2 gm. Within one half-life (1 day), body stores drop by 50%—from 2 gm down to 1 gm. At the beginning of day 2, the second 2-gm dose is given, causing body stores to rise from 1 gm up to 3 gm. Over the next 1-day half-life, body stores again drop by 50%, this time from 3 gm down to 1.5 gm. When the third dose is given, body stores go from 1.5 gm up to 3.5 gm. Over the next half-life, stores drop by 50% down to 1.75 gm. When the fourth dose is given, drug levels climb to 3.75 gm and, between doses, levels again drop by 50%, this time to approximately 1.9 gm. When the fifth dose is given (at the beginning of day 5), drug levels go up to about 3.9 gm. This process of accumulation continues until body stores reach 4 gm. When total body stores of this drug are 4 gm, 2 gm will be lost each day (i.e., over one half-life). Since a 2-gm dose is being administered each day, when body stores reach 4 gm, the amount lost between doses will equal the dose administered. At this point, body stores will simply alternate between 4 gm and 2 gm; average body stores will be stable; and plateau will have been reached. Note that the

reason that plateau is finally reached is that the actual amount of drug lost between doses gets larger each day. That is, although 50% of total body stores are lost each day, the amount in grams grows progressively larger because total body stores are getting larger day by day. Plateau is reached when the amount lost between doses grows to be as large as the amount administered.

Time to Plateau

When a drug is administered repeatedly in the same dose, *plateau will be reached in approximately four half-lives.* For the hypothetical agent illustrated in Figure 5–14, total body stores approached their peak near the beginning of day 5, or approximately 4 full days after treatment began. Since the half-life of this drug is 1 day, reaching plateau in 4 days is equivalent to reaching plateau in four half-lives.

As long as dosage remains constant, the time required to reach plateau is independent of dosage size. Put another way, the time required to reach plateau employing a large dose of a particular drug is identical to the time required to reach plateau employing a small dose of that drug. Referring to the drug in Figure 5–14, just as it took four half-lives (4 days) to reach plateau when a dose of 2 gm was administered daily, it would also take four half-lives to reach plateau if a dose of 4 gm were administered each day. It is true that the *height* of the plateau would be greater if a 4-gm dose were given, but the *time* required to reach plateau would not be altered by the increase in dosage. To confirm this statement, substitute a dose of 4 gm in the exercise we went through to demonstrate accumulation to plateau with a dose of 2 gm.

Techniques for Reducing Fluctuations in Drug Levels

As can be seen from Figure 5–14, when drugs are administered repeatedly, drug levels will fluctuate between doses. The degree of fluctuation that can be tolerated will depend upon a drug's therapeutic range: if there is not much difference between the toxic concentration and the MEC, then fluctuations must be kept to a minimum.

Two procedures can be employed to reduce fluctuations in drug levels. One technique is to administer drugs by *continuous infusion.* With this procedure, plasma levels can be kept nearly constant. The second procedure is to *reduce dosage size and increase the frequency of dosing* (keeping the total daily dose constant). For example, rather than giving the drug from Figure 5–14 in 2-gm doses once daily, we could give this drug in 1-gm doses twice daily. With this altered dosing schedule, the total daily dose would remain unchanged as would total body stores at plateau. However, instead of fluc-

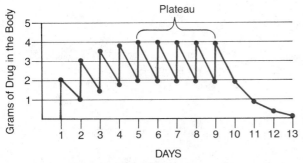

Figure 5–14. Drug accumulation with repeated administration. This figure illustrates the accumulation of a hypothetical drug during repeated administration. The drug has a half-life of 1 day and is being administered in a 2-gm dose once a day on days 1 through 9. Note that plateau is reached at about the beginning of day 5 (i.e., after 4 half-lives). Note also that when administration is discontinued, it takes about 4 days (4 half-lives) for most of the drug to leave the body.

tuating over a range of 2 gm between doses, levels would fluctuate over a range of 1 gm.

Loading Doses Versus Maintenance Doses

As discussed above, if we were to administer a drug in repeated doses of equal size, an interval equivalent to four half-lives would be required to achieve plateau. For drugs whose half-lives are long, achieving plateau could take days or even weeks. When plateau must be achieved more quickly, a large initial dose can be administered. This large initial dose is called a *loading dose*. Once high drug levels have been established with a loading dose, plateau can be maintained by giving smaller doses. These smaller doses are referred to as *maintenance doses*.

The claim that use of a loading dose will shorten the time to plateau may appear to contradict an earlier statement, which said that the time to plateau is not affected by dosage size. However, there is no contradiction. For any *specified* dosage, it will always take four half-lives to reach plateau. When a loading dose is administered followed by maintenance doses, we have not reached plateau *for the loading dose*. Rather, we have simply used the loading dose to rapidly produce a drug level equivalent to the plateau level *for a smaller dose*. If we wished to achieve plateau level *for the loading dose*, we would be obliged to either administer doses equivalent to the loading dose for a period of four half-lives or administer a dose even larger than the original loading dose.

Decline from Plateau

As discussed above, when a drug has been administered repeatedly and then withdrawn, a time equivalent to four half-lives is required for body stores of the drug to decline by 94%. This decline from plateau is illustrated in Figure 5–14. Note that a 50% reduction in drug stores occurs during each half-life.

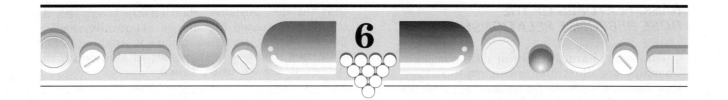

Pharmacodynamics

Pharmacodynamics is defined as the study of the biochemical and physiologic effects of drugs and the molecular mechanisms by which those effects are produced. In short, pharmacodynamics is the study of what drugs do to the body and how they do it.

In order to participate rationally in efforts to achieve the therapeutic objective, nurses need a basic understanding of pharmacodynamics. You must know about drug actions in order to educate patients about their medication. Knowledge of drug effects is also needed in order to make informed decisions on PRN orders. In addition, knowledge of pharmacodynamics is applied when evaluating patients for drug responses, both beneficial and harmful. You will also need to understand drug actions when conferring with the physician about drug therapy; the nurse who believes that a patient is receiving inappropriate medication or is being denied a required drug will need to support that conviction with arguments based at least in part on knowledge of pharmacodynamics.

DOSE-RESPONSE RELATIONSHIPS

The dose-response relationship (i.e., the relationship between the size of an administered dose and the intensity of the response produced) is a fundamental concern in therapeutics. Dose-response relationships determine the minimum amount of drug that we can use, the maximum response that a drug can elicit, and how much the dosage must be increased to produce the desired increase in response.

BASIC FEATURES OF THE DOSE-RESPONSE RELATIONSHIP

The basic characteristics of dose-response relationships are illustrated in Figure 6–1. Part A of this figure shows dose-response data plotted on *linear* coordinates. Part B shows the same data plotted on *semilogarithmic* coordinates (i.e., the scale on which dosage is plotted is logarithmic rather than linear). The most obvious and important characteristic revealed by these curves is that the dose-response relationship is *graded*. That is, as dosage is increased, the response becomes progressively larger. Because drug responses are graded, therapeutic effects can be adjusted to fit the needs of each patient. To tailor treatment to a particular patient, all we need do is raise or lower the dosage until a response of the desired intensity is achieved. If drug responses were *all-or-nothing* instead of graded, drugs could only produce one intensity of response. If that response were too strong or too weak for a particular patient, there would be nothing we could do to adjust the intensity to better suit the patient's needs. Clearly, the graded nature of the dose-response relationship is essential to successful drug therapy.

As indicated in Figure 6–1, the dose-response relationship can be viewed as having three phases. Phase 1 (see Fig. 6–1B) occurs at low doses; the curve is flat during this phase because doses are too low to elicit a measurable response. During phase 2, an increase in dose elicits a corresponding increase in the response; it is during this phase

that the dose-response relationship is graded. As the dose is raised higher, we eventually reach a point where an increase in dose is unable to elicit a further increase in response; at this point, the curve flattens out into phase 3.

MAXIMAL EFFICACY AND RELATIVE POTENCY

Dose-response curves can reveal two characteristic properties of drugs: *maximal efficacy* and *relative potency*. Curves that reflect these properties are shown in Figure 6–2.

Maximal Efficacy

Maximal efficacy is defined as *the largest effect that a drug can produce*. Maximal efficacy is indicated by the *height* of the dose-response curve.

The concept of maximal efficacy is illustrated by the dose-response curves for meperidine and pentazocine—two morphine-like pain relievers (Fig. 6–2A). As we can see, the curve for pentazocine levels off at a maximum height below that of the curve for meperidine. This tells us that the maximum degree of pain relief we can achieve with pentazocine is less than the maximum degree of pain relief we can achieve with meperidine. Put another way, no matter how much pentazocine we administer, we can never produce the degree of pain relief that we can with meperidine. Accordingly, we would say that meperidine has greater maximal efficacy than pentazocine.

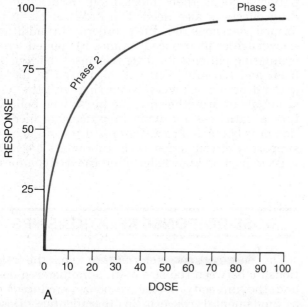

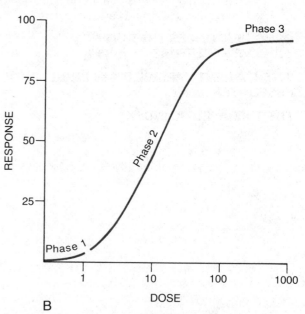

Figure 6–1. Basic components of the dose-response curve. *A*, A dose-response curve with dose plotted on a *linear scale*. *B*, The same dose-response relationship shown in *A* but with the dose plotted on a *logarithmic* scale. Note the three phases of the dose-response curve. *Phase 1,* The curve is relatively flat; doses are too low to elicit a significant response. *Phase 2,* The curve climbs upward as increases in dose elicit a corresponding increase in response. *Phase 3,* The curve levels off; increases in dose are unable to elicit further increases in response. (Phase 1 is not indicated in *A* because very low doses cannot be shown on a linear scale.)

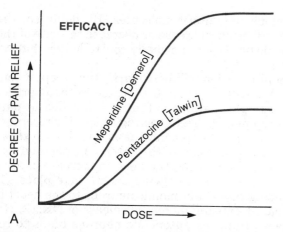

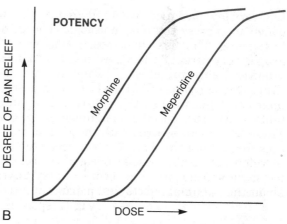

Figure 6–2. Dose-response curves demonstrating efficacy and potency. *A, Efficacy* or "maximal efficacy" is an index of the maximal response that a drug can produce. The efficacy of a drug is indicated by the *height* of its dose-response curve. In this example, meperidine has greater efficacy than pentazocine. Efficacy is an important quality in a drug. *B, Potency* is an index of *how* much drug must be administered to elicit a desired response. In this example, pain relief with meperidine requires higher doses than pain relief with morphine. We would say that morphine is more potent than meperidine. Note that if administered in sufficiently high doses, meperidine can produce just as much pain relief as morphine. Potency is usually not an important quality in a drug.

Despite what intuition might tell us, a drug with very high maximal efficacy is not always more desirable than a drug with lower efficacy. Recall that we want to match the intensity of the response to the patient's needs. This may be difficult to do with a drug that produces extremely intense responses. For example, certain diuretics (e.g., furosemide) have such high maximal efficacy that they can pose a danger of causing severe dehydration. If we only want to mobilize a modest volume of water, a diuretic with lower maximal efficacy (e.g., hydrochlorothiazide) would be preferred. Similarly, if a patient had a headache, we would not select a powerful analgesic (e.g., morphine) for relief; rather, we would select an analgesic with lower maximal efficacy, such as aspirin. Put another way, it is neither appropriate nor desirable to hunt squirrels with an atomic cannon.

Relative Potency

The term *potency* refers to the amount of drug that must be given to elicit an effect. Potency is indicated by the relative position of the dose-response curve along the X (dosage) axis.

The concept of potency is illustrated by the curves in Figure 6–2B. These curves plot doses for two analgesics—morphine and meperidine—versus the degree of pain relief achieved. As we can see, for any particular degree of pain relief, the required dose of meperidine is larger than the required dose of morphine. Since morphine produces pain relief at lower doses than meperidine, we would say that morphine is more potent than meperidine. That is, a potent drug is one that produces its effects at low doses.

Potency is rarely an important characteristic of a drug. The fact that morphine is more potent than meperidine does not mean that morphine is a superior medicine. In fact, the only consequence of morphine's greater potency is that morphine can be given in smaller doses. The difference between providing pain relief with morphine versus meperidine is much like the difference between purchasing candy with a dime instead of two nickels; although the dime is smaller (more potent) than the two nickels, the purchasing power of the dime and the two nickels is identical.

Not only is potency generally irrelevant, in certain cases high potency may actually be detrimental. When a drug is extremely potent, the doses required are very tiny. Such minuscule doses can be difficult to measure and dispense.

Although potency is usually of no clinical concern, it *can* be important if a drug is so lacking in potency that doses become inconveniently large. For example, if a drug were of extremely low potency, we might need to administer that drug in huge doses several times a day to achieve beneficial effects. In a case such as this, an alternative drug with higher potency would be desirable. Fortunately, it is rare for a drug to be so lacking in potency that doses of inconvenient magnitude need be given.

It is important to note that the potency of a drug implies nothing about its maximal efficacy! Potency and efficacy are completely independent qualities. Drug A can be more effective than drug B even though drug B may be more potent. Also, drugs A and B can be equally effective even though one may be more potent than the other. As we saw in Figure 6–2B, although meperidine happens to be less potent than morphine, the maximal degree of pain relief that we can achieve with these drugs is identical.

A final comment on the word *potency* is in order.

In everyday parlance, we tend to use the word *potent* to express the pharmacologic concept of effectiveness. That is, when most people say, "This drug is very potent," what they mean is, "This drug produces powerful effects." They do not mean, "This drug produces its effects at low doses." In pharmacology, we use the words potent and potency with the specific meanings given above. These words will be used with those specific meanings throughout this text. We will use potency only in reference to the dosage needed to produce effects; we will not use the term to imply anything about the maximal effects that a drug can produce.

DRUG-RECEPTOR INTERACTIONS

BASIC PROPERTIES OF DRUG RECEPTORS

Drugs are not "magic bullets"; they are simply chemicals. Being chemicals, all that drugs can do to produce their effects is interact with other chemicals. *Receptors* are the special "chemicals" in the body that drugs interact with to produce their effects.

We can define a receptor as *any functional macromolecule in a cell to which a drug binds to produce its effects.* Under this broad definition, many cellular components would be considered drug receptors, since drugs bind to many cellular components (e.g., DNA, enzymes, ribosomes) to produce their effects. However, although the formal definition of a receptor encompasses *all* functional macromolecules, *the term "receptor" is almost always reserved for what is arguably the most important group of macromolecules through which drugs act: the body's own receptors for hormones, neurotransmitters, and other regulatory molecules.* In this chapter and throughout the rest of this text, we will use the term *receptor* in this more limited sense. The other macromolecules to which drugs bind (e.g., DNA, enzymes) can be thought of simply as *target molecules*, rather than as true receptors.

The general equation for the interaction between drugs and their receptors is as follows:

DRUG + RECEPTOR ⇌
    DRUG-RECEPTOR COMPLEX → RESPONSE

As suggested by the equation, binding of drugs to their receptors is usually *reversible*.

A receptor is analogous to a light switch: like the switch, a receptor must be in the ON configuration to influence cellular function. Receptors are activated ("turned on") by interaction with other molecules. Under normal circumstances, receptor activity is regulated by endogenous compounds (neurotransmitters, hormones, other regulatory molecules). When a drug binds to a receptor, all that it can do is mimic or block the actions of endogenous regulatory molecules. By doing so, the drug will either increase or decrease the rate of the physiologic activity normally controlled by that receptor.

An illustration will help clarify the receptor concept. We will use receptors located in the heart for our example. Cardiac output is controlled in part by norepinephrine (NE) acting at specific receptors in the heart. Norepinephrine is supplied to those receptors by neurons of the autonomic nervous system (Fig. 6–3). When the need to increase cardiac output arises, the following events take place: (1) the firing rate of autonomic neurons to the heart is increased, causing increased release of NE; (2) NE released from the autonomic neurons binds to receptors on the heart; and (3) as a consequence of the interaction between NE and its receptors, both the rate and force of cardiac contractions are increased, thereby increasing cardiac output. When the demand for cardiac output subsides, the autonomic neurons reduce their firing rate, binding of NE to its receptors diminishes, and cardiac output returns to resting levels.

The same cardiac receptors whose function is regulated by endogenous NE can also serve as receptors for drugs. That is, just as endogenous molecules can bind to these receptors, so can compounds that enter the body as drugs. The binding of drugs to these receptors can have one of two effects: (1) drugs can *mimic* the action of NE supplied by nerves (and thereby increase cardiac output), or (2) drugs can *block* the action of endogenous NE (and thereby prevent stimulation of the heart).

Several important properties of receptors and drug-receptor interactions are illustrated by the example presented:

1. The receptors through which drugs act are nor-

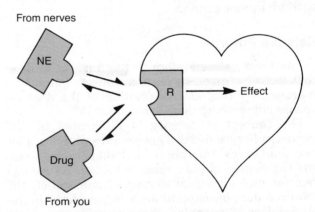

Figure 6–3. Interaction of drugs with receptors for norepinephrine. Under physiologic conditions, cardiac output can be increased by the binding of norepinephrine (NE) to receptors (R) on the heart. NE is supplied to these receptors by nerves. These same receptors can be acted upon by drugs. Drugs can act at these receptors to *mimic* endogenous NE (and thereby increase cardiac ouput), or drugs can *block* the actions of endogenous NE (and thereby reduce cardiac output).

mal points of control of physiologic processes. Under physiologic conditions, receptor function is regulated by molecules supplied by the body.

2. All that drugs can do at receptors is mimic or block the action of the body's own regulatory molecules.

3. Because drug action is limited to mimicking or blocking the body's own regulatory molecules, *drugs cannot give cells new functions.* Rather, drugs can only alter the rate of pre-existing processes. In other words, drugs cannot make the body do anything that it is not already capable of doing.

4. Drugs produce their therapeutic effects by helping the body use its pre-existing capacities to the patient's best advantage. Put another way, medications simply help the body help itself.

5. In theory, it should be possible to synthesize drugs that can alter the rate of any biologic process for which receptors exist.

RECEPTORS AND SELECTIVITY OF DRUG ACTION

In Chapter 1, we noted that selectivity is a highly desirable characteristic of a drug, since the more selective a drug is, the fewer side effects it will produce. Selective drug action is possible, in large part, because drugs act through specific receptors.

The body employs many different kinds of receptors to regulate its sundry physiologic activities. There are receptors for each neurotransmitter (e.g., norepinephrine, acetylcholine, dopamine); there are receptors for each hormone (e.g., progesterone, insulin, thyrotropin); and there are receptors for all of the other molecules that the body uses to regulate physiologic processes (e.g., histamine, prostaglandins, leukotrienes). As a rule, each type of receptor participates in the regulation of just a few processes.

Selective drug action is made possible by the existence of many types of receptors, each regulating just a few processes. Common sense tells us that if a drug interacts with only one kind of receptor, and if that receptor type regulates just a few processes, then the effects of the drug will be limited. Conversely, intuition also tells us that if a drug interacts with several different receptor types, then that drug is likely to elicit a wide variety of responses.

How can a drug interact with one receptor type and not with others? In some important ways, a receptor is analogous to a lock and a drug is analogous to a key for that lock: just as only those keys with the proper profile can fit a particular lock, only those drugs with the proper size, shape, and physical properties can bind to a particular receptor.

The binding of acetylcholine (a neurotransmit-

ter) to its receptor illustrates the lock and key analogy (Fig. 6–4). To bind with its receptor, acetylcholine must have a shape that is complementary to the shape of the receptor; in addition, acetylcholine must possess positive charges that are positioned so as to permit their interaction with corresponding negative sites on the receptor. If acetylcholine lacked these characteristics, it would be unable to interact with the receptor.

Like the acetylcholine receptor, all other receptors impose specific requirements on the molecules with which they will interact. Because receptors have such specific requirements, it is possible to synthesize drugs that will interact with just one receptor type to the exclusion of all others. Such medications will tend to elicit selective responses.

Even though a drug is selective for only one type of receptor, it is possible for that drug to produce nonselective effects. How can this be? If a single receptor type is responsible for regulating several physiologic processes, then drugs that interact with that receptor will also influence a variety of processes. For example, in addition to modulating perception of pain, morphine receptors help to regulate other processes, including respiration and motility of the bowel. Consequently, although morphine is selective for one class of receptor, the drug can still produce a variety of effects. In clinical practice, it is common for morphine to cause respiratory depression and constipation along with reduction of pain. Note that morphine produces these varied effects not because it lacks receptor selectivity, but because the receptor for which morphine is selective helps regulate a variety of physiologic processes.

One final comment on selectivity: *selectivity does not guarantee safety.* A compound can be highly selective for a particular receptor and yet still be extremely dangerous. For example, although botulinus toxin is highly selective for one type of receptor, the compound is anything but safe: this toxin can cause paralysis of the muscles of respiration, resulting in death from respiratory arrest.

THEORIES OF DRUG-RECEPTOR INTERACTION

In the discussion below, we will consider two theories of drug-receptor interaction: (1) the simple occupancy theory, and (2) the modified occupancy theory. These theories help explain dose-response relationships and the ability of drugs to mimic or block the actions of endogenous regulatory molecules.

Simple Occupancy Theory

The simple occupancy theory of drug-receptor interaction states that (1) the intensity of the re-

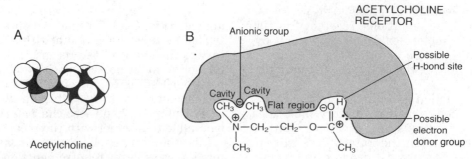

Figure 6–4. Interaction of acetylcholine with its receptor. *A,* Three-dimensional model of the acetylcholine molecule. *B,* Binding of acetylcholine to its receptor. Note how the shape of the acetylcholine molecule closely matches the shape of the receptor. Note also how the positive charges on acetylcholine align with the negative sites on the receptor. (Modified from Goldstein, A., Aronow, L., and Sumner, M.K. Principles of Drug Action: The Basis of Pharmacology, 2nd ed. New York, John Wiley & Sons, 1974. Copyright © 1974. Reprinted by permission of John Wiley & Sons, Inc.)

sponse to a drug is proportional to the number of receptors occupied by that drug and that (2) a maximal response will occur when *all* available receptors have been occupied. This relationship between receptor occupancy and the intensity of the response is shown graphically in Figure 6–5.

Although certain aspects of dose-response relationships can be explained by the simple occupancy theory, other important phenomena cannot. Specifically, there is nothing in this theory to explain why one drug should be more potent than another. In addition, this theory cannot explain how one drug can have higher maximal efficacy than another. That is, according to this theory, two drugs acting at the same receptor should produce the same maximal effect, providing that their dosages were high enough to produce 100% receptor occupancy. We have already seen, however, that this is not true. As shown in Figure 6–2A, there is a dose of pentazocine above which no further increase in response can be elicited. Presumably, all receptors are occupied when the dose-response curve levels off. However, at 100% receptor occupancy, the response elicited by pentazocine is less than that elicited by morphine. Simple occupancy theory cannot account for this observation.

Modified Occupancy Theory

The modified occupancy theory of drug-receptor interaction explains certain observations that cannot be accounted for with the simple occupancy theory. The simple occupancy theory assumes that all drugs acting at a particular receptor are identical with respect to (1) the ability to bind to the receptor and (2) the ability to influence receptor function once binding has taken place. The modified occupancy theory is based on different assumptions.

The modified theory ascribes two qualities to drugs: *affinity* and *intrinsic activity*. The term *affinity* refers to the strength of the attraction between a drug and its receptor. *Intrinsic activity* refers to the ability of a drug to activate the recep-

tor following binding. *Affinity and intrinsic activity are independent properties.*

Affinity. As noted, the term *affinity* refers to the strength of the attraction between a drug and its receptor. Drugs with *high* affinity are *strongly* attracted to their receptors. Conversely, drugs with *low* affinity are *weakly* attracted.

The affinity of a drug for its receptors is reflected in its *potency.* Because they are strongly attracted to their receptors, drugs with high affinity can bind their receptors when present in low concentrations. Because they bind receptors at low concentrations, drugs with high affinity are effective in low doses. That is, *drugs with high affinity are very potent.* Conversely, drugs with low affinity must be present in high concentrations to bind

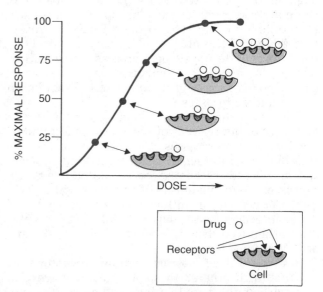

Figure 6–5. Model of simple occupancy theory. The simple occupancy theory states that the intensity of response to a drug is proportional to the number of receptors occupied; maximal response is reached with 100% receptor occupancy. Since the hypothetical cell in this figure has only four receptors, maximal response is achieved when all four receptors are occupied. (It should be noted that real cells have thousand of receptors.)

their receptors. Accordingly, these drugs are not very potent.

Intrinsic Activity. The term *intrinsic activity* refers to the ability of a drug to activate a receptor following binding. Drugs with high intrinsic activity cause intense receptor activation. Conversely, drugs with low intrinsic activity cause only slight activation.

The intrinsic activity of a drug is reflected in its *maximal efficacy*. Drugs with high intrinsic activity have high maximal efficacy. That is, by causing intense receptor activation, they are able to cause intense responses. Conversely, if intrinsic activity is low, maximal efficacy will be low as well.

It should be noted that under the modified occupancy theory, the intensity of the response to a drug is still related to the number of receptors occupied. The wrinkle added by the modified theory is that intensity is also related to the ability of the drug to activate receptors once binding has occurred. Under the modified theory, two drugs can occupy the same number of receptors but produce effects of different intensity; the drug with greater intrinsic activity will produce the more intense response.

AGONISTS, ANTAGONISTS, AND PARTIAL AGONISTS

As noted above, when drugs bind to receptors they can do one of two things: either they can *mimic* the action of endogenous regulatory molecules or they can *block* the action of endogenous regulators. Drugs that mimic the body's own regulatory molecules are called *agonists*. Drugs that block the actions of endogenous regulators are called *antagonists*. Like full agonists, *partial agonists* also mimic the actions of endogenous regulatory molecules, but they produce responses of reduced intensity.

Agonists

Agonists are molecules that activate receptors. Since neurotransmitters, hormones, and all other endogenous regulators of receptor function activate the receptors to which they bind, all of these compounds are considered agonists. When drugs act as agonists, they simply bind to receptors and mimic the actions of the body's own regulatory molecules.

In terms of the modified occupancy theory, an agonist is a drug that has both *affinity* and *high intrinsic activity*. Affinity allows the agonist to bind to receptors, while intrinsic activity allows the bound agonist to "activate" or "turn on" receptor function.

Many therapeutic agents produce their effects by functioning as agonists. Dobutamine, for example, is a drug that mimics the action of norepinephrine at receptors on the heart, thereby causing heart rate and force of contraction to increase. The insulin that we administer as a drug mimics the actions of endogenous insulin at receptors. Norethindrone, a component of many oral contraceptives, acts by "turning on" receptors for progesterone.

It is important to note that agonists do not necessarily make physiologic processes go faster; receptor activation can also slow a particular process down. For example, there are receptors on the heart that, when activated by acetylcholine (the body's own agonist for these receptors), will cause heart rate to decrease. Drugs that mimic the action of acetylcholine at these receptors will also decrease heart rate. Since such drugs produce their effects by causing receptor activation, they would be called agonists—despite the fact that their effect is to slow heart rate down.

Antagonists

Antagonists produce their effects by preventing receptor activation by endogenous regulatory molecules and drugs. Antagonists have virtually no effects of their own on receptor function.

In terms of the modified occupancy theory, an antagonist is a drug with *affinity* for a receptor but with *no intrinsic activity*. Affinity allows the antagonist to bind to receptors, but lack of intrinsic activity prevents the bound antagonist from causing receptor activation.

Although antagonists do not cause receptor activation, they most certainly *do* produce pharmacologic effects. Antagonists produce their effects by preventing the activation of receptors by agonists. Antagonists can produce beneficial effects by blocking the actions of endogenous regulatory molecules or by blocking the actions of other drugs. (The ability of antagonists to block the actions of other drugs is employed most commonly in the treatment of poisoning.)

It is important to note that the response to an antagonist will be determined by how much *agonist* is present. Since antagonists act by preventing receptor activation, *if there is no agonist present, administration of an antagonist will have no observable effect*; the drug will bind to its receptors but nothing will happen. On the other hand, if receptors are undergoing activation by agonists, administration of an antagonist will shut down the process, resulting in an observable response. This is an important concept; so think about it.

Many therapeutic agents produce their effects by acting as receptor antagonists. Antihistamines, for example, suppress allergy symptoms by binding to receptors for histamine, thereby preventing activation of these receptors by histamine released in response to allergens. The use of antagonists to treat drug toxicity is illustrated by naloxone, an agent that blocks receptors for morphine and re-

opioids; by preventing activation of opioid receptors, naloxone can completely reverse all symptoms of opioid overdosage.

Antagonists can be subdivided into two major classes: (1) noncompetitive antagonists and (2) competitive antagonists. Most antagonist drugs belong to the competitive class.

Noncompetitive (Insurmountable) Antagonists. Noncompetitive antagonists bind *irreversibly* to receptors. The effect of this irreversible binding is equivalent to reducing the total number of receptors available for activation by an agonist. Since the intensity of the response to an agonist is proportional to the total number of receptors occupied, and since noncompetitive antagonists decrease the number of receptors available for activation, a noncompetitive antagonist will *reduce the maximal response* that an agonist can elicit. If sufficient antagonist is present, agonist effects will be blocked completely. Dose-response curves illustrating inhibition by a noncompetitive antagonist are shown in Figure 6–6A.

Since the binding of noncompetitive antagonists is irreversible, inhibition by these agents cannot be overcome—no matter how much agonist may be available. Because inhibition by noncompetitive antagonists cannot be reversed, these agents are rarely used therapeutically. (Recall from Chapter 1 that reversibility is one of the properties of an ideal drug.)

The fact that noncompetitive antagonists bind irreversibly to receptors does *not* mean that the effects of these agents last forever. Cells are constantly breaking down "old" receptors and synthesizing new ones. Consequently, the effects of noncompetitive antagonists will wear off as the receptors to which they are bound are replaced. Since the life cycle of a receptor can be relatively short, the effects of noncompetitive antagonists may subside within a few days.

Competitive (Surmountable) Antagonists. Competitive antagonists bind *reversibly* to their receptors. As their name implies, competitive antagonists produce receptor blockade by competing with agonists for receptor binding. If an agonist and a competitive antagonist have equal affinity for a particular receptor, that receptor will be occupied by whichever agent—agonist or antagonist—is present in the highest concentration. If there are more antagonist molecules present than agonist molecules, antagonist molecules will occupy the receptors, and receptor activation will be blocked. Conversely, if agonist molecules outnumber the antagonists, receptors will be occupied mainly by the agonist, and little inhibition will occur.

Because competitive antagonists bind reversibly to receptors, the inhibition they cause is *surmountable*. In the presence of sufficiently high amounts of agonist, agonist molecules will occupy all receptors and inhibition will be completely overcome. The dose-response curves shown in Figure 6–6B illustrate the process of overcoming the effects of a competitive antagonist with large doses of an agonist.

Partial Agonists

A partial agonist is an agonist that has only *moderate intrinsic activity*. As a result, *the maximal effect that a partial agonist can produce is lower than that of a full agonist*. Pentazocine is an example of a partial agonist. As the curves in Figure 6–2A indicate, the degree of pain relief that can be achieved with pentazocine is much lower than the relief that can be achieved with meperidine (a full agonist).

Partial agonists are interesting in that they can act as *antagonists* as well as *agonists*. For example, when pentazocine is administered by itself, it will occupy opioid receptors and produce moderate relief of pain. In this situation, the drug will be

acting as an *agonist*. However, if a patient is already taking meperidine (a full agonist at opioid receptors) and is then given a large dose of pentazocine, pentazocine will occupy the opioid receptors and prevent their activation by meperidine. As a result, rather than experiencing the high degree of pain relief that meperidine can produce, the patient will experience only the limited relief that pentazocine can produce. In this situation, pentazocine will be acting as both an *agonist* (producing moderate pain relief) and as an *antagonist* (blocking the higher degree of relief that could have been achieved with meperidine by itself).

DRUG RESPONSES THAT DO NOT INVOLVE RECEPTORS

Although the effects of most drugs result from drug-receptor interactions, some drugs do not act through receptors. Rather, these drugs act through simple physical or chemical interactions with other small molecules.

Common examples of "receptorless drugs" include antacids, antiseptics, saline laxatives, and chelating agents. Antacids reduce gastric acidity by direct chemical interaction with stomach acid. The antiseptic action of ethyl alcohol results from precipitating bacterial proteins. Magnesium hydroxide, a powerful laxative, acts by retaining water in the intestinal lumen through an osmotic effect. Dimercaprol, a chelating agent, prevents toxicity from heavy metals (e.g., arsenic, mercury) by forming complexes with these compounds. All of these pharmacologic effects are the result of simple physical or chemical interactions, and not the result of interactions with cellular receptors.

INTERPATIENT VARIABILITY IN DRUG RESPONSES

The dose required to produce a therapeutic response can vary substantially among patients. The reason for this variability is that people differ from one another. The *specific* kinds of differences that underlie variability in drug responses are discussed in Chapter 9. In this chapter we will consider interpatient variation as a *general* issue.

In order to promote the therapeutic objective, you must be alert to interpatient variation in drug responses. Because of interpatient variation, it is not possible to predict just how an individual patient will respond to medication. Hence, each patient must be evaluated to determine his or her actual response to treatment. The nurse who appreciates the reality of interpatient variability will be better prepared to anticipate, evaluate, and re-

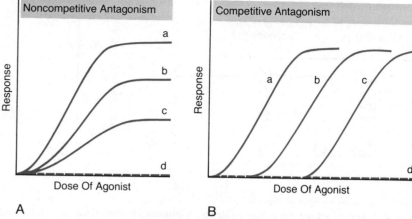

Figure 6–6. Dose–response curves in the presence of competitive and noncompetitive antagonists. *A,* Effect of a *noncompetitive* antagonist on the dose-response curve of an agonist. Note that noncompetitive antagonists decrease the maximal response achievable with an agonist. *B,* Effect of a *competitive* antagonist on the dose-response curve of an agonist. Note that the maximal response achievable with the agonist is not reduced. Competitive antagonists simply increase the amount of agonist required to produce any given intensity of response.

spond appropriately to each patient's therapeutic needs.

Measurement of Interpatient Variability

An example of how interpatient variability is measured will facilitate our discussion. Let's assume that we've just developed a new antacid and wish to evaluate variability in patient responses. To make this evaluation, we must first define a specific *therapeutic objective* or *endpoint*. For our antacid, an appropriate endpoint is elevation of gastric pH to a value of 5.

Having defined a therapeutic endpoint, we can now perform our study. Subjects for this study are 100 people with gastric ulcers. We begin our experiment by giving each subject a low initial dose (100 mg) of our drug. We then measure gastric pH to determine how many individuals achieved the therapeutic goal of pH 5. Let's assume that only two people responded to the initial dose. To the remaining 98 subjects, we give an additional 20-mg dose and again determine whose gastric pH rose to 5. Let's assume that six more subjects responded to this dose (120 mg total). We continue the experiment, administering doses in 20-mg increments, until all 100 people have responded with the desired elevation in gastric pH.

The data from our hypothetical experiment are tabulated and plotted in Figure 6–7. The plot is called a *frequency distribution curve.* We can see from the curve that a wide range of doses was required to produce the desired response in all subjects. For some subjects, a dose of only 100 mg was sufficient to produce the target response. For other subjects, the therapeutic endpoint was not achieved until a total dose of 240 mg had been given.

The ED50

The dose at the middle of the frequency distribution curve is termed the ED50 (see Fig. 6–7). (*ED* is an abbreviation for *effective dose.*) The ED50 is defined as *the dose that is required to produce a defined therapeutic response in 50% of the population.* In the case of our antacid, the ED50 was 170 mg—the dose needed to elevate gastric pH to a value of 5 in 50 of the 100 people tested.

The ED50 can be considered a "standard" dose and, as such, is frequently the dose selected for initiating treatment. After evaluating the patient's response to this "standard" dose, we can then adjust subsequent doses up or down in accordance with the patient's need.

Clinical Implications of Interpatient Variability

Interpatient variation has four important clinical consequences. As a nurse you should be aware of these implications:

1. *The initial dose of a drug is necessarily an approximation. Subsequent doses must be "fine tuned" based on the patient's response.* Because initial doses are approximations, it would be wise not to challenge the physician if the prescribed initial dose differs by a small amount (e.g., 10% to 20%) from recommended doses in a published drug reference. Rather, you should administer the medication as prescribed and evaluate the response; dosage adjustments can then be made as needed. (Of course, if the physician's order calls for a dose that differs from the recommended dose by a large amount, that order should be challenged.)

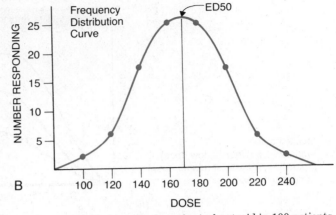

Dose of Drug (mg)	Number of Subjects Responding at Each Dose
100	2
120	6
140	17
160	25
180	25
200	17
220	6
240	2

A

Figure 6–7. Interpatient variation in drug responses. *A*, Data from clinical testing of a hypothetical antacid in 100 patients. The goal of the study was to determine the dosage of antacid required by each patient to elevate gastric pH to 5. Note the wide variability in doses needed to produce the target response for the 100 subjects. *B*, Frequency distribution curve for the data in *A*. The dose at the middle of the curve is termed the *ED50*—the dose that will produce a predefined intensity of response in 50% of the population.

2. *When given an average effective dose (ED50), some patients will have been undertreated, whereas others will have received more drug than they need.* Hence, when therapy is initiated with a dose equivalent to the ED50, it is especially important to evaluate the patient's response. Patients who fail to respond will need an increase in dosage. Conversely, patients who show signs of toxicity will need to have their dosage reduced.

3. *Since drug responses are not completely predictable, you must look at the patient (and not the Physicians' Desk Reference) to determine if too much or too little medication has been administered.* In other words, doses should be adjusted on the basis of the patient's response and not just on the basis of what some reference says is supposed to work. For example, although many postoperative patients will receive adequate pain relief with an "average" dose of morphine, this dose will not be appropriate for everyone: an average dose may be effective for some patients, ineffective for others, and toxic for still others. Clearly, dosage must be adjusted on the basis of the patient's response, and must not be given in blind compliance with the dosage recommended in a book.

4. *Because of variability in responses, nurses, patients, and other concerned persons must evaluate actual responses and be prepared to inform*

$$\text{THERAPEUTIC INDEX (TI)} = \frac{LD50}{ED50}$$

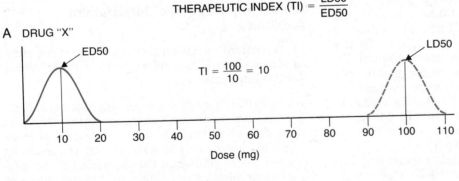

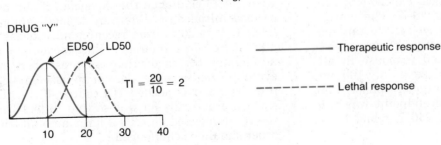

—————— Therapeutic response

- - - - - - - - - Lethal response

Figure 6–8. The therapeutic index. *A*, Frequency distribution curves indicating the ED50 and LD50 for drug "X." Because its LD50 is much greater than its ED50, drug X is relatively safe. *B*, Frequency distribution curves indicating the ED50 and LD50 for drug "Y." Because its LD50 is very close to its ED50, drug Y is not very safe. Also note the *overlap* between the effective-dose curve and the lethal-dose curve.

the prescribing physician about these responses so that proper adjustments in dosage can be made.

THE THERAPEUTIC INDEX

The therapeutic index is a measure of a drug's safety. The therapeutic index, which is determined using laboratory animals, is defined as *the ratio of a drug's LD50 to its ED50.* (The *LD50* is the dose that is *lethal* to 50% of the animals treated.) A *large* therapeutic index indicates that a drug is relatively *safe.* Conversely, a *small* therapeutic index indicates that a drug is relatively *unsafe.*

The concept of therapeutic index is illustrated by the frequency distribution curves in Figure 6–8. Part A of the figure shows curves for therapeutic and lethal responses to drug X. Part B shows equivalent curves for drug Y. We can see in Figure 6–8A that the average lethal dose (100 mg) for drug X is much larger than the average therapeu-

tic dose (10 mg). Since this drug's lethal dose is much larger than its therapeutic dose, common sense tells us that the drug should be relatively safe. The safety of this drug is reflected in its large therapeutic index, which is 10. In contrast, drug Y is unsafe. As shown in Figure 6–8B, the average lethal dose for drug Y (20 mg) is only twice the average therapeutic dose (10 mg). Hence, for drug Y, a dose only twice the ED50 could be lethal to 50% of those treated. Clearly, drug Y is not safe. This lack of safety is reflected in its small therapeutic index.

The curves for drug Y illustrate a phenomenon that is even more important than the therapeutic index. As we can see, there is *overlap* between the curve for therapeutic effects and the curve for lethal effects. This overlap tells us that the high doses needed to produce therapeutic effects in some people may be large enough to cause death. The message here is that if a drug is to be truly safe, the highest dose required to produce therapeutic effects must be substantially lower than the lowest dose capable of causing death.

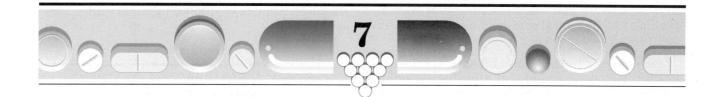
Drug Interactions

CONSEQUENCES OF DRUG INTERACTIONS
Intensification of Drug Effects
Reduction of Drug Effects

BASIC MECHANISMS OF DRUG INTERACTIONS
Direct Chemical or Physical Interaction
Pharmacokinetic Interaction
Pharmacodynamic Interaction

CLINICAL SIGNIFICANCE OF DRUG INTERACTIONS

The term *drug interactions* refers to the ability of one drug to alter the effects of another. Drug interactions may result whenever a patient takes two or more medications. Some drug interactions are beneficial; others are detrimental.

Our objective in this chapter is to establish an overview of drug interactions, emphasizing the basic mechanisms by which drugs interact. We will not attempt to catalogue and discuss the huge number of specific interactions that are known to occur. Information on the interactions of specific drugs can be found in the chapters in which those drugs are discussed.

CONSEQUENCES OF DRUG INTERACTIONS

In the most basic analysis, when drug A interacts with drug B, drug A can have one of two effects on the effects of drug B: drug A can either *intensify* the effects of drug B or drug A can *reduce* the effects of drug B.

INTENSIFICATION OF DRUG EFFECTS

When a patient is taking two medications, one drug may intensify the effects of the other. This type of interaction is often termed *potentiative* or *synergistic.* Potentiative interactions may be beneficial or detrimental. A potentiative interaction that enhances therapeutic effects is clearly beneficial. Conversely, a potentiative interaction that intensifies adverse responses is clearly detrimental. Examples of beneficial and detrimental potentiative interactions follow.

Increased Therapeutic Effects. The interaction between ampicillin and sulbactam is representative of beneficial potentiative interactions. When administered alone, ampicillin, an antibiotic, undergoes rapid inactivation by bacterial enzymes. By inhibiting those enzymes, sulbactam can prolong and intensify ampicillin's therapeutic effects.

Increased Adverse Effects. The interaction between aspirin and warfarin provides an example of a detrimental potentiative interaction. Warfarin, an anticoagulant, is used to suppress coagulation of blood. Unfortunately, if warfarin dosage is too high, the patient is at risk of spontaneous bleeding. Accordingly, for therapy to be safe and effective, the dosage must be high enough to suppress clot formation but not so high that spontaneous bleeding occurs. Like warfarin, aspirin also suppresses clot formation. As a result, if aspirin and warfarin are taken concurrently, the risk of spontaneous bleeding is significantly increased. Clearly, potentiative interactions such as this are undesirable.

REDUCTION OF DRUG EFFECTS

When two drugs are administered together, one drug may decrease the effects of the other. Interactions that result in reduced drug effects are often termed *inhibitory*. As with potentiative interactions, inhibitory interactions can be beneficial or detrimental. Inhibitory interactions that result in reduced toxicity are beneficial. Conversely, inhibitory interactions that result in reduced therapeutic effects are detrimental. Examples of these interactions follow.

Reduced Therapeutic Effects. The interaction between propranolol and terbutaline represents a detrimental inhibitory interaction. Terbutaline is taken by people with asthma to produce bronchial dilation. Propranolol, a drug used for cardiovascular disorders, can act in the lung to block the effects of terbutaline. Hence, if propranolol and terbutaline are taken together, propranolol will reduce terbutaline's therapeutic effects. Inhibitory actions such as this are clearly detrimental.

Reduced Adverse Effects. The use of naloxone to treat morphine overdosage is an excellent example of a beneficial inhibitory interaction. When administered in excessive dosage, morphine can produce coma and profound respiratory depression. Naloxone, a drug that blocks morphine's actions, can completely reverse all symptoms of tox-

icity. The benefits of such an inhibitory interaction are obvious.

BASIC MECHANISMS OF DRUG INTERACTIONS

Drugs can interact by way of three basic mechanisms: (1) direct chemical or physical interaction, (2) pharmacokinetic interaction, and (3) pharmacodynamic interaction.

DIRECT CHEMICAL OR PHYSICAL INTERACTION

Some drugs, because of their physical or chemical properties, can undergo direct interaction with other agents. Direct physical and chemical interactions usually render both drugs inactive.

Direct interactions occur most commonly when drugs are combined in intravenous (IV) solutions. Frequently, but not always, such interactions cause formation of a precipitate. If a precipitate appears when drugs are mixed together in an IV solution, that solution should be discarded. Remember, however, that direct drug interactions may not always leave visible evidence. Hence, simple inspection of the solution cannot be relied upon to reveal all direct interactions. Because drugs can interact in solution, you should adhere to the following rule when preparing an IV solution: *never combine two or more drugs in the same container unless it has been established that a direct interaction will not occur.*

The same kinds of interactions that can take place when drugs are mixed together in bottles can also occur when drugs come in contact with one another within the patient. However, since drugs are diluted in body water following administration, and since dilution decreases chemical interactions, direct interactions within the patient are much less likely than direct interactions within a bottle.

PHARMACOKINETIC INTERACTION

Drug interactions can affect all four of the basic pharmacokinetic processes. That is, when two drugs are taken together, one drug may alter the absorption, distribution, metabolism, or excretion of the other.

Altered Absorption

Drug absorption may be enhanced or reduced as a result of drug interactions. The impact of drug interactions on absorption can be of considerable clinical significance.

There are several mechanisms by which one drug can alter the absorption of another. (1) By elevating gastric pH, antacids can decrease the ionization of basic drugs present in the stomach, thereby increasing the ability of these agents to cross membranes and be absorbed. Antacids have the opposite effect on the absorption of weak acids. (2) Laxatives can reduce the absorption of other drugs by accelerating their passage through the intestine, which reduces the time available for absorption to occur. (3) In contrast to laxatives, drugs that depress peristalsis (e.g., morphine, atropine) prolong drug transit time in the intestine, thereby increasing the opportunity for absorption to occur. (4) Absorption of orally administered drugs can be reduced by drugs that induce vomiting. (5) Drugs that reduce regional blood flow can reduce absorption of other drugs from that region. For example, when epinephrine is injected together with a local anesthetic (as is often done), the epinephrine causes local vasoconstriction, thereby reducing regional blood flow and delaying absorption of the anesthetic.

Altered Distribution

There are two principal mechanisms by which one drug can alter the distribution of another: (1) competition for protein binding, and (2) alteration of extracellular pH. Of these two mechanisms, competition for protein binding is encountered most frequently.

Competition for Protein Binding. When two drugs have the ability to bind to the same sites on plasma albumin, coadministration of those drugs produces competition for binding. As a result, binding of one or both agents is reduced, causing plasma levels of free drug to rise. This increase in free drug intensifies drug effects, possibly to the point of toxicity. To prevent toxicity, the dosage of one or both drugs must be reduced.

The interaction between warfarin (an anticoagulant) and phenylbutazone (an aspirin-like drug) illustrates how one drug can intensify the effects of another through competition for protein binding. This interaction also provides a sobering example of the importance of considering drug interactions during multiple-drug therapy.

Let's consider a patient whose initial therapy consists of warfarin alone, in a dosage that is just sufficient to produce moderate anticoagulant effects. Under these conditions, about 99% of the warfarin in plasma is bound to albumin, leaving only 1% free to exert pharmacologic effects. Now let's see what happens when phenylbutazone is added to the regimen. Since phenylbutazone and warfarin both bind to albumin, these drugs will compete with each other for available binding sites. As a result, phenylbutazone will displace some of the bound warfarin. Let's assume that the amount of warfarin displaced is only 2% of the total bound. Although this amount may seem inconsequential, it isn't. Recall that only 1% of the warfarin in plasma was free prior to phenylbutazone administration. By displacing an additional 2%, phenylbutazone will raise the level of free warfarin to a total of 3%—a 200% increase in the level of free drug. This increase in free warfarin may be sufficient to change the pa-

tient's status from one of moderate suppression of coagulation to one of spontaneous hemorrhage. Put another way, as a result of competition between drugs for protein binding, the patient may end up bleeding to death. The nurse who is aware of the potential for this kind of interaction can take steps to prevent it.

Alteration of Extracellular pH. Because of the pH-partitioning effect (see Chapter 5), a drug with the ability to change extracellular pH can alter the distribution of other drugs. For example, if a drug were to increase extracellular pH, that drug would increase the ionization of acidic drugs present in extracellular fluids (i.e., plasma and interstitial fluid). As a result, acidic drugs would be drawn from within cells (where the pH was below that of the extracellular fluid) into the extracellular space. Hence, the alteration in pH would change drug distribution.

The ability of drugs to alter pH and thereby alter the distribution of other drugs can be put to practical use in the management of poisoning. For example, symptoms of aspirin toxicity can be reduced with sodium bicarbonate, a drug that elevates extracellular pH. By increasing the pH outside cells, bicarbonate causes aspirin to move from intracellular sites into the interstitial fluid and plasma, thereby minimizing injury to cells.

Altered Metabolism

Drug metabolism may be increased or decreased as a result of interactions between drugs. As a rule, drugs that *increase* the metabolism of other drugs do so through *induction of liver enzymes*. Drugs that *decrease* the metabolism of other drugs usually do so by *competing for the same metabolic pathway*.

Induction of Drug-Metabolizing Enzymes. As discussed in Chapter 5, some drugs can act in the liver to induce synthesis of hepatic drug-metabolizing enzymes. Drugs that promote induction are referred to as *inducing agents*. The classic example of an inducing agent is phenobarbital, a member of the barbiturate family. Inducing agents can stimulate their own metabolism as well as that of other drugs.

Inducing agents can increase the rate of drug metabolism by as much as two- to threefold. This increase develops over a period of several days. Rates of metabolism return to normal about 1 week after the inducing agent has been withdrawn.

When an inducing agent is taken concurrently with other medicines, dosage of the other medicines may require adjustment. For example, if a woman taking oral contraceptives were to begin taking phenobarbital, induction of drug metabolism by phenobarbital could accelerate metabolism of the contraceptive to such an extent that protection against pregnancy would be lost. To maintain contraceptive efficacy, dosage of the contraceptive should be increased. Conversely, when a patient *discontinues* an inducing agent, dosage of other drugs may need to be *lowered*. If dosage is not reduced, drug levels may climb dangerously high as rates of hepatic metabolism decline to noninduced values.

Competition for Metabolism. One drug may decrease the rate of metabolism of another by competing with that drug for the same metabolic pathway. Although such interactions have been reported, it should be noted that the effects of these interactions are rarely large enough to be of clinical significance.

Treatment of methanol (wood alcohol) poisoning provides an interesting example of how competition between drugs for the same metabolic pathway can be therapeutically relevant. When a person consumes methanol, toxicity is not caused by the methanol itself. Rather, injury results from conversion of methanol into toxic metabolites (formaldehyde and formic acid). By administering ethanol, a drug that competes with methanol for the same metabolic pathway, formation of methanol's harmful metabolites is prevented.

Altered Renal Excretion

Drugs can alter all three phases of renal excretion (filtration, reabsorption, and secretion). By doing so, one drug can alter the renal excretion of another. Glomerular filtration can be decreased by drugs that reduce cardiac output: a reduction in cardiac output decreases renal blood flow, which in turn decreases glomerular filtration; the decrease in filtration results in delayed drug excretion. By altering urinary pH, one drug can alter the ionization of another, thereby increasing or decreasing the extent to which that drug undergoes passive tubular reabsorption. Lastly, competition between two drugs for active tubular secretion can decrease the renal excretion of both agents.

PHARMACODYNAMIC INTERACTION

By influencing pharmacodynamic processes, one drug can alter the effects of another. Pharmacodynamic interactions are of two basic types: (1) interactions in which the interacting drugs act at the *same* site, and (2) interactions in which the interacting drugs act at *separate* sites. Pharmacodynamic interactions may be potentiative or inhibitory, and are of great clinical significance.

Interactions at the Same Receptor

Interactions that occur at the same receptor are almost always *inhibitory*. Inhibition occurs when an antagonist drug blocks access of an agonist drug to its receptor. These agonist-antagonist interactions are described in Chapter 6. There are many agonist-antagonist interactions of clinical importance. Some of these interactions result in reduced therapeutic effects and are therefore undesirable. Others result in reduced toxicity and are of obvious benefit. The interaction between naloxone and morphine noted above is an example of a beneficial inhibitory interaction: by blocking access of morphine to its receptors, naloxone can reverse all effects of morphine overdosage.

Interactions Resulting from Actions at Separate Sites

Even though two drugs have different mechanisms of action and act at separate sites, if both drugs influence the same physiologic process, then one drug can alter responses produced by the other. Interactions resulting from effects produced at different sites may be potentiative or inhibitory.

The interaction between morphine and diazepam [Valium] illustrates a potentiative interaction resulting from concurrent use of drugs that act at separate sites. Morphine and diazepam are central nervous system (CNS) depressants, but these drugs do not share the same mechanism of action. Hence, when these agents are administered together, the ability of each drug to depress CNS function reinforces the depressant effects of the other. This potentiative interaction can result in profound CNS depression.

The interaction between two diuretics—hydrochlorothiazide and spironolactone—illustrates how the effects of a drug acting at one site can counteract the effects of a second drug acting at a different site. Hydrochlorothiazide acts on the distal convoluted tubule of the nephron to *increase* excretion of potassium. Acting at a different site in the kidney, spironolactone works to *decrease* renal excretion of potassium. Consequently, when these two drugs are administered together, the potassium-sparing effects of spironolactone tend to balance the potassium-wasting effects of hydrochlorothiazide, leaving renal potassium excretion at about the same level it would have been had no drugs been given at all.

CLINICAL SIGNIFICANCE OF DRUG INTERACTIONS

From the foregoing discussion it should be clear that drug interactions have the potential to significantly affect the outcome of therapy. As a result of interactions between drugs, the intensity of drug responses may be increased or reduced. Interactions that increase therapeutic effects or reduce toxicity are desirable. In contrast, interactions that reduce therapeutic effects or increase toxicity are detrimental.

Common sense tells us that the risk of a serious drug interaction is proportional to the number of drugs that a patient is taking. That is, the more drugs the patient receives, the greater the risk of a detrimental interaction. Since the average hospitalized patient receives 6 to 10 drugs, interactions are common. Accordingly, you should always be alert for detrimental interactions.

Although a large number of drug interactions have been documented, there is no doubt that many interactions are yet to be discovered. Therefore, if a patient develops unusual symptoms, it is wise to suspect that a drug interaction may be the cause—especially since yet another drug might be given to control the new symptoms.

It is important that steps be taken to minimize adverse interactions. The most obvious step is to minimize the number of drugs a patient receives. Indiscriminate use of multiple-drug therapy does not constitute good treatment, and increases the risk of undesired interactions. A second and equally important means of avoiding detrimental interactions is to take a thorough medical history. A medical history that identifies all of the drugs that a patient is taking will allow the physician to adjust the regimen accordingly. Please note, however, that patients who are taking illicit drugs or over-the-counter preparations may fail to report such drug use. You should be aware of this possibility and should make a special effort to insure that the patient's drug-use profile is complete.

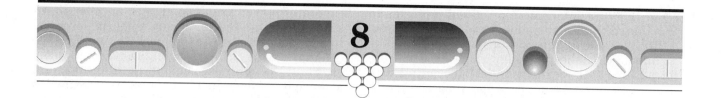

Adverse Drug Reactions

An adverse drug reaction is broadly defined as any undesired response to a drug. Adverse reactions can range in intensity from annoying to life-threatening.

Recall that *safety* is one of the most important characteristics of an ideal drug. A safe drug would be one that lacks the ability to produce severe adverse effects. There is no such thing as a safe drug: severe adverse reactions can occur with *all* medications. Fortunately, when drugs are chosen and used properly, many adverse reactions can be avoided, or at least kept to a low intensity. By understanding adverse drug reactions, you will be better prepared to help minimize undesired effects.

SCOPE OF THE PROBLEM

Drugs can produce many kinds of adverse reactions and in varying degrees of intensity. Among the more mild reactions are drowsiness, nausea, itching, and rash. Severe reactions include respiratory depression, neutropenia, anaphylaxis, and hemorrhage—all of which can result in death.

Although adverse reactions can occur in all patients, some individuals are more vulnerable than others. Neonates, the elderly, and the very sick are especially sensitive to the harmful effects of medications. In addition, patients taking several drugs are at greater risk than those taking only one drug.

Some data on adverse drug reactions will underscore the clinical significance of the problem. In the United States, the annual expense associated with adverse drug reactions may range as high as $3 billion. Of all hospital admissions, about 5% are for adverse reactions to drugs. Moreover, adverse drug reactions account for approximately 1 of 7 hospital days. A large fraction (10% to 20%) of hospitalized patients experience one or more adverse drug reactions during their stay. About 0.8% of hospitalized patients receive drug-induced injuries that are disabling. A significant number of drug-induced deaths occur annually.

DEFINITIONS

SIDE EFFECT

A side effect is formally defined as a *nearly unavoidable secondary drug effect produced at therapeutic doses.* Common examples include the drowsiness caused by antihistamines and the gastric irritation caused by low therapeutic doses of aspirin. Side effects are generally predictable, and their intensity is dose-dependent. Some side effects develop soon after the onset of drug use, whereas others may be delayed for weeks or months.

Although our formal definition of a side effect includes all undesired responses seen at therapeutic doses, in actual practice, *severe* drug effects are referred to as *toxicities*—even if these effects occur at therapeutic doses. For example, when administered in therapeutic doses, many anticancer drugs cause neutropenia (profound loss of neutrophilic white blood cells), thereby putting the patient at high risk of life-threatening infection. This neutropenia would be called a toxicity—not a side effect—even though it was produced when dosage was therapeutic.

TOXICITY

The formal definition of toxicity is *an adverse drug reaction caused by excessive dosing.* Examples include coma from overdosage with morphine and severe hypoglycemia from overdosage with insulin. Although the formal definition of toxicity includes only those severe reactions that occur when dosage is excessive, in everyday parlance the term *toxicity* has come to mean *any* severe adverse reaction, regardless of the dose by which it was produced.

ALLERGIC REACTION

An allergic reaction is an immune response. For an allergic reaction to occur, there must be prior sensitization of the immune system. Once the immune system has been sensitized to a drug, re-

exposure to that drug can trigger an allergic response. Allergic reactions can range in intensity from mild itching to severe rash to anaphylaxis. (Anaphylaxis is a life-threatening response characterized by bronchospasm, laryngeal edema, and a precipitous drop in blood pressure.) Estimates suggest that less than 10% of adverse drug reactions are of the allergic type.

The intensity of an allergic reaction is determined primarily by the degree of sensitization of the immune system. Hence, *the intensity of allergic reactions is largely independent of drug dosage.* Because the intensity of allergic reactions is not directly related to dosage, it is possible for a low dose to elicit a very strong allergic reaction in one patient while having little or no effect in another. Furthermore, since a patient's sensitivity to a drug can change over time, a dose that elicits a mild allergic reaction early in treatment may produce a more intense response as therapy progresses.

Very few medications cause severe allergic reactions. The drug family responsible for most serious reactions is the *penicillins*. Penicillin allergy is discussed in Chapter 74.

IDIOSYNCRATIC EFFECT

An idiosyncratic effect is defined as an *uncommon drug response resulting from a genetic predisposition.* Hence, susceptibility to a specific idiosyncratic reaction is determined by the patient's unique genetic makeup. To illustrate this concept, let's consider responses to succinylcholine, a drug used to produce flaccid paralysis of skeletal muscle. In most patients, paralysis from succinylcholine is brief, lasting only a few minutes. In contrast, genetically predisposed patients may become paralyzed for hours. Why the prolonged effect? In all patients, the effects of succinylcholine are terminated through enzymatic inactivation of the drug. Since most people have very high levels of the inactivating enzyme, paralysis is short-lived. However, in a small percentage of patients, the genes that code for succinylcholine-metabolizing enzymes are abnormal, producing enzymes that inactivate the drug very slowly. As a result, paralysis is greatly prolonged.

IATROGENIC DISEASE

The word *iatrogenic* is derived from *iatros*, the Greek word for physician, and from *-genic*, a combining form meaning *to produce*. Hence, an iatrogenic disease is *a disease produced by a physician.* The term iatrogenic disease is also used to denote *a disease produced by drugs.*

Iatrogenic diseases are nearly identical to idiopathic (naturally occurring) disease states. For example, when patients take glucocorticoids (e.g., cortisol) on a long-term basis, they frequently develop a syndrome whose symptoms are identical to those of Cushing's disease. Because this syndrome is (1) drug induced and (2) essentially identical to a naturally occurring pathology, we would call the syndrome an iatrogenic disease. Similarly, when patients take antipsychotic drugs, they can develop symptoms that resemble those of idiopathic Parkinson's disease. Accordingly, we would say that these parkinsonian symptoms represent an iatrogenic (drug-induced) disease.

PHYSICAL DEPENDENCE

Physical dependence develops during long-term use of certain drugs, such as opioids, barbiturates, and amphetamines. We can define physical dependence as a state in which the body has adapted to prolonged drug exposure in such a way that an abstinence syndrome will result if drug use is discontinued. The precise nature of the abstinence syndrome is determined by the drug upon which the individual is dependent.

Although physical dependence is usually associated with "narcotics" (heroin, morphine, other opioids), these are not the only dependence-inducing drugs. In addition to the opioids, a variety of other centrally acting drugs (e.g., ethanol, barbiturates, amphetamines) can promote dependence. Furthermore, some drugs that work outside the central nervous system (CNS) can cause physical dependence of a sort. Because a variety of drugs can cause physical dependence of one type or another, and because withdrawal reactions have the potential for harm, *patients should be warned against abrupt discontinuation of any medication without first consulting a knowledgeable health professional.*

CARCINOGENIC EFFECT

The term *carcinogenic effect* refers to the ability of certain medications and other chemicals to cause neoplastic diseases (cancers). Fortunately, although many carcinogenic chemicals exist, very few of our drugs are carcinogenic. Ironically, of those medicines that *can* cause cancer, several with the greatest carcinogenic potential are drugs used to *treat* neoplastic disease.

Evaluating drugs for their carcinogenic potential is extremely difficult. Evidence of neoplastic disease may not appear until 20 or more years after initial exposure to a cancer-causing compound. Consequently, it is unlikely that carcinogenic potential will be detected during preclinical and clinical trials of a new drug. Accordingly, when a new drug is released for general marketing, we cannot know with certainty that the drug will not eventually prove to be a carcinogen.

Experience with diethylstilbestrol (DES) illustrates the hazards posed by the delayed appearance of cancer following exposure to a carcinogenic drug. DES is a synthetic hormone with actions similar to those of estrogen. At one time, DES was used to prevent spontaneous abortion during high-risk pregnancies. It was not until years after DES had been used during pregnancy that the carcinogenic action of this drug became known: upon reaching maturity, a number of women who had been exposed to DES *in utero* developed vaginal and uterine cancers because of the drug.

TERATOGENIC EFFECT

A *teratogenic effect* can be defined as a drug-induced birth defect. Medicines and other chemicals capable of causing birth defects are called *teratogens*. Teratogenesis is discussed below.

ADVERSE REACTIONS ASSOCIATED WITH PREGNANCY

TYPES OF PREGNANCY-RELATED ADVERSE REACTIONS

Teratogenesis

The term *teratogenesis* is derived from *teras*, the Greek word for *monster*. Translated literally, *teratogenesis* means *to produce a monster*. Consistent with this derivation, we usually think of birth defects in terms of gross malformations, such as cleft palate, clubfoot, and hydrocephalus. However, birth defects are not limited to distortions of gross anatomy; birth defects also include behavioral and biochemical anomalies.

Because fetal sensitivity to teratogens changes during development, the response to a teratogen is highly dependent upon the timing of drug administration. *Gross malformations are most likely when exposure to a teratogen occurs during the first trimester.* Since the first trimester is the time during which the basic shape of internal organs and other structures is being established, it is not surprising that interference at this stage can result in conspicuous anatomic distortions. Because of fetal sensitivity to teratogens in the first trimester, expectant mothers must take special care to avoid exposure to teratogens during this period.

The types of birth defects that result from exposure to teratogens during the second and third trimesters differ from those caused during the first trimester. The second and third trimesters are the periods during which organ systems develop fine details of structure. As a result, exposure to teratogens during this time can injure the nervous system, endocrine system, immune system, and the developing teeth. Gross malformations are much less likely during late pregnancy than during the first trimester.

Physical Dependence

The pregnant woman who uses dependence-producing drugs (e.g., heroin, barbiturates, alcohol) can give birth to a drug-dependent infant. If the infant is not supplied with a drug that can support its dependence, an abstinence syndrome will ensue. Symptoms of withdrawal include shrill crying, vomiting, and extreme irritability. The physically dependent neonate should be weaned from dependence by giving progressively smaller doses of the drug on which it is dependent. Drug administration can cease when interruption of treatment fails to elicit signs of withdrawal.

Respiratory Depression

Certain pain relievers used during delivery can cause respiratory depression in the neonate. Newborn infants who were exposed to such drugs during delivery should be closely monitored until their respiration becomes normal.

REDUCING PREGNANCY-RELATED ADVERSE REACTIONS

The basic guideline for drug therapy of the pregnant woman is the same guideline applied to all other patients: the potential risks of treatment must be balanced by the expected benefits. Of course, when drugs are used during pregnancy, we must weigh the risks to the fetus as well as the risks to the expectant mother.

For many drugs, we lack conclusive data regarding their potential for fetal harm in humans. This lack of information complicates the task of balancing the risks of therapy versus the benefits. Why don't we know more about drug effects on the human fetus? The answer to this question is obvious: we cannot perform on pregnant women the types of drug studies that are done on animals. Hence, although the teratogenic effects of drugs on laboratory animals are generally understood, these effects have not and cannot be studied systematically in humans.

To facilitate decisions on drug therapy during pregnancy, the Food and Drug Administration (FDA) has established a system for classifying drugs according to their probable risks to the fetus. This classification scheme is summarized in Table 8–1. According to this scheme, drugs can be put into one of five categories: A, B, C, D, and X. Drugs in category A are the least dangerous: controlled studies have been done in pregnant women and have failed to demonstrate a risk of fetal harm. In

Table 8–1. FDA Pregnancy Categories	
Category	Category Description
A	*Remote Risk of Fetal Harm*: Controlled studies in women have been done and have failed to demonstrate a risk of fetal harm during the first trimester, and there is no evidence of risk in later trimesters.
B	*Slightly More Risk Than A*: Animal studies show no fetal risk, but controlled studies have not been done in women . . . *or* . . . animal studies do show a risk of fetal harm, but controlled studies in women have failed to demonstrate a risk during the first trimester, and there is no evidence of risk in later trimesters.
C	*Greater Risk Than B*: Animal studies show a risk of fetal harm, but no controlled studies have been done in women . . . *or* . . . no studies have been done in women or animals.
D	*Proven Risk of Fetal Harm*: Studies in women show proof of fetal damage, but the potential benefits of use during pregnancy may be acceptable despite the risks (e.g., treatment of life-threatening disease for which safer drugs are ineffective). A statement on risk will appear in the "WARNINGS" section of drug labeling.
X	*Proven Risk of Fetal Harm*: Studies in women or animals show definite risk of fetal abnormality . . . *or* . . . adverse reaction reports indicate evidence of fetal risk. The risks clearly outweigh any possible benefit. A statement on risk will appear in the "CONTRAINDICATIONS" section of drug labeling.

contrast, drugs in category X are the most dangerous; these drugs are known to cause human fetal harm, and their risk to the fetus outweighs any possible therapeutic benefit. Drugs in categories B, C, and D are progressively more dangerous than drugs in category A and less dangerous than drugs in category X.

Common sense tells us that the best way to reduce drug-induced fetal harm is to minimize drug use during pregnancy. If at all possible, pregnant women should avoid drugs entirely. At the least, all unnecessary drug use should be eliminated. Alcohol and cigarettes, for example, are known to harm the developing fetus (Table 8–2). These agents are completely unnecessary and there is no justification for their use by expectant mothers. Nurses and other health professionals should advise pregnant patients to avoid nonessential drugs.

Experience has shown that in some disease states failure to take medication may be worse for the fetus than taking the medication. Grand mal epilepsy is such a disease. If this form of epilepsy is left untreated, the risk to the fetus from maternal seizures is greater than the risk presented by anticonvulsant medication. However, even in dis-

Table 8–2. Selected Agents Known to Cause Fetal Harm	
Agent	**Type of Fetal Injury Produced**
Anticancer drugs	Many anomalies, including cranio-facial malformation, intrauterine growth retardation, mental retardation, abortion
Tobacco smoke	Intrauterine growth retardation, increased perinatal mortality, decreased fetal respiration
Ethanol	Intrauterine growth retardation, mental retardation, neonatal depression, other effects
Tetracycline	Inhibition of bone growth, staining of deciduous teeth
Testosterone	Masculinization of the female fetus
Diethylstilbestrol	Vaginal cancer
Lithium	Malformation of the heart
Thalidomide	Phocomelia and other gross malformations

orders like grand mal epilepsy, which require drug therapy to prevent disease-related fetal harm, we must still take steps to minimize fetal harm from the drugs. Accordingly, drugs that are known to cause fetal harm should be avoided and less toxic alternatives should be used in their place.

Rarely, a pregnant woman has a disease that requires treatment with drugs that have a high probability of causing severe fetal harm. Many anticancer drugs, for example, are highly toxic to the developing fetus (see Table 8–2), yet cannot be ethically withheld from the pregnant cancer patient. When such drugs must be used, termination of pregnancy should be considered.

ADVERSE REACTIONS ASSOCIATED WITH BREAST-FEEDING

Drugs taken by lactating women can be excreted in milk. Hence, breast-feeding is a potential source of drug exposure to the infant. If drug concentrations in milk are sufficiently high, toxicity to the nursing infant can result.

Although nearly all drugs can enter breast milk, the *extent* of entry depends on the specific drug. The factors that determine entry of a drug into breast milk are the same factors that determine drug passage across membranes. Accordingly, drugs that are lipid soluble will enter breast milk readily. Conversely, drugs that are ionized or highly polar will be excluded, as will drugs that are highly bound to plasma albumin.

For most drugs, the concentrations achieved in breast milk are too low to have significant effects on the nursing infant. Accordingly, it is usually safe for infants to breast-feed even though their

mothers are taking drugs. However, prudence is always in order: if the nursing mother can avoid taking drugs, she certainly should.

For some drugs, breast-feeding is absolutely contraindicated. Certain anticancer drugs, for example, accumulate in breast milk to levels that are toxic to the nursing infant. Other drugs that preclude breast-feeding include chloramphenicol (an antibiotic), lithium (used in manic-depressive illness), and certain radioactive pharmaceuticals.

ADVERSE REACTIONS FROM NEW DRUGS

As discussed in Chapter 4, preclinical and clinical trials of new drugs cannot detect all of the adverse reactions that a drug might be capable of causing. Consequently, when a new drug is released for general marketing, information regarding its adverse reactions is incomplete.

Because newly released drugs may have as yet unreported adverse effects, you should be alert for unusual responses when giving these agents. If the patient develops new symptoms, it is wise to suspect that the drug may be responsible—even if the symptoms are not described in the literature. If the drug is especially new, you may be the first clinician to have observed this particular effect.

When a drug is suspected of causing a previously unknown adverse effect, that effect should be reported to the FDA. It is only through voluntary reporting by alert clinicians that a drug's potential for harm can be made widely known. Accordingly, all suspected adverse effects should be reported, even if absolute proof of the drug's complicity has not been established. The form used for reporting adverse reactions is reproduced in Figure 8–1.

WAYS TO MINIMIZE ADVERSE DRUG REACTIONS

The responsibility for reducing adverse drug reactions lies with all persons associated with drug manufacture and use. The pharmaceutical industry must strive to produce the safest possible medicinal agents; the physician must select the least harmful medication for a particular patient; the nurse must evaluate patients for adverse drug reactions and must educate patients in ways to avoid or minimize them; and patients and their families must watch for signs that an adverse reaction may be developing, and should contact the physician if these signs appear.

Anticipation of adverse reactions can help minimize them. Both the nurse and the patient should know the major adverse reactions that a drug can

DEPARTMENT OF HEALTH AND HUMAN SERVICES PUBLIC HEALTH SERVICE FOOD AND DRUG ADMINISTRATION (HFN-730) ROCKVILLE, MD 20857 **ADVERSE REACTION REPORT** (Drugs and Biologics)	Form Approved: OMB No. 0910-0230.
	FDA CONTROL NO.
	ACCESSION NO.

I.   REACTION INFORMATION

1. PATIENT ID/INITIALS *(In Confidence)*	2. AGE YRS.	3. SEX	4.-6. REACTION ONSET	8.-12. CHECK ALL APPROPRIATE:
			MO. DA. YR.	

7. DESCRIBE REACTION(S)

☐ PATIENT DIED

☐ REACTION TREATED WITH Rx DRUG

☐ RESULTED IN, OR PROLONGED, INPATIENT HOSPITALIZATION

☐ RESULTED IN PERMANENT DISABILITY

13. RELEVANT TESTS/LABORATORY DATA

☐ NONE OF THE ABOVE

II.   SUSPECT DRUG(S) INFORMATION

14. SUSPECT DRUG(S) *(Give manufacturer and lot no. for vaccines/biologics)*

20. DID REACTION ABATE AFTER STOPPING DRUG?
☐ YES ☐ NO ☐ NA

15. DAILY DOSE | 16 ROUTE OF ADMINISTRATION

17. INDICATION(S) FOR USE

21. DID REACTION REAPPEAR AFTER REINTRODUCTION?

18. DATES OF ADMINISTRATION *(From/To)* | 19 DURATION OF ADMINISTRATION
☐ YES ☐ NO ☐ NA

III.   CONCOMITANT DRUGS AND HISTORY

22. CONCOMITANT DRUGS AND DATES OF ADMINISTRATION *(Exclude those used to treat reaction)*

23. OTHER RELEVANT HISTORY *(e.g. diagnoses, allergies, pregnancy with LMP, etc.)*

IV.   ONLY FOR REPORTS SUBMITTED BY MANUFACTURER | **V.   INITIAL REPORTER** *(In confidence)*

24. NAME AND ADDRESS OF MANUFACTURER *(Include Zip Code)* | 26.-26a. NAME AND ADDRESS OF REPORTER *(Include Zip Code)*

24a. IND/NDA. NO. FOR SUSPECT DRUG | 24b. MFR. CONTROL NO. | 26b. TELEPHONE NO. *(Include area code)*

24c. DATE RECEIVED BY MANUFACTURER | 24d. REPORT SOURCE *(Check all that apply)* ☐ FOREIGN ☐ STUDY ☐ LITERATURE ☐ HEALTH PROFESSIONAL ☐ CONSUMER | 26c. HAVE YOU ALSO REPORTED THIS REACTION TO THE MANUFACTURER? ☐ YES ☐ NO

25 15 DAY REPORT? ☐ YES ☐ NO | 25a. REPORT TYPE ☐ INITIAL ☐ FOLLOWUP | 26d. ARE YOU A HEALTH PROFESSIONAL? ☐ YES ☐ NO | Submission of a report does not necessarily constitute an admission that the drug caused the adverse reaction.

NOTE: Required of manufacturers by 21 CFR 314.80

FORM FDA 1639 (7 86)   PREVIOUS EDITION MAY BE USED

Figure 8–1. FDA adverse drug-reaction report form.

produce. This knowledge will allow early identification of adverse effects, thereby permitting timely implementation of measures to minimize harm.

Certain drugs are toxic to specific organs. When patients are using these drugs, function of the target organ should be monitored. The liver, kidneys, and bone marrow are important sites of drug toxicity. For drugs that are toxic to the liver, the patient should be monitored for signs and symptoms of liver damage (abdominal discomfort, jaundice, anorexia) and periodic tests of liver function should be performed. For drugs that are toxic to the kidneys, the patient should undergo routine urinalysis and measurement of serum creatinine content. In addition, periodic tests of creatinine clearance should be performed. For drugs that are toxic to the bone marrow, periodic blood cell counts are required.

Adverse effects can be reduced through individualization of therapy. When prescribing a drug for a particular patient, the physician must balance the risks of that drug versus its probable benefits. Drugs that are very likely to cause ill effects for a specific patient should obviously be avoided. For example, if a patient has a history of penicillin allergy, we can avoid a potentially severe reaction by withholding penicillin and administering a suitable substitute.

Lastly, we must be aware that patients being treated for chronic disorders are especially prone to developing adverse reactions. In this group are patients with hypertension, epilepsy, heart disease, and psychoses. When drugs must be used on a long-term basis, the patient should be informed about the adverse effects that may develop over time and should be monitored periodically for the their appearance.

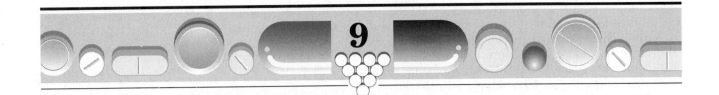

9

Sources of Individual Variation in Drug Responses

The issue of individual variation in drug responses has been a recurrent theme throughout the early chapters of this text. We have noted that because of individual variation, we must tailor drug therapy to each patient. In this chapter we will discuss the major factors that can cause one patient to react to drugs differently from another. With this information you will be better prepared to reduce individual variation in drug responses, thereby maximizing the benefits of treatment and reducing the potential for harm. In the process of discussing the sources of individual variation, we will review and integrate much of the information presented in previous chapters.

BODY WEIGHT AND COMPOSITION

In the absence of adjustments in dosage, body size can be a significant determinant of drug effects. Recall that the intensity of the response to a drug is determined in large part by the concentration of the drug at its sites of action—the higher the concentration the more intense the response will be. Common sense tells us that if a large person and a small person were given the same amount of the same drug, the drug would achieve a higher concentration in the small person and, therefore, would produce more intense effects. To compensate for this potential source of individual variation, dosage must be adapted to the size of the patient.

When adjusting dosage to account for size, the clinician may make the adjustment on the basis of *body surface area* rather than on the basis of body weight per se. The reason for this practice is that surface area determinations account not only for a patient's weight but also for how fat or lean he or she may be. Since percentage body fat can change drug distribution, and since altered distribution can change the concentration of a drug at its sites of action, dosage adjustments based on body surface area provide a more precise means of controlling drug responses than do adjustments made on the basis of weight alone.

AGE

Drug sensitivity varies with age. Infants are especially sensitive to drugs, as are the elderly. In the very young, heightened drug sensitivity is the result of organ system immaturity. In the elderly, heightened sensitivity is largely the result of progressive organ system degeneration. Other factors that affect drug sensitivity in the elderly are increased severity of illness, the presence of multiple pathologies, and treatment with multiple drugs. The clinical challenge created by heightened drug sensitivity in the very young and the elderly is discussed at length in Chapter 10 (Drug Therapy in Pediatric and Geriatric Patients).

PATHOPHYSIOLOGY

Abnormal physiology can alter responses to drugs. In this section we will examine the impact on drug responses produced by four pathophysiologic states: (1) kidney disease, (2) liver disease, (3) acid-base imbalance, and (4) altered electrolyte status.

KIDNEY DISEASE

In the patient with kidney disease, renal excretion of drugs can be reduced, causing them to accumulate in the body. If dosage is not lowered, drugs may accumulate to toxic levels. Consequently, if a patient is taking a drug whose elimination is dependent upon the kidneys, and if renal failure begins to develop, dosage must be de-

creased so that drug levels will remain within the therapeutic range.

The impact of renal disease on plasma drug levels is illustrated in Figure 9–1. The figure shows the decline in plasma levels of kanamycin (an antibiotic) following injection of the drug into two patients, one with healthy kidneys and one whose kidneys have failed. Elimination of kanamycin is exclusively renal. As shown in the figure, kanamycin levels fall off rapidly in the patient with good kidney function; the half-life of kanamycin in this patient is brief—only 1.5 hours. In contrast, drug levels decline very slowly in the patient with renal failure. Because of kidney disease, the half-life of kanamycin has increased by nearly 17-fold—from 1.5 hours to 25 hours. Under these conditions, if dosage is not reduced, kanamycin will quickly accumulate to toxic levels.

LIVER DISEASE

Like kidney disease, liver disease can cause drugs to accumulate. Recall that the liver is the major site of drug metabolism. Hence, if the liver ceases to function, rates of metabolism will fall and drug levels will climb. To prevent accumulation of drugs to toxic levels, patients with liver disease should be given their medication in reduced dosage. Of course, this guideline applies only to those drugs that are eliminated primarily by the liver. Liver dysfunction will not affect plasma levels of drugs that are eliminated largely by nonhepatic mechanisms (e.g., renal excretion).

ACID-BASE IMBALANCE

By altering pH partitioning (see Chapter 5), changes in acid-base status can alter the absorp-

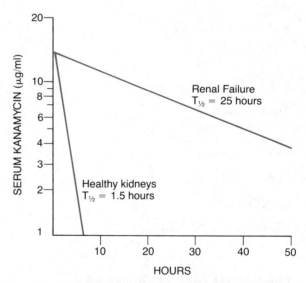

Figure 9–1. Effect of renal failure on kanamycin half-life. Kanamycin was administered at time "0" to two patients, one with healthy kidneys and one with renal failure. Note that drug levels decline very rapidly in the patient whose kidneys are healthy and extremely slowly in the patient whose kidneys have failed, indicating that renal failure greatly reduces the capacity to remove this drug from the body.

tion, distribution, metabolism, and excretion of drugs.

Figure 9–2 illustrates the impact of altered acid-base status on drug distribution. This figure summarizes the results of an experiment examining the effects of altered acid-base status on the distribution of phenobarbital (a weak acid). The experiment was performed in a dog. The upper curve shows plasma levels of phenobarbital. The lower curve indicates plasma pH. Acid-base status was altered by having the dog inhale a gas mixture rich in carbon dioxide (CO_2), a procedure that induces respiratory acidosis. In the figure, acidosis is indicated by the drop in plasma pH. Note that the decline in pH is associated with a parallel drop in plasma levels of phenobarbital. Upon discontinuation of CO_2 administration, plasma pH returned to normal and phenobarbital levels moved upward.

Why did acidosis alter plasma levels of phenobarbital? Recall that because of pH partitioning, if there is a difference in pH on two sides of a membrane, a drug will accumulate on the side where the pH most favors that drug's ionization—acidic drugs will accumulate in relatively alkaline media, whereas basic drugs will accumulate in relatively acidic media. Since phenobarbital is a weak acid, it tends to accumulate in alkaline environments. Accordingly, when the dog inhaled CO_2, causing extracellular pH to decline, phenobarbital left the plasma and entered cells, where the environment was less acidic (more alkaline) than that of the plasma. When CO_2 administration ceased, and plasma pH returned to normal, the pH-partitioning effect caused phenobarbital to leave cells and re-enter the blood; hence, the increase in plasma drug levels seen after CO_2 withdrawal.

ALTERED ELECTROLYTE STATUS

Electrolytes (e.g., potassium, sodium, calcium, magnesium) have important roles in cell physiology. Consequently, when electrolyte levels become disturbed, multiple cellular processes can be disrupted. Excitable tissues (nerves and muscles) are especially sensitive to alterations in electrolyte status. Given that disturbances in electrolyte balance can have widespread effects on cell physiology, one might expect that electrolyte imbalances

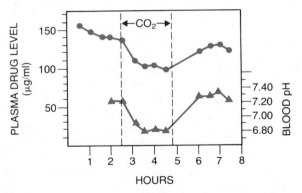

Figure 9–2. Altered drug distribution in response to altered plasma pH. *Lower curve,* Plasma (extracellular) pH. Note the decline in pH in response to inhalation of CO_2. *Upper curve,* Plasma levels of phenobarbital. Note the decline in plasma drug levels during the period of extracellular acidosis. This decline resulted from the redistribution of phenobarbital into cells. (See text for details.) (Redrawn from Waddell, W.J. and Butler, T.C. The distribution and excretion of phenobarbital. J. Clin. Invest. 36:1217, 1957, by copyright permission of the American Society for Clinical Investigation.)

would have a profound and widespread influence on responses to drugs. However, this does not seem to be the case; although disruption of electrolyte balance can change drug responses, examples of significant change are rare.

Perhaps the most important example of an altered drug effect occurring in response to electrolyte imbalance involves digoxin, a drug used to treat heart disease. The most serious toxicity of digoxin is the production of potentially fatal cardiac dysrhythmias. The tendency of digoxin to disturb cardiac rhythm is related to levels of potassium: when potassium levels are depressed, the ability of digoxin to induce dysrhythmias is greatly increased. Accordingly, all patients receiving digoxin must undergo regular measurement of serum potassium content to insure that levels remain within a safe range. Digoxin toxicity and its relationship to potassium levels are discussed at length in Chapter 42.

TOLERANCE

Tolerance can be defined as *decreased responsiveness to a drug as a result of repeated administration.* Patients who are tolerant to a drug require higher doses to produce the same effects that could be achieved with smaller doses before the tolerance developed. There are three categories of drug tolerance: (1) pharmacodynamic tolerance, (2) metabolic tolerance, and (3) tachyphylaxis.

PHARMACODYNAMIC TOLERANCE

The term *pharmacodynamic tolerance* refers to the familiar type of tolerance associated with long-term administration of drugs such as morphine and heroin. The person who is pharmacodynamically tolerant requires increased drug levels to produce effects that could formerly be elicited at lower concentrations of drug. Put another way, in the presence of pharmacodynamic tolerance, the minimum effective concentration (MEC) of a drug is abnormally high. Although the molecular mechanisms for pharmacodynamic tolerance are not fully understood, this form of tolerance is believed to result from an adaptive process occurring in response to chronic receptor stimulation.

METABOLIC TOLERANCE

Metabolic tolerance is defined as tolerance resulting from accelerated drug metabolism. This form of tolerance is brought about by the ability of certain drugs (e.g., barbiturates) to induce synthesis of hepatic drug-metabolizing enzymes, thereby causing rates of drug metabolism to increase. Because of increased metabolism, dosage must be increased to maintain drug effects. Unlike pharmacodynamic tolerance, which causes the MEC to increase, metabolic tolerance does not influence the level of drug required to elicit a response: in the person with metabolic tolerance, dosage is increased so that plasma drug levels can be maintained at pretolerance levels; the increase in dosage is not employed to produce drug levels that are above normal.

The experiment summarized in Table 9–1 demonstrates the development of metabolic tolerance in response to repeated administration of pentobarbital, a central nervous system (CNS) depressant. The experiment used two groups of rabbits, a control group and an experimental group. Rabbits in the experimental group were pretreated with pentobarbital for 3 days (60 mg/kg/day, SC) and then given an IV challenging dose (30 mg/kg) of this same drug; drug effect (sleeping time) and plasma drug levels were then measured. The control rabbits received the challenging dose of pentobarbital but did not receive any pretreatment. As indicated in Table 9–1, the challenging dose of pentobarbital had less effect on the pretreated rabbits than on the control animals. Specifically, whereas the control rabbits slept for an average of 67 minutes, the average sleeping time for the pretreated animals was only 30 minutes, an effect less than half that produced in the controls.

Why was pentobarbital less effective in the pretreated animals? The data on the plasma half-life of pentobarbital suggest an answer. As shown in the table, the half-life of pentobarbital was much shorter in the experimental animals than in the control group. Since elimination of pentobarbital is dependent primarily on metabolic conversion, the reduced half-life seen in the experimental animals indicates accelerated metabolism. This increase in metabolism, which was brought on by pentobarbital pretreatment, explains why the experimental rabbits were more tolerant to pentobarbital than were the control animals.

You might ask, "How do we know that the experimental rabbits had not developed *pharmacodynamic* tolerance?" The absence of pharmacodynamic tolerance is indicated by the plasma drug levels measured at the time the rabbits awoke. In the pretreated rabbits, the waking drug levels were slightly below the waking drug levels in the control group. Had the experimental animals developed pharmacodynamic tolerance, they would have required an increase in drug concentration to maintain sleep; hence, if pharmacodynamic tolerance were present, drug levels would have been abnormally *high* at the time of awakening rather than reduced.

TACHYPHYLAXIS

Tachyphylaxis is a form of tolerance that can be defined as a reduction in drug responsiveness brought on by repeated dosing *over a short period of time*. Hence, unlike pharmacodynamic and metabolic tolerance, which take days or longer to develop, tachyphylaxis occurs quickly. Tachyphylaxis is *not* a common mechanism of drug tolerance.

A good example of tachyphylaxis is the rapid loss of efficacy of nitroglycerin (often within 24 hours) following transdermal administration. As discussed in Chapter 41, this loss of effect is ascribed to rapid depletion of a co-factor needed to allow nitroglycerin to act. When nitroglycerin is administered on an intermittent schedule, rather than continuously, the co-factor can be replenished and no loss of effect occurs.

PLACEBO EFFECT

A *placebo* is a preparation that is devoid of intrinsic pharmacologic activity. Any response that a patient may have to a placebo is based solely on the patient's psychologic reaction to the idea of taking a medication and not to any direct physiologic or biochemical action of the placebo itself. The primary use of the placebo is as a control preparation during the testing of new medications.

The *placebo effect* is defined as that component of a drug response that is caused by psychologic factors and not by the biochemical or physiologic properties that a medication may have. Although it is impossible to assess with precision the contribution that psychologic factors make to the overall response to any particular drug, it is probably correct to say that with practically all medications some fraction of the total response results from a placebo effect.

Although placebo effects are determined by psychologic factors and not physiologic ones, the presence of a placebo response does not imply that a patient's original pathology was "all in his or her head." Placebo responses are *real*. Not only are placebo responses real, they can be of great therapeutic significance. For example, there is little doubt that some fraction of the pain relief experienced by patients taking nitroglycerin for angina pectoris is due to placebo effects. The fact that relief of anginal pain may be due in part to placebo effects and not entirely to the pharmacologic properties of nitroglycerin does not make the pain relief less real or less beneficial.

Not all placebo responses are beneficial; placebo responses can be negative as well as positive. If a patient believes that a medication is going to be effective, then placebo responses are likely to help promote recovery. Conversely, if a patient is convinced that a particular medication is ineffective or perhaps even harmful, then placebo effects are likely to detract from his or her progress.

Because the placebo effect is dependent upon a patient's attitude toward his or her medicine, fostering a positive attitude can help promote beneficial effects. In this regard, it is desirable that all members of the health team present the patient with an optimistic (but realistic) assessment of the effects that therapy is likely to produce. It is also

Table 9–1. Development of Metabolic Tolerance as a Result of Repeated Pentobarbital Administration		
	Type of Pretreatment	
Results	*None*	*Pentobarbital*
Sleeping time (minutes)	67 ± 4	30 ± 7
Pentobarbital half-life in plasma (minutes)	79 ± 3	26 ± 2
Plasma level of pentobarbital upon awakening (μg/ml)	9.9 ± 1.4	7.9 ± 0.6

Data from Remmer, H. Drugs as activators of drug enzymes. *In* Brodie, B.B. and Erdos, E.G. (eds.) Metabolic Factors Controlling Duration of Drug Action, Proceedings of First International Pharmacological Meeting, Vol. 6. New York, Macmillan, 1962, p. 235.

important that members of the team be consistent with one another. The intensity of beneficial placebo responses may well be decreased if, for example, nurses on the day shift repeatedly reassure a patient about the likely benefits of his or her regimen, while nurses on the night shift express pessimism about those same drugs.

GENETICS

A patient's unique genetic makeup can lead to drug responses that are qualitatively and quantitatively different from those of the population at large. Unique drug responses based on genetic heritage are often referred to as *idiosyncratic effects* (see Chapter 8).

The most common mechanism by which genetic differences can modify drug responses is by altering drug metabolism: genetic variations can result in increased or decreased metabolism of certain drugs. Some people, for example, have a genetically determined insufficiency in their ability to metabolize succinylcholine (a muscle relaxant). Hence, if succinylcholine is administered to these individuals, muscle relaxation is prolonged. Other drugs whose rate of metabolism is genetically determined include isoniazid (a drug for tuberculosis) and tolbutamide (a drug for diabetes). If genetically determined abnormalities in rates of drug metabolism are not too great, they can be compensated for by adjustments in dosage. However, when the alteration in metabolic rate is extremely large (as is the case with succinylcholine), then the drug should not be administered.

Some genetically determined drug responses are based on factors other than altered rates of metabolism. For example, some individuals produce red blood cells that are deficient in an enzyme called glucose-6-phosphate dehydrogenase. This deficiency renders the individual susceptible to hemolysis (red blood cell destruction) if given certain drugs, including aspirin, sulfanilamide (an antibiotic), and primaquine (an antimalarial agent). About 10% of African American males and many Near Eastern and Mediterranean males are subject to this idiosyncratic reaction.

VARIABILITY IN ABSORPTION

Both the rate and extent of drug absorption can vary from one patient to another. These variations in absorption can contribute to individual variation in drug responses. Differences in manufacturing processes are a major source of variability in drug absorption, although absorption may be altered by other factors as well. Several causes of variable absorption have been addressed previously, primarily in Chapter 5 (Pharmacokinetics) and Chapter 7 (Drug Interactions). Accordingly, discussion of information considered earlier will be brief.

BIOAVAILABILITY

The term *bioavailability* refers to the ability of a drug to reach the systemic circulation from its site of administration. Different preparations of the same drug can vary in their bioavailability. As discussed in Chapter 5, such factors as tablet disintegration time, enteric coating, and sustained-release formulation can alter bioavailability. These differences in bioavailability can result in variable drug responses.

Differences in bioavailability are associated primarily with orally administered drugs; differences in bioavailability are rare with drugs administered parenterally. Fortunately, even with oral agents, when differences in bioavailability do exist between preparations of the same drug, those differences are usually so small that they have no clinical significance.

Differences in bioavailability have their greatest clinical impact when they exist for drugs that have a narrow therapeutic range. When the therapeutic range is narrow, a relatively small change in drug level can produce a significant change in the response: a small decline in drug level may cause therapeutic failure, whereas a small increase in drug level may cause toxicity. Under these conditions, differences in bioavailability can have a significant impact. Because drugs produced by different manufacturers can vary in bioavailability, it is strongly recommended that patients taking drugs that have a narrow therapeutic range never switch from one brand to another without first consulting their physician.

The experiment summarized in Figure 9–3 illustrates the extent to which bioavailability can vary between different preparations of the same drug. In this experiment, a volunteer was given four different preparations of digoxin, a drug that has a narrow therapeutic range and that is used to treat cardiac disorders. For each of the four digoxin preparations (A, B₁, B₂, and C), bioavailability was determined by measuring levels of digoxin in blood following ingestion of two 0.25-mg tablets. As Figure 9–3 indicates, levels of digoxin varied widely. Although the dosage of all four preparations was identical, digoxin levels achieved with preparation A were twice as high as those achieved with preparation B₁; preparations B₂ and C were absorbed so poorly that blood levels were barely measurable. These data offer a dramatic demonstration of the differences in bioavailability that can exist between different preparations of the same drug.

OTHER CAUSES OF VARIABLE ABSORPTION

Several factors in addition to bioavailability can alter drug absorption and thereby lead to individ-

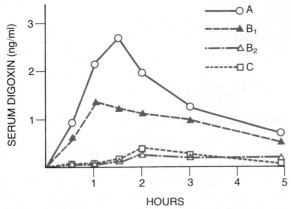

Figure 9–3. Variations in bioavailability among preparations of digoxin. On four separate occasions, the subject in this study was given two digoxin tablets (0.25 mg each) following an overnight fast. The tablets were from different sources (A, B$_1$, B$_2$, C). Blood levels of digoxin reveal clear differences in bioavailability among the different digoxin preparations. (See text for further details.) (Redrawn from Lindenbaum, J., Mellow, M.H., Blackstone, M.O., and Butler, V.P. Jr. Variation in biologic availability of digoxin from four preparations. N. Engl. J. Med. 285:1344, 1971.)

ual variations in drug responses. Alterations in gastric pH can affect absorption by altering the pH-partitioning effect. Prolongation of gastric emptying time can delay absorption of drugs that need to reach the intestine before they are absorbed. Diarrhea can reduce absorption by accelerating transport of drugs through the intestine. Conversely, constipation can enhance absorption by prolonging the time available for absorption to occur. The presence of food in the stomach tends to *delay* the absorption of most drugs. In some cases, food can decrease the *extent* of absorption as well. For example, absorption of tetracycline will be reduced substantially if this drug is ingested together with milk and other dairy products that contain calcium. Lastly, there are multiple mechanisms by which drug interactions can result in decreased or increased drug absorption (see Chapter 7).

FAILURE TO TAKE MEDICINE AS PRESCRIBED

Medications are not always administered as prescribed: dosage size and timing may be altered; doses may be omitted; and extra doses may be taken. Failure to administer medication as prescribed is a common explanation for variability in the response to a prescribed dose of a drug. As a rule, such failure results either from poor patient compliance or from medication errors made by hospital staff.

Patient compliance can be defined as cooperative and accurate participation in one's own drug ther-

apy. Multiple factors can influence compliance. These include manual dexterity, visual acuity, intellectual capacity, psychologic state, attitude toward drugs, and ability to pay for medication.

Patient education is an important means of promoting compliance. Instruction must be convincing and clear. In most cases, it is the responsibility of the nurse to provide this instruction. The nurse whose efforts at patient education succeed in promoting compliance will have contributed significantly to reducing variability in drug responses.

Medication errors are an obvious source of individual variation. Medication errors can originate with physicians, nurses, and pharmacists. However, since the nurse is usually the last member of the health team to check medications prior to administration, it is ultimately the nurse's responsibility to insure that medication errors are avoided.

DRUG INTERACTIONS

By definition, a drug interaction is a process in which one drug alters the effects of another. Drug interactions can be an important source of variability in drug responses. The mechanisms by which one drug can alter the effects of another and the clinical consequences of drug interactions are discussed at length in Chapter 7.

DIET

Diet can affect responses to drugs, primarily by affecting the patient's general health status. A diet that promotes good health will enable drugs to elicit therapeutic responses, and will increase the patient's capacity to tolerate adverse effects. Poor nutrition will have the opposite effect.

Starvation can have a significant impact on protein binding of drugs. Starvation causes plasma levels of albumin to fall. As a result, binding of drugs to albumin declines, levels of free drug rise, and drug responses become correspondingly more intense. For certain drugs (e.g., warfarin, an anticoagulant), the resultant increase in effects could be disastrous.

Although nutrition can affect drug responses by the general mechanisms noted, there are only a few examples of a specific nutritional factor affecting the response to a specific drug.

One important and well-documented illustration of the impact that diet can have on drug responses involves a drug family known as monoamine oxidase (MAO) inhibitors, medications used to treat depression. The principal adverse effect of these drugs is malignant hypertension, a reaction that can be triggered by foods that contain tyramine (a breakdown product of the amino acid tyrosine). Accordingly, patients taking MAO inhibitors must rigidly avoid all tyramine-rich foods (e.g., beef liver, ripe cheeses, yeast products, Chianti wine).

10

Drug Therapy in Pediatric and Geriatric Patients

The very young and the very old respond differently to drugs than the rest of the population. Most differences are *quantitative*. That is, patients in both age groups are more sensitive to drugs than other patients are, and they show greater individual variation. Drug sensitivity in the very young results largely from *organ system immaturity*. Drug sensitivity in the elderly results largely from *organ system degeneration*. Because of heightened drug sensitivity, patients in both age groups are at increased risk of adverse drug reactions. In this chapter we will discuss the physiologic and pathophysiologic factors that underlie heightened drug sensitivity in pediatric and geriatric patients, and will discuss ways to promote safe and effective drug use.

PEDIATRIC PATIENTS

Pediatrics covers all patients under the age of 16. Because of ongoing growth and development, pediatric patients of different ages present different therapeutic challenges. Traditionally, the pediatric population is subdivided into six groups: (1) premature infants (less than 36 weeks' gestational age), (2) full-term infants (36 to 40 weeks' gestational age), (3) neonates (first 4 postnatal weeks), (4) infants (weeks 5 to 52 postnatal), (5) children

(1 to 12 years), and (6) adolescents (12 to 16 years). Not surprisingly, as these patients grow older, they become more like adults with respect to drug therapy. Conversely, the very young—those less than 1 year old, and especially less than 1 month old—are very different from adults: because of the pharmacokinetic factors discussed below, neonates and infants are exquisitely sensitive to drugs. Our objectives in this section are to discuss (1) the pharmacokinetic factors that underlie drug sensitivity in the very young, (2) adverse drug reactions unique to pediatric patients, (3) dosage selection for young patients, and (4) ways to maximize benefits and minimize harm through promoting compliance with the prescribed regimen.

PHARMACOKINETICS: NEONATES AND INFANTS

As discussed in Chapter 5, pharmacokinetic factors determine the concentration of a drug at its sites of action and, hence, the intensity and duration of responses. If drug levels are elevated, responses will be more intense. If drug elimination is delayed, responses will be prolonged. Because the organ systems that regulate drug levels are not fully developed in the very young, these patients are at risk of both possibilities: drug effects that are unusually intense *and* prolonged. By accounting for pharmacokinetic differences in the very young, we can increase the chances that drug therapy will be both effective and safe.

Figure 10–1 illustrates how drug levels differ between infants and adults following administration of equivalent doses (i.e., doses adjusted for body weight). When a drug is administered *intravenously* (Fig. 10–1A), levels decline more slowly in the infant than in the adult. As a result, drug levels in the infant remain above the minimum effective concentration (MEC) longer than in the adult, thereby causing effects to be prolonged. When a drug is administered *subcutaneously* (Fig.

10–1B), not only do levels in the infant remain above the MEC *longer* than in the adult, these levels also rise *higher*, causing effects to be more intense as well as more prolonged. From these illustrations, it is clear that adjustment of dosage for infants on the basis of body size alone is not sufficient to achieve safe results.

If small body size is not the major reason for heightened drug sensitivity in infants, what is? The increased sensitivity of infants is due largely to the immature state of five pharmacokinetic processes: (1) drug absorption, (2) renal drug excretion, (3) hepatic drug metabolism, (4) protein binding of drugs, and (5) exclusion of drugs from the central nervous system (CNS) by the blood-brain barrier.

Absorption

Oral Administration. Gastrointestinal physiology in the infant is very different from that in the adult. Because of these differences, drug absorption may be enhanced or impeded, depending on the physicochemical properties of the drug involved.

Gastric emptying time is prolonged and irregular during early infancy, and gradually reaches adult values by 6 to 8 months. For drugs that are absorbed primarily from the stomach, delayed gastric emptying will enhance absorption. On the other hand, for drugs that are absorbed primarily from the intestine, absorption will be delayed. Because gastric emptying time is irregular, the precise impact on absorption is not predictable.

Gastric acidity is very low 24 hours after birth and does not reach adult values for 2 years. Because of low acidity, absorption of acid-labile drugs will be increased.

Intramuscular Administration. Drug absorption following IM injection in the *neonate* is *slow* and *erratic*. Delayed absorption is due in part to low blood flow through muscle during the first days of postnatal life. By early *infancy*, absorption

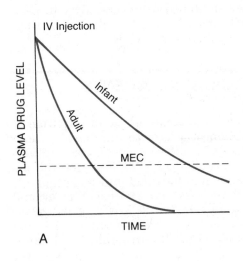

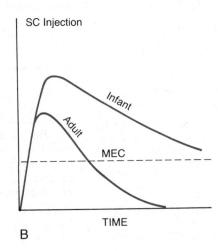

Figure 10–1. Comparison of plasma drug levels in adults and infants. *A*, Plasma drug levels following *intravenous* injection. Dosage was adjusted for body weight. Note that plasma levels remain above the minimum effective concentration (MEC) much longer in the infant. *B*, Plasma drug levels following *subcutaneous* injection. Dosage was adjusted for body weight. Note that both the maximum drug level as well as the duration of drug action are greater in the infant. (Redrawn from Levine, R.R. Pharmacology: Drug Actions and Reactions. Boston, Little, Brown, 1973.)

of IM drugs becomes *more rapid* than in neonates and adults.

Percutaneous Absorption. Because the skin of the very young is thin, percutaneous drug absorption is significantly greater than in older children and adults. This increases the risk of toxicity from topical drugs.

Distribution

Protein Binding. Binding of drugs to albumin and other plasma proteins is limited in the infant. This is because (1) the amount of albumin is relatively low, and because (2) endogenous compounds (e.g., fatty acids, bilirubin) compete with drugs for available binding sites. Consequently, drugs that ordinarily undergo extensive protein binding in adults undergo much less binding in infants. As a result, the concentration of *free* levels of such drugs is relatively high in the infant, thereby intensifying effects. To insure that effects are not too intense, dosages in infants should be reduced. Protein-binding capacity reaches adult values within 10 to 12 months.

Blood-Brain Barrier. The blood-brain barrier is not fully developed at birth. As a result, drugs and other chemicals have relatively easy access to the neonatal CNS, making the infant especially sensitive to drugs that can affect CNS function. Accordingly, all medicines employed for their CNS effects (e.g., morphine, phenobarbital) should be given in reduced dosage. Dosage should also be reduced for drugs used for actions *outside* the CNS if those drugs are capable of producing CNS toxicity as a side effect.

Hepatic Metabolism

The drug-metabolizing capacity of newborns is low. As a result, neonates are especially sensitive to drugs that are eliminated primarily by hepatic metabolism. When these drugs are used, dosages must be reduced. The capacity of the liver to metabolize many drugs increases rapidly about 1 month after birth, and approaches adult levels a few months later. Complete maturation of the liver develops by 1 year.

The minimal drug-metabolizing capacity of newborns is illustrated by the data in Table 10–1. These data are from experiments measuring the metabolism and the effect of hexobarbital (a CNS depressant) in newborn and adult animals. *Metabolism* was measured in microsomal enzyme preparations made from the livers of *guinea pigs*. The *effect* of hexobarbital—CNS depression—was assessed in *mice*. Duration of sleeping time following hexobarbital injection was used as the index of CNS depression.

As indicated in the table, the drug-metabolizing capacity of the adult liver is much greater than the drug-metabolizing capacity of the newborn liver: whereas the adult liver preparation metabolized an average of 33% of the hexobarbital presented to

Table 10–1. Comparison of the Metabolism and Effects of Hexobarbital in Adult versus Newborn Animals

Age	Percentage of Hexobarbital Metabolized (in 1 hour)	Duration of Drug-Induced Sleep 10 mg/kg Dose	50 mg/kg Dose
Newborn	"0"	6 hours	Eternal*
Adult	28 to 39	<5 minutes	12 to 22 minutes

Data from Jondorf, W.R., Maickel, R.P., and Brodie, B.B. Inability of newborn mice and guinea pigs to metabolize drugs. Biochem. Pharmacol. 1:352, 1958.
*The 50 mg/kg dose was lethal to newborn animals.

it, there was virtually no measurable metabolism performed by preparation made from newborn liver.

The overall consequence of the limited drug-metabolizing capacity of newborns is indicated by the effects of hexobarbital after injection. As shown in the table, a low dose (10 mg/kg) of hexobarbital caused adult mice to sleep less than 5 minutes. In contrast, the same dose caused newborns to sleep for 6 *hours*. The differential effects on adults and newborns are much more dramatic at a higher dose (50 mg/kg): whereas the adults merely slept for 20 minutes, this dose was *lethal* to the newborns.

Renal Excretion

Renal drug excretion is significantly reduced at birth. Renal blood flow, glomerular filtration, and active tubular secretion are all low during infancy. Because the drug-excreting capacity of infants is limited, drugs that are eliminated primarily by renal excretion must be given in reduced dosage. Adult levels of renal function are achieved by 1 year.

The relative inability of the infant kidney to excrete foreign compounds is illustrated by the data in Table 10–2. These data show rates of renal excretion for two compounds: inulin and

Table 10–2. Renal Function in Adults versus Infants

	Average Infant	Average Adult
Body Weight		
kilograms	3.5	70
Inulin Clearance		
ml/minute	3 (approximate)	130
T ½ (minutes)	630	120
Para-aminohippuric Acid (PAH) Clearance		
ml/minute	12 (approximate)	650
T ½ (minutes)	160	43

Adapted from Goldstein, A., Aronow, L., and Kalman, S.M. Principles of Drug Action: The Basis of Pharmacology, 2nd ed. New York, John Wiley & Sons, 1974. Copyright © 1974. Reprinted by permission of John Wiley & Sons, Inc.

para-aminohippuric acid (PAH). Inulin is excreted entirely by glomerular filtration. PAH is excreted by a combination of glomerular filtration and active tubular secretion. Note that the half-life for inulin is 630 minutes in infants but only 120 minutes in adults. Since inulin is eliminated by glomerular filtration alone, these data tell us that glomerular filtration in the infant is much slower than in the adult. From the data for clearance of PAH, taken together with the data for clearance of inulin, we can conclude that tubular secretion in infants is also much slower than in adults.

PHARMACOKINETICS: CHILDREN 1 YEAR AND OLDER

By the age of 1 year, most pharmacokinetic parameters are similar to those in adults. Hence, drug sensitivity in children over the age of 1 is more like that of adults than that of the very young. Although pharmacokinetically similar to adults, children do differ in one important way: they metabolize drugs *faster* than adults. Drug-metabolizing capacity is markedly elevated until the age of 2 years, and then gradually declines. A further sharp reduction takes place at puberty, when adult values are reached. Because of enhanced drug metabolism in children, an increase in dosage or a reduction in dosing interval may be needed for those drugs that are eliminated by hepatic metabolism.

ADVERSE DRUG REACTIONS

Like adults, pediatric patients are subject to adverse reactions when drug levels rise too high. In addition to these dose-related reactions, pediatric patients are vulnerable to unique adverse effects related to the immature state of organ systems and to ongoing growth and development. Among these age-related effects are growth suppression (caused by glucocorticoids), discoloration of developing teeth (caused by tetracyclines), and kernicterus (caused by sulfonamides). Table 10–3 presents a list of drugs that can cause unique adverse effects in the pediatric patient. Care should be taken to avoid these drugs in patients vulnerable to their actions. Adverse reactions that can affect the pediatric patient because of maternal drug use during pregnancy and lactation are discussed in Chapter 8.

DOSAGE

Because of the pharmacokinetic factors discussed above, dosage selection for pediatric patients is difficult. Dosing is a particular problem in the very young, since pharmacokinetic factors are undergoing rapid change.

Pediatric doses have been established for some drugs but not for others. For those drugs that do

Table 10–3. Adverse Drug Reactions Unique to Pediatric Patients

Drug	Adverse Effect
Androgens	Premature puberty in males; reduced adult height from premature epiphyseal closure
Aspirin and other salicylates	Severe intoxication from acute overdosage (acidosis, hyperthermia, respiratory depression); Reye's syndrome in children with chickenpox or influenza
Chloramphenicol	Gray syndrome (neonates and infants)
Glucocorticoids	Growth suppression with prolonged use
Hexachlorophene	CNS toxicity (infants)
Nalidixic acid	Cartilage erosion
Phenothiazines	Sudden infant death syndrome
Sulfonamides	Kernicterus (neonates)
Tetracyclines	Staining of developing teeth

not have an established pediatric dose, dosage can be extrapolated from adult doses. The method of conversion employed most commonly is based on body surface area:

$$\text{Approximate child's dose} = \frac{\text{Body surface area of the child}}{1.73 \text{ m}^2} \times \text{Adult dose}$$

Please note that initial pediatric doses—whether based on established pediatric doses or extrapolated from adult doses—are at best an *approximation*. Subsequent doses must be adjusted on the basis of clinical outcome, plasma drug concentrations, or both. These adjustments are especially important in neonates and younger infants. Clearly, if dosage adjustments are to be optimal, it is essential that we monitor the patient for therapeutic and adverse responses.

PROMOTING COMPLIANCE

Achieving accurate and timely dosing requires informed participation of the child's parents or guardian and, to the extent possible, active involvement of the child. Effective education is central. The following issues should be addressed:

1. Dosage size and timing
2. Route and technique of administration
3. Duration of treatment
4. Proper drug storage
5. The nature and time course of desired responses
6. The nature and time course of adverse responses

Written instructions should be provided. For techniques of administration that may be difficult to perform, a demonstration should be made, after which the parents should repeat the procedure to show their understanding. With young children, spills and spitting out are major causes of inaccurate dosing; parents should be taught to estimate the amount of drug lost to a spill or to spitting and to readminister that amount, being careful not to overcompensate. When more than one person is helping to medicate a child, all participants should be warned against multiple dosing. Multiple dosing can be avoided by maintaining a drug administration chart. With some disorders—especially infections—symptoms may resolve before the prescribed course of treatment has been completed. Parents should be instructed to complete the full treatment nonetheless. Additional ways to promote compliance include (1) selecting the most convenient dosage form and dosing schedule, (2) suggesting mixing oral drugs with food or juice (when allowed) to improve palatability, (3) providing a calibrated medicine spoon or syringe for measuring doses of liquid pediatric formulations, and (4) taking extra time with young or disadvantaged parents to help insure conscientious and skilled participation.

GERIATRIC PATIENTS

Drug use among the elderly is disproportionately high. Whereas the elderly (those over the age of 65) constitute only 12% of the United States population, they consume 31% of the nation's prescribed drugs. Reasons for this intensive use of drugs include increased severity of illness, the presence of multiple pathologies, and excessive prescribing.

Drug therapy in the elderly represents a special therapeutic challenge. As a rule, older patients are more sensitive to drugs than are younger adults, and they show wider individual variation in drug responses. In addition, the elderly experience more adverse drug reactions and drug-drug interactions. The principal factors underlying these complications of therapy are (1) altered pharmacokinetics (resulting from progressive organ system degeneration), (2) multiple and severe illnesses, (3) multiple drug therapy, and (4) poor compliance. To help insure that drug therapy is as safe and effective as possible, *individualization of treatment is essential: the patient must be monitored for desired and adverse responses, and the regimen must be adjusted accordingly.*

PHARMACOKINETIC CHANGES IN THE ELDERLY

The aging process can affect all phases of pharmacokinetics. From early adulthood on, there is a gradual, progressive decline in organ function. This decline can alter the absorption, distribution, metabolism, and excretion of drugs. As a rule, these pharmacokinetic changes result in increased drug sensitivity (largely from reduced hepatic and renal drug elimination). It should be noted, however, that the extent of change varies greatly among patients: pharmacokinetic changes may be minimal in patients who have remained physically fit, whereas they may be dramatic in patients who have aged less gracefully. Accordingly, the nurse should keep in mind that age-related changes in pharmacokinetics are not only a potential source of increased sensitivity to drugs, they are also a potential source of increased variability. Specific changes that occur with age are discussed below.

Absorption

Altered gastrointestinal absorption is not a major factor in drug sensitivity in the elderly. As a rule, the *percentage* of an oral dose that becomes absorbed does not change with age. However, the *rate* of absorption may be slowed (because of delayed gastric emptying and reduced gastrointestinal blood flow). As a result, drug responses may be somewhat delayed. Gastric acidity is reduced in the elderly and may alter the absorption of certain drugs. For example, some drug formulations require high acidity to dissolve. Absorption of these formulations may be reduced.

Distribution

Three primary factors can alter drug distribution in the elderly: (1) reduced concentration of serum albumin, (2) increased percent body fat, and (3) decreased percent lean body mass. Although albumin levels are only slightly reduced in healthy adults, these levels can be significantly reduced in adults who are malnourished. Because of reduced albumin levels, protein binding of drugs decreases, causing levels of free drug to rise. As a result, drug effects may be more intense. The increase in percent body fat seen in the elderly provides a storage depot for *lipid-soluble* drugs (e.g., thiopental). As a result, plasma levels of these drugs are reduced, causing a reduction in drug effects. Because of the decline in lean body mass, *water-soluble* drugs (e.g., ethanol) become distributed in a smaller volume than in younger adults. As a result, the concentration of these drugs is increased, causing their effects to be more intense.

Metabolism

Rates of hepatic drug metabolism tend to decline with age. Principal factors underlying the decline are (1) reduced hepatic blood flow, and (2) reduced liver size. Because liver function is diminished, the half-lives of certain drugs may be increased, thereby prolonging responses. Responses to oral drugs that ordinarily undergo extensive first-pass metabolism may be enhanced. It must be noted, however, that the degree of decline in drug metabolism varies greatly among individuals. As a result, we cannot predict whether drug responses will be altered in any particular patient.

Excretion

Renal drug excretion undergoes progressive decline from early adulthood on. The decline is the result of reductions in renal blood flow, glomerular filtration rate, and tubular secretion. Co-existence of renal pathology can further compromise kidney function. The degree of decline in renal function varies greatly among individuals. Accordingly, when patients are taking drugs that are eliminated primarily by the kidneys, renal function should be assessed. In the elderly, the proper index of renal function is *creatinine clearance*—not serum *creatinine levels*. Creatinine levels do not reflect kidney function in the elderly because the source of serum creatinine—lean muscle mass—declines in parallel with the decline in kidney function. As a result, creatinine levels may be normal even though renal function is greatly reduced.

PHARMACODYNAMIC CHANGES IN THE ELDERLY

Alterations in receptor properties may underlie altered sensitivity to some drugs. However, information on such pharmacodynamic changes is very limited. In support of the possibility of altered pharmacodynamics is the observation that beta-adrenergic blocking agents (drugs used for cardiac disorders) are *less* effective in the elderly than in younger adults when present at equivalent plasma concentrations. Possible explanations for this observation include (1) a reduction in the number of available beta receptors, and (2) a reduction in the affinity of beta receptors for beta-receptor blocking agents. Other drugs (certain CNS depressants, oral anticoagulants) produce effects that are *more* intense in the elderly than in younger adults when present at equivalent plasma concentrations, suggesting a possible increase in receptor number, receptor affinity, or both. Unfortunately, our knowledge of pharmacodynamic changes in the elderly is restricted to a few families of drugs.

ADVERSE DRUG REACTIONS

Adverse drug reactions (ADRs) are more common in the elderly than in younger adults, accounting for about 16% of hospital admissions among older individuals. The vast majority of these reactions are dose-related—not idiosyncratic. Perhaps surprisingly, the increase in ADRs seen in the elderly is not the direct result of aging per se. Rather, multiple factors predispose the older patient to ADRs. The most important of these factors are

1. Polypharmacy (treatment with multiple drugs)
2. Greater severity of illness
3. The presence of multiple pathologies
4. Altered pharmacokinetics and resulting increased individual variation
5. Greater use of drugs that have a low therapeutic index (e.g., digoxin, a drug for heart failure)
6. Inadequate supervision of long-term therapy
7. Poor patient compliance

The majority of ADRs in the elderly are avoidable. Measures that can can help reduce the incidence of ADRs include

1. Taking a thorough drug history, including over-the-counter medications
2. Accounting for the pharmacokinetic and pharmacodynamic changes that occur with aging
3. Initiating therapy with low doses
4. Monitoring clinical responses and plasma drug levels to provide a rational basis for dosage adjustment
5. Employing the simplest regimen possible
6. Monitoring for drug-drug interactions and iatrogenic illness
7. Periodically reviewing the need for continued drug therapy, and discontinuing medications as appropriate
8. Encouraging the patient to dispose of old medications
9. Taking steps to promote compliance (see below)

PROMOTING COMPLIANCE

As many as 40% or more of elderly patients fail to take their medicines as prescribed. This can result in therapeutic failure (from underdosing and erratic dosing) and toxicity (from overdosing). Underuse of drugs is by far (90%) the most common form of noncompliance.

Multiple factors underlie nonadherence to the prescribed regimen. Among these factors are forgetfulness, failure to comprehend instructions (because of intellectual, visual, or auditory impairment), inability to pay for medications, and use of complex regimens (several drugs taken several times a day). All of these factors can contribute to *unintentional* noncompliance. However, in the majority of cases (about 70%), noncompliance among the elderly is *intentional*. The principal reason given for intentional noncompliance is the patient's conviction that the drug was simply not needed in the dosage prescribed. Unpleasant side effects also contribute to intentional noncompliance.

A number of steps can be taken to promote adherence to the prescribed regimen. These include

1. Simplifying the regimen so that the number of drugs and doses per day is the smallest possible
2. Explaining the treatment plan using clear, concise verbal and written instructions
3. Choosing an appropriate dosage form (e.g., a liquid formulation if the patient has difficulty swallowing)
4. Labeling drug containers clearly, and avoiding containers that are difficult to open by patients with impaired dexterity (e.g., those with arthritis)
5. Suggesting the use of a calendar, diary, or pill counter to record drug administration
6. Asking the patient if he or she has access to a pharmacy and can afford the medication
7. Enlisting the aid of a friend, relative, or visiting health care professional
8. Monitoring for therapeutic responses, adverse reactions, and plasma drug levels

It must be noted that the benefits of these measures are restricted primarily to those patients whose nonadherence is *unintentional*. Unfortunately, these measures are generally inapplicable to the patient whose nonadherence is *intentional*. For these patients, intensive efforts at education may be beneficial.

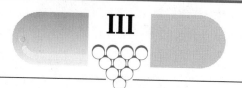

Peripheral Nervous System Drugs

Introduction

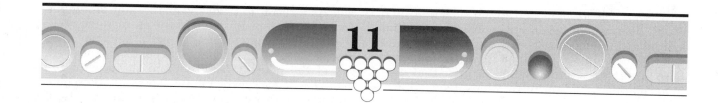

Basic Principles of Neuropharmacology

Neuropharmacology can be defined as *the study of drugs that alter processes controlled by the nervous system*. Neuropharmacologic drugs produce effects equivalent to those produced by excitation or suppression of neuronal activity. Neuropharmacologic agents can be divided into two broad categories: (1) peripheral nervous system drugs, and (2) central nervous system (CNS) drugs.

The neuropharmacologic drugs constitute a large and important family of therapeutic agents. These drugs are used to treat conditions that range from depression to epilepsy to hypertension to asthma. The clinical significance of neuropharmacologic agents is reflected in the fact that over 25% of the chapters in this text are dedicated to them.

Why do we have so many neuropharmacologic drugs? The answer can be found in a concept discussed in Chapter 6, namely, most therapeutic agents act by helping the body help itself. That is, most drugs produce their therapeutic effects by coaxing the body to perform its normal processes in a fashion that benefits the patient. Since the nervous system participates in the regulation of practically all bodily processes, practically all bodily processes can be influenced by drugs that alter neuronal regulation. By mimicking or blocking neuronal regulation, neuropharmacologic drugs can modify such diverse processes as skeletal muscle contraction, cardiac output, vascular tone, respiration, gastrointestinal function, uterine motility, glandular secretion, and functions unique to the CNS, such as pain perception, ideation, and mood. Given the broad spectrum of processes that neuropharmacologic drugs can alter, and given the potential benefits to be gained from manipulating those processes, it should be no surprise that neuropharmacologic drugs have widespread clinical applications.

We will begin our study of neuropharmacology by discussing peripheral nervous system drugs (Chapters 13 through 19), after which we will discuss central nervous system drugs (Chapters 20 through 34). The principal rationale for this order of presentation is that our understanding of peripheral nervous system pharmacology is much clearer than our understanding of central nervous system pharmacology. The reason for this discrepancy is that the peripheral nervous system is much less complex than the CNS, and also more accessible to experimentation. By placing our initial focus on the peripheral nervous system, we can establish a firm knowledge base in neuropharmacology before proceeding to the less definitive and vastly more complex realm of the CNS.

HOW NEURONS REGULATE PHYSIOLOGIC PROCESSES

As a rule, if we want to understand the effects of a drug on a particular physiologic process, we must first understand the process itself. Accordingly, if we wish to understand the impact of drugs on neuronal regulation of bodily function, we must first understand how neurons regulate bodily function when drugs are absent.

The primary steps in the process through which a neuron can elicit a response from another cell are illustrated in Figure 11–1. This figure depicts two cells: a neuron and a postsynaptic cell. The postsynaptic cell might be another neuron, a muscle cell, or a cell within a secretory gland. There are three basic steps in the process by which the neuron influences the behavior of the postsynaptic cell: (1) conduction of an action potential along the axon of the neuron, (2) release of neurotransmitter from the axon terminal, and (3) binding of transmitter molecules to receptors on the postsynaptic

cell. As a result of transmitter-receptor binding, a series of events is initiated in the postsynaptic cell, leading to a change in that cell's behavior. The precise nature of the change depends on the identity of the neurotransmitter and the type of cell involved. If the postsynaptic cell is another neuron, it may increase or decrease its firing rate; if the cell is within a muscle, it may contract or relax; and if the cell is glandular, it may increase or decrease its rate of secretion.

The three steps discussed above can be viewed as constituting two primary processes: *axonal conduction* and *synaptic transmission*. Axonal conduction is simply the process of conducting an action potential down the axon of the neuron. Synaptic transmission refers to steps 2 and 3 above—the steps by which information is carried across the gap between the neuron and the postsynaptic cell.

BASIC MECHANISMS BY WHICH NEUROPHARMACOLOGIC AGENTS ACT

SITES OF ACTION: AXONS VERSUS SYNAPSES

In order to influence a process under neuronal control, a drug can alter one of two basic neuronal activities: axonal conduction or synaptic transmission. *The vast majority of neuropharmacologic agents produce their effects by altering synaptic transmission;* axonal conduction is rarely a target for these drugs. Why do most neuropharmacologic agents act by altering synaptic transmission? Because drugs that affect this process can produce effects that are much more *selective* than those produced by drugs that alter axonal conduction.

Axonal Conduction

Drugs that act by altering axonal conduction are not very selective. Recall that the process of conducting an impulse along an axon is essentially the same in all neurons. As a consequence, a drug that alters axonal conduction can affect conduction in all nerves to which it has access. Such a drug cannot produce selective effects.

The *local anesthetics* and the *general anesthetics* are the only drugs whose therapeutic effects are the result of altered (decreased) axonal conduction. Since these agents produce nonselective inhibition of axonal conduction, they will suppress transmission in any nerve that they reach. Hence, although the anesthetics are certainly valuable, their indications are limited.

Synaptic Transmission

In contrast to drugs that alter axonal conduction, drugs that alter synaptic transmission can

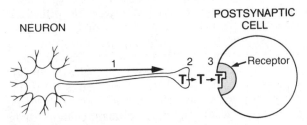

Figure 11–1. How neurons regulate other cells.
1. Action potential
2. Release of neurotransmitter (T) } Synaptic transmission
3. Interaction of T with receptor }

produce effects that are highly selective. These drugs can elicit selective responses because synapses, unlike axons, are not all the same. Synapses at different sites employ different transmitters. In addition, for many transmitters, the body employs more than one type of receptor. Hence, by using a drug that selectively influences a specific neurotransmitter or a specific type of receptor, we can alter one neuronally regulated process while leaving the majority of other neuronally regulated processes unaffected. Because of their ability to produce selective effects, drugs that act by altering synaptic transmission have numerous applications.

Receptors

The ability of a neuron to influence the behavior of another cell depends ultimately upon the ability of that neuron to alter receptor activity on the target cell. As discussed above, neurons alter receptor activity through release of transmitter molecules, which diffuse across the synaptic gap and bind to appropriate receptors on the postsynaptic cell. If the target cell lacked receptors for the type of transmitter that a particular neuron released, that neuron would have virtually no means by which to alter function in the target cell.

The effects of neuropharmacologic drugs, like those of neurons, are dependent on the production of altered receptor activity. That is, no matter what its precise mechanism of action, a neuropharmacologic drug ultimately produces its effects through influencing receptor activity on its target cells. Without altering receptor function, neuropharmacologic agents cannot produce effects. This common-sense concept is central to understanding the actions of neuropharmacologic drugs. In fact, this concept is so critical to our understanding of neuropharmacologic agents that I will repeat it: *The impact of a drug on a neuronally regulated process is dependent upon the ability of that drug to directly or indirectly influence receptor activity on target cells.*

STEPS IN SYNAPTIC TRANSMISSION

To understand how drugs alter receptor activity, we must first understand the steps by which synaptic transmission takes place, since it is by modifying these steps that neuropharmacologic drugs influence receptor function. The steps in synaptic transmission are summarized in Figure 11–2.

Step 1: Synthesis. For synaptic transmission to take place, molecules of transmitter must be present within the nerve terminal. Hence, we can look upon synthesis of transmitter as being the first step in transmission. In the figure, the letters Q, R, and S represent the precursor molecules from which the transmitter (T) is made.

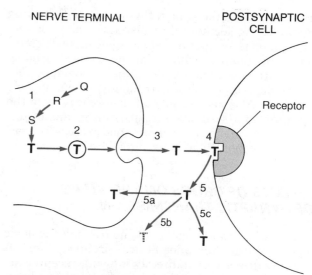

NERVE TERMINAL   POSTSYNAPTIC CELL

Figure 11–2. Steps in synaptic transmision. *Step 1,* Synthesis of transmitter (T) from precursor molecules (Q,R,S). *Step 2,* Storage of transmitter in vesicles. *Step 3,* Release of transmitter. In response to an action potential, vesicles fuse with the terminal membrane and discharge their contents into the synaptic gap. *Step 4,* Action at receptor. Transmitter binds (reversibly) to its receptor on the postsynaptic cell, causing a response in that cell. *Step 5,* Termination of transmission. Transmitter dissociates from its receptor and is then removed from the synaptic gap by *(a)* reuptake into the nerve terminal, *(b)* enzymatic degradation, or *(c)* diffusion away from the gap.

Step 2: Storage. Once transmitter is synthesized, it must be stored until the time of its release. Storage of transmitter molecules takes place within vesicles—tiny packets present in the axon terminal. Each nerve terminal contains a large number of transmitter-filled vesicles.

Step 3: Release. Release of transmitter is triggered by the arrival of an action potential at the axon terminal. The action potential initiates a process in which vesicles undergo fusion with the terminal membrane, causing release of vesicular contents into the synaptic gap. With each action potential, only a small fraction of all vesicles present in the axon terminal are caused to discharge their contents.

Step 4: Receptor Binding. Following their release, transmitter molecules diffuse across the synaptic gap and then undergo *reversible* binding to receptors on the postsynaptic cell. This binding initiates a series of events that result in altered behavior of the postsynaptic cell.

Step 5: Termination. Transmission is terminated by dissociation of transmitter from its receptors, followed by removal of free transmitter from the synaptic gap. Transmitter can be cleared from the synaptic gap by three processes: (1) reuptake, (2) enzymatic degradation, and (3) diffusion. In those synapses where transmission is terminated by reuptake, axon terminals contain "pumps" for the active transport of transmitter molecules back into the neuron (step 5a in Figure 11–2). Following reuptake, molecules of transmitter may be degraded, or they may be repackaged in vesicles for reuse. In synapses where transmitter is cleared by enzymatic degradation (step 5b), the synapse contains large quantities of transmitter-inactivating enzymes. Although simple diffusion away from the synaptic gap (step 5c) is a potential means of terminating transmitter action, this process is very slow and generally of little significance.

EFFECTS OF DRUGS ON THE STEPS OF SYNAPTIC TRANSMISSION

As stated previously, all neuropharmacologic agents (except for anesthetics) produce their effects by directly or indirectly altering receptor activity. We also noted that the way in which drugs alter receptor activity is by interfering with synaptic transmission. The reason that most neuropharmacologic drugs act by altering synaptic transmission (as opposed to axonal conduction) is that synaptic transmission, because of its multistepped nature, is a process that offers a number of opportunities for intervention with drugs. In this section, we will look at the specific ways in which drugs can alter the steps of synaptic transmission. By way of encouragement, although this information may appear complex, it isn't. In fact, most of it is self-evident.

Before discussing specific mechanisms by which drugs can alter receptor activity, we need to understand what drugs are capable of doing to receptors in general terms. From the broadest perspective, when a drug interacts with a receptor, that drug can do just one of two things: it can activate the receptor or it can prevent receptor activation. What do we mean by receptor activation? For our purposes, we can define *activation as an effect on receptor function equivalent to that produced by the natural neurotransmitter at a particular synapse.* Hence, a drug whose effects *mimic* the effects of a natural transmitter would be said to *increase* receptor activation. Conversely, a drug whose effects were equivalent to reducing the amount of natural transmitter available for receptor binding would be said to *decrease* receptor activation.

It should be noted that activation of a receptor does not necessarily mean that a physiologic process will go faster; receptor activation by drugs can also result in a process going slower. For example, a drug that mimicked the effects of acetylcholine at receptors on the heart would cause heart rate to slow down. Since the effect of this drug on receptor function mimicked that of the natural neurotransmitter, the drug would be said to *activate* acetylcholine receptors, despite the fact that this activation caused heart rate to decrease.

Having defined what we mean by receptor acti-

vation, we are now prepared to examine the impact on receptor activity that will be produced by drug-induced alterations in the steps of synaptic transmission. As we discussed, a drug can have one of two effects on a receptor: (1) increased activation or (2) decreased activation. Table 11–1 summarizes the mechanisms by which drugs, acting on the various steps of synaptic transmission, can increase or decrease the activation of receptors. As we consider these mechanisms one by one, their common-sense nature should become apparent.

Transmitter Synthesis. There are three different effects that drugs are known to have on transmitter synthesis. We can use drugs to (1) increase transmitter synthesis, (2) decrease transmitter synthesis, or (3) cause the synthesis of transmitter molecules that are more effective than the natural transmitter.

The impact of increased or decreased transmitter synthesis on receptor activity should be obvious. A drug that increases transmitter synthesis will cause receptor activation to be increased. That is, as a result of increased transmitter synthesis, storage vesicles will contain transmitter in abnormally high amounts. Hence, when an action potential reaches the axon terminal, more transmitter will be released and, therefore, more transmitter will be available to receptors on the postsynaptic cell, causing activation of those receptors to increase. Conversely, a drug that decreases transmitter synthesis will cause the transmitter content of vesicles to decline, resulting in reduced transmitter release and decreased activation of receptors.

Some drugs can cause neurons to synthesize

Table 11–1. Effects of Drugs on Synaptic Transmission and the Resulting Impact on Receptor Activation

Step of Junctional Transmission	Drug Action	Impact on Receptor Activation*
Synthesis of transmitter	Increased synthesis of T	Increase
	Decreased synthesis of T	Decrease
	Synthesis of "super" T	Increase
Storage of transmitter	Reduced storage of T	Decrease
Release of transmitter	Promotion of T release	Increase
	Inhibition of T release	Decrease
Binding to receptor	Direct receptor stimulation	Increase
	Blockade of T binding	Decrease
Termination of transmission	Blockade of T reuptake	Increase
	Prevention of T breakdown	Increase

*Receptor activation is defined as production of an effect equivalent to that produced by the natural transmitter that acts on a particular receptor. T = transmitter.

transmitter molecules whose structure is different from that of normal transmitter molecules. Drugs can, for example, cause enzymes present in the axon terminal to make "super" transmitters (molecules whose ability to activate receptors is greater than that of the naturally occurring transmitter at a particular site). Release of these super transmitters will obviously cause receptor activation to increase. In theory, it should be possible to cause the synthesis of *faulty* transmitter molecules (i.e., molecules with a reduced ability to activate a particular receptor). However, we have no drugs that are known to act by this mechanism.

Transmitter Storage. Drugs that interfere with transmitter storage will cause receptor activation to decrease. This is because disruption of storage depletes vesicles of their transmitter content, thereby decreasing the amount of transmitter available for release.

Transmitter Release. Drugs can have one of two effects on transmitter release: they can *promote* release or they can *inhibit* release. Drugs that promote release will increase receptor activation. Conversely, drugs that inhibit release will cause receptor activation to decrease. The amphetamines (CNS stimulants) are examples of drugs that act by promoting transmitter release. Botulinus toxin, in contrast, acts by inhibiting transmitter release. (Botulinus toxin blocks release of acetylcholine from the nerves that control movement of skeletal muscles, including the muscles of respiration. The potential for disaster is obvious.)

Receptor Binding. Many neuropharmacologic drugs act directly at receptors. Drugs in this category can act in one of two ways: (1) they can bind to receptors and cause receptor activation, or (2) they can bind to receptors and thereby prevent receptor activation by other agents. In the terminology introduced in Chapter 6, drugs that directly activate receptors would be called *agonists,* whereas drugs that prevent receptor activation would be called *antagonists.* The receptor agonists and antagonists constitute the largest and most important groups of neuropharmacologic drugs.

Examples of drugs that act directly at receptors are numerous. Drugs that bind to receptors and cause *activation* include morphine (used for its effects on the CNS), epinephrine (used mainly for its effects on the cardiovascular system), and bethanechol (used for its effects on the gastrointestinal system). Drugs that bind to receptors and *prevent* their activation include naloxone (used to treat overdosage with morphine-like drugs), succinylcholine (used to relax skeletal muscles), and haloperidol (used to treat schizophrenia).

Termination of Transmitter Action. Drugs can interfere with the termination of transmitter action by two mechanisms: (1) blockade of trans-

mitter reuptake, and (2) inhibition of transmitter degradation. Drugs that act by either mechanism will cause the concentration of transmitter in the synaptic gap to rise, thereby causing receptor activation to increase.

MULTIPLE RECEPTOR TYPES AND SELECTIVITY OF DRUG ACTION

As we discussed in Chapter 1, selectivity is one of the most desirable qualities a drug can have, since a selective drug is able to alter a disease process while leaving other physiologic processes largely unaffected.

Many neuropharmacologic agents display a high degree of selectivity. This selectivity is possible because the nervous system works through multiple types of receptors to regulate the organs under its control. If neurons had only one or two types of receptors through which to act, selective effects by neuropharmacologic drugs could not be achieved.

The relationship between multiple receptor types and selective drug actions is illustrated by the somewhat whimsical characters in Figure 11-3. Let's begin by considering critter 1. This critter can perform four functions: he can pump blood, digest food, shake hands, and empty his bladder. As indicated in the figure, all four functions are under neuronal control, and, in all cases, that control is exerted by activation of the same type of receptor (designated A).

As long as critter 1 remains healthy, the use of only one receptor type to regulate his various functions presents no problem. Selective *physiologic* regulation can be achieved simply by sending impulses down the appropriate nerves. When there is a need to increase cardiac output, impulses are sent down the nerve to the heart; when digestion is needed, impulses are sent down the nerve to the stomach; and so forth.

Although the use of only one receptor type is no disadvantage when all is well, if critter 1 gets sick, his use of only one receptor type creates a difficult therapeutic problem. Let's assume that this critter develops heart disease and that we need to give a drug that will help increase cardiac output. To stimulate cardiac function, we need to administer a drug that will activate receptors on his heart. Unfortunately, since the receptors on his heart are the same as the receptors on his other organs, a drug that stimulates cardiac function will stimulate all of his other organs as well. Consequently, any attempt to improve cardiac output with drugs will necessarily be accompanied by side effects. These effects will range from silly (compulsive handshaking) to embarrassing (enuresis) to hazardous (gastric ulcers). Such side effects are not likely to elicit either gratitude or compliance.

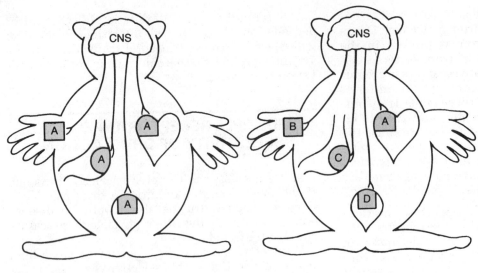

Figure 11-3. Multiple drug receptors and selective drug action. *Critter 1,* All organs are regulated through stimulation of type A receptors. Drugs that affect type A receptors on one organ will affect type A receptors on all other organs. Hence, selective drug action is impossible. *Critter 2,* This critter employs four types of receptors (A, B, C and D) to regulate his four organs. A drug that acts at one type of receptor will not affect the others. Hence, selective drug action can be achieved.

CRITTER 1

CRITTER 2

Please note that all of these undesirable effects are the direct result of the fact that this critter's nervous system works through only one type of receptor to regulate all of his organs. That is, the presence of only one receptor type has made selective drug action impossible.

Now let's consider critter 2. Although this critter might be the twin of critter 1, he differs in one important way: whereas all functions in critter 1 are regulated through just one type of receptor, critter 2 employs different receptors to control each of his four functions. Because of this simple but important difference, the selective drug action that was impossible with critter 1 can be achieved easily with critter 2. We can, for example, selectively enhance cardiac function in critter 2 without risking the side effects to which critter 1 was predisposed. This can be done simply by administering an agonist agent that binds selectively to receptors on the heart (type A receptors). If this medication is sufficiently selective for type A receptors, it will not interact with receptor types B, C, or D. Hence, function in structures regulated by those receptors will be unaffected. Note that our ability to produce selective drug action in critter 2 is made possible because his nervous system works through different types of receptors to regulate function in his different organs. The message from this example is: *the more types of receptors we have to work with, the greater our chances of producing selective drug effects.*

AN APPROACH TO LEARNING ABOUT PERIPHERAL NERVOUS SYSTEM DRUGS

As noted previously, to understand the ways in which drugs can alter a process under neuronal control, we must first understand how the nervous system itself regulates that process. Accordingly, when preparing to study peripheral nervous system pharmacology, we must first establish a working knowledge of the peripheral nervous system itself. In particular, we need to know two basic types of information about peripheral nervous system function. First, we need to know the types of receptors through which the peripheral nervous system works when influencing the function of a specific organ. Second, we need to know what the normal response to activation of those receptors is. All the pertinent information we will require regarding peripheral nervous system function is reviewed in Chapter 12.

Once we understand the peripheral nervous system itself, we can go on to learn about peripheral nervous system drugs. Although learning about these drugs will require significant effort, the learning process itself is remarkably straightforward. To understand any particular peripheral nervous system drug, we need to know three types of information: (1) the type (or types) of receptor through which the drug acts, (2) the normal response to activation of those receptors, and (3) what the drug in question does to receptor function (i.e., does the drug increase or decrease receptor activation). Armed with these three types of information, we can readily predict the major effects of any peripheral nervous system drug.

An example will serve to illustrate this learning process. Let's consider a drug named *isoproterenol* for our example. The first information we need is the identity of the receptors at which isoproterenol acts. Isoproterenol acts at two types of receptors, named beta$_1$ and beta$_2$. Next, we need to know the normal responses to activation of these receptors. The most prominent responses to activation of beta$_1$ receptors are *increased heart rate and increased force of cardiac contraction.* The primary responses to activation of beta$_2$ receptors are *bronchial dilation* and *elevation of glucose levels in blood*. Lastly, we need to know whether isoproterenol increases or decreases the activation of beta$_1$ and beta$_2$ receptors. At both types of receptor, isoproterenol causes *activation*. Armed with our three primary pieces of information about isoproterenol, we can now predict the principal effects of this drug. By *activating* beta$_1$ and beta$_2$ receptors, isoproterenol can elicit three major responses: (1) increased cardiac output (by increasing heart rate and force of contraction), (2) dilation of the bronchi, and (3) elevation of blood glucose levels. Depending on the patient to whom this drug is given, these responses may be beneficial or they may be detrimental.

Hopefully, the above example has communicated the ease with which we can predict the effects of a peripheral nervous system drug once we've mastered just three kinds of information. I strongly encourage you to take the approach suggested when studying peripheral nervous system agents. That is, for each peripheral nervous system drug, you should learn (1) the identity of the receptors at which that drug acts, (2) the normal responses to activation of those receptors, and (3) whether the drug increases or decreases receptor activation. With this information, you can predict most of the important effects of any peripheral nervous system drug.

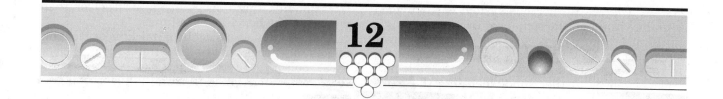

Physiology of the Peripheral Nervous System

To understand peripheral nervous system drugs, we must first understand the peripheral nervous system itself. The objective of this chapter is to provide that understanding.

It is not uncommon for students to be at least slightly apprehensive when approaching the study of the peripheral nervous system—especially the autonomic component. In fact, it is not uncommon for students who have studied this subject before to be thoroughly convinced that they will never, ever really understand it. This reaction is unfortunate in that although there is a lot to know about the peripheral nervous system, the information is not terribly difficult to grasp. In this chapter, information on the peripheral nervous system is presented in a fashion that differs from traditional methods of teaching this material. Hopefully, this new approach will facilitate learning.

Since our ultimate goal concerns pharmacology—and not physiology—we will not attempt to discuss everything there is to know about the peripheral nervous system. Rather, we will limit discussion to those aspects of peripheral nervous system physiology that have a direct bearing on our ability to understand drugs.

DIVISIONS OF THE NERVOUS SYSTEM

The nervous system has two main divisions, the *central nervous system* and the *peripheral nervous system*. The central nervous system is subdivided into the brain and the spinal cord.

The peripheral nervous system has two major subdivisions: (1) *the somatic motor system* and (2) the *autonomic nervous system*. The autonomic nervous system is further subdivided into the *parasympathetic nervous system* and the *sympathetic nervous system*. The somatic motor system controls movement of voluntary muscles, whereas the two subdivisions of the autonomic nervous system regulate many of the "involuntary" processes of the body.

The autonomic nervous system is the principal focus of this chapter. The somatic motor system is also considered, but discussion of it is limited.

OVERVIEW OF AUTONOMIC NERVOUS SYSTEM FUNCTIONS

The autonomic nervous system has three principal functions: (1) regulation of the heart, (2) regulation of secretory glands (salivary, gastric, sweat, and bronchial glands), and (3) regulation of smooth muscles (muscles of the bronchi, blood vessels, urogenital system, and gastrointestinal tract). These regulatory activities are shared between the sympathetic and parasympathetic divisions of the autonomic nervous system.

PRINCIPAL FUNCTIONS OF THE PARASYMPATHETIC NERVOUS SYSTEM

The parasympathetic nervous system performs seven regulatory functions that have particular relevance to the actions of peripheral nervous system drugs. Specifically, stimulation of appropriate parasympathetic nerves causes (1) slowing of heart rate, (2) increased gastric secretion, (3) emptying of the bladder, (4) emptying of the bowel, (5) focusing of the eye for near vision, (6) constriction of the pupil, and (7) contraction of bronchial smooth muscle. Just how the parasympathetic nervous system elicits these responses is discussed later under the heading *Functions of Cholinergic Receptor Subtypes*.

From the above we can see that the parasympathetic nervous system is concerned primarily with what might be called the "housekeeping" chores of the body (digestion of food and excretion of wastes). In addition, the system helps control vision and conserve energy (by reducing cardiac work).

As you might guess, therapeutic agents that work by altering parasympathetic nervous system function are used primarily for their effects on the gastrointestinal tract, the bladder, and the eye.

Occasionally, these drugs are also used for their effects on the heart and the lungs.

A variety of poisons act by mimicking or blocking effects of parasympathetic stimulation. Among these poisons are nerve gases, insecticides, and toxic compounds found in certain mushrooms and plants.

PRINCIPAL FUNCTIONS OF THE SYMPATHETIC NERVOUS SYSTEM

The main functions of the sympathetic nervous system are (1) regulation of the cardiovascular system, (2) regulation of body temperature, and (3) implementation of the "fight or flight" reaction.

The sympathetic nervous system exerts multiple influences on the heart and blood vessels. Stimulation of sympathetic nerves to the heart increases cardiac output. Stimulation of sympathetic nerves to arterioles and veins causes vasoconstriction. Release of epinephrine from the adrenal gland results in vasoconstriction in most vascular beds and vasodilation in certain others. By exerting its influence over blood vessels and the heart, the sympathetic nervous system can achieve three homeostatic objectives: (1) maintenance of blood flow to the brain, (2) redistribution of blood flow during exercise, and (3) compensation for blood loss (primarily by causing vasoconstriction).

The sympathetic nervous system helps regulate body temperature in three ways. (1) By regulating blood flow to the skin, sympathetic nerves can increase or decrease heat loss. By *dilating* surface vessels, sympathetic nerves increase blood flow to the skin and thereby accelerate heat loss. Conversely, *constriction* of cutaneous vessels conserves heat. (2) Sympathetic nerves to sweat glands promote secretion of sweat, thereby helping the body to cool. (3) By inducing piloerection (erection of hair), sympathetic nerves can increase heat conservation.

When we are faced with adversity, the sympathetic nervous system mobilizes various components of the body in preparation for fight or flight. The fight or flight response has several characteristic features. These are (1) increased heart rate and blood pressure, (2) shunting of blood away from the skin and viscera and into skeletal muscles, (3) dilation of the bronchi to improve oxygenation, (4) dilation of the pupils (perhaps to promote visual acuity), and (5) mobilization of stored energy, an action that provides glucose for the brain and fatty acids for muscle activity. The sensation of being "cold with fear" is brought on by the shunting of blood away from the skin. The phrase "wide-eyed with fear" may have pupillary dilation as its basis.

Many therapeutic agents produce their effects by altering functions under sympathetic control. These drugs are used primarily for their effects on the heart, vascular system, and lungs. Agents that alter cardiovascular function are used to treat hypertension, heart failure, angina pectoris, and other disorders. Drugs affecting the lungs are used primarily to treat asthma.

BASIC MECHANISMS BY WHICH THE AUTONOMIC NERVOUS SYSTEM REGULATES PHYSIOLOGIC PROCESSES

To understand how drugs influence processes under autonomic nervous system control, it is necessary to understand how the autonomic nervous system itself regulates those activities. The basic mechanisms by which the autonomic nervous system regulates physiologic processes are discussed below.

Patterns of Innervation and Control

Most structures under autonomic nervous system control are innervated by sympathetic nerves and parasympathetic nerves. The relative influence of the sympathetic nervous system versus that of the parasympathetic nervous system depends on the organ under consideration.

In many of the organs that receive *dual* innervation, the influence of sympathetic nerves *opposes* that of parasympathetic nerves. For example, whereas *sympathetic* nerves to the heart *increase* heart rate, *parasympathetic* nerves *slow* heart rate (Fig. 12–1).

In some organs that receive nerves from both divisions of the autonomic nervous system, the effects of sympathetic and parasympathetic nerves are *complementary*, rather than opposite. For example, in the male reproductive system, erection is regulated by parasympathetic nerves while sympathetic nerves control ejaculation; if attempts at reproduction are to succeed, cooperative interaction of both systems will be needed.

A few structures under autonomic control receive innervation from only one division of the system. The principal examples of such structures are the blood vessels, which are innervated exclusively by sympathetic nerves.

In summary, there are three basic patterns of autonomic innervation and regulation: (1) inner-

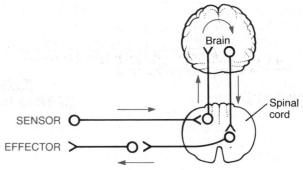

Figure 12–2. Feedback loop of the autonomic nervous system.

vation by *both* divisions of the autonomic nervous system in which the effects of the two divisions are *opposite*, (2) innervation by *both* divisions of the autonomic nervous system in which the effects of the two divisions are *complementary*, and (3) innervation and regulation by *only one* division of the autonomic nervous system.

Feedback Regulation

Feedback regulation is a process that allows a system to adjust itself by responding to incoming information. Practically all physiologic processes are regulated at least in part by feedback control.

Figure 12–2 depicts a feedback control loop typical of those used by the autonomic nervous system. The main elements of this system are (1) a *sensor*, (2) an *effector*, and (3) neurons connecting the sensor to the effector. The purpose of the sensor is to monitor the status of a process. Information picked up by the sensor is sent to the central nervous system (spinal cord and brain), where it is integrated with other relevant information. Signals (instructions for change) are then sent from the central nervous system along nerves of the autonomic nervous system to the effector. In response to the instructions it receives, the effector then produces appropriate adjustments in the process. The entire process of feedback regulation by the autonomic nervous system is termed a *reflex*.

From a pharmacologic perspective, the most important feedback loop of the autonomic nervous system is one that helps regulate *blood pressure*. This system is referred to as the *baroreceptor reflex*. (Baroreceptors are receptors that sense blood pressure.) You should be familiar with this feedback system because the reflexes that control blood pressure often oppose our attempts to modify blood pressure with drugs.

Feedback (reflex) control of blood pressure is achieved as follows: (1) Baroreceptors located in the carotid sinus and aortic arch monitor changes in blood pressure and send this information to the brain. (2) In response to alterations in blood pressure, the brain sends impulses along nerves of the

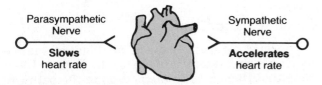

Figure 12–1. Opposing effects of parasympathetic and sympathetic nerves.

autonomic nervous system, instructing the heart and blood vessels to behave in such a way as to restore blood pressure to normalcy. Accordingly, when blood pressure *falls*, the baroreceptor reflex causes vasoconstriction and elevation of cardiac output so as to bring blood pressure back up. Conversely, when blood pressure *rises* too high, the baroreceptor reflex causes vasodilation and a reduction in cardiac output, thereby causing blood pressure to decline.

Autonomic Tone

The term *autonomic tone* refers to the steady, day-by-day influence exerted by the autonomic nervous system on a particular organ or organ system. Autonomic tone provides a basal level of control over which reflex regulation can be superimposed.

When an organ is innervated by both divisions of the autonomic nervous system, one division—either the sympathetic or the parasympathetic—provides most of the basal control, thereby obviating conflicting instructions. Recall that when an organ receives nerves from both divisions of the autonomic nervous system, it is common for those divisions to exert opposing influences. If both divisions were to send impulses simultaneously, the resultant conflicting instructions would interfere with productive function. By having only one division of the autonomic nervous system provide the basal control to an organ, this possible source of counterproductivity is avoided.

The branch of the autonomic nervous system that controls organ function most of the time is said to provide the *predominant tone* to that organ. *In most organs, the parasympathetic nervous system provides the predominant tone.* The *vascular system*, which is regulated almost exclusively by the *sympathetic* nervous system, is the principal exception to this general rule.

ANATOMIC CONSIDERATIONS

Although a great deal is known about the anatomy of the peripheral nervous system, very little of this information bears any meaningful relationship to our ability to understand peripheral nervous system drugs. The few details of peripheral nervous system anatomy that *do* pertain to pharmacology are summarized in Figure 12–3.

Parasympathetic Nervous System

Pharmacologically relevant aspects of parasympathetic anatomy are shown in Figure 12–3. Note that there are *two* neurons in the pathway leading from the spinal cord to the organs innervated by parasympathetic nerves. The junction (synapse) between these two neurons occurs within a structure called a *ganglion*. (A ganglion is simply a lump created by a group of nerve cell bodies.) Not surprisingly, the neurons that go from the spinal cord to the parasympathetic ganglia are called *preganglionic neurons*, whereas the neurons that go from the ganglia to effector organs are known as *postganglionic neurons*.

The anatomy of the parasympathetic nervous system offers two primary sites of action for drugs. These sites are (1) the synapses between preganglionic neurons and postganglionic neurons, and (2) the junctions between postganglionic neurons and their effector organs.

Sympathetic Nervous System

Pharmacologically relevant aspects of sympathetic nervous system anatomy are illustrated in Figure 12–3. As you can see, these features are nearly identical to those of the parasympathetic nervous system. Like the parasympathetic nervous system, the sympathetic nervous system employs *two* neurons in the pathways leading from the spinal cord to the organs under sympathetic control. The junctions between those neurons are located in *ganglia*. Neurons leading from the spinal cord to the sympathetic ganglia are termed *preganglionic neurons*, and neurons leading from ganglia to effector organs are termed *postganglionic neurons*.

The *medulla of the adrenal gland* is a feature of the sympathetic nervous system that requires comment. The adrenal medulla, although not a neuron per se, can be considered the functional equivalent of a postganglionic neuron of the sympathetic nervous system. (The adrenal medulla produces its effects by releasing epinephrine into the bloodstream. Epinephrine then produces responses much like those elicited by stimulation of postganglionic sympathetic nerves.) Since the adrenal medulla is very similar in function to a postganglionic neuron, it is appropriate to refer to the nerve leading from the spinal cord to this structure as *preganglionic*, even though there is no ganglion, as such, in this pathway.

As with the parasympathetic nervous system, drugs that affect sympathetic nervous system function have two primary sites of action: (1) the synapses between preganglionic and postganglionic neurons (including the adrenal medulla), and (2) the junctions between postganglionic neurons and their effector organs.

Somatic Motor System

Pharmacologically relevant anatomy of the somatic motor system is depicted in Figure 12–3. Note that there is *only one* neuron in the pathway from the spinal cord to the muscles innervated by somatic motor nerves. Because this pathway con-

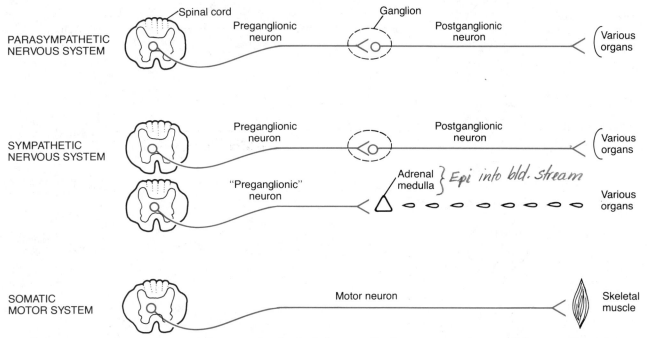

Figure 12–3. The basic anatomy of the parasympathetic and sympathetic nervous systems and the somatic motor system.

tains only one neuron, peripherally acting drugs that affect somatic motor system function have only one site of action: the *neuromuscular junction* (i.e., the junction between the somatic motor nerve and the muscle).

INTRODUCTION TO TRANSMITTERS OF THE PERIPHERAL NERVOUS SYSTEM

The peripheral nervous system employs three transmitters: *acetylcholine, norepinephrine, and epinephrine*. Any given junction in the peripheral nervous system uses only one of these transmitter substances. A fourth compound—*dopamine*—may also serve as a peripheral nervous system transmitter, but this role has not been demonstrated conclusively.

To understand peripheral nervous system pharmacology, it is necessary to know the identity of the transmitter employed at each of the junctions of the peripheral nervous system. This information is summarized in Figure 12–4.

As the figure indicates, *acetylcholine* is the transmitter employed at most junctions of the peripheral nervous system. Acetylcholine is the transmitter released by (1) all preganglionic nerves of the parasympathetic nervous system, (2) all preganglionic nerves of the sympathetic nervous system, (3) all postganglionic nerves of the parasympathetic nervous system, (4) all motor nerves to skeletal muscles, and (5) most postgan-

glionic nerves of the sympathetic nervous system that go to sweat glands.

Norepinephrine is the transmitter released by practically all postganglionic nerves of the sympathetic nervous system. The only exceptions to this rule are the postganglionic sympathetic nerves that go to sweat glands, which employ acetylcholine as their transmitter.

Epinephrine is the major transmitter released by the adrenal medulla. (The adrenal medulla also releases some norepinephrine.)

Much of what follows in this chapter is based on the information summarized in Figure 12–4. Accordingly, I strongly urge you to learn this information now.

INTRODUCTION TO RECEPTORS OF THE PERIPHERAL NERVOUS SYSTEM

The peripheral nervous system works through several different types of receptors. An understanding of these receptors is central to an understanding of peripheral nervous system pharmacology. All effort that you invest in learning about these receptors now will be richly rewarded as we discuss peripheral nervous system drugs in the chapters that follow.

Primary Receptor Types: Cholinergic Receptors and Adrenergic Receptors

There are two basic categories of receptors associated with the peripheral nervous system: *cholin-*

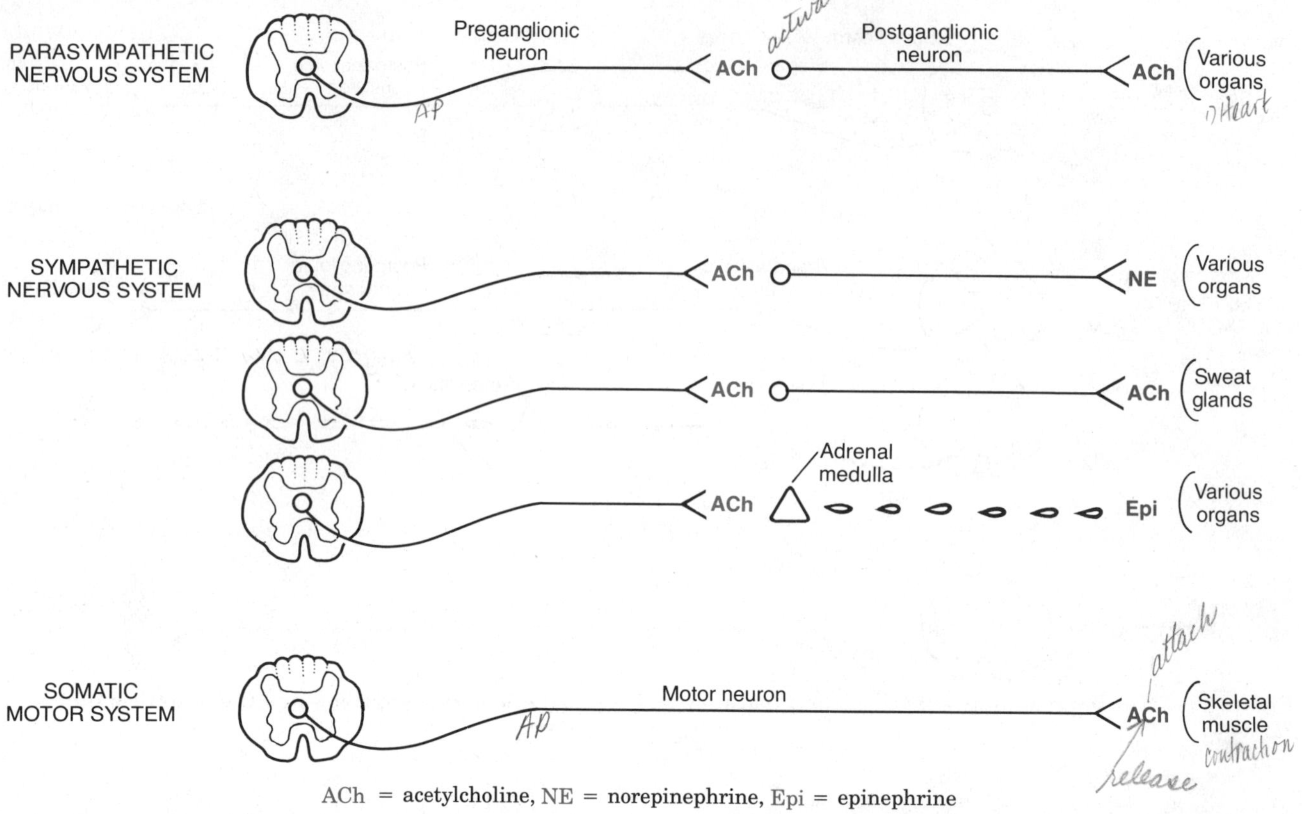

ACh = acetylcholine, NE = norepinephrine, Epi = epinephrine

Figure 12–4. Transmitters employed at specific junctions of the peripheral nervous system.
Summary
1. *All preganglionic* neurons of the *parasympathetic* and *sympathetic* nervous systems release *acetylcholine* as their transmitter.
2. *All postganglionic* neurons of the *parasympathetic* nervous system release *acetylcholine* as their transmitter.
3. *Most postganglionic* neurons of the *sympathetic* nervous system release *norepinephrine* as their transmitter.
4. *Postganglionic* neurons of the *sympathetic* nervous system that go to *sweat glands* release *acetylcholine* as their transmitter.
5. The principal transmitter released by the *adrenal medulla* is *epinephrine*.
6. All *motor neurons* to skeletal muscles release *acetylcholine* as their transmitter.

ergic receptors and *adrenergic receptors*. Cholinergic receptors are defined as receptors that mediate responses to acetylcholine. These receptors mediate responses at all junctions where acetylcholine is the transmitter. Adrenergic receptors are defined as receptors that mediate responses to epinephrine (adrenaline) and norepinephrine. These receptors mediate responses at all junctions where norepinephrine or epinephrine is the transmitter.

Subtypes of Cholinergic and Adrenergic Receptors

Not all cholinergic receptors are the same; likewise, not all adrenergic receptors are the same. For each of these two major receptor categories there are receptor subtypes. There are three major subtypes of cholinergic receptors, referred to as nicotinic$_N$, nicotinic$_M$, and muscarinic.* There are

four major subtypes of adrenergic receptors, referred to as alpha$_1$, alpha$_2$, beta$_1$, and beta$_2$.

In addition to the four major subtypes of adrenergic receptors, there is another adrenergic receptor type, referred to as the *dopamine* receptor. Although dopamine receptors are classified as adrenergic, these receptors do not respond to epinephrine or norepinephrine. Rather, they respond only to dopamine, a neurotransmitter found primarily in the central nervous system.

EXPLORING THE CONCEPT OF RECEPTOR SUBTYPES

The concept of receptor subtypes is important and potentially confusing. This section discusses what receptor subtypes are and why they matter to us as students of pharmacology.

What Do We Mean by the Term "Receptor Subtype"?

Receptors that respond to the same transmitter but which are, nonetheless, different from one an-

*Evidence gathered in recent years indicates that not all muscarinic receptors are the same. That is, like nicotinic receptors, muscarinic receptors come in subtypes. At least three subtypes have been identified. Since our understanding of these receptors is just beginning, and since drugs that can selectively alter their function are few, we will defer discussion of muscarinic subtypes to a future edition of this text.

other would be called receptor subtypes. For example, receptors that respond to acetylcholine can be found (1) within ganglia of the autonomic nervous system, (2) at neuromuscular junctions, and (3) on organs regulated by the parasympathetic nervous system. However, despite the fact that all of these receptors can be activated by acetylcholine, there is clear evidence that the receptors at these three sites are quite different from one another. Hence, although all of these receptors belong to the same major receptor category (cholinergic), they are sufficiently unlike one another as to constitute distinct receptor subtypes.

How Do We Know that Receptor Subtypes Exist?

Our knowledge of receptor subtypes comes from observing responses to drugs. In fact, were it not for drugs, we would not have any evidence to suggest that receptor subtypes exist at all.

The data in Table 12–1 illustrate the types of drug responses that have led to the realization that receptor subtypes exist. These data summarize the results of an experiment designed to study the effects of a natural transmitter (acetylcholine) and a series of drugs (nicotine, muscarine, *d*-tubocurarine, atropine) on two tissues: skeletal muscle and ciliary muscle. (The ciliary muscle is the muscle responsible for focusing the eye for near vision.) As these data indicate, although both skeletal muscle and ciliary muscle contract in response to acetylcholine, these tissues respond differently from each other to drugs. In the discussion below, we will examine the selective responses of these tissues to drugs and see how those responses point to the existence of receptor subtypes.

At synapses on skeletal muscle and ciliary muscle, acetylcholine is the transmitter employed by neurons to elicit contraction. Since both types of muscle respond to acetylcholine, it is safe to conclude that both muscles have receptors for this substance. Since acetylcholine is the natural transmitter for these receptors, we would classify these receptors as *cholinergic*.

What do the effects of nicotine on skeletal muscle and ciliary muscle suggest? The effects of nicotine on these muscles suggest four possible conclusions. (1) Since skeletal muscle contracts when nicotine is applied, we can conclude that skeletal muscle has receptors at which nicotine can act. (2) Since ciliary muscle does *not* respond to nicotine, we can tentatively conclude that ciliary muscle does not have receptors for nicotine. (3) Since nicotine mimics the effects of acetylcholine on skeletal muscle, we can conclude that nicotine may act at the same receptors on skeletal muscle that acetylcholine acts at. (4) Since both types of muscle have receptors for acetylcholine, and since nicotine appears to act only at the acetylcholine receptors on skeletal muscle, we can tentatively conclude that the acetylcholine receptors on skeletal muscle are different from the acetylcholine receptors on ciliary muscle.

What do the responses to muscarine suggest? The conclusions that can be drawn regarding responses to muscarine are exactly parallel to those drawn regarding nicotine. These conclusions are: (1) ciliary muscle has receptors that respond to muscarine; (2) skeletal muscle may not have receptors for muscarine; (3) muscarine may be acting at the same receptors on ciliary muscle as does acetylcholine; and (4) the receptors for acetylcholine on ciliary muscle may be different from the receptors for acetylcholine on skeletal muscle.

The responses of skeletal muscle and ciliary muscle to nicotine and muscarine suggest, but do not prove, that the cholinergic receptors on these two tissues are different from each other; the responses of these two tissues to *d-tubocurarine* and *atropine,* both of which are receptor blocking agents, eliminate any remaining doubts as to the presence of cholinergic receptor subtypes. When both muscle types are *pretreated* with *d*-tubocurarine and then exposed to acetylcholine, the response to acetylcholine is blocked—*but only in skeletal muscle.* Tubocurarine pretreatment does not reduce the ability of acetylcholine to stimulate ciliary muscle. Conversely, pretreatment with atropine selectively blocks the response to acetylcholine in the ciliary muscle; atropine does nothing to prevent acetylcholine from stimulating receptors on skeletal muscle. Since tubocurarine can selectively block cholinergic receptors in skeletal muscle, whereas atropine can selectively block cholinergic receptors in ciliary muscle, we can conclude with certainty that the receptors for acetylcholine in these two types of muscle must be different from each other.

The data just discussed illustrate the essential role of drugs in revealing the presence of receptor subtypes. If acetylcholine were the only probe that we had, all that we would have been able to observe is that both skeletal muscle and ciliary muscle can respond to this agent. This simple observation would provide no basis for suspecting that the

Table 12–1. Responses of Skeletal Muscle and Ciliary Muscle to a Series of Drugs

	Response	
Drug	**Skeletal Muscle**	**Ciliary Muscle**
Acetylcholine	Contraction	Contraction
Nicotine	Contraction	No response
Muscarine	No response	Contraction
Acetylcholine: after *d*-tubocurarine	No response	Contraction
Acetylcholine: after atropine	Contraction	No response

receptors for acetylcholine in these two tissues are different. It is only through the use of selectively acting drugs that the presence of receptor subtypes can be revealed.

Selective responses like those just described served as the basis for naming subtypes of cholinergic receptors: cholinergic receptor subtypes with the ability to respond to nicotine were given the name *nicotinic*. Receptor subtypes that responded selectively to muscarine were named *muscarinic*.

How Can Drugs Be More Selective than Transmitters at Receptor Subtypes?

Drugs achieve their selectivity for receptor subtypes by having structures that are different from those of natural transmitters. The relationship between structure and receptor selectivity is illustrated in Figure 12–5. In this figure, cartoon drawings are used to represent drugs (nicotine and muscarine), receptor subtypes (nicotinic and muscarinic), and acetylcholine (the natural transmitter at nicotinic and muscarinic receptors). From the structures shown, we can easily imagine how acetylcholine is able to interact with both kinds of receptor subtypes, whereas nicotine and muscarine can only interact with the receptor subtype whose structure is complementary to its own. It is by synthesizing chemicals of varied structure that pharmaceutical scientists have succeeded in producing drugs that are more selective for specific receptor subtypes than the natural transmitters that act at those sites.

Why Do Receptor Subtypes Exist?

It is not unreasonable for us to wonder why Mother Nature has bothered to create more than one type of receptor for any given transmitter. Unfortunately, definitive answers to questions along this line will have to come from Mother Nature herself. That is to say, the physiologic benefits of having multiple receptor subtypes for the same transmitter are not immediately obvious. In fact, as noted earlier, were it not for drugs, we probably wouldn't know that receptor subtypes existed at all.

Do Receptor Subtypes Matter to Us? You Bet!

Although receptor subtypes are of uncertain physiologic relevance, from the viewpoint of therapeutics, receptor subtypes are invaluable. The presence of receptor subtypes makes possible a dramatic increase in the selectivity of drug actions. For example, thanks to the existence of subtypes of cholinergic receptors (and the development of drugs selective for those receptor subtypes), it is possible to influence the activity of selected cholinergic receptors (e.g., receptors of the neuromuscular junction) without altering the activity of all other cholinergic receptors (i.e., the cholinergic receptors found in all autonomic ganglia and all target organs of the parasympathetic nervous system). Were it not for the existence of receptor subtypes, a drug that acted on cholinergic receptors at one site would alter the activity of cholinergic receptors at all other sites. Clearly, the existence of receptor subtypes for a particular transmitter makes possible drug actions that are much more selective than could be achieved if all of the receptors for that transmitter were the same.

LOCATIONS OF RECEPTOR SUBTYPES

Since many of the drugs that we will be discussing are selective for specific receptor subtypes, knowledge of the sites at which specific receptor subtypes are located will help us predict which organs a drug will affect. Accordingly, in laying our foundation for the study of peripheral nervous system drugs, it is important to learn the sites at which the subtypes of adrenergic and cholinergic receptors are located. This information is summarized in Figure 12–6. You will find it very helpful to master the contents of this figure before proceeding much further. (In the interest of minimizing confusion, subtypes of adrenergic receptors in Figure 12–6 are listed simply as alpha and beta rather than as alpha$_1$, alpha$_2$, beta$_1$, and beta$_2$. The locations of all four subtypes of adrenergic receptors are discussed in the section that follows.)

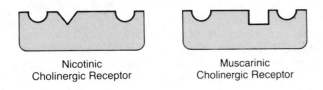

Nicotinic
Cholinergic Receptor

Muscarinic
Cholinergic Receptor

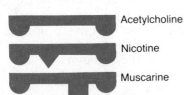

Acetylcholine

Nicotine

Muscarine

Figure 12–5. Drug structure and receptor selectivity. These cartoon figures illustrate the relationship between structure and receptor selectivity. The structure of acetylcholine allows this transmitter to interact with both receptor subtypes. In contrast, because of their unique configurations, nicotine and muscarine are selective for the cholinergic receptor subtypes whose structure complements their own.

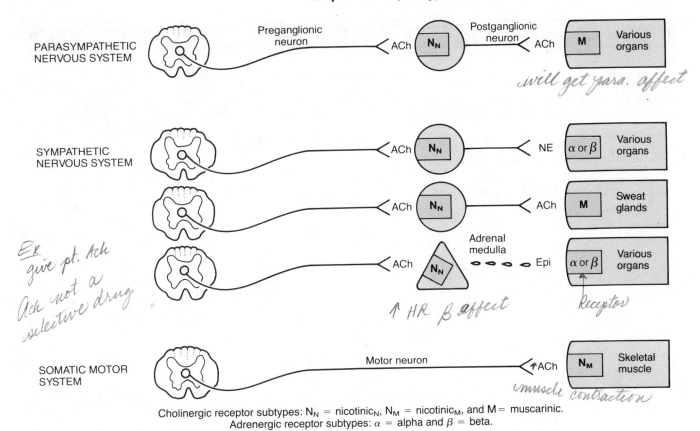

Cholinergic receptor subtypes: N_N = nicotinic$_N$, N_M = nicotinic$_M$, and M = muscarinic.
Adrenergic receptor subtypes: α = alpha and β = beta.

Figure 12–6. Locations of cholinergic and adrenergic receptor subtypes.
Summary
1. *Nicotinic$_N$* receptors are located on the *cell bodies* of *all postganglionic neurons* of the *parasympathetic* and *sympathetic* nervous systems. *Nicotinic$_N$* receptors are also located on cells of the *adrenal medulla*.
2. *Nicotinic$_M$* receptors are located on *skeletal muscle*.
3. *Muscarinic* receptors are located on *all organs* regulated by the *parasympathetic* nervous system (i.e., organs innervated by postganglionic parasympathetic nerves). *Muscarinic* receptors are also located on *sweat glands*.
4. *Adrenergic receptors—alpha, beta,* or both— are located on *all organs* (except sweat glands) regulated by the *sympathetic* nervous system (i.e., organs innervated by postganglionic sympathetic nerves). Adrenergic receptors are also located on organs regulated by epinephrine released from the *adrenal medulla*.

FUNCTIONS OF CHOLINERGIC AND ADRENERGIC RECEPTOR SUBTYPES

Knowledge of receptor function is an absolute requirement for understanding peripheral nervous system drugs. By knowing the receptors at which a drug acts and what those receptors do, we can predict the major effects of any peripheral nervous system drug.

Tables 12–2 and 12–3 summarize the pharmacologically relevant functions of peripheral nervous system receptors. Table 12–2 summarizes responses elicited by activation of cholinergic receptor subtypes. Table 12–3 summarizes responses to activation of adrenergic receptor subtypes. Before attempting to study specific peripheral nervous system drugs, you should master the contents of the appropriate table. Table 12–2 should be mastered before studying cholinergic drugs (Chapters 13 to 16). Table 12–3 should be mastered before studying adrenergic drugs (Chap-

ters 17 to 19). Students who study these tables in preparation for learning about peripheral nervous system drugs will find the process of learning the pharmacology relatively simple (and perhaps even enjoyable). Conversely, students who attempt to study the pharmacology without first mastering the appropriate table are likely to meet with frustration.

FUNCTIONS OF CHOLINERGIC RECEPTOR SUBTYPES

Table 12–2 summarizes the pharmacologically relevant responses to activation of the three subtypes of cholinergic receptors: nicotinic$_N$, nicotinic$_M$, and muscarinic. The information in this table should be committed to memory.

We can group responses to cholinergic receptor activation into three major categories based on the subtype of receptor involved:

1. Activation of *nicotinic$_N$* (neuronal) receptors

Table 12–2. Functions of Cholinergic Receptor Subtypes		
Receptor Subtype	**Location**	**Response to Receptor Activation**
*Nicotinic*_N	All autonomic nervous system ganglia and the adrenal medulla	Stimulation of parasympathetic and sympathetic postganglionic nerves and release of epinephrine from the adrenal medulla
*Nicotinic*_M	Neuromuscular junction	Contraction of skeletal muscle
Muscarinic	All parasympathetic target organs: Eye	Contraction of the ciliary muscle focuses the lens for near vision Contraction of the iris sphincter muscle causes miosis (decreased pupil diameter)
	Heart	Decreased rate
	Lung	Constriction of bronchi Promotion of secretions
	Bladder	Voiding
	GI tract	Salivation Increased gastric secretions Increased intestinal tone and motility Defecation
	Sweat glands*	Generalized sweating
	Sex organs	Erection
	Blood vessels†	Vasodilation

Radial muscle
Sphincter muscle
Pupil
Miosis

*Although sweating is due primarily to stimulation of muscarinic receptors by acetylcholine, the nerves that supply acetylcholine to sweat glands belong to the sympathetic nervous system rather than the parasympathetic nervous system.
†Cholinergic receptors on blood vessels are not associated with the nervous system.

promotes *ganglionic transmission* at all ganglia of the sympathetic and parasympathetic nervous systems. In addition, activation of nicotinic_N receptors promotes *release of epinephrine from the adrenal medulla*.

2. Activation of *nicotinic_M* (muscle) receptors causes *contraction of skeletal muscle*.

3. Activation of *muscarinic* receptors, which are located on target organs of the parasympathetic nervous system, elicits an appropriate response from the organ involved. Specifically, muscarinic activation causes (1) increased glandular secretions (from pulmonary, gastric, intestinal, and sweat glands); (2) contraction of smooth muscle in the bronchi, bladder, and gastrointestinal tract; (3) slowing of heart rate; (4) contraction of the sphincter muscle of the iris, resulting in miosis (reduction in pupillary diameter); and (5) contraction of the ciliary muscle of the eye, causing the lens to focus for near vision.

Muscarinic cholinergic receptors on blood vessels require additional comment. These receptors are not associated with the nervous system in any way. That is, no nerves terminate at vascular muscarinic receptors. It is not at all clear as to how, or even if, these receptors are activated physiologically. However, regardless of their physiologic relevance, the cholinergic receptors on blood vessels do have pharmacologic significance in that drugs that are able to activate these receptors will produce vasodilation. This vasodilation can cause blood pressure to fall.

FUNCTIONS OF ADRENERGIC RECEPTOR SUBTYPES

Adrenergic receptor subtypes and their functions are summarized in Table 12–3. This information should be committed to memory.

Alpha₁ Receptors

Alpha₁ receptors are located in blood vessels, sex organs, and the eyes.

Ocular alpha₁ receptors are present on the *ra-*

Table 12-3. Functions of Adrenergic Receptor Subtypes

Receptor Subtype	Location	Response to Receptor Activation	
Alpha₁	Eye	Contraction of the radial muscle of the iris causes mydriasis (increased pupil size)	
	Arterioles	Constriction	
	Skin		
	Viscera		
	Mucous membranes		
	Veins	Constriction	
	Sex organs	Ejaculation	
Alpha₂	Presynaptic nerve terminals	Inhibition of transmitter release	
Beta₁	Heart	Increased rate	
		Increased force of contraction	
		Increased A-V conduction velocity	
	Kidney	Renin release	
Beta₂	Arterioles	Dilation	
	Heart		
	Lung		
	Skeletal muscle		
	Bronchi	Dilation	
	Uterus	Relaxation	
	Skeletal muscle	Glycogenolysis	
	Liver	Glycogenolysis	
Dopamine	Kidney	Dilation of kidney vasculature	

dial muscle of the iris. Activation of these receptors leads to mydriasis (dilation of the pupil). As depicted in Table 12–3, the fibers of the radial muscle are arranged like the spokes of a wheel. It is because of this configuration that contraction of the radial muscle causes the pupil to enlarge. (If you have difficulty remembering that *mydriasis* means pupillary enlargement, whereas *miosis* means pupillary constriction, just remember that mydriasis [enlargement] is a larger word than miosis.)

Activation of alpha₁ receptors in *blood vessels* produces *vasoconstriction*. Alpha₁ receptors are present on veins and on arterioles in many—but not all—of the body's capillary beds.

Activation of alpha₁ receptors in the sexual apparatus of males causes *ejaculation*.

Alpha₂ Receptors

Alpha₂ receptors of the peripheral nervous system are located on *nerve terminals* (see Table 12–3) and not on the organs innervated by the autonomic nervous system. Because alpha₂ receptors are located on nerve terminals, these receptors are referred to as *presynaptic* or *prejunctional*. The function of

these receptors is to regulate transmitter release. As depicted in Table 12–3, norepinephrine can bind to alpha₂ receptors on the same neuron from which it was released. The consequence of this norepinephrine-receptor interaction is suppression of further norepinephrine release. Hence, presynaptic alpha₂ receptors can help reduce transmitter release when too much transmitter has accumulated in the synaptic gap. Drug effects resulting from activation of peripheral alpha₂ receptors are of minimal clinical significance.

Alpha₂ receptors are also present in the CNS. In contrast to peripheral alpha₂ receptors, central alpha₂ receptors are therapeutically relevant. We will consider these receptors in later chapters.

Beta₁ Receptors

Beta₁ receptors are located in the heart and in the kidney. *Cardiac* beta₁ receptors have great therapeutic significance. Activation of these receptors *increases heart rate, force of contraction,* and *velocity of impulse conduction through the atrioventricular (A-V) node.*

Activation of beta₁ receptors in the *kidney* causes *release of renin* into the blood. Since renin promotes synthesis of angiotensin, a powerful vasoconstrictor, activation of renal beta$_1$ receptors is a means by which the nervous system helps elevate blood pressure. (The role of renin in the regulation of blood pressure is discussed in depth in Chapter 37.)

Beta$_2$ Receptors

Beta$_2$ receptors mediate several important processes. Activation of beta$_2$ receptors in the lung leads to *bronchial dilation*. Activation of beta$_2$ receptors in the uterus causes *relaxation of uterine smooth muscle*. Activation of beta$_2$ receptors in arterioles of the heart, lungs, and skeletal muscles causes *vasodilation* (an effect opposite to that of alpha$_1$ activation). Activation of beta$_2$ receptors in the liver and in skeletal muscle promotes *glycogenolysis* (breakdown of glycogen into glucose), thereby increasing blood levels of glucose.

Dopamine Receptors

In the periphery, the only dopamine receptors of clinical significance are located in the vasculature of the kidney. Activation of these receptors *dilates renal blood vessels*, thereby enhancing renal perfusion.

In the central nervous system, receptors for dopamine are of great therapeutic significance. The functions of these receptors are discussed in Chapter 21 (Drugs for Parkinson's Disease) and Chapter 24 (Antipsychotic Agents).

RECEPTOR SPECIFICITY OF THE ADRENERGIC TRANSMITTERS

The receptor specificity of adrenergic transmitters is more complex than the receptor specificity of acetylcholine. Whereas acetylcholine can activate all three subtypes of cholinergic receptors, not every adrenergic transmitter (epinephrine, norepinephrine, dopamine) can interact with each of the five subtypes of adrenergic receptors.

Receptor specificity of adrenergic transmitters is as follows: (1) *epinephrine* can activate all alpha and beta receptors, but not dopamine receptors; (2) *norepinephrine* can activate alpha$_1$, alpha$_2$, and beta$_1$ receptors, but not beta$_2$ receptors or dopamine receptors; (3) *dopamine* can activate alpha$_1$, beta$_1$, and dopamine receptors. (Note that dopamine itself is the only transmitter capable of activating dopamine receptors.) Receptor specificity of the adrenergic transmitters is summarized in Table 12–4.

Knowing that epinephrine is the only transmitter that acts at beta$_2$ receptors can serve as an aid to remembering the functions of this receptor subtype. Recall that epinephrine is released from the

Table 12–4. Receptor Specificity of Adrenergic Transmitters

Transmitter	Adrenergic Receptor Subtype				
	Alpha$_1$	*Alpha$_2$*	*Beta$_1$*	*Beta$_2$*	*Dopamine*
Epinephrine	←――――――――――――――――→				
Norepinephrine	←――――――――→				
Dopamine	←――→		←――→		←――→

adrenal medulla (and not from nerves) and that the function of epinephrine is to prepare the body for fight or flight. Accordingly, since epinephrine is the only transmitter that activates beta$_2$ receptors, and since epinephrine is released only in preparation for fight or flight, times of fight or flight will be the only occasions on which beta$_2$ receptors will undergo significant activation. As it turns out, the physiologic changes elicited by beta$_2$ activation are precisely those needed for success in the fight or flight response. Specifically, activation of beta$_2$ receptors will cause (1) dilation of blood vessels in the heart, lungs, and skeletal muscles, thereby increasing blood flow to these organs; (2) dilation of the bronchi, thereby increasing oxygenation; (3) glycogenolysis, thereby increasing available energy; and (4) relaxation of uterine muscle, thereby preventing delivery, a process that would be inconvenient for anyone preparing for fight or flight. Hence, if we think of the physiologic requirements for success during fight or flight, we will have a good picture of the responses that beta$_2$ activation can bring about.

TRANSMITTER LIFE CYCLES

In this section we will consider the life cycles of acetylcholine, norepinephrine, and epinephrine. Since a number of drugs produce their effects by interfering with specific phases of the transmitter life cycle, knowledge of these cycles will help us understand drug actions.

Life Cycle of Acetylcholine

The life cycle of acetylcholine (ACh) is depicted in Figure 12–7. This cycle begins with the synthesis of ACh from two precursors: choline and acetyl coenzyme A. Following synthesis, ACh is stored in vesicles and is later released in response to an action potential. Following release, ACh binds to receptors (nicotinic$_N$, nicotinic$_M$, or muscarinic) located on the postjunctional cell. Upon dissociating from its receptors, ACh is destroyed almost instantaneously by *acetylcholinesterase* (AChE), an enzyme present in abundance on the surface of the postjunctional cell. AChE degrades ACh into two

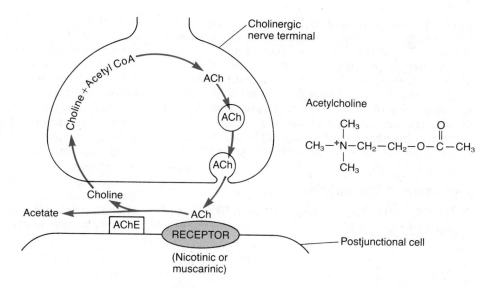

Figure 12–7. Life cycle of acetylcholine. Note that transmission is terminated by enzymatic degradation of ACh and not by uptake of intact ACh back into the nerve terminal. (ACh = acetylcholine, AChE = acetylcholinesterase, and Acetyl CoA = acetyl coenzyme A.)

inactive products—acetate and choline. Uptake of choline into the cholinergic nerve terminal completes the life cycle of ACh. Note that an inactive substance (choline), and not the active transmitter (acetylcholine), is taken back up for reuse.

Therapeutic and toxic agents can interfere with the ACh life cycle at several points. Botulinus toxin produces its effects by inhibiting ACh release. A number of medicines and poisons act at cholinergic receptors to mimic or block the actions of ACh. Several therapeutic and toxic agents act by inhibiting AChE, thereby causing ACh to accumulate in the junctional gap.

Life Cycle of Norepinephrine

The life cycle of norepinephrine is depicted in Figure 12–8. As indicated, this cycle begins with

the synthesis of norepinephrine from a series of precursors. The final step of synthesis takes place within vesicles, where norepinephrine is stored until the time of its release. Following release, norepinephrine binds to adrenergic receptors. As shown in the figure, norepinephrine can interact with postsynaptic alpha$_1$ and beta receptors and with presynaptic alpha$_2$ receptors. Transmission is terminated by *reuptake* of norepinephrine back into the nerve terminal. (Note that the termination process for norepinephrine differs from that for acetylcholine, whose effects are terminated by enzymatic degradation and not by reuptake.) Following reuptake, norepinephrine can undergo one of two fates: (1) uptake into vesicles for reuse, or (2) inactivation by monoamine oxidase (MAO), an enzyme present within the nerve terminal.

Practically every step in the life cycle of norepi-

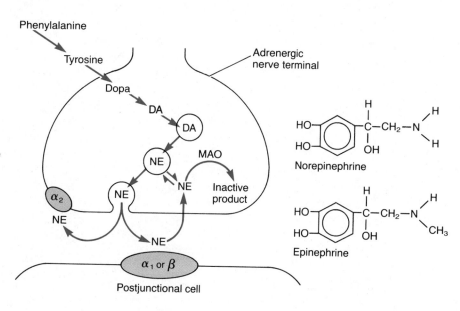

Figure 12–8. Life cycle of norepinephrine. Note that transmission is terminated by reuptake of NE into the nerve terminal and not by enzymatic degradation. Note also the structural similarity between epinephrine and norepinephrine. (DA = dopamine, NE = norepinephrine, and MAO = monoamine oxidase.)

nephrine can be altered by therapeutic agents: we have drugs that alter the synthesis, storage, and release of norepinephrine; we have drugs that act at adrenergic receptors to mimic or block the effects of norepinephrine; we have drugs, such as cocaine and certain antidepressants, that inhibit the reuptake of norepinephrine (and thereby intensify transmission); and we have drugs that inhibit the breakdown of norepinephrine by MAO, causing an increase in the amount of transmitter available for release.

Life Cycle of Epinephrine

The life cycle of epinephrine is much like that of norepinephrine—although there are some significant differences. This life cycle begins with the synthesis of epinephrine within chromaffin cells of the adrenal medulla. These cells produce epinephrine by first making norepinephrine, which is then converted enzymatically to epinephrine. (Since sympathetic neurons lack the enzyme needed to convert norepinephrine to epinephrine, epinephrine is not produced in sympathetic nerves.) Following synthesis, epinephrine is stored in vesicles until the time of its release. Once released from the adrenal medulla, epinephrine travels via the bloodstream to target organs throughout the body. Termination of epinephrine's actions is accomplished primarily via hepatic metabolism, and not by uptake into nerves.

Cholinergic Drugs

The cholinergic drugs are agents that influence the activity of cholinergic receptors. Most of these drugs act directly at cholinergic receptors to either mimic or block the actions of acetylcholine. Some of these drugs (the cholinesterase inhibitors) influence cholinergic receptors indirectly by preventing the breakdown of acetylcholine.

The cholinergic drugs have both therapeutic and toxicologic significance. The therapeutic applications of cholinergic drugs are limited but valuable. The toxicology of the cholinergic drugs is extensive, encompassing such agents as nicotine, insecticides, and compounds designed for chemical warfare.

There are six categories of cholinergic drugs. These categories, along with representative agents, are summarized in Table 1. The *muscarinic agonists*, represented by bethanechol, are drugs that selectively mimic the effects of acetylcholine at muscarinic receptors. The *muscarinic antagonists*, represented by atropine, selectively block the effects of acetylcholine at muscarinic receptors. *Ganglionic stimulating agents*, of which nicotine is the major representative, selectively mimic the effects of acetylcholine at nicotinic$_N$ receptors of autonomic ganglia. *Ganglionic blocking agents*, represented by trimethaphan, selectively

block ganglionic nicotinic$_N$ receptors. *Neuromuscular blocking agents*, represented by d-tubocurarine and succinylcholine, selectively block the effects of acetylcholine at nicotinic$_M$ receptors of the neuromuscular junction. The *cholinesterase inhibitors*, represented by neostigmine, prevent the breakdown of acetylcholine by acetylcholinesterase, and can thereby increase the stimulation of practically all cholinergic receptors in the body.

Table 2 is your master key to understanding the cholinergic drugs. This table lists the three subtypes of cholinergic receptors (muscarinic, nicotinic$_N$, and nicotinic$_M$) and indicates for each receptor type: (1) location, (2) responses to activation, (3) drugs that produce activation (agonists), and (4) drugs that prevent activation (antagonists). This information, along with the detailed information on cholinergic receptor function summarized in Table 12–2, is just about all that you need in order to predict the actions of cholinergic drugs.

An example will demonstrate the combined value of Table 2 and Table 12–2. Let's consider *bethanechol* for our example. As indicated in Table 2, bethanechol is a selective agonist at *muscarinic* cholinergic receptors. Referring to Table 12–2, we see that activation of muscarinic receptors can produce the following: ocular effects (miosis and ciliary muscle contraction), lowering of heart rate, bronchial constriction, urination, glandular secretion, stimulation of the gastrointestinal tract, penile erection, and vasodilation. Since bethanechol *activates* muscarinic receptors, the drug is capable of eliciting all of these responses. Hence, by knowing which receptors bethanechol stimulates (from Table 2) and by knowing what those receptors do (from Table 12–2), we can predict the kinds of responses we might expect bethanechol to produce.

In the chapters that follow, we will employ the approach just described for understanding peripheral nervous system drugs. That is, for each drug discussed, you will want to know (1) the receptors that the drug affects, (2) the normal responses to

Table 1. Categories of Cholinergic Drugs

Category	Representative Drugs
Muscarinic agonists	Bethanechol
Muscarinic antagonists	Atropine
Ganglionic stimulating agents	Nicotine
Ganglionic blocking agents	Trimethaphan
Neuromuscular blocking agents	d-Tubocurarine, succinylcholine
Cholinesterase inhibitors	Neostigmine, physostigmine, DFP

Table 2. Summary of Cholinergic Drugs and Their Receptors

	Receptor Subtype		
	Muscarinic	*Nicotinic$_N$*	*Nicotinic$_M$*
Receptor Location	Sweat glands Blood vessels All organs regulated by the parasympathetic nervous system	All ganglia of the autonomic nervous system	Neuromuscular junctions (NMJ)
Effects of Receptor Activation	Many, including: ↓ Heart rate ↑ Gland secretion Smooth muscle contraction	Promotes ganglionic transmission	Skeletal muscle contraction
Receptor Agonists	Bethanechol Cholinesterase inhibitors: physostigmine, neostigmine, DFP (these drugs indirectly stimulate all cholinergic receptors)	Nicotine	(Nicotine*)
Receptor Antagonists	Atropine	Trimethaphan	*d*-Tubocurarine, succinylcholine

*The doses of nicotine needed to stimulate nicotinic$_M$ receptors of the NMJ are much higher than the doses needed to stimulate nicotinic$_N$ receptors in autonomic ganglia.

activation of those receptors, and (3) whether the drug in question increases or decreases receptor activation. All of this information is contained in Table 2 and Table 12–2. Accordingly, if you master the information in these tables now, you will be prepared to follow discussions in succeeding chapters with relative ease – and perhaps even pleasure. In contrast, if you postpone mastery of Table 2 and Table 12–2, you are likely to find it both difficult and dissatisfying to proceed.

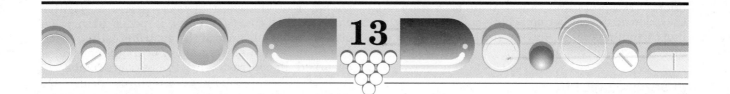

Muscarinic Agonists and Antagonists

The muscarinic agonists and muscarinic antagonists produce their effects through direct interaction with muscarinic receptors. The muscarinic agonists cause receptor activation, whereas the muscarinic antagonists prevent receptor activation.

MUSCARINIC AGONISTS

The muscarinic agonists are drugs that bind to muscarinic receptors and thereby cause their activation. Since nearly all muscarinic receptors are associated with the parasympathetic nervous system, the responses to muscarinic agonists closely resemble those produced by stimulation of parasympathetic nerves. Because their effects resemble those of parasympathetic stimulation, muscarinic agonists are known alternatively as *parasympathomimetic agents*.

BETHANECHOL

Bethanechol embodies the characteristics that typify all muscarinic agonists and will serve as our prototype for the group.

Mechanism of Action

Bethanechol is a direct-acting muscarinic agonist. The drug binds reversibly to muscarinic cholinergic receptors and causes their activation. At therapeutic doses, bethanechol acts selectively at muscarinic receptors, having little or no effect on nicotinic cholinergic receptors.

Pharmacologic Effects

Bethanechol can elicit all of the responses typical of muscarinic receptor activation. Accordingly, we can readily predict the effects of bethanechol by knowing the information on muscarinic responses summarized in Table 12–2.

The major structures affected by muscarinic activation are the *heart, exocrine glands, smooth muscles,* and the *eye.* Muscarinic agonists act on the heart to cause *bradycardia* (decreased heart rate) and on exocrine glands to increase *sweating, salivation, bronchial secretions,* and *secretion of gastric acid.* In most smooth muscles, muscarinic agonists promote *contraction,* causing *constriction of the bronchi, increased tone and motility of gastrointestinal smooth muscle,* and *contraction of the bladder.* In vascular smooth muscle, these drugs cause *relaxation;* the resultant vasodilation can produce hypotension. Activation of muscarinic receptors in the eye has two effects: (1) *miosis* (pupillary constriction), and (2) *contraction of the ciliary muscle,* resulting in accommodation for near vision. (The ciliary muscle, which is attached to the lens, focuses the eye for near vision by altering lens curvature.)

Pharmacokinetics

Bethanechol is administered orally and by subcutaneous (SC) injection. Following oral drug administration, effects begin in 30 to 60 minutes and persist for approximately 1 hour. With SC injection, effects begin more rapidly (in 5 to 15 minutes).

To produce an equivalent therapeutic response, oral doses of bethanechol must be about 40 times greater than SC doses. As indicated in Figure 13–1, bethanechol is a *quaternary ammonium compound,* and therefore always carries a positive charge. This charge greatly impedes absorption across the membranes of the gastrointestinal tract. Hence, only a small fraction of oral bethanechol is absorbed. In contrast, since the barriers to absorption of subcutaneously administered drugs are minimal, bethanechol is readily absorbed following SC injection. These differences in absorption underlie the differences in dosage for the two routes.

Therapeutic Uses

Although bethanechol can produce a broad range of pharmacologic effects, its therapeutic uses are limited. The principal indication is urinary retention.

Urinary Retention. Bethanechol relieves urinary retention by activating muscarinic receptors of the urinary tract. Muscarinic stimulation increases voiding pressure (by contracting the detrusor muscle of the bladder) and relaxes the urinary sphincters. Bethanechol is used to treat urinary retention in postoperative and postpartum patients. The drug should not be used to treat urinary retention caused by physical obstruction of the urinary tract, since increased pressure in the tract in the presence of blockage could cause injury. When patients are treated with bethanechol, a bedpan or urinal should be readily available.

Gastrointestinal Uses. Bethanechol has been used on an investigational basis to treat *gastroesophageal reflux.* Benefits may result from increased esophageal motility and increased pressure in the lower esophageal sphincter.

Bethanechol can be used for disorders associated with gastrointestinal paralysis. Beneficial effects are due to increased tone and motility of gastrointestinal smooth muscle. Specific applications are *adynamic ileus, gastric atony,* and *postoperative abdominal distention.* Bethanechol should not be given if physical obstruction of the gastrointestinal tract is present, since, in the presence of blockage, increased propulsive contractions might result in damage to the intestinal wall.

Adverse Effects

In theory, bethanechol can produce the full range of muscarinic responses as side effects. How-

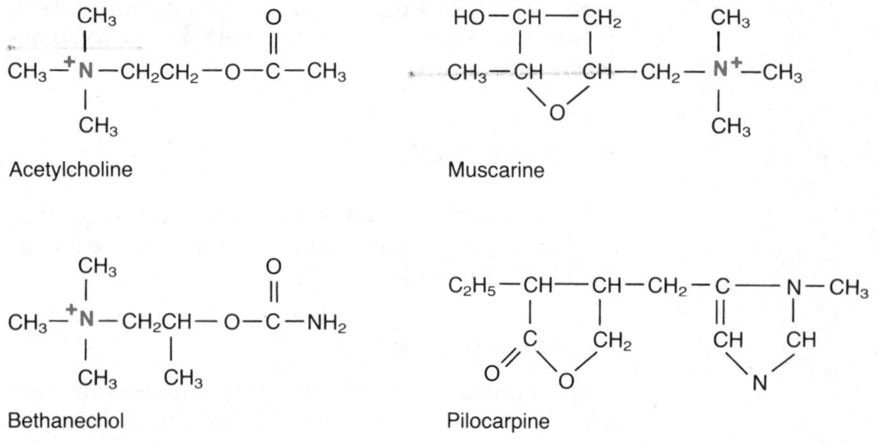

Acetylcholine

Muscarine

Bethanechol

Pilocarpine

Figure 13–1. Structures of muscarinic agonists. Note that with the exception of pilocarpine, all of these agents are quaternary ammonium compounds and therefore always carry a positive charge. Because of this charge, these compounds cross membranes poorly.

ever, in actual practice, side effects are relatively rare, and their incidence depends on route of administration. With *oral* administration, side effects are uncommon. In contrast, when bethanechol is given *subcutaneously*, the incidence of side effects is relatively high.

Cardiovascular System. Bethanechol can cause *hypotension* (secondary to vasodilation) and *bradycardia*. Accordingly, the drug is contraindicated for patients with low blood pressure or low cardiac output.

Alimentary System. At usual therapeutic doses, bethanechol can cause *excessive salivation, increased secretion of gastric acid, abdominal cramps*, and *diarrhea*. Higher doses can cause *involuntary defecation*. Bethanechol is contraindicated in patients with gastric ulcers, since stimulation of acid secretion could intensify gastric erosion, causing bleeding and possibly perforation. The drug is also contraindicated for patients with *intestinal obstruction* and for those recovering from *recent surgery of the bowel*. In both cases, the ability of bethanechol to increase the tone and motility of intestinal smooth muscle could result in rupture of the bowel wall.

Urinary Tract. Because of its ability to contract the bladder and thereby increase pressure within the urinary tract, bethanechol can be hazardous to patients with *urinary tract obstruction* or *weakness of the bladder wall*. In both groups of patients, elevation of pressure within the urinary tract could cause the bladder to rupture. Accordingly, bethanechol is contraindicated for patients with either disorder.

Exacerbation of Asthma. By stimulating muscarinic receptors in the lungs, bethanechol can cause bronchoconstriction. Accordingly, *the drug is contraindicated for patients with latent or active asthma*.

Dysrhythmias in Hyperthyroid Patients. Bethanechol can cause *dysrhythmias* in hyperthyroid patients. Hence, the drug is contraindicated for these individuals. The mechanism of dysrhythmia induction is explained below.

If given to hyperthyroid patients, bethanechol may increase heart rate to the point of causing a dysrhythmia. (Note that increased heart rate is opposite to the effect that muscarinic agonists have on most patients.) When hyperthyroid patients are given bethanechol, their initial cardiovascular responses are like those of anyone else: bradycardia and hypotension. In reaction to hypotension, the baroreceptor reflex attempts to return blood pressure to normal. Part of this reflex involves the release of increased amounts of norepinephrine from the sympathetic nerves that regulate the heart. In patients who are not hyperthyroid, this increase in norepinephrine availability serves to increase cardiac output, and thereby helps restore blood pressure. However, in hyperthyroid patients, increased amounts of norepinephrine can induce cardiac dysrhythmias. The reason for this unusual response is that in hyperthyroid patients the heart is exquisitely sensitive to the effects of nor-

epinephrine; hence, relatively small amounts of norepinephrine can cause stimulation that is sufficient to elicit a dysrhythmia.

Preparations, Dosage, and Administration

Preparations. Bethanechol [Urecholine, Duvoid, Myotonachol] is available in tablets (5, 10, 25, and 50 mg) and as an injection (5 mg/ml).

Dosage and Administration. *Oral.* Adult dosages range from 10 to 50 mg 3 to 4 times a day. Administration with meals can cause nausea and vomiting. To avoid this problem, oral doses should be administered 1 hour before meals or 2 hours after.

Subcutaneous. The usual adult dosing schedule is 5 mg administered up to 4 times a day. (Note that this dosage is significantly *lower* than the oral dosage.) The injectable form of bethanechol is intended for *subcutaneous* administration only. *Bethanechol must never be injected intramuscularly or intravenously*, since the resulting high drug levels can cause severe toxicity (bloody diarrhea, bradycardia, profound hypotension, cardiovascular collapse).

OTHER MUSCARINIC AGONISTS

Pilocarpine

Pilocarpine is a muscarinic agonist used only in the treatment of glaucoma, an ophthalmic disorder characterized by elevated intraocular pressure with subsequent injury to the optic nerve. The basic pharmacology of pilocarpine and its use in glaucoma are discussed in Chapter 69 (Drugs for Disorders of the Eye).

Acetylcholine

Clinical use of acetylcholine is restricted to dilation of the pupil in ophthalmic surgery. Two factors explain the limited utility of this drug. First, acetylcholine lacks selectivity: in addition to stimulating muscarinic cholinergic receptors, acetylcholine can also stimulate all nicotinic cholinergic receptors. Second, because of rapid destruction by cholinesterases, acetylcholine has a half-life that is extremely short—too short for most clinical applications.

Muscarine

Although muscarine is not used clinically, this agent has historic and toxicologic significance. Muscarine is of historic interest because of the role it played in the discovery of cholinergic receptor subtypes. The drug has toxicologic significance because of its presence in certain poisonous mushrooms.

TOXICOLOGY OF MUSCARINIC AGONISTS

Sources of Muscarinic Poisoning. Muscarinic poisoning can result from ingestion of certain mushrooms and from overdosage with two kinds of medications: (1) direct-acting muscarinic agonists (bethanechol, pilocarpine) and (2) cholinesterase inhibitors (see Chapter 16).

Of the mushrooms that cause poisoning, only a few do so through muscarinic stimulation. Mushrooms of the *Inocybe* and *Clitocybe* species have especially high concentrations of muscarine, and ingestion of these mushrooms can produce typical signs of muscarinic toxicity. Interestingly, *Amanita muscaria*, the mushroom from which muscarine was originally extracted, actually contains very little muscarine; poisoning by this mushroom is due to toxins other than muscarinic agonists.

Symptoms. Manifestations of muscarinic poisoning result from excessive stimulation of muscarinic receptors. Prominent symptoms are profuse salivation, lacrimation (tearing), visual disturbances, bronchospasm, diarrhea, bradycardia, and hypotension. Severe poisoning can produce cardiovascular collapse.

Treatment. Management is direct and specific: administer *atropine* (a selective muscarinic blocking agent) and provide supportive therapy. By blocking access of muscarinic agonists to their receptors, atropine can reverse most signs of toxicity.

MUSCARINIC ANTAGONISTS

Muscarinic antagonists are drugs that competitively block the actions of acetylcholine at muscarinic receptors. Because the majority of muscarinic receptors are located on structures innervated by parasympathetic nerves, the muscarinic antagonists are also known as *parasympatholytic* drugs. Additional names for these agents are *antimuscarinic drugs*, *muscarinic blockers*, and *anticholinergic drugs*.

The term *anticholinergic* can be a source of confusion and requires comment. This term is unfortunate in that it implies blockade at *all* cholinergic receptors. However, as normally used, the term anticholinergic only indicates blockade of *muscarinic* receptors. Therefore, when a drug is described as being anticholinergic, you can take this to mean that the drug produces muscarinic blockade—and not blockade of all other cholinergic receptors.

ATROPINE

Atropine is the best known muscarinic antagonist and will serve as our prototype for the group. The actions of all other muscarinic antagonists are qualitatively similar to those of this drug.

Atropine is found naturally in a variety of plants, including *Atropa belladonna* (deadly nightshade) and *Datura stramonium* (also known as Jimson weed, stinkweed, and devil's apple). Because of its presence in *A. belladonna*, atropine is referred to as a *belladonna alkaloid*.

Mechanism of Action

Atropine produces its effects through competitive blockade at muscarinic receptors. Like all other receptor antagonists, atropine has no *direct* effects of its own. Rather, all responses to atropine result from *preventing receptor activation* by endogenous acetylcholine (or by drugs that act as muscarinic agonists).

At therapeutic doses, atropine produces selective blockade of muscarinic cholinergic receptors. However, if the dosage is sufficiently high, the drug will

produce some blockade of nicotinic receptors as well.

Pharmacologic Effects

Since atropine acts by causing muscarinic receptor blockade, its effects are opposite to those caused by muscarinic activation. Accordingly, we can readily predict the effects of atropine by knowing the normal responses to muscarinic receptor activation (see Table 12–2) and by knowing that atropine will reverse those responses. Like the muscarinic agonists, the muscarinic antagonists exert their influence primarily on the *heart, exocrine glands, smooth muscles*, and the *eye*.

Heart. Atropine *increases heart rate*. Since *stimulation* of cardiac muscarinic receptors decreases heart rate, *blockade* of these receptors with atropine will cause heart rate to increase.

Exocrine Glands. Atropine *decreases secretion* from salivary glands, bronchial glands, sweat glands, and the acid-secreting cells of the stomach. Note that these effects are opposite to those of muscarinic agonists, which increase secretion from exocrine glands.

Smooth Muscle. By preventing activation of muscarinic receptors on smooth muscle, atropine causes *relaxation of the bronchi, decreased tone of the urinary bladder*, and *decreased tone and motility of the gastrointestinal tract*. In the absence of an exogenous muscarinic agonist (e.g., bethanechol), muscarinic blockade has no effect on vascular smooth muscle tone.

Eye. Blockade of muscarinic receptors on the iris sphincter causes *mydriasis* (dilation of the pupil). Blockade of muscarinic receptors on the ciliary muscle produces *cycloplegia* (relaxation of the ciliary muscle), thereby focusing the lens for far vision.

Central Nervous System (CNS). At therapeutic doses, atropine can cause mild CNS *excitation*. Toxic doses can cause *hallucinations* and *delirium*, which can resemble psychosis. Extremely high doses can result in coma, respiratory arrest, and death.

Dose Dependency of Muscarinic Blockade. It is important to note that not all muscarinic receptors are equally sensitive to blockade by atropine and most other muscarinic antagonists: at some sites, muscarinic receptors can be blocked with relatively low doses, whereas at other sites much higher doses are needed. Table 13–1 indicates the order in which specific muscarinic receptors will be blocked as the dose of atropine is increased.

Differences in receptor sensitivity to muscarinic blockers are of clinical significance. As indicated in

Table 13–1. Relationship Between Dosage and Responses to Atropine

Dosage of Atropine	Response Produced
Low Doses ↓ High Doses	Salivary glands—decreased secretion Sweat glands—decreased secretion Bronchial glands—decreased secretion
	Heart—increased rate Eye—mydriasis, blurred vision
	Urinary tract—interference with voiding Intestine—decreased tone and motility Lung—dilation of bronchi
	Stomach—decreased acid secretion

Note that doses of atropine that are high enough to decrease gastric acid secretion or dilate the bronchi will also affect all other structures under muscarinic control. As a result, atropine and most other muscarinic antagonists are not very desirable for treating peptic ulcer disease or asthma.

Table 13–1, the doses needed to block muscarinic receptors in the stomach and bronchial smooth muscle are higher than the doses needed to block muscarinic receptors at all other locations. Accordingly, if we want to use atropine to treat peptic ulcer disease (by suppressing gastric acid secretion) or asthma (by dilating the bronchi), we cannot do so without also affecting the heart, exocrine glands, many smooth muscles, and the eye. Because of these obligatory side effects, atropine and most other muscarinic antagonists are not preferred drugs for treating peptic ulcers or asthma.

Pharmacokinetics

Atropine may be administered orally, topically (to the eye), and by injection (IM, SC, and IV). The drug is rapidly absorbed following oral administration and distributes to all tissues, including the CNS. Elimination is by a combination of hepatic metabolism and urinary excretion. Atropine has a half-life of approximately 3 hours.

Therapeutic Uses

Preanesthetic Medication. The cardiac effects of atropine can be helpful during surgery. Procedures that stimulate baroreceptors of the carotid body can initiate reflex slowing of the heart, resulting in profound bradycardia. Since this reflex is mediated by muscarinic receptors on the heart, pretreatment with atropine can prevent dangerous reductions in heart rate.

Certain anesthetics (especially ether, which is obsolete) irritate the respiratory tract, and thereby stimulate secretion from salivary, nasal, pharyngeal, and bronchial glands. If these secretions are sufficiently profuse, they can interfere with respiration. By blocking muscarinic receptors on secretory glands, atropine can help prevent excessive secretions. Fortunately, modern anesthetics are much less irritating than ether. The availability of these new anesthetics has greatly reduced the use of atropine as an antisecretagogue during anesthesia.

Disorders of the Eye. By blocking muscarinic receptors in the eye, atropine can cause mydriasis and paralysis of the ciliary muscle. Both actions can be helpful during eye examinations and ocular surgery. The ophthalmic uses of atropine and other muscarinic antagonists are discussed in Chapter 69.

Bradycardia. Atropine can accelerate heart rate in certain patients with bradycardia. Heart rate is increased because blockade of cardiac muscarinic receptors prevents the parasympathetic nervous system from slowing the heart.

Biliary Colic. Biliary colic is characterized by intense abdominal pain brought on by passage of a gallstone through the bile duct. This condition is usually treated with morphine. In some cases, atropine may be combined with morphine. By relaxing biliary tract smooth muscle, atropine can help alleviate discomfort.

Intestinal Hypertonicity and Hypermotility. By blocking muscarinic receptors in the intestine, atropine can decrease both the tone and motility of intestinal smooth muscle. This action can be beneficial in conditions characterized by excessive intestinal motility, such as mild dysentery and diverticulitis. When taken for these disorders, atropine can reduce both the frequency of bowel movements and associated abdominal cramps.

Muscarinic Agonist Poisoning. Atropine is a specific antidote to poisoning by agents that activate muscarinic receptors. By blocking muscarinic receptors, atropine can reverse all signs of muscarinic poisoning. As discussed previously, muscarinic poisoning can result from an overdose with medications that promote muscarinic activation (e.g., bethanechol, cholinesterase inhibitors) and from ingestion of certain mushrooms.

Peptic Ulcer Disease. Because it can suppress secretion of gastric acid, atropine has been used to treat peptic ulcer disease. Unfortunately, when administered in doses that are strong enough to block the muscarinic receptors that regulate secretion of gastric acid, atropine also blocks most other muscarinic receptors. Hence, treatment of ulcers is necessarily associated with a broad range of antimuscarinic side effects (dry mouth, blurred vision, urinary retention, constipation, and so forth). Because of these side effects, atropine is not a first choice drug for ulcer therapy. Rather, atropine is reserved for those cases in which symptoms cannot be relieved with preferred medications (e.g., histamine₂ receptor antagonists, sucralfate).

Asthma. By blocking bronchial muscarinic receptors, atropine can promote bronchial dilation, thereby improving respiration in patients with asthma. Unfortunately, in addition to dilating the bronchi, atropine also causes drying and thickening of bronchial secretions, effects that can be harmful to the asthmatic patient. Furthermore, when given in the doses needed to dilate the bronchi, atropine will cause a variety of antimuscarinic side effects. Because of the potential for harm, and because superior medicines are available, atropine has a very limited role in asthma therapy.

Adverse Effects

Most side effects of atropine and other muscarinic antagonists are the direct consequence of muscarinic receptor blockade and, therefore, can be predicted from your knowledge of muscarinic receptor function.

Dry Mouth (Xerostomia). Blockade of muscarinic receptors on salivary glands can inhibit salivation to such an extent that the mouth becomes dry. Not only is xerostomia uncomfortable, it can impede swallowing. Patients should be informed that dryness can be alleviated by chewing gum, sucking on hard candy, and sipping fluids.

Blurred Vision and Photophobia. Blockade of muscarinic receptors on the ciliary muscle and the sphincter of the iris can paralyze both muscles. Paralysis of the ciliary muscle focuses the eye for far vision, causing nearby objects to appear blurred. Patients should be forewarned about this effect and advised to avoid hazardous activities if their vision is significantly impaired.

Paralysis of the iris sphincter prevents constriction of the pupil, thereby rendering the eye unable to adapt to bright light. Patients should be advised to wear dark glasses if photophobia (intolerance to light) is a problem. Room lighting for hospitalized patients should be kept low.

Elevation of Intraocular Pressure. Paralysis of the iris sphincter can cause intraocular pressure (IOP) to rise. The mechanism of this effect is discussed in Chapter 69 (Drugs for Disorders of the Eye). Because they can raise IOP, muscarinic blockers are contraindicated for patients with glaucoma, a disease characterized by abnormally high IOP. In addition, antimuscarinic drugs should be used with caution in patients who may not have glaucoma per se but for whom a predisposition to glaucoma may be present; included in the group are all individuals older than 40.

Urinary Retention. Blockade of muscarinic receptors in the urinary tract reduces pressure within the bladder and increases the tone of the urinary sphincter. These effects can produce urinary hesitancy or urinary retention. In the event of severe urinary retention, catheterization or treatment with a muscarinic agonist (e.g., bethanechol) may be required. Patients should be advised that urinary retention can be minimized by voiding just prior to taking their medication.

Constipation. Muscarinic blockade decreases the tone and motility of intestinal smooth muscle. The resultant delay in transit through the intestine can produce constipation. Patients should be informed that constipation can be minimized by increasing dietary fluids and fiber. A laxative may be needed if constipation is severe. Because of their ability to decrease smooth muscle tone, muscarinic antagonists are contraindicated for patients with intestinal atony, a condition in which intestinal tone is already low.

Anhidrosis. Blockade of muscarinic receptors on sweat glands can produce anhidrosis (a deficiency or absence of sweat). Since sweating is necessary for cooling the body, patients who cannot sweat are at risk of hyperthermia. Patients should be warned of this possibility and advised to avoid activities that might lead to overheating (e.g., exercising on a hot day).

Tachycardia. Blockade of cardiac muscarinic receptors eliminates the parasympathetic influence on the heart. By removing the "braking" influence of parasympathetic nerves, muscarinic antagonists can cause tachycardia (excessive heart rate). Caution must be exercised in patients with pre-existing tachycardia.

Asthma. Administration of antimuscarinic drugs to patients with asthma can cause thickening and drying of bronchial secretions, which can result in bronchial plugging. Consequently, although muscarinic antagonists have been used to treat asthma, these drugs have the potential to be detrimental.

Drug Interactions

A number of drugs that are not classified as muscarinic antagonists can nonetheless produce significant muscarinic blockade. These drugs include *antihistamines*, *phenothiazine antipsychotics*, and *tricyclic antidepressants*. Because of their prominent antimuscarinic actions, these drugs can greatly enhance the antimuscarinic effects of atropine and related agents. Accordingly, it is wise to avoid combined use of atropine with other drugs capable of causing muscarinic blockade.

Preparations, Dosage, and Administration

Atropine sulfate is dispensed in oral tablets (0.4 and 0.6 mg); as an ointment or solution for ophthalmic use; and in solution for SC, IM, and IV injection. The average systemic dose for adults is 0.5 mg.

OTHER MUSCARINIC ANTAGONISTS

Scopolamine. Scopolamine is a muscarinic antagonist with actions much like those of atropine, but with two exceptions: (1) whereas therapeutic doses of atropine produce mild CNS excitation, therapeutic doses of scopolamine produce *sedation*, and (2) scopolamine *suppresses emesis and motion sickness*, whereas atropine does not. Principal uses for scopolamine are motion sickness (see Chapter 68), production of cycloplegia and mydriasis for ophthalmic procedures (see Chapter 69), and production of preanesthetic sedation and obstetric amnesia.

Ipratropium Bromide. Ipratropium [Atrovent] is an antimuscarinic drug used to treat asthma and chronic obstructive pulmonary disease. The drug is administered by inhalation, and systemic absorption is minimal. As a result, therapy is not associated with typical antimuscarinic side effects (dry mouth, blurred vision, urinary hesitancy, constipation, and so forth). The pharmacology and applications of ipratropium are discussed further in Chapter 64.

Pirenzepine and Telenzepine. These drugs produce selective blockade of M_1-muscarinic receptors – the subtype of muscarinic receptor involved in regulating the secretion of gastric acid. Both drugs can effectively suppress acid secretion in patients with peptic ulcer disease, but neither is available in the United States. Because these drugs are selective blockers of M_1-muscarinic receptors, the incidence of dry mouth, blurred vision, and other typical antimuscarinic side effects is minimal.

Dicyclomine. This drug is indicated for irritable bowel syndrome (spastic colon, mucous colitis) and functional bowel disorders (diarrhea, hypermotility). Administration may be oral (40 mg 4 times a day) or by IM injection (20 mg 4 times a day). Dicyclomine has many trade names, including Bentyl, Byclomine, Di-Spaz, and Antispas.

Centrally Acting Anticholinergics. Several anticholinergic drugs, including *trihexyphenidyl* [Artane] and *benztropine* [Cogentin], are employed to treat Parkinson's disease and drug-induced parkinsonism. Benefits derive from blockade of muscarinic receptors in the CNS. The centrally acting anticholinergics and their use in parkinsonism are discussed in Chapter 21.

Mydriatic Cycloplegics. Five muscarinic antagonists – *atropine, homatropine, scopolamine, cyclopentolate,* and *tropicamide* – are employed to produce mydriasis and cycloplegia in ophthalmic procedures. These applications are discussed in Chapter 69.

Antisecretory Anticholinergics. A number of muscarinic blockers are available for suppressing gastric acid secretion in patients with peptic ulcer disease. However, since superior antiulcer drugs are available, and since the anticholinergic agents produce significant side effects (dry mouth, blurred vision, urinary retention, and so forth), these drugs are used only rarely. Trade names and dosages for the antisecretory anticholinergics are summarized in Table 13–2. All of these agents are administered orally, and one—glycopyrrolate—may also be administered IM and IV.

TOXICOLOGY OF MUSCARINIC ANTAGONISTS

Sources of Antimuscarinic Poisoning. Sources of poisoning include natural products (e.g., *Atropa belladonna, Datura stramonium*), selective antimuscarinic drugs (e.g., atropine, scopolamine), and other drugs with pronounced antimuscarinic properties (e.g., antihistamines, phenothiazines, tricyclic antidepressants).

Symptoms. Symptoms of antimuscarinic poisoning, which are the direct result of excessive muscarinic blockade, include dry mouth, blurred vision, photophobia, hyperthermia, CNS effects (hallucinations, delirium), and skin that is hot, dry, and flushed. Death results from respiratory depression secondary to blockade of cholinergic receptors in the brain.

Treatment. Treatment consists of (1) minimizing absorption of the antimuscarinic agent, and (2) administering an antidote. Absorption can be re-

Table 13–2. Antisecretory Anticholinergics

Generic Names	Trade Names	Usual Adult Dose (mg)
Anisotropine methylbromide	Valpin 50	50
Clidinium bromide	Quarzan	2.5–5
Glycopyrrolate	Robinul	1–2
Hexocyclium methylsulfate	Tral Filmtabs	25
Isopropamide iodide	Darbid	5–10
Mepenzolate bromide	Cantil	25–50
Methantheline bromide	Banthine	1–2
Methscopolamine bromide	Pamine	2.5–5
Oxyphencyclimine hydrochloride	Daricon	1–2
Oxyphenonium bromide	Antrenyl Bromide	10
Propantheline bromide	Pro-Banthine	7.5–15
Tridihexethyl chloride	Pathilon	25–50

duced by giving an emetic (e.g., syrup of ipecac) followed by activated charcoal. The emetic will induce vomiting, thereby removing unabsorbed poison from the stomach. The charcoal will adsorb poison within the intestine, thereby preventing its absorption into the blood.

The most effective antidote to antimuscarinic poisoning is *physostigmine*, an inhibitor of acetylcholinesterase. By inhibiting cholinesterase, physostigmine causes acetylcholine to accumulate at all cholinergic junctions. As acetylcholine builds up, it competes with the antimuscarinic agent for receptor binding, and thereby reverses excessive muscarinic blockade. The pharmacology of physostigmine is discussed in Chapter 16 (Cholinesterase Inhibitors).

Warning. It is important to differentiate between antimuscarinic poisoning, which can resemble psychosis (hallucinations, delirium), and an actual psychotic episode. Since a true psychotic episode is not ordinarily associated with signs of excessive muscarinic blockade (dry mouth, hyperthermia, dry skin, and so forth), differentiating is not usually difficult. We need to make the differential diagnosis because antipsychotic drugs, which have antimuscarinic properties of their own, will intensify symptoms if given to a victim of antimuscarinic poisoning.

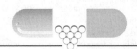

Summary of Major Nursing Implications

BETHANECHOL

 Preadministration Assessment

Therapeutic Goal

Treatment of nonobstructive urinary retention.

Baseline Data

Record fluid intake and output.

Identifying High-Risk Patients

Bethanechol is *contraindicated* for patients with *peptic ulcer disease, urinary tract obstruction, intestinal obstruction, coronary insufficiency, hypotension, asthma,* and *hyperthyroidism.*

 Implementation: Administration

Routes

Oral, SC
Never administer IM or IV!

Administration

Oral. Administer 1 hour before meals or 2 hours after to reduce gastric upset.

Subcutaneous. Subcutaneous doses are much smaller than oral doses. Check SC doses carefully.

Both Routes. Since effects on the intestine and urinary tract can be rapid and dramatic, insure that a bedpan or bathroom is readily accessible.

 Ongoing Evaluation and Interventions

Evaluating Therapeutic Effects

Monitor fluid intake and output to evaluate treatment of urinary retention.

Minimizing Adverse Effects

Excessive muscarinic stimulation can cause salivation, sweating, urinary urgency, bradycardia, and hypotension. Monitor blood pressure and pulse rate. Observe for signs of muscarinic excess and report these to the physician. Inform patients about manifestations of muscarinic excess and advise them to notify the nurse or physician if these occur.

Management of Acute Toxicity

Overdosage produces manifestations of excessive muscarinic stimulation (salivation, sweating, involuntary urination and defecation, bradycardia, severe hypotension). Treat with supportive measures and atropine (SC or IV).

ATROPINE AND OTHER MUSCARINIC ANTAGONISTS

 Preadministration Assessment

Therapeutic Goal

Atropine has many applications, including *preanesthetic medication* and treatment of *bradycardia*, *biliary colic*, *intestinal hypertonicity* and *hypermotility*, and *muscarinic agonist poisoning*.

Identifying High-Risk Patients

Atropine and other muscarinic antagonists are *contraindicated* for patients with *glaucoma*, *intestinal atony*, *urinary tract obstruction*, and *tachycardia*. Use with caution in patients with *asthma*.

 Implementation: Administration

Routes

Atropine is administered PO, IV, IM, and SC.

Administration

Dry mouth from muscarinic blockade may interfere with swallowing. Advise the patient to moisten the mouth by sipping water prior to oral administration.

 Ongoing Evaluation and Interventions

Minimizing Adverse Effects

Dry Mouth (Xerostomia). Decreased salivation can dry the mouth. Inform the patient that xerostomia can be relieved by chewing gum, sucking on hard candy, and sipping fluids.

Blurred Vision. Paralysis of the ciliary muscle may reduce visual acuity. Warn the patient against participation in hazardous activities if vision is impaired.

Photophobia. Muscarinic blockade prevents the pupil from constricting in response to bright light. Keep hospital room lighting low to reduce visual discomfort. Advise the patient to wear sunglasses outdoors.

Urinary Retention. Muscarinic blockade in the bladder and urinary sphincter can cause urinary hesitancy or retention. Advise the patient that urinary retention can be minimized by voiding just prior to taking anticholinergic medication. If urinary retention is severe, catheterization or treatment with bethanechol (a muscarinic agonist) may be required.

Constipation. Reduced tone and motility of the gut may cause constipation. Advise the patient that constipation can be reduced by increasing dietary fiber and fluids. A laxative may be needed if constipation is severe.

Hyperthermia. Suppression of sweating may result in hyperthermia. Advise the patient to avoid vigorous exercise in warm environments.

Tachycardia. Blockade of cardiac muscarinic receptors can accelerate heart rate. Monitor pulse rate and report significant increases to the physician.

Minimizing Adverse Interactions

Antihistamines, tricyclic antidepressants, and *phenothiazines* have prominent antimuscarinic actions. Coadministration of these agents with atropine and other muscarinic antagonists can lead to excessive muscarinic blockade.

Management of Acute Toxicity

Symptoms. Overdosage produces dry mouth, blurred vision, photophobia, hyperthermia, hallucinations, and delirium; the skin becomes hot, dry, and flushed. Poisoning with a muscarinic antagonist must be distinguished from psychosis!

Treatment. Treatment centers on removing ingested poison with an emetic (e.g., syrup of ipecac); adsorbing ingested poison onto activated charcoal; and administering *physostigmine*, an inhibitor of acetylcholinesterase.

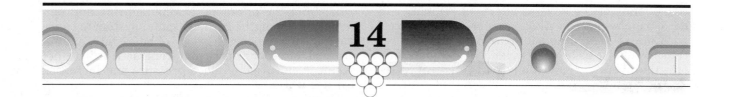

14

Ganglionic Stimulants and Blocking Agents

Nonselective - limited clinical application

GANGLIONIC STIMULANTS
　　Nicotine

GANGLIONIC BLOCKING AGENTS
　　Trimethaphan
　　Mecamylamine

Ganglionic stimulants and blocking agents are drugs that produce their effects by stimulating or blocking nicotinic receptors in autonomic ganglia. Since nicotinic receptors are the same in sympathetic and parasympathetic ganglia, ganglionic drugs alter transmission through all ganglia of the autonomic nervous system. Because ganglionic agents are so nonselective, their clinical applications are very limited.

GANGLIONIC STIMULANTS

Ganglionic stimulants activate nicotinic receptors in autonomic ganglia, causing generation of action potentials in postganglionic neurons. By stimulating postganglionic neurons, these drugs can influence virtually all processes regulated by the sympathetic and the parasympathetic nervous systems. Because they activate both divisions of the autonomic nervous system, ganglionic stimulants have virtually no ability to produce selective effects. Consequently, these drugs have practically no therapeutic value.

NICOTINE

Nicotine is the prototype of the ganglionic stimulants. This compound is of interest primarily be-

135

cause many of the adverse effects of smoking can be attributed to the nicotine content of tobacco. Nicotine is of additional toxicologic interest because of its use as an insecticide. Nicotine has only one therapeutic application: facilitation of withdrawal from smoking.

Mechanism of Action

Nicotine produces its effects by acting on nicotinic receptors. Whether receptor function will be stimulated or inhibited depends upon nicotine dosage. At *low* doses nicotine *stimulates* receptor function, whereas *high* doses cause receptor *blockade*. The amount of nicotine received from cigarettes is relatively low. Accordingly, cigarette smoking causes *stimulation* of nicotinic receptors.

Nicotine can stimulate nicotinic receptors at several locations. Most of nicotine's effects result from stimulation of nicotinic receptors in autonomic ganglia and the adrenal medulla. In addition, nicotine can stimulate nicotinic receptors in the aortic arch, the carotid body, and the central nervous system (CNS). When present at the levels produced by smoking, nicotine has no significant effect on nicotinic receptors of the neuromuscular junction.

Pharmacokinetics

Nicotine in tobacco smoke can be absorbed from the lungs and the mouth. When tobacco smoke is inhaled, absorption of nicotine is nearly complete: between 90% and 98% of nicotine in the lungs enters the blood. Absorption from the mouth is less extensive—but still sufficient to produce pharmacologic effects. Consequently, smokers who do not inhale are still subject to the drug's effects.

Nicotine can cross membranes easily and is widely distributed throughout the body. The drug readily enters breast milk, reaching levels that can be toxic to the nursing infant. It also crosses the placental barrier and can cause fetal harm.

Nicotine is rapidly metabolized to inactive products. Nicotine and its metabolites are excreted by the kidney. The drug's half-life is 1 to 2 hours.

Pharmacologic Effects

The pharmacologic effects discussed in this section are associated with *low* doses of nicotine. These are the effects caused by smoking cigarettes. Responses to *high* doses of nicotine are discussed under *Acute Poisoning*.

Cardiovascular Effects. The cardiovascular effects of nicotine result from stimulating nicotinic receptors in *sympathetic ganglia* and the *adrenal medulla*. Stimulation of these receptors promotes release of norepinephrine from sympathetic nerves and release of epinephrine (and some norepineph-

rine) from the adrenals. Norepinephrine and epinephrine act on the cardiovascular system to cause vasoconstriction, acceleration of heart rate, and increased force of ventricular contraction. The net result is elevation of blood pressure and increased cardiac work.

Of all deaths associated with tobacco use, the greatest number are due to cardiovascular disease. In the United States, smoking-related cardiovascular diseases (e.g., coronary artery disease, peripheral vascular disease, cerebrovascular disease) cause an estimated 225,000 deaths per year. In contrast, smoking-related lung cancer and other cancers cause approximately 145,000 deaths per year—about 60% of the number caused by cardiovascular disorders. Respiratory diseases (e.g., pneumonia, bronchitis, emphysema, chronic airway obstruction) account for another 80,000 deaths annually.

Gastrointestinal Effects. Nicotine influences gastrointestinal function primarily by stimulating nicotinic receptors in *parasympathetic* ganglia. This results in increased secretion of gastric acid and increased tone and motility of gastrointestinal smooth muscle. In addition, nicotine can promote vomiting. Nicotine-induced vomiting results from a complex process that involves nicotinic receptors in the aortic arch, the carotid sinus, and the CNS.

Central Nervous System Effects. Nicotine is a CNS stimulant. The drug stimulates respiration and produces an arousal pattern on the electroencephalogram (EEG). Moderate doses can cause tremors, and high doses can cause convulsions.

Nicotine has multiple psychologic effects. The drug increases alertness, facilitates memory, improves cognitive function, reduces aggression, and suppresses appetite. It may also activate a "pleasure system" located in the limbic system of the brain. These psychologic effects contribute to the addiction potential of nicotine.

Effects During Pregnancy and Lactation. Administration of nicotine during pregnancy can cause fetal harm. Nicotine in breast milk can harm the nursing infant. Accordingly, therapeutic formulations of nicotine (nicotine chewing gum, nicotine transdermal patches) are contraindicated during pregnancy, and their use by nursing mothers is not recommended.

Tolerance and Dependence

Tolerance. Tolerance develops to some effects of nicotine but not to others. Tolerance usually develops to the dizziness, nausea, and vomiting that can occur when individuals first begin smoking. In contrast, *very little tolerance develops to the cardiovascular actions of nicotine*: chronic smokers continue to experience increased blood pressure and increased cardiac work in response to nicotine in tobacco.

Dependence. Chronic cigarette smoking results in dependence. By definition, this means that individuals who discontinue smoking will experience an abstinence syndrome. The tobacco withdrawal syndrome is characterized by craving, nervousness, restlessness, irritability, impatience, increased hostility, insomnia, impaired concentration, increased appetite, and weight gain. Symptoms begin about 24 hours after smoking has ceased, and can last for weeks to months. Since symptoms can be suppressed to some degree by nicotine, at least part of this syndrome can be attributed to dependence upon nicotine itself.

Acute Poisoning

Nicotine is highly toxic. Doses as low as 40 mg can be fatal. The drug's toxicity is attested to by its use in insecticides. Common causes of nicotine poisoning include ingestion of tobacco by children and exposure to nicotine-containing insecticides.

Symptoms. The most prominent symptoms of nicotine poisoning involve the cardiovascular, gastrointestinal (GI), and central nervous systems. Specific symptoms include nausea, salivation, vomiting, diarrhea, cold sweat, disturbed hearing and vision, confusion, and faintness; pulses may be rapid, weak, and irregular. Death results from respiratory paralysis, which is caused by direct effects of nicotine on the muscles of respiration and by effects exerted within the CNS.

Treatment. Management centers on reducing nicotine absorption and supporting respiration; there is no specific antidote to nicotine poisoning. To minimize absorption, patients should be given syrup of ipecac followed by activated charcoal. Ipecac induces vomiting, thereby removing any nicotine remaining in the stomach. Activated charcoal adsorbs nicotine, thereby preventing any nicotine that remains in the GI tract from being absorbed into the blood. If respiration is depressed, ventilatory assistance should be provided. Since nicotine undergoes rapid metabolic inactivation, recovery from the acute phase of poisoning can occur within hours.

Therapeutic Use

The Food and Drug Administration has approved the use of nicotine as an aid to individuals who are trying to quit smoking. Prior to this approval, nicotine had virtually no therapeutic applications. Nicotine can facilitate cessation of smoking by suppressing those aspects of the tobacco withdrawal syndrome that are due to the absence of nicotine. Two nicotine formulations are available: *nicotine chewing gum* and *nicotine transdermal patches*. Unfortunately, long-term success rates with both formulations have been unimpressive.

Nicotine Chewing Gum (Nicotine Polacrilex)

Description. Nicotine chewing gum [Nicorette] is composed of a gum base plus nicotine polacrilex, an ion exchange resin to which nicotine is bound. The gum must be chewed to release the nicotine. Following its release, nicotine is absorbed across the oral mucosa into the systemic circulation.

Adverse Effects. The most common adverse effects are mouth and throat soreness, jaw muscle ache, eructation (belching), and hiccoughs. Use of an optimal chewing technique should minimize all of these effects. Nicotine gum and all other nicotine-containing products should be avoided during pregnancy and lactation.

Dosage and Administration. Nicotine gum is available in two dosage strengths: 2 mg/piece and 4 mg/piece. Patients should be advised to chew the gum slowly and intermittently for about 30 minutes. Rapid chewing can release too much nicotine at one time, resulting in effects similar to those of excessive smoking (e.g., nausea, throat irritation, hiccoughs). Since foods and beverages can reduce nicotine absorption, patients should not eat or drink for 15 minutes before chewing and while chewing.

Dosing is individualized and based on the degree of nicotine dependence. For initial therapy, patients with low-to-moderate nicotine dependence should use the 2-mg strength; highly dependent patients (those who smoke more than 25 cigarettes a day) should use the 4-mg strength. The average adult dosage is 9 to 12 pieces of gum/day. The maximum daily dosage is 30 pieces of the 2-mg strength or 20 pieces of the 4-mg strength. Experience indicates that dosing on a fixed schedule (one piece every 2 to 3 hours) is more effective than PRN dosing for achieving abstinence.

After 3 months without cigarettes, patients should discontinue nicotine use. Withdrawal should be done gradually. Use of nicotine gum beyond 6 months is not recommended.

Nicotine Transdermal Systems

Description. Nicotine transdermal systems are nicotine-containing adhesive patches that, after application to the skin, slowly release their nicotine content. The nicotine is absorbed into the skin and then into the blood, producing steady blood levels of the drug.

Four systems are available: Habitrol, Nicoderm, Nicotrol, and ProStep. As indicated in Table 14–1, each is available in two or three sizes. The larger patches release larger amounts of nicotine.

Dosage and Administration. Nicotine transdermal systems are applied once a day to clean, dry, non-hairy skin of the upper body or upper

Table 14–1. Nicotine Transdermal Systems

Trade Name	Surface Area (cm^2)	Nicotine Content (mg)	Dose Absorbed	Duration of Use For Each Patch	Total
Habitrol	30	52.5	21 mg/24 hr	First 4–8 wk	8–12 wk
	20	35.0	14 mg/24 hr	Next 2–4 wk	
	10	17.5	7 mg/24 hr	Last 2–4 wk	
Nicoderm	22	114.0	21 mg/24 hr	First 4–8 wk	8–12 wk
	15	78.0	14 mg/24 hr	Next 2–4 wk	
	7	36.0	7 mg/24 hr	Last 2–4 wk	
Nicotrol	30	24.9	15 mg/16 hr	First 10–12 wk	14–20 wk
	20	16.6	10 mg/16 hr	Next 2–4 wk	
	10	8.3	5 mg/16 hr	Last 2–4 wk	
ProStep	7	30.0	22 mg/24 hr	First 4–8 wk	6–12 wk
	3.5	15.0	11 mg/24 hr	Next 2–4 wk	

arm. The site should be changed daily and not reused for at least 1 week. With three products (Habitrol, Nicoderm, and ProStep) the patch is left in place for 24 hours and then immediately replaced with a fresh patch. With one product (Nicotrol) the patch is applied in the morning and removed 16 hours later at bedtime. This pattern is intended to simulate nicotine dosing produced by smoking.

Most patients begin treatment with a large patch and then progress to smaller patches over a period of weeks (see Table 14–1). Certain patients (those with cardiovascular disease, those who weigh less than 100 pounds, or those who smoke less than one-half pack of cigarettes a day) should begin treatment with a smaller patch.

Adverse Effects. Short-lived erythema, itching, and burning occur under the patch in 35% to 50% of users. In 14% to 17% of users, persistent erythema occurs, lasting up to 24 hours after patch removal. Patients who experience severe, persistent local reactions (e.g., severe erythema, itching, edema) should discontinue the patch and contact the physician. Nicotine patches and all other nicotine-containing products should be avoided during pregnancy and lactation.

GANGLIONIC BLOCKING AGENTS

Ganglionic blocking agents produce a broad spectrum of pharmacologic effects. Because they lack selectivity, the ganglionic blockers have limited applications. These drugs are used only to lower blood pressure—and then only in special circumstances. In the United States, two ganglionic blockers are available: *trimethaphan* and *mecamylamine*. Trimethaphan will serve as our prototype.

TRIMETHAPHAN

Mechanism of Action

Trimethaphan [Arfonad] interrupts impulse transmission through ganglia of the autonomic nervous system. The drug blocks transmission by competitive antagonism with acetylcholine at ganglionic nicotinic receptors. Since the nicotinic receptors of sympathetic and parasympathetic ganglia are the same, trimethaphan blocks transmission at all autonomic ganglia. By blocking all ganglionic transmission, the drug can, in effect, shut down the entire autonomic nervous system, thereby depriving organs of all autonomic regulation.

In addition to blocking ganglionic transmission, trimethaphan has two other actions: (1) vasodilation (from a direct effect on blood vessels) and (2) release of histamine. Both actions tend to reduce blood pressure.

Pharmacologic Effects

Since trimethaphan acts by depriving organs of autonomic regulation, to predict the drug's effects, we need to know how the autonomic nervous system is affecting specific organs at the time of drug administration. That is, we need to know which branch of the autonomic nervous system is providing the predominant tone to specific organs. By knowing the source of predominant tone to an organ, and by knowing that ganglionic blockade will remove that tone, we can predict the effects that ganglionic blockade will produce.

Table 14–2 indicates (1) the major structures innervated by autonomic nerves, (2) the branch of the autonomic nervous system that provides the predominant tone to those structures, and (3) the responses to ganglionic blockade. As the table shows, *the predominant autonomic tone to most organs is provided by the parasympathetic nervous system.* The *sympathetic* branch provides the predominant tone only to *sweat glands, arterioles,* and *veins.*

Since the parasympathetic nervous system provides the predominant tone to most organs, and since the parasympathetic nervous system works through muscarinic receptors to influence organ function, *most responses to ganglionic blockade resemble those produced by muscarinic antagonists.* These responses include dry mouth, blurred vision, photophobia, urinary retention, constipation, tachycardia, and anhidrosis.

In addition to their parasympatholytic effects, ganglionic blockers produce *hypotension*. These drugs lower blood pressure by causing dilation of arterioles and veins. Vasodilation results primarily from blocking sympathetic nerve traffic to vascular smooth muscle.

Pharmacokinetics

Trimethaphan is a quaternary ammonium compound and therefore always carries a positive charge. As a result, this drug cannot readily cross membranes. Accordingly, trimethaphan must be administered parenterally. The drug has a brief duration of action and is eliminated by renal excretion.

Therapeutic Uses

Hypertensive Crisis. A hypertensive crisis is a condition in which blood pressure has risen so high as to constitute an

Location	Predominant Tone	Response to Ganglionic Blockade
Table 14–2. Predominant Autonomic Tone and Responses to Ganglionic Blockade		
Salivary glands	Parasympathetic	Dry mouth
Ciliary muscle	Parasympathetic	Blurred vision
Iris sphincter	Parasympathetic	Photophobia (from mydriasis)
Urinary bladder	Parasympathetic	Urinary retention
Gastrointestinal tract	Parasympathetic	Constipation
Heart	Parasympathetic	Tachycardia
Sweat glands	Sympathetic*	Anhidrosis
Arterioles	Sympathetic	Hypotension (from vasodilation)
Veins	Sympathetic	Orthostatic hypotension (from pooling of blood in veins secondary to venous dilation)

*Sympathetic nerves to sweat glands release acetylcholine as their transmitter, which acts at muscarinic receptors on the sweat glands.

immediate danger. Trimethaphan is one of several drugs that can be used to reduce blood pressure in patients with acute, severe hypertension.

Controlled Hypotension in Surgery. Trimethaphan can produce controlled hypotension during surgery. Controlled reductions in blood pressure can (1) reduce blood loss and (2) facilitate surgery by decreasing the amount of blood in the surgical field.

Adverse Effects

Trimethaphan produces a broad spectrum of undesired effects, all of which are the predictable consequence of generalized inhibition of the autonomic nervous system. Side effects fall into two groups: (1) antimuscarinic effects (caused by parasympathetic blockade), and (2) hypotension (caused largely by sympathetic blockade).

Antimuscarinic Effects. Blockade of parasympathetic ganglia produces typical antimuscarinic responses: dry mouth, blurred vision, photophobia, urinary retention, constipation, tachycardia, and anhidrosis. Antimuscarinic responses are discussed in detail in Chapter 13.

Hypotension. By causing arteriolar dilation, ganglionic blockers can produce a profound reduction in blood pressure. Excessive hypotension can be the most serious adverse effect of ganglionic blockade. If blood pressure drops too low, it may be necessary to administer a vasoconstrictor (e.g., norepinephrine) to restore pressure to a safe level.

Orthostatic Hypotension. Orthostatic hypotension is defined as a drop in blood pressure that occurs upon assuming an upright posture. Ganglionic blockers promote orthostatic hypotension by dilating *veins*. Venous dilation causes blood to "pool" in veins when the patient moves from a recumbent to an upright posture. As a result, return of blood to the heart is significantly reduced, causing a reduction in cardiac output and a subsequent fall in blood pressure.

Since much of the hypotension that results from ganglionic blockade is dependent upon posture, patients who are supine or in Trendelenburg's position (head down) experience less hypotension than patients in reverse Trendelenburg's position (head up). Consequently, the blood pressure of patients receiving tri-

methaphan can be raised or lowered (within limits) by the simple expedient of changing body position: if blood pressure is too low, the head should be lowered and the feet raised; if blood pressure is too high, the head should be raised and the feet lowered.

Preparations, Dosage, and Administration

Trimethaphan camsylate [Arfonad] is available in solution (50 mg/ml) for IV infusion. The drug must be diluted to 1 mg/ml with 5% dextrose prior to use. The average infusion rate is 3 to 4 ml/min (3 to 4 mg/min). The rate is adjusted to achieve the desired reduction in blood pressure. No other drugs should be added to the infusion fluid.

MECAMYLAMINE

Mecamylamine is a ganglionic-blocking agent with pharmacologic properties much like those of trimethaphan. The principal difference between the two drugs is pharmacokinetic: mecamylamine can cross membranes with ease, whereas trimethaphan cannot. Because it crosses membranes, mecamylamine can be administered orally. In addition, the drug can cross the blood-brain barrier to produce CNS effects (mental aberrations, weakness, fatigue, and sedation).

Therapeutic Use. Mecamylamine is indicated for *essential hypertension* in selected patients. The drug is reserved for those rare cases in which blood pressure cannot be reduced with more desirable medications.

Adverse Effects. The principal concern is *orthostatic hypotension*. Patients should be informed that hypotension can be minimized by moving slowly when assuming an upright posture. Patients should also be warned that hypotension can cause fainting and, consequently, they should sit or lie down if they become dizzy or lightheaded. In addition to hypotension, mecamylamine can cause typical antimuscarinic effects (dry mouth, blurred vision, photophobia, urinary retention, tachycardia, constipation, anhidrosis).

Preparations, Dosage, and Administration. Mecamylamine hydrochloride [Inversine] is available in 2.5-mg tablets for oral use. The dosage is 2.5 mg twice daily initially and then gradually increased until the target blood pressure has been achieved. The average daily maintenance dose is 25 mg.

15

Neuromuscular Blocking Agents

Neuromuscular blocking agents are drugs that competitively block cholinergic receptors on skeletal muscles and thereby cause muscle relaxation. These drugs are used to produce muscle relaxation during surgery, endotracheal intubation, mechanical ventilation, and other procedures.

CONTROL OF MUSCLE CONTRACTION

Before we discuss the neuromuscular blockers themselves, it will be helpful to review physiologic control of muscle contraction. In particular, we need to understand *excitation-contraction coupling*, the process by which an action potential in a motor neuron leads to contraction of a muscle.

Basic Concepts: Polarization, Depolarization, and Repolarization

The concepts of *polarization*, *depolarization*, and *repolarization* are important to our understanding of muscle contraction as well as the neuromuscular blockers. In *resting* muscle there is uneven distribution of electrical charge between the inner and outer surfaces of the cell membrane. As shown in Figure 15–1, positive charges cover the outer surface of the membrane and negative charges cover the inner surface. Because of this uneven charge

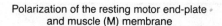

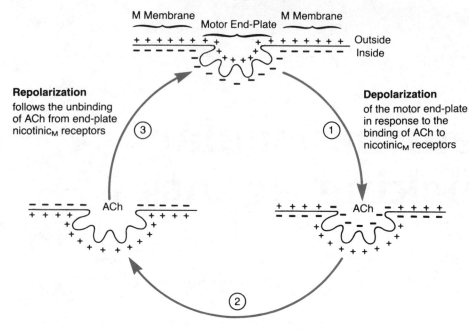

Figure 15–1. The depolarization-repolarization cycle of the motor end-plate and muscle membrane.

distribution, the resting membrane is said to be *polarized*.

When the membrane *depolarizes,* positive charges move from outside the membrane to the inside. So many positive charges move inward that the inside of the membrane becomes more positive than the outside (see Fig. 15–1).

Under physiologic conditions, depolarization of the muscle membrane is followed almost instantaneously by *repolarization*. Repolarization is accomplished by pumping positively charged ions out of the cell. Repolarization restores the original resting membrane state, with positive charges on the outer surface and negative charges on the inner surface.

Steps in Muscle Contraction

The steps leading to muscle contraction are summarized in Figure 15–2. The process begins with the arrival of an action potential at the terminal of a motor neuron, causing acetylcholine (ACh) to be released into the subneural space. Acetylcholine then binds reversibly to nicotinic_M receptors on the motor end-plate (a specialized region of the muscle membrane that contains the receptors for ACh) and causes the end-plate to *depolarize*. This depolarization initiates a muscle action potential (i.e., a wave of depolarization that spreads rapidly over the entire muscle membrane), which, in turn, triggers the release of calcium from the sarcoplasmic

reticulum (SR) of the muscle. This calcium permits the interaction of actin and myosin, thereby causing contraction. Very rapidly, ACh dissociates from the motor end-plate, the motor end-plate repolarizes, the muscle membrane repolarizes, and calcium is taken back up into the SR. Because there is no longer any calcium available to support the interaction of actin and myosin, the muscle relaxes.

Sustained muscle contraction requires a continuous series of motor neuron action potentials. These action potentials cause repeated release of ACh, which causes repeated activation of nicotinic receptors on the motor end-plate. As a result, the end-plate goes through repeating cycles of depolarization and repolarization, which results in sufficient release of calcium to sustain contraction. If, for some reason, the motor end-plate fails to repolarize, that is, if the end-plate remains in a *depolarized* state, the signal for calcium release will stop, calcium will undergo immediate reuptake into the SR, and contraction will cease.

CLASSIFICATION OF NEUROMUSCULAR BLOCKING AGENTS

The neuromuscular blockers can be classified according to *mechanism of action* and *time course of*

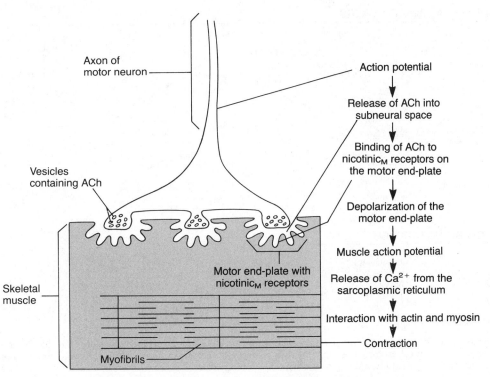

Figure 15–2. Steps in excitation-contraction coupling.

action. When classified by mechanism of action, these drugs fall into two categories: *nondepolarizing agents* and *depolarizing agents*. When classified by time course of action, these drugs fall into four categories: *long-acting, intermediate-acting, short-acting,* and *ultrashort-acting*.

NONDEPOLARIZING NEUROMUSCULAR BLOCKING AGENTS

In the United States, nine nondepolarizing neuromuscular blockers are approved for clinical use. All share the same mechanism of action. The principal differences among these drugs relate to cardiovascular effects and duration of action.

TUBOCURARINE

Tubocurarine is the oldest nondepolarizing neuromuscular blocker and will serve as our prototype for the group.

The pharmacologic powers of tubocurarine were known to primitive hunters long before coming to the attention of modern scientists. Tubocurarine is one of several active principles found in *curare*, an arrow poison used for hunting by South American Indians. When shot into a monkey or other small animal, curare-tipped arrows cause relaxation (pa-

ralysis) of skeletal muscles. Death results from paralyzing the muscles of respiration.

The clinical utility of tubocurarine is based on the same action that is useful in hunting: production of skeletal muscle relaxation. Relaxation of skeletal muscles is helpful in patients undergoing surgery, endotracheal intubation, mechanical ventilation, and other procedures.

Chemistry

Tubocurarine and all other neuromuscular blocking agents contain a *quaternary nitrogen atom* (Fig. 15–3). As a result, these drugs always carry a positive charge, and therefore cannot readily cross membranes.

The inability to cross membranes has three clinical consequences. First, neuromuscular blockers cannot be administered orally. Instead, they must all be administered parenterally (almost always IV). Second, these drugs cannot cross the blood-brain barrier and, hence, have no effect on the central nervous system (CNS). Third, neuromuscular blockers cannot readily cross the placenta. Hence, effects on the fetus are minimal.

Mechanism of Action

Tubocurarine acts by competing with ACh for binding to nicotinic$_M$ receptors on the motor end-plate (Fig. 15–4). Since tubocurarine does not activate these receptors, binding does not result in contraction. Muscle relaxation will persist as long

NONDEPOLARIZING BLOCKERS

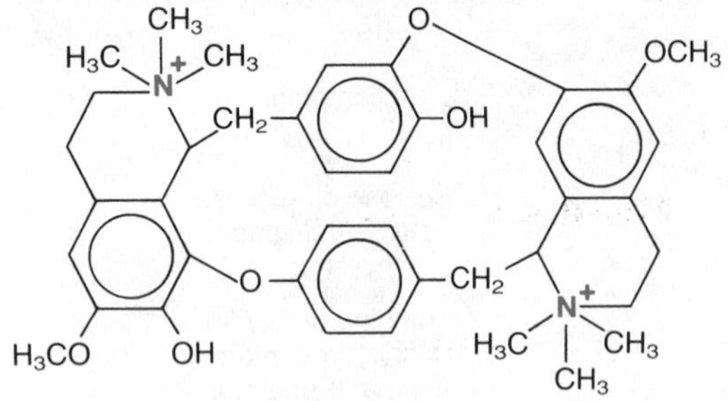

Tubocurarine

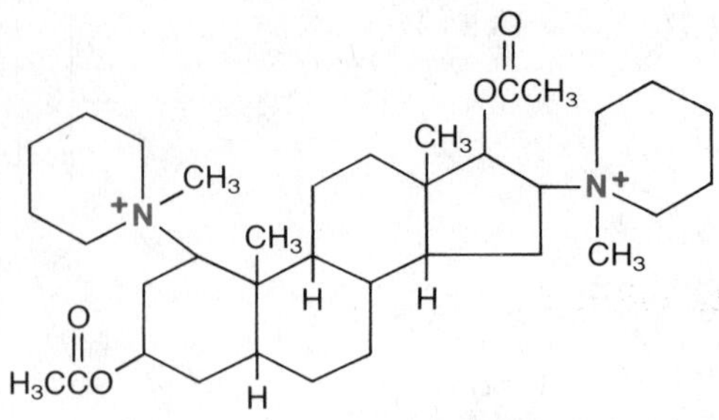

Pancuronium

DEPOLARIZING BLOCKER

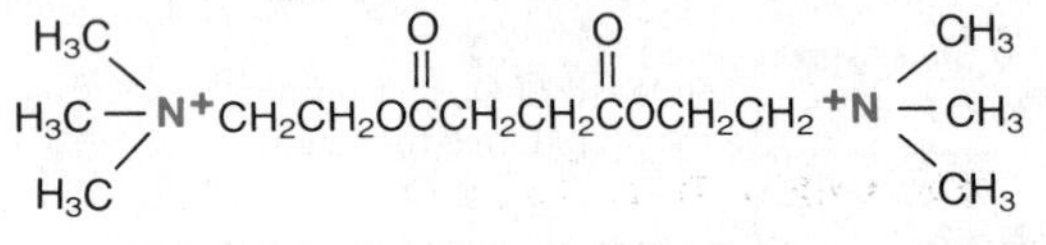

Succinylcholine

Figure 15–3. Structural formulas of representative neuromuscular blocking agents. Note that all of these agents contain quaternary nitrogen atoms and therefore cross membranes poorly. Consequently, these drugs must be administered parenterally and have little effect on the central nervous system or the developing fetus.

as the amount of tubocurarine at the neuromuscular junction (NMJ) is sufficient to prevent receptor occupation by ACh. Muscle function can be restored by eliminating tubocurarine from the body or by increasing the amount of ACh at the NMJ.

Pharmacologic Effects

Muscle Relaxation. The primary effect of tubocurarine is relaxation of skeletal muscles. Muscle relaxation produces a state of *flaccid paralysis.*

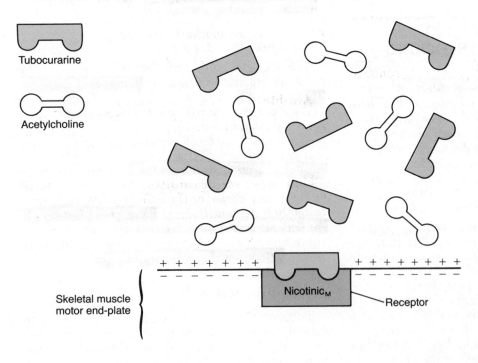

Tubocurarine

Acetylcholine

Skeletal muscle motor end-plate

Nicotinic$_M$

Receptor

Figure 15–4. Mechanism of nondepolarizing neuromuscular blockade. Tubocurarine competes with ACh for binding to nicotinic$_N$ receptors on the motor end-plate. Binding of tubocurarine does not depolarize the end-plate, and therefore causes no contraction. At the same time, the presence of tubocurarine prevents ACh from binding to the receptor to produce contraction.

Although tubocurarine can paralyze all skeletal muscles, not all muscles are affected at the same time. The first muscles to become paralyzed are the levator muscle of the eyelid and the muscles of mastication. Paralysis occurs next in muscles of the limbs, abdomen, and glottis. The last muscles affected are the muscles of respiration—the intercostals and the diaphragm.

Hypotension. Tubocurarine can lower blood pressure by two mechanisms: (1) release of histamine, and (2) partial ganglionic blockade. Histamine lowers blood pressure by promoting vasodilation. Ganglionic blockade lowers blood pressure by decreasing sympathetic tone to arterioles and veins. Tubocurarine suppresses ganglionic transmission by causing partial blockade of nicotinic$_N$ receptors in autonomic ganglia.

Central Nervous System. As noted above, tubocurarine and the other neuromuscular blocking agents are unable to cross the blood-brain barrier. Consequently these drugs have no effect on the CNS. Please note: *neuromuscular blockers do not diminish consciousness or perception of pain—even when administered in doses that produce complete paralysis.*

Pharmacokinetics

Paralysis develops rapidly (in minutes) following IV injection. Peak effects persist for 35 to 60 minutes and then decline. Complete recovery may take several hours. Tubocurarine is eliminated by a combination of hepatic metabolism and renal excretion.

Therapeutic Uses

Tubocurarine can be used for muscle relaxation during surgery, mechanical ventilation, endotracheal intubation, and electroconvulsive therapy. These applications are discussed later under *Therapeutic Uses of Neuromuscular Blocking Agents.*

Adverse Effects

The principal adverse effects of tubocurarine concern the respiratory and cardiovascular systems.

Respiratory Depression. Paralysis of respiratory muscles can produce respiratory arrest. Because of this risk, facilities for artificial ventilation must be immediately available. Patients must be monitored closely and continuously. When tubocurarine is withdrawn, vital signs must be monitored until muscle function has fully recovered.

Cardiovascular Effects. As noted above, tubocurarine can cause *hypotension* secondary to histamine release and partial ganglionic blockade. In

addition, the drug can cause *bradycardia, dysrhythmias,* and *cardiac arrest.* The mechanism underlying these latter effects is not clear.

Precautions and Contraindications

Myasthenia Gravis. Neuromuscular blocking agents must be used with special care in patients with myasthenia gravis, a condition characterized by skeletal muscle weakness. The cause of weakness is a reduction in the number of nicotinic$_M$ receptors on the motor end-plate. Because receptor number is reduced, neuromuscular blockade occurs very readily in these patients; doses that would have a minimal effect on other patients can produce complete paralysis in patients with myasthenia. Accordingly, dosing must be done with great care. Myasthenia gravis is discussed further in Chapter 16.

Electrolyte Disturbances. Responses to tubocurarine can be altered by electrolyte abnormalities. For example, low potassium levels can enhance paralysis, whereas high potassium levels can reduce paralysis. Because electrolyte status can influence the depth of neuromuscular blockade, an effort should be made to maintain normal electrolyte balance.

Drug Interactions

Tubocurarine can interact with many other drugs. Interactions of primary interest are discussed below.

General Anesthetics. All inhalation anesthetics produce some degree of skeletal muscle relaxation and can thereby enhance the actions of tubocurarine and the other neuromuscular blockers. Consequently, when general anesthetics and neuromuscular blockers are combined (as they often are), the dosage of the neuromuscular blocker should be reduced so as to avoid excessive neuromuscular blockade.

Antibiotics. Several antibiotics can intensify responses to neuromuscular blockers. Included in this group are *aminoglycosides* (e.g., gentamicin), *tetracyclines,* and certain other nonpenicillin antibiotics.

Cholinesterase Inhibitors. Cholinesterase inhibitors can *decrease* the effects of tubocurarine and other *nondepolarizing* neuromuscular blockers. (As discussed later in the chapter, cholinesterase inhibitors have the opposite effect on responses to succinylcholine, a *depolarizing* neuromuscular blocker.)

How do cholinesterase inhibitors decrease the effects of tubocurarine? Recall that nondepolarizing blockers compete with ACh for binding to nicotinic$_M$ receptors. By decreasing the degradation of ACh, cholinesterase inhibitors increase the amount of ACh available to compete with tubocurarine for receptor binding. As more ACh (and less tubocurarine) occupies nicotinic$_M$ receptors, the degree of neuromuscular blockade will decline.

The ability of cholinesterase inhibitors to decrease responses to nondepolarizing neuromuscular blockers has two clinical applications: (1) management of overdosage with a nondepolarizing neuromuscular blocker, and (2) reversal of neuromuscular blockade following surgery and other procedures.

Toxicology

Overdosage with tubocurarine has three major effects: (1) prolonged apnea, (2) massive histamine release, and (3) cardiovascular collapse. Apnea is managed with respiratory support along with a cholinesterase inhibitor (e.g., neostigmine) to reverse neuromuscular blockade. Antihistamines are given to counteract histamine. Cardiovascular toxicity must be assessed and treated as appropriate.

Preparations, Dosage, and Administration

Tubocurarine is always administered parenterally. The usual route is intravenous. Intramuscular injections are employed on occasion.

Because of their potential for harm, neuromuscular blocking agents are administered only by clinicians with special training in their use. Whenever these drugs are given, facilities for artificial respiration and management of cardiovascular complications must be at hand.

Tubocurarine is dispensed in solution (20 units/ml) for IM and IV injection. The dosage depends on the indication. A typical dosage for the adult surgical patient is 40 to 60 units IV at the time of the initial incision, followed by 20 to 30 units a few minutes later. During long operations, additional doses of 20 to 30 units may be administered as needed.

OTHER NONDEPOLARIZING NEUROMUSCULAR BLOCKERS

In addition to tubocurarine, eight other nondepolarizing blockers are approved for use in the United States. Like tubocurarine, these drugs cause muscle relaxation by competing with acetylcholine at nicotinic$_M$ receptors on the motor endplate. Differences among these drugs relate primarily to time course of action (Table 15–1) and cardiovascular effects. With all of these drugs, respiratory depression secondary to neuromuscular blockade is the major concern. Respiratory depression can be reversed with a cholinesterase inhibitor.

Long-Acting Agents

Metocurine. Metocurine [Metubine] is a semisynthetic derivative of tubocurarine with a similar time course of action. The drug is used primarily for muscle relaxation during surgery. Metocurine causes less histamine release than tubocurarine and less ganglionic blockade. As a result, the risk of hypotension is low.

Doxacurium. Doxacurium [Nuromax] is a long-acting neuromuscular blocker used for muscle relaxation during general anesthesia and intubation. The drug is eliminated by the kidneys and, hence, actions will be prolonged in patients with renal failure. Doxacurium is devoid of adverse cardiovascular effects.

Pipercuronium. Pipercuronium [Arduan] is indicated for muscle relaxation during surgery and intubation. Because its effects are long-lasting, pipercuronium is not recommended for procedures of less than 90 minutes' duration. Pipercuronium does not release histamine, does not cause vagal block, and is generally free of adverse cardiovascular effects. Duration of paralysis may be prolonged and unpredictable in obese patients and in those with renal failure.

Intermediate-Acting Agents

Atracurium. Atracurium [Tracrium] is approved for muscle relaxation during surgery, intubation, and mechanical ventilation. The drug can cause hypotension secondary to histamine release. Atracurium may be desirable for patients with renal or hepatic dysfunction since these disorders do not prolong the drug's effects.

Gallamine. Gallamine [Flaxedil] is used for muscle relaxation during general anesthesia and mechanical ventilation. The drug does not cause histamine release or ganglionic blockade and, therefore, does not induce hypotension. Gallamine can cause tachycardia by blocking vagal input to the heart. The drug is excreted entirely by the kidneys; hence, effects will be prolonged in patients with renal failure.

Pancuronium. Pancuronium [Pavulon] is approved for muscle relaxation during general anesthesia, intubation, and mechanical ventilation. The drug does not cause histamine release, ganglionic blockade, or hypotension. Vagolytic effects may produce tachycardia. Elimination is primarily renal.

Vecuronium. Vecuronium [Norcuron], an analogue of pancuronium, is used for muscle relaxation during general anesthesia and intubation. The drug does not produce ganglionic or vagal block and does not release histamine. Consequently, cardiovascular effects are minimal. Vecuronium is excreted primarily in the bile. Hence, paralysis may be prolonged in patients with liver dysfunction. Paralysis may also be prolonged in obese patients.

Short-Acting Agent

Mivacurium. Mivacurium [Mivacron] is the shortest-acting *nondepolarizing* neuromuscular blocker. Paralysis is maximal 2 to 5 minutes after IV injection and persists for 10 to 15 minutes. The only neuromuscular blocker with a shorter duration of action is succinylcholine, a *depolarizing* neuromuscular blocker. Like succinylcholine, mivacurium is metabolized by plasma cholinesterases. As a result, effects will be prolonged in patients with low levels of that enzyme. Mivacurium can cause cutaneous facial flushing secondary to histamine release. Other cardiovascular effects are minimal.

DEPOLARIZING NEUROMUSCULAR BLOCKING AGENTS

SUCCINYLCHOLINE

Succinylcholine, an ultrashort-acting drug, is the only depolarizing neuromuscular blocker in

Table 15–1. Neuromuscular Blockers: Time Course of Action*

Generic Name [Trade Name]	Route	Time to Maximum Paralysis (min)	Duration of Effective Paralysis (min)	Time to Nearly Full Spontaneous Recovery†
Long-acting				
Doxacurium [Nuromax]	IV	4–10	100	Hours
Metocurine [Metubine]	IV	3–5	25–90	Hours
Pipercuronium [Arduan]	IV	3–5	90–120	Hours
Tubocurarine	IV, IM‡	2–5	35–60	Hours
Intermediate-acting				
Atracurium [Tracrium]	IV	2–5	20–35	60–70 min
Gallamine [Flaxedil]	IV	2–5	15–30	—
Pancuronium [Pavulon]	IV	3–4	35–45	60–70 min
Vecuronium [Norcuron]	IV	3–5	25–30	45–60 min
Short-acting				
Mivacurium [Mivacron]	IV	2–5	10–15	21–34 min
Ultrashort-acting				
Succinylcholine [Anectine, others]	IV, IM‡	1	4–6	—

*Time course of action can vary widely with dosage and route of administration. The values presented are for an average adult dose administered as a single IV injection.
†Because spontaneous recovery can take a long time, recovery from the *nondepolarizing* agents (all of the drugs listed except succinylcholine) is often accelerated by giving a cholinesterase inhibitor.
‡Intramuscular administration is rare.

clinical use. This drug differs from the nondepolarizing blockers with regard to mechanism of action, mode of elimination, interaction with cholinesterase inhibitors, and management of toxicity.

Mechanism of Action

Succinylcholine produces a state known as depolarizing neuromuscular blockade. Like acetylcholine, succinylcholine binds to nicotinic$_M$ receptors on the motor end-plate and thereby causes depolarization. This depolarization produces transient muscle contractions (fasciculations). Then, instead of dissociating rapidly from the receptor, succinylcholine remains bound. By remaining bound, the drug prevents the end-plate from repolarizing. That is, succinylcholine maintains the end-plate in a state of *constant depolarization.* Since the end-plate must repeatedly depolarize and repolarize to maintain muscle contraction, succinylcholine's ability to keep the end-plate depolarized causes paralysis (following the brief initial period of contraction). Paralysis will persist until plasma levels of succinylcholine decline, thereby allowing the drug to dissociate from its receptors.

Pharmacologic Effects

Muscle Relaxation. The muscle-relaxant effects of succinylcholine are much like those of tubocurarine; both drugs produce a state of flaccid paralysis. However, despite this similarity, it should be noted that the effects of succinylcholine differ from those of tubocurarine in two ways: paralysis from succinylcholine (1) is preceded by transient contractions and (2) abates much more rapidly.

Central Nervous System. Like tubocurarine, succinylcholine has no effect on the CNS. The drug can produce complete paralysis without decreasing consciousness or the ability to feel pain.

Pharmacokinetics

Succinylcholine has an extremely short duration of action. Paralysis peaks about 1 minute after IV injection and fades completely 4 to 10 minutes later.

Paralysis is brief because succinylcholine is rapidly degraded by *pseudocholinesterase*, an enzyme present in the plasma. (This enzyme is called pseudocholinesterase to distinguish it from "true" cholinesterase, the enzyme present at synapses where ACh is the transmitter.) Because of its presence in plasma, pseudocholinesterase is also known as *plasma cholinesterase.* In most individuals, pseudocholinesterase is highly active and can eliminate succinylcholine in minutes.

Therapeutic Uses

Succinylcholine is used primarily for muscle relaxation during endotracheal intubation, electroconvulsive therapy, endoscopy, and other short procedures. Because of its brief duration of action, succinylcholine is less desirable than tubocurarine for use during surgery and mechanical ventilation. Clinical applications are discussed further under *Therapeutic Uses of Neuromuscular Blocking Agents.*

Adverse Effects

Prolonged Apnea in Patients with Low Pseudocholinesterase Activity. A few people, because of their genetic makeup, produce a form of pseudocholinesterase that has extremely low activity. As a result, they are unable to degrade succinylcholine rapidly. If succinylcholine is given to these people, paralysis can persist for hours, instead of just a few minutes. Not surprisingly, succinylcholine is contraindicated for these individuals.

Patients suspected of having low pseudocholinesterase activity should be tested for this possibility before receiving full succinylcholine doses. Pseudocholinesterase activity can be assessed by direct measurement of a blood sample or by administering a tiny test dose of succinylcholine. If the test dose produces muscle relaxation that is unexpectedly intense and prolonged, it can be assumed that pseudocholinesterase activity is low.

Malignant Hyperthermia. Malignant hyperthermia is a rare and potentially fatal condition that can be triggered by succinylcholine (and all inhalation anesthetics). The condition is characterized by muscle rigidity associated with a profound elevation of temperature—sometimes to as high as 43°C. Temperature becomes elevated as a result of excessive and uncontrolled metabolic activity in muscle. Left untreated, the condition can rapidly prove fatal. Malignant hyperthermia is a genetically determined reaction that has an incidence of about 1 in 25,000. Individuals with a family history of the reaction should not receive succinylcholine.

Treatment of malignant hyperthermia includes (1) immediate discontinuation of succinylcholine and the accompanying anesthetic, (2) cooling of the patient with ice or an infusion of iced saline, and (3) administering *dantrolene*, a drug that stops heat generation by acting directly on skeletal muscle to reduce its metabolic activity. The pharmacology of dantrolene is discussed in Chapter 23.

Postoperative Muscle Pain. Between 10% and 70% of patients receiving succinylcholine experience postoperative muscle pain, most commonly in the neck, shoulder, and back. Pain develops 12 to 24 hours after surgery and may persist for several hours or days. The cause of pain may be the muscle contractions that occur during the initial phase of succinylcholine action.

Drug Interactions

Cholinesterase Inhibitors. These drugs *potentiate* the effects of succinylcholine. Potentiation occurs because cholinesterase inhibitors decrease the activity of pseudocholinesterase, the enzyme that inactivates succinylcholine. It should be noted that the effect of cholinesterase inhibitors on succinylcholine is opposite to the effect of these drugs on *nondepolarizing* neuromuscular blockade.

Antibiotics. The effects of succinylcholine, like those of tubocurarine, can be potentiated by certain antibiotics, including *aminoglycosides*, *tetracyclines*, and certain other nonpenicillin antibiotics.

Toxicology

Overdosage can produce prolonged apnea. Since there is no specific antidote to succinylcholine poisoning, management is purely supportive. Recall that with tubocurarine overdosage, paralysis can be reversed with a cholinesterase inhibitor. Since cholinesterase inhibitors delay the degradation of succinylcholine, use of these agents would prolong—not reverse—succinylcholine toxicity.

Preparations, Dosage, and Administration

Succinylcholine chloride [Anectine, Quelicin, Sucostrin] is available in solution and as a powder. The drug is usually administered IV but can also be injected IM. Solutions of succinylcholine are unstable and should be used within 24 hours. Multidose vials are stable for up to 2 weeks.

Dosage must be individualized and depends on the specific application. A typical adult dose for brief procedures is 25 to 75 mg administered as a single IV injection. For prolonged procedures, succinylcholine may be administered by infusion at a rate of 2.5 to 4.3 mg/min.

THERAPEUTIC USES OF NEUROMUSCULAR BLOCKING AGENTS

The primary applications of the neuromuscular blocking agents are discussed below. No one agent is used for all of these applications.

Muscle Relaxation During Surgery

Production of muscle relaxation during surgery offers two benefits. First, relaxation of skeletal muscles, especially those of the abdominal wall, makes the surgeon's job easier. Second, muscle relaxants allow us to decrease the dosage of the general anesthetic, thereby decreasing the risks associated with anesthesia. Before neuromuscular blockers became available, surgical muscle relaxation had to be achieved with the general anesthetic alone, often requiring high levels of the anesthetic. (As noted earlier, inhalation anesthetics have muscle relaxant properties of their own.) By combining a neuromuscular blocker with the general anesthetic, we can achieve adequate surgical muscle relaxation with less anesthetic than was possible when paralysis had to be achieved with an anesthetic alone. By allowing a reduction in anesthetic levels, neuromuscular blockers have decreased the risk of respiratory depression from anesthesia. In addition, since less anesthetic is administered, recovery from anesthesia occurs more quickly.

Whenever neuromuscular blockers are employed during surgery, it is extremely important that anesthesia be maintained at a level sufficient to produce unconsciousness. Recall that neuromuscular blockers do not enter the CNS and, therefore, have no effect on hearing, thinking, or the ability to feel pain; all that these drugs do is produce paralysis. Neuromuscular blockers are obviously and definitely not a substitute for anesthesia. It does not require a great deal of imagination to appreciate the horror of the surgical patient who is completely paralyzed from neuromuscular blockade yet fully awake thanks to inadequate anesthesia. Clearly, full anesthesia must be provided whenever surgery is performed on a patient who is under neuromuscular blockade.

Full recovery from neuromuscular blockade may take from one to several hours. During the recovery period, patients must be monitored closely to insure adequate ventilation. A patent airway should be maintained until the patient can swallow or speak. Recovery from the effects of *nondepolarizing* neuromuscular blockers (e.g., tubocurarine) can be accelerated with a cholinesterase inhibitor.

Facilitation of Mechanical Ventilation

Some patients who require mechanical ventilation still have some spontaneous respiratory movements—movements that can fight the rhythm of the respirator. By suppressing these movements, neuromuscular blocking agents can reduce resistance to ventilation.

When neuromuscular blockers are used to facilitate mechanical ventilation, patients should be treated as if they were awake—even though they will appear to be sleeping. (Remember that the patient is paralyzed and, hence, there is no way to assess state of consciousness.) Because the patient may be fully awake, steps should be taken to insure comfort at all times. Furthermore, since neuromuscular blockade does not affect hearing, nothing should be said in the patient's presence that might be inappropriate for him or her to hear.

Being fully awake but completely paralyzed can be a very stressful and generally horrific experience. (Think about it.) Accordingly, many clinicians do not recommend routine use of neuromuscular blockers during prolonged mechanical ventilation in intensive care units.

Adjunct to Electroconvulsive Therapy

Electroconvulsive therapy is an effective treatment for severe depression (see Chapter 25). Benefits derive strictly from the effects of electroshock on the brain; the convulsive movements that can accompany electroshock do not help relieve depression. Since convulsions per se serve no useful purpose, and since electroshock-induced convulsions can be harmful, neuromuscular blockers are now used to prevent convulsive movements during electroshock therapy. Because of its short duration of action, *succinylcholine* is the preferred neuromuscular blocker for this application.

Endotracheal Intubation

An endotracheal tube is a large catheter that is inserted past the glottis and into the trachea to facilitate ventilation. Gag reflexes can fight tube insertion. By suppressing these reflexes, neuromuscular blockers can make intubation easier. Because of its short duration of action, *succinylcholine* is the preferred neuromuscular blocker for this use.

Diagnosis of Myasthenia Gravis

Tubocurarine can be used to diagnose myasthenia gravis when safer diagnostic procedures have been inconclusive. To diagnose myasthenia, a very small test dose of tubocurarine is administered. Since this test dose is too small to affect individuals who do not have myasthenia, a significant reduction in muscle strength would be diagnostic of myasthenia. If the test dose does decrease strength, neostigmine (a cholinesterase inhibitor) should be administered immediately; the resultant elevation in ACh at the NMJ will reverse neuromuscular blockade. It must be stressed that use of tubocurarine to diagnose myasthenia gravis is not without risk: if the patient does have myasthenia, the challenging dose may be sufficient to cause severe respiratory depression. Consequently, facilities for artificial ventilation must be immediately available.

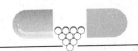

Summary of Major Nursing Implications

NEUROMUSCULAR BLOCKING AGENTS

Except where noted otherwise, the implications summarized below apply to all of the neuromuscular blocking agents.

 Preadministration Assessment

Therapeutic Goal

Provision of muscle relaxation during surgery, endotracheal intubation, mechanical ventilation, electroconvulsive therapy, and other procedures.

Identifying High-Risk Patients

Use *all* neuromuscular blockers with *caution* in patients with *myasthenia gravis*.

Succinylcholine is contraindicated for patients with *low pseudocholinesterase activity* or a *personal or familial history of malignant hyperthermia*.

 Implementation: Administration

Routes

Intravenous: *all* neuromuscular blockers.
Intramuscular: *tubocurarine* and *succinylcholine*.

Administration

Neuromuscular blockers are dangerous drugs that should be administered only by clinicians skilled in their use.

 Implementation: Measures to Enhance Therapeutic Effects

Neuromuscular blockers do not affect consciousness or perception of pain. When used during surgery, these drugs must be accompanied by adequate anesthesia. When neuromuscular blockers are used for prolonged paralysis during mechanical ventilation, care should be taken to insure comfort (e.g., positioning the patient comfortably, moistening the mouth periodically). Since patients may be awake (but won't appear to be), conversations held in their presence should convey only information that is appropriate for them to hear.

Minimizing Adverse Effects

 Ongoing Evaluation and Interventions

Apnea. All neuromuscular blockers can cause respiratory arrest. Facilities for intubation and mechanical ventilation should be immediately available.

Monitor respiration constantly during the period of peak drug action. When drug administration is discontinued, take vital signs at least every 15 minutes until recovery is complete.

Cholinesterase inhibitors can be used to reverse respiratory depression caused by *nondepolarizing* neuromuscular blockers—but not by succinylcholine, a *depolarizing* blocker.

Malignant Hyperthermia. Succinylcholine can trigger malignant hyperthermia. Predisposition to this reaction is genetic. Assess for a family history of the reaction.

Muscle Pain. *Succinylcholine* may cause muscle pain. Reassure the patient that this response, although unpleasant, is not unusual.

Hypotension. Several neuromuscular blockers can cause hypotension secondary to ganglionic blockade or release of histamine. Antihistamines may help counteract this effect.

Minimizing Adverse Interactions

Antibiotics. Certain antibiotics, including *aminoglycosides* and *tetracyclines*, can intensify neuromuscular blockade. Use these antibiotics with caution.

Cholinesterase Inhibitors. These drugs will delay inactivation of *succinylcholine*, thereby greatly prolonging paralysis. Accordingly, cholinesterase inhibitors are contraindicated for patients receiving succinylcholine.

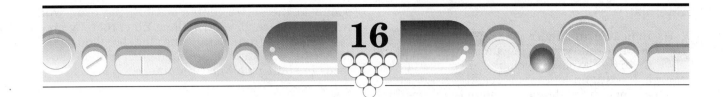

16

Cholinesterase Inhibitors

REVERSIBLE CHOLINESTERASE INHIBITORS
Neostigmine
Physostigmine
Other Reversible Cholinesterase Inhibitors
Treatment of Myasthenia Gravis

"IRREVERSIBLE" CHOLINESTERASE INHIBITORS
Isoflurophate
Toxicology of the Irreversible Cholinesterase Inhibitors

Cholinesterase inhibitors are drugs that prevent the degradation of acetylcholine (ACh) by acetylcholinesterase (cholinesterase). By preventing the inactivation of ACh, the cholinesterase inhibitors enhance the actions of ACh released from cholinergic nerves. Hence, the cholinesterase inhibitors can be looked upon as indirect-acting cholinergic agonists. Since cholinesterase inhibitors can intensify transmission at all cholinergic junctions (muscarinic, ganglionic, and neuromuscular), these drugs can elicit a wide variety of responses. Because of this relative lack of selectivity, the cholinesterase inhibitors have limited therapeutic applications. An alternative name for the cholinesterase inhibitors is *anticholinesterase agents.*

There are two basic categories of cholinesterase inhibitors: (1) *reversible* inhibitors, and (2) *"irreversible"* inhibitors. The reversible inhibitors produce effects of moderate duration. In contrast, the effects of the irreversible inhibitors are prolonged.

REVERSIBLE CHOLINESTERASE INHIBITORS

NEOSTIGMINE

Neostigmine [Prostigmin] typifies the reversible cholinesterase inhibitors and will serve as our prototype for the group. The principal indication for neostigmine is *myasthenia gravis.*

Chemistry

As indicated in Figure 16–1, neostigmine contains a quaternary nitrogen atom and therefore always carries a positive charge. Because of this charge, neostigmine cannot readily cross membranes, including those of the gastrointestinal tract, the blood-brain barrier, and the placenta. Consequently, neostigmine is absorbed poorly following oral administration and has minimal effects on the brain and the developing fetus.

Mechanism of Action

Neostigmine and the other reversible cholinesterase inhibitors can be envisioned as poor substrates for cholinesterase (ChE). As indicated in Figure 16–2, the normal function of ChE is to break down acetylcholine into choline and acetic acid. This process is termed a *hydrolysis* reaction because of the water molecule involved. As depicted in Figure 16–3A, hydrolysis of ACh takes place in two steps: (1) binding of ACh to the active center of ChE, followed by (2) splitting of ACh, which regenerates free ChE. The overall reaction between ACh and ChE takes place *extremely* rapidly. As a result, one molecule of ChE can inactivate a huge amount of ACh in a very short time.

As depicted in Figure 16–3B, the reaction between neostigmine and ChE is very similar to the reaction between ACh and ChE. The difference between the two reactions is simply that the splitting of neostigmine by ChE occurs more *slowly* than the splitting of ACh. Hence, once neostigmine becomes

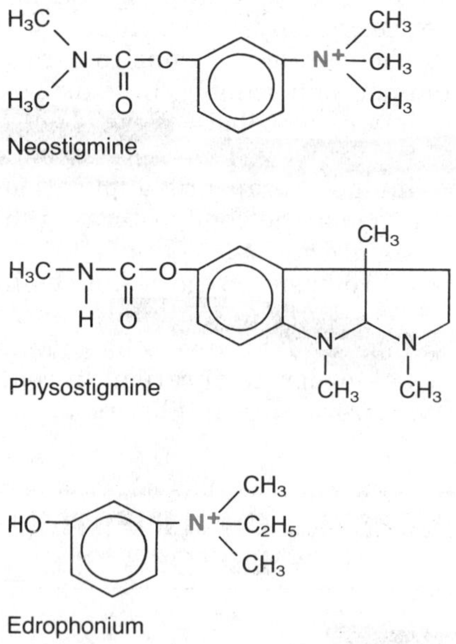

Figure 16–1. Structural formulas of reversible cholinesterase inhibitors. Note that neostigmine and edrophonium are quaternary ammonium compounds, whereas physostigmine is not. What does this difference in structures imply about the relative abilities of these drugs to cross membranes, including those of the blood-brain barrier?

bound to the active center of ChE, the drug will remain in place for a fairly long time, thereby preventing ChE from catalyzing the breakdown of ACh. ChE will remain inhibited until it finally succeeds in splitting off neostigmine.

Pharmacologic Effects

By preventing inactivation of ACh, neostigmine and the other cholinesterase inhibitors can intensify transmission at virtually all junctions where ACh is the transmitter. In sufficient doses, the cholinesterase inhibitors can produce skeletal muscle stimulation, activation of muscarinic receptors, ganglionic stimulation, and activation of cholinergic receptors within the central nervous system (CNS). However, when used therapeutically, the cholinesterase inhibitors usually affect only muscarinic receptors and nicotinic receptors of the neuromuscular junction. Ganglionic transmission is usually not altered.

Muscarinic Responses. Muscarinic effects of the cholinesterase inhibitors are identical to those of the direct-acting muscarinic agonists. By preventing breakdown of ACh, cholinesterase inhibitors can cause increased glandular secretions, increased tone and motility of gastrointestinal smooth muscle, bradycardia, urinary urgency, bronchial constriction, miosis, and focusing of the lens for near vision.

Neuromuscular Effects. The effects of cholinesterase inhibitors on skeletal muscle are dose dependent. At *therapeutic* doses, these drugs *increase* force of contraction. In contrast, *toxic* doses *reduce* force of contraction. Reductions in strength occur because the presence of excessive amounts of ACh at the neuromuscular junction (NMJ) keeps the motor end-plate in a state of constant depolarization, resulting in depolarizing neuromuscular blockade (see Chapter 15).

Central Nervous System. Effects on the CNS vary with drug concentration. Therapeutic drug levels can produce mild *stimulation*, whereas toxic levels *depress* the CNS, including the areas that regulate respiration. However, it must be noted that for CNS effects to occur, the inhibitor must first penetrate the blood–brain barrier; some cholinesterase inhibitors can do this only when present in very high concentrations.

Pharmacokinetics

Neostigmine may be administered orally and by injection (SC, IM, IV). Because neostigmine carries a positive charge, the drug is poorly absorbed following oral administration. Hence, oral doses must be much greater than parenteral doses to produce equivalent effects. Once absorbed, neostigmine can reach sites of action at the NMJ and at peripheral muscarinic receptors, but cannot cross the blood–brain barrier to produce effects within the CNS. Duration of action is 2 to 4 hours. Neostigmine is

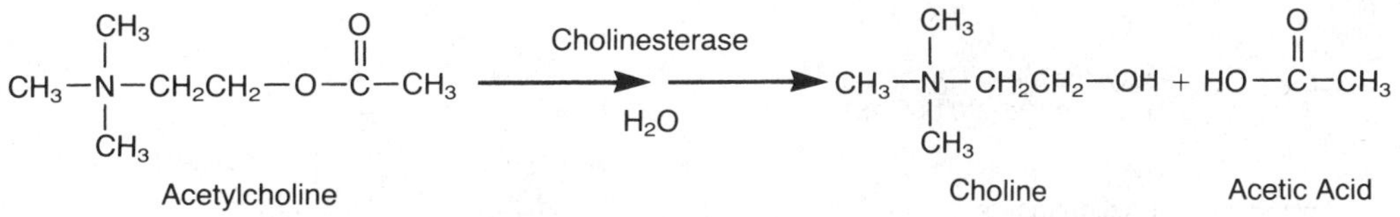

Figure 16–2. Hydrolysis of acetylcholine by cholinesterase.

eliminated by enzymatic degradation: cholinesterase, the enzyme that neostigmine inhibits, eventually converts neostigmine itself into an inactive product.

Therapeutic Uses

Myasthenia Gravis. Myasthenia gravis is a major indication for neostigmine and several other reversible cholinesterase inhibitors. Treatment of myasthenia is discussed separately later in this chapter.

Reversal of Nondepolarizing Neuromuscular Blockade. By causing accumulation of ACh at neuromuscular junctions, cholinesterase inhibitors can reverse the effects of nondepolarizing neuromuscular blocking agents (e.g., tubocurarine). The ability of cholinesterase inhibitors to counteract nondepolarizing neuromuscular blockade has two clinical applications: (1) reversal of neuromuscular blockade in postoperative patients, and (2) treatment of overdosage with nondepolarizing neuromuscular blockers. When neostigmine is used to treat neuromuscular blocker overdosage, artificial respiration must be maintained until muscle function has fully recovered. At the doses employed to reverse neuromuscular blockade, neostigmine is likely to elicit substantial muscarinic responses; symptoms of excessive muscarinic stimulation can be reduced with atropine. It is important to note that cholinesterase inhibitors cannot be employed to counteract the effects of succinylcholine, a *depolarizing* neuromuscular blocker.

Adverse Effects

Excessive Muscarinic Stimulation. Accumulation of ACh at muscarinic receptors can result in excessive salivation, increased gastric secretions, increased tone and motility of the gastrointestinal tract, urinary urgency, bradycardia, sweating, miosis, and spasm of accommodation (focusing of the lens for near vision). If necessary, these responses can be suppressed with atropine.

Neuromuscular Blockade. If administered in toxic doses, cholinesterase inhibitors can cause accumulation of ACh in amounts sufficient to produce depolarizing neuromuscular blockade. Paralysis of respiratory muscles can be fatal.

Precautions and Contraindications

Most of the precautions and contraindications regarding the cholinesterase inhibitors are the same as those that apply to the direct-acting muscarinic agonists. These include (1) obstruction of the gastrointestinal tract, (2) obstruction of the urinary tract, (3) peptic ulcer disease, (4) asthma, (5) coronary insufficiency, and (6) hyperthyroidism. The rationales underlying these precautions are discussed in Chapter 13. In addition to precautions related to muscarinic stimulation, cholinesterase inhibitors are contraindicated for patients receiving *succinylcholine*.

Drug Interactions

Muscarinic Antagonists. The effects of cholinesterase inhibitors at muscarinic junctions are opposite to those of atropine and other muscarinic antagonists. Consequently, atropine can be used to reduce muscarinic stimulation caused by cholinesterase inhibitors. Conversely, cholinesterase inhibitors can be used to overcome muscarinic blockade caused by atropine.

Nondepolarizing Neuromuscular Blockers. By causing accumulation of ACh at the NMJ, cholinesterase inhibitors can reverse muscle relaxation brought on by tubocurarine and other nondepolarizing neuromuscular blocking agents.

Depolarizing Neuromuscular Blockers. Cholinesterase inhibitors do not reverse the muscle-relaxant effects of succinylcholine, a depolarizing neuromuscular blocker. In fact, since cholinesterase inhibitors will decrease the breakdown of succinylcholine by cholinesterase, cholinesterase inhibitors will actually *intensify* neuromuscular blockade caused by succinylcholine.

Acute Toxicity

Symptoms. Overdosage with cholinesterase inhibitors causes *excessive muscarinic* stimulation and *respiratory depression*. (Respiratory depression results from a combination of depolarizing neuromuscular blockade and depression of the CNS.) The state produced by cholinesterase inhibitor poisoning is sometimes referred to as *cholinergic crisis*.

Treatment. Intravenous *atropine* will alleviate the muscarinic effects of cholinesterase inhibition. Since repiratory depression from cholinesterase in-

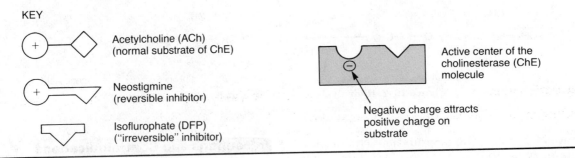

KEY

⊕— ◇   Acetylcholine (ACh)
       (normal substrate of ChE)

⊕—⬦   Neostigmine
       (reversible inhibitor)

▽   Isoflurophate (DFP)
       ("irreversible" inhibitor)

Active center of the
cholinesterase (ChE)
molecule

Negative charge attracts
positive charge on
substrate

A   REACTION BETWEEN ACh and ChE

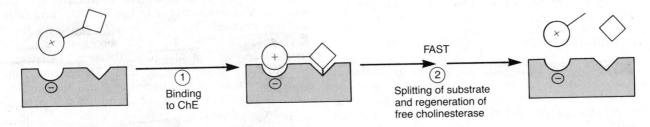

FAST

① Binding
to ChE

② Splitting of substrate
and regeneration of
free cholinesterase

B   REVERSIBLE INHIBITION OF ChE (BY NEOSTIGMINE)

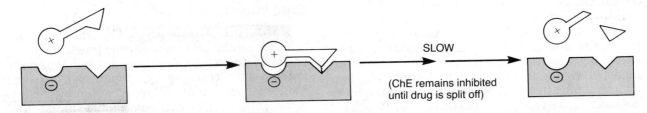

SLOW

(ChE remains inhibited
until drug is split off)

C   "IRREVERSIBLE" INHIBITION OF ChE (BY DFP)

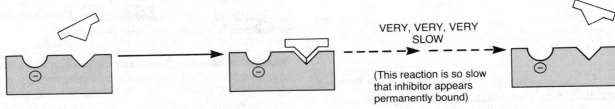

VERY, VERY, VERY
SLOW

(This reaction is so slow
that inhibitor appears
permanently bound)

Figure 16–3. Inhibition of cholinesterase by reversible and "irreversible" inhibitors.

---

hibitors cannot be managed with drugs, treatment consists of *mechanical ventilation* with oxygen. Suctioning may be necessary if atropine fails to suppress bronchial secretions.

Preparations, Dosage, and Administration

Preparations. Neostigmine [Prostigmin] is available as two salts: *neostigmine bromide* (for oral use) and *neostigmine methylsulfate* (for IM, SC, and IV injection). Neostigmine bromide is dispensed in 15-mg tablets. Neostigmine methylsulfate is available in solutions containing 0.25, 0.5, and 1.0 mg/ml.

Dosage and Administration. Dosages for *myasthenia gravis* are highly individualized. *Oral dosages range from 15 to 375 mg/day administered in divided doses every 3 to 4 hours. It is important to note that oral doses of neostigmine are usually about 30 times greater than parenteral doses.*

For treatment of *poisoning by nondepolarizing neuromuscu-*

lar blockers, the initial dose is 0.5 to 2.0 mg administered by slow IV injection. Additional doses totaling a maximum of 5 mg may be administered as required.

PHYSOSTIGMINE

The pharmacology of physostigmine is similar to that of neostigmine. The major differences between these two drugs stem from differences in their chemistry. As indicated in Figure 16–1, neostigmine is a quaternary ammonium compound and always carries a positive charge. In contrast, physostigmine is not a quaternary ammonium compound and does not carry a charge. Because physostigmine is uncharged, this drug crosses membranes much more readily than neostigmine. This ability to cross membranes makes physostigmine superior to neostigmine for certain applications.

Therapeutic Uses

Treatment of Muscarinic Antagonist Poisoning. Physostigmine is the drug of choice for treating poisoning by atropine and other drugs that cause muscarinic blockade (e.g., antihistamines, tricyclic antidepressants, phenothiazine antipsychotics). Physostigmine counteracts antimuscarinic poisoning by causing ACh to build up at muscarinic junctions. The accumulated ACh competes with the muscarinic blocker for receptor binding, and thereby reverses the blockade. Physostigmine is preferred to neostigmine for treating antimuscarinic poisoning because, lacking a charge, physostigmine is able to cross the blood–brain barrier to reverse muscarinic blockade in the CNS. The usual dosage for treatment of antimuscarinic poisoning is 2 mg given by IM or slow IV injection.

Glaucoma. Physostigmine and several other cholinesterase inhibitors can lower intraocular pressure in patients with glaucoma. However, superior drugs are available. The role of anticholinesterase agents in treating glaucoma is discussed in Chapter 69 (Drugs for Disorders of the Eye).

OTHER REVERSIBLE CHOLINESTERASE INHIBITORS

In addition to neostigmine and physostigmine, four other reversible cholinesterase inhibitors—*ambenonium, demecarium, edrophonium,* and *pyridostigmine*—are approved for use in the United States. The pharmacology of these agents is much like that of neostigmine. One of these drugs—edrophonium—is noteworthy for its very brief duration of action. Routes of administration and indications for the reversible cholinesterase inhibitors are summarized in Table 16–1.

TREATMENT OF MYASTHENIA GRAVIS

Pathophysiology. Myasthenia gravis is a disease characterized by muscle weakness and a predisposition to rapid fatigue. Common symptoms include difficulty in swallowing and ptosis (drooping eyelids). Patients with severe myasthenia may experience difficulty in breathing due to weakness of the muscles of respiration.

The symptoms of myasthenia gravis are caused by an *autoimmune* process in which the patient's immune system produces antibodies directed against nicotinic$_M$ receptors on skeletal muscle. As a result of attack by these antibodies, the number of receptors at the neuromuscular junction is reduced by 70% to 90%, resulting in the muscle weakness that characterizes myasthenia.

Treatment. Reversible cholinesterase inhibitors (e.g., neostigmine) are the mainstay of myasthenia therapy. By preventing ACh inactivation, anticholinesterase agents can intensify the effects of ACh released from motor neurons, and can thereby increase muscle strength. Cholinesterase inhibitors do not cure myasthenia; these drugs only produce symptomatic relief. Consequently patients with myasthenia are likely to require therapy lifelong.

When working with the hospitalized myasthenic patient, you should keep in mind that muscle strength can sometimes be so inadequate as to make swallowing impossible. Accordingly, the patient's ability to swallow should be assessed prior to administration of oral medications. Assessment can be accomplished by determining if the patient can swallow a few sips of water. If the patient is unable to swallow, a parenteral drug will be needed.

Side Effects of Treatment. Since cholinesterase inhibitors can inhibit acetylcholinesterase at any location, these drugs will cause ACh to accumulate at muscarinic junctions as well as at the neuromuscular junction. If muscarinic responses are excessive, atropine may be given to suppress them. However, atropine should not be employed *routinely* since this drug can mask the early signs (e.g., excessive salivation) of overdosage with anticholinesterase agents.

Dosage Adjustment. In the treatment of myasthenia gravis, establishing an optimal dosage for cholinesterase inhibitors can be a challenge. Dosage determination is accomplished by administering a small initial dose followed by additional small doses until an optimal level of muscle function has been produced. Important signs of improvement include increased ease of swallowing and increased ability to raise the eyelids. You can contribute to the process of dosage determination by keeping records of (1) times of drug administration, (2) times at which fatigue occurs, (3) state of muscle strength before and after drug administration, and (4) signs of excessive muscarinic stimulation.

To maintain optimal responses, patients will occasionally need to modify dosage themselves. To do this properly, patients must be taught to recognize signs of undermedication (difficulty in swallowing, ptosis) and signs of overmedication (excessive salivation, other muscarinic responses). Patients may also need to modify dosage in anticipation of exertion. For example, patients may find it necessary to take supplementary medication 30 to 60 min-

Table 16–1. Clinical Applications of Cholinesterase Inhibitors						
Generic Name [Trade Name]	Routes	Myasthenia Gravis		Glaucoma	Reversal of Nondepolarizing Neuromuscular Blockade	Antidote to Poisoning by Muscarinic Antagonists
		Diagnosis	*Treatment*			
Reversible Inhibitors						
Ambenonium [Mytelase Caplets]	PO		√			
Demecarium [Humorsol]	Topical			√		
Edrophonium [Tensilon, Enlon, Reversol]	IM,IV	√			√	
Neostigmine [Prostigmin]	PO,IM,IV,SC	√	√		√	
Physostigmine [Eserine, Antilirium]	Topical, IM,IV			√		√
Pyridostigmine [Mestinon, Regonol]	PO,IM,IV		√		√	
Irreversible Inhibitors						
Echothiophate [Phospholine Iodide]	Topical			√		
Isoflurophate (DFP) [Floropryl]	Topical			√		

utes prior to such activities as eating and shopping.

Myasthenic Crisis. Patients who are inadequately medicated may experience *myasthenic crisis*, a state characterized by extreme muscle weakness and caused by insufficient ACh at the neuromuscular junction. Left untreated, myasthenic crisis can result in death owing to paralysis of the muscles of respiration. A cholinesterase inhibitor (e.g., neostigmine) is used to relieve the crisis.

Cholinergic Crisis. As noted previously, overdosage with a cholinesterase inhibitor can produce cholinergic crisis. Like myasthenic crisis, cholinergic crisis is characterized by extreme muscle weakness or frank paralysis. In addition, cholinergic crisis is accompanied by signs of excessive muscarinic stimulation. Treatment consists of respiratory support plus atropine. The offending cholinesterase inhibitor should be withheld until muscle strength has returned.

Distinguishing Myasthenic Crisis from Cholinergic Crisis. Since myasthenic crisis and cholinergic crisis share similar symptoms (muscle weakness or paralysis), but are treated very differently, it is essential to distinguish between these conditions so that appropriate treatment can be provided. A history of medication use or signs of excessive muscarinic stimulation are usually sufficient to permit a differential diagnosis. If these

clues are inadequate, the differential diagnosis can be made by administering a challenging dose of *edrophonium*, an ultrashort-acting cholinesterase inhibitor. If edrophonium-induced elevation of ACh levels alleviates symptoms, the crisis was myasthenic. Conversely, if edrophonium intensifies symptoms, the crisis was cholinergic. Since the symptoms of cholinergic crisis will be made even worse by edrophonium, atropine and oxygen should be immediately available whenever edrophonium is used to distinguish myasthenic crisis from cholinergic crisis.

Use of Identification by the Patient. Because of the possibility of experiencing either myasthenic crisis or cholinergic crisis, and because both of these crises can be fatal, myasthenic patients should be encouraged to wear a Medic Alert bracelet or some other form of identification to inform emergency medical personnel of their condition.

"IRREVERSIBLE" CHOLINESTERASE INHIBITORS

The "irreversible" cholinesterase inhibitors are highly toxic. These agents are employed primarily as *insecticides*. During World War II, huge quantities of irreversible cholinesterase inhibitors were produced for possible use as nerve gases. Fortunately, these deadly weapons were never deployed.

The only clinical indication for the irreversible inhibitors is *glaucoma*.

The spectrum of effects produced by the irreversible cholinesterase inhibitors is nearly identical to that of the reversible inhibitors. The major difference between responses to these two groups of drugs is that responses to the irreversible inhibitors persist for a very long time, whereas responses to the reversible inhibitors are relatively short lived.

ISOFLUROPHATE

Isoflurophate (di*iso*propyl fluorophosphate, DFP) is one of two irreversible cholinesterase inhibitors in clinical use. DFP will serve as our prototype of the irreversible inhibitors.

Chemistry

DFP and the other irreversible cholinesterase inhibitors contain an atom of *phosphorus* (Fig. 16–4). Because of this phosphorus atom, the irreversible inhibitors are known as *organophosphate* cholinesterase inhibitors.

All of the irreversible cholinesterase inhibitors are *highly lipid soluble*. As a result, these drugs are readily absorbed from all routes of administration. They can even be absorbed directly through the skin. Ease of absorption is a contributing factor to the use of the irreversible inhibitors as insecticides and to their potential use as agents of chemical warfare. Once absorbed, the organophosphate inhibitors have ready access to all tissues and organs, including the CNS.

Mechanism of Action

DFP and the other irreversible cholinesterase inhibitors produce their effects by binding to the active center of cholinesterase, thereby preventing the enzyme from hydrolyzing ACh. Although it is possible for bound DFP to be split from ChE, this splitting reaction takes place *extremely* slowly (see Fig. 16–3C). Hence, under normal conditions, the binding of DFP to ChE can be considered permanent. Because binding is permanent, effects will persist until new molecules of cholinesterase can be synthesized.

Although we normally consider the binding of DFP to cholinesterase to be irreversible, this binding can, in fact, be reversed. To produce reversal, we must administer *pralidoxime* (see below).

Therapeutic Uses

The only indication for DFP is *glaucoma*. The use of DFP and other cholinesterase inhibitors in glaucoma is discussed in Chapter 69 (Drugs for Disorders of the Eye).

TOXICOLOGY OF THE IRREVERSIBLE CHOLINESTERASE INHIBITORS

Sources of Poisoning. Poisoning by the organophosphate cholinesterase inhibitors is not uncommon. Agricultural workers have been poisoned by accidental ingestion of organophosphate insecticides and by absorption of these lipid-soluble compounds directly through the skin. In addition, because organophosphate insecticides are readily available to the general public, poisoning occurs from attempts at homicide and suicide.

Symptoms. Toxic doses of irreversible cholinesterase inhibitors produce a state of *cholinergic crisis*, a condition characterized by *excessive muscarinic stimulation* and by *depolarizing neuromuscular blockade*. Overstimulation of muscarinic receptors results in profuse secretions from salivary and bronchial glands, involuntary urination and defecation, laryngospasm, and bronchoconstriction. Neuromuscular blockade can result in death from respiratory paralysis.

Treatment. Treatment involves the following: (1) *mechanical ventilation* using oxygen, (2) giving *atropine* to reduce muscarinic stimulation, and (3) giving *pralidoxime* to reverse inhibition of cholinesterase.

Pralidoxime. Pralidoxime [Protopam] is a specific antidote to poisoning by the *irreversible* (organophosphate) cholinesterase inhibitors. This drug is *not* effective against poisoning by *reversible* cholinesterase inhibitors. Pralidoxime reverses

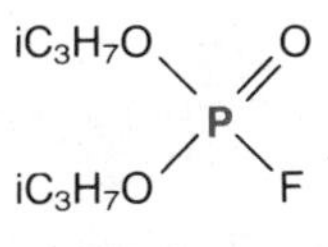

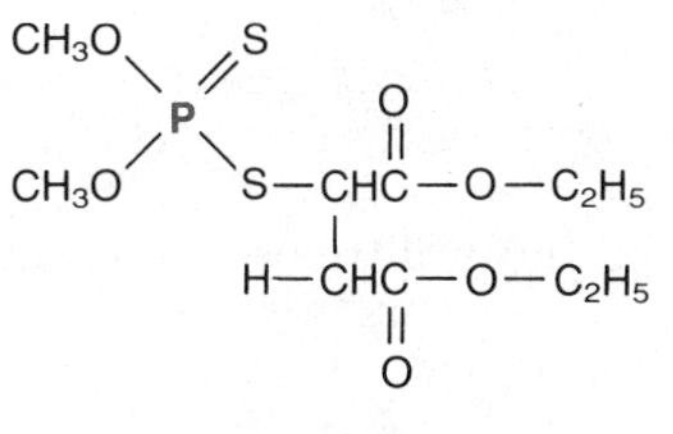

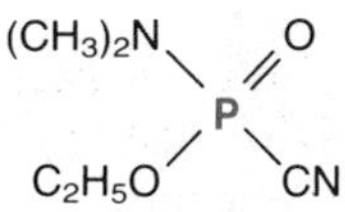

Figure 16–4. Structural formulas of "irreversible" cholinesterase inhibitors. Note that all of the irreversible cholinesterase inhibitors contain an atom of phosphorus. Because of this atom, these drugs are known as *organophosphate* cholinesterase inhibitors. All of the organophosphate inhibitors are highly lipid soluble and can therefore move throughout the body with ease.

poisoning by causing organophosphate inhibitors to dissociate from the active center of cholinesterase. Pralidoxime is a quaternary ammonium compound and, therefore, cannot cross the blood-brain barrier. As a result, the drug cannot reverse cholinesterase inhibition within the CNS.

To be effective, pralidoxime must be administered soon after organophosphate poisoning has occurred. If too much time is allowed to elapse, a process called *aging* will take place. In this aging process, the bond between the organophosphate inhibitor and cholinesterase increases in strength. Once aging has occurred, pralidoxime will no longer be able to cause the inhibitor to dissociate from the enzyme.

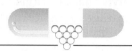 # Summary of Major Nursing Implications

REVERSIBLE CHOLINESTERASE INHIBITORS

Neostigmine Demecarium

Physostigmine Edrophonium

Ambenonium Pyridostigmine

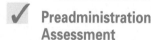 ✓ **Preadministration Assessment**

Therapeutic Goal

These drugs are used to treat *myasthenia gravis* and *glaucoma*, to *reverse nondepolarizing neuromuscular blockade*, and to *treat muscarinic antagonist poisoning*. Applications of individual agents are summarized in Table 16–1.

Baseline Data

Myasthenia Gravis. Determine the extent of neuromuscular dysfunction by assessing muscle strength, fatigue, ptosis, and ability to swallow.

Identifying High-Risk Patients

Cholinesterase inhibitors are *contraindicated* for patients with *mechanical obstruction of the intestine or urinary tract*. Exercise *caution* in patients with *peptic ulcer disease, bradycardia, asthma, or hyperthyroidism.*

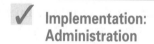 ✓ **Implementation: Administration**

Routes

These drugs are given orally, topically, and by IM, IV, and SC injection. Routes for individual agents are summarized in Table 16–1.

Administration and Dosage in Myasthenia Gravis

Administration. Assess the patient's ability to swallow before giving oral medication. If swallowing is impaired, parenteral medication is required.

Optimization of Dosage. Monitor for therapeutic responses (see below) and adjust dosage accordingly. Teach patients to distinguish between insufficient and excessive dosing to enable their participation in dosage adjustment.

Oral versus Parenteral Doses. Oral doses of *neostigmine* are about 30 times greater than parenteral doses. If a patient is switched from oral to parenteral medication, the dosage must be greatly reduced.

Reversing Nondepolarizing Neuromuscular Blockade

To reverse toxicity from overdosage with tubocurarine and other nondepolarizing neuromuscular blocking agents, administer *neostigmine* by slow IV infusion. Support respiration until muscle strength has recovered fully.

Treating Muscarinic Antagonist Poisoning

Physostigmine is the drug of choice for this indication. The usual dose is 2 mg given by IM or slow IV injection.

✓ Implementation: Measures to Enhance Therapeutic Effects

✓ Ongoing Evaluation and Interventions

Patients with Myasthenia Gravis

Promoting Compliance. Inform patients that myasthenia gravis is not curable and, hence, treatment will be lifelong. Encourage patients to take their medication as prescribed.

Use of Identification. Since myasthenic patients are at risk of fatal complications (cholinergic crisis, myasthenic crisis), encourage them to wear a MedicAlert bracelet or similar form of identification to inform emergency medical personnel of their condition.

Evaluating Therapeutic Effects

Myasthenia Gravis. Monitor and record (1) times of drug administration; (2) times at which fatigue occurs; (3) state of muscle strength, ptosis, and ability to swallow; and (4) signs of excessive muscarinic stimulation. Dosage is increased or decreased based on these observations.

Monitor for *myasthenic crisis* (extreme muscle weakness, paralysis of respiratory muscles), which can occur when cholinesterase inhibitor dosage is insufficient. Manage with respiratory support and an increase in dosage.

Be certain to distinguish myasthenic crisis from cholinergic crisis. This is done by observing for signs of excessive muscarinic stimulation, which will accompany cholinergic crisis but not myasthenic crisis. If necessary, these crises can be distinguished by administering *edrophonium*, which will reduce symptoms of myasthenic crisis but will intensify symptoms of cholinergic crisis.

Minimizing Adverse Effects

Excessive Muscarinic Stimulation. Accumulation of ACh at muscarinic receptors can cause profuse salivation, increased tone and motility of the gut, urinary urgency, sweating, miosis, spasm of accommodation, bronchoconstriction, and bradycardia. Inform patients about signs of excessive muscarinic stimulation and advise them to notify the physician if these occur. Excessive muscarinic responses can be reduced with *atropine*.

Cholinergic Crisis. This condition results from cholinesterase inhibitor overdosage. Manifestations are *skeletal muscle paralysis* (from depolarizing neuromuscular blockade) and *signs of excessive muscarinic stimulation* (e.g., salivation, sweating, miosis, bradycardia).

Manage with mechanical ventilation and *atropine*. Cholinergic crisis must be distinguished from myasthenic crisis.

Adrenergic Drugs

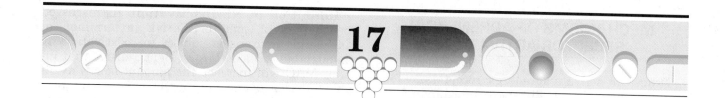

Adrenergic Agonists

The adrenergic agonists are drugs that produce their effects by causing activation of adrenergic receptors. Since the sympathetic nervous system acts through these same receptors, responses to adrenergic agonists and responses to stimulation by the sympathetic nervous system are very similar. Because of this similarity, the adrenergic agonists are often referred to as *sympathomimetics*. The adrenergic agonists have a broad spectrum of clinical applications, ranging from treatment of heart failure to relief of asthma to delay of preterm labor.

Learning about the adrenergic agonists can be a challenge. To facilitate learning, we will approach these drugs in four stages. First, we will discuss the general mechanisms by which drugs can activate adrenergic receptors. Next, we will establish an overview of the major adrenergic agonists, focusing on their receptor specificity and chemical classification. After that, we will address the adrenergic receptors themselves; for each receptor type (alpha$_1$, alpha$_2$, beta$_1$, beta$_2$, dopamine), we will discuss the beneficial and harmful effects that can result from receptor activation. Lastly, we will integrate all of this information by discussing the characteristic properties of individual sympathomimetic drugs.

It should be noted that this chapter is intended only as an *introduction* to the adrenergic agonists. Our objective here is to discuss the basic properties of the sympathomimetic drugs and establish an overview of their applications and adverse effects. Virtually all the drugs addressed in this chapter are discussed again in later chapters. In the subsequent chapters, the clinical applications of the adrenergic agonists are considered in greater depth than they are here.

MECHANISMS OF ADRENERGIC RECEPTOR ACTIVATION

Drugs can activate adrenergic receptors by four basic mechanisms: (1) direct receptor binding, (2) promotion of norepinephrine (NE) release, (3) blockade of NE reuptake, and (4) inhibition of NE inactivation. Note that only the first mechanism is *direct*. With the other three mechanisms, receptor activation occurs by an *indirect* process. Examples of drugs that act by these four mechanisms are presented in Table 17–1.

Direct Receptor Binding. Direct interaction with receptors is the most common mechanism by which drugs activate peripheral adrenergic receptors. The direct-acting receptor stimulants produce their effects by binding to adrenergic receptors and mimicking the actions of natural transmitters (NE, epinephrine, dopamine). In this chapter, all of the drugs discussed activate adrenergic receptors directly.

Promotion of NE Release. By acting on terminals of sympathetic nerves to cause release of NE, drugs can bring about activation of adrenergic receptors. Agents that promote receptor activation by this indirect mechanism include the amphetamines and ephedrine. (Ephedrine is also a direct-acting receptor stimulant.)

Inhibition of NE Reuptake. Recall that reuptake of NE into terminals of sympathetic nerves is the major mechanism by which adrenergic transmission is terminated. Hence, by blocking NE reuptake, drugs can cause NE to accumulate within the synaptic gap, and can thereby increase receptor activation. Agents that act by blocking NE reuptake include cocaine and the tricyclic antidepressants.

Inhibition of NE Inactivation. As discussed in Chapter 12, some of the NE in terminals of adrenergic neurons is subject to inactivation by monoamine oxidase (MAO). Hence, drugs that inhibit MAO will increase the amount of NE available for release, and will thereby enhance receptor activation. (It should be noted that in addition to being present in sympathetic nerves, MAO is present in the liver and the intestinal wall. The significance of MAO at these other sites is considered later in the chapter.)

In this chapter, which is dedicated to *peripherally* acting sympathomimetics, practically all of the drugs discussed act exclusively by *direct* receptor activation. The only exception is *ephedrine*, an agent that works by a combination of direct receptor activation and promotion of NE release.

Most of the *indirect-acting* adrenergic agonists are used for their ability to activate adrenergic receptors in the *central nervous system* (CNS)—not for their effects in the periphery. The indirect-acting sympathomimetics (e.g., amphetamine, cocaine) are mentioned here to emphasize the fact that although these agents are employed for their effects on the brain, they can and will cause activation of adrenergic receptors in the periphery. Peripheral activation is responsible for certain toxicities of these drugs (e.g., cardiac dysrhythmias, hypertension).

OVERVIEW OF THE ADRENERGIC AGONISTS

CHEMICAL CLASSIFICATION: CATECHOLAMINES VERSUS NONCATECHOLAMINES

The adrenergic agonists fall into two major chemical classes: catecholamines and noncatechol-

---

Table 17–1. Mechanisms of Adrenergic Receptor Activation	
Mechanism of Stimulation	**Examples**
Direct Mechanism	
Binding to receptor to cause activation	Epinephrine Isoproterenol Ephedrine*
Indirect Mechanisms	
Promotion of NE release	Ephedrine* Amphetamines
Inhibition of NE reuptake	Cocaine Tricyclic antidepressants
Inhibition of MAO	MAO inhibitors

NE = norepinephrine, MAO = monamine oxidase
*Ephedrine is a mixed-acting drug that activates adrenergic receptors directly and also promotes release of norepinephrine.

amines. As we shall see, the catecholamines and noncatecholamines differ from each other in three important respects: (1) oral usability, (2) duration of action, and (3) ability to act in the CNS. Accordingly, if we know which category a particular adrenergic agonist belongs to, we will know three of that drug's prominent characteristics.

Catecholamines

The catecholamines are so named because they contain a *catechol* group and an *amine* group. A catechol group is simply a benzene ring that has hydroxyl groups on two adjacent carbons (Fig. 17–1). The amine component of the catecholamines is *ethylamine*. Structural formulas for each of the major catecholamines—epinephrine, norepinephrine, isoproterenol, dopamine, and dobutamine—are presented in Figure 17–1. Because of their chemistry, all of the catecholamines have three characteristics in common: (1) they cannot be taken orally, (2) they have a brief duration of action, and (3) they cannot cross the blood-brain barrier.

The actions of two enzymes—*monoamine oxidase* (MAO) and *catechol-o-methyltransferase* (COMT)—explain why the catecholamines have short half-lives and cannot be used orally. MAO and COMT are located in the liver and in the intestinal wall. Both enzymes are very active and quickly destroy catecholamines administered by any route. Because these enzymes are located in the liver and intestinal wall, catecholamines that are administered orally will be inactivated before they can reach the systemic circulation. Hence, catecholamines are ineffective if given by mouth. Because of rapid inactivation by MAO and COMT, several catecholamines (norepinephrine, dopamine, dobutamine) are effective only if administered by continuous infusion. Administration by other parenteral routes (e.g., SC, IM) will not permit adequate blood levels to be achieved.

The catecholamines cannot cross the blood-brain barrier because they are polar molecules. (Recall from Chapter 5 that polar compounds penetrate membranes poorly.) The polar nature of the catecholamines is due to the hydroxyl groups on the catechol portion of the molecule. Because they cannot cross the blood-brain barrier, catecholamines have minimal effects on the CNS.

You should be aware that catecholamine-containing solutions, which are normally colorless when first prepared, will turn pink or brown over time. This pigmentation is caused by oxidation of the catecholamine molecule. As a rule, *catecholamine solutions should be discarded as soon as discoloration appears*. The only exception to this rule applies to *dobutamine*, which can be used up to 24 hours after solution preparation, even if discoloration has developed.

Noncatecholamines

The noncatecholamines have ethylamine in their structure (see Fig. 17–1) but do not contain the catechol portion that characterizes the catecholamines. The noncatecholamines considered in this chapter are ephedrine, phenylephrine, and terbutaline.

The noncatecholamines differ from the catecholamines in several important respects. First, because they lack a catechol group, noncatecholamines are not substrates for COMT, and are metabolized slowly by MAO. As a result, the noncatecholamines have half-lives that are much longer than those of the catecholamines. Furthermore, since they do not undergo rapid degradation by MAO and COMT, the noncatecholamines can be given orally, whereas the catecholamines cannot. Lastly, the noncatecholamines are considerably less polar than the catecholamines. As a result, the noncatecholamines are more able to penetrate the blood-brain barrier and influence the CNS.

RECEPTOR SPECIFICITY

Understanding the actions of individual adrenergic agonists requires knowledge of their receptor specificity. Since the sympathomimetic drugs differ widely from one another with respect to the receptors they can activate, learning the receptor specificity of these drugs will take some effort.

Variability in receptor specificity among the adrenergic agonists can be illustrated with three drugs: terbutaline, isoproterenol, and epinephrine. Terbutaline is highly selective, acting at beta$_2$ receptors only. Isoproterenol is less selective, acting at beta$_2$ receptors as well as beta$_1$ receptors. Epinephrine is less selective yet, acting at all four subtypes (alpha$_1$, alpha$_2$, beta$_1$, beta$_2$) of adrenergic receptors.

The receptor specificities of the major adrenergic agonists are summarized in Table 17–2. In the *upper* part of this table, receptor specificity is presented in *tabular* format. In the *lower* part of the table, the same information is presented *schematically*. By learning (memorizing) the content of Table 17–2, you will have taken a major step toward understanding the pharmacology of the sympathomimetic drugs.

It should be noted that the concept of receptor specificity is *relative*—not absolute: the ability to selectively activate certain receptors to the exclusion of others is dependent upon dosage. At low doses, selectivity is maximal; as dosage increases, selectivity declines. For example, when terbutaline is administered in low-to-moderate doses, the drug is highly selective for beta$_2$-adrenergic receptors. However, if the dosage is high, terbutaline will activate beta$_1$ receptors as well. The information on receptor specificity in Table 17–2 relates to

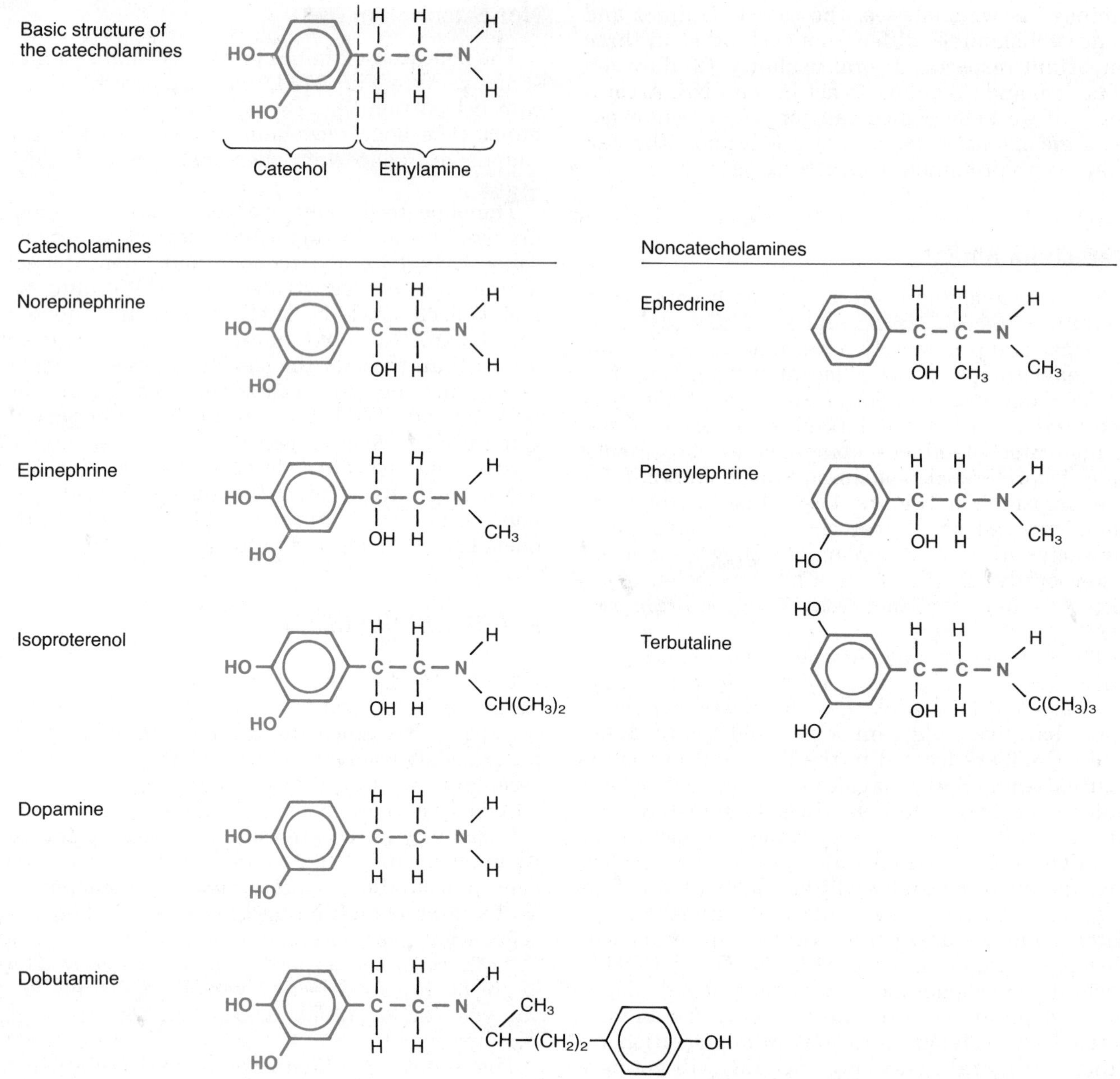

Basic structure of
the catecholamines

Catechol   Ethylamine

Catecholamines

Norepinephrine

Epinephrine

Isoproterenol

Dopamine

Dobutamine

Noncatecholamines

Ephedrine

Phenylephrine

Terbutaline

Figure 17–1. Structures of catecholamines and noncatecholamines. *Catecholamines.* Note that all of the catecholamines share the same basic chemical formula. Because of their biochemical properties, the catecholamines cannot be used orally, cannot cross the blood-brain barrier, and have short half-lives (owing to rapid inactivation by MAO and COMT).

Noncatecholamines. Although structurally similar to catecholamines, noncatecholamines differ from catecholamines in three important ways: (1) the noncatecholamines are usable orally; (2) they are able to cross the blood-brain barrier; and (3) since they are not rapidly metabolized by MAO or COMT, they have much longer half-lives than the catecholamines.

usual therapeutic doses. So-called "selective" agents will activate additional adrenergic receptors if dosage is abnormally high.

THERAPEUTIC APPLICATIONS AND ADVERSE EFFECTS OF ADRENERGIC RECEPTOR ACTIVATION

In this section we will discuss the responses, both therapeutic and undesired, that can be elic-

ited with sympathomimetic drugs. Since most of the adrenergic agonists activate more than one type of receptor (see Table 17–2), it could be quite confusing if we were to talk about the effects of the sympathomimetics employing specific drugs as examples. Consequently, rather than attempting to structure this presentation around representative drugs, we will discuss the actions of the adrenergic agonists one receptor at a time. Our discussion will begin with alpha$_1$ receptors, and then move sequentially to alpha$_2$ receptors, beta$_1$ receptors, beta$_2$ receptors, and dopamine receptors. For each receptor type, we will discuss both the therapeutic

Table 17–2. Receptor Specificity of Representative Adrenergic Agonists			
Catecholamines		**Noncatecholamines**	
Drug	*Receptors Activated*	*Drug*	*Receptors Activated*
Epinephrine	α_1, α_2, β_1, β_2	Ephedrine*	α_1, α_2, β_1, β_2
Norepinephrine	α_1, α_2, β_1	Phenylephrine	α_1
Isoproterenol	β_1, β_2	Terbutaline	β_2
Dobutamine	β_1		
Dopamine†	α_1, β_1, dopamine		

α = alpha
β = beta

Receptors Activated‡				
Alpha₁	*Alpha₂*	*Beta₁*	*Beta₂*	*Dopamine*
←————————————————— Epinephrine —————————————————→				
←————————————————— Ephedrine* —————————————————→				
←——————————— Norepinephrine ———————————→				
←— Phenylephrine →		←——————— Isoproterenol ———————→		
		←— Dobutamine†→←— Terbutaline —→		
←— Dopamine† ——→		←— Dopamine†→		←— Dopamine†→

*Ephedrine is a mixed-acting agent that causes NE release and also activates alpha and beta receptors directly.
†Receptor activation by dopamine is dose dependent.
‡This chart presents the same information on receptor specificity given above in tabular form. Arrows indicate the range of receptors that the drugs can stimulate (at usual therapeutic doses).

and the adverse responses that can result from receptor activation.

To understand the effects of any specific adrenergic agonist, all that you need is two types of information: (1) the identity of the receptor type at which the drug acts and (2) the effects produced by activating those receptors. Combining these two types of information will reveal a profile of drug action. This is the same approach to understanding neuropharmacologic agents that we discussed in Chapter 11.

Before proceeding, you are advised to review Table 12–3. Since we are about to discuss the clinical consequences of adrenergic receptor activation, and since Table 12–3 summarizes the responses to activation of these receptors, the benefits of being familiar with Table 12–3 should be obvious. If you choose not to memorize Table 12–3 at this time, at least be prepared to refer to the table as we discuss the clinical consequences of receptor activation.

CLINICAL CONSEQUENCES OF ALPHA₁ ACTIVATION

In this section we will discuss the therapeutic and adverse effects that can result from activation of alpha₁-adrenergic receptors. As indicated in Table 17–2, drugs capable of activating alpha₁ receptors include epinephrine, norepinephrine, phenylephrine, ephedrine, and dopamine.

Therapeutic Applications of Alpha₁ Activation

Activation of alpha₁ receptors elicits two responses that can be of therapeutic use: (1) *vasoconstriction* (in blood vessels of the skin, viscera, and mucous membranes) and (2) *mydriasis*. Of these two responses, vasoconstriction is the one for which alpha₁ activation is most often employed. Use of alpha₁-activating agents to produce mydriasis is relatively rare.

Hemostasis. Hemostasis is defined as the arrest of bleeding. Drugs capable of alpha₁ activation produce hemostasis by causing vasoconstriction. Alpha₁ stimulants are given to stop bleeding primarily in the skin and mucous membranes. Epinephrine, applied topically, is the alpha₁-activating agent used most often for this purpose.

Nasal Decongestion. Nasal congestion results from dilation and engorgement of blood vessels in the nasal mucosa. Drugs can relieve congestion by causing alpha₁-mediated vasoconstriction. Specific alpha₁-activating agents employed as nasal decongestants include phenylephrine (applied topically) and ephedrine (taken orally).

Adjunct to Local Anesthesia. Alpha₁ agonists are frequently combined with local anesthetics to delay anesthetic absorption. Absorption is delayed because alpha₁-mediated vasoconstriction reduces blood flow to the site of anesthetic administration. Delay of anesthetic absorption has three benefits:

(1) it prolongs anesthesia, (2) it allows a reduction in anesthetic dosage, and (3) it reduces the systemic effects that a local anesthetic might produce. The drug used most frequently to delay anesthetic absorption is epinephrine.

Elevation of Blood Pressure. Because of their ability to cause vasoconstriction, alpha$_1$ agonists can be used to elevate blood pressure in hypotensive states. It must be noted, however, that alpha$_1$ agonists are not the primary therapy for hypotension; these drugs should be reserved for situations in which other measures, including fluid replacement, have failed to restore blood pressure to a satisfactory level.

Mydriasis. Activation of alpha$_1$ receptors on the radial muscle of the iris causes mydriasis (dilation of the pupil). Production of mydriasis can facilitate eye examinations and ocular surgery. The use of alpha$_1$-agonists in ophthalmology is discussed further in Chapter 69 (Drugs for Disorders of the Eye). Note that the ophthalmic applications of alpha$_1$ activation are the only applications that are not based on vasoconstriction.

Adverse Effects of Alpha$_1$ Activation

All of the adverse effects associated with alpha$_1$ activation result directly or indirectly from vasoconstriction.

Hypertension. Alpha$_1$ agonists can produce hypertension by causing widespread vasoconstriction. Severe hypertension is most likely with parenteral administration. Accordingly, when an alpha$_1$ agonist is given parenterally, cardiovascular status must be monitored continuously; the patient must never be left unattended.

Necrosis. If the intravenous line employed to administer an alpha$_1$ agonist becomes extravasated, local seepage of the drug may result in necrosis (tissue death). The cause of necrosis is lack of blood flow secondary to excessive local vasoconstriction. If extravasation occurs, the area should be infiltrated with an alpha$_1$-blocking agent (e.g., phentolamine). By counteracting alpha$_1$-mediated vasoconstriction, the antagonist will help minimize injury.

Bradycardia. Alpha$_1$ agonists can cause reflex slowing of the heart. The mechanism is as follows: alpha$_1$-mediated vasoconstriction elevates blood pressure, which triggers the baroreceptor reflex, causing heart rate to decline. In patients with marginal cardiac reserve, the decrease in blood flow caused by reflex bradycardia may compromise tissue perfusion.

CLINICAL CONSEQUENCES OF ALPHA$_2$ ACTIVATION

As discussed in Chapter 12, alpha$_2$ receptors in the periphery are located *presynaptically* and their activation inhibits norepinephrine release. Several adrenergic agonists (e.g., epinephrine, norepinephrine, ephedrine) are capable of causing alpha$_2$ activation. However, the ability of drugs to activate alpha$_2$ receptors in the periphery has only minimal clinical significance. There are no *therapeutic* applications related to activation of peripheral alpha$_2$ receptors. Furthermore, activation of these receptors does not produce adverse effects of any consequence. Please note, however, that clinically significant effects *can* result from the activation of alpha$_2$ receptors in the *CNS*. These responses are discussed in Chapter 40 (Drug Therapy of Hypertension).

CLINICAL CONSEQUENCES OF BETA$_1$ ACTIVATION

All of the clinically relevant responses to activation of beta$_1$ receptors result from activating beta$_1$ receptors in the *heart*; activation of *renal* beta$_1$ receptors is not associated with either beneficial or adverse effects. As indicated in Table 17–2, beta$_1$ receptors can be activated by epinephrine, norepinephrine, isoproterenol, dopamine, dobutamine, and ephedrine.

Therapeutic Applications of Beta$_1$ Activation

Cardiac Arrest. By activating cardiac beta$_1$ receptors, drugs can initiate contraction in a heart that has stopped beating. It should be noted, however, that drugs are not the preferred treatment for cardiac arrest; rather, drugs should be used only after more desirable procedures (mechanical thumping, DC cardioversion) have failed to restart the heart. When a beta$_1$ agonist is indicated, epinephrine—injected directly into the heart—is the preferred agent.

Heart Failure. Heart failure is characterized by a reduction in the force of myocardial contraction, resulting in insufficient cardiac output. Since activation of beta$_1$ receptors in the heart has a positive inotropic effect (i.e., increases the force of contraction), drugs that activate these receptors can improve cardiac performance. Drug therapy of heart failure is discussed at length in Chapter 42.

Shock. This condition is characterized by profound hypotension and greatly reduced tissue perfusion. The primary goal of treatment is to maintain blood flow to vital organs. By increasing heart rate and force of contraction, beta$_1$ stimulants can increase cardiac output and can thereby improve tissue perfusion.

Atrioventricular Heart Block. Atrioventricular (A-V) heart block is a condition in which impulse conduction from the atria to the ventricles is impeded—or blocked entirely. As a consequence, the ventricles are no longer driven at an appropriate rate. Since activation of cardiac beta$_1$ receptors can enhance impulse conduction through the A-V node, beta$_1$ stimulants can help overcome A-V block. It should be noted, however, that drugs are only a temporary form of treatment; for long-term management, a pacemaker should be implanted.

Adverse Effects of Beta$_1$ Activation

All of the adverse effects of beta$_1$ activation result from activating beta$_1$ receptors in the *heart*; activating *renal* beta$_1$ receptors is not associated with untoward effects.

Altered Heart Rate or Rhythm. Overstimulation of cardiac beta$_1$ receptors can produce *tachycardia* (excessive heart rate) and *dysrhythmias* (irregular heart beat).

Angina Pectoris. In some patients, drugs that activate beta$_1$ receptors can precipitate an attack of angina pectoris, a condition characterized by substernal pain in the region of the heart. Anginal pain occurs when oxygen supply (blood flow) to the heart is insufficient to meet the heart's oxygen demand. The most common cause of angina is coronary atherosclerosis (accumulation of lipids and other substances in coronary arteries). Since beta$_1$ agonists increase cardiac oxygen demand (by increasing heart rate and force of contraction), patients with compromised coronary blood flow are at risk of an anginal attack. Angina pectoris and its treatment are discussed at length in Chapter 41.

CLINICAL CONSEQUENCES OF BETA$_2$ ACTIVATION

Therapeutic Applications of Beta$_2$ Activation

Therapeutic applications of beta$_2$ activation are limited to the lung and the uterus. Drugs used for their beta$_2$-activating ability include epinephrine, isoproterenol, terbutaline, and ephedrine.

Asthma. Asthma is a chronic condition characterized by bronchoconstriction occurring in response to a variety of stimuli. During a severe attack, airflow can be reduced so greatly as to threaten life. Since drugs that activate beta$_2$ receptors in the lung promote *bronchodilation*, these agents can help relieve or prevent asthma attacks.

For therapy of asthma, adrenergic agonists that are *selective for beta$_2$ receptors* (e.g., terbutaline) are preferred to less selective agents (e.g., epinephrine, isoproterenol). This is especially true for patients who suffer from *angina pectoris* or *tachycardia* in addition to asthma; we do not want to give

these patients drugs that can activate beta$_1$ receptors since these drugs could aggravate their cardiac disorder.

Several of the beta$_2$ agonists used to treat asthma are administered by *inhalation*. This route is desirable in that it helps minimize adverse systemic effects. It should be noted, however, that inhalation does not guarantee safety: serious systemic toxicity can result from overdosage with inhaled sympathomimetics. Accordingly, patients must be warned against inhaling too much medication. Asthma and its therapy are discussed at length in Chapter 64.

Delay of Preterm Labor. Activation of beta$_2$ receptors in the uterus relaxes uterine smooth muscle. This action can be exploited to delay preterm labor. The use of beta$_2$ agonists to delay delivery is discussed in Chapter 58 (Uterine Stimulants and Relaxants).

Adverse Effects of Beta$_2$ Activation

The most noteworthy adverse response to beta$_2$ activation is *hyperglycemia* (elevation of blood glucose). Beta$_2$ agonists can cause hyperglycemia by acting on the liver and skeletal muscles to promote breakdown of glycogen into glucose. As a rule, these drugs produce hyperglycemia only in patients with *diabetes*; in patients with normal pancreatic function, insulin will be released in response to glucose elevation, thereby reducing blood glucose to an appropriate level. If hyperglycemia develops in the diabetic patient, insulin dosage should be increased.

CLINICAL CONSEQUENCES OF DOPAMINE RECEPTOR ACTIVATION

Activation of peripheral dopamine receptors causes dilation of the vasculature of the kidneys. This effect is exploited in the treatment of *shock*: by dilating renal blood vessels, we can improve renal perfusion and can thereby reduce the risk of kidney failure. *Dopamine* itself is the only drug available that can activate dopamine receptors. It should be noted that when dopamine is given to treat shock, the drug will also enhance cardiac performance (by virtue of its ability to activate beta$_1$ receptors in the heart).

MULTIPLE RECEPTOR ACTIVATION: TREATMENT OF ANAPHYLACTIC SHOCK

Pathophysiology of Anaphylaxis. Anaphylactic shock is a manifestation of severe allergy. This reaction is characterized by *hypotension* (from widespread vasodilation), *bronchoconstriction*, and *edema of the glottis.* Although histamine contributes to these responses, symptoms are due largely to release of other mediators (e.g., leukotrienes). Anaphylaxis can be triggered by a variety of substances, including bee venom, wasp venom, and certain drugs (e.g., penicillins).

Treatment. *Epinephrine*, injected subcutaneously, is the treatment of choice for anaphylactic shock. Beneficial responses derive from the ability of epinephrine to activate three types of adrenergic receptors: $alpha_1$, $beta_1$, and $beta_2$. By activating these receptors, epinephrine can reverse the most severe manifestations of the anaphylactic reaction. By activating $beta_1$ receptors, epinephrine increases cardiac output, thereby helping to elevate blood pressure. Blood pressure is also increased because of epinephrine's ability to promote $alpha_1$-mediated vasoconstriction. In addition to increasing blood pressure, vasoconstriction helps suppress glottal edema. By activating $beta_2$ receptors, epinephrine can counteract bronchoconstriction. Individuals who are prone to severe allergic responses should be advised to carry a syringe of epinephrine at all times. (Antihistamines are not especially useful against anaphylaxis because histamine is only a minor contributor to the overall reaction.)

PROPERTIES OF REPRESENTATIVE ADRENERGIC AGONISTS

Our objective of this section is to establish an overview of the adrenergic agonists. This overview is presented in the form of "drug digests" that highlight characteristic features of representative sympathomimetic agents.

As noted previously, there are two major keys to understanding individual adrenergic agonists: (1) knowledge of the receptors that the drug can activate and (2) knowledge of the therapeutic and adverse effects that receptor activation can elicit. Integrating these two types of information will reveal the spectrum of effects that a particular drug can produce.

Unfortunately, knowing the effects that a drug is *capable* of producing does not always allow us to predict the *actual clinical applications* of that drug. Why? Because some adrenergic agonists are not used for all of the effects that they are able to produce. Norepinephrine, for example, can activate $alpha_1$ receptors and can therefore produce mydriasis; however, although norepinephrine can produce mydriasis, the drug is not actually used for this purpose. Similarly, although isoproterenol is capable of producing uterine relaxation (through $beta_2$ activation), isoproterenol is not employed clinically for this effect. Because receptor specificity is not always a predictor of the therapeutic applications of a particular adrenergic agonist, for

each of the drugs discussed below, approved clinical applications are indicated.

EPINEPHRINE

Receptor specificity: Alpha$_1$, alpha$_2$, beta$_1$, beta$_2$. *Chemical classification:* Catecholamine.

Epinephrine [Adrenalin] was among the first adrenergic agonists employed clinically and can be considered the prototype of the sympathomimetic drugs. Because of its prototypic status, epinephrine is discussed in detail.

Therapeutic Uses

Epinephrine can activate all four subtypes of adrenergic receptors. As a consequence, the drug can produce a broad spectrum of beneficial sympathomimetic effects.

Because of its ability to cause $alpha_1$-mediated vasoconstriction, epinephrine is used to (1) delay absorption of local anesthetics, (2) control superficial bleeding, (3) reduce nasal congestion, and (4) elevate blood pressure.

Activation of $alpha_1$ receptors on the iris is employed to produce mydriasis during ophthalmologic procedures.

Because of its ability to activate $beta_1$ receptors, epinephrine is used to (1) overcome A-V heart block and (2) restore cardiac function in patients with cardiac arrest.

Activation of $beta_2$ receptors in the lung promotes bronchodilation in patients with asthma.

Because of its ability to activate a combination of alpha and beta receptors, epinephrine is the treatment of choice for anaphylactic shock.

Pharmacokinetics

Absorption. Epinephrine may be administered topically, by injection, and by inhalation. The drug cannot be given orally; as discussed previously, catecholamines cannot be given orally because they undergo destruction by MAO and COMT before reaching the systemic circulation. With subcutaneous injection, absorption is slow because of epinephrine-induced local vasoconstriction. Absorption is more rapid following intramuscular injection. When epinephrine is inhaled (to treat asthma), systemic absorption is usually minimal; however, if dosing is excessive, systemic absorption can be sufficient to cause serious toxicity.

Inactivation. Epinephrine has a short plasma half-life because of two processes: (1) enzymatic inactivation and (2) uptake into adrenergic nerves. The enzymes that inactivate epinephrine and other catecholamines are MAO and COMT.

Adverse Effects

Because of its ability to activate the four major adrenergic receptor subtypes, epinephrine can produce multiple adverse effects.

Hypertensive Crisis. Vasoconstriction secondary to excessive alpha$_1$ activation can produce a dramatic and dangerous increase in blood pressure. Cerebral hemorrhage can occur. Because of the potential for severe hypertension, patients receiving *parenteral* epinephrine must undergo continuous monitoring of cardiovascular status.

Dysrhythmias. Excessive activation of beta$_1$ receptors in the heart can produce dysrhythmias. Because of their sensitivity to catecholamines, hyperthyroid patients are at high risk for epinephrine-induced dysrhythmias.

Angina Pectoris. By activating beta$_1$ receptors in the heart, epinephrine can increase both the work and the oxygen demands of the heart. If the increase in oxygen demand is sufficiently large, an anginal attack may ensue. Precipitation of angina is especially likely in patients with coronary atherosclerosis.

Necrosis Following Extravasation. If an IV line containing epinephrine becomes extravasated, the resultant localized vasoconstriction may cause necrosis. Because of this possibility, patients receiving IV epinephrine should be monitored closely. If extravasation occurs, injury can be minimized by local injection of phentolamine, an alpha-adrenergic antagonist.

Hyperglycemia. In diabetics, epinephrine can cause hyperglycemia. Hyperglycemia results from breakdown of glycogen in response to activation of beta$_2$ receptors in liver and skeletal muscle. If hyperglycemia develops, insulin dosage should be increased.

Drug Interactions

Monoamine Oxidase Inhibitors. The MAO inhibitors are drugs that suppress the activity of MAO. These agents are used primarily in the treatment of depression (see Chapter 25). Since MAO is one of the enzymes that inactivate epinephrine and other catecholamines, inhibition of MAO will prolong and intensify epinephrine's effects. As a rule, patients receiving an MAO inhibitor should not be given epinephrine.

Tricyclic Antidepressants. As discussed in Chapter 25, tricyclic antidepressants block the uptake of catecholamines into adrenergic neurons. Since neuronal uptake is one mechanism by which the actions of norepinephrine and other catecholamines are terminated, blockade of uptake can intensify and prolong epinephrine's effects. Accord-

ingly, patients receiving a tricyclic antidepressant may require a reduction in epinephrine dosage.

General Anesthetics. Several inhalation anesthetics render the myocardium hypersensitive to activation by beta$_1$ agonists. When the heart is in this hypersensitive state, exposure to epinephrine and other beta$_1$ agonists can cause dysrhythmias. These dysrhythmias may respond to a beta-adrenergic blocker (e.g., propranolol).

Alpha-Adrenergic Blocking Agents. Drugs that block alpha-adrenergic receptors can prevent their activation by epinephrine. Alpha blockers (e.g., phentolamine) can be used to treat toxicity (e.g., hypertension, local vasoconstriction) stemming from excessive epinephrine-induced alpha activation.

Beta-Adrenergic Blocking Agents. Drugs that block beta-adrenergic receptors can prevent their activation by epinephrine. Beta-blocking agents (e.g., propranolol) can reduce adverse effects (e.g., dysrhythmias, anginal pain) caused by epinephrine and other beta$_1$ agonists.

Preparations, Dosage, and Administration

Epinephrine [Adrenalin] is dispensed in solution for administration by various routes: intravenous, subcutaneous, intramuscular, intracardiac, intraspinal, inhalation, and topical. As indicated in Table 17–3, the strength of the epinephrine solution employed depends in large part on the route of administration. Note that solutions intended for *intravenous* administration are *less concentrated* than solutions intended for administration by most other routes. The reason that epinephrine must be diluted for intravenous use is that *intravenous administration of a concentrated epinephrine solution can produce potentially fatal reactions* (severe dysrhythmias and hypertension). Therefore, *before*

Table 17–3. Epinephrine Solutions: Concentrations for Different Routes of Administration	
Concentration of Epinephrine Solution	**Route of Administration**
1% (1:100)	Oral inhalation
0.1% (1:1,000)	Subcutaneous Intramuscular Intraspinal
0.01% (1:10,000)	Intravenous Intracardiac
0.001% (1:100,000)	In combination with local anesthetics

epinephrine is administered intravenously, the solution should be carefully checked to insure that its concentration is appropriate for intravenous use! Aspirate prior to IM or SC injection to avoid inadvertent injection into a vein.

Patients receiving intravenous epinephrine should be monitored constantly. They should be observed for signs of excessive cardiovascular activation (e.g., dysrhythmias, hypertension) and for possible extravasation of the IV line. If systemic toxicity develops, epinephrine should be discontinued; if indicated, an alpha-adrenergic blocker, a beta-adrenergic blocker, or both should be given to suppress symptoms. If an epinephrine-containing IV line becomes extravasated, administration should be discontinued and the region of extravasation infiltrated with an alpha-adrenergic blocker.

NOREPINEPHRINE

Receptor specificity: Alpha$_1$, alpha$_2$, beta$_1$.
Chemical classification: Catecholamine.

Norepinephrine (NE) is similar to epinephrine in many respects. With regard to receptor specificity, NE differs from epinephrine only in that NE does not activate beta$_2$ receptors. Accordingly, NE can elicit all of the responses that epinephrine can except those that are beta$_2$ mediated. Because NE is a catecholamine, the drug cannot be given orally and is subject to rapid inactivation by MAO and COMT. Adverse effects are nearly identical to those of epinephrine: dysrhythmias, angina, hypertension, and local necrosis upon extravasation. In contrast to epinephrine, NE does not promote hyperglycemia, a response that is mediated by beta$_2$ receptors. As with epinephrine, responses to NE can be modified by MAO inhibitors, tricyclic antidepressants, general anesthetics, and adrenergic blocking agents.

Despite its similarities with epinephrine, NE has limited clinical applications. The only recognized indications are *hypotensive states* and *cardiac arrest*.

Norepinephrine [Levophed] is dispensed in solution (1 mg/ml) for administration by intravenous infusion only. Patients should never be left unattended. Cardiovascular status should be monitored continuously. Care must be taken to avoid extravasation.

ISOPROTERENOL

Receptor specificity: Beta$_1$ and beta$_2$.
Chemical classification: Catecholamine.

Isoproterenol [Isuprel] differs significantly from NE and epinephrine in that isoproterenol acts only at beta-adrenergic receptors. Isoproterenol was the first beta-selective agent employed clinically and will serve as our prototype of the beta-selective adrenergic agonists.

Therapeutic Uses

Cardiovascular. By activating beta$_1$ receptors on the heart, isoproterenol can benefit patients with several cardiovascular disorders. The drug can help overcome A-V heart block; it can restart the heart following cardiac arrest; and it can increase cardiac output during shock.

Asthma. By activating beta$_2$ receptors in the lung, isoproterenol can cause bronchodilation, thereby decreasing airway resistance. Following its introduction, isoproterenol became a mainstay of asthma therapy. However, because of the development of more selective adrenergic agonists (drugs that activate beta$_2$ receptors only), use of isoproterenol has declined.

Adverse Effects

Since isoproterenol does not activate alpha-adrenergic receptors, the drug produces fewer adverse effects than norepinephrine or epinephrine. The major undesired responses are cardiac. Excessive activation of beta$_1$ receptors in the heart can cause *dysrhythmias* and *angina pectoris*. In addition to its cardiac effects, isoproterenol can cause *hyperglycemia in diabetics* by promoting beta$_2$-mediated glycogenolysis.

Drug Interactions

The major drug interactions of isoproterenol are nearly identical to those of epinephrine. Effects of isoproterenol are *enhanced by MAO inhibitors* and *tricyclic antidepressants* and *reduced by beta-adrenergic blocking agents*. Like epinephrine, isoproterenol can cause dysrhythmias in patients receiving certain *inhalation anesthetics*.

Receptor Specificity

Isoproterenol activates beta$_1$ and beta$_2$ receptors, but not alpha-adrenergic receptors. Because it can activate beta$_1$ as well as beta$_2$ receptors, when used to treat asthma, isoproterenol will cause beta$_1$ activation of the heart as a side effect. Accordingly, isoproterenol should not be used to treat asthma in patients who also have angina, tachycardia, or any other cardiac disorder that might be aggravated by beta$_1$ activation. Because isoproterenol is unable to distinguish between beta$_1$ and beta$_2$ receptors, and because beta$_2$-selective adrenergic agonists (e.g., terbutaline) are now available, use of isoproterenol to treat asthma has greatly declined.

Preparations and Administration

Preparations. Isoproterenol hydrochloride [Isuprel] is available in solution (0.2 mg/ml) for parenteral administration and in glossets (10 and 15 mg) for sublingual and rectal administration. In addition, the drug is available in a metered-dose aerosol device [Isuprel Mistometer, Medihaler-Iso] for treatment of asthma.

Administration. For therapy of *asthma*, isoproterenol can be administered by oral inhalation, sublingually, and intravenously. For routine therapy, oral inhalation is preferred. Drug therapy of asthma is discussed in depth in Chapter 64.

When used to *stimulate the heart*, isoproterenol can be administered IV, IM, and by direct intracardiac injection. The dosage for intramuscular administration is about ten times greater than the dosage employed by the other two routes.

DOPAMINE

Receptor specificity: Dopamine, beta$_1$, and, at high doses, alpha$_1$.
Chemical classification: Catecholamine.

Receptor Specificity

The degree of receptor specificity displayed by dopamine is dose dependent. When administered in low therapeutic doses, dopamine acts on dopamine receptors only. At moderate therapeutic doses, dopamine activates beta$_1$ receptors in addition to dopamine receptors. At very high doses, dopamine activates alpha$_1$ receptors along with beta$_1$ receptors and dopamine receptors.

Therapeutic Uses

Shock. The major indication for dopamine is shock. Benefits derive from effects on the heart and the renal vasculature. By activating beta$_1$ receptors in the heart, dopamine can increase cardiac output, thereby improving tissue perfusion. By activating dopamine receptors in the kidney, dopamine can dilate renal blood vessels, thereby improving renal perfusion, which, in turn, reduces the risk of renal failure. Treatment can be evaluated by monitoring output of urine.

Heart Failure. Heart failure is characterized by reduced tissue perfusion secondary to reduced cardiac output. Dopamine can help alleviate symptoms by activating beta$_1$ receptors on the heart, which increases cardiac output by increasing myocardial contractility.

Adverse Effects

The most common adverse effects of dopamine—*tachycardia, dysrhythmias,* and *anginal pain*—result from activation of beta$_1$ receptors in the heart. Because of its cardiac actions, dopamine is contraindicated for patients with tachydysrhythmias or ventricular fibrillation. Since high concentrations of dopamine will cause alpha$_1$ activation, extravasation may result in *necrosis* from localized vasoconstriction; tissue injury can be minimized by local administration of phentolamine (an alpha-adrenergic blocking agent).

Drug Interactions

MAO inhibitors can intensify the effects of dopamine on the heart and blood vessels. If a patient is receiving an MAO inhibitor, the dosage of dopamine must be reduced by at least 90%. *Tricyclic antidepressants* can also intensify dopamine's actions, but not to the extent seen with MAO inhibitors. Certain *general anesthetics* can sensitize the myocardium to the stimulant actions of dopamine

and other catecholamines, thereby creating a risk of dysrhythmias. *Diuretics* can complement the beneficial effects of dopamine on the kidney.

Preparations, Dosage, and Administration

Preparations. Dopamine hydrochloride [Dopastat, Intropin] is dispensed in aqueous solutions that range in concentration from 40 to 320 mg/ml.

Dosage. Dopamine must be diluted prior to infusion. For treatment of *shock*, a dilution of 400 μg/ml can be used. The recommended initial rate of infusion is 2 to 5 μg/kg/min. If needed, the infusion rate can be gradually increased to a maximum of 20 to 50 μg/kg/min.

Administration. Administration is intravenous. Because of extremely rapid inactivation by MAO and COMT, dopamine must be given by *continuous infusion*. A metering device (e.g., Microdrip) is needed to control the flow rate. Cardiovascular status must be closely monitored. If extravasation occurs, the infusion should be stopped and the region of extravasation infiltrated with an alpha-adrenergic antagonist.

DOBUTAMINE

Receptor specificity: Beta$_1$.
Chemical classification: Catecholamine.

Actions and Uses. At therapeutic doses, dobutamine causes selective activation of beta$_1$-adrenergic receptors. The only indication for the drug is *heart failure*.

Adverse Effects. The major adverse effect is tachycardia. Blood pressure and the electrocardiogram (EKG) should be monitored closely.

Drug Interactions. Effects of dobutamine on the heart and blood vessels are intensified greatly by *MAO inhibitors*. In patients receiving an MAO inhibitor, the dosage of dobutamine must be reduced by at least 90%. Concurrent use of *tricyclic antidepressants* may cause a moderate increase in the cardiovascular effects of dobutamine. Certain *general anesthetics* can sensitize the myocardium to the stimulant actions of dobutamine, thereby increasing the risk of dysrhythmias.

Preparations, Dosage, and Administration. Dobutamine hydrochloride [Dobutrex] is dispensed as a sterile powder (250 mg) in 20-ml vials. The powder is reconstituted in 10 or 20 ml of either sterile water or 5% dextrose. This concentrated solution must be diluted to at least 50 ml prior to use. Because of rapid inactivation by MAO and COMT, dobutamine is administered by IV infusion only. Rates of infusion usually range from 2.5 to 10 μg/kg/min.

PHENYLEPHRINE

Receptor specificity: Alpha$_1$.
Chemical classification: Noncatecholamine.

Phenylephrine is a selective alpha$_1$ agonist. The drug can be administered locally to alleviate nasal congestion (see Chapter 65) and parenterally to elevate blood pressure. In addition, phenylephrine can be applied to the eye to dilate the pupil (see Chapter 69). Lastly, phenylephrine can be coadministered with local anesthetics to retard absorption of the anesthetic.

TERBUTALINE

Receptor specificity: Beta$_2$.
Chemical classification: Noncatecholamine.

Therapeutic Uses

Asthma. Terbutaline can reduce airway resistance in asthma by causing beta$_2$-mediated bronchodilation. Since terbutaline is "selective" for beta$_2$ receptors, it produces much less activation of the heart than does isoproterenol. Accordingly, terbutaline is preferred to isoproterenol and related drugs for therapy of asthma. It must be remembered, however, that receptor selectivity is only relative: if administered in large doses, terbutaline will lose selectivity and activate beta$_1$ receptors as well as beta$_2$ receptors. Accordingly, patients should be warned not to exceed recommended doses, since doing so may cause undesired cardiac stimulation. The use of terbutaline and other beta$_2$ agonists to treat asthma is discussed fully in Chapter 64.

Delay of Preterm Labor. By activating beta$_2$ receptors in the uterus, terbutaline can relax uterine smooth muscle, thereby delaying labor. However, although terbutaline can be employed to delay labor, a different beta$_2$ agonist—ritodrine—is the drug of choice for this indication. The use of ritodrine and terbutaline to delay preterm labor is discussed in detail in Chapter 58 (Uterine Stimulants and Relaxants).

Adverse Effects

Adverse effects are minimal at therapeutic doses. However, if the dosage is excessive, terbu-taline can cause tachycardia by activating beta$_1$ receptors in the heart.

EPHEDRINE

Receptor specificity: Alpha$_1$, alpha$_2$, beta$_1$, beta$_2$.
Chemical classification: Noncatecholamine.

Ephedrine is referred to as a *mixed-acting* drug because it activates adrenergic receptors by *direct* and *indirect* mechanisms. *Direct* activation results from binding of the drug to alpha and beta receptors. *Indirect* activation results from release of NE from adrenergic neurons.

Therapeutic Uses

Nasal Congestion. Ephedrine can reduce nasal congestion by causing alpha$_1$-mediated vasoconstriction. When used for this indication, the drug can be administered topically or orally. As a rule, topical administration is preferred. This is because systemic reactions to topical administration are minimal, whereas oral administration results in activation of adrenergic receptors throughout the body.

Narcolepsy. Narcolepsy is a CNS disorder characterized by sudden and irresistible "attacks" of sleep. Ephedrine is one of several medications employed for treatment. (As discussed in Chapter 32, the principal drugs for narcolepsy are the amphetamines and ritodrine.) Benefits of ephedrine are thought to result from activation of adrenergic receptors in the brain. Ephedrine has access to CNS receptors because, being a noncatecholamine, the drug is able to cross the blood-brain barrier.

Adverse Effects

Since ephedrine activates the same receptors as epinephrine, these drugs share the same adverse effects: *hypertension, dysrhythmias, angina,* and *hyperglycemia.* In addition to these shared effects, ephedrine can act in the CNS to cause *insomnia.*

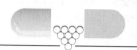

Summary of Major Nursing Implications

EPINEPHRINE

 Preadministration Assessment

Therapeutic Goal

Epinephrine has multiple uses. Major applications include treatment of *anaphylaxis* and *cardiac arrest*. Other uses include *control of superficial bleeding, delay of local anesthetic absorption,* and *reduction of nasal congestion.*

Identifying High-Risk Patients

Epinephrine must be used with *great caution* in patients with *hyperthyroidism, cardiac dysrhythmias, organic heart disease,* or *hypertension. Caution* is also needed in patients with *angina pectoris* or *diabetes* and in those receiving *MAO inhibitors, tricyclic antidepressants,* or *general anesthetics.*

 Implementation: Administration

Routes

Topical, oral inhalation, and parenteral (IV, IM, SC, intracardiac, intraspinal). Rapid inactivation by MAO and COMT prohibits oral use.

Administration

The concentration of epinephrine solutions varies with the route of administration (see Table 17–3). To avoid serious injury, check solutions carefully to insure that their concentration is appropriate for the intended route. Aspirate prior to SC and IM administration to avoid inadvertent injection into a vein.

Epinephrine solutions oxidize over time, causing them to turn pink or brown. Discard discolored solutions.

 Ongoing Evaluation and Interventions

Evaluating Therapeutic Effects

In patients receiving intravenous epinephrine, monitor cardiovascular status continuously.

Minimizing Adverse Effects

Cardiovascular Effects. By stimulating the heart, epinephrine can cause *anginal pain, tachycardia,* and *dysrhythmias*. These reactions can be decreased with a beta-adrenergic blocking agent (e.g., propranolol).

By stimulating alpha₁ receptors on blood vessels, epinephrine can cause intense vasoconstriction, which can result in *severe hypertension*. Blood pressure can be lowered with an alpha-adrenergic blocking agent (e.g., phentolamine).

Necrosis. If an IV line delivering epinephrine becomes extravasated, necrosis may result. Exercise care to avoid extravasation. If extravasation occurs, infiltrate the region with phentolamine to minimize injury.

Hyperglycemia. Epinephrine may cause hyperglycemia in diabetics. If hyperglycemia develops, insulin dosage should be increased.

Minimizing Adverse Interactions

MAO Inhibitors and Tricyclic Antidepressants. These drugs can prolong and intensify the actions of epinephrine. Patients taking these antidepressants will require a reduction in epinephrine dosage.

General Anesthetics. When combined with certain general anesthetics, epinephrine can induce cardiac dysrhythmias. These may respond to a beta$_1$-adrenergic blocker.

DOPAMINE

 Preadministration Assessment

Therapeutic Goal

Improvement of hemodynamic status in patients with shock or heart failure. Benefits derive from enhanced cardiac performance and increased renal perfusion.

Baseline Data

Full assessment of cardiac, hemodynamic, and renal status is needed.

Identifying High-Risk Patients

Dopamine is *contraindicated* for patients with *tachydysrhythmias or ventricular fibrillation*. Use with *extreme caution* in patients with *organic heart disease, hyperthyroidism,* or *hypertension* and in patients receiving *MAO inhibitors. Caution* is also needed in patients with *angina pectoris* and in those receiving *tricyclic antidepressants* or *general anesthetics.*

 Implementation: Administration

Route

Intravenous.

Administration

Administer by continuous infusion, employing a metering device (e.g., Microdrip) to control the flow rate.

If extravasation occurs, stop the infusion immediately and infiltrate the region with an alpha-adrenergic antagonist.

 Ongoing Evaluation and Interventions

Evaluating Therapeutic Effects

Monitor cardiovascular status continuously. Increased urine output is one index of success. Diuretics may complement the beneficial effects of dopamine on the kidney.

Minimizing Adverse Effects

Cardiovascular Effects. By stimulating the heart, dopamine may cause *anginal pain, tachycardia,* or *dysrhythmias.* These reactions can be decreased with a beta-adrenergic blocking agent (e.g., propranolol).

Necrosis. If the IV line delivering dopamine becomes extravasated, necrosis may result. Exercise care to avoid extravasation. If extravasation occurs, infiltrate the region with phentolamine.

Minimizing Adverse Interactions

MAO Inhibitors. Concurrent use of MAO inhibitors and dopamine can result in severe cardiovascular toxicity. If a patient is taking an MAO inhibitor, dopamine dosage must be reduced by at least 90%.

Tricyclic Antidepressants. These drugs can prolong and intensify the actions of dopamine. Patients receiving them may require a reduction in dopamine dosage.

General Anesthetics. When combined with certain general anesthetics, dopamine can induce dysrhythmias. These may respond to a beta$_1$-adrenergic blocker.

DOBUTAMINE

 Preadministration Assessment

Therapeutic Goal

Improvement of hemodynamic status in patients with heart failure.

Baseline Data

Full assessment of cardiac, renal, and hemodynamic status is needed.

Identifying High-Risk Patients

Use with *great caution* in patients with *organic heart disease, hyperthyroidism, tachydysrhythmias,* or *hypertension* and in those taking an *MAO inhibitor. Caution* is also needed in patients with *angina pectoris* and in those receiving *tricyclic antidepressants* and *general anesthetics.*

 Implementation: Administration

Route

Intravenous.

Administration

Administer by continuous infusion. Dilute concentrated solutions prior to use. Infusion rates usually range from 2.5 to 10 µg/kg/min. Adjust the infusion rate on the basis of the cardiovascular response.

 Ongoing Evaluation and Interventions

Evaluating Therapeutic Effects

Monitor cardiac function (heart rate, EKG), blood pressure, and urine output. When possible, monitor central venous pressure and pulmonary wedge pressure as well.

Minimizing Adverse Effects

Major adverse effects are *tachycardia* and *dysrhythmias.* Monitor the EKG and blood pressure closely. Adverse cardiac effects can be reduced with a beta-adrenergic antagonist.

Minimizing Adverse Interactions

MAO Inhibitors. Concurrent use of an MAO inhibitor with dobutamine can cause severe cardiovascular toxicity. If a patient is taking an MAO inhibitor, dobutamine dosage must be reduced by at least 90%.

Tricyclic Antidepressants. These drugs can prolong and intensify the actions of dobutamine. Patients receiving them may require a reduction in dobutamine dosage.

General Anesthetics. When combined with certain general anesthetics, dobutamine can cause cardiac dysrhythmias. These may respond to a beta$_1$-adrenergic antagonist.

18

Adrenergic Antagonists

The adrenergic antagonists cause direct blockade of adrenergic receptors. With only one exception (phenoxybenzamine), all of the adrenergic antagonists produce *reversible* (competitive) receptor blockade.

In contrast to some adrenergic agonists (e.g., epinephrine), the adrenergic antagonists display a high degree of receptor specificity. Because of this specificity, the adrenergic-blocking agents can be neatly divided into two major groups: (1) *alpha-adrenergic blocking agents* (drugs that produce selective blockade of alpha-adrenergic receptors) and (2) *beta-adrenergic blocking agents* (drugs that produce selective blockade of beta receptors). The drugs that belong to these two groups are listed in Table 18–1.

Our approach to the adrenergic antagonists will mirror the approach we took to the adrenergic agonists. That is, we will begin by discussing the therapeutic and adverse effects that can result from alpha- and beta-receptor blockade, after which we will discuss the individual drugs that block these receptors.

I remind you that it is much easier to understand responses to the adrenergic drugs if you first understand the responses to activation of adrenergic receptors. Accordingly, if you have not yet mastered (memorized) Table 12–3, you should do so now (or at least be prepared to consult that table as we proceed).

181

Table 18–1. Receptor Specificity of Adrenergic Antagonists		
Category	**Drugs**	**Receptors Blocked**
Alpha-Adrenergic Blocking Agents	Phentolamine	alpha$_1$, alpha$_2$
	Phenoxybenzamine	alpha$_1$, alpha$_2$
	Prazosin	alpha$_1$
	Terazosin	alpha$_1$
	Doxazosin	alpha$_1$
Beta-Adrenergic Blocking Agents	Carteolol	beta$_1$, beta$_2$
	Labetalol*	beta$_1$, beta$_2$
	Nadolol	beta$_1$, beta$_2$
	Penbutolol	beta$_1$, beta$_2$
	Pindolol	beta$_1$, beta$_2$
	Propranolol	beta$_1$, beta$_2$
	Sotalol	beta$_1$, beta$_2$
	Timolol	beta$_1$, beta$_2$
	Acebutolol	beta$_1$
	Atenolol	beta$_1$
	Betaxolol	beta$_1$
	Bisoprolol	beta$_1$
	Esmolol	beta$_1$
	Metoprolol	beta$_1$

*Labetalol also blocks alpha$_1$-adrenergic receptors.

ALPHA-ADRENERGIC ANTAGONISTS I: THERAPEUTIC AND ADVERSE RESPONSES TO ALPHA BLOCKADE

In this section we will discuss the beneficial and adverse responses that can result from blockade of alpha-adrenergic receptors. Properties of individual blocking agents are discussed later.

THERAPEUTIC APPLICATIONS OF ALPHA BLOCKADE

Virtually all of the clinically useful responses to alpha-adrenergic antagonists result from *blockade of alpha$_1$ receptors on blood vessels*. Blockade of alpha$_2$ receptors and blockade of alpha$_1$ receptors in the eye have no recognized therapeutic applications.

Essential Hypertension. Hypertension (high blood pressure) can be treated with a variety of drugs, including the alpha-adrenergic antagonists. Alpha antagonists lower blood pressure by blocking alpha$_1$ receptors on arterioles and veins, thereby causing vasodilation. Dilation of arterioles reduces arterial pressure directly. Dilation of veins lowers arterial pressure by an indirect process: in response to venous dilation, return of blood to the heart decreases, thereby decreasing cardiac output, which, in turn, reduces arterial pressure. The role of alpha-adrenergic blockers in essential hypertension is discussed further in Chapter 40 (Drug Therapy of Hypertension).

Reversal of Toxicity from Alpha$_1$ Agonists. Overdosage with an alpha-adrenergic agonist (e.g., epinephrine) can produce *hypertension* secondary to excessive stimulation of alpha$_1$ receptors on blood vessels. When this occurs, blood pressure can be lowered by reversing the vasoconstriction with an alpha-adrenergic antagonist. If an IV line containing an alpha agonist becomes extravasated, necrosis can occur secondary to intense local vasoconstriction. By infiltrating the region with phentolamine (an alpha-adrenergic antagonist), we can block the vasoconstriction and can thereby prevent injury.

Treatment of Pheochromocytoma. A pheochromocytoma is a catecholamine-secreting tumor derived from cells of the sympathetic nervous system. These tumors are usually located in the adrenal medulla. If secretion of catecholamines (epinephrine, norepinephrine) is sufficiently great, persistent hypertension can result. The principal cause of hypertension is activation of alpha$_1$ receptors on blood vessels, although activation of beta$_1$ receptors on the heart can also contribute. The preferred treatment is surgical removal of the tumor, but alpha-adrenergic blockers can also be employed.

Alpha-blocking agents have two roles in managing pheochromocytoma. First, in patients with inoperable tumors, alpha blockers are given chronically to suppress hypertension. Second, when surgery is indicated, alpha blockers are administered preoperatively to reduce the risk of acute hypertension during the procedure. (The surgical patient is at risk of acute hypertension because manipulation of the tumor can cause massive release of catecholamines.)

Raynaud's Disease. Raynaud's disease is a peripheral vascular disorder characterized by vasospasm in the toes and fingers. Prominent symptoms are local sensations of pain and cold. Alpha-adrenergic blocking agents can suppress symptoms by preventing alpha₁-mediated vasoconstriction. It should be noted, however, that although alpha blockers can relieve symptoms of Raynaud's disease, these drugs are generally ineffective against other peripheral vascular disorders that involve inappropriate vasoconstriction.

ADVERSE EFFECTS OF ALPHA BLOCKADE

The most significant adverse effects of the alpha-adrenergic antagonists result from blockade of alpha₁ receptors. Detrimental effects associated with alpha₂ blockade are minor.

Adverse Effects of Alpha₁ Blockade

Orthostatic Hypotension. This is the most serious adverse response to alpha-adrenergic blockade. Orthostatic hypotension can reduce blood flow to the brain, thereby causing dizziness, lightheadedness, and even syncope (fainting).

The cause of orthostatic hypotension is blockade of alpha receptors on *veins*, resulting in reduced muscle tone in the venous wall. Because of reduced venous tone, blood tends to pool (accumulate) in veins when the patient assumes an erect posture. (This redistribution of blood is analogous to the movement of water within a long, skinny balloon. When the balloon is horizontal, the water distributes evenly. However, when the balloon is suspended by one end, fluid pressure stretches the balloon, causing water to pool at the low end.) Because of venous pooling, return of blood to the heart is reduced. This reduction in venous return decreases cardiac output, which in turn causes blood pressure to fall.

Patients should be informed about the symptoms of hypotension (lightheadedness, dizziness) and advised to sit or lie down if these occur. In addition, patients should be informed that orthostatic hypotension can be minimized by avoiding abrupt transitions from a supine or sitting position to an erect posture.

Reflex Tachycardia. Alpha-adrenergic antagonists can increase heart rate by triggering the baroreceptor reflex. Activation of the reflex occurs as follows: (1) blockade of vascular alpha₁ receptors causes vasodilation; (2) vasodilation reduces blood pressure; and (3) baroreceptors sense the reduction in blood pressure and, in an attempt to restore normal pressure, initiate a reflexive increase in heart rate via the autonomic nervous system. If necessary, reflex tachycardia can be suppressed with a beta-adrenergic blocking agent.

Nasal Congestion. Alpha blockade can dilate the blood vessels of the nasal mucosa, producing nasal congestion.

Inhibition of Ejaculation. Since activation of alpha₁ receptors is required for ejaculation (see Table 12–3), blockade of these receptors can cause impotence. This form of drug-induced impotence is reversible, and resolves when the alpha blocker is withdrawn.

The ability of alpha blockers to inhibit ejaculation can be a major cause of noncompliance. If a patient deems the adverse sexual effects of alpha blockade unacceptable, a change in medication will be required. Since males may be reluctant to discuss their concerns, a tactful interview will be needed to discern if drug-induced impotence is discouraging compliance.

Sodium Retention and Increased Blood Volume. By reducing blood pressure, alpha blockers can promote retention of sodium and water by the kidney, thereby causing blood volume to increase. The steps in this process are as follows: (1) by reducing blood pressure, alpha₁ blockers decrease renal blood flow; (2) in response to reduced perfusion, the kidney excretes less sodium and water; and (3) the resultant retention of sodium and water increases blood volume. As a result of these events, blood pressure is elevated, blood flow to the kidney is increased, and, as far as the kidney is concerned, all is well. Unfortunately, this compensatory elevation in blood pressure tends to negate the effects for which alpha-blocking drugs are often given. That is, alpha antagonists are often used to treat hypertension; by increasing blood volume and blood pressure, the kidney effectively counteracts the blood pressure–lowering action of alpha blockade. In order to prevent the kidney from "neutralizing" the hypotensive actions of alpha-blocking agents, these drugs are usually combined with a diuretic when employed to treat hypertension.

Adverse Effects of Alpha₂ Blockade

The most significant adverse effect associated with alpha₂ blockade is *potentiation of the reflex tachycardia that can occur in response to blockade of alpha₁ receptors.* How does alpha₂ blockade intensify reflex tachycardia? Recall that peripheral alpha₂ receptors are located presynaptically and that activation of these receptors inhibits neurotransmitter (norepinephrine) release. Hence, if alpha₂ receptors are blocked, release of transmitter will increase. Since the reflex tachycardia caused by alpha₁ blockade is ultimately the result of increased firing of the sympathetic nerves to the heart, and since alpha₂ blockade will cause each nerve impulse to release a greater amount of norepinephrine, alpha₂ blockade will potentiate cardiac stimulation resulting from the reflexes initiated by blockade of alpha₁ receptors. Because alpha₂ blockade potentiates the reflex tachycardia induced by alpha₁ blockade, drugs such as phentolamine, which block alpha₂ as well as alpha₁ receptors, cause greater reflex tachycardia than the drugs that block alpha₁ receptors only.

ALPHA-ADRENERGIC ANTAGONISTS II: PROPERTIES OF INDIVIDUAL ALPHA BLOCKERS

Only five alpha-adrenergic antagonists are employed clinically. Because the alpha blockers often cause postural hypotension, therapeutic uses for these drugs are limited.

As can be seen from Table 18–1, the alpha-adrenergic blocking agents can be subdivided into two groups. One subgroup—the *nonselective* alpha-blocking agents—contains drugs that block alpha$_1$ *and* alpha$_2$ receptors. *Phentolamine* is the prototype for this group. The second subgroup, represented by *prazosin*, contains drugs that produce *selective alpha$_1$ blockade*.

PRAZOSIN

Actions and Uses. Prazosin [Minipress] is a competitive antagonist that produces selective blockade of alpha$_1$-adrenergic receptors. By blocking alpha$_1$ receptors, prazosin can cause dilation of arterioles and veins. The principal indication for prazosin is *hypertension*.

Pharmacokinetics. Prazosin is administered orally. Antihypertensive effects peak in 1 to 3 hours and persist for 10 hours. The drug undergoes extensive hepatic metabolism followed by excretion in the bile. Only about 10% is eliminated in the urine. The drug's half-life is 2 to 3 hours.

Adverse Effects. Blockade of alpha$_1$ receptors can cause *orthostatic hypotension, reflex tachycardia, inhibition of ejaculation,* and *nasal congestion*. The most serious of these effects is postural hypotension. Patients should be educated about the symptoms of hypotension (dizziness, lightheadedness) and advised to sit or lie down if these occur. Patients should also be informed that orthostatic hypotension can be minimized by moving slowly when making the transition from a supine or sitting position to an upright position.

About 1% of patients lose consciousness 30 to 60 minutes after receiving their first prazosin dose. This "first-dose" effect is the result of severe postural hypotension. To minimize the first-dose effect, the initial dose should be small (1 mg or less). After this low initial dose, the dosage can be gradually increased with little risk of fainting. Patients who are starting treatment should be forewarned about the first-dose effect and advised to avoid driving and other hazardous activities for 12 to 24 hours. Administering the initial dose at bedtime eliminates the risk of a first-dose effect.

Preparations, Dosage, and Administration. Prazosin hydrochloride [Minipress] is available in capsules (1, 2, and 5 mg) for oral use. The initial adult dosage for essential hypertension is 1 mg administered two or three times a day. For maintenance therapy, the dosage is 6 to 15 mg/day administered in divided doses.

TERAZOSIN

Actions and Uses. Like prazosin, terazosin is a selective, competitive antagonist at alpha$_1$ adrenergic receptors. The only indication for the drug is hypertension.

Pharmacokinetics. Terazosin is administered orally, and peak effects develop in 1 to 2 hours. The drug has a half-life of 9 to 12 hours; hence, antihypertensive effects can be sustained with once-a-day dosing. Terazosin undergoes hepatic metabolism followed by excretion in the bile and urine.

Adverse Effects. Like other alpha-blocking agents, terazosin can cause *orthostatic hypotension, reflex tachycardia, nasal congestion,* and *inhibition of ejaculation*. In addition, terazosin is associated with a high incidence (16%) of *headache*. As with

prazosin, the first dose of terazosin can cause profound hypotension. To minimize this first-dose effect, the initial dose should be administered at bedtime.

Preparations, Dosage, and Administration. Terazosin [Hytrin] is available in tablets (1, 2, 5, and 10 mg) for oral use. Therapy is initiated with a 1-mg dose administered at bedtime (to minimize the first-dose effect). Dosage can be gradually increased as needed and tolerated. The recommended dosage range for maintenance therapy is 1 to 5 mg once daily.

DOXAZOSIN

Actions and Uses. Doxazosin is a selective, competitive inhibitor of alpha$_1$-adrenergic receptors. The drug is indicated only for treatment of hypertension.

Pharmacokinetics. Doxazosin is administered orally, and peak effects develop in 2 to 3 hours. The drug has a prolonged half-life (22 hours); hence, treatment can be accomplished with once-a-day dosing. Most (98%) of the drug in blood is bound to plasma proteins. Doxazosin undergoes extensive hepatic metabolism followed by biliary excretion.

Adverse Effects. Like prazosin and terazosin, doxazosin can cause *orthostatic hypotension, reflex tachycardia, nasal congestion,* and *inhibition of ejaculation*. As with prazosin, the first dose of terazosin can cause profound hypotension. First-dose hypotension can be minimized by giving the initial dose at bedtime.

Preparations, Dosage, and Administration. Doxazosin [Cardura] is dispensed in tablets (1, 2, 4, and 8 mg) for oral administration. The initial dosage is 1 mg once daily. The dosage may be gradually increased as needed up to a maximum of 16 mg once daily.

PHENTOLAMINE

Actions and Uses. Like prazosin, phentolamine is a competitive adrenergic antagonist. However, in contrast to prazosin, phentolamine blocks alpha$_2$ as well as alpha$_1$ receptors. Phentolamine has two applications: (1) treatment of pheochromocytoma and (2) prevention of tissue necrosis following extravasation of drugs that produce alpha$_1$-mediated vasoconstriction (e.g., norepinephrine).

Adverse Effects. Like prazosin, phentolamine can produce the typical adverse effects associated with alpha-adrenergic blockade: *orthostatic hypotension, reflex tachycardia, nasal congestion,* and *inhibition of ejaculation*. Because of its ability to block alpha$_2$ receptors, *phentolamine produces greater reflex tachycardia than prazosin*. If reflex tachycardia is especially severe, heart rate can be reduced with a beta-adrenergic blocker. Since tachycardia can aggravate angina pectoris and myocardial infarction, phentolamine is contraindicated for patients with either disorder.

Overdosage can produce profound hypotension. If necessary, blood pressure can be elevated with *norepinephrine. Epinephrine* should *not* be used, because the drug can cause blood pressure to drop even further! Why? Because in the presence of alpha$_1$ blockade, the ability of epinephrine to promote vasodilation (via activation of vascular beta$_2$ receptors) may outweigh the ability of epinephrine to cause vasoconstriction (via activation of vascular alpha$_1$ receptors). Further lowering of blood pressure is not a problem with norepinephrine because norepinephrine does not cause beta$_2$ stimulation.

Preparations, Dosage, and Administration. Phentolamine [Regitine] is available in solution (5 mg/25 ml) for IM and IV administration. The dosage for preventing hypertension during surgical excision of a pheochromocytoma is 5 mg (IM or IV). For preventing necrosis following extravasation of IV norepinephrine, the region should be infiltrated with 5 to 10 mg of phentolamine diluted in 10 ml of saline.

PHENOXYBENZAMINE

Actions and Uses. Like phentolamine, phenoxybenzamine blocks alpha$_1$ and alpha$_2$ receptors. However, unlike all of the other alpha-adrenergic antagonists, phenoxybenzamine is a *noncompetitive* receptor antagonist. Hence, receptor blockade is *not reversible.* As a result, the effects of phenoxybenzamine are long lasting. (Responses to a single dose can persist for several days.) Effects subside as newly synthesized receptors replace the ones that have been irreversibly blocked. Phenoxybenzamine has only two indications: pheochromocytoma and peripheral vascular disease.

Adverse Effects. Like the other alpha-adrenergic antagonists, phenoxybenzamine can produce *orthostatic hypotension, reflex tachycardia, nasal congestion,* and *inhibition of ejaculation.* Reflex tachycardia is greater than that caused by prazosin but about equal to that caused by phentolamine.

If administered in excessive amounts, phenoxybenzamine, like phentolamine, will cause profound hypotension. Furthermore, since hypotension is the result of *irreversible* alpha$_1$ blockade, phenoxybenzamine-induced hypotension cannot be corrected with an alpha$_1$ agonist. To restore blood pressure, patients must be given IV fluids, which elevate blood pressure by increasing blood volume.

Preparations, Dosage, and Administration. Phenoxybenzamine hydrochloride [Dibenzyline] is available in 10-mg capsules for oral use. The initial adult dosage is 10 mg per day. The dosage can be increased every 4 days until the desired level of alpha blockade has been achieved. Daily maintenance dosages for adults range from 20 to 60 mg.

BETA-ADRENERGIC ANTAGONISTS I: THERAPEUTIC AND ADVERSE RESPONSES TO BETA BLOCKADE

In this section we will consider the beneficial and adverse responses that can result from blockade of beta-adrenergic receptors. Properties of individual beta-blocking agents are discussed later.

THERAPEUTIC APPLICATIONS OF BETA BLOCKADE

Practically all of the therapeutic effects of the beta-adrenergic antagonists result from blockade of beta$_1$ receptors in the heart. The major consequences of blocking these receptors are (1) reduced heart rate, (2) reduced force of contraction, and (3) reduced velocity of impulse conduction through the atrioventricular (A-V) node. Because of these effects, the beta blockers are useful in a variety of pathologic states.

Hypertension. Beta-adrenergic blocking agents are drugs of choice for many patients with hypertension. Because of their use in this common disorder, the beta blockers are one of our most widely prescribed families of drugs.

The exact mechanism by which beta blockers reduce blood pressure is not known. Proposed mechanisms include (1) reduction of cardiac output through blockade of beta$_1$ receptors in the heart, (2) suppression of renin release through blockade of beta$_1$ receptors in the kidney (the role of renin

in control of blood pressure is discussed in Chapter 37), and (3) suppression of reflex tachycardia caused by the vasodilators (e.g., alpha$_1$ antagonists) used to treat hypertension. The role of beta-adrenergic blocking agents in hypertension is discussed further in Chapter 40 (Drug Therapy of Hypertension).

Angina Pectoris. Angina pectoris (paroxysmal pain in the region of the heart) occurs when oxygen supply (blood flow) to the heart is insufficient to meet cardiac oxygen demand. Anginal attacks can be precipitated by exertion, intense emotion, and other factors. Beta-adrenergic blockers are a mainstay of antianginal therapy. By blocking beta$_1$ receptors in the heart, these drugs decrease cardiac work. This brings oxygen demand back into balance with oxygen supply, and thereby prevents pain. Angina pectoris and its treatment are the subject of Chapter 41.

Cardiac Dysrhythmias. Beta-adrenergic blocking agents are especially useful for treating dysrhythmias that involve excessive electrical activity in the sinus node and atria. By blocking cardiac beta$_1$ receptors, these drugs can (1) decrease the rate of sinus nodal discharge and (2) suppress conduction of atrial impulses through the A-V node, thereby preventing the ventricles from being driven at an excessive rate. The use of beta-adrenergic blockers to treat dysrhythmias is discussed in Chapter 44 (Antidysrhythmic Drugs).

Myocardial Infarction. A myocardial infarction (MI) is a region of myocardial necrosis caused by localized interruption of blood flow to the heart wall. Treatment with a beta blocker can reduce pain, infarct size, mortality, and the risk of reinfarction. To be effective, therapy with a beta-blocker must commence soon after an MI has occurred and should be continued for several years. The role of beta blockers in treating MI is discussed further in Chapter 43 (Management of Myocardial Infarction).

Hyperthyroidism. Hyperthyroidism (excessive production of thyroid hormone) is associated with an increase in the sensitivity of the heart to catecholamines (e.g., norepinephrine, epinephrine). As a result, normal levels of sympathetic activity to the heart can generate tachydysrhythmias and angina pectoris. Blockade of cardiac beta$_1$ receptors suppresses these responses.

Migraine. When taken prophylactically, beta-adrenergic blocking agents can reduce the frequency of migraine attacks. However, although beta blockers are effective as prophylaxis, these drugs are not able to abort a migraine headache once it has begun. The mechanism by which beta blockers prevent migraine is not known. Treatment of migraine and other headaches is the subject of Chapter 29.

Stage Fright. Public speakers and other performers sometimes experience "stage fright." Prominent symptoms are tachycardia and sweating brought on by generalized discharge of the sympathetic nervous system. Beta blockers help by preventing the beta$_1$-mediated tachycardia.

Pheochromocytoma. As discussed previously, a pheochromocytoma secretes large amounts of catecholamines, which can cause excessive stimulation of the heart. Cardiac stimulation can be counteracted by beta$_1$ blockade.

Glaucoma. Beta blockers are important drugs for treating glaucoma, a condition characterized by elevated intraocular pressure with subsequent injury to the optic nerve. The group of beta blockers used in glaucoma (see Table 69–2) is different from the group of beta blockers discussed in this chapter. Glaucoma and its treatment are addressed in Chapter 69 (Drugs for Disorders of the Eye).

ADVERSE EFFECTS OF BETA BLOCKADE

Although *therapeutic* responses to beta blockers are due almost entirely to blockade of *beta$_1$* receptors, adverse effects involve both beta$_1$ *and* beta$_2$ blockade. Consequently, the *nonselective* beta-adrenergic blocking agents (drugs that block beta$_1$ and beta$_2$ receptors) produce a broader spectrum of adverse effects than do the *"cardioselective"* beta-adrenergic antagonists (drugs that selectively block beta$_1$ receptors at usual therapeutic doses).

Adverse Effects of Beta$_1$ Blockade

All of the adverse effects of beta$_1$ blockade are the result of blocking beta$_1$ receptors in the heart. Blockade of renal beta$_1$ receptors does not produce adverse effects of clinical significance.

Bradycardia. Blockade of cardiac beta$_1$ receptors can produce bradycardia (excessively slow heart rate). If necessary, heart rate can be increased using a combination of isoproterenol (a beta-adrenergic agonist) and atropine (a muscarinic antagonist). Isoproterenol will compete with the beta blocker for cardiac beta$_1$ receptors, thereby promoting cardiac stimulation. By blocking muscarinic receptors on the heart, atropine will prevent slowing of the heart by the parasympathetic nervous system.

Reduced Cardiac Output. Beta$_1$ blockade can reduce cardiac output by (1) decreasing heart rate and (2) decreasing the force of myocardial contraction. Because they can decrease cardiac output, *beta blockers are contraindicated for patients with heart failure and should be used with great caution in patients with reduced cardiac reserve.* In both cases, any further decrease in cardiac output could result in insufficient tissue perfusion.

Precipitation of Congestive Heart Failure. In some patients, suppression of cardiac function with a beta blocker can be so great as to cause outright congestive heart failure (CHF), a condition in which the heart is unable to pump a sufficient amount of blood to maintain adequate perfusion of tissues. Patients should be informed about the early signs of heart failure (shortness of breath, night coughs, swelling of the extremities) and instructed to notify the physician if these occur. As noted above, beta-adrenergic blocking agents are contraindicated for most patients who already have CHF.

A-V Heart Block. A-V heart block is defined as suppression of impulse conduction through the A-V node. In its most severe form, A-V block prevents *all* atrial impulses from reaching the ventricles. Since blockade of cardiac beta$_1$ receptors can suppress A-V conduction, production of A-V block is a potential complication of beta-blocker therapy. These drugs are contraindicated for patients with pre-existing A-V block.

Rebound Cardiac Excitation. Long-term use of beta blockers can sensitize the heart to catecholamines. As a result, if a beta blocker is withdrawn *abruptly*, anginal pain or ventricular dysrhythmias may develop. This phenomenon of increased cardiac activity in response to abrupt cessation of beta-blocker therapy is referred to as *rebound excitation*. The risk of rebound excitation can be minimized by the simple expedient of withdrawing these drugs gradually (e.g., by tapering the dosage over a period of 1 to 2 weeks). If rebound excitation occurs, dosing should be temporarily resumed. Patients should be warned against abrupt cessation of treatment. Also, they should be advised to carry an adequate supply of their beta blocker when traveling.

Adverse Effects of Beta$_2$ Blockade

Bronchoconstriction. Blockade of beta$_2$ receptors in the lungs can cause constriction of the bronchi. (Recall that activation of these receptors promotes bronchodilation.) For most people, the degree of bronchoconstriction is insignificant. However, when bronchial beta$_2$ receptors are blocked in patients with *asthma*, the resulting increase in airway resistance can be life-threatening. Accordingly, *drugs that block beta$_2$ receptors are contraindicated for people with asthma*. If these individuals must use a beta blocker, they should use only those agents that are beta$_1$ selective (e.g., metoprolol).

Inhibition of Glycogenolysis. As noted in Chapter 12, epinephrine, acting at beta$_2$ receptors in skeletal muscle and the liver, can stimulate glycogenolysis (breakdown of glycogen into glucose). Beta$_2$ blockade will inhibit this process. Although suppression of beta$_2$-mediated glycogenolysis is inconsequential for most people, interference with this process *can* be detrimental to diabetics. This is because diabetics are especially dependent on beta$_2$-mediated glycogenolysis as a way to overcome severe reductions in blood glucose levels. If the diabetic patient requires a beta blocker, a beta$_1$-selective agent should be chosen.

BETA ADRENERGIC ANTAGONISTS II: PROPERTIES OF INDIVIDUAL BETA BLOCKERS

The beta-adrenergic antagonists can be subdivided into two groups: *nonselective* beta blockers and *cardioselective* beta blockers. The *nonselective* agents, represented by *propranolol,* block beta$_1$ and beta$_2$ receptors. The *cardioselective* agents, represented by *metoprolol,* produce selective blockade of beta$_1$ receptors (at usual therapeutic doses). Our discussion of the individual beta blockers will focus on the two prototypes: propranolol and metoprolol.

PROPRANOLOL

Propranolol [Inderal] was the first beta-adrenergic blocker to receive widespread clinical use and remains one of our most important beta-blocking agents. Propranolol blocks beta$_1$ and beta$_2$ receptors, and is the prototype of the nonselective beta-adrenergic antagonists.

Pharmacologic Effects

By blocking cardiac beta$_1$ receptors, propranolol can *reduce heart rate, decrease the force of ventricular contraction,* and *suppress impulse conduction through the A-V node.* The net response to these effects is a reduction in cardiac output.

By blocking beta$_1$ receptors in the kidney, propranolol can *suppress secretion of renin.*

Blockade of beta$_2$ receptors has three major effects: (1) blockade of beta$_2$ receptors in the lung can cause *bronchoconstriction,* (2) blockade of beta$_2$ receptors on certain blood vessels can produce *vasoconstriction,* and (3) blockade of beta$_2$ receptors in skeletal muscle and the liver can cause *inhibition of glycogenolysis.*

Pharmacokinetics

Propranolol is *highly lipid soluble* and, therefore, can readily cross membranes. The drug is well absorbed following oral administration, but, because of extensive metabolism on its first pass through the liver, less than 30% of each dose reaches the systemic circulation. Because of its ability to cross membranes, propranolol is widely distributed to all tissues and organs, including the CNS. Propranolol is inactivated by hepatic metabolism, and the metabolites are excreted in the urine.

Therapeutic Uses

Practically all of the applications of propranolol are based on blockade of beta$_1$ receptors in the heart. The drug's most important indications are *hypertension, angina pectoris,* and *cardiac dysrhythmias.* The role of propranolol and other beta blockers in these disorders is discussed in Chapter 40 (Drug Therapy of Hypertension), Chapter 41 (Drug Therapy of Angina Pectoris), and Chapter 44 (Antidysrhythmic Drugs). Additional indica-

tions include *myocardial infarction, migraine headache,* and *"stage fright."*

Adverse Effects

The most serious adverse effects of propranolol result from blockade of beta$_1$ receptors in the heart and blockade of beta$_2$ receptors in the lung.

Bradycardia. Beta$_1$ blockade in the heart can cause bradycardia. Heart rate should be assessed before each dose. If necessary, heart rate can be increased by administering atropine and isoproterenol.

A-V Heart Block. By slowing conduction of impulses through the A-V node, propranolol can cause A-V heart block. The drug is contraindicated for patients with pre-existing A-V block if it is greater than first degree.

Congestive Heart Failure. In patients with cardiac disease, suppression of myocardial contractility by propranolol can result in congestive heart failure (CHF). Patients should be informed about the early signs of CHF (shortness of breath, night coughs, swelling of the extremities) and instructed to notify the physician if these occur. Propranolol is contraindicated for patients with pre-existing heart failure.

Rebound Cardiac Excitation. Abrupt withdrawal of propranolol can cause rebound excitation of the heart, resulting in tachycardia or ventricular dysrhythmias. To avoid rebound excitation, propranolol should be withdrawn slowly by giving progressively smaller doses over 1 to 2 weeks. Patients should be warned against abrupt cessation of drug use. In addition, they should be advised to carry an adequate supply of the drug when traveling.

Bronchoconstriction. Blockade of beta$_2$ receptors in the lung can cause bronchoconstriction. As a rule, increased airway resistance is hazardous only to patients with asthma and other obstructive pulmonary disorders.

Inhibition of Glycogenolysis. Blockade of beta$_2$ receptors in skeletal muscle and the liver can inhibit glycogenolysis. This effect can be dangerous for people with diabetes (see below).

CNS Effects. Because of its lipid solubility, propranolol can readily cross the blood-brain barrier to reach sites in the CNS. Primary neuropsychiatric responses are *insomnia* and *depression.* The drug may also cause *nightmares* and *hallucinations.* Propranolol should be used with caution in patients with a history of major depression.

Precautions, Warnings, and Contraindications

Severe Allergy. Propranolol should be avoided in patients with a history of severe allergic reactions (anaphylaxis). Recall that epinephrine, the drug of choice for anaphylaxis, relieves symptoms in large part by activating beta$_1$ receptors in the heart and beta$_2$ receptors in the lung. If these receptors are blocked by propranolol, the ability of epinephrine to act will be dangerously impaired.

Diabetes. Propranolol can be detrimental to the diabetic in two ways. First, by blocking beta$_2$ receptors in muscle and the liver, propranolol can suppress glycogenolysis, thereby eliminating an important mechanism for correcting hypoglycemia (which can occur when insulin dosage is excessive). Second, by blocking beta$_1$ receptors, propranolol can suppress tachycardia, which normally serves as an early warning signal that blood glucose levels are falling too low. (When blood glucose drops below a safe level, the sympathetic nervous system is activated, causing an increase in heart rate.) By "masking" tachycardia, propranolol can delay awareness of hypoglycemia, thereby compromising the diabetic's ability to correct the problem in a timely fashion. Diabetic patients who are taking propranolol should be warned that tachycardia may no longer be a reliable indication of hypoglycemia. In addition, they should be taught to recognize alternative signs (sweating, hunger, fatigue, poor concentration) that blood glucose is falling perilously low. Because of its ability to suppress glycogenolysis and mask tachycardia, propranolol must be used with caution by diabetic patients. Also, patients may need to reduce their dosage of insulin.

Cardiac, Respiratory, and Psychiatric Disorders. Propranolol can exacerbate *congestive heart failure, A-V heart block, sinus bradycardia, asthma,* and *bronchospasm.* The drug is contraindicated for patients with these disorders. In addition, propranolol should be used with caution in patients with a history of *depression.*

Drug Interactions

Calcium Channel Blockers. The cardiac effects of certain calcium channel blockers (e.g., verapamil) are identical to those of propranolol: reduction of heart rate, suppression of A-V conduction, and suppression of myocardial contractility. When propranolol and calcium channel blockers are used concurrently, there is a risk of excessive cardiac suppression.

Insulin. As discussed above, propranolol can impede early recognition of insulin-induced hypoglycemia. In addition, propranolol can block glycogenolysis, the body's mechanism for correcting hypoglycemia.

Preparations, Dosage, and Administration

General Dosing Considerations. Establishing an effective propranolol dosage is difficult for two reasons: (1) patients vary widely in their requirements for propranolol, and (2) there is a poor correlation between blood levels of propranolol and the response produced. The explanation for these observations is that responses to propranolol are dependent on the activity of the sympathetic nervous system. If sympathetic activity is high, then the dose needed to reduce receptor activation will be high as well. Conversely, if sympathetic activity is low, then low doses will be sufficient to produce receptor blockade. Since sympathetic activity varies among patients, propranolol requirements vary as well. Accordingly, the dosage must be adjusted by monitoring the patient's response, and not by relying on dosing information in drug references.

Preparations. Propranolol hydrochloride [Inderal] is available in three oral formulations: (1) tablets (10 to 90 mg), (2) sustained-release capsules (60 to 160 mg), and (3) oral solutions (4, 8, and 80 mg/ml). The drug is also available in solution (1 mg/ml) for IV administration.

Dosage. For treatment of *hypertension*, the initial dosage is 40 mg twice a day. Daily maintenance dosages usually range from 120 to 240 mg (in divided doses), although some patients may need as much as 640 mg a day. The usual adult dosage for *angina pectoris* is 160 mg per day.

METOPROLOL

Metoprolol [Lopressor, Toprol XL] is the prototype of the "cardioselective" beta-adrenergic antagonists. At usual therapeutic doses, metoprolol blocks beta$_1$ receptors only. Please note, however, that selectivity for beta$_1$ receptors is not absolute: at higher doses, metoprolol and the other "cardioselective" agents will block beta$_2$ receptors as well as beta$_1$ receptors. Because their effects on beta$_2$ receptors are normally minimal, the cardioselective agents are not likely to cause bronchoconstriction or suppression of glycogenolysis. As a result, these drugs are preferred to the nonselective beta blockers for use by patients with asthma and diabetes.

Pharmacologic Effects. By blocking cardiac beta$_1$ receptors, metoprolol has the same impact on the heart as propranolol: the drug reduces heart rate, force of contraction, and conduction of impulses through the A-V node. Also like propranolol, metoprolol reduces secretion of renin by the kidney. In contrast to propranolol, metoprolol does not block bronchial beta$_2$ receptors (at usual therapeutic doses) and, therefore, does not increase airway resistance.

Pharmacokinetics. Metoprolol is moderately lipid soluble and is well absorbed following oral administration. Like propranolol, metoprolol undergoes extensive metabolism on its first pass through the liver. As a result, only about 40% of an oral dose reaches the systemic circulation. Elimination is by a combination of hepatic metabolism and renal excretion.

Therapeutic Uses. The primary indication for metoprolol is *hypertension*. The drug is also approved for management of *angina pectoris* and *myocardial infarction*.

Adverse Effects. The major adverse effects of metoprolol involve the heart. Like propranolol, metoprolol can cause *bradycardia, reduction of cardiac output, A-V heart block, congestive heart failure,* and *rebound cardiac excitation following abrupt withdrawal.* In contrast to propranolol, metoprolol causes minimal bronchoconstriction and does not interfere with beta$_2$-mediated glycogenolysis.

Precautions, Warnings, and Contraindications. Like propranolol, metoprolol is contraindicated for patients with *congestive heart failure, sinus bradycardia,* and *A-V heart block that is greater than first degree.* Because metoprolol produces only minimal blockade of beta$_2$ receptors, the drug is safer than propranolol for use by patients with asthma or a history of severe allergic reactions. In addition, since metoprolol does not suppress beta$_2$-mediated glycogenolysis, the drug can be used more safely than propranolol by diabetics. It should be noted, however, that metoprolol, like propranolol, will "mask" tachycardia, thereby depriving the diabetic of an early indication that hypoglycemia is developing.

Preparations, Dosage, and Administration. Metoprolol is available in standard oral tablets (50 and 100 mg) under the trade name Lopressor and in sustained-release oral tablets (50, 100, and 200 mg) under the trade name Toprol XL. The drug is also available in solution (1 mg/ml) for IV administration. The initial dosage for hypertension is 100 mg/day in single or divided doses. The dosage for maintenance therapy ranges from 100 to 400 mg/day in divided doses. Intravenous administration is reserved for treating myocardial infarction.

OTHER BETA-ADRENERGIC BLOCKERS

In the United States, fourteen beta blockers are approved for treatment of cardiovascular disorders (hypertension, angina pectoris, cardiac dysrhythmias, myocardial infarction). Principal differences among these drugs concern receptor specificity, pharmacokinetics, indications, and side effects.

In addition to the agents used for cardiovascular disorders, there is a group of beta blockers used to treat glaucoma. These drugs are discussed in Chapter 69 (Drugs for Disorders of the Eye).

Pharmacologic properties of the beta blockers employed for cardiovascular disorders are discussed below.

Receptor Specificity. As noted previously, the beta blockers fall into two major groups: *nonselective* agents and *cardioselective* agents. The nonselective agents block beta$_1$ *and* beta$_2$ receptors, whereas the cardioselective agents block *beta$_1$ receptors only* (at usual therapeutic doses). Because of their limited side effects, the cardioselective agents are preferred for patients with asthma or diabetes. One beta blocker—*labetalol*—differs from all the others in that it blocks *alpha* adrenergic receptors in addition to beta receptors. The receptor specificity of individual beta blockers is indicated in Tables 18–1 and 18–2.

Pharmacokinetics. Pharmacokinetic properties of the beta blockers are summarized in Table 18–2. The relative *lipid solubility* of these agents is of particular importance. The drugs with the *highest* lipid solubility—propranolol and penbutolol—have two prominent features: they penetrate the blood-brain barrier with ease, and they are eliminated primarily by *hepatic metabolism*. The drugs with *low* lipid solubility (e.g., acebutolol, atenolol) penetrate the blood-brain barrier poorly, and are eliminated primarily by *renal excretion*. The drugs with *moderate* lipid solubility—metoprolol, labetalol, and pindolol—are able to penetrate the blood-brain barrier, and are eliminated by a combination of *hepatic metabolism and renal excretion*.

Therapeutic Uses. Principal indications for the beta-adrenergic blockers are *hypertension, angina pectoris,* and *cardiac dysrhythmias.* Other uses include prophylaxis of migraine headache, treatment of myocardial infarction, and suppression

Table 18–2. Clinical Pharmacology of the Beta-Adrenergic Blocking Agents

Generic Name	Trade Name	Receptors Blocked	ISA	Lipid Solubility	Half-Life (hr)	Route*	Maintenance Dosage in Hypertension†
Acebutolol	Sectral		+	Low	3–4	PO	400 mg once/day
Atenolol	Tenormin		0	Low	6–9	PO, IV	50 mg once/day
Betaxolol	Kerlone		0	Low	14–22	PO	10 mg once/day
Bisoprolol	Zebeta	Beta$_1$	0	Low	9–12	PO	5 mg once/day
Esmolol	Brevibloc		0	Low	0.15	IV	Not for hypertension
Metoprolol	Lopressor		0	Moderate	3–7	PO, IV	100 mg once/day
slow release	Toprol XL					PO	100 mg once/day
Carteolol	Cartrol		+ +	Low	6	PO	2.5 mg once/day
Labetalol‡	Normodyne, Trandate		0	Moderate	6–8	PO, IV	300 mg twice/day
Nadolol	Corgard	Beta$_1$	0	Low	20–24	PO	40 mg once/day
Penbutolol	Levatol	and	+	High	5	PO	20 mg once/day
Pindolol	Visken	Beta$_2$	+ + +	Moderate	3–4	PO	10 mg twice/day
Propranolol	Inderal		0	High	3–5	PO, IV	60 mg twice/day
slow release	Inderal LA		0	High	3–5	PO	120 mg once/day
Sotalol	Betapace		0	Low	12	PO	Not for hypertension
Timolol	Blocadren		0	Low	4	PO	20 mg twice/day

ISA = intrinsic sympathomimetic activity (partial agonist activity)
*Oral administration is used for essential hypertension. Intravenous administration is reserved for acute myocardial infarction (atenolol, metoprolol), cardiac dysrhythmias (esmolol, propranolol), and severe hypertension (labetalol).
†These are the lowest doses normally used for maintenance in hypertension.
‡Labetalol blocks alpha$_1$-adrenergic receptors in addition to blocking beta receptors.

Table 18–3. Beta-Adrenergic Blocking Agents: Summary of Therapeutic Uses

	Hyper-tension	Angina Pectoris	Cardiac Dysrhythmias	Myocardial Infarction	Migraine Prophylaxis	Stage Fright
Acebutolol	A		A			
Atenolol	A	A	I	A	I	I
Betaxolol	A					
Bisoprolol	A	I	I			
Carteolol	A	I				
Esmolol		I	A			
Labetalol	A					
Metoprolol	A	A	I	A	I	
Nadolol	A	A	I		I	I
Penbutolol	A					
Pindolol	A		I			I
Propranolol	A	A	A	A	A	I
Sotalol			A			
Timolol	A		I	A	A	I

A = FDA-approved use, I = investigational use.
A group of beta blockers not discussed in this chapter is used to treat glaucoma. These beta blockers are discussed in Chapter 69 (Drugs for Disorders of the Eye).

of symptoms in individuals with situational anxiety (e.g., stage fright).

Approved and investigational uses of the beta blockers are summarized in Table 18–3. With the exception of *esmolol*, all of the drugs in the table are approved for oral therapy of *essential hypertension*. Because of its very short half-life (15 minutes), esmolol is clearly unsuited for treating hypertension, which requires that blood levels be maintained throughout the day, every day, for an indefinite time. The only approved indication for *esmolol* is emergency intravenous therapy of *supraventricular tachycardia*.

Adverse Effects. By blocking cardiac beta$_1$ receptors, *all* of the beta blockers can cause *bradycardia, A-V heart block*, and, rarely, *congestive heart failure*. By blocking beta$_2$ receptors in the lung, the *nonselective* agents can cause significant *bronchoconstriction* in patients with asthma and chronic obstructive pulmonary disease. In addition, by blocking beta$_2$ receptors in the liver and skeletal muscle, the *nonselective* agents can *inhibit glycogenolysis*, thereby compromising the ability of diabetic patients to compensate for insulin-induced hypoglycemia. Because of its ability to block alpha-adrenergic receptors, *labetalol* can cause *postural hypotension*. Although *CNS effects* (insomnia, depression) can occur with all beta blockers, these effects may be more prominent with the highly lipid-soluble agents. Abrupt discontinuation of any beta blocker can produce *rebound cardiac excitation*. Accordingly, all beta blockers should be withdrawn slowly (by tapering the dosage over 1 to 2 weeks).

Intrinsic Sympathomimetic Activity (Partial Agonist Activity). The term *intrinsic sympathomimetic activity* (ISA) refers to the ability of certain beta blockers—especially *pin-*

dolol—to act as *partial agonists* at beta-adrenergic receptors. (As discussed in Chapter 6, a partial agonist is a drug whose binding to a receptor produces a limited degree of receptor activation, while at the same time preventing strong agonists from binding to the receptor to cause full activation.)

In contrast to other beta blockers, agents with ISA have very little effect on *resting* heart rate and cardiac output. When patients are at rest, stimulation of the heart by the sympathetic nervous system is low. If an ordinary beta blocker is given, it will block sympathetic stimulation, causing heart rate and cardiac output to decline. However, if a beta blocker has ISA, its own ability to cause limited receptor activation will compensate for blocking receptor activation by the sympathetic nervous system; consequently, resting heart rate and cardiac output will not be reduced.

Because of their ability to provide a low level of cardiac stimulation, beta blockers with ISA are preferred to other beta blockers for use in patients with bradycardia or borderline CHF. Conversely, these agents should not be given to patients with myocardial infarction, since their ability to cause even limited cardiac stimulation can be detrimental.

Dosage and Administration. With the exception of esmolol, all of the beta blockers discussed in this chapter can be administered *orally*. Three drugs—*atenolol, labetalol,* and *propranolol*—may be given *intravenously* as well as by mouth. *Esmolol* is administered only by IV injection.

Maintenance dosages for hypertension are summarized in Table 18–2. For most beta blockers, dosing can be done just once a day. For the drugs with especially short half-lives, twice-a-day dosing is required (unless an extended-release formulation is available).

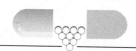 **Summary of Major Nursing Implications**

ALPHA₁-ADRENERGIC ANTAGONISTS

Doxazosin

Prazosin

Terazosin

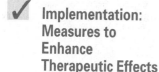 **Preadministration Assessment**

Therapeutic Goal

Reduction of blood pressure in patients with essential hypertension.

Baseline Data

Determine blood pressure.

Identifying High-Risk Patients

The only contraindication is hypersensitivity to these drugs.

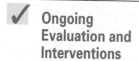 **Implementation: Administration**

Route

Oral.

Administration

Instruct patients to take the initial dose at bedtime to minimize the "first-dose" effect. All three drugs may be taken with food.

Implementation: Measures to Enhance Therapeutic Effects

For supportive measures in the treatment of hypertension, refer to the *Summary of Major Nursing Implications* in Chapter 40.

Ongoing Evaluation and Interventions

Evaluating Therapeutic Effects

Evaluate treatment by monitoring blood pressure.

Minimizing Adverse Effects

Orthostatic Hypotension. Alpha₁ blockade can cause postural hypotension. Inform patients about the symptoms of hypotension (dizziness, light-headedness), and advise them to sit or lie down if these occur. Advise patients to move slowly when changing from a supine or sitting position to an upright posture.

First-Dose Effect. The first dose of prazosin, terazosin, or doxazosin may cause fainting from severe orthostatic hypotension. Forewarn patients about this effect, and advise them to avoid driving and other hazardous activities for 12 to 24 hours after receiving the initial dose. To minimize risk, advise patients to take the first dose at bedtime.

BETA-ADRENERGIC ANTAGONISTS

Except where noted, the implications summarized here apply to all beta-adrenergic blocking agents.

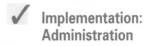

Preadministration Assessment

Therapeutic Goal

Principal indications are *hypertension, angina pectoris,* and *cardiac dysrhythmias.* Indications for individual agents are summarized in Table 18–3.

Baseline Data

For Hypertension. Determine standing and supine blood pressure.

For Angina Pectoris. Determine the incidence, severity, and circumstances of anginal attacks.

For Cardiac Dysrhythmias. Obtain a baseline EKG.

Identifying High-Risk Patients

All beta blockers are *contraindicated* for patients with *congestive heart failure, sinus bradycardia,* and *A-V heart block* (greater than first degree). Use with *caution* (especially the nonselective agents) in patients with *asthma, bronchospasm, diabetes,* and *history of severe allergic reactions.* Use *all* beta blockers with *caution* in patients taking *calcium channel blockers.*

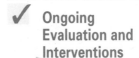

Implementation: Administration

Routes

Oral. All beta blockers except esmolol.

Intravenous. *Atenolol, esmolol, labetalol, metoprolol, propranolol.*

Administration

For maintenance therapy of hypertension, administration is done once or twice daily (see Table 18–2).

Warn patients against abrupt discontinuation of treatment.

Ongoing Evaluation and Interventions

Evaluating Therapeutic Effects

Hypertension. Monitor blood pressure and heart rate prior to each dose. Advise outpatients to monitor blood pressure and heart rate daily.

Angina Pectoris. Advise patients to record the incidence, circumstances, and severity of anginal attacks.

Cardiac Dysrhythmias. Monitor for improvement in the EKG.

Minimizing Adverse Effects

Bradycardia. Beta$_1$ blockade can reduce heart rate. If bradycardia is severe, withhold medication and notify the physician. If necessary, administer atropine and isoproterenol to restore heart rate.

A-V Heart Block. Beta$_1$ blockade can decrease A-V conduction. Do not give beta blockers to patients with A-V block greater than first degree.

Congestive Heart Failure. Suppression of myocardial contractility can cause CHF. Inform patients about early signs of CHF (shortness of breath, night coughs, swelling of the extremities), and instruct them to notify the physician if these occur.

Rebound Cardiac Excitation. Abrupt withdrawal of beta blockers can cause tachycardia and ventricular dysrhythmias. Warn patients against abrupt discontinuation of drug use. Advise patients to carry an adequate supply of medication when traveling.

Postural Hypotension. By blocking alpha-adrenergic receptors, *labetalol* can cause postural hypotension. Inform patients about signs of hypotension (lightheadedness, dizziness), and advise them to sit or lie down if these develop. Advise patients to move slowly when changing from a supine or sitting position to an upright posture.

Bronchoconstriction. Beta$_2$ blockade can cause substantial airway constriction in patients with asthma. The risk of bronchoconstriction is much lower with the cardioselective agents than with the nonselective agents.

Effects in Diabetics. Beta$_1$ blockade can "mask" tachycardia, an early sign of hypoglycemia. Warn patients that tachycardia cannot be relied on as an indicator of impending hypoglycemia, and teach them to recognize other indicators (sweating, hunger, fatigue, poor concentration) that blood glucose is becoming dangerously low. Beta$_2$ blockade can prevent glycogenolysis, an emergency means of increasing blood glucose. Patients may need to reduce their insulin dosage. Cardioselective beta blockers are preferred to nonselective agents in patients with diabetes.

CNS Effects. Beta blockers can cause insomnia, depression, and nightmares. If these effects occur, it may be helpful to switch to a beta-blocker with low lipid solubility (see Table 18–2).

Minimizing Adverse Interactions

Calcium Channel Blockers. Two of these drugs (verapamil, nifedipine) can intensify the cardiosuppressant effects of the beta blockers. Use the combination with caution.

Insulin. Beta blockers can prevent the compensatory glycogenolysis that normally occurs in response to insulin-induced hypoglycemia. Diabetic patients may need to reduce their insulin dosage.

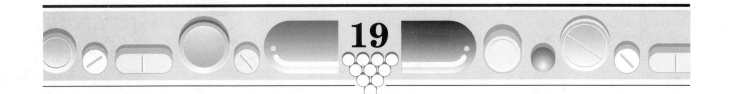

19

Indirect-Acting Antiadrenergic Agents

ADRENERGIC NEURON BLOCKING AGENTS
Reserpine
Guanethidine

CENTRALLY ACTING ANTIADRENERGIC AGENTS
Clonidine
Methyldopa

The indirect-acting antiadrenergic agents are drugs that prevent the stimulation of peripheral adrenergic receptors, but they do so by mechanisms that do not involve direct receptor interaction. There are two categories of indirect-acting antiadrenergic drugs. The first group—*adrenergic neuron blocking agents*—consists of drugs that act within the terminals of sympathetic neurons to decrease norepinephrine release. The second group, known as *centrally acting antiadrenergic agents,* consists of drugs that act within the central nervous system (CNS) to reduce the outflow of impulses along sympathetic nerves. With both groups, the net result of drug actions is a reduction in the stimulation of peripheral adrenergic receptors. Hence, the pharmacologic effects of the indirect-acting adrenergic blocking agents are similar to those of drugs that block adrenergic receptors directly.

ADRENERGIC NEURON BLOCKING AGENTS

The adrenergic neuron blocking agents are drugs that act presynaptically to reduce the release of norepinephrine from sympathetic neurons. (These drugs have very little effect on the release of epinephrine from the adrenal medulla.) Our discussion of the adrenergic neuron blockers will focus on two agents: reserpine and guanethidine.

RESERPINE

Reserpine [Serpasil, Serpalan] is a naturally occurring compound prepared from the root of *Rauwolfia serpentina*, a shrub indigenous to India. Because of its source, reserpine is classified as a *Rauwolfia alkaloid*.* The primary indication for reserpine is hypertension. When employed clinically, the drug can produce several serious side effects, the most important being severe mental depression. Surprisingly, despite its adverse effects, and despite the availability of superior alternatives, reserpine remains a widely prescribed drug.

Mechanism of Action

Reserpine produces its pharmacologic effects by causing *depletion of norepinephrine (NE) from postganglionic sympathetic neurons*. By doing so, the drug can decrease the stimulation of practically all adrenergic receptors. Hence, the effects of reserpine closely resemble those produced by a combination of alpha- and beta-adrenergic blockade.

There are two mechanisms by which reserpine depletes NE from neurons. First, *reserpine acts on vesicles within the nerve terminal to cause displacement of stored NE,* thereby exposing the transmitter to destruction by monoamine oxidase (MAO). Second, *reserpine suppresses norepinephrine synthesis.* As depicted in Figure 19–1, reserpine decreases NE synthesis by blocking the uptake of dopamine (the immediate precursor of NE) into presynaptic vesicles, the structures that contain the enzymes needed to convert dopamine into NE. A week or two may be required for maximal transmitter depletion to develop.

In addition to its peripheral effects, reserpine can cause depletion of transmitters (serotonin, catecholamines) from neurons within the CNS. Depletion of these CNS transmitters underlies the most serious side effect of reserpine—deep emotional depression—and also explains the occasional use of reserpine in psychiatry.

Pharmacologic Effects

Peripheral Effects. By depleting sympathetic neurons of norepinephrine, reserpine decreases

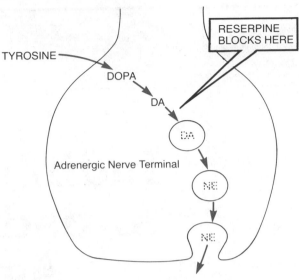

Figure 19–1. Mechanism of reserpine action. Reserpine depletes neurons of norepinephrine (NE) by two mechanisms. (1) As indicated in this figure, reserpine blocks the uptake of dopamine (DA) into vesicles, thereby preventing NE synthesis. (2) Reserpine displaces NE from vesicles, thereby allowing degradation of NE by monoamine oxidase present in the nerve terminal (not shown).

the activation of alpha- and beta-adrenergic receptors. Decreased activation of beta receptors slows heart rate and reduces cardiac output. Decreased alpha activation promotes vasodilation. All three effects cause a *decrease in blood pressure.*

Effects on the CNS. Reserpine produces sedation and a state of indifference to the environment. In addition, the drug can cause severe depression. These effects are thought to result from depletion of certain neurotransmitters (catecholamines, serotonin) from neurons within the brain.

Therapeutic Uses

Hypertension. The principal indication for reserpine is hypertension. Antihypertensive effects result from vasodilation and reduced cardiac output. Since these effects occur secondary to depletion of NE, and since transmitter depletion occurs slowly, full antihypertensive responses can take a week or more to develop. Conversely, when reserpine is discontinued, effects may persist for several weeks as the NE content of sympathetic neurons becomes replenished. Because its side effects can be severe, and because more desirable drugs are available (see Chapter 40), reserpine is not a drug of choice for hypertension.

Psychotic States. Reserpine can be used to treat agitated psychotic patients, such as those suffering from certain forms of schizophrenia. However, since superior drugs are available (e.g., phenothiazine antipsychotics), reserpine is rarely employed in psychotherapy.

---

*In addition to reserpine, four other Rauwolfia derivatives are available: whole root rauwolfia [Raudixin, Rauverid, Wolfina], deserpidine [Harmonyl], rescinnamine [Moderil], and alseroxylon [Rauwiloid]. All four preparations have pharmacologic effects and uses similar to those of reserpine.

Adverse Effects

Depression. Reserpine can produce severe depression that may persist for months after the drug is withdrawn. Suicide has occurred. All patients should be informed about the risk of depression. Also, they should be educated about signs of depression (e.g., early morning insomnia, loss of appetite, change in mood) and instructed to notify the physician immediately if these develop. Because of the risk of suicide, patients who develop depression may require hospitalization. *Reserpine is contraindicated for patients with a history of depressive disorders.*

Cardiovascular Effects. Depletion of norepinephrine from sympathetic neurons can result in *bradycardia, orthostatic hypotension,* and *nasal congestion.* Bradycardia is caused by decreased activation of beta$_1$ receptors in the heart. Hypotension and nasal congestion are caused by reduced activation of alpha receptors on blood vessels. Patients should be informed that orthostatic hypotension, the most serious cardiovascular effect, can be minimized by moving slowly when changing from a supine to an upright posture. In addition, patients should be advised to sit or lie down if lightheadedness or dizziness occurs.

Gastrointestinal Effects. By mechanisms that are not understood, reserpine can stimulate several aspects of gastrointestinal function. The drug can increase secretion of gastric acid, which may result in ulcer formation. In addition, reserpine can increase the tone and motility of intestinal smooth muscle, thereby causing cramps and diarrhea.

Preparations, Dosage, and Administration

Reserpine [Serpasil, Serpalan] is available in tablets (0.1, 0.25, and 1 mg) for oral use. The drug may be administered with food if gastrointestinal upset occurs. The initial dosage for hypertension in adults is 0.5 mg/day. For maintenance therapy, the dosage should be reduced to 0.1 to 0.25 mg/day.

GUANETHIDINE

Guanethidine [Ismelin] is an adrenergic neuron blocking agent that has hypotensive actions similar to those of reserpine. However, in contrast to reserpine, guanethidine cannot cross the blood-brain barrier and, hence, does not adversely affect the CNS. The drug's most serious adverse effect is profound orthostatic hypotension. Because of this effect, indications for guanethidine are limited.

Mechanism of Action

Primary Action: Inhibition of Norepinephrine Release. Guanethidine acts presynaptically to inhibit the release of NE from sympathetic neurons. (The drug does not decrease the release of catecholamines from the adrenal medulla.) In order to inhibit NE release, guanethidine must first be taken up into terminals of sympathetic nerves

(Figure 19–2A). Uptake occurs by way of the same transport system employed for reuptake of NE. Once inside the nerve terminal, guanethidine acts to prevent NE release. The precise mechanism by which the drug inhibits release is not known (hence the nonscientific nature of Figure 19–2B).

Secondary Actions. In addition to blocking NE release, guanethidine has two other actions. First, during *initial* use, guanethidine can *promote NE release*. As a result, the early phase of therapy may be associated with a brief period of *sympathomimetic effects* and not with sympathetic blockade. Second, with chronic use, guanethidine, like reserpine, *depletes NE from sympathetic nerves*. Since the hypotensive effects of guanethidine can be seen before transmitter depletion occurs, it would appear that this secondary action is unrelated to the drug's hypotensive effects.

Pharmacologic Effects

The pharmacologic effects of guanethidine, like those of reserpine, result from decreased activation of alpha- and beta-adrenergic receptors. By reducing receptor activation, guanethidine can cause *bradycardia*, a *decrease in cardiac output*, and a *great reduction in venous smooth muscle tone*. As a result, systolic blood pressure falls, especially when the patient is standing.

Therapeutic Use

The only indication for guanethidine is *hypertension.* Because of its tendency to cause severe orthostatic hypotension, guanethidine is not used routinely. Rather, the drug is reserved for those patients whose blood pressure cannot be controlled with more desirable agents.

Adverse Effects

Orthostatic Hypotension. Guanethidine-induced orthostatic hypotension can be severe. Blood pressure may fall so low that perfusion of the heart and brain is seriously compromised. Supine and standing blood pressure should be monitored. If

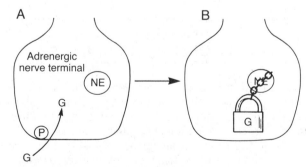

Figure 19–2. Mechanism of guanethidine action. *A,* Uptake. Before it can act, guanethidine must be taken up into terminals of sympathetic neurons. *B,* Action. Once inside the nerve terminal, guanethidine inhibits NE release (by a process that is not understood). (G = guanethidine, NE = norepinephrine, P = uptake pump)

standing blood pressure drops too low, guanethidine should be withheld and the physician notified. Patients should be warned about orthostatic hypotension and informed that this response can be minimized by moving slowly when assuming an erect posture. Also, patients should be made aware that factors that promote vasodilation (e.g., alcohol consumption, warm environments, strenuous exercise) can intensify orthostatic hypotension and should be avoided.

Gastrointestinal Effects. Like reserpine, guanethidine can stimulate the gastrointestinal system; *diarrhea* is the most common result. In most cases, guanethidine-induced diarrhea can be managed with antidiarrheal drugs (e.g., diphenoxylate, loperamide, anticholinergic agents). The mechanism by which guanethidine stimulates the gastrointestinal tract is unknown.

Hypertension. Although used to treat hypertension, guanethidine can *cause* hypertension in the patient with a pheochromocytoma (a catecholamine-secreting tumor). Recall that guanethidine stimulates NE release during the initial phase of treatment. Since pheochromocytomas contain massive amounts of NE, guanethidine-induced NE release can result in a dramatic rise in blood pressure.

Drug Interactions

The effects of guanethidine are *decreased* by *tricyclic antidepressants*. As discussed in Chapter 25, tricyclic antidepressants can block the uptake of NE into adrenergic neurons. Since guanethidine and NE share the same mechanism for uptake, tricyclic antidepressants will block the uptake of guanethidine, thereby preventing the drug from reaching its site of action.

Preparations, Dosage, and Administration

Guanethidine monosulfate [Ismelin Sulfate] is available in 10 and 25 mg tablets for oral use. The initial dosage for hypertension in adults is 10 mg administered once daily. The dosage can be increased every 5 to 7 days to a maintenance level of 25 to 50 mg administered once daily. Dosage should be reduced in patients who develop orthostatic hypotension or severe diarrhea.

CENTRALLY ACTING ANTIADRENERGIC AGENTS

The centrally acting antiadrenergic agents are drugs that act within the CNS to reduce the firing of sympathetic neurons. These drugs are used primarily in the treatment of hypertension. Two centrally acting antiadrenergic agents—clonidine and methyldopa—will be the focus of our discussion.

Why are centrally acting drugs being discussed in a unit on peripheral nervous system pharmacology? Because the effects of these drugs are ultimately the result of decreased activation of alpha- and beta-adrenergic receptors in the periphery.

That is, by inhibiting the firing of sympathetic neurons, the centrally acting agents decrease the release of NE from sympathetic nerves, thereby reducing activation of peripheral adrenergic receptors. Hence, although the centrally acting antiadrenergic agents act within the CNS, their effects are like those of the direct-acting adrenergic receptor blockers. Accordingly, it seems appropriate to discuss the centrally acting antiadrenergic agents in the context of peripheral nervous system pharmacology—rather than presenting these agents in the context of CNS drugs.

CLONIDINE

Clonidine [Catapres] is an antihypertensive agent whose site of action lies within the CNS. Except for rare instances of rebound hypertension, the drug is generally free of serious adverse effects. Because it is both effective and safe, clonidine is widely used.

Mechanism of Action

Clonidine is an alpha$_2$-adrenergic agonist whose effects result primarily from stimulating alpha$_2$ receptors in the brain—not in the periphery. The central alpha$_2$ receptors at which clonidine acts are located *post*synaptically. (This contrasts with peripheral alpha$_2$ receptors, which are *pre*synaptic.) By stimulating CNS alpha$_2$ receptors, clonidine exerts an inhibitory influence on regions of the brain that help regulate sympathetic nervous system activity. The net result is a reduction in sympathetic outflow to blood vessels and the heart.

Pharmacologic Effects

The most significant effects of clonidine occur in the heart and the vascular system. By suppressing the firing of sympathetic nerves to the heart, clonidine can cause *bradycardia* and a *decrease in cardiac output*. By suppressing sympathetic regulation of blood vessels, the drug promotes *vasodilation*. The net result of cardiac suppression and vasodilation is a *decrease in blood pressure*. Blood pressure is reduced in supine and standing subjects. (Note that the effect of clonidine on blood pressure is unlike that of the peripheral alpha-adrenergic blockers, which tend to decrease blood pressure only when the patient is standing.) Since the hypotensive effects of clonidine are not posture dependent, orthostatic hypotension with this drug is minimal.

Pharmacokinetics

Clonidine is very lipid soluble. As a result, the drug is readily absorbed following oral administration and undergoes wide distribution throughout the body, including the CNS. Hypotensive responses begin 30 to 60 minutes after administration and peak in approximately 4 hours. Effects of a single dose may persist for as long as 1 day. Clonidine is eliminated by a combination of hepatic metabolism and renal excretion.

Therapeutic Uses

Clonidine is *approved* only for treatment of *hypertension*. The drug has been used on an *investigational basis* to treat various conditions, including menopausal flushing, opioid withdrawal, alcohol withdrawal, migraine headache, and Tourette's syndrome (a CNS disease characterized by uncontrollable jerking and verbal outbursts that are frequently obscene).

Adverse Effects

Rebound Hypertension. Rebound hypertension is defined as a large increase in blood pressure occurring in response to abrupt clonidine withdrawal. This rare but serious reaction is caused by overactivity of the sympathetic nervous system, and can be accompanied by nervousness, tachycardia, and sweating. Left untreated, the reaction may persist for a week or more. If blood pressure climbs dangerously high, it should be lowered with a combination of alpha- and beta-adrenergic blocking agents. Rebound effects can be avoided by withdrawing clonidine slowly (over 2 to 4 days). Patients should be informed about rebound hypertension and warned not to discontinue clonidine without consulting the physician.

Xerostomia. Xerostomia (dry mouth) is common, occurring in about 40% of those treated. The reaction usually diminishes over the first 2 to 4 weeks of clonidine therapy. Although not dangerous, xerostomia can be sufficiently annoying as to discourage drug use. Patients should be advised that discomfort can be reduced by chewing gum, sucking on hard candy, and taking frequent sips of fluids.

Drowsiness. CNS depression occurs frequently. About 35% of patients experience drowsiness, and an additional 8% experience outright sedation. These responses become less intense with continued drug use. Patients in their early weeks of treatment should be advised to avoid hazardous activities if alertness is significantly impaired.

Use in Pregnancy. Clonidine is embryotoxic in animals. Because of the possibility of fetal harm, clonidine is not recommended for use by pregnant women. Pregnancy should be ruled out before therapy is instituted.

Other Adverse Effects. Clonidine can cause a variety of adverse effects in addition to those discussed above. Notable among these are *constipation, impotence, gynecomastia,* and ad-

verse *CNS effects* (e.g., vivid dreams, nightmares, anxiety, depression). *Localized skin reactions* occur frequently with the transdermal clonidine formulation.

Preparations, Dosage, and Administration

Preparations. Clonidine hydrochloride [Catapres] is available in tablets (0.1, 0.2, and 0.3 mg) for oral use and in transdermal systems [Catapres-TTS] that contain 2.5, 5, or 7.5 mg of drug.

Dosage and Administration

Oral. For treatment of hypertension, the initial adult dosage is 0.1 mg twice a day. The usual maintenance dosage is 0.2 to 0.8 mg a day administered in divided doses. By taking the majority of the daily dose at bedtime, adverse consequences of sedation can be minimized.

Transdermal. Transdermal patches are applied to a region of hairless, intact skin on the upper arm or torso. A new patch is applied every 7 days.

METHYLDOPA

Methyldopa [Aldomet, Amodopa] is a widely used antihypertensive agent. Like clonidine, the drug lowers blood pressure by acting at sites within the CNS. Certain side effects (hemolytic anemia, hepatic necrosis) can be severe. Given the potential hazards of the drug, its frequent usage is difficult to understand.

Mechanism of Action

The mechanism of action of methyldopa is similar to that of clonidine. Like clonidine, methyldopa inhibits sympathetic outflow from the CNS by causing alpha$_2$ stimulation in the brain. Methyldopa differs from clonidine in that methyldopa itself is not an effective alpha$_2$ agonist. In order to cause alpha$_2$ stimulation, methyldopa must first be taken up by neurons within the brain and then converted to methylnorepinephrine, a compound that is an effective alpha$_2$ agonist. Release of methylnorepinephrine results in alpha$_2$ stimulation.

Pharmacologic Effects

The most prominent response to methyldopa is a drop in blood pressure. The drug reduces blood pressure primarily by causing vasodilation—and not by effects on the heart. Vasodilation occurs because of reduced sympathetic traffic to blood vessels. At usual therapeutic doses, methyldopa does not decrease heart rate or cardiac output. Hence, hypotensive actions cannot be ascribed to cardiac depression. The hemodynamic effects of methyldopa are very much like those of clonidine: both drugs lower blood pressure in supine and standing subjects, and both produce relatively little orthostatic hypotension.

Therapeutic Use

The only indication for methyldopa is *hypertension*. Methyldopa was one of the earliest antihypertensive agents available and remains in wide use.

Adverse Effects

Positive Coombs' Test and Hemolytic Anemia. A positive Coombs' test* develops in 10% to 20% of patients taking methyldopa chronically. The Coombs' test usually turns positive between the sixth and twelfth month of treatment. Of those patients with a positive test result, only a few (about 5%) develop hemolytic anemia. Coombs'-positive patients who do not have hemolytic anemia may continue methyldopa treatment. However, if hemolytic anemia develops, drug use should cease immediately. For most patients, hemolytic anemia resolves soon after methyldopa withdrawal—although the Coombs' test may remain positive for months. A Coombs' test should be performed prior to treatment and 6 to 12 months later. Blood counts (hematocrit, hemoglobin or red cell count) should be obtained prior to treatment and periodically thereafter.

---

*The Coombs' test detects the presence of antibodies directed against the patient's own red blood cells. These antibodies can cause hemolysis (i.e., red cell lysis).

Hepatotoxicity. Methyldopa treatment has been associated with hepatitis, jaundice, and, rarely, fatal hepatic necrosis. All patients should undergo periodic assessment of liver function. If signs of hepatotoxicity appear, methyldopa should be discontinued immediately. Liver function usually normalizes following drug withdrawal.

Other Adverse Effects. Methyldopa can cause *xerostomia, sexual dysfunction, orthostatic hypotension,* and a variety of *CNS effects,* including drowsiness, reduced mental acuity, nightmares, and depression. These responses are not usually dangerous, but they can detract from compliance.

Preparations, Dosage, and Administration

Preparations. *Methyldopa* [Aldomet, Amodopa] is available in tablets (125, 250, and 500 mg) and in a suspension (50 mg/ml) for oral use. In addition, a derivative of methyldopa, named *methyldopate,* is available as an injection (50 mg/ml in 5-ml vials) for IV use.

Oral Therapy. For treatment of hypertension, the initial adult dosage is 250 mg 2 to 3 times a day. Daily maintenance dosages usually range from 0.5 to 2 gm administered in two to four divided doses.

Intravenous Therapy. Methyldopate, administered by slow IV infusion, is indicated for hypertensive emergencies. However, since faster-acting drugs are available, use of methyldopate is rare. Methyldopate for infusion should be diluted in 5% dextrose to a concentration of 10 mg/ml. The usual adult dose is 250 to 500 mg infused over 30 to 60 minutes. Dosing may be repeated every 6 hours as required.

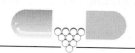 # Summary of Major Nursing Implications

---

RESERPINE

 ✓ **Preadministration Assessment**

Therapeutic Goal
Lowering of blood pressure in hypertensive patients.

Baseline Data
Determine blood pressure.

Identifying High-Risk Patients
Reserpine is *contraindicated* for patients with *active peptic ulcer disease* or a *history of depression*.

 ✓ **Implementation: Administration**

Route
Oral.

Administration
Administer with food to reduce gastric upset.

 ✓ **Ongoing Evaluation and Interventions**

Evaluating Therapeutic Effects
Full antihypertensive effects may take a week or more to develop. Monitor blood pressure to evaluate treatment.

Minimizing Adverse Effects
Depression. Reserpine can cause profound depression that may last for months after the drug is withdrawn; suicide has occurred. Inform patients about signs of depression (e.g., early morning insomnia, loss of appetite, change in mood), and instruct them to notify the physician if these develop. If depression occurs, hospitalization may be required. Avoid reserpine in patients with a history of depression.

Cardiovascular Effects. Reserpine can cause *orthostatic hypotension, bradycardia,* and *nasal congestion.* Inform patients that orthostatic hypotension can be minimized by moving slowly when changing from a seated or supine position to an upright posture. Advise patients to sit or lie down if dizziness or lightheadedness occurs.

Gastrointestinal Effects. Reserpine can promote *peptic ulcer disease* by increasing secretion of gastric acid. Advise patients to notify the physician if gastric pain develops.

GUANETHIDINE

 ✓ **Preadministration Assessment**

Therapeutic Goal
Lowering of blood pressure in hypertensive patients.

Baseline Data

Determine blood pressure in supine position, standing position, and, if possible, immediately after exercise.

Identifying High-Risk Patients

Guanethidine is contraindicated for patients with *pheochromocytoma*.

Implementation: Administration

Route

Oral.

Administration

For ambulatory patients, the entire daily dose is usually taken at one time. Prolonged treatment may be required; encourage patients to take the medication as prescribed.

Ongoing Evaluation and Interventions

Evaluating Therapeutic Effects

Monitor supine and standing blood pressure. Dosage is adjusted on the basis of the therapeutic response.

Minimizing Adverse Effects

Orthostatic Hypotension. Orthostatic hypotension can be severe. Monitor supine and standing blood pressure. If standing blood pressure falls too low, withhold medication and notify the physician. Educate patients about the signs of hypotension (dizziness, lightheadedness), and advise them to sit or lie down if these occur. Advise patients to move slowly when changing from a supine or sitting position to an upright posture. Warn patients to avoid factors that can promote hypotension (e.g., alcohol consumption, warm environments, strenuous exercise).

Diarrhea. Stimulation of the gastrointestinal tract can cause diarrhea. This response can be managed with antidiarrheal drugs.

Hypertension. Guanethidine can promote severe hypertension in patients with *pheochromocytoma*. The drug is contraindicated for these patients.

Minimizing Adverse Interactions

Tricyclic antidepressants can decrease the effects of guanethidine and should be avoided.

CLONIDINE

Preadministration Assessment

Therapeutic Goal

Lowering of blood pressure in hypertensive patients.

Baseline Data

Determine blood pressure.

Identifying High-Risk Patients

Clonidine is embryotoxic to animals and should not be used during *pregnancy*. Rule out pregnancy before initiating treatment.

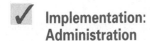 **Implementation: Administration**

Routes

Oral, transdermal.

Administration

Oral. Advise the patient to take the major portion of the daily dose at bedtime to minimize the adverse consequences of sedation.

Transdermal. Instruct the patient to apply transdermal patches to hairless, intact skin on the upper arm or torso. A new patch is applied every 7 days.

 Ongoing Evaluation and Interventions

Evaluating Therapeutic Effects

Monitor blood pressure to evaluate treatment.

Minimizing Adverse Effects

Rebound Hypertension. Severe hypertension, accompanied by nervousness, tachycardia, and sweating, occurs rarely following abrupt clonidine withdrawal. If necessary, blood pressure can be lowered with a combination of alpha- and beta-adrenergic blocking agents. To avoid rebound hypertension, withdraw clonidine slowly (over 2 to 4 days). Inform patients about rebound hypertension and warn them against abrupt discontinuation of treatment.

Xerostomia. Dry mouth occurs in about 40% of patients during the first few weeks of treatment. Inform patients that discomfort can be reduced by chewing gum, sucking on hard candy, and taking frequent sips of fluids.

Drowsiness and Sedation. During the early weeks of treatment, about 35% of patients experience drowsiness, and an additional 8% experience outright sedation. Inform patients about CNS depression, and warn them against participation in hazardous activities if alertness is impaired.

METHYLDOPA

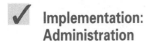 **Preadministration Assessment**

Therapeutic Goal

Lowering of blood pressure in hypertensive patients.

Baseline Data

Obtain baseline values for blood pressure, blood counts (hematocrit, hemoglobin or red cell count), Coombs' test, and liver function tests.

Identifying High-Risk Patients

Methyldopa is *contraindicated* for patients with active *liver disease* and for those with a *history of methyldopa-induced liver dysfunction*.

Implementation: Administration

Routes

Oral (for routine management of hypertension).
Intravenous (for hypertensive emergencies).

Administration

Most patients on oral therapy require divided (two to four) daily doses. For some patients, blood pressure can be controlled with a single daily dose at bedtime.

Evaluating Therapeutic Effects

Monitor blood pressure to evaluate therapy.

✓ **Ongoing Evaluation and Interventions**

Minimizing Adverse Effects

Positive Coombs' Test and Hemolytic Anemia. A positive Coombs' test develops in 10% to 20% of those treated; about 5% of Coombs'-positive patients develop hemolytic anemia. If hemolysis occurs, withdraw methyldopa immediately. In most cases, hemolytic anemia resolves soon after drug withdrawal (although the Coombs' test may remain positive for months). Obtain a Coombs' test prior to treatment and 6 to 12 months later. Obtain blood counts (hematocrit, hemoglobin or red cell count) prior to treatment and periodically thereafter.

Hepatotoxicity. Methyldopa can cause hepatitis, jaundice, and fatal hepatic necrosis. Assess liver function prior to treatment and periodically thereafter. If liver dysfunction develops, discontinue methyldopa immediately. In most cases, liver function returns to normal following drug withdrawal.

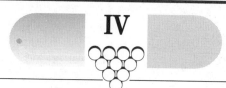

Central Nervous System Drugs

Introduction

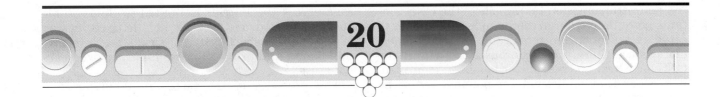

20

Introduction to Central Nervous System Pharmacology

The central nervous system (CNS) drugs—agents that act on the brain and spinal cord—are used widely for medical and nonmedical purposes. Medical applications include treatment of mental illness, suppression of seizures, relief of pain, and production of anesthesia. CNS drugs are used nonmedically for their stimulant, depressant, euphoriant, and other "mind-altering" abilities.

Despite the widespread use of CNS drugs, knowledge of these agents is limited. Much of our ignorance stems from the anatomic and neurochemical complexity of the brain and spinal cord. (There are more than 50 billion neurons in the cerebral hemispheres alone.) Because of this complexity, we are a long way from fully understanding both the CNS itself and the drugs used to influence its function.

TRANSMITTERS OF THE CNS

In contrast to the peripheral nervous system, in which only three compounds—acetylcholine, norepinephrine, and epinephrine—mediate most of the neurotransmission taking place, the CNS contains more than a dozen compounds that appear to serve as neurotransmitters (Table 20–1). Furthermore, since there are numerous sites within the CNS for which no transmitter has been identified, it is clear that additional compounds, yet to be discovered, also mediate neurotransmission in the brain and spinal cord.

It is important to note that none of the compounds that are thought to be CNS neurotransmitters have actually been proved to serve this function. The reason for uncertainty lies with the technical difficulties involved in CNS research. However, although absolute proof may be lacking, the evidence supporting a neurotransmitter role for several compounds (e.g., dopamine, norepinephrine, serotonin, enkephalins) is convincing.

Although much is known about the actions of CNS transmitters at various sites in the brain and spinal cord, it is not usually possible to relate these known actions in a precise way to behavioral or psychologic processes. For example, although we know the locations of specific CNS sites at which norepinephrine appears to act as a transmitter, and although we know the effect of norepinephrine at most of these sites (suppression of neuronal excitability), we do not know the precise relationship between suppression of neuronal excitability at each of these sites and the impact of that suppression on the overt function of the organism. This example illustrates the general state of our knowledge of CNS transmitter function: we have a great deal of detailed information about the biochemistry and electrophysiology of CNS transmitters, but we are as yet unable to assemble those details into a completely meaningful picture.

THE BLOOD-BRAIN BARRIER

As discussed in Chapter 5, the blood-brain barrier impedes the entry of drugs into the brain. Pas-

sage across the barrier is limited to lipid-soluble agents and to drugs that are able to cross by way of specific transport systems. Drugs that are protein bound and drugs that are highly ionized cannot cross.

The presence of the blood-brain barrier is a mixed blessing. On the positive side, the barrier protects the brain from injury by potentially toxic substances. On the negative side, the barrier can be a significant obstacle in therapeutics.

The blood-brain barrier is not fully developed at birth. Accordingly, newborn infants are much more sensitive to CNS drugs than are older children and adults.

HOW DO CNS DRUGS PRODUCE THERAPEUTIC EFFECTS?

Although much is known about the biochemical and electrophysiologic effects of CNS drugs, in most cases we cannot state with certainty the relationship between these effects and production of beneficial responses. Why is this so? In order to fully understand how a drug alters symptoms, we need to understand, at a biochemical and physiologic level, the pathophysiology of the disorder being treated. In the case of most CNS disorders, this knowledge is deficient. That is, we do not fully understand the brain in either health or disease. Given our incomplete understanding of the CNS itself, we must exercise caution when attempting to assign a precise mechanism for a drug's therapeutic effects.

Although we can't state with certainty how CNS drugs act, we do have sufficient data to permit the formulation of plausible hypotheses. Consequently, as we study the CNS drugs, proposed mechanisms of action will be presented. However, keep in mind that these mechanisms are tentative, representing our best guess based on data available today. As we learn more, it is almost certain that these concepts will need to be modified, if not discarded entirely.

ADAPTATION OF THE CNS TO PROLONGED DRUG EXPOSURE

When CNS drugs are taken chronically, effects may differ from those observed during initial use. These altered effects are the result of adaptive changes that occur in the brain in response to prolonged drug exposure. The brain's ability to adapt to drugs can produce alterations in therapeutic effects and in side effects. Adaptive changes are often beneficial, although they can also be detrimental.

Table 20–1. Neurotransmitters of the CNS	
Monoamines	**Amino Acids**
Norepinephrine	Aspartate
Epinephrine	Glutamate
Dopamine	GABA
Serotonin	Glycine
Peptides	**Other Compounds**
Enkephalins	Acetylcholine
Endorphins	Histamine
Substance P	
Oxytocin	
Vasopressin	

All the compounds listed above are thought (but not proved) to act as neurotransmitters within the CNS. For some of these compounds, the evidence supporting a role in transmission is quite strong; for others, the evidence is more tentative.

Increased Therapeutic Effects. Certain drugs used in psychiatry—antipsychotics and antidepressants—must be taken for several weeks before full therapeutic effects develop. It has been suggested that beneficial responses are delayed because these responses result from adaptive changes and not from the direct effects of drugs on synaptic function. Hence, full therapeutic effects will not be seen until the CNS has had time to modify itself in response to prolonged drug exposure.

Decreased Side Effects. When CNS drugs are taken chronically, the intensity of their side effects may decrease (while therapeutic effects remain undiminished). For example, phenobarbital (an anticonvulsant) produces sedation during the initial phase of therapy; however, with continued treatment, sedation declines while full protection from seizures is retained. Similarly, when morphine is given to control pain, nausea is a common side effect early on; however, as treatment continues, nausea diminishes while analgesic effects persist. Adaptations within the brain may explain these observations.

Tolerance and Physical Dependence. Tolerance and physical dependence are special manifestations of CNS adaptation. (Tolerance is defined as a decreased response occurring in the course of prolonged drug use. Physical dependence is defined as a state in which abrupt discontinuation of drug use will precipitate a withdrawal syndrome.) Research indicates that the kinds of adaptive changes that underlie tolerance and dependence are such that, once they have taken place, continued drug use is required for the brain to function "normally." If drug use is stopped, the drug-adapted brain can no longer function properly, and a withdrawal syndrome ensues. The withdrawal reaction will continue until the adaptive changes have had time to revert, thereby restoring the CNS to its predrug-use status.

DEVELOPMENT OF NEW PSYCHOTHERAPEUTIC DRUGS

Because of deficiencies in our knowledge of the neurochemical and physiologic changes that underlie mental disease, it is impossible to take a rational approach to the development of truly new (nonderivative) psychotherapeutic agents. History bears this out: virtually all of the major advances in psychopharmacology have been happy accidents.

In addition to our relative ignorance about the neurochemical and physiologic correlates of mental illness, two other factors contribute to the difficulty in generating new truly psychotherapeutic agents. (1) In contrast to many other diseases, we have no adequate animal models of mental illness. Accordingly, animal research is not likely to reveal new types of psychotherapeutic agents. (2) Mentally healthy individuals cannot be used as subjects to assess potential psychotherapeutic agents, since, as a rule, psychotherapeutic drugs either have no effect on healthy individuals or produce paradoxical effects.

Once a new drug has been stumbled upon, variations on that agent can be developed systematically. The following process is employed: (1) structural analogues of the new agent are synthesized, (2) these analogues are run through biochemical and physiologic screening tests to determine whether or not they possess activity similar to that of the parent compound, and (3) after serious toxicity has been ruled out, promising agents are tested in humans for possible psychotherapeutic activity. By following this procedure, it is possible to develop drugs that have fewer side effects than the original drug and perhaps even have superior therapeutic effects. However, although this procedure may produce small advances, it is not likely to yield a major therapeutic breakthrough.

APPROACHING THE STUDY OF CNS DRUGS

Because our understanding of the CNS is less complete than our understanding of the peripheral nervous system, our approach to studying CNS drugs will differ from the approach we took with peripheral nervous system agents. When we studied the pharmacology of the peripheral nervous system, we emphasized the importance of understanding transmitters and their receptors prior to embarking on a study of drugs. Since our knowledge of CNS transmitters is insufficient to allow this approach, rather than making a detailed examination of CNS transmitters before we study CNS drugs, we will discuss drugs and transmitters concurrently. Hence, for now, all that you need know about CNS transmitters is that (1) there are a lot of them, (2) their precise functional roles are not clear, and (3) their complexity makes it difficult for us to know with any certainty just how CNS drugs produce their effects.

Neurologic Drugs

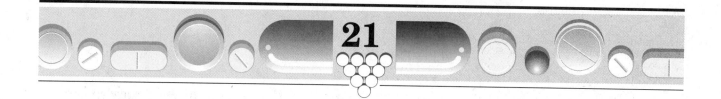

Drugs for Parkinson's Disease

Parkinson's disease is <u>a neurologic disorder</u> characterized by <u>disturbance of movement</u>. This disease is the rare example of a central nervous system (CNS) disorder for which both the underlying pathophysiology and the mechanisms by which drugs provide relief are understood with some precision.

PATHOPHYSIOLOGY OF PARKINSON'S DISEASE

Parkinson's disease is a disorder of the *extrapyramidal system*, a complex neuronal network that helps regulate movement. When extrapyramidal function is disrupted, *dyskinesias* (disorders of movement) result. The dyskinesias that characterize Parkinson's disease are *tremor, rigidity, postural instability*, and *bradykinesia* (slowed movement) or *akinesia* (complete absence of movement). In addition to movement disorders, patients frequently experience *psychologic disturbances*, including dementia, depression, and impaired memory. Onset of symptoms usually occurs in middle age.

Symptoms of Parkinson's disease result from disruption of neurotransmission within the *striatum*, an important component of the extrapyramidal system. A model of striatal neurotransmission is depicted in Figure 21–1A. As indicated, proper functioning of the striatum requires a balance between two neurotransmitters: *dopamine* (DA) and

A   HEALTHY STRIATUM

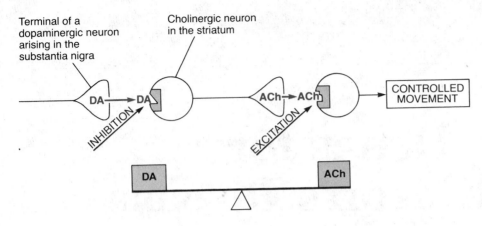

B   PARKINSONIAN STRIATUM

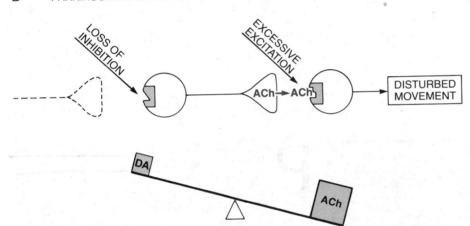

Figure 21–1. A model of neurotransmission in the healthy striatum and parkinsonian striatum.
A, In the healthy striatum, dopamine (DA) released from neurons originating in the substantia nigra inhibits the firing of neurons in the striatum that release acetylcholine (ACh) as their transmitter. Since ACh is excitatory, suppression of ACh release reduces excitation. Hence, under normal conditions, the excitatory actions of ACh are balanced by the inhibitory actions of DA, and controlled movement results.
B, In Parkinson's disease there is degeneration of the neurons that supply DA to the striatum. In the absence of DA, the excitatory effects of ACh go unopposed. This imbalance between DA's inhibitory actions and ACh's excitatory actions results in disturbance of movement.

acetylcholine (ACh). Dopamine is an *inhibitory* transmitter; ACh is an *excitatory* transmitter. According to the model, the neurons that release DA regulate the neurons that release ACh. By suppressing discharge of the cholinergic neurons, the dopaminergic neurons can prevent excessive excitation. Movement is normal when the excitatory effects of ACh are balanced by the inhibitory influence of DA.

In Parkinson's disease, there is an imbalance between DA and ACh in the striatum (Fig. 21–1B). The cause of the imbalance is degeneration of the neurons that supply DA to the striatum. (Why these neurons degenerate is not known.) Since, according to our model, DA serves to inhibit discharge of striatal cholinergic neurons, DA deficiency will release those neurons from inhibition, causing their rate of discharge to increase. The resultant increase in ACh-mediated excitation is thought to be responsible for the movement disorders of Parkinson's disease.

As discussed in Chapter 24, movement disorders similar to those of Parkinson's disease can occur as side effects of therapy with antipsychotic agents. These dyskinesias, which are referred to as

extrapyramidal side effects, result from blockade of dopamine receptors in the striatum. This drug-induced parkinsonism can be managed with some of the drugs used to treat Parkinson's disease.

OVERVIEW OF DRUG THERAPY

Therapeutic Goal

The goal of treatment is to improve the patient's ability to carry out activities of daily life. Drug selection and dosage are determined by the extent to which Parkinson's disease interferes with such activities as work, walking, dressing, eating, bathing, and arising from bed or a chair. Improving the capacity for these activities is primarily a function of decreasing bradykinesia, gait disturbance, and postural instability. Tremor and rigidity, although disturbing, are less disabling.

It is important to note that drug therapy of Parkinson's disease provides only symptomatic relief, not cure. Furthermore, with only one possible exception—selegiline—the drugs employed do not alter the progression of the disease.

Therapeutic Strategy

Given the neurochemical basis of parkinsonism—too little striatal DA and too much ACh—the strategy for treatment is self-evident: therapy must be directed at restoring the functional balance between DA and ACh. To restore this balance, two pharmacologic approaches are used: (1) activation of DA receptors, and (2) blockade of ACh receptors.

Overview of Drugs Employed

Table 21–1 presents an overview of the drugs used to treat Parkinson's disease. As indicated, these drugs fall into two major categories: (1) *dopaminergic drugs* (drugs that promote activation of dopamine receptors), and (2) *anticholinergic drugs* (drugs that prevent activation of cholinergic receptors). The dopaminergic agents act by a variety of mechanisms, including promotion of dopamine synthesis, direct activation of dopamine receptors, and prevention of dopamine degradation. In contrast, all of the anticholinergic agents act by the same mechanism: blockade of cholinergic receptors in the striatum.

BASIC PHARMACOLOGY OF THE DRUGS USED TO TREAT PARKINSON'S DISEASE

LEVODOPA

Use in Parkinson's Disease

Levodopa [Dopar, Larodopa] is the drug of choice for treating Parkinson's disease. With initial treatment, about 75% of patients experience a 50% reduction in severity of symptoms. Levodopa is so effective, in fact, that a diagnosis of Parkinson's

disease should be questioned if the patient fails to respond to this drug.

Full therapeutic responses may take several months to develop. Consequently, although the effects of levodopa can be significant, the patient should not expect improvement immediately. Rather, the patient should be informed that beneficial effects are likely to increase steadily over the first few months of treatment.

In contrast to the dramatic improvements seen during initial therapy, long-term therapy with levodopa has been disappointing. Although symptoms may be well-controlled during the first 2 years of treatment, by the end of 5 years the patient's ability to function may deteriorate to pretreatment levels. This loss of effectiveness over time is thought to reflect progression of the underlying disease and not development of tolerance to levodopa.

Mechanism of Action

Levodopa reduces symptoms of Parkinson's disease by promoting synthesis of dopamine in the striatum (Fig. 21–2). Once in the bloodstream, levodopa is transported across the blood-brain barrier and taken up by the few dopaminergic nerve terminals that remain in the striatum. Following uptake, levodopa, which has no direct effects of its own, is converted into dopamine (DA), its active form. By promoting synthesis of DA, levodopa helps restore a proper balance between DA and ACh.

The enzymatic conversion of levodopa to dopamine is depicted in Figure 21–3. As indicated, the enzyme that catalyzes this reaction is called a *decarboxylase* (because it removes a carboxyl group from levodopa). The activity of decarboxylases is enhanced by *pyridoxine* (vitamin B_6).

Why is Parkinson's disease treated with levodopa and not with dopamine itself? Dopamine can-

Table 21–1. Overview of Drugs for Parkinson's Disease

Drug Class	Drug	Mechanism of Action
Dopaminergic drugs	Levodopa	Increases synthesis of dopamine
	Carbidopa	Used with levodopa to prevent destruction of levodopa in the periphery
	Selegiline	Used with levodopa to prevent destruction of dopamine in the CNS; may retard progression of disease
	Amantadine	Promotes release of dopamine
	Bromocriptine	Activates dopamine receptors directly
	Pergolide	Activates dopamine receptors directly
Anticholinergic drugs	Benztropine	All of these drugs act by blocking receptors for acetylcholine in the CNS
	Biperidin	
	Diphenhydramine	
	Ethopropazine	
	Procyclidine	
	Trihexyphenidyl	

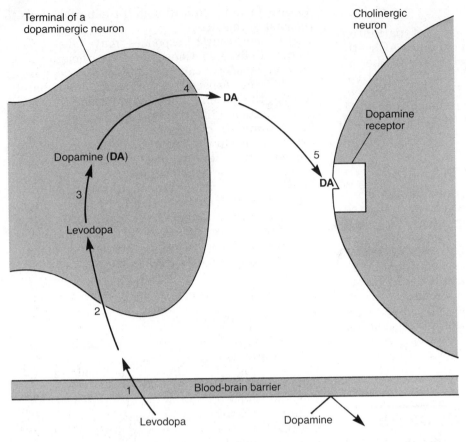

Figure 21–2. Steps leading to alteration of CNS function by levodopa. To produce its beneficial effects in parkinsonism, levodopa must be (1) transported across the blood-brain barrier; (2) taken up by a dopaminergic nerve terminal in the striatum; (3) converted into dopamine; (4) released into the synaptic space; and (5) bound to a dopamine receptor on a striatal cholinergic neuron, causing that neuron to decrease its firing rate. Note that dopamine itself is unable to cross the blood-brain barrier and, hence, cannot be used to treat parkinsonism.

not be employed because this compound is unable to cross the blood-brain barrier (see Fig. 21–3). As noted, levodopa crosses the barrier by means of an active transport system; this system will not transport dopamine.

Pharmacokinetics

Only a small fraction of an administered dose of levodopa reaches the brain. The majority of each dose is converted to dopamine in the periphery by

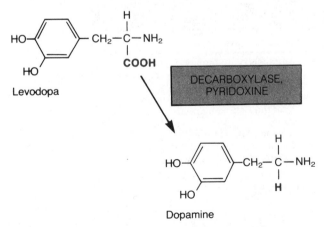

Figure 21–3. Conversion of levodopa to dopamine. Decarboxylases present in the brain, liver, and intestine convert levodopa into dopamine. Pyridoxine (vitamin B₆) accelerates the reaction.

decarboxylases present in the liver and intestine (Fig. 21–4A). Less than 1% of an administered dose escapes peripheral decarboxylation and enters the brain. Like the enzymes that decarboxylate levodopa within the brain, peripheral decarboxylases work faster in the presence of pyridoxine.

Adverse Effects

Most untoward effects of levodopa are dose dependent. The elderly are especially sensitive to adverse effects.

Nausea and Vomiting. Most patients experience nausea and vomiting early in treatment. These effects result from activation of dopamine receptors in the chemoreceptor trigger zone (CTZ) of the medulla. Nausea and vomiting can be reduced by administering levodopa in low initial doses and with meals. (The presence of food retards levodopa absorption, causing a decrease in peak plasma drug levels and a corresponding decrease in stimulation of the CTZ.) However, since administration with food can reduce therapeutic effects (by decreasing levodopa absorption), administration with meals should be avoided if possible.

Dyskinesias. Ironically, levodopa, a drug given to *alleviate* movement disorders, *causes* movement disorders in many patients. About 80% of those treated develop involuntary movements (head bobbing, tics, grimacing) within the first year of ther-

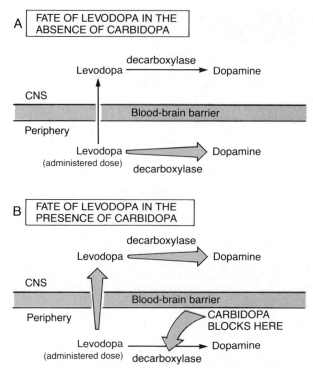

Figure 21–4. Fate of levodopa in the presence and absence of carbidopa. *A,* In the absence of carbidopa, most of an administered dose of levodopa is converted to dopamine by decarboxylases in the *periphery* (liver, intestine), leaving little levodopa for actions within the CNS.

B, By inhibiting peripheral decarboxylases, carbidopa increases the amount of levodopa available for actions within the CNS. Since carbidopa cannot cross the blood-brain barrier, it does not interfere with conversion of levodopa to its active form (dopamine) by decarboxylases in the brain.

apy. These dyskinesias develop just before or soon after optimal levodopa dosage has been achieved. The only treatment is to reduce levodopa dosage. Unfortunately, dosage reduction may lead to re-emergence of parkinsonian symptoms.

"On-Off" Phenomenon. The "on-off" phenomenon, which may be seen in the course of prolonged treatment, is characterized by periods in which symptoms of parkinsonism are controlled ("on" times) and periods in which loss of control occurs ("off" times). Oscillations between "on" and "off" times may occur rapidly (e.g., several times a day) or they may occur more slowly, with patients being "on" one day and "off" the next.

Cardiovascular Effects. Conversion of levodopa to dopamine in the periphery can result in excessive activation of beta$_1$ receptors in the heart. Activation of these receptors can cause *dysrhythmias,* particularly in patients with cardiac disease.

Patients may experience *postural hypotension* early in treatment. The mechanism of this paradoxical effect is not known.

Psychiatric Effects. Psychologic disturbances (anxiety, hallucinations, vivid dreams, irritability) are common. These reactions are seen most frequently in elderly patients who are taking levo-dopa along with other drugs that have psychologic effects (e.g., anticholinergic drugs, amantadine, dopamine agonists). Adverse psychologic effects may respond to a reduction in levodopa dosage or a reduction in the dosage of other drugs taken concurrently.

Other Adverse Effects. Levodopa drug may *darken sweat and urine*; patients should be forewarned of this harmless effect. The drug can *activate malignant melanoma* and, consequently, should be avoided in patients with undiagnosed skin lesions.

Drug Interactions

Interactions between levodopa and other drugs can (1) decrease beneficial effects of levodopa, (2) increase beneficial effects of levodopa, and (3) increase toxicity from levodopa. Major interactions are summarized in Table 21–2. Several interactions are discussed immediately below; others are discussed later in the chapter.

Pyridoxine. Pyridoxine (vitamin B$_6$) stimulates decarboxylase activity. By accelerating decarboxylation of levodopa in the periphery, pyridoxine can decrease the amount of levodopa that reaches the CNS. As a result, therapeutic effects of levodopa are reduced. Patients should be informed about this interaction and instructed to avoid vitamin preparations that contain pyridoxine.

Antipsychotic Drugs. All of the antipsychotic drugs in current use (e.g., chlorpromazine, haloperidol) block receptors for dopamine. By blocking dopamine receptors in the striatum, antipsychotic agents will decrease therapeutic effects of levodopa. Accordingly, concurrent use of antipsychotic agents with levodopa should be avoided.

Anticholinergic Drugs. Since excessive stimulation of cholinergic receptors contributes to the dyskinesias of Parkinson's disease, drugs that block cholinergic receptors can help reduce symptoms. Hence, anticholinergic agents will enhance the therapeutic effects of levodopa.

Monoamine Oxidase Inhibitors. Levodopa can cause a hypertensive crisis if administered to an individual undergoing treatment with a monoamine oxidase (MAO) inhibitor. The mechanism of this interaction is as follows. (1) Levodopa elevates neuronal stores of DA and norepinephrine (NE) by promoting synthesis of both compounds. (2) Since intraneuronal MAO serves to inactivate DA and NE, inhibition of MAO allows elevated neuronal stores of these transmitters to grow even larger. (3) Since both DA and NE promote vasoconstriction, release of these agents in supranormal amounts can lead to massive vasoconstriction, thereby causing blood pressure to rise dangerously high. To avoid hypertensive crisis, MAO inhibitors should be withdrawn at least 2 weeks prior to initiating levodopa.

Table 21–2. Major Drug Interactions of Levodopa

Drug Category	Drug	Mechanism of Interaction
Drugs that decrease beneficial effects of levodopa	Pyridoxine (vitamin B$_6$)	Enhanced destruction of levodopa
	Antipsychotics	Blockade of dopamine receptors
Drugs that increase beneficial effects of levodopa	Carbidopa	Inhibition of the peripheral decarboxylation of levodopa
	Anticholinergics	Blockade of cholinergic receptors in the CNS
	Amantadine	Promotion of dopamine release
	Bromocriptine	Stimulation of dopamine receptors
	Pergolide	Stimulation of dopamine receptors
	Selegiline	Inhibition of dopamine breakdown
Drugs that increase levodopa toxicity	MAO inhibitors	Inhibition of MAO increases the risk of severe levodopa-induced hypertension

Preparations, Dosage, and Administration

Levodopa [Dopar, Larodopa] is dispensed in tablets and capsules (100, 250, and 500 mg) for oral administration. To minimize adverse effects, especially drug-induced movement disorders, dosage must be individualized. The usual initial dosage is 0.5 to 1.0 gm/day administered in two or more divided doses. The total daily dosage can be increased gradually to a maximum of 8 gm. Full therapeutic responses may take 6 months to develop.

CARBIDOPA PLUS LEVODOPA

The combination of carbidopa plus levodopa is our most effective therapy for Parkinson's disease. This combination is considerably more effective than levodopa alone.

Mechanism of Action

Carbidopa is used to enhance the effects of levodopa. Carbidopa has no therapeutic effects of its own, and is always taken together with levodopa. As indicated in Figure 21–4B, carbidopa inhibits decarboxylases in the *periphery*. By suppressing peripheral decarboxylation, carbidopa makes more levodopa available to the CNS. Carbidopa does not prevent the conversion of levodopa to dopamine by decarboxylases within the brain because carbidopa is unable to cross the blood-brain barrier.

Advantages of Carbidopa

The combination of carbidopa plus levodopa is superior to levodopa alone in four ways.

1. By increasing the fraction of levodopa available for actions within the CNS, carbidopa allows the dosage of levodopa to be reduced by about 75%.
2. By inhibiting peripheral decarboxylation, carbidopa allows the administration of levodopa in a single daily dose rather than in multiple doses. This can facilitate compliance.
3. By reducing production of dopamine in the periphery, carbidopa reduces cardiovascular responses to levodopa, and also reduces nausea and vomiting.
4. By causing direct inhibition of decarboxylase, carbidopa obviates stimulation of decarboxylase by pyridoxine. As a result, carbidopa eliminates concern about decreasing the effects of levodopa through inadvertent use of vitamin preparations that contain pyridoxine.

Disadvantages of Carbidopa

Carbidopa has no adverse effects of its own; any adverse responses associated with treatment are due to potentiation of levodopa's effects. When levodopa is combined with carbidopa, abnormal movements and psychiatric disturbances may occur sooner and may be more intense than when levodopa is employed alone.

Preparations, Dosage, and Administration

Carbidopa is almost always administered together with levodopa in a single formulation that contains both drugs. These combination products (tablets and sustained-release capsules) are marketed under the trade name Sinemet. Sinemet tablets are available in three strengths: (1) 10 mg carbidopa/100 mg levodopa, (2) 25 mg carbidopa/100 mg levodopa, and (3) 25 mg carbidopa/250 mg levodopa. The sustained-release capsules [Sinemet CR] contain 50 mg carbidopa and 200 mg levodopa.

Carbidopa without levodopa, dispensed under the trade name Lodosyn, is available by special request for investigational use. This preparation is employed when dosages of levodopa and carbidopa must be titrated separately.

When patients who have been taking levodopa alone are switched over to the combination of carbidopa plus levodopa, at least 8 hours should elapse between the last dose of levodopa and the first dose of the combination. This delay is needed to prevent excessive potentiation of levodopa by carbidopa. Also, when switching from therapy with levodopa alone to the combination, the total daily dose of levodopa must be reduced substantially: the dose of levodopa within the combination regimen should be only 25% of the dose employed when levodopa was being administered alone. For patients who are not currently receiving levodopa, therapy can be initiated with either 10 mg carbidopa/100 mg levodopa or 25 mg carbidopa/100 mg levodopa, each taken 3 times a day.

AMANTADINE

Actions and Uses. Amantadine, an antiviral agent (see Chapter 84), is also effective in the therapy of Parkinson's disease. This agent relieves symptoms of parkinsonism by promoting release of dopamine from dopaminergic terminals in the striatum. Responses develop rapidly (often within 2 to 3 days) but are less profound than those seen with levodopa. Furthermore, responses may begin to diminish within 3 to 6 months. Amantadine may be employed alone in the early stages of Parkinson's disease, and in combination with other drugs (levodopa/carbidopa, anticholinergic agents) in later stages of the disease.

Adverse Effects. Amantadine can cause adverse *CNS effects* (confusion, lightheadedness, anxiety) and effects that resemble those caused by *muscarinic blockade* (blurred vision, urinary retention, dry mouth, constipation). These responses are generally mild when amantadine is used alone. However, if amantadine is combined with an anticholinergic agent, both the CNS and peripheral responses will be intensified.

Patients taking amantadine for 1 month or longer often develop *livedo reticularis*, a condition characterized by mottled discoloration of the skin. Livedo reticularis is a benign condition that gradually subsides following amantadine withdrawal.

Preparations, Dosage, and Administration. Amantadine [Symmetrel] is dispensed in 100-mg capsules and in a syrup (10 mg/ml) for oral use. The usual dosage is 100 mg twice daily. Since amantadine is eliminated primarily by the kidneys, dosage must be reduced in patients with renal impairment.

Amantadine often loses effectiveness after several months of use. If effects diminish they can be restored by either (1) increasing the dosage, or (2) interrupting treatment for several weeks.

Amantadine can enhance responses to levodopa and to anticholinergic agents. When combined with these drugs, amantadine is administered in the same doses employed when taken alone.

DOPAMINE RECEPTOR AGONISTS

Bromocriptine

Actions and Uses. Bromocriptine [Parlodel] is a direct-acting dopamine agonist. Beneficial effects result from *activation of dopamine receptors in the striatum*. Responses are superior to those of amantadine and the centrally acting anticholinergic drugs, but inferior to those of levodopa. Although bromocriptine can be used as monotherapy, the drug is usually employed as an adjunct to levodopa. When combined with levodopa, bromocriptine can prolong therapeutic responses and reduce motor fluctuations. In addition, since bromocriptine allows the dosage of levodopa to be reduced, the incidence of levodopa-induced dyskinesias may be reduced as well.

Adverse Effects. Adverse effects are dose dependent and occur in 30% to 50% of patients. *Nausea* is most common, occurring in over 50% of those treated. The most common dose-limiting effects are *psychologic reactions* (confusion, nightmares, agitation, hallucinations, paranoid delusions). These reactions occur in about 30% of patients and are most likely when the dosage is high. Like levodopa, bromocriptine can cause *dyskinesias* and *postural hypotension.*

Preparations, Dosage, and Administration. Bromocriptine mesylate [Parlodel] is available in 2.5-mg tablets and 5-mg capsules for oral use. The initial dosage is 1.25 mg twice daily, administered with meals. Dosage is gradually increased until the desired level of response has been achieved. Maintenance dosages range from 30 to 100 mg/day.

Pergolide

Actions, Uses, and Adverse Effects. Pergolide is similar to bromocriptine with respect to actions, uses, and adverse effects. Like bromocriptine, pergolide reduces symptoms of Parkinson's disease by causing direct activation of dopamine receptors in the striatum. When used as an adjunct to levodopa, pergolide can prolong symptomatic control, reduce fluctuations in motor responses, and reduce the incidence of levodopa-induced dyskinesias. Like bromocriptine, pergolide can cause nausea, postural hypotension, and adverse psychologic reactions (hallucinations, confusion, sedation, paranoid delusions).

Preparations, Dosage, and Administration. Pergolide mesylate [Permax] is dispensed in tablets (0.05, 0.25, and 1 mg) for oral administration. The recommended initial dosage is 0.05 mg once daily. Dosage is gradually increased to a maximum of 5 mg/day (in three divided doses).

SELEGILINE

Actions and Uses. Selegiline [Eldepryl] is a *selective inhibitor of type A monoamine oxidase* (MAO-A), an enzyme that inactivates dopamine in the brain. Another form of MAO, known as MAO-B, inactivates norepinephrine and serotonin. As discussed in Chapter 25, drugs that inhibit MAO-B can relieve symptoms of depression and create a risk of hypertensive crisis. Since selegiline is a selective inhibitor of MAO-A, the drug is *not* an antidepressant and does *not* present a risk of severe hypertension (at usual doses).

Selegiline appears to benefit patients with Parkinson's disease in two ways. When used as an adjunct to levodopa, *selegiline can delay destruction of dopamine derived from levodopa.* By doing so, selegiline can prolong the effects of levodopa and can decrease fluctuations in motor control. Unfortunately, these benefits decline dramatically within 12 to 24 months.

In addition to enhancing the effects of levodopa, selegiline may actually *retard progression of Parkinson's disease.* When recently diagnosed patients are treated with selegiline (in the absence of levodopa), the need for treatment with levodopa is delayed for about 12 months. That is, the rate at which symptoms intensify appears to slow down. Because of its apparent ability to delay progression of Parkinson's disease, selegiline is recommended for all patients with newly diagnosed disease. In these patients, the therapeutic objective is protection rather than relief of symptoms, although some symptomatic improvement may occur.

In experimental animals, selegiline can prevent development of parkinsonism following exposure to MPTP, a neurotoxin that causes selective degeneration of dopaminergic neurons. (Humans accidentally exposed to MPTP develop severe parkinsonism.) Neuronal degeneration is caused *not* by MPTP itself, but rather by a *toxic metabolite* of MPTP. Formation of this metabolite is catalyzed by MAO-B. By inhibiting MAO-B, selegiline prevents formation of the toxic metabolite, and thereby protects against neuronal injury.

The ability of selegiline to protect against MPTP-induced injury in animals may help explain the drug's ability to delay progression of Parkinson's disease in humans. That is, just as selegiline protects animals by suppressing formation of a neurotoxic metabolite of MPTP, the drug may retard progression of Parkinson's disease by suppressing formation of a neurotoxic metabolite of an as-yet unidentified compound. Just what that compound might be is under investigation.

Pharmacokinetics. Selegiline is rapidly absorbed following oral administration and readily penetrates the blood-brain barrier. Irreversible inhibition of MAO-B follows. Selegiline undergoes hepatic metabolism followed by renal excretion.

Two metabolites—*amphetamine* and *methamphetamine*—are *CNS stimulants*. These metabolites do not appear to contribute to the drug's therapeutic effects, but can contribute to toxicity.

Adverse Effects. When selegiline is used alone, the principal adverse effect is *insomnia* (presumably because of CNS excitation by amphetamine and methamphetamine). Insomnia can be minimized by administering the last daily dose at noon.

When used with levodopa, selegiline can intensify adverse responses to levodopa-derived dopamine. These reactions—orthostatic hypotension, dyskinesias, and psychologic disturbances (hallucinations, confusion)—can be reduced by decreasing the dosage of levodopa.

Preparations, Dosage, and Administration. Selegiline [Eldepryl] is available in 5-mg tablets for oral administration. The usual dosage is 5 mg taken with breakfast and lunch. Since a total daily dose of 10 mg is sufficient to produce complete inhibition of MAO-B, doses greater than this are unnecessary.

CENTRALLY ACTING ANTICHOLINERGIC DRUGS

The classic anticholinergic agents (e.g., atropine) were the first anticholinergic drugs employed to treat Parkinson's disease. Although these drugs were effective, they also caused intense anticholinergic effects in the periphery (dry mouth, blurred vision, photophobia, constipation, urinary retention, tachycardia). With the advent of newer cholinergic blockers, referred to as *centrally acting anticholinergic agents*, use of the classic cholinergic blockers for parkinsonism has become obsolete. The centrally acting agents are just as effective as the older agents and have the advantage of producing fewer anticholinergic effects in the periphery.

Mechanism of Action

As discussed earlier, excessive stimulation of striatal cholinergic receptors contributes to the symptoms of Parkinson's disease. The centrally acting anticholinergic drugs help control symptoms by blocking access of acetylcholine to these receptors.

Table 21–3. Dosages of Centrally Acting Anticholinergic Drugs

Generic Name	Trade Name	Dosage Range (mg/day)
Benztropine	Cogentin	0.5–6
Biperidin	Akineton	2–16
Diphenhydramine	Benadryl, others	25–100
Ethopropazine	Parsidol	50–600
Procyclidine	Kemadrin	2.5–20
Trihexyphenidyl	Artane, others	1–15

Therapeutic Use

When used to treat Parkinson's disease, the centrally acting anticholinergics are less effective than levodopa but also produce fewer serious adverse effects. These drugs may be employed alone or in combination with levodopa.

The anticholinergic drugs are often preferred agents for treating mild parkinsonism in *younger* patients. These drugs are effective enough to control mild symptoms, and their use avoids exposing the patient to the more serious adverse effects of levodopa. Anticholinergic drugs are generally avoided in the *elderly* because of the risk of severe CNS effects.

Adverse Effects

Peripheral Effects. Like the classic anticholinergic drugs, the centrally acting agents are able to block cholinergic receptors in the periphery. As a result, these drugs can cause *dry mouth, blurred vision, photophobia, urinary retention, constipation,* and *tachycardia.* These effects are usually dose limiting. Blockade of cholinergic receptors in the eye may precipitate or aggravate *glaucoma.* Accordingly, intraocular pressure should be determined periodically. For a more complete discussion of peripheral anticholinergic responses, refer to Chapter 13 (Muscarinic Agonists and Antagonists).

CNS Effects. Anticholinergic agents may cause confusion, delusions, depression, and hallucinations. These responses are most likely in the elderly.

Withdrawal. If anticholinergic agents are discontinued abruptly, symptoms of parkinsonism may be intensified. Accordingly, these drugs should be withdrawn gradually.

Preparations, Dosage, and Administration

The anticholinergic drugs used in parkinsonism are listed in Table 21–3. Trade names and dosage ranges are given. Dosing is initiated with the lower value in the table, and then gradually increased until the desired therapeutic response has been achieved or until side effects have become intolerable. These drugs are administered in two or three divided daily doses.

DRUG SELECTION

Drug selection is based on the severity of symptoms and the patient's ability to tolerate the side effects of specific drugs.

For patients with *mild* symptoms, an *anticholinergic* agent or *amantadine* is indicated. (Anticholinergic drugs should be used only in younger patients because CNS effects can be severe in the elderly.) Because *selegiline* may be able to retard progression of Parkinson's disease, this drug is recommended for all newly diagnosed patients.

For patients with *advanced* disease, *levodopa/ carbidopa* is the treatment of choice. If levodopa/ carbidopa is inadequate, selegiline, amantadine, or a dopamine agonist (bromocriptine, pergolide) may be added to the regimen. In addition, levodopa/ carbidopa may be combined with an anticholinergic agent (except in elderly patients and those with a history of psychosis, since the risk of adverse psychologic reactions is high).

Summary of Major Nursing Implications

LEVODOPA/CARBIDOPA [SINEMET]

✓ **Preadministration Assessment**

Therapeutic Goal

Treatment is directed at improving the patient's ability to carry out activities of daily life. Levodopa does not cure Parkinson's disease.

Baseline Data

Assess overt manifestations of Parkinson's disease (bradykinesia, akinesia, postural instability, tremor, rigidity) and the extent to which these manifestations interfere with activities of daily living (ability to work, dress, bathe, walk, etc.).

Identifying High-Risk Patients

Levodopa is *contraindicated* for patients with *malignant melanoma* (the drug can activate this neoplasm) and for patients taking *MAO inhibitors*. Exercise *caution* in patients with *cardiac disease* and *psychiatric disorders*.

✓ **Implementation: Administration**

Route

Oral.

Administration

Inform the patient that levodopa may be taken with food to reduce nausea and vomiting.

Parkinsonism may render self-medication impossible. Assist the patient with dosing when needed. If appropriate, involve family members in medicating the outpatient.

If the patient has been taking levodopa alone, allow at least 8 hours to elapse between the last dose of levodopa and the first dose of levodopa/carbidopa. The dosage of levodopa in the combination should be reduced to no more than 25% the dosage employed when levodopa was being taken alone.

So that expectations may be realistic, inform the patient that effects of levodopa may be delayed for weeks to months. This knowledge will facilitate compliance.

✓ **Ongoing Evaluation and Interventions**

Evaluating Therapeutic Effects

Evaluate for improvements in activities of daily living and for reductions in bradykinesia, postural instability, tremor, and rigidity.

Minimizing Adverse Effects

Nausea and Vomiting. Inform the patient that nausea and vomiting can be reduced by taking levodopa with food. Instruct the patient to notify the physician if nausea and vomiting persist or become severe.

Dyskinesias. Inform patients about possible levodopa-induced movement disorders (tremor, dystonic movements, twitching) and instruct them to notify the physician if these develop.

If the hospitalized patient develops dyskinesias, withhold levodopa and consult with the physician about a possible reduction in dosage.

"On-Off" Phenomenon. Forewarn patients about possible abrupt loss of therapeutic effects and instruct them to notify the physician if this occurs.

Dysrhythmias. Inform patient about signs of excessive cardiac stimulation (palpitations, tachycardia, irregular heartbeat) and instruct them to notify the physician if these occur.

Orthostatic Hypotension. Inform patients about symptoms of hypotension (dizziness, lightheadedness) and advise them to sit or lie down if these occur. Advise patients to move slowly when assuming an erect posture.

Psychiatric Disturbances. Inform patients about possible adverse psychiatric effects (hallucinations, delusions, agitation, anxiety, malaise, depression) and instruct them to notify the physician if these develop.

Discoloration of Urine and Sweat. Forewarn the patient that levodopa may cause harmless darkening of urine and sweat.

Minimizing Adverse Interactions

Antipsychotic Drugs. These drugs can block responses to levodopa and should be avoided.

MAO Inhibitors. Concurrent use of levodopa and an MAO inhibitor can produce severe hypertension. Withdraw MAO inhibitors at least 2 weeks before initiating levodopa.

Anticholinergic Drugs. These agents can enhance therapeutic responses to levodopa, but they also increase the risk of adverse psychiatric effects.

CENTRALLY ACTING ANTICHOLINERGIC DRUGS

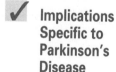

General Implications

Implications Specific to Parkinson's Disease

Centrally acting anticholinergic drugs have the same pharmacologic properties as the "classic" anticholinergic agents. Relevant nursing implications are summarized in Chapter 13.

Therapeutic Goal

Treatment is directed at improving the patient's ability to carry out activities of daily life. Anticholinergic drugs do not cure Parkinson's disease.

Baseline Data

Assess overt manifestations of Parkinson's disease (bradykinesia, akinesia, postural instability, tremor, rigidity) and the extent to which these manifestations interfere with activities of daily living.

Minimizing Adverse Effects

Many patients with Parkinson's disease are elderly, and therefore highly susceptible to the ability of anticholinergic drugs to induce *glaucoma* and *psychologic disturbances.* Intraocular pressure should be monitored periodically. Observe the patient for alteration of intellectual or emotional status.

Discontinuation of Treatment

Abrupt withdrawal of anticholinergics can intensify symptoms of parkinsonism. Warn the patient against abrupt discontinuation of treatment.

Drugs for Epilepsy

The term *epilepsy* refers to a group of disorders characterized by excessive excitability of neurons within the central nervous system (CNS). This abnormal neuronal activity can produce a variety of symptoms, ranging from brief periods of unconsciousness to violent convulsions. The incidence of epilepsy in the United States is about 5 in 1000. Approximately 60% of those who have the disorder can be rendered seizure free with drugs; another 25% can expect significant improvement.

The terms *seizure* and *convulsion* are not synonymous and require clarification. *Seizure* is a general term that applies to all types of epileptic events. In contrast, the term *convulsion* has a more limited meaning, applying only to abnormal motor phenomena (e.g., the jerking muscle movements that occur during a grand mal attack). Accordingly, although all convulsions may be called seizures, it is not appropriate to call all seizures convulsions. Absence seizures, for example, manifest as brief periods of unconsciousness, which may or may not be accompanied by involuntary movements.

Since not all epileptic seizures involve convulsions, we will refer to the agents used to treat epilepsy as *antiseizure drugs*, rather than *anticonvulsants*. It should be noted, however, that other texts may use the term *anticonvulsants* when referring to this group of drugs.

Our discussion of the antiseizure drugs will be done in four phases. We will begin by reviewing the pathophysiology of epilepsy. Next we will discuss the mechanisms by which antiseizure drugs are thought to act. After that, we will discuss general issues in the drug therapy of epilepsy. Lastly, we will discuss the antiseizure drugs themselves.

227

PATHOPHYSIOLOGY OF EPILEPSY

SEIZURE GENERATION

Seizures are initiated by synchronous, high-frequency discharge from a group of abnormally hyperexcitable neurons, called a *focus*. A focus may result from several causes, including congenital defects, hypoxia at birth, head trauma, and cancer. Seizures result when discharge from a focus spreads to other brain areas, thereby recruiting normal neurons to discharge abnormally along with the focus.

The overt manifestations of a particular seizure disorder depend upon the location of the seizure focus and the neuronal connections to that focus. (The connections to the focus determine the brain areas to which seizure activity can spread.) If seizure activity invades a very limited part of the brain, a partial or local seizure will result. In contrast, if seizure activity spreads to a large portion of the brain, a generalized seizure will result.

An experimental procedure referred to as *kindling* may explain how a focal discharge is eventually able to generate a seizure. Experimental kindling is performed by implanting a small electrode into the brain of an experimental animal. The electrode is used to deliver localized stimuli for a brief interval once each day. When stimuli are first administered, no seizures result. However, after repeated once-a-day delivery, these stimuli eventually elicit a seizure. If the procedure of brief, daily stimulation is continued for a long enough time, spontaneous seizures will begin to occur.

The process of kindling may be telling us something about seizure development in humans. For example, kindling may account for the delay that can take place between injury to the head and the eventual development of seizures. Furthermore, kindling may explain why the seizures associated with some forms of epilepsy become more frequent as time passes. Also, the progressive nature of kindling would suggest that early treatment might prevent seizure disorders from becoming more severe with time.

TYPES OF SEIZURES

Seizure can be divided into two broad categories: (1) *partial (focal) seizures* and (2) *generalized seizures*. In partial seizures, seizure activity usually begins in the cerebral cortex and spreads only to adjacent cortical areas. In generalized seizures, seizure activity usually begins beneath the cortex and spreads bilaterally to distant areas of the brain.

Partial Seizures

Partial seizures fall into two major groups: (1) *simple partial seizures* and (2) *complex partial seizures*. Complex partial seizures involve *impairment of consciousness*, whereas simple partial seizures do not. Simple partial seizures may appear as convulsions in a single limb or muscle group, but with no effect on consciousness. Complex partial seizures may manifest as an attack of confused or bizarre behavior during which consciousness is impaired.

Generalized Seizures

The major subtypes of generalized seizures are listed in Table 22–1. Three of these subtypes— tonic-clonic seizures, absence seizures, and status epilepticus—are described below.

Tonic-Clonic Seizures (Grand Mal). In tonic-clonic seizures, neuronal discharge spreads throughout the entire brain. These seizures manifest as major convulsions, characterized by a period of muscle rigidity (tonic phase) followed by synchronous muscle jerks (clonic phase). Tonic-clonic seizures are accompanied by marked impairment of consciousness and are followed by a period of CNS depression, referred to as the *postictal state*.

Absence Seizures (Petit Mal). Absence seizures are characterized loss of consciousness for a brief time (10 to 30 seconds). Seizures usually involve mild, symmetric motor activity (e.g., eye blinking) but may occur with no motor activity at all. The patient may experience hundreds of absence attacks per day. Absence seizures occur primarily in children and usually cease during the early teens.

Status Epilepticus. *Status epilepticus* (SE) is defined as a seizure that persists for a "long" time. (For purposes of diagnosis, a "long" time is generally accepted as 30 minutes or more.) There are

Table 22–1. Seizure Types and Their Treatment		
Seizure Type	**Drugs of Choice**	**Alternatives**
Partial Seizures (focal seizures)		
Simple partial seizures and complex partial seizures	Carbamazepine Phenytoin	Phenobarbital Primidone Valproic acid
Generalized Seizures (convulsive and nonconvulsive)		
Tonic-clonic seizures (grand mal)	Carbamazepine Phenytoin Valproic acid	Phenobarbital Primidone
Absence seizures (petit mal)	Ethosuximide Valproic acid	Clonazepam
Status epilepticus (convulsive)	Diazepam (IV) Phenytoin (IV) Phenobarbital (IV)	Lorazepam Lidocaine
Myoclonic seizures and atonic seizures	Valproic acid	Clonazepam

several types of SE, including absence SE, myoclonic SE, and tonic-clonic SE.

The most dangerous form of SE is the generalized convulsive type, in which the patient experiences an unrelenting series of tonic-clonic seizures. Consciousness is lost during the entire attack. Generalized convulsive SE is a life-threatening condition that requires immediate treatment.

A common cause of SE is failure to take antiseizure medication as prescribed. In addition, SE can be triggered by fever and by abrupt withdrawal of general CNS depressants (e.g., alcohol, barbiturates).

HOW ANTISEIZURE DRUGS WORK

There are two ways by which drugs can control seizures: (1) drugs can act on neurons within a focus to reduce excessive rates of discharge, and (2) drugs can prevent the propagation of seizure activity from a focus to other brain regions. Most antiseizure drugs appear to act at least in part by preventing the spread of seizure activity.

Although we don't know with certainty just how antiseizure medications alter neuronal excitability, several hypotheses have been offered. One hypothesis suggests that some antiseizure drugs act by "stabilizing" neuronal membranes. This would reduce excitability, which in turn would suppress seizure generation.

A number of antiseizure medications are able to potentiate the actions of *gamma-aminobutyric acid (GABA)*, an inhibitory neurotransmitter that is widely distributed throughout the brain. By potentiating the inhibitory actions of GABA, these drugs can decrease neuronal excitability and may thereby help suppress seizures.

GENERAL THERAPEUTIC CONSIDERATIONS

THERAPEUTIC GOAL

The goal in treating epilepsy is to reduce seizures to an extent that will enable the patient to live a normal or near-normal life. Ideally, treatment should eliminate seizures entirely. However, this may not be possible without causing intolerable side effects. Hence, we must balance the desire for complete seizure control against the acceptability of undesired drug effects.

DIAGNOSIS AND DRUG SELECTION

Control of seizures requires proper drug selection. As indicated in Table 22–1, most antiseizure medications are selective for specific seizure disorders. Phenytoin, for example, is useful for treating tonic-clonic and partial seizures, but is ineffective against absence seizures. Conversely, ethosuximide is active against absence seizures, but does not work against tonic-clonic or partial seizures. The only drug that appears effective against practically all forms of epilepsy is valproic acid. Since most antiseizure drugs are selective for specific seizure disorders, effective treatment requires a proper match between the drug and the seizure. This match can be made only if the seizure type has been accurately diagnosed.

Making a diagnosis requires physical, neurologic, and laboratory evaluations along with a thorough history. The history should determine the age of onset of seizure activity, the frequency and duration of seizure events, precipitating factors, and times when seizures occur. Physical and neurologic evaluations may reveal signs of head injury or other disorders that could underlie seizure activity, although, in many patients, the physical and neurologic evaluations may be normal. An electroencephalogram (EEG) is essential for diagnosis of seizure type. Other tests that may be employed for diagnosis include computerized axial tomography (CAT), positron emission tomography (PET), and magnetic resonance imaging (MRI).

DRUG EVALUATION

Once an antiseizure drug has been selected, a trial period is needed to determine its effectiveness. During this time there is no guarantee that seizures will not occur. Accordingly, until certainty of seizure control has been established, the patient should be warned against participation in activities that could be hazardous if a seizure were to occur (e.g., driving, operating dangerous machinery).

During the process of drug evaluation, adjustments in dosage are often needed. No drug should be considered ineffective until it has been tested in sufficiently high dosage and for a reasonable period of time. Measurement of plasma drug levels can be a valuable tool for establishing dosage and evaluating the effectiveness of a specific drug.

Maintenance of a seizure-frequency chart is essential for evaluating treatment. The chart should be maintained by the patient or a family member and should contain a complete record of all seizure events. This record will enable the physician to determine if treatment has been effective. The nurse should teach the patient how to create and use a seizure-frequency chart.

MONITORING PLASMA DRUG LEVELS

Monitoring plasma drug levels is a common practice in epilepsy therapy. For most antiseizure drugs, the plasma drug levels that produce therapeutic and toxic effects have been established. Hence, knowledge of drug levels can serve as a useful guide for adjusting dosage. Table 22–2 indicates the plasma drug levels that define the therapeutic range for the major antiseizure drugs.

Monitoring plasma drug levels is especially helpful when treating major convulsive disorders (e.g., tonic-clonic seizures). Since these seizures can be dangerous, and since delay of therapy may allow the condition to worsen, rapid control of seizures is desirable. However, since these seizures occur infrequently, a long time may be needed to establish control if clinical outcome is relied on as the only means of determining an effective dosage. By adjusting initial doses on the basis of plasma drug levels (rather than on the basis of seizure control), we can readily achieve drug levels that are likely to be effective, thereby increasing our chances of establishing control quickly.

Measurements of plasma drug levels are not especially important for determining effective dosages for *absence* seizures. Because absence seizures occur very frequently (up to several hundred a day), simple observation of the patient is the best means for establishing an effective dosage: if seizures stop, dosage is sufficient; if seizures continue, more drug is probably needed.

In addition to serving as a guide for dosage adjustment, knowledge of plasma drug levels can serve as an aid to (1) monitoring compliance, (2) determining the cause of loss of seizure control, and (3) identifying the causes of toxicity, especially in patients receiving multidrug therapy.

PROMOTING COMPLIANCE

Epilepsy is a chronic condition that requires regular and continuous therapy. As a result, seizure control is highly dependent on patient compliance. In fact, it is estimated that noncompliance accounts for about 50% of all treatment failures. Accordingly, promoting compliance should be a priority for all members of the health care team.

Several measures can help promote compliance. These are (1) educating the patient and family about the chronic nature of epilepsy and the importance of adhering to the prescribed regimen, (2) monitoring plasma drug levels as a means of encouraging and evaluating compliance, and (3) deepening patient and family involvement by having them maintain a seizure-frequency chart.

GUIDELINES FOR TREATMENT DURING PREGNANCY AND LACTATION

Although most pregnant women who take antiseizure medication give birth to normal babies, *in utero* exposure to these drugs does carry some risk. The dilemma, therefore, is to balance the risk of drug-induced fetal injury against the risk of injury from convulsions that might occur if antiseizure medication were withdrawn. Most clinicians agree that the risk to the fetus from uncontrolled convulsions is greater than the risk from antiseizure medications. Hence, as a general rule, women with major seizure disorders should continue to take antiseizure drugs throughout pregnancy.

One antiseizure medicine—*trimethadione*—should *not* be taken during pregnancy. This drug has been associated with a high incidence (80%) of birth defects and spontaneous abortions. Women who became pregnant while taking trimethadione should be counseled about possible therapeutic abortion. (Trimethadione is prescribed infrequently and is not discussed further in this chapter.)

Several antiseizure medications interfere with vitamin K metabolism and can thereby disrupt clotting mechanisms. Antiseizure drugs that interfere with vitamin K are *phenytoin, phenobarbital,* and *primidone.* Women who take these medicines during pregnancy should receive vitamin K injections early in labor to reduce bleeding tendencies in the newborn.

Use of antiseizure drugs does not constitute an absolute prohibition against breast-feeding. How-

		Daily Maintenance Dosage		Therapeutic Serum Concentration (µg/ml)
Generic Name	**Trade Name**	*Adults (mg)*	*Children (mg/kg)*	
Carbamazepine	Tegretol, Epitol	600–1200	15–30	4–12
Clonazepam	Klonopin	1.5–20	0.1–0.2	0.02–0.08
Ethosuximide	Zarontin	750–2000	20–40	40–100
Phenobarbital	Many names	120–250	3–5	15–40
Phenytoin	Dilantin	300–400	4–7	10–20
Primidone	Mysoline	750–1500	10–25	5–12
Valproic acid	Depakene	1000–3000	15–60	50–150

Table 22–2. Clinical Pharmacology of Major Antiseizure Medications

ever, since several of these medications can readily enter breast milk, the nursing infant should be monitored closely for possible drug effects (e.g., sedation). Breast-feeding should cease if adverse effects are suspected.

WITHDRAWAL OF ANTISEIZURE MEDICATION

Some forms of epilepsy undergo spontaneous remission; hence, at some point, discontinuation of antiseizure medication must be considered. Unfortunately, there are no firm guidelines to indicate the most appropriate time to withdraw treatment. However, once the decision to discontinue treatment has been made, agreement does exist on how drug withdrawal should be accomplished. *The most important rule governing discontinuation of antiseizure medication is that withdrawal be done slowly (over a period of several months).* Failure to gradually reduce dosage is a frequent cause of status epilepticus. If the patient is taking two drugs to control seizures, these drugs should be withdrawn sequentially, not simultaneously.

CHEMICAL CLASSIFICATION OF ANTISEIZURE DRUGS

The antiseizure drugs fall into five major chemical classes: (1) hydantoins, (2) barbiturates, (3) succinimides, (4) benzodiazepines, and (5) oxazolidinediones. The drugs that belong to these classes are listed in Table 22–3. Of the drugs in the table, only nine are used frequently; these agents are discussed below. The other 10 drugs are employed less commonly and will not be considered further.

Table 22–3. Chemical Classification of Antiseizure Drugs

Hydantoins	Benzodiazepines
Phenytoin	Diazepam
Mephenytoin*	Clonazepam
Ethotoin*	Clorazepate*
Barbiturates	Oxazolidinediones
Phenobarbital	Trimethadione*
Mephobarbital*	Paramethadione*
Succinimides	Miscellaneous
Ethosuximide	Primidone
Methsuximide*	Valproic acid
Phensuximide*	Carbamazepine
	Felbamate
	Phenacemide*
	Acetazolamide*

*This agent is used infrequently to treat seizures and is not discussed in the text.

BASIC PHARMACOLOGY OF THE MAJOR ANTISEIZURE DRUGS

The antiseizure drugs used most frequently are *phenytoin, phenobarbital, carbamazepine,* and *valproic acid.* Most of the discussion below focuses on these four drugs. Five other drugs are also considered: *primidone, ethosuximide, diazepam, clonazepam,* and *felbamate.*

PHENYTOIN

Phenytoin [Dilantin] is a broad-spectrum antiseizure agent. This drug is active against all forms of epilepsy except absence seizures. Phenytoin is of historic note in that it was the first drug known to suppress seizure activity without producing generalized depression of the entire CNS. Hence, phenytoin heralded the development of selective medications that could treat epilepsy while leaving most normal CNS functions undiminished.

Mechanism of Action

Phenytoin suppresses seizures primarily by preventing the spread of seizure activity from the focus to other regions of the brain. The drug is not very effective at suppressing discharge of the focus itself. Phenytoin appears to prevent the propagation of seizure activity by "stabilizing" neuronal membranes, thereby rendering neurons outside the focus less responsive to stimulation by hyperactive focal cells.

Pharmacokinetics

Phenytoin has unusual pharmacokinetic properties that must be accounted for in therapy. Both the absorption and metabolism of the drug vary substantially among patients. In addition, small changes in dosage can produce disproportionately large changes in plasma drug levels. Because of these kinetic characteristics, a dosage that is both effective and safe is difficult to establish, and, once determined, must be adhered to rigidly.

Absorption. Absorption of oral phenytoin is variable. Variability exists between *different formulations* of phenytoin (e.g., tablets versus extended-release capsules) and between preparations made by *different manufacturers.*

Metabolism. Individuals differ widely in the rate at which they metabolize phenytoin. As a result, the half-life of phenytoin varies substantially among patients, ranging from 8 to 60 hours. The capacity of the liver to metabolize phenytoin is very limited. As a result, the relationship between dosage and plasma levels of phenytoin is unusual. Therapeutic doses of phenytoin are only slightly smaller than those needed to saturate the hepatic enzymes that metabolize the drug. Consequently, if phenytoin is administered in doses only slightly greater than those needed for therapeutic effects, the liver's capacity to metabolize the drug will be overwhelmed, causing plasma levels of phenytoin to rise dramatically.

The unusual relationship between phenytoin dosage and plasma levels is illustrated in Figure 22–1A. As can be seen, once plasma levels of phenytoin have reached the therapeutic range, small changes in dosage produce large changes in drug levels. As a result, small increases in dosage can cause toxicity, and small decreases can cause therapeutic failure. This relationship makes it difficult to establish and maintain a dosage that is both safe and effective.

Figure 22–1B indicates the relationship between dosage and plasma drug levels that exists for most drugs. As can be seen, this relationship is *linear*, in contrast to the nonlinear relationship that exists for phenytoin. Accordingly, for most drugs, if the patient is taking doses that produce plasma drug levels that are within the therapeutic range, small deviations from that dosage produce only small deviations in plasma drug levels. Because of this relationship, it is relatively easy to maintain drug levels that are safe and effective.

Therapeutic Uses

Epilepsy. Phenytoin can be used to treat all major forms of epilepsy except absence seizures. The drug is especially effective against tonic-clonic seizures, and is the drug of first choice for treating these seizures in adults and older children. (Carbamazepine is preferred to phenytoin for treating tonic-clonic seizures in young children.) Although phenytoin can be used to treat simple and complex partial seizures, the drug is less effective against these seizures than it is against tonic-clonic seizures. Phenytoin can be administered intravenously to treat generalized convulsive status epilepticus.

Cardiac Dysrhythmias. Phenytoin is active against certain types of dysrhythmias. Antidysrhythmic applications are discussed in Chapter 44.

Adverse Effects

Effects on the CNS. Although phenytoin acts on the CNS in a relatively selective fashion to suppress seizures, the drug is not completely devoid of CNS side effects—especially when dosage is excessive. At therapeutic drug levels, sedation and other CNS effects are mild. At plasma levels above 20 μg/ml, toxic effects can occur. *Nystagmus* (continuous back-and-forth movements of the eyes) is relatively common. Other manifestations of excessive dosage include *sedation*, *ataxia* (staggering gait), *diplopia* (double vision), and *cognitive impairment*.

Gingival Hyperplasia. Gingival hyperplasia (excessive growth of gum tissue) is characterized by swelling, tenderness, and bleeding of the gums. This effect occurs in about 20% of patients. Gingival hyperplasia can be minimized by good oral hygiene, including dental flossing and gum massage. Patients should be given instruction on these techniques and encouraged to practice them. In some cases, gingival hyperplasia is so great as to require gingivectomy (surgical removal of excess gum tissue).

Skin Rash. Between 2% and 5% of patients develop a *morbilliform (measles-like) rash*. Rarely, morbilliform rash progresses to exfoliative dermatitis or Stevens-Johnson syndrome (an inflammatory skin disease characterized by red macules, papules, and tubercles). If a rash develops, phenytoin should be discontinued.

Cardiovascular Effects. When phenytoin is administered by IV injection (to treat status epilepticus), cardiac dysrhythmias and hypotension may result. These dangerous responses can be minimized by injecting phenytoin slowly and in dilute solution.

Other Adverse Effects. *Hirsutism* (overgrowth of hair in unusual places) can be a disturbing response, especially in young women. Interference with vitamin D metabolism may cause *rickets* and *osteomalacia* (softening of the bones). Interference with vitamin K metabolism can lower prothrombin levels, thereby causing *bleeding tendencies in newborns* whose mothers took phenytoin during pregnancy.

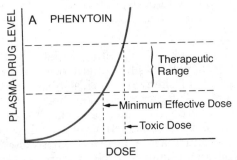 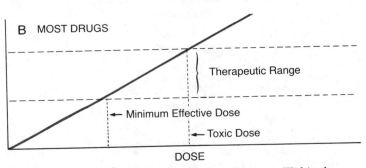

Figure 22–1. Relationship between dose and plasma level for phenytoin versus most other drugs. *A,* Within the therapeutic range, small increments in phenytoin dosage produce *sharp* increases in plasma drug levels. This relationship makes it difficult to maintain plasma phenytoin levels within the therapeutic range.

B, Within the therapeutic range, small increments in dosage produce *small* increases in drug levels. With this relationship, moderate fluctuations in dosage are unlikely to result in either toxicity or loss of therapeutic effects.

Drug Interactions

Phenytoin interacts with a large number of drugs. The more important interactions are discussed below.

Drugs That Increase Plasma Levels of Phenytoin. Since the therapeutic range of phenytoin is narrow, slight increases in phenytoin levels can cause toxicity. Consequently, caution must be exercised when phenytoin is used concurrently with drugs that can increase phenytoin levels. Drugs known to elevate phenytoin levels include *diazepam* (an antianxiety agent and antiseizure drug), *isoniazid* (a drug used to treat tuberculosis), *cimetidine* (a drug used to treat gastric ulcers), and *ethanol* (when taken acutely). These agents increase phenytoin levels by reducing the rate at which phenytoin is metabolized. *Valproic acid* (an antiseizure drug) elevates levels of free phenytoin by displacing phenytoin from binding sites on plasma proteins.

Drugs That Decrease Plasma Levels of Phenytoin. Drugs known to decrease phenytoin levels include *folic acid* (vitamin B₉), *carbamazepine* and *phenobarbital* (antiseizure drugs), and *ethanol* (when used chronically). These agents reduce phenytoin levels by accelerating phenytoin metabolism. By lowering phenytoin levels, these drugs can increase the risk of seizures.

Interactions Resulting from Induction of Hepatic Drug-Metabolizing Enzymes. Phenytoin stimulates synthesis of hepatic drug-metabolizing enzymes. By increasing drug metabolism, phenytoin can *decrease* the effects of other drugs, including *oral anticoagulants, oral contraceptives,* and *glucocorticoids* (anti-inflammatory/immunosuppressive drugs). Because it is desirable to avoid pregnancy while taking antiseizure medication, and because phenytoin can decrease the effectiveness of oral contraceptives, women who are taking these drugs should increase the dosage of the contraceptive.

CNS Depressants. The depressant effects of *alcohol, barbiturates,* and *other CNS depressants* will add to those of phenytoin. Patients should be advised to avoid alcohol and other drugs with CNS-depressant properties.

Preparations, Dosage, and Administration

Preparations. Phenytoin [Dilantin] is available in an *injectable* form and in four *oral* formulations: chewable tablets, oral suspension, prompt-acting capsules, and extended-release capsules.

As noted previously, phenytoin products differ significantly in bioavailability. *Differences in bioavailability exist among different formulations of phenytoin (e.g., tablets versus capsules) and be-* tween the same formulations produced by different manufacturers. Because of differences in bioavailability, and because small changes in phenytoin dosage can produce large changes in plasma drug levels, *patients should not switch from one formulation of phenytoin to another or from one brand of phenytoin to another without the physician's approval and supervision.* (It should be noted that phenytoin is one of the rare examples of a drug for which there are significant differences among preparations produced by different manufacturers.)

Dosage. Because patients vary widely in their ability to metabolize phenytoin, *dosing is highly individualized.* Initial doses are usually given twice daily. Once a maintenance dosage has been established, once-a-day dosing is often possible (using an extended-release formulation). For *adults,* a typical *initial* dosage is 150 mg twice a day; *maintenance* dosages usually range between 300 and 400 mg/day. For *children,* a typical *initial* dosage is 2.5 mg/kg twice a day; *maintenance* dosages usually range between 4 and 7 mg/kg/day.

Plasma drug levels are often monitored as an aid to dosage determination. *The dosing objective is to produce phenytoin levels between 10 and 20 μg/ml.* Levels below 10 μg/ml are too low to control seizures; at levels above 20 μg/ml, signs of toxicity begin to appear. Because phenytoin has a relatively narrow therapeutic range (between 10 and 20 μg/ml), and because of the nonlinear relationship between phenytoin dosage and phenytoin plasma levels, *once a safe and effective dosage has been established, the patient should adhere to it rigidly, since even small deviations from the established dosage can cause toxicity or therapeutic failure.*

When treatment with phenytoin is discontinued, dosage should be reduced gradually. Abrupt withdrawal may precipitate seizures.

Administration. *Oral* preparations may cause gastric discomfort. The patient should be informed that gastric upset can be reduced by administering phenytoin with meals or immediately after meals. Patients using the oral suspension of phenytoin should be instructed to shake the preparation well before dispensing, since failure to do so may result in uneven dosing.

Intravenous administration is used to treat generalized convulsive status epilepticus. *It is imperative that infusions be performed slowly* (no faster than 50 mg per minute), since rapid administration can cause cardiovascular collapse. Phenytoin should not be added to an existing IV infusion, since mixing phenytoin with other solutions is likely to produce a precipitate. Solutions of phenytoin are highly alkaline and can cause local venous irritation; irritation can be reduced by flushing the IV needle or catheter with sterile saline immediately after completing the phenytoin infusion.

PHENOBARBITAL

Phenobarbital is one of our oldest antiseizure medications. The drug is effective, inexpensive, and has few serious side effects. Because of these qualities, phenobarbital remains one of our most commonly used antiseizure drugs.

Phenobarbital belongs to the barbiturate family. However, in contrast to most barbiturates, which produce generalized depression of the CNS, phenobarbital is able to suppress seizures at doses that produce minimal disruption of CNS function. Because it can reduce seizures without causing sedation, phenobarbital is classified as an *anticonvulsant barbiturate* (to distinguish it from most other barbiturates, which are employed as daytime sedatives or as "sleeping pills").

The basic pharmacology of the barbiturates is discussed in Chapter 27. Discussion here is limited to the use of phenobarbital to treat seizure disorders.

Mechanism of Antiseizure Action

The mechanism by which phenobarbital reduces seizures is not known with certainty. Suggested mechanisms are (1) potentiation of the inhibitory effects of GABA, and (2) inhibition of the excitatory effects of glutamate (an excitatory neurotransmitter). Although the mechanism by which phenobarbital suppresses seizures is unclear, what does seem clear is that this mechanism must be different from the mechanism by which phenobarbital produces sedation. This conclusion is based on the observation that phenobarbital can control seizures at doses that are significantly lower than those needed to produce generalized depression of the CNS.

Pharmacokinetics

Phenobarbital is absorbed completely following oral administration. The half-life of the drug is approximately 4 days. Because of this prolonged half-life, 2 to 3 weeks are required for plasma levels of phenobarbital to reach a plateau. (Recall that in the absence of a loading dose an interval equivalent to four half-lives is required for plateau levels to be achieved.) Phenobarbital is eliminated by a combination of hepatic metabolism and renal excretion.

Therapeutic Uses

Epilepsy. Phenobarbital is effective against all major forms of epilepsy except absence seizures. Until recently, phenobarbital had been a drug of choice for tonic-clonic seizures and partial seizures in older children and adults. However, many clinicians now prefer to treat these epilepsies with carbamazepine, phenytoin, or valproic acid—drugs that cause fewer neuropsychologic effects than phenobarbital. Intravenous phenobarbital is indicated for control of generalized convulsive status epilepticus, although IV diazepam is generally preferred.

Sedation and Induction of Sleep. Like other barbiturates, phenobarbital can be used to produce daytime sedation and to treat insomnia. These applications are discussed in Chapter 27.

Adverse Effects

Neuropsychologic Effects. *Drowsiness* is the most common CNS effect. During the initial phase of therapy, sedation develops in practically all patients. With continued drug use, tolerance to sedation develops. Some *children* experience paradoxical responses: instead of becoming sedated, they may become *irritable* and *hyperactive*. *Depression* may occur in adults. Elderly patients may experience *agitation* and *confusion*.

Physical Dependence. Like all other barbiturates, phenobarbital can cause physical dependence. However, at the doses employed to treat epilepsy, significant dependence is unlikely.

Exacerbation of Intermittent Porphyria. Phenobarbital and other barbiturates can increase the risk of acute intermittent porphyria. Accordingly, barbiturates are absolutely contraindicated for patients with a history of this disorder. The relationship of barbiturates to intermittent porphyria is discussed further in Chapter 27.

Use in Pregnancy. Use of barbiturates during pregnancy has been associated with congenital abnormalities. Women who take phenobarbital during pregnancy or become pregnant while taking the drug should be informed of the potential risk to the fetus.

Other Adverse Effects. Like phenytoin, phenobarbital can interfere with the metabolism of vitamins D and K. Disruption of vitamin D metabolism can cause *rickets* and *osteomalacia*. Disruption of vitamin K metabolism can cause *bleeding tendencies in neonates* whose mothers took phenytoin during pregnancy.

Toxicity

When taken in moderately excessive doses, phenobarbital causes *nystagmus* and *ataxia*. Severe overdosage produces generalized *CNS depression*; death results from depression of respiration. Barbiturate toxicity and its treatment are discussed at length in Chapter 27.

Drug Interactions

Induction of Drug-Metabolizing Enzymes. Phenobarbital acts on the liver to induce (stimulate) the synthesis of drug-metabolizing enzymes. By doing so, phenobarbital can increase the rate at which many drugs are inactivated, thereby decreasing their effects. Of particular concern are reduced effects of *oral contraceptives* and *oral anticoagulants*.

CNS Depressants. Being a CNS depressant itself, phenobarbital will intensify CNS depression caused by other drugs (e.g., alcohol, benzodiazepines, opioids, antihistamines), possibly resulting in severe respiratory depression and coma. Patients should be warned against combining phenobarbital with other drugs that have CNS-depressant properties.

Valproic Acid. Valproic acid is an anticonvulsant that has been used in combination with phenobarbital. By competing with phenobarbital for drug-metabolizing enzymes, valproic acid can increase plasma levels of phenobarbital by approximately 40%. Hence, when this combination is used, dosage of phenobarbital must be reduced.

Drug Withdrawal

When phenobarbital is withdrawn, *dosage should be reduced gradually,* since abrupt withdrawal from patients with epilepsy can precipitate status epilepticus. Patients should be warned of this danger and instructed not to discontinue phenobarbital abruptly.

Preparations, Dosage, and Administration

Preparations. Phenobarbital is dispensed in three oral formulations: tablets, capsules, and elixir. The drug is also available in formulations for IM and IV administration.

Dosage. *Maintenance dosages* for *adults* range from 50 to 100 mg/day administered in two or three divided doses. Maintenance dosages for *children* range from 3 to 5 mg/kg/day administered in two or three divided doses. When dosage is being established, plasma drug levels may be used as a guide; target levels are 15 to 40 μg/ml.

Loading doses may sometimes be needed. Because phenobarbital has a long half-life, several weeks are required for drug levels to reach plateau. If plateau must be reached sooner, a loading schedule can be employed. For example, doses that are twice normal can be given for 4 days. Unfortunately, these large doses are likely to produce substantial CNS depression.

Administration. Phenobarbital may be administered orally, IV, and IM. Oral administration is employed for routine therapy of epilepsy. Intravenous administration is needed for status epilepticus.

Intravenous injection must be done slowly. If administration is too rapid, excessive CNS depression may result. Phenobarbital is highly alkaline and may cause local tissue injury if extravasation occurs.

PRIMIDONE

Primidone is active against all major seizure disorders except absence seizures. The drug is nearly identical in structure to phenobarbital. As a result, the pharmacology of both agents is very similar.

Pharmacokinetics

Primidone is readily absorbed following oral administration. In the liver, much of the drug undergoes conversion to two active metabolites: phenobarbital and phenylethylmalonamide (PEMA). Seizure control is produced by primidone itself and by these metabolites.

Therapeutic Uses

Primidone is effective against tonic-clonic, simple partial, and complex partial seizures. The drug is not active against absence seizures.

As a rule, primidone is employed in combination with another antiseizure drug, usually phenytoin or carbamazepine. Primidone is never taken together with phenobarbital; since phenobarbital is one of the active metabolites of primidone, concurrent use of these drugs would be irrational.

Adverse Effects

Sedation, ataxia, and dizziness are common during the initial phase of treatment but diminish with continued drug use. Like phenobarbital, primidone can cause confusion in the elderly and paradoxical hyperexcitability in children. A sense of acute intoxication can occur shortly after administration. As with phenobarbital, primidone is absolutely contraindicated for patients with acute intermittent porphyria. Serious adverse reactions (acute psychosis, leukopenia, thrombocytopenia, systemic lupus erythematosus) have occurred but are rare.

Drug Interactions

Drug interactions for primidone are similar to those for phenobarbital. Primidone can induce hepatic drug-metabolizing enzymes and can thereby reduce the effects of oral contraceptives, oral anticoagulants, and other drugs. In addition, primidone can intensify responses to other CNS depressants.

Preparations, Dosage, and Administration

Primidone [Mysoline] is available in tablets (50 and 250 mg) and in suspension (250 mg/5 ml) for oral use. Therapy in *adults* is initiated with a dose of 100 to 125 mg at bedtime. Dosage is gradually increased over the next 10 days to a maintenance amount of 250 mg 3 or 4 times a day. The maximum dosage is 500 mg 4 times a day.

CARBAMAZEPINE

Carbamazepine [Tegretol, Epitol] is a mainstay of antiseizure therapy. The drug is effective against all common forms of epilepsy except absence seizures.

Mechanism of Action

Carbamazepine appears to act by suppressing high-frequency neuronal discharge in and around seizure foci. Exactly how the drug does this is not known. Suggested mechanisms include (1) potentiation of the inhibitory effects of GABA and (2) acceleration of the firing rate of noradrenergic neurons.

Pharmacokinetics

Absorption of oral carbamazepine is delayed and variable. Peak levels are achieved in 4 to 12 hours. Overall bioavailability is about 80%. The drug distributes well to tissues.

Elimination is by hepatic metabolism. Carbamazepine is unusual in that its half-life decreases as therapy progresses. During the initial phase of treatment, the drug's half-life is approximately 40 hours. The half-life decreases to about 15 hours with continued treatment. The explanation for this phenomenon is that carbamazepine, like phenytoin and phenobarbital, is an inducer of hepatic drug-metabolizing enzymes; by increasing the rate of its own metabolism, carbamazepine causes its own half-life to shorten.

Therapeutic Uses

Epilepsy. Carbamazepine is effective against tonic-clonic, simple partial, and complex partial seizures. Because the drug causes fewer adverse effects than phenytoin and phenobarbital, it is often preferred to these agents. Many clinicians consider carbamazepine the drug of first choice for partial seizures. Carbamazepine is not effective against absence, myoclonic, or atonic seizures.

Trigeminal and Glossopharyngeal Neuralgias. A neuralgia is a severe, stabbing pain that occurs along the course of a nerve. Carbamazepine can reduce neuralgia associated with the trigeminal and glossopharyngeal nerves. The mechanism of this analgesic effect is unknown. It should be noted that although carbamazepine can reduce pain in these specific neuralgias, the drug is not generally effective as an analgesic, and is not indicated for other kinds of pain.

Bipolar Disorder (Manic-Depressive Illness). Carbamazepine can provide symptomatic control in patients with manic-depressive illness, although the drug is not labeled for this application. The role of carbamazepine in manic-depressive illness is discussed in Chapter 26.

Adverse Effects

CNS Effects. In contrast to phenytoin and phenobarbital, carbamazepine has minimal effects on cognitive function. This is a primary reason for selecting carbamazepine over these other drugs.

Carbamazepine can cause a variety of neurologic effects, including visual disturbances (nystagmus, blurred vision, diplopia), ataxia, vertigo, unsteadiness, and headache. These reactions are common during the first weeks of treatment, affecting between 35% and 50% of patients. Fortunately, tolerance usually develops with continued drug use. These effects can be minimized by initiating therapy at low doses and by giving the largest portion of the daily dose at bedtime.

Hematologic Effects. Carbamazepine-induced bone marrow suppression can cause *leukopenia, anemia,* and *thrombocytopenia.* However, serious reactions are rare. Thrombocytopenia and anemia, which have an incidence of 5%, respond to discontinuation of drug use. Leukopenia, which has an incidence of 10%, is usually transient and subsides even with continued drug use. Accordingly, carbamazepine should not be withdrawn unless the white blood cell count drops below 2500/mm³.

Fatal *aplastic anemia* has occurred during carbamazepine therapy. This reaction is extremely rare, having an incidence of 1 in 200,000. Very few cases have been reported since 1964, and in many of these a direct cause-and-effect relationship could not be established.

To reduce the risk of serious hematologic effects, complete blood counts should be performed before treatment and periodically thereafter. Patients with pre-existing hematologic abnormalities should not

be given carbamazepine. Patients should be informed about manifestations of hematologic abnormalities (fever, sore throat, pallor, weakness, infection, easy bruising, petechiae) and instructed to notify the physician if these occur.

Hypo-osmolarity. Carbamazepine can inhibit renal excretion of water, apparently by promoting secretion of antidiuretic hormone. Water retention can reduce the osmolarity of blood and other body fluids, thereby posing a threat to patients with heart failure. Periodic monitoring of serum sodium content is recommended.

Dermatologic Effects. Carbamazepine has been associated with a number of dermatologic effects, including rashes, photosensitivity reactions, Stevens-Johnson syndrome, and exfoliative dermatitis. Mild reactions can often be treated with prednisone (an anti-inflammatory agent) or with an antihistamine. Severe reactions necessitate drug withdrawal.

Drug Interactions

Induction of Drug-Metabolizing Enzymes. Carbamazepine is an effective inducer of hepatic drug-metabolizing enzymes. By promoting synthesis of these enzymes, carbamazepine can increase the rate at which it and other drugs are inactivated. Accelerated inactivation of oral contraceptives and oral anticoagulants is of particular concern.

Phenytoin and Phenobarbital. Both phenytoin and phenobarbital are effective inducers of hepatic drug metabolism. Hence, if either drug is taken with carbamazepine, induction of metabolism is likely to be greater than with carbamazepine alone. Accordingly, phenytoin and phenobarbital can further accelerate the metabolism of carbamazepine, thereby decreasing its effects.

Preparations, Dosage, and Administration

Carbamazepine [Tegretol, Epitol] is available in standard tablets (200 mg), chewable tablets (100 mg), and an oral suspension (100 mg/5 ml). The drug should be administered with meals to reduce gastric upset. Administering the largest portion of the daily dose at bedtime can help reduce adverse CNS effects.

Therapy is initiated with small doses (100 to 200 mg twice a day) to minimize side effects. The dosage is then increased gradually (every 1 to 3 weeks) until control of seizures is achieved. Maintenance dosages for adults range from 600 to 1200 mg/day, administered in divided doses. Maintenance dosages for children range from 15 to 30 mg/kg/day, administered in divided doses.

ETHOSUXIMIDE

Actions and Uses

Ethosuximide is the drug of first choice for absence seizures, the only seizures for which this drug is indicated. Absence seizures are abolished in 60% of patients, and, in newly diagnosed patients, practical control is achieved in 80% to 90%. Beneficial effects derive from elevation of seizure threshold and reduced synaptic responses to repetitive low-frequency stimulation. Ethosuximide is inactive against tonic-clonic, simple partial, and complex partial seizures.

Pharmacokinetics

Ethosuximide is well absorbed following oral administration. Therapeutic effects occur at plasma drug levels of 40 to 100 μg/ml. The drug is eliminated by a combination of hepatic metabolism and renal excretion. Ethosuximide does not induce hepatic drug-metabolizing enzymes.

Adverse Effects and Drug Interactions

Ethosuximide is generally devoid of significant adverse effects and interactions. During the initial phase of treatment, the drug may cause *drowsiness, dizziness,* and *lethargy.* These responses diminish with continued drug use. *Nausea* and *vomiting* may occur and can be reduced by administering ethosuximide with food. Rare but serious reactions include systemic lupus erythematosus, leukopenia, and aplastic anemia.

Preparations, Dosage, and Administration

Ethosuximide [Zarontin] is available in capsules (250 mg) and in a syrup (250 mg/5 ml) for oral use. For children aged 3 to 6 years, the initial dosage is 250 mg/day. For older children and adults, the initial dosage is 500 mg/day. Dosage should be gradually increased until control of seizures is obtained. Maintenance dosages range from 750 to 2000 mg/day for adults, and from 20 to 40 mg/kg/day for children.

Since absence seizures occur many times each day, monitoring the clinical response (rather than plasma drug levels) is the preferred method for determining dosage. Dosage should be increased until seizures have been controlled or until adverse effects become too great.

When withdrawal of ethosuximide is indicated, dosage should be reduced gradually.

VALPROIC ACID

Valproic acid [Depakene, Depakote] is approved by the Food and Drug Administration (FDA) only for treatment of absence seizures. However, the drug is also active against tonic-clonic, atonic, and myotonic seizures, and is used widely to treat these disorders. In addition, valproic acid provides protection against partial seizures. The drug is generally devoid of serious side effects. Death from liver toxicity has occurred rarely.

Mechanism of Action

The mechanism by which valproic acid reduces seizures is not known. One hypothesis suggests that the drug increases the availability of GABA at synapses within the CNS. Two mechanisms for increasing GABA have been proposed: (1) inhibition of GABA breakdown, and (2) inhibition of GABA reuptake. Another hypothesis suggests that valproic acid may act at receptor sites to mimic or potentiate the actions of GABA. The drug may also act by "stabilizing" neuronal membranes.

Pharmacokinetics

Valproic acid is readily absorbed following oral administration and is widely distributed throughout the body. The drug undergoes extensive hepatic metabolism followed by renal excretion.

Therapeutic responses are often seen at plasma drug levels of 50 to 150 μg/ml. However, the correlation between plasma levels and therapeutic effects is not very tight.

Therapeutic Uses

Absence Seizures. Absence seizures are the only FDA-approved indication for valproic acid. For these seizures, valproic acid provides the same degree of control as ethosuximide. Some clinicians consider valproic acid to be the drug of first choice for absence seizures. Others believe that valproic acid, because of its ability to cause liver injury (see below), should be reserved for patients who have failed to respond to ethosuximide.

Other Seizures. Although labeled only for absence seizures, valproic acid can provide effective control of most other seizures. The drug can suppress tonic-clonic seizures, partial seizures, myoclonic seizures, and atonic seizures. Because valproic acid causes fewer serious adverse effects than phenobarbital and phenytoin, the drug is increasingly preferred.

Manic-Depressive Illness. Like carbamazepine, valproic acid can provide symptomatic control in patients with manic-depressive illness. This application is discussed in Chapter 26.

Adverse Effects

Valproic acid is generally well tolerated and causes minimal sedation and cognitive impairment. Gastrointestinal effects are most common. Hepatotoxicity is rare but serious.

Gastrointestinal Effects. Nausea, vomiting, and indigestion are common, occurring in 16% of those treated. These effects are transient and rarely require drug withdrawal. Gastrointestinal effects can be minimized by administering valproic acid with food and by using an enteric-coated formulation.

Hepatotoxicity. Rarely, valproic acid has been associated with fatal liver failure. Most deaths have occurred within the first few months of therapy. The overall incidence of fatal hepatotoxicity is about 1 in 30,000. However, in high-risk patients—children under the age of 2 years who are receiving multidrug therapy—the incidence is 1 in 500. To minimize the risk of fatal liver injury, the following guidelines have been established.

1. Don't use valproic acid in conjunction with other drugs in children under the age of 3 years.
2. Don't use valproic acid in patients with pre-existing liver dysfunction.
3. Evaluate liver function before initiating treatment and periodically thereafter. (Unfortunately, monitoring liver function may fail to provide advance warning of severe hepatotoxicity: in some patients, fatal liver failure devel-

oped so rapidly that it was not preceded by abnormal test results.)

4. Inform patients about signs and symptoms of liver injury (reduced appetite, malaise, nausea, abdominal pain, jaundice) and instruct them to notify the physician if these develop.
5. Use valproic acid in the lowest effective dosage.

Teratogenic Effects. Valproic acid can adversely affect the developing fetus. In laboratory animals the drug has caused intrauterine growth retardation, fetal resorption, and major developmental abnormalities. Available data suggest, but do not prove, that the drug may also be teratogenic in humans. Valproic acid is classified in FDA Pregnancy Category D: there is evidence of human fetal risk, but the drug may be used during pregnancy if the potential benefits are considered to outweigh the potential risks.

Other Adverse Effects. Valproic acid may cause rash, weight gain, hair loss, and blood dyscrasias (leukopenia, thrombocytopenia, red blood cell aplasia). Significant CNS effects are uncommon.

Drug Interactions

Phenobarbital. Valproic acid decreases the rate at which phenobarbital is metabolized. Blood levels of phenobarbital may rise by 40%, resulting in significant CNS depression. When the combination is used, levels of phenobarbital should be monitored. If levels rise too high, phenobarbital dosage should be reduced.

Phenytoin. Valproic acid can displace phenytoin from binding sites on plasma proteins. The resultant increase in the concentration of free phenytoin may lead to toxicity. Phenytoin levels and clinical status should be monitored.

Preparations, Dosage, and Administration

Preparations. Valproic acid is available in three closely related chemical forms: (1) valproic acid itself, (2) the sodium salt of valproic acid, and (3) divalproex sodium, which is a combination of valproic acid plus its sodium salt. All three forms have identical antiseizure actions.

Valproic acid [Depakene] is available in 250-mg tablets. The sodium salt of valproic acid [Depakene] is available in a syrup (50 mg/ml). Divalproex sodium [Depakote] is available in enteric-coated tablets (125, 250, and 500 mg). Gastric irritation is less with the enteric-coated tablets than with the regular tablets or syrup.

Dosage and Administration. Daily doses are small initially and then gradually increased to a maintenance level. For *adults,* the initial dosage is 5 to 15 mg/kg/day, usually administered in two divided doses. The usual adult maintenance dosage is 10 to 20 mg/kg/day. For *children* aged 1 to 12 years, the initial dosage is 10 to 30 mg/kg/day, usually administered in divided doses. The usual pediatric maintenance dosage is 20 to 30 mg/kg/day. For both adults and children, the dosage should be increased if phenobarbital or another inducer of hepatic drug metabolism is taken concurrently.

Patients should be instructed to swallow the tablets and capsules intact, without chewing or crushing. Gastric discomfort can be decreased by administering valproic acid with meals and by using enteric-coated tablets.

CLONAZEPAM

Clonazepam belongs to the benzodiazepine family of drugs. The basic pharmacology of the benzodiazepines is discussed in Chapter 27. Consideration here is limited to the use of clonazepam in epilepsy.

Mechanism of Action

Benzodiazepines act by preventing the spread of seizure activity throughout the brain. These drugs do not suppress abnormal excitability within the seizure focus. Although the mechanism by which benzodiazepines decrease seizure spread has not been firmly established, a likely mechanism is enhancement of the inhibitory actions of GABA.

Therapeutic Uses

Clonazepam is indicated for absence, myoclonic, and atonic seizures. (Atonic seizures are characterized by a loss of all muscle tone.) The drug is not used to treat tonic-clonic or partial seizures. For therapy of absence seizures, ethosuximide and valproic acid are preferred to clonazepam. Some patients develop tolerance to clonazepam within months, causing loss of seizure control.

Adverse Effects

Like other benzodiazepines, clonazepam is generally devoid of serious adverse effects. *CNS depression* (drowsiness, lethargy, fatigue) is common early in therapy, but diminishes with continued drug use. Like phenobarbital, clonazepam can cause *paradoxical excitement* (hyperactivity, aggression, decreased ability to concentrate) in children. Clonazepam may stimulate secretion from salivary glands and glands of the upper respiratory tract; these secretions may compromise breathing in patients with respiratory diseases.

Drug Interactions

Depressant effects of clonazepam will add with those of other *CNS depressants* (e.g., alcohol, opioids, barbiturates, antihistamines). Accordingly, concurrent use of these drugs should be avoided.

Combined treatment with clonazepam and *valproic acid* has caused tonic seizures and should be avoided. The mechanism of this interaction is not known.

Preparations, Dosage, and Administration

Clonazepam [Klonopin] is dispensed in tablets (0.5, 1, and 2 mg) for oral administration. The initial dosage for *adults* is 0.5 mg 3 times/day. The maximum dosage is 20 mg/day. The initial dosage for *infants and children* is 0.01 to 0.03 mg/kg/day. Dosage may be gradually increased to a maximum of 0.2 mg/kg/day.

As with other drugs used to treat epilepsy, abrupt discontinuation may trigger seizures. Accordingly, withdrawal of clonazepam should be done slowly.

FELBAMATE

Felbamate [Felbatol] is the first antiseizure drug to receive FDA approval since 1978, the year that valproic acid was introduced. The new drug has a broad spectrum of antiseizure activity and appears to be very safe. Its ultimate therapeutic niche is yet to be determined.

Mechanism of Action. Felbamate increases seizure threshold and suppresses seizure spread. The mechanism underlying these effects is not known. Unlike some antiseizure drugs (e.g., phenobarbital, benzodiazepines), felbamate does not interact with GABA receptors and does not enhance the inhibitory actions of GABA.

Pharmacokinetics. Felbamate is well absorbed following oral administration, even in the presence of food. Peak plasma levels are achieved in 1 to 4 hours. The drug readily penetrates to the CNS. Although therapeutic plasma levels have not been established, levels of 20 to 120 µg/ml have been measured dur-

Table 22–4. Drugs for Generalized Convulsive Status Epilepticus

Drug	Usual Initial Dose	Usual Rate of Administration	Repeat Doses PRN	Maximum Dose per 24 Hours
Diazepam, IV				
Adults	5–10 mg	1–2 mg/min	5–10 mg q20–30 min	100 mg
Children	0.25–0.4 mg/kg*	<1–2 mg/min	0.25–0.4 mg/kg q20–30 min*	40 mg
Phenytoin, IV				
Adults	15–20 mg/kg	30–50 mg/min	100–150 mg q30 min	1.5 gm
Children	15–20 mg/kg	0.5–1.5 mg/kg/min	1.5 mg/kg q30 min	20 mg/kg
Phenobarbital, IV				
Adults	300–800 mg	25–50 mg/min	120–240 mg q20 min	1–2 gm
Children	20 mg/kg	25–50 mg/min	6 mg/kg q20 min	40 mg/kg

*To a maximum of 5 to 10 mg.

ing clinical trials. Felbamate is eliminated in the urine, primarily unchanged. The drug's half-life is 14 to 23 hours.

Therapeutic Uses. Felbamate is approved for (1) adjunctive or monotherapy in adults with partial seizures (with or without generalization), and (2) adjunctive therapy in children with Lennox-Gastaut syndrome. Clinical trials to assess efficacy in other seizure disorders are in progress. There are no data comparing felbamate with other antiseizure drugs.

Adverse Effects. Felbamate is generally well tolerated. The most common adverse effects are gastrointestinal disturbances (anorexia, nausea, vomiting) and CNS effects (insomnia, somnolence, dizziness, headache, diplopia). These effects occur more frequently when felbamate is combined with other drugs than when used alone. To date, felbamate has not been associated with the severe adverse effects—cardiac dysrhythmias, blood dyscrasias, hepatotoxicity, teratogenesis—seen occasionally with certain other antiseizure drugs. However, since these effects are relatively rare, and since experience with felbamate is limited, it is too soon to know if the drug is truly devoid of serious toxocity. Felbamate has no major contraindications.

Drug Interactions. Felbamate can alter plasma levels of other antiseizure drugs, and vice versa. Felbamate increases levels of phenytoin and valproic acid. Levels of felbamate are increased by valproic acid and reduced by phenytoin and carbamazepine. Increased levels of phenytoin and valproic acid (and possibly felbamate) could lead to toxicity; reduced levels of felbamate could lead to therapeutic failure. Therefore, to keep levels of these drugs within the therapeutic range, they should be monitored and dosages should be adjusted accordingly.

Preparations, Dosage, and Administration. Felbamate [Felbatol] is available in tablets (400 and 600 mg) and an oral suspension (600 mg/5 ml). For *older children* (over 14 years old) *and adults,* the initial dosage is 1200 mg/day in divided doses; the maximum dosage is 3600 mg/day. For *younger children* (2 to 14 years old), the initial dosage is 15 mg/kg/day in divided doses; the maximum dosage is 45 mg/kg/day or 3600 mg/day, whichever is less.

DRUGS FOR GENERALIZED CONVULSIVE STATUS EPILEPTICUS

Generalized convulsive status epilepticus is a life-threatening medical emergency. Intravenous antiseizure medication is required. Effective drugs include diazepam, phenobarbital, and phenytoin.

In addition to antiseizure medication, supportive measures (intravenous fluids, mechanical ventilation) may be needed.

DIAZEPAM

Diazepam belongs to the benzodiazepine family of drugs. The basic pharmacology of these agents is discussed in Chapter 27. Discussion here is limited to the use of diazepam in status epilepticus.

Use in Status Epilepticus

Of the drugs employed to treat convulsive status epilepticus, diazepam is frequently selected first. Intravenous diazepam controls convulsions in 80% to 90% of patients. It must be stressed, however, that the effects of diazepam are short lived. Consequently, as soon as seizures have been controlled, an intravenous dose of phenytoin (whose effects persist longer than those of diazepam) should be given.

Adverse Effects

Although *oral* diazepam is extremely safe, *intravenous* diazepam can cause serious harm. Adverse responses to IV diazepam include *venous thrombosis, apnea* (secondary to CNS depression), and *cardiac arrest.* The risks of IV therapy can be minimized by (1) injecting diazepam slowly, (2) avoiding injection into small veins and all arteries, and (3) having facilities available for mechanical ventilation.

Preparations, Dosage, and Administration

Preparations and Dosage. Diazepam [Valium] for parenteral administration is dispensed in ampuls (1, 2, 5, and 10 ml) and prefilled syringes (1 and 2 ml). Both the ampuls and syringes contain the drug in a 5 mg/ml solution. Adult and pediatric dosages for intravenous therapy are summarized in Table 22–4.

Administration. For treatment of convulsive status epilepticus, diazepam is usually administered IV. Injections should be done *slowly* (no faster than 5 mg/min). Small veins and all arteries must be avoided. Facilities for ventilatory assistance should be available.

To insure effectiveness, diazepam should not be added to other solutions. If the drug cannot be injected directly into a vein (and therefore must be administered through a pre-existing IV line), it should be injected into the line as close to the venous insertion as possible.

For some patients, IV administration will not be possible. These patients should receive diazepam by deep IM injection.

OTHER DRUGS FOR STATUS EPILEPTICUS

The most common alternatives to diazepam are *phenobarbital* and *phenytoin*. Dosages for these drugs are presented in Table 22–4. *Lorazepam,* a benzodiazepine similar to diazepam, has also been employed. All of these drugs should be administered intravenously. If diazepam and the alternative antiseizure drugs fail to suppress convulsions, general anesthesia may be tried as a last resort.

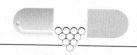

Summary of Major Nursing Implic

NURSING IMPLICATIONS THAT APPLY TO ALL ANTISEIZURE MEDICATIONS

 Preadministration Assessment

Therapeutic Goal

The goal of treatment is to minimize or eliminate seizure events, thereby allowing the patient to live a normal or near normal life.

Baseline Data

Before initiating treatment, it is essential to know the type of seizure involved (e.g., absence, tonic-clonic) and the frequency of seizure events.

 Implementation: Dosage and Administration

Dosage Determination

Dosages are often highly individualized and difficult to establish. Clinical evaluation of therapeutic and adverse effects is essential to establish a dosage that is both safe and effective. For several antiseizure drugs (especially those used to treat tonic-clonic seizures), knowledge of plasma drug levels can be a significant aid to dosage determination.

 Implementation: Measures to Enhance Therapeutic Effects

Minimizing Danger from Uncontrolled Seizures

Advise the patient to avoid potentially hazardous activities (e.g., driving, operating dangerous machinery) until seizure control has been established. Also, since seizures may recur after they are largely under control, advise the patient to carry some form of identification (e.g., Medic-Alert bracelet) to aid in diagnosis and treatment if a seizure occurs.

Promoting Compliance

Seizure control requires rigid adherence to the prescribed regimen; non-compliance is a major cause of therapeutic failure. To promote compliance, educate the patient about the importance of taking antiseizure medication exactly as prescribed. Monitoring plasma drug levels can motivate compliance and can facilitate assessment of compliance.

 Ongoing Evaluation and Interventions

Evaluating Therapeutic Effects

Teach the patient (or a family member) to maintain a seizure-frequency chart, indicating the date, time, and nature of all seizure events. The physician will use this record to evaluate treatment and make dosage adjustments and drug selections.

Minimizing Adverse Effects

CNS Depression. Practically all antiseizure medications depress the CNS. Signs of CNS depression (sedation, drowsiness, lethargy) are most prominent during the initial phase of treatment and decline with continued drug use. Forewarn patients about CNS depression and advise them to avoid driving and other hazardous activities if CNS depression is significant.

Withdrawal Seizures. Abrupt discontinuation of antiseizure medication can lead to status epilepticus. Consequently, withdrawal of medication should be done slowly (over several months). Forewarn patients about the dangers of abrupt drug withdrawal and instruct them never to discontinue drug use without consulting the physician. Advise patients who are planning to travel to carry extra medication to insure a continued supply in the event they become stranded where medication is unavailable.

Usage in Pregnancy and Lactation. When antiseizure medication is to be used during pregnancy, the risk of fetal harm from the medication must be weighed against the risk of fetal harm from uncontrolled seizures. In most cases, the risk from uncontrolled seizures exceeds the risk from medication. Accordingly, most women with major seizure disorders should continue to take antiseizure drugs during pregnancy.

Antiseizure therapy does not constitute an automatic contraindication to breast-feeding. However, if the infant experiences toxicity (e.g., excessive CNS depression), breast-feeding should cease.

Minimizing Adverse Interactions

CNS Depressants. Drugs with CNS-depressant actions (e.g., alcohol, antihistamines, barbiturates, opioids) will intensify the depressant effects of antiseizure drugs, thereby posing a risk of excessive CNS depression. Warn the patient against using alcohol and other CNS depressants.

PHENYTOIN

In addition to the nursing implications presented below, *see also* the nursing implications presented above for all antiseizure drugs.

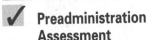

Therapeutic Goal

Oral phenytoin is used to treat partial seizures (simple and complex) and tonic-clonic seizures. *Intravenous* phenytoin is used to treat convulsive status epilepticus.

Identifying High-Risk Patients

Intravenous phenytoin is contraindicated for patients with *sinus bradycardia, S-A block, second- or third-degree A-V block,* and *Stokes-Adams syndrome.*

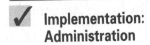

Routes

Oral, IV, and (rarely) IM.

Administration

Oral. Instruct the patient to take phenytoin exactly as prescribed. Inform the patient that once a safe and effective dosage has been established, small deviations in dosage can lead to toxicity or to loss of seizure control.

Advise the patient to take phenytoin with meals to reduce gastric discomfort.

Instruct the patient to shake the phenytoin oral suspension before dispensing in order to provide consistent dosing.

Warn the patient not to switch formulations or brands of phenytoin without the physician's approval and oversight.

Intravenous. To minimize the risk of severe reactions (e.g., cardiovascular collapse) infuse phenytoin *slowly* (no faster than 50 mg/min).

Do not mix phenytoin solutions with other drugs.

To minimize venous inflammation at the site of injection, flush the needle or catheter employed for phenytoin administration with saline immediately after completing the infusion.

✓ **Ongoing Evaluation and Interventions**

Minimizing Adverse Reactions

CNS Effects. Inform the patient that excessive doses can produce sedation, ataxia, diplopia, and interference with cognitive function. Instruct the patient to notify the physician if these occur.

Gingival Hyperplasia. Inform the patient that phenytoin often promotes overgrowth of gum tissue. To minimize harm and discomfort, instruct the patient in proper techniques of brushing, flossing, and gum massage.

Skin Rash. Inform the patient that phenytoin can cause a morbilliform (measles-like) rash that may progress to a more serious reaction. Instruct the patient to notify the physician immediately if a rash develops. Use of phenytoin should stop.

Withdrawal Seizures. Abrupt discontinuation of phenytoin can trigger convulsive status epilepticus. Warn the patient against abrupt cessation of treatment.

Minimizing Adverse Interactions

Phenytoin is subject to a large number of significant interactions with other drugs; some are summarized below. Warn the patient against use of any drugs not specifically approved by the physician.

CNS Depressants. Warn the patient against use of alcohol and all other drugs with CNS-depressant properties, including opioids, barbiturates, and antihistamines.

Oral Anticoagulants and Oral Contraceptives. Phenytoin can decrease the effects of these agents (and other drugs) by inducing hepatic drug-metabolizing enzymes. Dosages of oral anticoagulants and oral contraceptives may need to be increased.

PHENOBARBITAL

Nursing implications that apply to the antiseizure applications of phenobarbital include those presented below and those presented above for all antiseizure drugs. Nursing implications that apply to the barbiturates as a group are summarized in Chapter 27.

**Preadministration
Assessment**

**Implementation:
Administration**

**Ongoing
Evaluation and
Interventions**

Therapeutic Goal

Oral phenobarbital is used to treat partial seizures (simple and complex) and tonic-clonic seizures. *Intravenous* therapy is used for convulsive status epilepticus.

Identifying High-Risk Patients

Phenobarbital is *contraindicated* for patients with a history of *acute intermittent porphyria*. The drug should be used with *extreme caution* during *pregnancy*.

Routes

Oral and IV.

Administration

Oral. A loading schedule using larger than normal doses may be employed to initiate treatment. Monitor the patient for excessive CNS depression while these large doses are used.

Intravenous. Rapid IV infusion can cause severe adverse effects. Perform infusions slowly.

Minimizing Adverse Effects

Neuropsychologic Effects. Warn the patient that sedation may occur during the initial phase of treatment. Advise the patient to avoid hazardous activities if sedation is significant.

Inform parents that children may become irritable and hyperactive. Instruct parents to notify the physician if these behaviors occur.

Exacerbation of Intermittent Porphyria. Phenobarbital can exacerbate acute intermittent porphyria. Accordingly, the drug is absolutely contraindicated for patients with a history of this disorder.

Use in Pregnancy. Warn women of child-bearing age that barbiturates may cause birth defects.

Withdrawal Seizures. Abrupt withdrawal of phenobarbital can trigger seizures. Warn the patient against abrupt discontinuation of treatment.

Minimizing Adverse Interactions

Interactions Due to Induction of Drug Metabolism. Phenobarbital can decrease responses to other drugs by inducing hepatic drug-metabolizing enzymes. Effects on *oral contraceptives* and *oral anticoagulants* are of particular concern. Patients using these drugs will require increased dosages to maintain therapeutic responses.

CNS Depressants. Warn the patient against use of alcohol and all other drugs with CNS-depressant properties, including opioids, benzodiazepines, and antihistamines.

Valproic Acid. Valproic acid increases blood levels of phenobarbital. To avoid toxicity, the dosage of phenobarbital should be reduced.

CARBAMAZEPINE

In addition to the nursing implications summarized below, *see above* for nursing implications that apply to all antiseizure drugs.

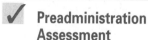
Preadministration Assessment

Therapeutic Goal

Carbamazepine is used to treat partial seizures (simple and complex) and tonic-clonic seizures.

Baseline Data

Obtain complete blood counts prior to treatment.

Identifying High-Risk Patients

Carbamazepine is *contraindicated* for patients with a *history of bone marrow depression* or *adverse hematologic reactions to other drugs.*

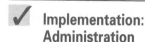
Implementation: Administration

Route

Oral.

Administration

Advise the patient to administer carbamazepine with meals to decrease gastric upset.

Use of low initial doses and administering the largest portion of the daily dose at bedtime can minimize adverse CNS effects.

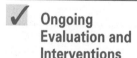
Ongoing Evaluation and Interventions

Minimizing Adverse Effects

CNS Effects. Carbamazepine can cause headache, visual disturbances (nystagmus, blurred vision, diplopia), ataxia, vertigo, and unsteadiness. To minimize these effects, initiate therapy with low doses and have the patient take the largest portion of the daily dose at bedtime.

Hematologic Effects. Carbamazepine can cause leukopenia, anemia, thrombocytopenia, and, very rarely, fatal aplastic anemia. To reduce the risk of serious hematologic effects (1) obtain complete blood counts prior to treatment and periodically thereafter, (2) avoid carbamazepine in patients with pre-existing hematologic abnormalities, and (3) inform patients about manifestations of hematologic abnormalities (fever, sore throat, pallor, weakness, infection, easy bruising, petechiae) and instruct them to notify the physician if these occur.

Minimizing Adverse Interactions

Interactions Due to Induction of Drug Metabolism. Carbamazepine can decrease responses to other drugs by inducing hepatic drug-metabolizing enzymes. Effects on *oral contraceptives* and *oral anticoagulants* are of particular concern. Patients using these drugs will require increased dosages to maintain therapeutic responses.

Phenytoin and Phenobarbital. These drugs can decrease responses to carbamazepine by inducing drug-metabolizing enzymes (beyond the degree of induction caused by carbamazepine itself). Dosage of carbamazepine may need to be increased.

ETHOSUXIMIDE

In addition to the nursing implications summarized below, *see above* for implications that apply to all antiseizure drugs.

 Preadministration Assessment

Therapeutic Goal

Ethosuximide is used only for absence seizures.

Identifying High-Risk Patients

The only contraindication to ethosuximide is hypersensitivity to ethosuximide itself.

 Implementation: Administration

Route

Oral.

Administration

Advise patients to administer ethosuximide with food or milk if gastric upset occurs.

 Ongoing Evaluation and Interventions

Minimizing Adverse Effects and Interactions

Ethosuximide is generally devoid of serious adverse effects and interactions. Warn patients against abrupt discontinuation of treatment.

VALPROIC ACID

Nursing implications for valproic acid include those presented below as well as those presented above for all antiseizure drugs.

 Preadministration Assessment

Therapeutic Goal

Valproic acid is labeled only for treatment of absence seizures. However, the drug is also used widely to treat tonic-clonic seizures, myoclonic seizures, atonic seizures, and partial seizures (simple and complex).

Baseline Data

Obtain baseline tests of liver function.

Identifying High-Risk Patients

Valproic acid is *contraindicated* for patients with *significant hepatic dysfunction* and for *children under the age of 3 years who are taking other antiseizure drugs*.

 Implementation: Administration

Route

Oral.

Administration

Advise patients to take valproic acid with meals to reduce gastric upset. Gastric upset can be further reduced by using an enteric-coated formulation.

Instruct patients to ingest tablets and capsules intact, without crushing or chewing.

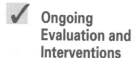

Ongoing Evaluation and Interventions

Minimizing Adverse Effects

Hepatotoxicity. Rarely, valproic acid has caused fatal liver injury. To minimize the risk of hepatotoxicity (1) don't use valproic acid in conjunction with other drugs in children under the age of 3 years, (2) don't use valproic acid in patients with pre-existing liver dysfunction, (3) evaluate liver function before initiating treatment and periodically thereafter, (4) inform patients about signs and symptoms of liver injury (reduced appetite, malaise, nausea, abdominal pain, jaundice) and instruct them to notify the physician if these develop, and (5) use valproic acid in the lowest effective dosage.

Teratogenesis. Valproic acid may cause birth defects. Advise women of child-bearing age to avoid pregnancy. If pregnancy occurs, the risks to the fetus must be weighed against the benefits of continued drug use.

Minimizing Adverse Interactions

Anticonvulsants. Valproic acid can elevate plasma levels of *phenytoin* and *phenobarbital*. Levels of phenobarbital and phenytoin should be monitored and their dosage adjusted accordingly.

INTRAVENOUS DIAZEPAM FOR CONVULSIVE STATUS EPILEPTICUS

The implications summarized below pertain only to the treatment of status epilepticus. Implications that apply to the benzodiazepines as a group are summarized in Chapter 27.

Route

Intravenous.

Administration

Inject diazepam slowly (no faster than 1 to 2 mg/min). Rapid injection can cause severe adverse effects (venous thrombosis, apnea, cardiac arrest) and must be avoided.

Avoid making injections into small veins and all arteries.

Do not mix diazepam solutions with other solutions.

Monitor blood pressure, pulse, and respiration.

Have facilities for mechanical ventilation immediately available.

23

Drugs for Muscle Spasm and Spasticity

I n this chapter we will consider two groups of drugs used to affect skeletal muscle function. One group is used to treat localized muscle spasm. The other group is used to treat spasticity. With only one exception, these drugs produce their therapeutic effects through actions exerted within the central nervous system (CNS). As a rule, the drugs used to treat spasticity do not relieve acute muscle spasm and vice versa. Hence, these two groups of drugs are not therapeutically interchangeable.

DRUG THERAPY OF MUSCLE SPASM: CENTRALLY ACTING MUSCLE RELAXANTS

Muscle spasm is defined as involuntary contraction of a muscle or muscle group. Muscle spasm is often painful and decreases the patient's level of functioning. Spasm can result from a variety of causes, including epilepsy, hypocalcemia, acute and chronic pain syndromes, and trauma (localized skeletal muscle injury). Discussion in this chapter is limited to spasm resulting from muscle injury.

Treatment of spasm involves physical measures as well as pharmacologic therapy. Physical measures include immobilization of the affected muscle, application of cold compresses, whirlpool baths, and physical therapy. For drug therapy, two groups of medicines are used: (1) analgesic anti-inflammatory agents (e.g., aspirin), and (2) centrally acting skeletal muscle relaxants. The analgesic anti-inflammatory agents are discussed in Chapter 61 (Aspirin-like Drugs). The centrally acting skeletal muscle relaxants are discussed below.

The family of centrally acting muscle relaxants consists of eight drugs (Table 23–1). All share similar pharmacologic properties. Hence, we will consider these drugs as a group.

Mechanism of Action

The mechanism by which the centrally acting muscle relaxants relieve spasm is not clear. In laboratory animals, high doses of these drugs can depress spinal reflexes. However, these doses are much higher than those used to relieve spasm in humans. Hence, many investigators believe that relaxation of spasm results from the sedative properties of these drugs, and not from specific actions exerted on CNS pathways involved in the control of muscle tone.

Therapeutic Use

The centrally acting muscle relaxants are used to treat localized spasm resulting from muscle injury. These agents can decrease local pain and tenderness and can increase range of motion. Treatment is almost always associated with sedation. The ability of central muscle relaxants to relieve discomfort of muscle spasm appears about equal to that of aspirin and the other analgesic anti-inflammatory drugs. Since there are no studies to indicate the superiority of one centrally acting muscle relaxant over another, drug selection is based largely on the physician's preference and the patient's response. With the exception of diazepam, the central muscle relaxants are not useful for treating spasticity or other muscle disorders resulting from CNS pathology.

Adverse Effects

CNS Depression. All of the centrally acting muscle relaxants can produce generalized depression of the CNS; drowsiness, dizziness, and light-headedness are common. Patients should be warned against participating in hazardous activities (e.g., driving) if CNS depression is significant.

Depression of the CNS caused by central muscle relaxants can be additive with that produced by other drugs. Hence, the patient should be warned against concurrent use of drugs with CNS-depressant properties (e.g., opioids, antihistamines, alcohol, barbiturates).

Like other CNS depressants, the centrally acting muscle relaxants can produce physical dependence if taken chronically in high doses. An abstinence syndrome will result if these agents are abruptly withdrawn from the physically dependent patient. Accordingly, withdrawal should always be done slowly.

Other Adverse Effects. Certain central muscle relaxants cause unique toxicities. *Chlorzoxazone* is hepatotoxic. If signs of liver dysfunction appear, the drug should be withdrawn. *Carisoprodol* can be hazardous to patients predisposed to intermittent porphyria and, therefore, is contraindicated for these people. *Cyclobenzaprine* has significant anticholinergic (atropine-like) properties; possible effects include dry mouth, blurred vision, photophobia, urinary retention, and constipation.

Dosage and Administration

All of the centrally acting skeletal muscle relaxants can be administered orally. In addition, two agents—methocarbamol and diazepam—can be administered by injection (IM and IV). Average oral maintenance dosages for adults are listed in Table 23–1.

DRUGS USED TO TREAT SPASTICITY

The term *spasticity* refers to a group of movement disorders of CNS origin. These disorders are characterized by heightened muscle tone, spasm, and loss of dexterity. The most common causes of

Table 23–1. Drugs for Muscle Spasm: Centrally Acting Muscle Relaxants

Generic Name	Trade Names	Usual Adult Oral Maintenance Dosage
Baclofen	Lioresal	15 to 20 mg 3 to 4 times/day
Carisoprodol	Rela, Soma, others	350 mg 4 times/day
Chlorphenesin	Maolate	400 to 800 mg 4 times/day
Chlorzoxazone	Paraflex, Parafon Forte	250 mg 3 to 4 times/day
Cyclobenzaprine	Flexeril	10 mg 3 times/day
Diazepam	Valium, others	2 to 10 mg 3 to 4 times/day
Metaxalone	Skelaxin	800 mg 3 to 4 times/day
Methocarbamol	Delaxin, Robaxin, others	1000 mg 4 times/day
Orphenadrine	Norflex, Banflex, others	100 mg morning and evening

spasticity are multiple sclerosis and cerebral palsy. Other causes include traumatic spinal cord lesions and stroke. Spasticity is managed with a combination of drugs and physical therapy.

Three drugs—baclofen, diazepam, and dantrolene—have proved effective in the treatment of spasticity. Two of these agents—baclofen and diazepam—relieve spasticity through actions exerted within the CNS. The third drug—dantrolene—acts directly on skeletal muscle to produce its effects. With the exception of diazepam, the drugs employed to treat muscle spasm (i.e., the centrally acting muscle relaxants) are ineffective against spasticity.

BACLOFEN

Mechanism of Action

Baclofen acts within the spinal cord to suppress reflexes involved in regulating muscle movement. The precise mechanism of reflex attenuation is not known. Since baclofen is a structural analogue of the inhibitory neurotransmitter gamma-aminobutyric acid (GABA) (Fig. 23–1), there is speculation that baclofen may act by mimicking the actions of GABA on spinal neurons. Baclofen has no direct effects on skeletal muscle.

Therapeutic Use

Baclofen can reduce spasticity associated with multiple sclerosis and spinal cord injury (but not with stroke). The drug decreases flexor and extensor spasms and suppresses resistance to passive movement. These actions reduce the discomfort of spasticity and allow increased performance. Since baclofen has no direct muscle relaxant action, and hence does not decrease muscle strength, baclofen is preferred to dantrolene in patients whose spasticity is associated with significant muscle weakness. Baclofen is not useful in treating the spasticity of Parkinson's disease or Huntington's chorea.

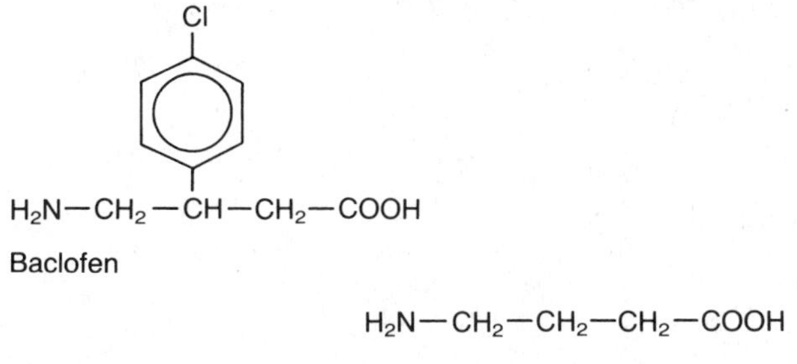

$H_2N—CH_2—CH—CH_2—COOH$ (with Cl-substituted benzene ring)

Baclofen

$H_2N—CH_2—CH_2—CH_2—COOH$

GABA

Figure 23–1. Structural similarity between baclofen and gamma-aminobutyric acid (GABA).

Adverse Effects

The most common side effects of baclofen involve the CNS and the gastrointestinal tract. Serious adverse reactions are rare.

CNS Effects. Baclofen is a CNS depressant and frequently causes drowsiness, dizziness, weakness, and fatigue. These responses are most intense during the early phase of therapy and diminish with continued drug use. CNS depression can be minimized with doses that are small initially and then gradually increased. Patients should be cautioned against use of alcohol and other CNS depressants, since baclofen potentiates the depressant actions of these drugs.

Overdosage with baclofen can produce coma and respiratory depression. There is no specific antidote to baclofen poisoning. Hence, treatment is supportive.

Although baclofen does not appear to cause physical dependence, abrupt discontinuation of the drug has been associated with adverse reactions, including visual hallucinations, paranoid ideation, and seizures. Accordingly, withdrawal of baclofen should be done slowly (over 1 to 2 weeks).

Other Adverse Effects. Baclofen frequently causes *nausea, constipation,* and *urinary retention.* Patients should be forewarned about these possible reactions.

Preparations, Dosage, and Administration

Baclofen [Lioresal] is dispensed in tablets (10 and 20 mg) for oral use. Dosages are low initially (e.g., 5 mg 3 times a day) and then gradually increased. Maintenance dosages range from 15 to 20 mg administered 3 to 4 times a day.

DIAZEPAM

Diazepam is a member of the benzodiazepine family. Although diazepam is the only benzodiazepine labeled for treating spasticity, there is no reason to believe that other benzodiazepines would not be effective as well. The basic pharmacology of the benzodiazepines is discussed in Chapter 27. The use of diazepam in spasticity is considered below.

Actions. Like baclofen, diazepam acts within the CNS to suppress spasticity. Beneficial effects appear to result from mimicking the actions of GABA at receptors in the spinal cord and brain. Diazepam does not affect skeletal muscle directly. Since diazepam has no direct effects on muscle strength, the drug is preferred to dantrolene in patients whose strength is marginal.

Adverse Effects. *Sedation* is common when diazepam is used to treat spasticity. This effect can be minimized by initiating therapy with low doses. Other adverse effects are discussed in Chapter 27.

Preparations, Dosage, and Administration

For oral use, diazepam [Valium, others] is dispensed in tablets (2, 5, and 10 mg), sustained-release capsules (15 mg), and in solution (1 and 5 mg/ml). The drug is available as an injection (5 mg/ml) for IM and IV administration. The usual oral dosage for adults is 2 to 10 mg 3 to 4 times a day.

DANTROLENE

Mechanism of Action

Unlike baclofen and diazepam, which act within the CNS, dantrolene acts directly on skeletal muscle to relieve spasticity. The drug's primary action is suppression of calcium release from the sarcoplasmic reticulum (SR). This, in turn, decreases the ability of skeletal muscle to contract. Fortunately, therapeutic doses have only minimal effects on smooth muscle and cardiac muscle.

Therapeutic Uses

Spasticity. Dantrolene can relieve spasticity associated with multiple sclerosis, cerebral palsy, and spinal cord injury. Unfortunately, since dantrolene suppresses spasticity by causing a generalized reduction in the ability of skeletal muscle to contract, treatment may be associated with a significant decrease in strength. As a result, for some patients, overall function may be reduced rather than improved. Accordingly, care must be taken to insure that the benefits of therapy (reduced spasticity) outweigh the harm (reduced strength).

Malignant Hyperthermia. Malignant hyperthermia is a rare, life-threatening syndrome that can be triggered by any general anesthetic and by succinylcholine, a neuromuscular blocking agent. Onset of symptoms is most abrupt with succinylcholine (when used alone or in combination with an anesthetic). Prominent symptoms are muscle rigidity and profound elevation of temperature. The heat of malignant hyperthermia is generated by muscle contraction occurring secondary to massive release of calcium from the SR. Dantrolene relieves symptoms of malignant hyperthermia, apparently by acting on the SR to block calcium release. Malignant hyperthermia is discussed further in Chapter 15.

Adverse Effects

Hepatotoxicity. Dose-related liver damage is dantrolene's most serious adverse effect. Liver injury has an incidence of 1 in 1000. Death has occurred. Hepatotoxicity is most common in women over age 35. In contrast, liver injury is rare in children under age 10. To reduce the risk of liver damage, tests of liver function should be performed prior to treatment and throughout the treatment interval. Because of the potential for liver damage, dantrolene should be administered in the lowest effective dosage and for the shortest time necessary.

Other Adverse Effects. *Muscle weakness, drowsiness,* and *diarrhea* are the most common side effects. Muscle weakness is a direct extension of dantrolene's pharmacologic action. Other disturbing reactions include *anorexia, nausea, vomiting,* and *acne-like rash.*

Preparations, Dosage, and Administration

Preparations. Dantrolene sodium [Dantrium] is dispensed in capsules (25, 50, and 100 mg) for oral use, and as a powder to be reconstituted for IV injection.

Use in Spasticity. For treatment of spasticity, the drug is administered orally. The initial dosage in adults is 25 mg once daily. The usual maintenance dosage is 100 mg 2 to 4 times a day. If beneficial effects do not develop within 45 days, dantrolene therapy should cease.

Use in Malignant Hyperthermia. *Preoperative Prophylaxis.* Patients with a history of malignant hyperthermia can be given dantrolene for prophylaxis prior to elective surgery. The dosage is 4 to 8 mg/kg/day in 4 divided doses for 1 to 2 days preceding surgery.

Treatment of an Ongoing Crisis. For treatment of malignant hyperthermia, dantrolene is administered by IV push. The initial dose is 2 mg/kg. Administration is repeated until symptoms are controlled or until a total dose of 10 mg/kg has been given. Other measures for management of malignant hyperthermia as discussed in Chapter 15.

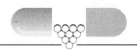 # Summary of Major Nursing Implications

DRUGS USED TO TREAT MUSCLE SPASM: CENTRALLY ACTING SKELETAL MUSCLE RELAXANTS

The nursing implications summarized here apply to all centrally acting muscle relaxants used to treat muscle spasm. Specific agents are listed in Table 23–1.

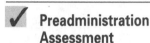 **✓ Preadministration Assessment**

Therapeutic Goal

Relief of signs and symptoms of muscle spasm.

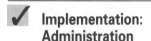 **✓ Implementation: Administration**

Routes

Oral. Used for *all* central skeletal muscle relaxants.

Parenteral. Methocarbamol and *diazepam* may be given IM and IV as well as PO.

Dosage

See Table 23–1.

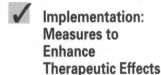 **✓ Implementation: Measures to Enhance Therapeutic Effects**

The treatment plan should include appropriate physical measures (e.g., immobilization of the affected muscle, application of cold compresses, whirlpool baths, and physical therapy).

 ✓ Ongoing Evaluation and Interventions

Minimizing Adverse Effects

CNS Depression. All central muscle relaxants cause CNS depression. Inform patients about possible effects (drowsiness, dizziness, lightheadedness, fatigue) and advise them to avoid hazardous activities (e.g., driving) if significant impairment occurs.

Minimizing Adverse Interactions

CNS Depressants. Caution the patient against use of CNS depressants (e.g., alcohol, benzodiazepines, opioids, antihistamines) since these will intensify depressant effects of the muscle relaxants.

Avoiding Withdrawal Reactions

Central muscle relaxants can cause physical dependence. To avoid an abstinence syndrome, withdraw gradually. Warn the patient against abrupt discontinuation of treatment.

BACLOFEN

 Preadministration Assessment

Therapeutic Goal

Relief of signs and symptoms of spasticity.

Baseline Data

Assess for muscle rigidity, muscle spasm, pain, range of motion, and dexterity.

 Implementation: Administration

Route

Oral.

Administration

The spastic patient may have difficulty with self-medication. Provide assistance if needed.

 Ongoing Evaluation and Interventions

Evaluating Therapeutic Effects

Monitor for reductions in rigidity, muscle spasm, and pain, and for improvements in dexterity and range of motion.

Minimizing Adverse Effects

CNS Depression. Baclofen is a CNS depressant. Inform patients about possible depressant effects (drowsiness, dizziness, lightheadedness, fatigue) and advise them to avoid hazardous activities (e.g., driving) if significant impairment occurs.

Minimizing Adverse Interactions

CNS Depressants. Caution the patient against use of CNS depressants (e.g., alcohol, benzodiazepines, opioids, antihistamines) since these will intensify depressant effects of baclofen.

Avoiding Withdrawal Reactions

Abrupt withdrawal can cause visual hallucinations, paranoid ideation, and seizures. Caution the patient against abrupt discontinuation of treatment.

DANTROLENE

The nursing implications summarized here apply only to the use of dantrolene for spasticity.

 Preadministration Assessment

Therapeutic Goal

Relief of signs and symptoms of spasticity.

Baseline Data

Assess for muscle rigidity, muscle spasm, pain, range of motion, and dexterity. Obtain laboratory tests of liver function.

Identifying High-Risk Patients

Dantrolene is contraindicated for patients with active hepatic disease (e.g., cirrhosis, hepatitis).

Implementation: Administration

Route

Oral.

Administration

The spastic patient may have difficulty with self-medication. Provide assistance if needed.

Ongoing Evaluation and Interventions

Summary of Monitoring

Therapeutic Effects. Monitor for reductions in rigidity, muscle spasm, and pain, and for improvements in dexterity and range of motion.

Adverse Effects. Monitor liver function tests and for reductions in muscle strength.

Minimizing Adverse Effects

CNS Depression. Dantrolene is a CNS depressant. Inform patients about possible depressant effects (drowsiness, dizziness, lightheadedness, fatigue) and advise them to avoid hazardous activities (e.g., driving) if significant impairment occurs.

Hepatotoxicity. Dantrolene is hepatotoxic. Assess liver function prior to treatment and periodically thereafter. If signs of liver dysfunction develop, withdraw dantrolene. Inform patients about signs of liver dysfunction (e.g., jaundice, abdominal pain, malaise) and instruct them to notify the physician if these develop.

Muscle Weakness. Dantrolene can decrease muscle strength. Evaluate muscle function to insure that benefits of therapy (decreased spasticity) are not outweighed by reductions in strength.

Minimizing Adverse Interactions

CNS Depressants. Caution the patient against use of CNS depressants (e.g., alcohol, benzodiazepines, opioids, antihistamines), since these will intensify depressant effects of dantrolene.

DIAZEPAM

Nursing implications for diazepam and the other benzodiazepines are summarized in Chapter 27.

Psychotherapeutic Drugs

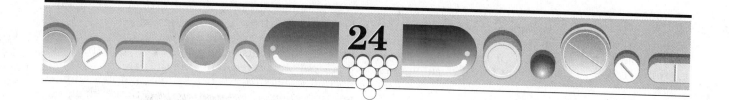

24

Antipsychotic Agents and Their Use in Schizophrenia

The antipsychotic agents are a chemically diverse group of compounds employed to treat a broad spectrum of psychotic disorders. Specific indications include schizophrenia, delusional disorders, acute mania, depressive psychoses, and drug-induced psychoses. In addition to their psychiatric applications, the antipsychotics are used to suppress emesis and to treat Tourette's syndrome and Huntington's chorea.

Since their introduction in the early 1950's, the antipsychotic agents have catalyzed revolutionary change in the management of psychotic illnesses. Before these drugs became available, psychoses were largely untreatable and patients were fated to a life of institutionalization. With the advent of antipsychotic medications, many patients with schizophrenia and other severe psychiatric disorders have been able to leave psychiatric hospitals and return to the community. Others have been spared hospitalization entirely. For those who must remain institutionalized, antipsychotic drugs have at least been able to reduce suffering.

The antipsychotic drugs fall into two major groups: *traditional antipsychotics* and *atypical antipsychotics*. All of the *traditional* agents block receptors for dopamine in the central nervous system (CNS), and they all can cause serious *movement disorders*, referred to as *extrapyramidal reactions*. Although the *atypical* agents also block dopamine receptors, the pattern of blockade differs from that of the traditional agents. As a result, the risk of extrapyramidal reactions with the atypical agents is low.

TRADITIONAL ANTIPSYCHOTIC AGENTS I: GROUP PROPERTIES

In this section we will discuss pharmacologic properties shared by all of the traditional agents. Much of our attention will focus on adverse effects. Of these, the extrapyramidal reactions are of particular concern. Because of these neurologic side effects, the traditional antipsychotics are known alternatively as *neuroleptics*.

CLASSIFICATION

The traditional antipsychotics can be classified according to potency or chemical structure. From a clinical viewpoint, classification by potency is more informative.

Classification by Potency

Traditional antipsychotic agents can be classified as *low potency, medium potency,* or *high potency* (Table 24–1). The low-potency drugs, represented by chlorpromazine [Thorazine], and the high-potency drugs, represented by haloperidol [Haldol], are of particular interest.

It is important to note that although the neuroleptics differ from one another in *potency*, all of these drugs are essentially *equal* in their ability to relieve symptoms of psychoses. Recall that the term potency refers only to the *size* of the dose needed to elicit a given response; potency implies nothing about the *maximal effect* that a drug can produce. Hence, when we say that haloperidol has a higher potency than chlorpromazine, we mean only that the dose of haloperidol required to relieve psychotic symptoms is smaller than the required dose of chlorpromazine; we do not mean that haloperidol can produce greater effects. If administered in therapeutically equivalent doses, both drugs will elicit an equivalent antipsychotic response.

If the low-potency and high-potency neuroleptics possess the same therapeutic ability, why should we distinguish between them? The answer is that although these agents produce identical *antipsychotic* effects, they differ significantly in their *side effects*. Hence, by knowing the potency category to which a particular neuroleptic belongs, we can better predict that drug's undesired responses. This knowledge is useful in drug selection and providing patient care and education.

Chemical Classification

The traditional antipsychotic agents can be placed into six major groups based on their chemical structures (Table 24–2). One of these groups, the phenothiazines, has three subdivisions. Drugs in all groups are equivalent with respect to antipsychotic actions. Because of this equivalence, chemical classification will not be emphasized.

Two chemical categories—the *phenothiazines*

Table 24–1. Traditional Antipsychotic Drugs: Relative Potency and Major Side Effects

Potency Class	Drug	Equivalent Oral Dose (mg)*	Sedation	Orthostatic Hypotension	Anticholinergic Effects	Extrapyramidal Effects†
				Incidence of Major Side Effects		
Low	Chlorpromazine	100	High	High	Medium	Low
	Thioridazine	100	High	High	High	Low
	Chlorprothixene	100	High	High	High	Low
	Mesoridazine	50	High	Medium	Medium	Low
Medium	Triflupromazine	25	High	High	Medium	Medium
	Acetophenazine	20	Medium	Low	Low	Medium
	Loxapine	10	Medium	Medium	Medium	High
	Molindone	10	Medium	Low	Medium	Medium
	Perphenazine	8	Low	Low	Low	High
High	Trifluoperazine	5	Low	Low	Low	High
	Thiothixene	4	Low	Low	Low	High
	Fluphenazine	2	Low	Low	Low	High
	Haloperidol	2	Low	Low	Low	High
	Pimozide	1	Low	Low	Low	High

*Doses listed are the therapeutic equivalent of 100 mg of oral chlorpromazine.
†Incidence refers to *early* extrapyramidal reactions (acute dystonia, parkinsonism, akathisia). Incidence of *late* reactions (tardive dyskinesia) is the same for all of these drugs.

Table 24–2. Traditional Antipsychotic Drugs: Chemical Classification, Routes, and Dosages

Chemical Class and Generic Name	Trade Name	Routes	Dosage Range (mg/day)
Phenothiazine: aliphatic			
Chlorpromazine	Thorazine, Ormazine	PO, IM, R	30–800
Triflupromazine	Vesprin	IM	60–150
Phenothiazine: piperidine			
Mesoridazine	Serentil	PO, IM	30–400
Thioridazine	Mellaril	PO	150–800
Phenothiazine: piperazine			
Acetophenazine	Tindal	PO	60–120
Fluphenazine	Prolixin, Permitil	PO, IM	2–40
Perphenazine	Trilafon	PO, IM	12–64
Trifluoperazine	Stelazine	PO, IM	2–40
Thioxanthene			
Chlorprothixene	Taractan	PO, IM	75–600
Thiothixene	Navane	PO, IM	8–30
Butyrophenone			
Haloperidol	Haldol	PO, IM	1–15
Dihydroindolone			
Molindone	Moban	PO	15–225
Dibenzoxazepine			
Loxapine	Loxitane	PO, IM	20–250

PO = oral; IM = intramuscular, R = rectal (suppository).

and the *butyrophenones*—deserve special attention. The phenothiazines were the first of the modern antipsychotic agents. Chlorpromazine, our prototype of the low-potency neuroleptics, is a member of the phenothiazine family. The butyrophenones stand out because they are the family to which haloperidol belongs. Haloperidol is the prototype of the high-potency antipsychotics.

MECHANISM OF ACTION

The traditional antipsychotic drugs block a variety of receptors within and outside the CNS. To varying degrees, these drugs produce blockade at receptors for dopamine, acetylcholine (muscarinic), histamine, and norepinephrine (alpha$_1$). There is little question that blockade at these receptors is responsible for the major *adverse effects* of the antipsychotics. However, since the etiology of psychotic illness is entirely unknown, the relationship of receptor blockade to *therapeutic effects* can only be guessed. One theory suggests that neuroleptics suppress symptoms of psychosis by blocking specific subtypes of *dopamine* receptors in the mesolimbic and mesocortical areas of the brain, regions thought to be involved in the expression of psychotic symptoms. In support of this theory is the observation that all of the traditional antipsychotics produce dopamine receptor blockade.

THERAPEUTIC USES

Schizophrenia. Schizophrenia is the most common indication for antipsychotic drugs. These agents effectively suppress symptoms during acute psychotic episodes, and, when taken chronically, can greatly decrease the risk of relapse. Initial effects are seen in 1 to 2 days, but full effects develop gradually—over 6 to 8 weeks. So-called *positive symptoms* (e.g., agitation, tension, delusions, hallucinations) generally respond better than *negative symptoms* (social withdrawal, blunted affect, motor retardation). All of the traditional antipsychotic agents are equally effective, although individual patients may respond better to one drug than to another. Consequently, selection among these drugs is based primarily on their side-effect profiles, rather than on their therapeutic effects. It must be noted that antipsychotic drugs do not alter the underlying pathology of schizophrenia. Hence, treatment is not curative—it offers only symptomatic relief. Schizophrenia and its management are discussed further later in the chapter.

Bipolar Disorder (Manic-Depressive Illness). Most patients with bipolar disorder are managed with lithium, the drug of choice for this disease. Neuroleptics may be employed acutely (in combination with lithium) to help manage patients going through a severe manic phase. Bipolar disorder and its treatment are the subject of Chapter 26.

Tourette's Syndrome. This rare, inherited disorder is characterized by severe motor tics, barking cries, grunts, and outbursts of obscene language, all of which are spontaneous and beyond the control of the patient. At least two antipsychotic drugs—haloperidol and pimozide—can help suppress symptoms.

Prevention of Emesis. Neuroleptics suppress emesis by blocking dopamine receptors in the chemoreceptor trigger zone of the medulla. These drugs can be employed to suppress vomiting associated with cancer chemotherapy, gastroenteritis, uremia, and other conditions.

Other Applications. Neuroleptics can be used for *organic mental syndromes* (psychiatric syndromes resulting from organic causes, such as infection, metabolic disorders, poisoning, and structural injury to the brain), *delusional disorders*, and *schizoaffective disorder*. In addition, these agents can relieve symptoms of *Huntington's chorea*.

ADVERSE EFFECTS

Although antipsychotic agents produce a variety of undesired effects, these drugs are, on the whole, very safe; death by overdose is practically unheard of. Of the many side effects these drugs can produce, the most troubling are the extrapyramidal reactions—especially tardive dyskinesia.

Extrapyramidal Reactions

Extrapyramidal reactions are movement disorders resulting from effects of antipsychotic drugs on the extrapyramidal motor system. The extrapyramidal system is the same neuronal network whose malfunction is responsible for the movement disorders of Parkinson's disease.

Four types of extrapyramidal reactions occur. These differ from one another with respect to time of onset and management. Three of these reactions—*acute dystonia, parkinsonism,* and *akathisia*—occur *early* in therapy and can be managed with a variety of drugs. The fourth reaction—*tardive dyskinesia*—occurs *late* in therapy and has no satisfactory treatment. Characteristics of the four extrapyramidal reactions are summarized in Table 24–3.

The *early* reactions occur *less frequently* with *low-potency* agents (e.g., chlorpromazine) than with high-potency agents (e.g., haloperidol). In contrast, the risk of *tardive dyskinesia* is *equal* with *all* antipsychotics.

Acute Dystonia. Acute dystonia develops within the first few days of therapy and can be both disturbing and dangerous. Typically, the patient develops severe spasm of the muscles of the tongue, face, neck, or back. Oculogyric crisis (involuntary upward deviation of the eyes) and opisthotonus (tetanic spasm of the back muscles causing the trunk to arch forward, while the head and lower limbs are thrust backward) may also occur. Severe cramping can cause joint dislocation. Laryngeal dystonia can impair respiration. The cause of acute dystonia is unknown.

Intense dystonia constitutes a crisis that requires rapid intervention. Initial treatment consists of anticholinergic medication (e.g., benztropine, diphenhydramine) administered IM or IV. As a rule, symptoms resolve within 5 minutes of IV administration and within 15 to 20 minutes of IM administration.

It is important to differentiate between acute dystonia and psychotic hysteria. Misdiagnosis of acute dystonia as hysteria could result in escalation of antipsychotic dosage, thereby causing the acute dystonia to become even worse.

Parkinsonism. Antipsychotic-induced parkinsonism is characterized by bradykinesia, mask-like facies, drooling, tremor, rigidity, shuffling gait, cogwheeling, and stooped posture. Symptoms develop within the first month of therapy and are indistinguishable from those of idiopathic Parkinson's disease.

Neuroleptics cause parkinsonism by blocking dopamine receptors in the striatum. Since idiopathic Parkinson's disease is also due to reduced activation of striatal dopamine receptors (see Chapter 21), it is no wonder that Parkinson's disease and neuroleptic-induced parkinsonism share the same symptoms.

Neuroleptic-induced parkinsonism is treated with some—but not all—of the drugs used to treat Parkinson's disease. Specifically, centrally acting *anticholinergic drugs* (e.g., benztropine, diphenhydramine) and *amantadine* [Symmetrel] may be employed. Levodopa, however, should be avoided, since this drug promotes activation of dopamine

Type of Reaction	Time of Onset	Features	Management
Early Reactions			
Acute dystonia	1 to 5 days	Spasm of muscles of tongue, face, neck, and back; opisthotonus	Anticholinergic drugs (e.g., benztropine) IM or IV
Parkinsonism	5 to 30 days	Bradykinesia, mask-like facies, tremor, rigidity, shuffling gait, drooling, cogwheeling, stooped posture	Anticholinergics (e.g., benztropine, diphenhydramine), amantadine, or both
Akathisia	5 to 60 days	Compulsive, restless movement; symptoms of anxiety, agitation	Reduce dosage or switch to a low-potency antipsychotic. Anticholinergic drugs, beta blockers, and benzodiazepines may help
Late Reaction			
Tardive dyskinesia	Months to years	Oral-facial dyskinesias, choreoathetoid movements	Best approach is prevention; no reliable treatment

Table 24–3. Extrapyramidal Reactions to Antipsychotic Drugs

receptors, and might thereby counteract the beneficial effects of antipsychotic treatment.

Use of antiparkinsonian drugs should not continue indefinitely. Antipsychotic-induced parkinsonism tends to resolve spontaneously, usually within a few months after its appearance. Hence, antiparkinsonian drugs should be withdrawn after a few months to determine if they are still required.

Akathisia. Akathisia is characterized by pacing and squirming brought on by an uncontrollable need to be in motion. This profound sense of restlessness can be very disturbing. The syndrome usually develops within the first 2 months of treatment. The cause is unknown. Like other early extrapyramidal reactions, akathisia occurs most frequently with high-potency antipsychotics.

Three types of drugs have been used to suppress symptoms: (1) anticholinergic agents, (2) beta-adrenergic blockers, and (3) benzodiazepines. Although drugs can be helpful, a reduction in antipsychotic dosage or switching to a low-potency agent may be more effective.

It is important to differentiate akathisia from worsening of psychosis. If akathisia were to be confused with anxiety or psychotic agitation, it is likely that antipsychotic dosage would be increased, thereby making akathisia more intense.

Tardive Dyskinesia. Tardive dyskinesia (TD) develops in 20% of patients during long-term therapy and is the most troubling of the extrapyramidal reactions. The risk increases with duration of treatment and dosage size. For many patients, symptoms are irreversible.

Tardive dyskinesia is characterized by involuntary choreoathetoid (twisting, writhing, worm-like) movements of the tongue and face. Patients may also present with lip-smacking movements, and their tongues may flick out in a "fly-catching" motion. One of the earliest manifestations is the appearance of slow, worm-like movements of the tongue. Involuntary movements that involve the tongue and mouth can interfere with chewing, swallowing, and speaking. Eating difficulties can result in malnutrition and weight loss. Over time, TD produces involuntary movements of the limbs, toes, fingers, and trunk. For some patients, symptoms decline following a dosage reduction or drug withdrawal. For others, TD is irreversible.

The cause of TD is complex and incompletely understood. One theory suggests that symptoms result from excessive *activation* of dopamine receptors. It is postulated that, in response to chronic receptor blockade, dopamine receptors of the extrapyramidal system undergo a functional change such that their sensitivity to activation is increased. Stimulation of these "supersensitive" receptors produces an imbalance in favor of dopamine, and thereby produces abnormal movement. In support of this theory is the observation that

symptoms of TD can be reduced (temporarily) by *increasing* antipsychotic drug dosage, which will cause greater receptor blockade. (Since symptoms will eventually return even though antipsychotic dosage is kept at an elevated level, dosage elevation cannot be used to manage TD.)

Tardive dyskinesia has no reliable means of treatment; hence, prevention is the best approach. Antipsychotic drugs should be used in the lowest effective dosage for the shortest time required. After 12 months, the need for continued therapy should be assessed. If drug use must continue, a neurologic evaluation should be done at least every 3 months to detect early signs of TD. For patients with chronic schizophrenia, dosage should be tapered periodically (at least annually) to determine the need for continued treatment.

If signs of TD appear but the patient requires continued antipsychotic therapy, what should be done? Unfortunately, this question has no easy answer. If drug use continues, TD may become progressively worse; hence, discontinuation would seem desirable. However, if treatment ceases, relapse of psychosis may occur; hence, discontinuation may well be harmful. In the face of this dilemma, the clinician should discuss the options with the patient and a family member so that the patient can make an informed decision regarding continued treatment.

Other Adverse Effects

Neuroleptic Malignant Syndrome. Neuroleptic malignant syndrome (NMS) is a rare but serious reaction that carries a 4% risk of mortality (down from 20% just a decade ago thanks to early recognition and treatment). Primary symptoms are "lead-pipe" rigidity, fever (temperature may exceed 41°C), sweating, and autonomic instability, manifested as dysrhythmias and fluctuations in blood pressure. Level of consciousness may rise and fall; the patient may appear confused or mute; and seizures or coma may develop. Death can result from respiratory failure, cardiovascular collapse, dysrhythmias, and other causes. NMS is more likely with high-potency agents than with low-potency agents.

Treatment consists of supportive measures, drug therapy, and immediate withdrawal of antipsychotic medication. Hyperthermia should be controlled with antipyretics and cooling blankets. Hydration should be maintained with fluids. Two drugs—*dantrolene* and *bromocriptine*—are helpful. Dantrolene is a direct-acting muscle relaxant (see Chapter 23). In patients with NMS, this drug reduces rigidity and hyperthermia. Bromocriptine is a dopamine-receptor agonist (see Chapter 21). In patients with NMS, the drug helps relieve CNS toxicity.

Resumption of antipsychotic therapy following an episode of NMS carries a significant risk that

NMS will recur. Since NMS has a high rate of morbidity and mortality, the decision to resume treatment must be made with great care. If continued treatment with an antipsychotic is clearly required, the lowest effective dosage should be employed, and high-potency agents should be avoided.

Anticholinergic Effects. Antipsychotic drugs produce varying degrees of muscarinic cholinergic blockade (see Table 24–1). By blocking muscarinic receptors, these drugs can elicit a full spectrum of anticholinergic responses (dry mouth, blurred vision, photophobia, urinary hesitancy, constipation, tachycardia). Patients should be informed about these responses and taught how to minimize danger and discomfort. As indicated in Table 24–1, anticholinergic effects are more likely with low-potency agents than with high-potency agents. Anticholinergic effects and their management are discussed in detail in Chapter 13.

Orthostatic Hypotension. Antipsychotic drugs promote orthostatic hypotension by blocking alpha$_1$-adrenergic receptors on blood vessels. Alpha-adrenergic blockade prevents compensatory vasoconstriction when the patient stands; hence, blood pressure falls. Patients should be informed about signs of hypotension (lightheadedness, dizziness) and advised to sit or lie down if these occur. In addition, patients should be informed that hypotension can be minimized by moving slowly when assuming an erect posture. With hospitalized patients, blood pressure and pulses should be checked before drug administration and 1 hour after. Measurements should be made while the patient is lying down and again after he or she has been sitting or standing for 1 to 2 minutes. If blood pressure is low, the drug should be withheld and the physician consulted. Hypotension is more likely with low-potency antipsychotics than with the high-potency drugs (see Table 24–1). Tolerance to hypotension develops in 2 to 3 months.

Sedation. Sedation is common during the early days of treatment but subsides within a week or so. Neuroleptic-induced sedation is thought to result from blockade of histamine receptors in the CNS. Daytime sedation can be minimized by administering the entire daily dose at bedtime. Patients should be warned against participation in hazardous activities (e.g., driving) until sedative effects diminish.

Seizures. Antipsychotic drugs can reduce seizure threshold, thereby increasing the risk of seizure activity. The risk of seizures is greatest in patients with epilepsy and other seizure disorders. These patients should be monitored, and, if loss of seizure control occurs, the dosage of their antiseizure medication must be increased.

Sexual Dysfunction. Antipsychotics can cause sexual dysfunction in women and men. In women, these drugs can suppress libido and impair the ability to achieve orgasm. In men, neuroleptics can suppress libido and cause erectile and ejaculatory dysfunction; the incidence of these effects is 25% to 60%. Drug-induced sexual dysfunction can make treatment unacceptable to sexually active patients, thereby leading to poor compliance. A reduction in dosage or switching to a high-potency antipsychotic may reduce effects on sexual function. Patients should be counseled about possible sexual dysfunction and encouraged to report problems.

Dermatologic Effects. Drugs in the *phenothiazine* class can sensitize the skin to ultraviolet light, thereby increasing the risk of severe sunburn. Patients should be warned against excessive exposure to sunlight and advised to apply a sunscreen or wear protective clothing. Phenothiazines can also produce pigmentary deposits in the skin, cornea, and lens of the eye.

Handling antipsychotics can cause contact dermatitis in patients and health care personnel. Dermatitis can be prevented by avoiding direct contact with these drugs.

Neuroendocrine Effects. Antipsychotics increase levels of circulating prolactin by blocking the inhibitory action of dopamine on prolactin release. Elevation of prolactin levels promotes *gynecomastia* (breast growth) and *galactorrhea* in up to 57% of women. Up to 97% experience menstrual irregularities. Gynecomastia and galactorrhea can also occur in males. Since prolactin can promote growth of prolactin-dependent carcinoma of the breast, neuroleptics should be avoided in patients with this form of cancer. (It should be noted that although antipsychotic drugs can *promote* the growth of cancers that already exist, there is no evidence that antipsychotic drugs actually *cause* cancer.)

Agranulocytosis. Agranulocytosis is a rare but serious reaction. Among the traditional antipsychotics, the risk is highest with chlorpromazine and certain other phenothiazines. Since agranulocytosis severely compromises the ability to fight infection, white blood cell counts should be assessed whenever signs of infection (e.g., fever, sore throat) appear. If agranulocytosis is diagnosed, the neuroleptic should be withdrawn. Agranulocytosis reverses upon discontinuation of treatment.

PHYSICAL AND PSYCHOLOGIC DEPENDENCE

Development of physical and psychologic dependence is rare. Patients should be reassured that addiction and dependence are not likely to occur.

Although physical dependence is minimal, abrupt withdrawal of antipsychotics *can* precipitate a mild abstinence syndrome. Symptoms result from chronic cholinergic blockade and include restlessness, insomnia, headache, gastric distress, and sweating. This syndrome can be avoided by withdrawing antipsychotic medication gradually.

DRUG INTERACTIONS

Anticholinergic Drugs. Drugs with anticholinergic properties will intensify anticholinergic responses to neuroleptics. Patients should be advised to avoid all drugs with anticholinergic actions, including antihistamines and certain over-the-counter sleeping aids.

CNS Depressants. Neuroleptics can intensify CNS depression caused by other drugs. Patients should be warned against using alcohol and all other drugs with CNS-depressant actions (e.g., antihistamines, opioids, barbiturates).

Levodopa. Levodopa (a drug used to treat Parkinson's disease) may counteract the antipsychotic effects of neuroleptics. Conversely, neuroleptics may counteract the therapeutic effects of levodopa. These interactions occur because levodopa and neuroleptics have opposing effects on receptors for dopamine: levodopa activates these receptors, whereas neuroleptics cause blockade.

TOXICITY

The traditional antipsychotic drugs are very safe; death by overdose is extremely rare. With chlorpromazine, for example, the therapeutic index is about 200. That is, the lethal dose of this drug is 200 times greater than the therapeutic dose.

Overdosage produces hypotension, CNS depression, and extrapyramidal reactions. Extrapyramidal reactions can be treated with antiparkinsonian drugs. Hypotension can be treated with IV fluids plus an alpha-adrenergic agonist (e.g., phenylephrine). There is no specific antidote to CNS depression. Excess drug should be removed from the stomach by gastric lavage. (Emetics cannot be used because their effects would be blocked by the antiemetic action of the neuroleptic.)

TRADITIONAL ANTIPSYCHOTIC AGENTS II: PROPERTIES OF INDIVIDUAL AGENTS

All of the traditional antipsychotic drugs are equally effective at suppressing symptoms of schizophrenia, although individual patients may respond better to one drug than to another. Hence,

differences among these agents relate primarily to their side-effect profiles (see Table 24–1).

LOW-POTENCY AGENTS

Chlorpromazine

Chlorpromazine [Thorazine, Ormazine] was the first modern antipsychotic medication and is the prototype for all that followed. None of the newer agents is superior at relieving symptoms of psychotic illnesses. Chlorpromazine is a low-potency neuroleptic and belongs to the phenothiazine family of compounds.

Therapeutic Uses. Principal indications for chlorpromazine are schizophrenia and other psychotic disorders. Additional psychiatric indications are schizoaffective disorder and the manic phase of bipolar disorder. Other uses include suppression of emesis and relief of intractable hiccoughs.

Pharmacokinetics. Chlorpromazine may be administered orally, IM, and by rectal suppository. Following oral administration, the drug is well absorbed but undergoes extensive metabolism on its first pass through the liver. As a result, oral bioavailability is only 30%. When chlorpromazine is given by IM injection, peak plasma levels are 10 times those achieved with an equal oral dose. Excretion is renal, almost entirely as metabolites.

Adverse Effects. The most common adverse effects are *sedation, orthostatic hypotension*, and *anticholinergic effects* (dry mouth, blurred vision, urinary retention, photophobia, constipation, tachycardia). Neuroendocrine effects—*galactorrhea, gynecomastia*, and *menstrual irregularities*—occur occasionally. *Photosensitivity reactions* are possible and patients should be warned to minimize unprotected exposure to sunlight. Because chlorpromazine is a low-potency neuroleptic, the risk of *early extrapyramidal reactions* (dystonia, akathisia, parkinsonism) is relatively low. However, the risk of *tardive dyskinesia* is the same as with all other traditional agents. Chlorpromazine *lowers seizure threshold*; hence, patients with seizure disorders should be especially diligent about taking antiseizure medication. *Agranulocytosis* and *neuroleptic malignant syndrome* occur rarely.

Drug Interactions. Chlorpromazine can intensify responses to *CNS depressants* (e.g., antihistamines, opioids, benzodiazepines) and *anticholinergic drugs* (e.g., antihistamines, tricyclic antidepressants, atropine-like drugs).

Preparations, Dosage, and Administration. Chlorpromazine [Thorazine, Ormazine] is available in six formulations: *tablets* (10, 25, 50, 100, and 200 mg), *sustained-release capsules* (30, 75, 150, 200, and 300 mg), *syrup* (2 mg/ml), *liquid concentrate* (30 and 100 mg/ml), *rectal suppositories* (25 and 100 mg), and *injection* (25 mg/ml).

Oral Therapy. The initial dosage for adults is 25 mg 3 times a day. Dosage should be gradually increased until symptoms are controlled. The usual maintenance dosage is 400 mg/day. Elderly patients require less drug than younger patients. Patients with severe psychosis may require doses that are unusually high.

Parenteral Therapy. Parenteral therapy is indicated for the acutely psychotic, hospitalized patient. Intramuscular administration is preferred to intravenous. (Intravenous chlorpromazine is highly irritating and is generally avoided.) The initial dose is 25 to 50 mg. Dosage may be increased gradually to a maximum of 400 mg every 4 to 6 hours. Once symptoms are controlled, oral therapy should be substituted for parenteral.

Other Low-Potency Agents

Thioridazine. Thioridazine [Mellaril] is a low-potency agent indicated for schizophrenia and other psychotic disorders. The drug belongs to the piperidine subclass of phenothiazines. The most common adverse effects are sedation, orthostatic hypotension, anticholinergic effects, weight gain, and inhibition of ejaculation. Effects seen occasionally include extrapyramidal reactions (dystonia, parkinsonism, akathisia, tardive dyskinesia), galactorrhea, gynecomastia, menstrual irregularities, and photosensitivity reactions. Neuroleptic malignant syndrome, convulsions, agranulocytosis, and pigmentary retinopathy occur rarely. Principal interactions are with anticholinergic drugs and CNS depressants. Thioridazine is dispensed in tablets (10, 15, 25, and 50 mg) for oral use. The initial dosage is 50 to 100 mg 3 times a day. Dosage may be gradually increased until symptoms are controlled, but should not exceed 800 mg/day. The usual maintenance dosage is 200 to 800 mg/day in 2 to 4 divided doses.

Chlorprothixene. Chlorprothixene [Taractan] is a low-potency agent used to treat schizophrenia and other psychotic disorders. The drug's side-effect profile is like that of chlorpromazine. Administration is oral and by IM injection. Three formulations are available: tablets (10, 25, 50, and 100 mg), liquid concentrate (20 mg/ml), and injection (12.5 mg/ml). The initial *oral dosage* is 25 to 50 mg 3 or 4 times daily. Dosage is then increased until a maximal response is achieved. Dosages above 600 mg/day are rarely needed. The *intramuscular dosage* is 75 to 200 mg/day in divided doses.

MEDIUM-POTENCY AGENTS

Loxapine. Loxapine [Loxitane] is a medium-potency agent indicated for schizophrenia and other psychotic disorders. The drug's side-effect profile is similar to that of fluphenazine (see below). Administration is oral and intramuscular. Three formulations are available: capsules (5, 10, 25, and 50 mg), liquid concentrate (25 mg/ml), and injection (50 mg/ml). The initial *oral dosage* is 10 mg twice daily. Dosage is increased until symptoms are controlled, typically with 60 to 100 mg/day in divided doses. The dosage should be reduced for maintenance therapy; the usual range is 20 to 60 mg/day. The *intramuscular dosage* is 12.5 to 50 mg every 4 to 6 hours.

Molindone. Molindone [Moban] is a medium-potency agent used to treat schizophrenia and other psychotic disorders. The most common adverse effects are early extrapyramidal reactions (dystonia, parkinsonism, akathisia) and anticholinergic effects (dry mouth, blurred vision, photophobia, urinary retention, constipation, tachycardia). Effects seen occasionally include sedation, menstrual irregularities, weight loss, and tardive dyskinesia. Orthostatic hypotension and neuroleptic malignant syndrome occur rarely. Molindone is available in tablets (5, 10, 25, 50, and 100 mg) for oral administration. The initial dosage is 50 to 75 mg/day in divided doses. Dosage is then increased until symptoms are controlled. As much as 225 mg/day has been given. Dosage should be reduced to the lowest effective amount for maintenance.

Perphenazine. Perphenazine [Trilafon] is a medium-potency agent used to treat schizophrenia and other psychotic disorders. The drug's side-effect profile is like that of fluphenazine (see below). For therapy of psychotic disorders, perphenazine is given orally and by IM injection. Three formulations are

available: tablets (2, 4, 8, and 16 mg), liquid concentrate (16 mg/5 ml), and injection (5 mg/ml). The initial oral dosage is 4 to 8 mg 3 times daily. Once symptoms have been controlled the dosage should be reduced to the lowest effective amount. The initial *intramuscular dosage* is 5 mg every 6 hours. Parenteral dosage should should not exceed 15 mg/24 hours in ambulatory patients or 30 mg/24 hours in hospitalized patients.

HIGH-POTENCY AGENTS

Haloperidol

Actions and Uses. Haloperidol [Haldol], a member of the *butyrophenone* family, is the prototype of the high-potency neuroleptics. Antipsychotic actions are equivalent to those of chlorpromazine. Principal indications are schizophrenia and acute psychoses. In addition, haloperidol is a preferred drug for Tourette's syndrome.

Pharmacokinetics. Haloperidol may be administered orally and by IM injection. Oral bioavailability is about 60%. Hepatic metabolism is extensive. Parent drug and metabolites are excreted in the urine.

Adverse Effects. As indicated in Table 24–1, *early extrapyramidal reactions* (dystonia, parkinsonism, akathisia) occur *frequently*, whereas *sedation, hypotension,* and *anticholinergic effects* are *uncommon.* Note that the incidence of these reactions is exactly opposite to that seen with chlorpromazine and other low-potency agents. The incidence of *tardive dyskinesia* with haloperidol is the same as with the low-potency drugs. Like chlorpromazine, haloperidol occasionally causes *gynecomastia, galactorrhea,* and *menstrual irregularities.* Neuroleptic malignant syndrome, photosensitivity, convulsions, and impotence are rare.

Preparations, Dosage, and Administration. Haloperidol [Haldol] is dispensed in tablets (0.5, 1, 2, 5, 10, and 20 mg) and in a liquid concentrate (2 mg/ml) for oral use. Two injectable forms—*haloperidol lactate* and *haloperidol decanoate*—are available for parenteral (IM) administration. Haloperidol *lactate* is employed for *acute* therapy. Haloperidol *decanoate* is a depot preparation employed for *long-term* treatment.

Oral Therapy. The initial dosage for adults is 0.5 to 2 mg taken 2 or 3 times a day. For severe illness, daily doses of up to 100 mg may be needed. Once symptoms have been controlled, the dosage should be reduced to the lowest effective amount.

Intramuscular Therapy. For acute therapy of severe psychosis, haloperidol lactate is administered IM in doses of 2 to 5 mg. Dosing may be repeated at intervals of 30 minutes to 8 hours. Once symptoms are under control, treatment should be changed to oral therapy. Long-term therapy with haloperidol decanoate is discussed later in the chapter under *Depot Preparations.*

Other High-Potency Agents

Fluphenazine. Fluphenazine [Prolixin, Permitil] is a high-potency agent indicated for schizophrenia and other psychotic disorders. The drug belongs to the piperazine subclass of phenothiazines. As with other high-potency agents, the most common adverse effects are early extrapyramidal reactions (dystonia, parkinsonism, akathisia). The risk of tardive dyskinesia is the same as with all other traditional antipsychotics. Effects seen occasionally include sedation, orthostatic hypotension, anticholinergic effects, gynecomastia, galactorrhea, and menstrual irregularities. Neuroleptic malignant syndrome, convulsions, and agranulocytosis are rare.

Fluphenazine is administered orally and by IM injection. Oral preparations are tablets (1, 2.5, and 5 mg), elixir (0.5 mg/ml), and a liquid concentrate (5 mg/ml). The liquid concentrate should be diluted with water, fruit juice, or some other suitable liquid—but *not* with beverages that contain caffeine, tannics (tea), or pectinates (apple juice) because of physical incompatibilities. The initial *oral dosage* is 2.5 to 10 mg/day given in divided doses every 6 to 8 hours. Daily dosages greater than 3 mg are rarely needed, although some patients may require as much as 30 mg. Once symptoms have been controlled, the dosage should be reduced to the lowest effective amount, typically 1 to 5 mg/day taken as a single dose.

Three injectable preparations are available: *fluphenazine* (2.5 mg/ml), *fluphenazine decanoate* (25 mg/ml), and *fluphenazine enanthate* (25 mg/ml). Fluphenazine itself is used for acute therapy. Fluphenazine enanthate and fluphenazine decanoate are depot preparations used for long-term therapy (see below). *Intramuscular dosages* for acute therapy are usually one-third to one-half the oral dosage.

Trifluoperazine. Trifluoperazine [Stelazine] is a high-potency agent used for schizophrenia and other psychotic disorders. The drug belongs to the piperazine subclass of phenothiazines. The most common adverse effects are early extrapyramidal reactions (dystonia, parkinsonism, akathisia). Effects seen occasionally include sedation, orthostatic hypotension, anticholinergic effects, gynecomastia, galactorrhea, menstrual irregularities, and tardive dyskinesia. Neuroleptic malignant syndrome, convulsions, and agranulocytosis are rare.

Trifluoperazine is administered orally and by deep IM injection. Three formulations are available: tablets (1, 2, 5, and 10 mg), liquid concentrate (10 mg/ml), and injection (2 mg/ml). *Oral dosing* is begun at 2 to 5 mg twice daily. Dosage is then increased until an optimal response has been produced, usually with 15 to 20 mg/day. Intramuscular therapy is employed acutely. The usual *intramuscular dosage* is 1 to 2 mg every 4 to 6 hours as needed.

Thiothixene. Thiothixene [Navane] is a high-potency agent approved for schizophrenia and other psychotic disorders. The most common adverse effects are early extrapyramidal reactions (dystonia, parkinsonism, akathisia) and anticholinergic responses. Side effects seen occasionally include galactorrhea, gynecomastia, menstrual irregularities, sedation, orthostatic hypotension, and tardive dyskinesia. Agranulocytosis, neuroleptic malignant syndrome, and convulsions are rare.

Thiothixene is administered orally and by IM injection. Three formulations are available: capsules (1, 2, 5, 10, and 20 mg), liquid concentrate (5 mg/ml), and IM solution (2 and 5 mg/ml). The initial *oral dosage* is 2 mg 3 times daily. Dosage is increased until an optimal response has been achieved, usually with 20 to 30 mg/day. The initial *intramuscular dosage* is 4 mg 2 to 4 times daily. Dosage is increased until symptoms are controlled, but should not exceed 30 mg/day.

Pimozide. Pimozide [Orap] is a high-potency neuroleptic used only for suppressing symptoms of *Tourette's syndrome*, a rare disorder characterized by severe motor tics and uncontrollable grunts, barking cries, and outbursts of obscene language. Like other neuroleptics, pimozide can cause sedation, postural hypotension, and extrapyramidal reactions (dystonia, parkinsonism, akathisia, tardive dyskinesia). The drug is available in 2-mg tablets for oral therapy. The initial dosage is 1 to 2 mg/day in divided doses. Dosage should be slowly increased to a maintenance amount of 10 mg/day or 0.2 mg/kg/day (whichever is less).

DEPOT PREPARATIONS

The depot antipsychotics are long-acting, injectable preparations used to treat patients with chronic schizophrenia. The objective is to prevent relapse and maintain the highest possible level of functioning. The rate of relapse is lower with depot therapy than with oral therapy. Depot preparations are valuable for all patients who need long-term treatment—not just for those who have difficulty with compliance. There is no evidence that depot preparations pose an increased risk of side effects, including neuroleptic malignant syndrome.

Three depot preparations are available: *haloperidol decanoate, fluphenazine decanoate, and fluphenazine enanthate.* Following IM or SC injection, active drug (fluphenazine or haloperidol) is slowly absorbed into the blood. Because of this slow, steady absorption, plasma drug levels remain relatively constant between injections. The dosing interval is 2 to 4 weeks. Typical maintenance dosages are presented in Table 24–4.

ATYPICAL ANTIPSYCHOTIC AGENTS

Atypical antipsychotic agents differ from traditional agents in that they cause few or no extrapyramidal symptoms, including tardive dyskinesia. In fact, tardive dyskinesia may actually remit when patients are switched from a traditional antipsychotic drug to an atypical one. At this time, clozapine is the only atypical antipsychotic drug available in the United States. Several others are in clinical trials.

CLOZAPINE

Clozapine [Clozaril] is a relatively new antipsychotic drug indicated for patients with schizophrenia who have not responded to traditional agents, or who cannot tolerate their extrapyramidal effects. The drug's major adverse effect is agranulocytosis; a few deaths have occurred despite weekly hematologic monitoring.

Mechanism of Action

Like traditional antipsychotic agents, clozapine blocks receptors for dopamine. However, the pattern of blockade is unique: compared with traditional agents, clozapine produces relatively high blockade of dopamine$_1$ receptors and relatively low blockade of dopamine$_2$ receptors. This pattern of receptor blockade may explain the drug's relative lack of extrapyramidal effects, and may also underlie its therapeutic effects. In addition to blocking receptors for dopamine, clozapine blocks receptors for serotonin, norepinephrine (alpha$_1$), histamine, and acetylcholine.

Table 24–4. Depot Antipsychotic Preparations		
Generic Name [Trade Name]	**Route**	**Typical Maintenance Dosage**
Haloperidol decanoate [Haldol Decanoate]	IM	50 to 200 mg every 4 weeks
Fluphenazine decanoate [Prolixin Decanoate]	IM, SC	2.5 to 25 mg every 2 weeks
Fluphenazine enanthate [Prolixin Enanthate]	IM, SC	2.5 to 25 mg every 2 weeks

Therapeutic Use

Because of the risk of fatal agranulocytosis, clozapine should be reserved for patients with severe schizophrenia who have not responded to traditional antipsychotic drugs. In this treatment-resistant group, clozapine has had a 40% to 60% success rate. Furthermore, not only have patients responded, the quality of the response is often superior to that seen with traditional drugs: patients are more animated, behavior is more socially acceptable, and rates of rehospitalization are lower. Because the incidence of extrapyramidal effects with clozapine is low, the drug is well suited for patients who have experienced severe extrapyramidal symptoms with a traditional antipsychotic drug.

Pharmacokinetics

Clozapine is rapidly absorbed following oral administration. Peak plasma levels develop in 3.2 hours. In the blood, about 95% of the drug is bound to plasma proteins. Clozapine undergoes extensive metabolism followed by excretion in the urine and feces. The drug's half-life is approximately 12 hours.

Adverse Effects and Interactions

In contrast to traditional antipsychotics, clozapine carries a low risk of extrapyramidal effects. Tardive dyskinesia has not been reported. In fact, tardive dyskinesia may improve when patients switch to clozapine from a traditional agent. Neuroendocrine effects (galactorrhea, gynecomastia, amenorrhea) and interference with sexual function are minimal.

Agranulocytosis. Clozapine produces agranulocytosis in 1% to 2% of patients. The overall risk of death is about 1 in 5000, the usual cause being gram-negative septicemia. Agranulocytosis typically occurs during the first 6 months of treatment, and the onset is usually gradual. Why agranulocytosis occurs in not known.

Because of the risk of fatal agranulocytosis, *weekly* hematologic monitoring is mandatory. If the total white blood cell (WBC) count falls below 3000/mm³ or if the granulocyte count falls below 1500/mm³, treatment should be interrupted. When subsequent *daily* monitoring indicates that counts

have risen above these values, clozapine can be resumed. If the total WBC count falls below 2000/mm³ or if the granulocyte count falls below 1000/mm³, clozapine should be permanently discontinued. Blood counts should be monitored for 4 weeks after drug withdrawal.

Patients should be informed about the risk of agranulocytosis and told that clozapine will not be dispensed if the weekly blood test has not been made. Also, patients should be informed about early signs of infection (fever, sore throat, fatigue, mucous membrane ulceration) and instructed to report these immediately.

Seizures. Generalized tonic-clonic convulsions occur in 3% of patients. The risk of seizures is dose related. Patients should be warned not to drive or to participate in other potentially hazardous activities.

Other Adverse Effects. The most common side effects are *drowsiness and sedation* (40%), *dizziness* (20%), *hypersalivation* (30%), *tachycardia* (25%), and *constipation* (14%). Additional effects include *postural hypotension* (9%) and *elevation of body temperature* (5%).

Drug Interactions. Because of its ability to cause agranulocytosis, clozapine is contraindicated for patients taking other drugs that can suppress bone marrow function (e.g., many anticancer drugs).

Preparations, Dosage, and Administration

Clozapine [Clozaril] is dispensed in tablets (25 and 100 mg) for oral administration. To minimize side effects, treatment should begin with a 12.5-mg dose, followed by 25 mg once or twice daily. Dosage is then increased by 25 mg/day until it reaches 300 to 450 mg/day. Further increases can be made once or twice weekly, in increments no larger than 100 mg. The usual maintenance dosage is 300 to 600 mg/day in 3 divided doses. The maximum dosage is 900 mg/day. If therapy is interrupted, it should resume with a 12.5-mg dose and then follow the original build-up guidelines.

INVESTIGATIONAL AGENTS

Remoxipride. Remoxipride [Roxiam] produces weak but selective blockade of dopamine₂ receptors. This action may underlie the drug's antipsychotic effects. In patients with chronic schizophrenia, remoxipride is as effective as haloperidol. The drug improves positive symptoms (e.g., thought disturbances, hostility, hallucinations, delusions) as well as negative symptoms (e.g., social withdrawal, blunted affect, motor retardation). Administration is oral and absorption is essentially complete. Following partial hepatic metabolism, parent drug and metabolites are excreted in the urine. Like clozapine, remoxipride causes fewer extrapyramidal symptoms than traditional antipsychotic drugs. There have been no reports of tardive dyskinesia. Postural hypotension is minimal and sedation is less than with haloperidol. An initial therapeutic response occurs at a dosage of 300 to 450 mg/day. Dosage can be reduced to 150 to 300 mg/day for maintenance therapy.

Sulpiride. Like remoxipride, sulpiride causes selective blockade of dopamine₂ receptors. Antipsychotic effects are equivalent to those of chlorpromazine and haloperidol. Extrapyramidal reactions are less common and less severe than with traditional antipsychotics. The incidence of sedation, orthostatic hypotension, and anticholinergic effects is low, but neuroendocrine effects (galactorrhea, gynecomastia, menstrual irregularities) occur frequently.

Risperidone. This drug blocks dopamine₂ receptors and serotonin₂ receptors. Antipsychotic effects are equivalent to those of haloperidol and may have a more rapid onset. Both positive and negative symptoms are improved. Like other atypical antipsychotics, risperidone causes fewer extrapyramidal symptoms than the traditional agents.

SCHIZOPHRENIA AND ITS MANAGEMENT

CLINICAL PRESENTATION

Schizophrenia is a chronic psychotic illness characterized by thought disorders and a reduced ability to comprehend reality. Symptoms usually emerge during adolescence or early adulthood. In the United States, the incidence of schizophrenia is 1% to 3%.

Acute Episodes. During an acute psychotic episode, delusions (fixed false beliefs) and hallucinations are frequently prominent. Delusions are typically religious, grandiose, or persecutory. Auditory hallucinations, which are more common than visual hallucinations, may consist of voices arguing or commenting on one's behavior. The patient may feel that he or she is under the control of external influences. Disordered thinking and loose association may render rational conversation impossible. Affect may be blunted or labile. Misperception of reality may result in hostility and uncooperativeness. Impaired self-care skills may leave the patients disheveled and dirty. Patterns of sleeping and eating are usually disrupted.

Residual Symptoms. After florid symptoms (e.g., hallucinations, delusions) of an acute episode remit, less vivid symptoms may remain. These include suspiciousness; poor anxiety management; and diminished judgement, insight, motivation, and capacity for self-care. As a result, patients frequently find it difficult to establish close relationships, maintain employment, and function independently in society. Suspiciousness and poor anxiety management contribute to social with-

drawal. An inability to appreciate the need for continued drug therapy may cause noncompliance, resulting in relapse and, possibly, hospital readmission.

Long-term Course. The long-term course of schizophrenia is characterized by episodic acute exacerbations separated by intervals of partial remission. As the years pass, some patients experience progressive decline in mental status and social functioning, whereas others may stabilize. Maintenance therapy with antipsychotic drugs reduces the risk of acute relapse, but may not prevent long-term deterioration.

Positive versus Negative Symptoms. The symptoms of schizophrenia can be divided into two major groups: *positive symptoms* and *negative symptoms*. Positive symptoms can be viewed as an exaggeration or distortion of normal function, whereas negative symptoms can be viewed as a loss or diminution of normal function. Positive symptoms include hallucinations, delusions, agitation, tension, and paranoia. Negative symptoms include lack of motivation, poverty of speech, blunted affect, poor self-care, and social withdrawal. In general, antipsychotic drugs have a greater impact on positive symptoms than on negative symptoms.

ETIOLOGY

Although there is strong evidence that schizophrenia has a genetic component, the specific etiology of the disease is unknown. Possible primary defects include (1) excessive activation of CNS receptors for dopamine, and (2) insufficient activation of CNS receptors for glutamate. Although psychosocial stressors can precipitate acute exacerbations in susceptible patients, these stressors are not considered causative.

NONDRUG THERAPY

Although drugs can be of great benefit in schizophrenia, it is important to appreciate that medication alone does not constitute optimal treatment. The acutely ill patient needs care, support, and protection; a period of hospitalization may be essential. Counseling can offer the patient and family insight into the nature of schizophrenia and can facilitate adjustment and rehabilitation. Although traditional psychotherapy is of little value in schizophrenia, establishing a good therapeutic relationship can promote compliance and can help the clinician acquire information on the patient's status that is needed to make adjustments in dosage. Behavioral therapy can help reduce stress. Vocational training in a sheltered environment offers the hope of productivity and some measure of independence. Ideally, the patient will be provided with a comprehensive therapeutic program to complement the benefits of medication. Unfortunately, ideal situations don't always exist, leaving many patients to rely on drugs as their sole treatment modality.

DRUG THERAPY

Drug therapy of schizophrenia has three major objectives: (1) suppression of acute episodes, (2) prevention of acute exacerbations, and (3) maintenance of the highest possible level of functioning.

Drug Selection

Treatment is usually initiated with one of the traditional antipsychotic agents. Although all of the traditional agents produce equivalent therapeutic effects, some patients may respond better to one agent than to another. Accordingly, if treatment with one traditional agent is unsuccessful, a trial with a drug from a different chemical class should be made.

Selection among the traditional antipsychotic drugs is based largely on side effects: the patient should not be given a drug that, because of its side-effect profile, is especially likely to cause discomfort, inconvenience, or harm. For example, certain patients (e.g., those with prostatism or glaucoma) are especially sensitive to anticholinergic drugs. Accordingly, these patients should not be treated with low-potency neuroleptics. By similar logic, if the patient has a history of extrapyramidal reactions, high-potency agents should be avoided. By properly matching patients and drugs, side effects can be minimized, comfort can be maximized, and compliance can be promoted. Table 24–5 indicates the neuroleptics that should be avoided in specific groups of patients.

In the United States, *clozapine* is currently the only alternative to the traditional antipsychotic agents. If trials with at least two of the traditional agents have been unsuccessful, therapy with clozapine should be considered. Clozapine is also indicated for patients who have experienced severe extrapyramidal reactions to traditional agents. Since clozapine can cause fatal agranulocytosis, it is not considered a drug of first choice. However, as other atypical agents become available, these may well replace the traditional agents as preferred drugs for initial therapy.

Dosing

Dosing with neuroleptics is highly individualized. Unresponsive patients may need doses 10 to 20 times greater than those employed for highly responsive patients. Elderly patients require rela-

Table 24–5. Neuroleptics that Should be Avoided in the Presence of Certain Predisposing Factors

Predisposing Factor	Neuroleptic Agents to Avoid
Glaucoma, prostatism, adynamic ileus, urinary hesitancy	Low-potency agents (anticholinergic actions can exacerbate these disorders)
Use of anticholinergic drugs (e.g., tricyclic antidepressants)	Low-potency agents (anticholinergic effects will intensify muscarinic blockade)
Old age	Low-potency agents (the elderly are especially sensitive to the anticholinergic and sedative effects of these drugs)
Active life-style	Low-potency agents (sedative effects can interfere with function)
Delirium	Low-potency agents (anticholinergic action can exacerbate delirium)
Cardiovascular disorders	Low-potency agents (anticholinergic and hypotensive actions can exacerbate these disorders)
History of extrapyramidal reactions	High-potency agents (disruption of extrapyramidal function is greatest with these drugs)
Active sex life in males	Thioridazine (this agent inhibits ejaculation)

tively small doses—typically 30% to 50% of those taken by younger patients.

Dosage size and timing are likely to change over the course of therapy. During the early phase of treatment, antipsychotics should be administered in divided daily doses. Once an effective dosage has been determined, the entire daily dose may be given at bedtime. Since antipsychotics cause sedation, this practice can promote sleep and decrease drowsiness during the day. During long-term therapy, the dosage should be gradually reduced to the lowest effective amount.

Routes

Oral. Oral administration is preferred for most patients. Antipsychotics are available in tablets, capsules, and liquids for oral use.

The liquid formulations require special handling. These preparations are concentrated and must be diluted prior to use. Dilution may be performed with a variety of fluids, including fruit juices, milk, and carbonated beverages. The oral liquids are light sensitive and must be stored in amber or opaque containers. Liquid formulations of *phenothiazines* can cause contact dermatitis; nurses and patients should take care to avoid skin contact with these preparations.

Intramuscular. Intramuscular injection is generally reserved for patients with severe, acute schizophrenia and for long-term maintenance therapy. Depot preparations are given every 2 to 4 weeks (see Table 24–4).

Initial Therapy

With adequate dosing, symptoms begin to resolve within 1 to 2 days. However, the full therapeutic response develops gradually—over 6 to 8 weeks.

Some symptoms resolve sooner than others. During the first week, the goal is to reduce agitation, hostility, anxiety, and tension, and to normalize sleeping and eating patterns. Over the next 6 to 8 weeks, symptoms should continue to steadily improve. The goals over this interval are increased socialization, improved self-care and mood, and improved formal thought processes. Of the patients who have not responded within 6 weeks, 50% are likely to respond by the end of 12 weeks.

It is important to note that not all symptoms respond equally. As discussed above, positive symptoms generally respond better than negative symptoms.

Maintenance Therapy

Schizophrenia is usually chronic, requiring prolonged treatment. The purpose of long-term therapy is to reduce the recurrence of acute florid episodes and to maintain the highest possible level of functioning. Unfortunately, although long-term treatment can be very effective, it also carries a risk of adverse effects, especially tardive dyskinesia.

Following control of an acute episode, antipsychotic therapy should continue for at least 12 months. Withdrawal of medication prior to this time is associated with a 55% incidence of relapse, compared to only 20% in patients who continue drug use. Accordingly, patients must be convinced to continue therapy for the entire 12-month course, even though they may be symptom free and consider themselves "cured."

After 12 months, an attempt should be made to discontinue drug use, provided that symptoms are absent. About 25% of patients will not need drugs beyond this time. To avoid adverse reactions to drug withdrawal, dosage should be reduced gradually. It is important that medication not be withdrawn at a time of stress (e.g., when the patient is being discharged following hospitalization). If relapse occurs in response to withdrawal, treatment should be reinstituted. For many patients, resumption controls symptoms and prevents further relapse.

When long-term therapy is conducted, dosage should be adjusted with care. To reduce the risk of tardive dyskinesia and other adverse effects, a minimum effective dosage should be established. Annual attempts should be made to lower the dosage or to discontinue treatment entirely.

Long-acting (depot) antipsychotics are especially well suited for long-term therapy. Depot therapy has two major advantages over oral therapy: (1) the relapse rate is lower with depot therapy, and (2) depot therapy maintains steady drug levels between doses. There is no evidence that depot preparations pose an increased risk of side effects, including tardive dyskinesia and neuroleptic malignant syndrome. In the United States, only 10% of patients receive depot therapy. This low rate of use is based in large part on the widely held (but incorrect) perception that depot therapy is for "losers"—patients who suffer recurrent relapse because of persistent noncompliance with oral therapy.

Promoting Compliance

Poor compliance is a common cause of therapeutic failure, and is responsible for a substantial number of hospital re-admissions. Compliance can be difficult to achieve because treatment is prolonged and because patients may fail to appreciate the need for therapy, or they may be unwilling or unable to take medicine as prescribed. In addition, side effects can discourage compliance.

Compliance can be enhanced by:

1. Insuring that the medication given to hospitalized patients is actually swallowed and not "cheeked."
2. Encouraging family members to oversee medication by outpatients.
3. Providing patients with written and verbal instructions on dosage size and timing, and encouraging them to take their medicine exactly as prescribed.
4. Informing patients and their families that antipsychotics must be taken on a regular schedule to be effective and, hence, cannot be used on a PRN basis.
5. Informing patients about side effects of treatment and teaching them how to minimize undesired responses.
6. Assuring patients that antipsychotic drugs do not cause addiction.
7. Establishing a good therapeutic relationship with the patient and his or her family.
8. Using a depot preparation (e.g., fluphenazine decanoate, haloperidol decanoate) for long-term therapy.

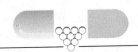

Summary of Major Nursing Implications

TRADITIONAL ANTIPSYCHOTIC AGENTS: CHLORPROMAZINE, HALOPERIDOL, AND ALL OTHERS

Except where indicated otherwise, the nursing implications summarized here apply to all of the traditional antipsychotic drugs.

Preadministration Assessment

Therapeutic Goal

Treatment of schizophrenia has three goals: suppression of acute episodes, prevention of acute exacerbations, and maintenance of the highest possible level of functioning.

Baseline Data

Patients should receive a thorough mental status examination and a physical examination.

Observe and record such factors as overt behavior (e.g., gait, pacing, restlessness, volatile outbursts), emotional state (e.g., depression, agitation, mania), intellectual function (e.g., stream of thought, coherence, hallucinations, delusions), and responsiveness to the environment.

Obtain a complete family and social history.

Determine vital signs and obtain complete blood counts, electrolytes, and evaluations of hepatic, renal, and cardiovascular function.

Identifying High-Risk Patients

Traditional antipsychotic agents are *contraindicated* for patients who are *comatose* or *severely depressed* and for patients with *Parkinson's disease, prolactin-dependent carcinoma of the breast, bone marrow depression*, and *severe hypotension or hypertension*. Use with *caution* in patients with *glaucoma, adynamic ileus, prostatic hypertrophy, cardiovascular disease, hepatic or renal dysfunction*, and *seizure disorders*.

Implementation: Administration

Routes

Oral, IM, SC, rectal (suppository). Routes for individual agents are summarized in Tables 24–2 and 24–4.

Administration

Dosing. Divided daily doses are employed initially. Once an effective dosage has been determined, the entire daily dose is usually administered at bedtime, thereby promoting sleep and minimizing daytime sedation. For long-term therapy, the smallest effective dosage should be employed.

Oral Liquids. Oral liquid formulations must be protected from light. Concentrated formulations should be diluted just prior to use. Dilution in fruit juice improves palatability.

Oral liquids can cause *contact dermatitis*. Warn patients against making skin contact with these drugs, and instruct them to flush the affected area if a spill occurs. Take care to avoid skin contact with these preparations yourself.

Intramuscular. Make injections into the deltoid or gluteal muscle. Rotate the injection site. Depot preparations are administered every 2 to 4 weeks (see Table 24–4).

✓ Implementation: Measures to Enhance Therapeutic Effects

Promoting Compliance

Poor compliance is a common cause of therapeutic failure and rehospitalization. Compliance can be improved by:

1. Insuring that medication is actually swallowed and not "cheeked."
2. Encouraging family members to oversee medication by outpatients
3. Providing patients with written and verbal instructions on dosage size and timing, and encouraging them to take their medicine as prescribed.
4. Informing patients and their families that antipsychotic drugs must be taken on a regular schedule to be effective and, hence, cannot be used on a PRN basis.
5. Informing patients about side effects of treatment and teaching them how to minimize undesired responses.
6. Assuring patients that neuroleptics do not cause addiction.
7. Establishing a good therapeutic relationship with the patient and his or her family.
8. Using a depot preparation (e.g., fluphenazine decanoate, haloperidol decanoate) for long-term therapy.

Nondrug Therapy

Acutely ill patients need care, support, and protection; hospitalization may be essential. Educate patients and their families about the nature of schizophrenia to facilitate adjustment and rehabilitation. Behavioral therapy can help reduce stress. Vocational training in a sheltered environment offers the hope of productivity and some measure of independence.

✓ Ongoing Evaluation and Interventions

Evaluating Therapeutic Effects

Success is indicated by improvement in psychotic symptoms. Evaluate for suppression of hallucinations, delusions, agitation, tension, and hostility, and for improvement in judgment, insight, motivation, affect, self-care, social skills, anxiety management, and patterns of sleeping and eating.

Minimizing Adverse Effects

Early Extrapyramidal Reactions: Acute Dystonia, Parkinsonism, and Akathisia. These reactions develop within days to months of the onset of treatment. The risk is greatest with high-potency agents. Take care to differentiate these reactions from worsening of psychotic symptoms. Inform patients and their families about symptoms (e.g., muscle spasm of tongue, face, neck, or back; tremor; rigidity; restless movement) and instruct them to notify the physician if these appear. Symptoms can be suppressed with anticholinergic drugs (e.g., benztropine) and other medications (see Table 24–3).

Late Extrapyramidal Reaction: Tardive Dyskinesia. Tardive dyskinesia develops after months or years of continuous therapy. The risk is equal with all neuroleptics. Inform patients and their families about early signs (e.g., fine, worm-like movements of the tongue) and instruct them to notify the physician if these develop. The physician may suggest a dosage reduction, discontinuation of neuroleptic treatment, or a switch to clozapine. Tardive dyskinesia has no satisfactory treatment.

Neuroleptic Malignant Syndrome. NMS is a rare reaction that carries a 4% risk of mortality. Symptoms include rigidity, fever, sweating, dysrhythmias, and fluctuations in blood pressure. NMS is most likely with high-potency agents.

Treatment consists of supportive measures (use of cooling blankets, rehydration), drug therapy (dantrolene, bromocriptine), and immediate withdrawal of the neuroleptic. If neuroleptic therapy is resumed after symptoms have subsided, the lowest effective dosage of a low-potency drug should be employed.

Anticholinergic Effects. Inform patients about possible anticholinergic reactions (dry mouth, blurred vision, photophobia, urinary hesitancy, constipation, tachycardia, suppression of sweating) and teach them how to minimize discomfort. A complete summary of nursing implications for anticholinergic effects is given in Chapter 13. Anticholinergic effects are most likely with the low-potency neuroleptics.

Orthostatic Hypotension. Inform patients about signs of hypotension (lightheadedness, dizziness) and advise them to sit or lie down if these occur. Inform patients that hypotension can be minimized by moving slowly when assuming an erect posture. Orthostatic hypotension is most likely with low-potency neuroleptics.

When medicating the hospitalized patient, measure blood pressure and pulses before drug administration and 1 hour after. Make these measurements while the patient is lying down and again after he or she has been sitting or standing for 1 to 2 minutes. If blood pressure is low, withhold medication and consult the physician.

Sedation. Sedation is most intense during the first weeks of therapy and declines with continued drug use. Warn patients about sedative effects and advise them to avoid hazardous activity until sedation subsides. Sedation is most likely with the low-potency agents.

Seizures. Neuroleptics reduce seizure threshold, thereby increasing the risk of seizures, especially in patients with epilepsy and other seizure disorders. For patients with seizure disorders, adequate doses of antiseizure medication must be employed. Monitor the patient for seizure activity; if loss of seizure control occurs, dosage of antiseizure medication must be increased.

Sexual Dysfunction. In women, antipsychotics can suppress libido and impair the ability to achieve orgasm. In men, these drugs can suppress libido and cause erectile and ejaculatory dysfunction. Counsel patients about possible sexual dysfunction and encourage them to report problems. Dosage reduction or switching to a high-potency neuroleptic may be helpful.

Dermatologic Effects. Inform patients that *phenothiazines* can sensitize the skin to ultraviolet light, thereby increasing the risk of sunburn. Advise them to avoid excessive exposure to sunlight and to apply a sunscreen or wear protective clothing.

Oral liquid formulations of neuroleptics can cause contact dermatitis. Warn patients to avoid skin contact with these drugs.

Neuroendocrine Effects. Inform patients that neuroleptics can cause galactorrhea, gynecomastia, and menstrual irregularities.

Neuroleptics can promote growth of prolactin-dependent carcinoma of the breast and must not be used by patients with this cancer.

Agranulocytosis. Agranulocytosis greatly diminishes the ability to fight infection. Inform patients about early signs of infection (fever, sore throat) and instruct them to notify the physician if these develop. If blood tests indicate agranulocytosis, the neuroleptic should be withdrawn.

Minimizing Adverse Interactions

Anticholinergics. Drugs with anticholinergic properties will intensify anticholinergic responses to neuroleptics. Instruct patients to avoid all drugs with anticholinergic properties, including the antihistamines and certain over-the-counter sleeping aids.

CNS Depressants. Antipsychotics will intensify CNS depression caused by other drugs. Warn patients against use of alcohol and all other drugs with CNS-depressant properties (e.g., barbiturates, opioids, antihistamines, benzodiazepines).

Levodopa. Levodopa promotes activation of dopamine receptors and may thereby diminish the therapeutic effects of neuroleptics. These drugs should not be used concurrently.

CLOZAPINE (AN ATYPICAL ANTIPSYCHOTIC)

Preadministration Assessment

Therapeutic Goal and Baseline Data

See *Traditional Antipsychotic Agents.*

Identifying High-Risk Patients

Clozapine is *contraindicated* for patients with a *history of clozapine-induced agranulocytosis* and for patients with *bone marrow suppression* and for those taking *myelosuppressive drugs* (e.g., many anticancer drugs). Use with *caution* in patients with *seizure disorders.*

Implementation: Administration

Route

Oral.

Dosing

To minimize side effects, dosage must be low initially and then gradually increased. If treatment is interrupted, it should resume at the original low dosage.

Ongoing Evaluation and Interventions

Evaluating Therapeutic Effects

See *Traditional Antipsychotic Agents.*

Minimizing Adverse Effects

In contrast to traditional antipsychotic drugs, clozapine carries a low risk of sexual dysfunction, neuroendocrine effects, and extrapyramidal reactions, including tardive dyskinesia.

Agranulocytosis. Clozapine produces agranulocytosis in 1% to 2% of patients, typically during the first 6 months of treatment. Deaths have occurred, usually from gram-negative septicemia.

Weekly hematologic monitoring is mandatory. If the total white blood cell (WBC) count falls below 3000/mm³ or if the granulocyte count falls below 1500/mm³, treatment should be interrupted. When subsequent *daily* monitoring indicates that cell counts have risen above these values, clozapine can be resumed. If the total WBC count falls below 2000/mm³ or if the granulocyte count falls below 1000/mm³, clozapine should be permanently discontinued. Continue monitoring blood counts for 4 weeks.

Warn patients about the risk of agranulocytosis and inform them that clozapine will not be dispensed without weekly proof of blood counts. Inform patients about early signs of infection (fever, sore throat, fatigue, mucous membrane ulceration) and instruct them to report these immediately.

Seizures and Sedation. Generalized tonic-clonic seizures occur in 3% of patients. Drowsiness and sedation occur in 40%. Warn patients against driving and participation in other potentially hazardous activities.

Minimizing Adverse Interactions

Myelosuppressive Drugs. Clozapine must not be given to patients taking other drugs that can suppress bone marrow function (e.g., many anticancer agents).

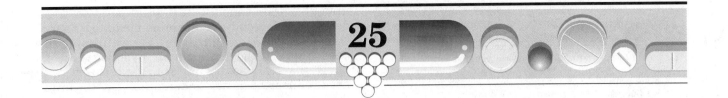

Antidepressants

As their name suggests, antidepressants are drugs used to treat depression. These agents fall into four major groups: (1) tricyclic antidepressants, (2) monoamine oxidase inhibitors, (3) selective serotonin reuptake blockers, and (4) miscellaneous antidepressants. The principal indication for these drugs is major depression. As a rule, antidepressants are not indicated for uncomplicated bereavement. It should be noted that antidepressants are not merely general psychic stimulants. Rather, these drugs act selectively to alleviate symptoms of depression.

MAJOR DEPRESSION: CHARACTERISTICS, PATHOGENESIS, AND TREATMENT MODALITIES

Characteristics

The diagnostic criteria for major depression are summarized in Table 25–1. As indicated, the principal symptoms are (1) *depressed mood* and (2) *loss of pleasure or interest in all or nearly all of one's usual activities and pastimes.* Associated symptoms include insomnia (or sometimes hypersomnia); anorexia and weight loss (or sometimes hyperphagia and weight gain); mental slowing and loss of concentration; feelings of guilt, worthlessness, and helplessness; thoughts of death and suicide; and overt suicidal behavior. For a diagnosis to be made, symptoms must be present most of the day, nearly every day, for at least 2 weeks.

Major depression is a frustrating illness in that symptoms seldom bear correspondence to external

277

Table 25–1. Diagnostic Criteria for Major Depressive Disorder

For a diagnosis of major depression, at least five of the following symptoms must be present for 2 weeks or more, and one of the symptoms must be (1) depressed mood or (2) loss of interest or pleasure:

1. Depressed mood
2. Loss of interest or pleasure in all (or almost all) activities
3. Significant weight loss or weight gain without dieting *or* decrease or increase in appetite
4. Insomnia or hypersomnia
5. Psychomotor agitation or retardation
6. Fatigue or loss of energy
7. Feelings of worthlessness or excessive or inappropriate guilt
8. Diminished ability to think or concentrate *or* indecisiveness
9. Recurrent thoughts of death, recurrent suicidal ideation, or a suicide attempt or a specific suicide plan

Modified from American Psychiatric Association. Diagnostic and Statistical Manual of Mental Disorders, 3rd ed, revised (DSM-III-R). Washington, D.C., American Psychiatric Association, 1987.

events. That is, rather than occurring in response to life's tragedies, symptoms of major depression just descend "out of the blue"; otherwise healthy individuals—unexpectedly and without apparent cause—find themselves feeling profoundly depressed.

It is important to distinguish between major depression and normal grief or sadness. Whereas major depression is an illness, grief or sadness is not. Rather, grief and sadness are appropriate reactions to a major life stressor (e.g., death of a loved one, loss of a job). In most cases, grief and sadness resolve spontaneously over several weeks, and do not require medical intervention. If, however, symptoms are unusually intense, and if they fail to abate within an appropriate time, a major depressive episode may have been superimposed. In these cases, treatment is indicated.

Pathogenesis

The etiology of major depression is undoubtedly complex and not yet known. Since depressive episodes can be triggered by stressful life events in some individuals but not in others, it would appear that, for some individuals, a predisposition to depression exists. Social, developmental, and biologic factors, including genetic heritage, may all contribute to that predisposition.

Clinical observations made in the 1960's led to formulation of the *monoamine hypothesis of depression*, which asserts that depression is caused by a functional insufficiency of monoamine neurotransmitters (norepinephrine, serotonin, or both) in the brain. This hypothesis is based in large part on two observations: (1) depression can be induced with reserpine, a drug that depletes monoamines

from the brain, and (2) the drugs used to treat depression intensify monoamine-mediated neurotransmission. Although these observations do indeed support the monoamine hypothesis, it is likely that this somewhat simplistic theory will need refinement as our understanding of the brain deepens. However, despite its shortcomings, the monoamine hypothesis does provide a useful conceptual framework for understanding the antidepressant drugs.

Treatment Modalities

Depression can be treated with three modalities: (1) drugs, (2) electroconvulsive therapy, and (3) psychotherapy. Each modality has a legitimate role.

Drugs are the primary therapy for major depression. Currently available antidepressants are listed in Table 25–2. For many patients, the *tricyclic antidepressants* are drugs of first choice. These agents are effective, relatively safe, and can be administered with ease. Fluoxetine, a selective serotonin reuptake blocker, is as effective as the tricyclics and better tolerated. As a result, fluoxetine has achieved rapid and widespread popularity. *Monoamine oxidase inhibitors* (MAOIs) are generally reserved for patients who have not responded to tricyclics or to one of the newer antidepressants. However, for patients with atypical depression, MAOIs are drugs of choice. *Antianxiety agents* (e.g., diazepam) can be employed in depression, but their use is not routine. As a rule, CNS stimulants (amphetamines, methylphenidate) are without benefit in depression. As discussed in Chapter 26, patients with *bipolar depression* can be treated prophylactically with *lithium*.

Electroconvulsive therapy (ECT) is a valuable tool for treating depression. This procedure is effective, and beneficial responses develop more rapidly than with drugs. Accordingly, ECT is indicated when speed is critical (i.e., in severely depressed, suicidal patients) or when a patient has failed to respond to antidepressants.

The role of psychotherapy in major depression is largely supportive; symptoms do not respond nearly as well to psychotherapy as they do to medication. However, although of less direct benefit than drugs, psychotherapy can help relieve suffering by providing insight, reassurance, and caring.

TRICYCLIC ANTIDEPRESSANTS

The tricyclic antidepressants are drugs of first choice for many patients with major depression. The first tricyclic agent—imipramine—was introduced to psychiatry in the late 1950's. Since then, the ability of the tricyclics to relieve depressive symptoms has been firmly established. The most

		Table 25-2. Adult Dosages for Antidepressants		
Generic Name	**Trade Name**	**Initial Dose*† (mg/day)**	**Dose After 4–8 weeks* (mg/day)**	**Maximum Dose‡ (mg/day)**
Tricyclic Antidepressants				
Amitriptyline	Elavil, Endep	50–150	100–200	300
Desipramine	Norpramin, Pertofrane	50–150	75–200	300
Doxepin	Adapin, Sinequan	50–150	100–200	300
Imipramine	Tofranil	50–150	100–200	300
Nortriptyline	Aventyl, Pamelor	25–100	75–150	150
Protriptyline	Vivactil	10–40	15–40	60
Trimipramine	Surmontil	50–150	75–250	250
Monoamine Oxidase Inhibitors				
Isocarboxazid	Marplan	20–30	20–30	30
Phenelzine	Nardil	45–75	45–75	75
Tranylcypromine	Parnate	20–30	20–30	30
Selective Serotonin Reuptake Blockers				
Fluoxetine	Prozac	20	20–40	80
Fluvoxamine§	Floxyfral	50–100	50–300	300
Paroxetine	Paxil	20	20–50	50
Sertraline§	Zoloft	50	50–200	200
Trazodone	Desyrel	150	150–200	400
Miscellaneous Antidepressants				
Amoxapine	Asendin	50–150	200–300	400
Bupropion	Wellbutrin	200	300	450
Maprotiline	Ludiomil	50–100	100–150	225

*Doses listed are *total daily doses*. Depending on the drug and the patient, the total dose may be given in a single dose or in divided doses.
†Initial doses are employed for 4–8 weeks, the time required for most symptoms to respond. The smaller dose within the range listed is used initially. Dosage is gradually increased as required.
‡Doses higher than these may be needed for some patients with severe depression.
§Investigational agent.

common adverse effects of the tricyclics are sedation, orthostatic hypotension, and anticholinergic effects. The most hazardous adverse effect is cardiac toxicity. Because all of the tricyclic agents have similar properties, we will discuss these drugs as a group, rather than focusing on a representative prototype.

Chemistry

The structure of imipramine (a representative agent) is shown in Figure 25–1. As can be seen, the nucleus of this drug has three rings—hence the classification *tricyclic* antidepressant.

As can be seen in Figure 25–1, the three-ringed nucleus of the tricyclic antidepressants is very similar to the three-ringed nucleus of the phenothiazine antipsychotics. Because of this structural similarity, the tricyclic antidepressants and the phenothiazines have several actions in common. Specifically, both groups of drugs produce varying degrees of *sedation, orthostatic hypotension,* and *anticholinergic effects.*

Mechanism of Action

The proposed mechanism of action of the tricyclic antidepressants is depicted in Figure 25–2. As

indicated, the tricyclic drugs are blockers of monoamine (norepinephrine and serotonin) reuptake. By blocking reuptake of these neurotransmitters, the tricyclics can intensify their effects. Such a mechanism would be consistent with the monoamine hypothesis of depression. That is, the monoamine hypothesis, which asserts that depression stems from a *deficiency* in monoamine-mediated neurotransmission, would predict that drugs capable of *increasing* the effects· of monoamines would reduce symptoms of depression. This predic-

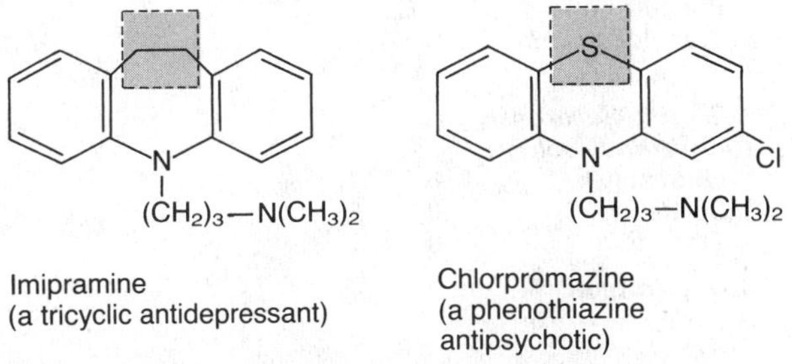

Imipramine (a tricyclic antidepressant)

Chlorpromazine (a phenothiazine antipsychotic)

Figure 25–1. Structural similarities between tricyclic antidepressants and phenothiazine antipsychotics. Except for the areas highlighted, the phenothiazine nucleus is nearly identical to that of the tricyclic antidepressants. Because of their structural similarities, the tricyclic antidepressants and the phenothiazines have several pharmacologic properties in common.

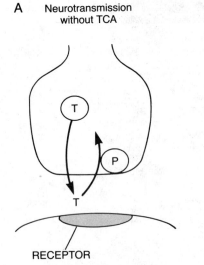

A   Neurotransmission without TCA

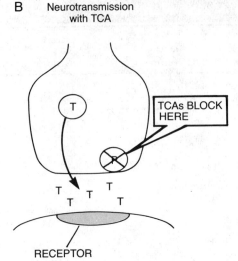

B   Neurotransmission with TCA

TCAs BLOCK HERE

RECEPTOR

Figure 25-2. Mechanism of action of tricyclic antidepressants. *A,* Under drug-free conditions, the actions of norepinephrine and serotonin are terminated by active uptake of these transmitters back into the nerve terminals from which they were released.

B, By inhibiting the uptake pumps for norepinephrine and serotonin, tricyclic antidepressants cause these transmitters to accumulate in the synaptic space, thereby intensifying transmission.

(T = transmitter [norepinephrine or serotonin], P = uptake pump, TCA = tricyclic antidepressant)

tion is fulfilled by the tricyclic drugs. The relative abilities of individual tricyclics to block reuptake of norepinephrine and serotonin are summarized in Table 25–3.

We should note that blockade of reuptake, by itself, cannot fully account for the therapeutic ef-

fects of the tricyclic drugs. This statement is based on the observation that clinical responses to the tricyclics (relief of depressive symptoms) and the biochemical effects of the tricyclics (blockade of transmitter uptake) do not occur in the same time frame. That is, whereas the tricyclic drugs block

Table 25–3. Antidepressants: Adverse Effects and Effects on Neurotransmitters

	Transmitter Reuptake Antagonism		Anti-cholinergic Activity	Sedation	Hypo-tension	Seizure Risk	Cardiac Toxicity	Other Side Effects
	NE	5-HT						
Tricyclic Antidepressants								
Amitriptyline	+ +	+ + + +	+ + + +	+ + + +	+ + +	+ + +	+ + + +	
Desipramine	+ + + +	+	+ +	+ +	+ +	+ +	+ + +	
Doxepin	+ +	+ +	+ + +	+ + + +	+ +	+ + +	+ +	
Imipramine	+ + +	+ + +	+ + +	+ + +	+ + +	+ + +	+ + + +	
Nortriptyline	+ + +	+ +	+ +	+ + +	+	+ +	+ + +	
Protriptyline	+ + + +	+ +	+ + +	+	+ +	+ + +	+ + + +	
Trimipramine	+	+	+ + +	+ + + +	+ + +	+ + +	+ + + +	
Monoamine Oxidase Inhibitors								
Isocarboxazid	a	a	0	+	+ +	0	0	Hypertensive crisis from tyramine in food
Phenelzine	a	a	0	+	+ +	0	0	
Tranylcypromine	a	a	0	b	+ +	0	0	
Selective Serotonin Reuptake Blockers								
Fluoxetine	0	+ + + +	0	b	0	+	0	Skin rash
Sertraline	0	+ + + +	0	b	0	+	0	
Trazodone	0	+ +	0	+ + +	+ + +	+ +	+	Priapism
Miscellaneous Antidepressants								
Amoxapine	+ + +c	+ +c	+ + +	+ +	+	+ + +	+	Parkinsonism
Bupropion	d	d	+ +	b	+	+ + + + +	+	Seizures
Maprotiline	+ + +	+	+ + +	+ + +	+ +	+ + + +	+ + +	Seizures

NE = norepinephrine, 5-HT = serotonin, DA = dopamine
aMAOIs do not block transmitter reuptake. Rather, they increase intraneuronal stores at NE, 5-HT, and DA.
bProduces moderate *stimulation*, not sedation.
cIn addition to blocking NE and 5-HT *reuptake*, amoxapine blocks *receptors* for DA.
dBupropion primarily inhibits reuptake of DA rather than NE or 5-HT.

transmitter uptake within *hours* of administration, relief of depression takes several *weeks* to develop. Hence, it would appear that in the interval between the onset of uptake blockade and the onset of a therapeutic response, intermediary neurochemical events must be taking place. Just what these events might be is not known.

Pharmacokinetics

Tricyclic antidepressants have half-lives that are long and variable. Because their half-lives are long, the tricyclic antidepressants can usually be administered in a single daily dose. Because their half-lives are variable, the tricyclic drugs require individualization of dosage.

Therapeutic Uses

Depression. Tricyclic antidepressants are preferred drugs for treatment of major depression. These medicines can elevate mood, increase activity and alertness, decrease morbid preoccupation, improve appetite, and normalize sleep patterns.

It is important to note that the tricyclic agents, and all other antidepressants, do not relieve symptoms immediately. *Initial* responses take from 1 to 3 weeks to develop. One or 2 months may be needed before a *maximal* response is achieved. Because therapeutic effects are delayed, tricyclic antidepressants cannot be used on a PRN basis. Furthermore, because responses are delayed, a therapeutic trial should not be considered a failure until medication has been administered for at least 1 month without success.

Suicide is always a concern during the treatment of depression, since the patient may be so despondent as to perceive suicide as the only means of relieving his or her suffering. To reduce the chances of suicide, several precautions can be taken. First, since antidepressants take several weeks to alleviate symptoms, the patient presenting with suicidal tendencies should be hospitalized until treatment has had time to produce remission. In addition, since the antidepressants themselves can be vehicles for suicide, the patient should not be given access to a large supply of these drugs. Accordingly, you should insure that each dose is actually swallowed and not "cheeked." This precaution will prevent the patient from accumulating multiple doses that might be taken with suicidal intent.

Manic-Depressive Illness. Manic-depressive illness (bipolar disorder) is characterized by alternating episodes of mania and depression (see Chapter 26). Tricyclic antidepressants can be helpful during the depressive phase of this illness.

Panic Disorder. Panic disorder is characterized by spontaneous panic attacks. Primary associated symptoms are anticipatory anxiety and phobic avoidance (agoraphobia). Tricyclic antidepressants can eliminate panic attacks in about 75% of those treated. The associated symptoms (anticipatory anxiety and phobic avoidance) are not affected.

Adverse Effects

The most common undesired responses to tricyclics are orthostatic hypotension, sedation, and anticholinergic effects. The most serious adverse effect is cardiac toxicity. Adverse effects of individual tricyclics are summarized in Table 25–3.

Orthostatic Hypotension. Orthostatic hypotension is the most serious of the common adverse responses to treatment. Hypotension is due in large part to blockade of alpha$_1$-adrenergic receptors on blood vessels. The patient should be informed that orthostatic hypotension can be minimized by moving slowly when assuming an upright posture. Also, the patient should be instructed to sit or lie down if symptoms of hypotension (dizziness, lightheadedness) occur. For the hospitalized patient, blood pressure and pulse rate should be monitored on a regular schedule (e.g., four times daily). These measurements should be taken while the patient is lying down and again after the patient has been sitting or standing for 1 to 2 minutes. If blood pressure is low, medication should be withheld and the physician notified.

Anticholinergic Effects. The tricyclic antidepressants can block muscarinic-cholinergic receptors, thereby causing an array of anticholinergic effects (dry mouth, blurred vision, photophobia, constipation, urinary hesitancy, and tachycardia). The patient should be informed about possible anticholinergic responses and instructed in ways to minimize discomfort. A detailed discussion of anticholinergic effects and their management is presented in Chapter 13.

Diaphoresis. Despite their anticholinergic properties, tricyclic antidepressants often cause diaphoresis (sweating). The mechanism of this paradoxical effect is unknown.

Sedation. Sedation is a common response to the tricyclic drugs. This response is probably due to blockade of histamine receptors in the central nervous system (CNS). The patient should be advised to avoid hazardous activity if prominent sedation occurs.

Cardiac Toxicity. Tricyclics can adversely affect cardiac function. However, in the absence of overdosage or pre-existing cardiac impairment, serious cardiotoxicity is rare. These drugs affect the heart by (1) decreasing vagal influence on the heart (secondary to muscarinic blockade) and by (2) acting directly on the bundle of His to slow conduction. Both effects increase the risk of dysrhythmias. To minimize adverse cardiac effects, patients over the age of 40 and those with heart disease should undergo electrocardiographic evaluation prior to treatment and periodically thereafter.

Seizures. Tricyclic antidepressants lower seizure threshold. Caution must be exercised in patients with epilepsy and other seizure disorders.

Hypomania. Occasionally, the tricyclics produce too much of a good thing, elevating mood from depression all the way to hypomania (mild mania). If hypomania develops, the patient should be evaluated to determine whether elation is drug induced or symptomatic of manic-depressive illness.

Drug Interactions

Monoamine Oxidase Inhibitors (MAOIs). The combination of a tricyclic antidepressant and an MAOI can lead to *severe hypertension* from excessive adrenergic stimulation of the heart and blood vessels. Excessive adrenergic stimulation occurs because (1) inhibition of MAO causes accumulation of norepinephrine in adrenergic neurons and (2) blockade of norepinephrine reuptake by the tricyclics decreases norepinephrine inactivation. Because of the potential for hypertensive crisis, combined therapy with tricyclic antidepressants and MAOIs is generally avoided.

Direct-Acting Sympathomimetic Drugs. Tricyclic antidepressants *potentiate* responses to direct-acting sympathomimetics (i.e., drugs such as epinephrine and norepinephrine that produce their effects by direct interaction with adrenergic receptors). Stimulation by these drugs is increased because tricyclics block their uptake into adrenergic terminals, thereby prolonging their presence in the synaptic space.

Indirect-Acting Sympathomimetic Drugs. Tricyclic antidepressants *decrease* responses to indirect-acting sympathomimetics (i.e., drugs such as ephedrine and amphetamine that produce their effects by promoting release of transmitter from adrenergic nerves). Effects of indirect-acting sympathomimetics are reduced because tricyclics block uptake of these agents into adrenergic nerves, thereby preventing them from reaching their site of action within the nerve terminal.

Anticholinergic Agents. Since the tricyclic antidepressants exert anticholinergic actions of their own, these drugs will intensify the effects of other medications that exert anticholinergic actions. Consequently, patients receiving tricyclic agents should be advised to avoid all other drugs with anticholinergic properties, including antihistamines and certain over-the-counter sleeping aids.

CNS Depressants. Depression of the CNS caused by the tricyclics will add with that caused by other drugs that have CNS-depressant proper-

ties. Accordingly, the patient should be warned against taking all other CNS depressants, such as alcohol, antihistamines, opioids, and barbiturates.

Toxicity

Overdosage with tricyclic antidepressants is often life threatening. (The lethal dose is only eight times the average daily dose.) To minimize the risk of death by suicide, the acutely depressed patient should be given no more than a 1-week supply of medication at one time.

Clinical Manifestations. Symptoms result primarily from *anticholinergic* and *cardiotoxic* actions. The combination of cholinergic blockade and direct cardiotoxicity can produce *dysrhythmias*, including tachycardia, intraventricular blocks, complete atrioventricular block, ventricular tachycardia, and ventricular fibrillation. Responses to peripheral muscarinic blockade include hyperthermia, flushing, dry mouth, and dilation of the pupils.

CNS symptoms are prominent. Early responses are confusion, agitation, and hallucinations. Seizures and coma may follow.

Treatment. Absorption of ingested drug can be reduced with gastric lavage followed by administration of activated charcoal. Physostigmine (a cholinesterase inhibitor) is given to counteract anticholinergic actions. Propranolol, lidocaine, or phenytoin can be given to control dysrhythmias. Dysrhythmias should not be treated with procainamide or quinidine, because these drugs will aggravate cardiac depression.

Dosage and Routes of Administration

Dosage. Dosages for individual tricyclics are summarized in Table 25–2. General guidelines on dosing are discussed below.

Initial doses of tricyclic antidepressants should be kept *low* (e.g., 50 mg of imipramine/day for the adult outpatient). Low initial doses will minimize adverse reactions and, as a result, will help promote compliance. High initial doses are both undesirable and unnecessary. High initial doses are undesirable in that they pose an increased risk of adverse reactions. High initial doses are unnecessary in that onset of therapeutic effects is delayed, and, therefore, aggressive initial dosing offers no benefit.

Because of interpatient variability in metabolism of tricyclics, dosing is highly individualized. As a rule, dosage is adjusted on the basis of *clinical response*. However, in the absence of a therapeutic response, *plasma drug levels* can be used as a guide for dosage determination. Levels of imipramine, for example, must be above 225 ng/ml for antidepressant effects to occur. If a patient has not responded to imipramine, measurements should be made to insure that plasma drug levels are greater than 225 ng/ml. If drug levels are below this value, the dosage should be increased.

Once an effective dosage has been established, most patients can take their entire daily dose at bedtime, since the long half-lives of the tricyclic antidepressants make divided daily doses unnecessary. Once-daily dosing at bedtime has several advantages: (1) it is simple to perform and, hence, facilitates compliance; (2) it promotes sleep by causing maximal sedation at night; and (3) it reduces the intensity of side effects during the day. Although once-a-day dosing is generally desirable, not all patients can use this schedule. The elderly, for example, can be especially sensitive to the cardiotoxic actions of the tricyclics. As a result, if the entire daily dose were taken at one time, effects on the heart might be intolerable.

Once remission has been produced, therapy should continue for at least 6 months. Failure to take medication for this period is likely to result in relapse. Patients should be encouraged to continue drug therapy even if they are symptom free and feel that further medication is not needed.

Routes of Administration. *All* of the tricyclic agents can be administered by mouth, the usual route for these drugs. Two agents—*amitriptyline* and *imipramine*—may be given by IM injection. Intravenous administration is not used. Since effects take weeks to develop, there would be no advantage to this route.

Preparations and Drug Selection

Preparations. In the United States, seven tricyclic antidepressants are available (see Tables 25–2 and 25–3). When administered in adequate doses, all seven are equally effective at reducing symptoms of depression and panic disorder. Principal differences among these agents concern side effects (see Table 25–3).

Drug Selection. Selection among tricyclic agents is made on the basis of side effects. For example, if the patient has been experiencing insomnia, a drug with prominent sedative properties (e.g., doxepin) might be selected. Conversely, if daytime sedation is undesirable, a weakly sedative agent (e.g., desipramine) might be preferred. Elderly patients with glaucoma or constipation and males with prostatic hypertrophy can be especially sensitive to anticholinergic effects; for these patients, a drug with weak anticholinergic properties (e.g., desipramine) would be appropriate.

MONOAMINE OXIDASE INHIBITORS

The MAO inhibitors (MAOIs) are second- or third-choice antidepressants for most patients. Al-though these drugs are as effective as the tricyclics, they are more dangerous. Of particular concern is the risk of hypertensive crisis in response to ingestion of certain foods. With the advent of newer alternatives to the tricyclic antidepressants, indications for the MAOIs continue to decline.

Only three MAOIs are approved for use in the United States (see Tables 25–2 and 25–3). One of these drugs—isocarboxazid—is essentially obsolete. Hence, only two MAOIs—phenelzine and tranylcypromine—are employed to any significant degree.

Mechanism of Action

Before discussing the MAOIs, we need to discuss MAO itself. MAO is an enzyme present in the liver, the intestinal wall, and the terminals of adrenergic nerves. The function of MAO in nerve terminals is to convert monoamine transmitters (norepinephrine, epinephrine, serotonin) into inactive products. In the liver and intestine, MAO serves to inactivate biogenic amines present in food; in addition, these enzymes inactivate biogenic amines administered as drugs.

Antidepressant effects of the MAOIs appear to result from inhibition of MAO within nerve terminals (Fig. 25–3). By inhibiting intraneuronal MAO, these drugs increase the amount of norepinephrine and serotonin available for release from neurons of the CNS. The intensified transmission that occurs when these transmitters are released in supranormal amounts is thought to be responsible for relief of depression.

The MAOIs can act on MAO in two ways: reversibly and irreversibly. Phenelzine and isocarboxazid produce *irreversible* inhibition. Tranylcypromine produces *reversible* inhibition. Recovery from irreversible inhibition requires synthesis of new enzyme, a somewhat slow process. Hence, the effects of the irreversible inhibitors persist for about 2 weeks after drug withdrawal. Recovery from reversible inhibition is more rapid, occurring in 3 to 5 days.

It should be noted that antidepressant effects of the MAOIs cannot be fully accounted for by MAO inhibition alone. This statement is based on the fact that the biochemical action of these drugs (inhibition of MAO) takes place rapidly, whereas the clinical response (relief of depression) takes weeks to develop. Hence, it would appear that in the interval between initial inhibition of MAO and alleviation of depression, additional neurochemical events must be taking place. It is these as yet unknown events that are ultimately responsible for the beneficial response to treatment.

Therapeutic Uses

Depression. The MAOIs are as effective as the tricyclic agents for relieving depression. However, because their use can be hazardous, MAOIs are generally reserved for patients who have not responded to tricyclics or the newer antidepressants. For one group of patients—those with *atypical depression*—MAOIs are drugs of first choice. As with the tricyclic agents, beneficial effects take a week or more to develop.

Other Uses. MAOIs have been used with some success in the treatment of *bulimia* and other *obsessive-compulsive disorders*. Like the tricyclics, MAOIs can eliminate spontaneous *panic attacks* in patients with panic disorder.

Adverse Effects

CNS Stimulation. Unlike the tricyclic agents, MAOIs cause direct CNS stimulation (in addition to acting as antidepressants). Excessive stimulation can produce anxiety, agitation, hypomania, and even mania.

Orthostatic Hypotension. Despite their ability to increase the norepinephrine content of peripheral sympathetic nerves, the MAOIs *reduce blood pressure* when administered in usual therapeutic doses. The patient should be informed about signs

A   Neurotransmission
without MAO Inhibitors

B   Neurotransmission
with MAO Inhibitors

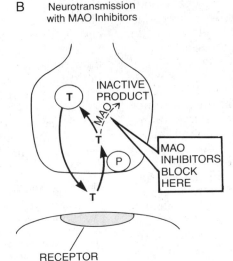

Figure 25–3. Mechanism of action of monoamine oxidase inhibitors. *A,* Under drug-free conditions, much of the norepinephrine or serotonin that undergoes reuptake into nerve terminals becomes inactivated by MAO. This inactivation process helps maintain an appropriate concentration of transmitter within the terminal.

B, MAO inhibitors prevent inactivation of norepinephrine and serotonin, thereby increasing the amount of transmitter available for release. Release of supranormal amounts of transmitter intensifies transmission.

(T = transmitter [norepinephrine or serotonin], P = uptake pump, MAO = monoamine oxidase)

of hypotension (dizziness, lightheadedness) and advised to sit or lie down if these occur. Also, the patient should be informed that hypotension can be minimized by moving slowly when assuming an erect posture. For the hospitalized patient, blood pressure and pulse rate should be monitored on a regular schedule (e.g., four times daily). These measurements should be taken while the patient is lying down and after the patient has been sitting or standing for 1 to 2 minutes.

MAOIs are thought to lower blood pressure through actions exerted in the CNS. The following sequence has been proposed: (1) inhibition of MAO increases the norepinephrine (NE) content of neurons within the vasomotor center of the brain; (2) when NE is released, it binds to postsynaptic alpha receptors on neurons within the vasomotor center, causing a reduction in the firing rate of sympathetic nerves that control vascular tone; and (3) this reduction in sympathetic activity results in vasodilation, causing blood pressure to fall.

Hypertensive Crisis from Dietary Tyramine. Although the MAOIs normally produce *hypotension*, these drugs can be the cause of severe *hypertension* if the patient should ingest foods that contain *tyramine*, a substance that promotes the release of norepinephrine from sympathetic nerves. Hypertensive crisis is characterized by headache, tachycardia, hypertension, nausea, and vomiting.

Before considering the mechanism by which hypertensive crisis is produced, let's consider the effect of tyramine under drug-free conditions. In the absence of MAO inhibition, dietary tyramine does not represent a threat. Much of the tyramine in food is metabolized by MAO in the intestinal wall. Furthermore, as shown in Figure 25–4A, any dietary tyramine that does get absorbed passes directly to the liver via the hepatic portal circulation. Once in the liver, tyramine is immediately inactivated by MAO. Hence, as long as hepatic MAO is functioning, dietary tyramine is prevented from reaching the general circulation and, therefore, is devoid of adverse effects.

In the presence of MAOIs, the picture is very different: dietary tyramine can produce a life-threatening hypertensive crisis. The mechanism of this reaction has three components (Fig. 25–4B). First, inhibition of *neuronal* MAO augments NE levels within the terminals of sympathetic neurons that regulate cardiac function and vascular tone. Second, inhibition of *hepatic* MAO allows dietary tyramine to pass directly through the liver and enter the systemic circulation intact. Third, upon reaching peripheral sympathetic nerves, tyramine stimulates the release of the accumulated NE, thereby causing massive vasoconstriction and excessive stimulation of the heart; hypertensive crisis results.

To reduce the risk of tyramine-induced hypertensive crisis, the following precautions must be taken:

1. MAOIs must not be dispensed to patients considered incapable of rigid adherence to dietary restrictions.
2. Before an MAOI is dispensed, the patient must be fully informed about the hazard of ingesting tyramine-rich foods.
3. The patient must be provided with a list of specific foods and beverages to avoid. These foods—which include most cheeses, yeast extracts, fermented sausages (e.g., salami, pepperoni, bologna), and aged fish or meat—are listed in Table 25–4.
4. The patient should be instructed to avoid all drugs not specifically approved by the physician.

The patient should be informed about the symptoms of hypertensive crisis (headache, tachycardia, palpitations, nausea, vomiting) and instructed to notify the physician immediately if these develop. If the physician is unavailable, the patient should go directly to an emergency room. In the event of hypertensive crisis, blood pressure can be lowered with *phentolamine*, a short-acting alpha-adrenergic antagonist; blood pressure declines because of vasodilation secondary to blockade of alpha₁ receptors on blood vessels.

In addition to tyramine, several other dietary constituents (e.g., caffeine, phenylethylamine) can precipitate hypertension if ingested by patients taking MAOIs. Foods that contain these compounds are listed in Table 25–4. The patient should be instructed to avoid them.

Drug Interactions

The MAOIs can interact with many drugs to cause potentially disastrous results. Accordingly, the patient should be instructed to avoid all medications—prescription agents and over-the-counter drugs—that have not been specifically approved by the physician.

Indirect-Acting Sympathomimetic Agents. Indirect-acting sympathomimetics (e.g., ephedrine, amphetamine) are drugs that promote the release of NE from sympathetic nerves. Use of these agents by patients taking MAOIs can result in *hypertensive crisis.* The mechanism of this interaction is the same as that described for tyramine. The patient should be instructed to avoid all sympathomimetic drugs, including ephedrine, methylphenidate, amphetamines, and cocaine. Sympathomimetic agents may be present in cold remedies, nasal decongestants, and asthma medications; all of these preparations should be avoided unless approved by the physician.

Interactions Secondary to Inhibition of Hepatic MAO. Inhibition of MAO in the liver can decrease the metabolism of several drugs, including epinephrine, norepinephrine, and dopamine. These drugs must be used with caution since their effects will be intensified and prolonged.

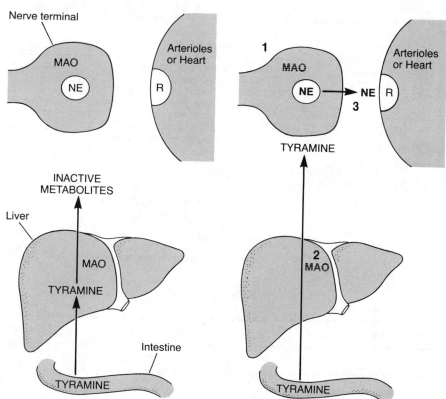

A Influence of Dietary Tyramine in the Absence of MAO Inhibitors

B Influence of Dietary Tyramine in the Presence of MAO Inhibitors

Figure 25–4. Interaction between dietary tyramine and monoamine oxidase inhibitors. *A,* In the absence of MAO inhibitors, dietary tyramine is absorbed from the intestine, transported to the liver, and then immediately inactivated by hepatic MAO. No tyramine reaches the general circulation intact.

B, Three events occur in the presence of MAO inhibitors. (1) Inhibition of *neuronal* MAO elevates levels of norepinephrine (NE) in sympathetic nerve terminals. (2) Inhibition of *hepatic* MAO allows dietary tyramine to pass through the liver and enter the systemic circulation intact. (3) Upon reaching peripheral sympathetic nerve terminals, tyramine promotes the release of accumulated NE stores, thereby causing massive vasoconstriction and excessive stimulation of the heart.

(MAO = monoamine oxidase, R = receptor for norepinephrine)

Tricyclic Antidepressants. The combination of tricyclic antidepressants with MAOIs may produce hypertensive episodes or hypertensive crisis. As a result, this combination is not employed routinely. However, although potentially dangerous, the combination can benefit certain patients. If this combination is employed, caution must be exercised.

Antihypertensive Drugs. Combined use of MAOIs and antihypertensive agents may result in excessive lowering of blood pressure. This response should be no surprise considering that MAOIs, by themselves, can cause hypotension.

Meperidine. Meperidine [Demerol] can cause hyperpyrexia (excessive elevation of temperature) in patients receiving MAOIs. Accordingly, if a strong analgesic is required, an agent other than meperidine should be chosen. Furthermore, the analgesic should be administered in its lowest effective dosage.

Preparations, Dosage, and Administration

MAOIs are dispensed in tablets for oral administration. Dosages are summarized in Table 25–2.

SELECTIVE SEROTONIN REUPTAKE BLOCKERS

In recent years, drugs that produce selective blockade of serotonin reuptake have become available (see Tables 25–2 and 25–3.) These new drugs are as effective as the tricyclic antidepressants and appear to be safer, although possible long-term effects are not yet known. Fluoxetine, the most pop-

ular of these drugs, will serve as our prototype for the group.

FLUOXETINE

Since its introduction a few years ago, fluoxetine [Prozac] has become the most widely prescribed antidepressant in the United States. The drug is as effective as the tricyclic agents, causes fewer side effects, and is less dangerous when taken in overdosage.

Mechanism of Action. Fluoxetine causes selective inhibition of serotonin reuptake. This action is thought to underlie its antidepressant effects. The drug has no effect on dopamine or norepinephrine. In contrast to the tricyclic agents, fluoxetine does not block cholinergic, histaminergic, or alpha-adrenergic receptors. Furthermore, fluoxetine produces CNS excitation rather than sedation.

Therapeutic Uses. Fluoxetine is approved for treatment of *major depression.* Antidepressant effects begin in 1 to 3 weeks and are equivalent to those produced by the tricyclics. The drug has been used on an investigational basis to treat *obsessive-compulsive disorders* and *bulimia* and to *suppress appetite in obese patients.*

Table 25–4. Foods That Can Interact with MAO Inhibitors

Foods That Contain Tyramine

Category	Unsafe Foods (High Tyramine Content)	Safe Foods (Little or No Tyramine)
Vegetables	Avocados, especially if overripe; fermented bean curd; fermented soybean; soybean paste	Most vegetables
Fruits	Figs, especially if overripe; bananas, in large amounts	Most fruits
Meats	Meats that are fermented, smoked, or otherwise aged; spoiled meats; liver, unless *very* fresh	Meats that are known to be fresh (exercise caution in restaurants; meat may not be fresh)
Sausages	Fermented varieties: bologna, pepperoni, salami, others	Nonfermented varieties
Fish	Dried or cured fish; fish that is fermented, smoked, or otherwise aged; spoiled fish	Fish that is known to be fresh; vacuum-packed fish, if eaten promptly or refrigerated only briefly after opening
Milk, milk products	Practically all cheeses	Milk, yogurt, cottage cheese, cream cheese
Foods with yeast	Yeast extract (e.g., Marmite, Bovril)	Baked goods that contain yeast
Beer, wine	Some imported beers; Chianti wine	Major domestic brands of beer; most wines
Other foods	Protein dietary supplements; soups (may contain protein extract); shrimp paste; soy sauce	

Foods That Contain Other Vasopressors

Food	Comments
Chocolate	Contains phenylethylamine, a pressor agent; large amounts can cause a reaction.
Fava beans	Contain dopamine, a pressor agent; reactions are most likely with overripe beans.
Ginseng	Headache, tremulousness, and manic-like reactions have occurred.
Caffeinated beverages	Caffeine is a weak pressor agent; large amounts may cause a reaction.

Pharmacokinetics. Fluoxetine is well absorbed following oral administration, even in the presence of food. The drug is widely distributed throughout the body and is highly bound (94%) to plasma proteins. Fluoxetine undergoes extensive hepatic conversion to norfluoxetine, a metabolite with pharmacologic actions like those of fluoxetine itself. Norfluoxetine is eventually converted to inactive metabolites that are excreted in the urine. The drug has a long half-life (about 7 days). As a result, about 4 weeks are required to produce steady-state plasma drug levels.

Adverse Effects. The most common reactions are *nausea* (21%), *headache* (20%), and manifestations of CNS stimulation, including *nervousness* (15%), *insomnia* (14%), and *anxiety* (10%). Fluoxetine can cause *dizziness* and *fatigue*; patients should be warned against participation in hazardous activities (e.g., driving). *Skin rash*, which can be severe, has occurred in 4% of patients; in most cases, rashes readily respond to drug therapy (antihistamines, glucocorticoids) or to withdrawal of fluoxetine. Other common reactions include *diarrhea* (12%), *excessive sweating* (8%), and *anorexia with associated weight loss* (11%).

In contrast to the tricyclic agents, fluoxetine pro-duces little or no cardiotoxicity, hypotension, or muscarinic blockade.

Overdosage causes nausea, vomiting, and signs of CNS stimulation (agitation, restlessness, hypomania, seizures). Because fluoxetine is not cardiotoxic, overdosage is less dangerous than with the tricyclics.

Drug Interactions. Fluoxetine should not be combined with *monoamine oxidase inhibitors* (MAOIs), since severe adverse effects have been reported. MAOIs should be withdrawn at least 14 days before starting fluoxetine. When fluoxetine is discontinued, at least 5 weeks should elapse before giving an MAOI.

Because fluoxetine is highly bound to plasma proteins, it may displace other highly bound drugs. Displacement of *warfarin* (an anticoagulant) is of particular concern. Monitor responses to warfarin closely.

Fluoxetine can elevate plasma levels of tricyclic antidepressants and lithium (a drug for bipolar depression). Caution should be exercised if these combinations are used.

Preparations, Dosage, and Administration. Fluoxetine [Prozac] is dispensed in solution (20 mg/5 ml) and pulvules (20 mg) for oral administration. The drug may be taken with or without food. The initial dosage recommended by the manufacturer is 20 mg/day. If needed, the dosage may be increased gradually to a maximum of 80 mg/day; however, doses greater than 20 mg/day are likely to increase toxicity more than they increase beneficial effects. If daily doses above 20 mg are used, they should be divided. Elderly patients and patients with impaired liver function should use lower doses.

SERTRALINE

Actions, Adverse Effects, and Drug Interactions. Sertraline [Zoloft] is a new antidepressant similar to fluoxetine. Both drugs produce selective blockade of serotonin reuptake; both relieve symptoms of major depression; both cause CNS stimulation rather than sedation; and both have minimal effects on seizure threshold or the electrocardiogram (EKG). Common side effects include headache, tremor, insomnia, agitation, nervousness, nausea, and diarrhea. Because of the risk of a "serotonin syndrome" (autonomic instability, hyperthermia, rigidity, myoclonus, confusion, delirium, coma), sertraline must not be combined with MAO inhibitors; at least 14 days should separate use of these drugs.

Pharmacokinetics. Sertraline is slowly absorbed following oral administration. Food increases the extent of absorption. Once in the blood, the drug is highly bound (99%) to plasma proteins. Sertraline undergoes extensive hepatic metabolism followed by elimination in the urine and feces. The plasma half-life is approximately 1 day.

Dosage. The initial adult dosage is 50 mg/day administered in the morning or evening. After 4 to 8 weeks, the dosage may be increased by 50-mg increments to a maximum of 200 mg/day.

TRAZODONE

Trazodone [Desyrel] produces selective blockade of serotonin reuptake and may also act directly to stimulate serotonin receptors. Antidepressant effects take several weeks to develop and are equivalent to those of the tricyclic agents.

Common side effects are sedation, orthostatic hypotension, nausea, and vomiting. In contrast to the tricyclic agents, trazodone lacks anticholinergic actions and is not cardiotoxic. Accordingly, trazodone may be preferred for elderly patients and other individuals for whom the cardiac and anticholinergic effects of the tricyclics may be intolerable.

Trazodone can cause *priapism* (prolonged, painful erection of the penis). In some cases, surgical intervention has been required. Priapism itself or the procedures required for relief can result in permanent impotence. Patients should be instructed to notify the physician or to go to an emergency room if persistent erection occurs. (Prolonged clitoral erection has not been reported.)

Overdosage with trazodone is considered safer than overdosage with tricyclic agents or MAO inhibitors. Death from overdosage with trazodone alone has not been reported (although death has occurred following overdosage with trazodone plus other CNS depressants).

Trazodone is dispensed in tablets (50 mg to 300 mg) for oral administration. The initial dosage is 150 mg/day. Dosage may be gradually increased to a maximum of 400 mg/day (for outpatients) and 600 mg/day (for hospitalized patients).

INVESTIGATIONAL AGENTS

Fluvoxamine

Fluvoxamine [Floxyfral], another selective serotonin reuptake blocker, is under investigation for use in major depression and obsessive-compulsive disorder. Clinical trials indicate that the drug is equal to tricyclic antidepressants for relieving symptoms of major depression.

Common side effects include nausea and vomiting (37%), dry mouth (26%), headache (22%), constipation (18%), and insomnia (15%). Some patients have developed abnormal liver function tests. Hence, liver function should be assessed prior to treatment and weekly during the first month of therapy. When fluvoxamine was given to patients taking propranolol (a beta-adrenergic blocking agent), plasma levels of propranolol rose five fold; patients taking beta blockers should be followed closely.

Administration is oral. Absorption is rapid and unaffected by food. Fluvoxamine undergoes extensive hepatic metabolism followed by excretion in the urine. The half-life is 15 hours.

Treatment is initiated with daily doses of 50 to 100 mg for 1 week. Dosage is then gradually increased to a maximum of 300 mg/day. Side effects are minimized by giving the entire daily dose at bedtime.

Paroxetine

Paroxetine [Paxil] is yet another selective inhibitor of serotonin reuptake with marked antidepressant effects. The drug does not block norepinephrine reuptake and has no influence on dopaminergic or cholinergic transmission.

Paroxetine is well absorbed following oral administration, even in the presence of food. The drug is widely distributed throughout the body and is highly bound (95%) to plasma proteins. Concentrations in breast milk equal those in plasma. The drug undergoes hepatic metabolism followed by renal excretion.

Side effects are dose dependent and generally mild. Early reactions include nausea, somnolence, sweating, tremor, and fatigue. These tend to diminish over time. After 5 to 6 weeks, the major complaints are headache and weight gain. Like fluoxetine, paroxetine causes signs of CNS stimulation (increased awakenings, reduced time in REM sleep, insomnia). In contrast to the tricyclic agents, paroxetine has no effect on heart rate, blood pressure, or the EKG.

In clinical trials, dosing has been initiated at 20 mg/day. The daily dose is administered in the morning (to minimize sleep disturbance) and with food (to minimize gastrointestinal upset). Dosage may be increased gradually (every 3 to 4 weeks) to a maximum of 50 mg/day.

MISCELLANEOUS ANTIDEPRESSANTS

AMOXAPINE

Actions, Use, and Dosage. Amoxapine [Asendin], which is similar in structure to the antipsychotic agent loxapine, has both antidepressant and neuroleptic properties. Antidepressant effects are equivalent to those of the tricyclics. Usual dosages range from 200 to 300 mg/day.

Adverse Effects. Amoxapine has relatively weak anticholinergic and sedative properties. Following overdosage, the risk of seizures with this drug is greater than with the tricyclics. Caution should be exercised in patients with epilepsy.

Like loxapine and the other antipsychotics, amoxapine can block receptors for dopamine. As a result, the drug can cause *extrapyramidal side effects* (e.g., parkinsonism, akathisia). Because of the risk of tardive dyskinesia (an extrapyramidal effect that develops with prolonged use of dopamine antagonists), long-term use of amoxapine should be avoided.

BUPROPION

Actions and Use. Bupropion [Wellbutrin] is a unique antidepressant similar in structure to the amphetamines. Like the amphetamines, this agent has stimulant properties and suppresses appetite. Bupropion is devoid of the anticholinergic, antiadrenergic, and cardiotoxic effects associated with the tricyclic agents. Antidepressant effects begin in 1 to 3 weeks and are equivalent to those of amitriptyline (a tricyclic antidepressant). The mechanism by which depression is relieved is unknown.

Adverse Effects. Bupropion is generally well tolerated. The most common adverse effects are weight loss, dry mouth, and dizziness. Other undesired responses include tremor, agitation, and insomnia.

At doses greater than 450 mg/day, bupropion produces *seizures* in about 0.4% of patients. The risk of seizures is greatly increased in patients with predisposing factors, such as head trauma, pre-existing seizure disorder, CNS tumor, and use of other drugs that lower seizure threshold.

Preparations, Dosage, and Administration. Bupropion [Wellbutrin] is dispensed in 75- and 100-mg tablets for oral use. Dosing must be done carefully to minimize the risk of seizures. Dosage escalation must be done slowly. The initial dosage is 100 mg twice a day. After 4 days, the dosage can be increased to 100 mg three times a day. If necessary, the dosage can be increased to a maximum of 150 mg three times a day.

MAPROTILINE

Although maprotiline [Ludiomil] is structurally different from the tricyclic antidepressants (maprotiline has four rings rather than three), this drug is very similar to the tricyclics with respect to therapeutic effects and side effects. The principal difference between these drugs is that maprotiline is more likely to cause *seizures*, even when used in moderate doses; following overdosage, about 30% of patients experience seizures. Because of the risk of seizures, maprotiline should not be taken by patients with a history of seizure disorders. The drug's side effect profile is summarized in Table 25–3. Usual dosages are shown in Table 25–2.

ELECTROCONVULSIVE THERAPY

Although outside the realm of pharmacology, electroconvulsive therapy (ECT) is a valuable treatment for depression and deserves our consideration. Electroconvulsive therapy has two characteristics that are especially desirable: (1) *effectiveness,* and (2) *rapid onset* (relative to antidepressant drugs). Because of these properties, ECT is indicated for two types of patients: (1) those who have failed to respond to pharmacologic treatment for depression, and (2) severely depressed, suicidal patients who need rapid relief of symptoms.

Modern electroconvulsive therapy is much less dramatic and traumatic than ECT was in the past. Improvements in ECT have resulted in large part from the adjunctive use of drugs. Prior to the delivery of electroshock, patients are now treated with a combination of *thiopental* and *succinylcholine*. Thiopental is an injectable, ultrashort-acting anesthetic that prevents conscious awareness of the ECT procedure (without interfering with beneficial actions). Succinylcholine is a short-acting neuromuscular blocking agent that prevents shock-induced convulsive movements—movements that are both hazardous and unnecessary for a therapeutic response.

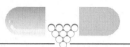 # Summary of Major Nursing Implications

IMPLICATIONS THAT APPLY TO ALL ANTIDEPRESSANT DRUGS

Psychologic Assessment

Observe and record the patient's behavior. Factors to assess include affect, thought content, interest in environment, appetite, sleep patterns, and appearance.

Reducing the Risk of Suicide

Severely depressed patients should be hospitalized until symptoms are under control. To prevent patients from accumulating a potentially lethal supply of medication, insure that each dose is swallowed and not "cheeked." Provide outpatients with no more than a 1-week supply of medication at a time.

Promoting Compliance

Inform the patient that antidepressant effects usually develop slowly, over 1 to 3 weeks. This knowledge will make expectations more realistic, and that realism should help promote compliance.

Premature discontinuation of therapy can result in relapse. Educate patients about the importance of taking their medication as prescribed—despite the fact that they may be symptom free and therefore feel "cured." In general, treatment should continue for 6 months after symptoms have subsided.

Nondrug Therapy

Treatment of depression with drugs alone is not optimal. Emotional support and traditional psychotherapy can complement and reinforce responses to antidepressants.

Evaluating Therapeutic Effects

Assess patients for improvement in symptoms, especially depressed mood and loss of interest or pleasure in usual activities.

TRICYCLIC ANTIDEPRESSANTS

Amitriptyline	Maprotiline
Desipramine	Nortriptyline
Doxepin	Protriptyline
Imipramine	Trimipramine

In addition to the implications summarized below, *see above* for implications that apply to all antidepressants.

Preadministration Assessment

Therapeutic Goal

Alleviation of symptoms of major depression.

Baseline Data

Assess psychologic status. Arrange for an EKG for patients with cardiac disease and for patients over the age of 40.

Identifying High-Risk Patients

All tricyclic antidepressants are generally *contraindicated* for patients taking *MAOIs*.

All tricyclic antidepressants must be used with *caution* in patients with *cardiac disorders* (e.g., coronary heart disease, progressive heart failure, paroxysmal tachycardia), *closed-angle glaucoma, elevated intraocular pressure, history of urinary retention, hyperthyroidism, seizure disorders,* and *liver or kidney dysfunction.*

Doxepin is *contraindicated* for patients with *glaucoma* or a tendency to *urinary retention.*

Maprotiline is *contraindicated* for patients with *seizure disorders.*

 Implementation: Administration

Routes

Oral (usual).
IM (occasional).

Administration

Instruct the patient to take medication daily as prescribed and not on a PRN basis. Warn the patient not to discontinue treatment once mood has improved, since doing so may result in relapse. Once an effective dosage has been established, the entire daily dose can usually be taken at bedtime.

 Ongoing Evaluation and Interventions

Minimizing Adverse Effects

Orthostatic Hypotension. Inform patients about symptoms of hypotension (dizziness, lightheadedness), and advise them to sit or lie down if these occur. Inform patients that hypotension can be minimized by moving slowly when assuming an erect posture. For the hospitalized patient, monitor blood pressure and pulse rate on a regular schedule; take measurements while the patient is lying down and again after the patient has been sitting or standing for 1 to 2 minutes. If blood pressure is low, withhold medication and inform the physician.

Anticholinergic Effects. Forewarn patients about possible anticholinergic effects (dry mouth, blurred vision, photophobia, urinary hesitancy, constipation, tachycardia), and advise them to notify the physician if these are troublesome. A detailed summary of nursing implications for anticholinergic drugs is presented in Chapter 13.

Diaphoresis. Tricyclics promote sweating (despite their anticholinergic properties). Excessive sweating may necessitate frequent changes of bedding and clothing.

Sedation. Sedation is most intense during the first weeks of therapy and declines with continued drug use. Advise the patient to avoid hazardous activities (e.g., driving, operating dangerous machinery) if sedation is significant.

Administration at bedtime will minimize daytime sedation and will promote sleep.

Cardiotoxicity. Tricyclics can disrupt cardiac function, but usually only when taken in excessive doses or by patients with heart disease. Elderly patients and those with heart disease should receive an EKG prior to treatment and periodically thereafter.

Seizures. Tricyclics decrease seizure threshold. Exercise caution in patients with seizure disorders.

Hypomania. Tricyclics may cause mood to shift from depression to hypomania. If hypomania develops, the patient must be evaluated to determine if elation is drug induced or indicative of manic-depressive disorder.

Minimizing Adverse Interactions

MAO Inhibitors. Rarely, the combination of a tricyclic and an MAO inhibitor has produced hypertensive episodes and hypertensive crisis. Exercise caution if this combination is employed.

Sympathomimetic Agents. Tricyclics *decrease* the effects of *indirect-acting* sympathomimetics (e.g., ephedrine, amphetamine), but *potentiate* the actions of *direct-acting* sympathomimetics (e.g., epinephrine, dopamine). If sympathomimetics are to be used, these effects must be accounted for.

Anticholinergic Agents. Drugs capable of blocking muscarinic receptors will enhance the anticholinergic effects of tricyclics. Warn the patient against concurrent use of other anticholinergic drugs (e.g., scopolamine, antihistamines, phenothiazines).

CNS Depressants. CNS depressants will enhance the depressant effects of the tricyclics. Warn the patient against the use of alcohol and all other drugs with CNS-depressant properties (e.g., opioids, antihistamines, barbiturates, benzodiazepines).

MONOAMINE OXIDASE INHIBITORS

Isocarboxazid

Phenelzine

Tranylcypromine

In addition to the implications summarized below, *see above* for implications that apply to all antidepressants.

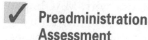 **Preadministration Assessment**

Therapeutic Goal

Alleviation of symptoms of major depression.

Identifying High-Risk Patients

MAOIs are *contraindicated* for patients with *pheochromocytoma, congestive heart failure, liver disease, severe renal impairment, cerebrovascular defect (known or suspected), cardiovascular disease,* and *hypertension* and for patients *over the age of 60* (because of possible cerebral sclerosis associated with vessel damage).

Implementation: Administration

Route

Oral.

Administration

Instruct the patient to take MAOIs every day as prescribed and not on a PRN basis. Warn the patient not to discontinue treatment once mood has improved, since doing so may result in relapse.

Ongoing Evaluation and Interventions

Minimizing Adverse Effects

Hypertensive Crisis. Dietary tyramine, certain other dietary constituents (see Table 25–4), and indirect-acting sympathomimetics (e.g., amphetamine, methylphenidate, ephedrine, cocaine) can precipitate a hypertensive crisis in patients taking MAOIs.

Inform patients about symptoms of hypertensive crisis (headache, palpitations, tachycardia, nausea, vomiting), and instruct them to notify the physician or report to an emergency room if these develop.

To reduce the risk of hypertensive crisis, the following precautions must be observed: (1) MAOIs must not be prescribed for patients who are suicidal or who are considered incapable of rigid adherence to dietary constraints; (2) prior to treatment, forewarn the patient about the hazard of hypertensive crisis and the need to avoid tyramine-rich foods and sympathomimetic drugs; (3) provide the patient with a list of specific foods to be avoided (see Table 25–4); and (4) instruct the patient to avoid all drugs not approved by the physician.

If hypertensive crisis develops, blood pressure can be lowered with *phentolamine*, a short-acting alpha-adrenergic antagonist.

Orthostatic Hypotension. Inform patients about signs of hypotension (dizziness, lightheadedness), and advise them to sit or lie down if these occur. Inform patients that hypotension can be minimized by moving slowly when assuming an erect posture. For the hospitalized patient, monitor blood pressure and pulse rate on a regular schedule. Take these measurements while the patient is lying down and again after the patient has been sitting or standing for 1 to 2 minutes. If blood pressure is low, withhold medication and inform the physician.

Minimizing Adverse Interactions

All Drugs. The MAOIs can interact adversely with many other drugs. Instruct the patient to avoid all medications—prescription and nonprescription—that have not been specifically approved by the physician.

Indirect-Acting Sympathomimetics. Concurrent use with MAOIs can precipitate a hypertensive crisis. Warn the patient against use of any indirect-acting sympathomimetics (e.g., ephedrine, methylphenidate, amphetamines, cocaine).

Tricyclic Antidepressants. Concurrent use with MAOIs can produce hypertensive episodes and hypertensive crisis. Use this combination with caution.

Antihypertensive Drugs. These drugs will potentiate the hypotensive effects of MAOIs. If these agents are combined, monitor blood pressure periodically.

Meperidine. Meperidine can produce hyperthermia in patients taking MAOIs and should be avoided.

FLUOXETINE

In addition to the implications summarized below, *see above* for implications that apply to all antidepressants.

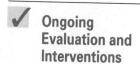
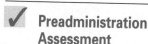
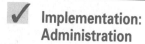

Preadministration Assessment

Therapeutic Goal

Alleviation of symptoms of major depression.

Identifying High-Risk Patients

Use with *caution* in patients with *liver disease, the elderly,* and in *women who are pregnant or breast-feeding.*

Implementation: Administration

Route

Oral.

Administration

Inform the patient that fluoxetine may be taken with meals. If the dosage exceeds 20 mg/day, instruct the patient to take part of the dose in the morning and part later in the day. Warn the patient not to discontinue treatment once mood has improved, since doing so could result in relapse.

Ongoing Evaluation and Interventions

Minimizing Adverse Effects

CNS Stimulation. Fluoxetine can cause nervousness, insomnia, and anxiety. These reactions may respond to a decrease in dosage.

Skin Rash. Inform patients about the risk of skin rash and instruct them to notify the physician if rash develops. Treatment consists of drug therapy (antihistamines, glucocorticoids) or withdrawal of fluoxetine.

Dizziness and Fatigue. Inform patients about possible dizziness and fatigue, and advise them to exercise caution while performing hazardous tasks (e.g., driving).

Minimizing Adverse Interactions

Monoamine Oxidase Inhibitors (MAOIs). Don't combine fluoxetine with MAOIs. Withdraw MAOIs at least 14 days before starting fluoxetine. When fluoxetine is discontinued, wait at least 5 weeks before initiating MAOI therapy.

Warfarin. Fluoxetine may displace warfarin from binding sites on plasma proteins, thereby increasing free levels of the drug. Monitor responses to warfarin carefully.

Tricyclic Depressants and Lithium. Fluoxetine can increase levels of these drugs. Exercise caution.

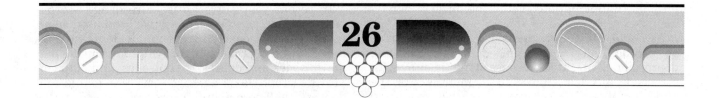

Drugs for Bipolar Disorder

Our topic in this chapter is drug therapy of bipolar disorder, which is also known as manic-depressive illness. The mainstay of therapy is lithium, and discussion will focus largely on this agent.

BIPOLAR DISORDER (MANIC-DEPRESSIVE ILLNESS)

CLINICAL MANIFESTATIONS

Manic-depressive illness is a cyclic disorder characterized by recurrent fluctuations in mood. Typically, patients experience alternating episodes of mania and depression separated by periods in which mood is normal. The characteristics of depressive episodes are described in Chapter 25 and won't be repeated here.

Manic episodes are characterized by heightened mood (euphoria), hyperactivity, excessive enthusiasm, and flight of ideas. Manic individuals display overactivity at work and at play and have a reduced need for sleep. Mania produces excessive sociability and talkativeness. Extreme self-confidence, grandiose ideas, and delusions of importance are common. Manic individuals frequently indulge in high-risk activities (e.g., questionable business deals, reckless driving, gambling, sexual indiscretions), giving no forethought to the consequences. Symptoms in the late stages of a manic episode may resemble those of paranoid schizophrenia (hallucinations, delusions, bizarre behavior).

As noted, most individuals with bipolar disorder go through alternating episodes of mania and depression. Untreated episodes of mania or depression generally last from 4 to 13 months. For the majority (about 70%) of patients, periods of normal mood separate the episodes of mania and depression. As time passes, manic and depressive episodes tend to occur more frequently.

TREATMENT STRATEGY

Nondrug Therapy

Ideally, bipolar disorder should be treated with a combination of drugs and adjunctive psychotherapy (individual, group, or family); drug therapy alone is not optimal. Bipolar disorder is a chronic illness that requires supportive therapy and education for the patient and family. Counseling can help patients cope with the sequelae of manic episodes, such as strained relationships, reduced self-confidence, and a sense of shame regarding uncontrolled behavior. Certain life stresses (e.g., moving, job loss, bereavement, childbirth) can precipitate a mood change; therapy can help reduce the destabilizing impact of these events. Patients should be taught to recognize early symptoms of mood change, and encouraged to contact the physician immediately if these develop.

Drug Therapy

Overview of Treatment. Drug therapy of bipolar disorder is summarized in Table 26–1. As indicated, the mainstay of therapy is *lithium*. Lithium can provide symptomatic control during both the manic phase and the depressed phase. In addition, when taken *prophylactically*, lithium can reduce the frequency and severity of recurrent manic and depressive episodes. When used to control acute mania, lithium is often combined with a *benzodiazepine* (if symptoms are mild) or with an *antipsychotic agent* (if symptoms are severe). When used during the depressive phase, lithium is usually combined with a *tricyclic antidepressant*.

In recent years, two antiseizure drugs—*carbamazepine* and *valproic acid*—have been used on an investigational basis to treat manic-depressive illness. Both drugs can control symptoms during manic episodes and depressive episodes, and both can provide prophylaxis against recurrent mania and depression. These agents represent an alternative to lithium for patients who fail to respond to lithium, or who find its side effects intolerable.

Promoting Compliance. Poor patient compliance can frustrate attempts to treat acute manic episodes. Patients may resist treatment because they fail to see anything wrong with their thinking or behavior. Furthermore, the experience is not necessarily unpleasant. In fact, individuals going through a manic episode may well enjoy it. As a result, in order to insure adequate treatment, hospitalization is often needed. To achieve this, collaboration with the patient's family may be required. Since hospitalization per se won't guarantee compliance, lithium administration should be observed to insure that each dose is actually taken.

After an acute manic episode has been controlled, long-term prophylactic therapy is indicated, making compliance an ongoing concern. To promote compliance, the patient and family should be educated about the nature of manic-depressive illness and the importance of taking medication as prescribed. Family members can help insure compliance by overseeing medication use, and by urging the patient to visit a physician or psychiatric clinic if a pattern of noncompliance develops.

LITHIUM

Lithium can provide symptomatic control in patients with manic-depressive illness. Beneficial effects were first described by John Cade, an Australian, in 1949. However, because of concerns about toxicity, lithium was not approved for use in the United States until 1970. Since lithium has a low therapeutic index, toxicity is a concern. Because significant injury can occur when plasma drug levels are only slightly greater than therapeutic, monitoring lithium levels is mandatory.

Table 26–1. Drug Therapy of Manic-Depressive Illness	
Illness Phase	**Drugs**
Manic phase	
Moderate symptoms	Lithium* + a benzodiazepine
Severe symptoms	Lithium* + an antipsychotic agent
Depressive phase	Lithium + a tricyclic antidepressant
Normalized mood	Lithium (for prophylaxis against recurrence of mania or depression)

*For lithium nonresponders, addition or substitution of carbamazepine or valproic acid may be helpful.

Chemistry

Lithium is a simple inorganic ion that carries a single positive charge. In the periodic table of elements, lithium falls within the same group as potassium and sodium. Accordingly, lithium has properties in common with these two elements. Lithium occurs naturally in animal tissues, but has no known physiologic function.

Pharmacokinetics

Absorption and Distribution. Lithium is well absorbed following oral administration. The drug distributes evenly to all tissues and body fluids.

Excretion. Lithium has a short half-life, owing to rapid renal excretion. Because of its short half-life (and high toxicity), the drug must be administered in divided daily doses; large, single daily doses cannot be used. Because lithium is excreted by the kidneys, it must be used with great care in patients with renal impairment.

Sodium depletion will *decrease* renal excretion of lithium, thereby causing the drug to accumulate. Toxicity may result. Accordingly, it is important that sodium levels remain normal. Patients should be instructed to maintain normal sodium intake; a sodium-free diet cannot be used. Since diuretics promote sodium loss, these agents must be employed with caution. Sodium loss secondary to diarrhea can be sufficient to cause lithium accumulation, and the patient should be forewarned of this possibility.

Plasma Lithium Levels. Measurement of plasma lithium levels is an essential feature of treatment. *Lithium levels must be kept below 1.5 mEq/L; levels greater than this can produce significant toxicity.* For *initial* therapy of a manic episode, lithium levels should range from 0.8 to 1.4 mEq/L. Once the desired therapeutic effect has been achieved, the dosage should be reduced to produce *maintenance* drug levels of 0.4 to 1.0 mEq/L. Blood for lithium determinations should be drawn in the morning, 12 hours after the evening dose.

Therapeutic Uses

Manic-Depressive Illness. Lithium is the drug of choice for controlling manic episodes in patients with manic-depressive illness and for long-term prophylaxis against recurrent mania and depression in these patients.

In manic patients, lithium reduces euphoria, hyperactivity, and other symptoms, but does not cause sedation. Antimanic effects begin 5 to 7 days after the onset of treatment. However, full effects may not be seen until 2 to 3 weeks. For many patients, adjunctive therapy with a benzodiazepine or an antipsychotic agent can be helpful. Benzodiazepines (e.g., diazepam) are used to provide sedation in patients with relatively mild symptoms of mania. Antipsychotics (e.g., haloperidol) may be required to provide rapid control in patients with severe symptoms.

Prophylaxis with lithium may not prevent episodes of depression. If depression occurs, adjunctive therapy with an antidepressant is indicated.

Other Uses. Although approved only for treatment of manic-depressive illness, lithium has been used with varying degrees of success in other psychiatric disorders, including *alcoholism, bulimia, schizophrenia, premenstrual syndrome,* and *glucocorticoid-induced psychosis.* Nonpsychiatric uses include *hyperthyroidism, cluster headache, migraine,* and *syndrome of inappropriate secretion of antidiuretic hormone.* In addition, lithium can *raise neutrophil counts* in children with chronic neutropenia and in patients receiving anticancer drugs or zidovudine (AZT).

Mechanism of Action in Manic-Depressive Illness

We do not know the underlying cause of manic-depressive illness, nor do we know how lithium stabilizes mood. Lithium has multiple effects on the nervous system. The drug can alter the synthesis, storage, release, and reuptake of neurotransmitters (norepinephrine, serotonin, dopamine, acetylcholine, GABA). Also, lithium can alter the distribution of neuronally important ions (calcium, sodium, and magnesium). In addition, lithium can influence the function of second-messenger systems. Which, if any, of these actions underlies lithium's therapeutic effects is unknown.

Adverse Effects

Adverse effects of lithium can be divided into two categories: (1) effects that occur at excessive drug levels, and (2) effects that occur at therapeutic drug levels. Adverse effects produced at excessive lithium levels are considered as a group. Effects produced at therapeutic levels are considered individually.

Adverse Effects That Occur When Lithium Levels are Excessive. Certain toxicities are closely correlated with the concentration of lithium in plasma. As indicated in Table 26–2, mild responses (e.g., fine hand tremor, gastrointestinal upset, thirst, muscle weakness) can develop at lithium levels that are still within the therapeutic range (i.e., below 1.5 mEq/L). When plasma levels exceed 1.5 mEq/L, more serious toxicities begin to appear. At drug levels above 2.5 mEq/L, death has resulted. Patients should be informed about early signs of toxicity and instructed to interrupt lithium use if these appear. The most common cause of lithium accumulation in compliant patients is sodium depletion.

To keep lithium levels within the therapeutic range, plasma drug levels should be monitored routinely. Levels should be measured every 2 to 3 days at the beginning of treatment and every 1 to 3 months during maintenance therapy.

Treatment of acute overdosage is primarily supportive; there is no specific antidote to lithium toxicity. The severely intoxicated patient should be

Table 26–2. Toxicities Associated with Excessive Plasma Levels of Lithium	
Plasma Lithium Level	**Signs of Toxicity**
<1.5 mEq/L	Nausea, vomiting, diarrhea, thirst, polyuria, lethargy, slurred speech, muscle weakness, fine hand tremor
1.5 to 2.0 mEq/L	Persistent GI upset, coarse hand tremor, confusion, hyperirritability of muscles, EKG changes, sedation, incoordination
2.0 to 2.5 mEq/L	Ataxia, giddiness, high output of dilute urine, serious EKG changes, fasciculations, tinnitus, blurred vision, clonic movements, seizures, stupor, severe hypotension, coma, death (usually secondary to pulmonary complications)
>2.5 mEq/L	Symptoms may progress rapidly to generalized convulsions, oliguria, and death

hospitalized. Hemodialysis is an effective means of lithium removal, and it should be considered whenever drug levels exceed 2.5 mEq/L.

Tremor. Patients may develop a fine hand tremor, especially in the fingers, that can interfere with writing and other motor skills. Lithium-induced tremor can be augmented by stress, fatigue, and certain drugs (antidepressants, antipsychotics, caffeine). Tremor can be reduced with a beta-adrenergic blocking agent (e.g., propranolol) and by measures that reduce peak levels of lithium (i.e., dosage reduction, use of divided doses, or use of sustained-release formulations).

Renal Toxicity. Chronic administration of lithium has occasionally been associated with degenerative changes in the kidney. The risk of renal injury can be reduced by keeping the dosage low and, when possible, avoiding long-term lithium therapy. Kidney function should be assessed prior to treatment and once a year thereafter.

Goiter. Long-term use of lithium can cause goiter (enlargement of the thyroid gland). Although usually benign, lithium-induced goiter is sometimes associated with hypothyroidism. Treatment with thyroid hormone or withdrawal of lithium will reverse thyroid hypertrophy. Measurement of thyroid hormones (T_3 and T_4) and thyroid-stimulating hormone (TSH) should be obtained prior to treatment and annually thereafter.

Teratogenesis. Use of lithium during the first trimester of pregnancy is associated with an 11% incidence of birth defects (usually malformations of the heart). Accordingly, *lithium is contraindi-*

cated during the first trimester of pregnancy. Furthermore, unless the benefits of therapy clearly outweigh the potential risk to the fetus, lithium should be avoided during the remainder of pregnancy as well. Women of child-bearing age should be counseled about the importance of avoiding pregnancy while taking lithium.

Use in Lactation. Lithium readily enters breast milk and can achieve concentrations that are potentially harmful to the nursing infant. Consequently, breast-feeding during lithium therapy should be discouraged.

Polyuria. Polyuria occurs in 50% to 70% of patients taking lithium chronically. In some patients, daily urine output may exceed 3 L. Lithium promotes polyuria by antagonizing the effects of antidiuretic hormone. To maintain adequate hydration, patients should be instructed to drink 8 to 12 glasses of fluids daily. Polyuria, nocturia, and excessive thirst can discourage patients from complying with the prescribed regimen.

Lithium-induced polyuria can be *reduced* with a thiazide *diuretic.* The mechanism of this paradoxical effect is not known. Unfortunately, thiazides can increase plasma levels of lithium (perhaps by promoting sodium excretion). Accordingly, a reduction in lithium dosage will be required.

Early Adverse Effects. Several responses occur early in treatment, and then usually subside. *Gastrointestinal effects* (e.g., nausea, diarrhea, abdominal bloating, anorexia) are common but transient. About 30% of patients experience transient *fatigue, muscle weakness, headache, confusion,* and *memory impairment. Polyuria* and *thirst* occur in 30% to 50% of those treated, and, in many cases, these effects persist.

Other Effects. Lithium can cause mild, reversible *leukocytosis* (10,000 to 18,000 WBC/mm³); complete blood counts with a differential should be obtained prior to treatment and annually thereafter. Possible *dermatologic reactions* include psoriasis, acne, folliculitis, and alopecia.

Drug Interactions

Diuretics. Diuretics promote sodium loss, and can thereby increase the risk of lithium toxicity. Toxicity can occur because, in the presence of low sodium, renal excretion of lithium is reduced, causing lithium levels to rise.

Anticholinergic Drugs. Anticholinergic drugs can cause urinary hesitancy. Coupled with lithium-induced polyuria, this effect can result in considerable discomfort. Unfortunately, the combination of lithium plus an anticholinergic drug cannot always be avoided: patients frequently require concurrent therapy with agents that have prominent anticholinergic properties (antipsychotics, tricyclic antidepressants).

Preparations, Dosage, and Administration

Preparations and Administration. Lithium is available as two salts: *lithium carbonate* and *lithium citrate.* With either salt, administration is oral. Lithium *carbonate* is dispensed in capsules, standard tablets, and slow-release tablets. Lith-

Table 26–3. Lithium Preparations

Lithium Salt	Formulation	Lithium Content*	Trade Name
Lithium carbonate (Li_2CO_3)	Capsules	4.06 mEq lithium (150 mg Li_2CO_3) 8.12 mEq lithium (300 mg Li_2CO_3) 16.24 mEq lithium (600 mg Li_2CO_3)	Eskalith, Lithonate
	Tablets	8.12 mEq lithium (300 mg Li_2CO_3)	Eskalith, Lithane, Lithotabs
	Tablets: slow-release	8.12 mEq lithium (300 mg Li_2CO_3)	Lithobid
	Tablets: controlled release	12.18 mEq lithium (450 mg Li_2CO_3)	Eskalith CR
Lithium citrate	Syrup	8 mEq lithium/5 ml (equivalent to 300 mg Li_2CO_3)	Cibalith-S

*Lithium content is expressed in two ways: (1) mEq of lithium ion and (2) mg of the particular lithium salt of which the preparation is composed.

ium *citrate* is dispensed in a syrup. Lithium formulations and trade names are summarized in Table 26–3.

Lithium can cause gastric upset. This response can be reduced by administering lithium with meals or with milk.

Dosing. Dosing with lithium is highly individualized. Dosage adjustments are based on plasma drug levels and clinical response.

Plasma drug levels should be kept within the therapeutic range. Levels between 0.8 and 1.4 mEq/L are generally appropriate for *acute* therapy of manic episodes. For *maintenance* therapy, lithium levels should range from 0.4 to 1.0 mEq/L. (Levels of 0.6 to 0.8 mEq/L are effective for most patients.) To avoid serious toxicity, *lithium levels should not exceed 1.5 mEq/L.*

Knowledge of plasma drug levels is not the only guide to lithium dosing; consideration of the clinical response is at least as important. That is, when evaluating the appropriateness of a lithium dosage, we must not forget to look at the patient. Laboratory tests are all well and good, but they are not a substitute for clinical assessment. If, for example, blood levels of lithium appear proper, but clinical evaluation indicates toxicity, there is no question as to the action that should be taken: the dosage should be reduced—despite the apparent acceptability of the dosage as reflected by plasma drug levels.

Because of its short half-life and low therapeutic index, *lithium cannot be administered in a single daily dose;* with once-a-day dosing, peak drug levels would be excessive. Hence, a typical dosage is 300 mg (of lithium carbonate) taken three or four times a day. A dosage of 600 mg twice daily is acceptable, provided that an extended-release formulation is employed; however, even these preparations cannot be given on a once-daily basis.

CARBAMAZEPINE AND VALPROIC ACID

Carbamazepine [Tegretol] and valproic acid [Depakene, Depakote] were originally developed and marketed for treatment of seizure disorders. In recent years, these drugs have been used with success to treat patients with bipolar disorder. At this time, carbamazepine and valproic acid are reserved for patients who have failed to respond to lithium or who cannot tolerate lithium's side effects. The basic pharmacology of these drugs and their use in seizure disorders is discussed in Chapter 22.

Carbamazepine was the first drug to be widely studied as an alternative to lithium for patients with manic-depressive illness. Like lithium, carbamazepine reduces symptoms during manic episodes and depressive episodes. In addition, the drug appears to provide effective prophylaxis against recurrence of mania and depression. For patients with severe mania, and for those who cycle rapidly, carbamazepine may be superior to lithium. When given to manic patients who have failed to respond to lithium, carbamazepine has had a success rate of about 60%. For treatment of acute manic episodes, the dosage should be low initially (200 to 400 mg/day) and then gradually increased to as much as 1.6 to 2.2 gm/day. Lower doses should be employed when carbamazepine is used together with lithium, valproic acid, or antipsychotic drugs. The mechanism by which carbamazepine stabilizes mood is unknown.

Valproic acid is another promising alternative to lithium for manic-depressive patients who have failed to respond to lithium or who cannot tolerate its side effects. Clinical studies indicate that valproic acid can control symptoms in acute manic episodes and can provide prophylaxis against recurrent episodes of mania and depression. Like carbamazepine, valproic acid appears especially useful for patients with rapid-cycling bipolar disorder. Dosing should be initiated at 300 to 500 mg/day and then gradually increased to between 750 and 3000 mg/day. Valproic acid alters GABA-mediated neurotransmission, and this action may underlie the drug's mood-stabilizing effects.

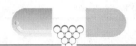

Summary of Major Nursing Implications

LITHIUM

Preadministration Assessment

Therapeutic Goal

Control of acute manic episodes in patients with manic-depressive illness, and prophylaxis against recurrent mania and depression in these patients.

Baseline Data

Obtain baseline measurements of cardiac status (EKG, blood pressure, pulse), hematologic status (complete blood counts with differential), serum electrolytes, renal function (serum creatinine, creatinine clearance, urinalysis), and thyroid function (T_3, T_4, and TSH).

Identifying High-Risk Patients

Lithium is *contraindicated* during the *first trimester of pregnancy,* and should be avoided later in pregnancy whenever possible. Use with *caution* in the presence of *renal disease, cardiovascular disease, dehydration, sodium depletion,* and *concurrent therapy with diuretics.*

Implementation: Administration

Route

Oral.

Administration

Advise the patient to administer lithium with meals or a glass of milk to decrease gastric upset. Instruct the patient to swallow slow-release and controlled-release tablets intact, without crushing or chewing.

Promoting Compliance

Rigid adherence to the prescribed regimen is important: deviations in dosage size and timing can cause toxicity, and inadequate dosing may cause relapse.

To promote compliance, educate the patient and his or her family about the nature of manic-depressive illness and the importance of taking lithium as prescribed. Encourage family members to oversee lithium use, and advise them to urge the patient to visit the physician or a psychiatric clinic if a pattern of noncompliance develops.

When medicating the hospitalized patient, make sure that each lithium dose is ingested.

Ongoing Evaluation and Interventions

Monitoring Summary

Lithium Levels. Monitor lithium levels to insure that they remain within the therapeutic range (0.8 to 1.4 mEq/L for initial therapy, and 0.4 to 1.0 mEq/L for maintenance therapy). Levels should be measured every 2 to 3 days during initial therapy, and every 1 to 3 months during maintenance. Blood for lithium determination should be drawn in the morning, 12 hours after the evening dose.

Other Parameters to Monitor. Evaluate the patient at least once a year for hematologic status (complete blood counts with differential), serum electrolytes, renal function (serum creatinine, creatinine clearance, urinalysis), and thyroid function (T_3, T_4, and TSH).

Evaluating Therapeutic Effects

Evaluate the patient for abatement of manic symptoms (e.g., flight of ideas, pressure of speech, hyperactivity) and for mood stabilization.

Minimizing Adverse Effects

Effects Caused by Excessive Drug Levels. Excessive lithium levels can result in serious adverse effects (see Table 26–2). Lithium levels must be monitored (see *Monitoring Summary*) and the dosage adjusted accordingly.

Teach the patient about signs of toxicity, and instruct him or her to withhold medication and notify the physician if these develop.

Renal impairment can cause lithium accumulation. Kidney function should be assessed prior to treatment and once yearly thereafter.

Sodium deficiency can cause lithium to accumulate. Instruct the patient to maintain normal sodium intake. Forewarn the patient that diarrhea can cause significant sodium loss. Diuretics promote sodium excretion and must be used with caution.

In the event of severe toxicity, hospitalization may be required. If lithium levels exceed 2.5 mEq/L, hemodialysis should be considered.

Tremor. Lithium can cause fine hand tremor that can interfere with motor skills. Tremor can be reduced with a beta-adrenergic blocker (e.g., propranolol) and by measures that reduce peak lithium levels (dosage reduction, use of divided doses, or use of sustained-release formulations).

Goiter. Lithium can promote goiter. Plasma levels of T_3, T_4, and TSH should be measured prior to treatment and yearly thereafter. Treat hypothyroidism with thyroid hormone.

Renal Toxicity. Lithium can cause renal damage. Kidney function should be assessed prior to treatment and once a year thereafter. If renal impairment develops, lithium dosage must be reduced.

Polyuria. Lithium increases urine output. Polyuria can be suppressed with a thiazide diuretic; the mechanism of this paradoxical effect is not known. Instruct the patient to drink 8 to 12 glasses of fluid daily to maintain hydration.

Use in Pregnancy and Lactation. Lithium is associated with a high incidence of serious birth defects. The drug should be avoided during pregnancy, especially in the first trimester. Counsel women of child-bearing age about the importance of avoiding pregnancy.

Lithium enters breast milk. Breast-feeding should be avoided.

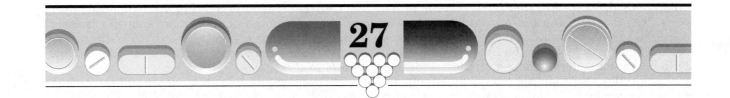

Benzodiazepines and Other Drugs for Anxiety and Insomnia

A nxiety and insomnia are common complaints, and the drugs employed for treatment are prescribed widely. Drugs used to relieve anxiety are called *antianxiety agents* or *anxiolytics*; an older term for these drugs is *tranquilizer*. Drugs that promote sleep are referred to as *hypnotics*. The distinction between antianxiety effects and hypnotic effects is frequently a matter of dosage: some drugs relieve anxiety in low doses and induce sleep in higher doses. Hence, a single drug may be considered both an antianxiety agent and a hypnotic agent, depending upon the reason for its use and the dosage employed.

Before the benzodiazepines became available, anxiety and insomnia were treated with barbiturates and other *general central nervous system (CNS) depressants*—drugs with multiple undesirable qualities: (1) These drugs are *powerful respiratory depressants* that can readily prove *fatal* in overdosage. As a result, they are "drugs of choice" for *suicide*. (2) Because they produce subjective effects that many individuals find desirable, general CNS depressants often have a *high potential for abuse*. (3) With prolonged use, most general CNS depressants produce significant *tolerance and physical dependence*. (4) Barbiturates and certain other CNS depressants *stimulate synthesis of hepatic drug-metabolizing enzymes,* and can thereby decrease responses to other drugs. Since the benzodiazepines are just as effective as the general CNS depressants, but do not share their undesirable properties, benzodiazepines have largely replaced the general CNS depressants for managing anxiety and insomnia.

BENZODIAZEPINES

Benzodiazepines are drugs of first choice for treating anxiety and insomnia. In addition, these agents are used to induce general anesthesia and to manage seizure disorders, muscle spasm, panic disorder, and withdrawal from alcohol.

Benzodiazepines were introduced in the early 1960's and are among the most widely prescribed drugs in the United States. Perhaps the most familiar member of the family is diazepam [Valium]. The most frequently prescribed members are lorazepam [Ativan] and alprazolam [Xanax].

The popularity of the benzodiazepines as sedatives and hypnotics stems from their clear superiority over the alternatives: barbiturates and other general CNS depressants. The benzodiazepines are safer than the general CNS depressants and have a lower potential for abuse. In addition, benzodiazepines produce less tolerance and physical dependence and are subject to fewer drug interactions. Contrasts between the benzodiazepines and barbiturates are summarized in Table 27–1.

Since all of the benzodiazepines produce nearly identical effects, we will consider the family as a group, rather than selecting a representative member as a prototype.

Overview of Pharmacologic Effects

Practically all responses to benzodiazepines result from actions in the CNS. Benzodiazepines have few direct actions outside the CNS. All of the benzodiazepines produce a similar spectrum of responses. However, because of pharmacokinetic differences, individual benzodiazepines may differ in their clinical applications.

Central Nervous System. All beneficial effects of benzodiazepines and most adverse effects result from depressant actions in the CNS. With increasing dosage, effects progress from *sedation* to *hypnosis* to *stupor*.

Benzodiazepines depress neuronal function at multiple sites throughout the CNS. These drugs *reduce anxiety* through effects on the limbic system, a neuronal network associated with emotionality. They *promote sleep* through effects on cortical areas and on the sleep-wakefulness clock. They *induce muscle relaxation* through effects on supraspinal motor areas, including the cerebellum. Two important side effects—*confusion* and *amnesia*—result from effects on the hippocampus and cerebral cortex.

Cardiovascular System. When taken *orally,* benzodiazepines have negligible effects on the heart and blood vessels. In contrast, when administered *intravenously*—even in therapeutic doses—benzodiazepines can produce profound hypotension and cardiac arrest.

Respiratory System. In contrast to the barbiturates, the benzodiazepines are weak respiratory depressants. When taken alone in therapeutic doses, these drugs produce little or no depression of respiration; and with toxic doses, respiratory depression is moderate at most. With oral therapy, clinically significant respiratory depression occurs only when benzodiazepines are combined with other CNS depressants (e.g., opioids, barbiturates, alcohol).

Molecular Mechanism of Action

Benzodiazepines *potentiate the actions of gamma-aminobutyric acid* (GABA), an inhibitory neurotransmitter found throughout the CNS. These drugs enhance the actions of GABA by binding to specific receptors in a supramolecular structure known as the GABA receptor–chloride channel complex (Fig. 27–1). Benzodiazepines do *not* act as direct GABA agonists.

Because benzodiazepines act by amplifying the actions of endogenous GABA, rather than by directly mimicking GABA, there is a limit to how much CNS depression these drugs can produce.

Table 27–1. Contrasts Between Benzodiazepines and Barbiturates		
Area of Comparison	**Benzodiazepines**	**Barbiturates**
Relative safety	High	Low
Maximal ability to depress CNS function	Low	High
Respiratory depressant ability	Low	High
Suicide potential	Low	High
Ability to cause physical dependence	Low	High
Ability to cause tolerance	Low	High
Abuse potential	Low	High
Ability to induce drug metabolism	Low	High

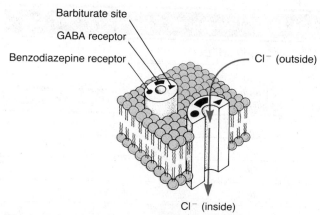

Barbiturate site
GABA receptor
Benzodiazepine receptor
Cl⁻ (outside)
Cl⁻ (inside)

Figure 27–1. Schematic model of the GABA receptor–chloride channel complex showing binding sites for benzodiazepines and barbiturates. The GABA receptor–chloride channel complex, which spans the neuronal cell membrane, can exist in an open or closed configuration. Binding of GABA to its receptor causes the chloride channel to *open*. The resulting inward flow of chloride ions hyperpolarizes the neuron (makes the cell highly negative inside) and thereby decreases the cell's ability to fire. Hence, GABA is an *inhibitory* neurotransmitter. Binding of a *benzodiazepine* to its receptor on the complex prolongs the time that the chloride channel remains open. Hence, benzodiazepines enhance the inhibitory effects of GABA. In the absence of GABA, benzodiazepines have no effect on channel opening. Effects of *barbiturates* on the chloride channel are dose dependent: at low doses, barbiturates enhance the actions of GABA (by increasing the frequency of channel opening); at high doses, barbiturates directly mimic the actions of GABA.

This explains why benzodiazepines are so much safer than the barbiturates—drugs that can directly mimic GABA. Since benzodiazepines simply potentiate the inhibitory effects of endogenous GABA, and since the amount of GABA in the CNS is finite, there is a built-in limit to the depth of CNS depression the benzodiazepines can produce. In contrast, since the barbiturates are direct-acting CNS depressants, maximal effects are limited only by the amount of barbiturate administered.

Pharmacokinetics

Absorption and Distribution. Most benzodiazepines are well absorbed following oral administration. Because of their high lipid solubility, benzodiazepines readily cross the blood-brain barrier to reach sites within the CNS.

Metabolism. Most benzodiazepines undergo extensive metabolic alterations. With few exceptions, the *metabolites are pharmacologically active*. As a result, responses produced by administering a particular benzodiazepine often persist long after the parent drug has disappeared from the plasma. Hence, there may be a poor correlation between the plasma half-life of the parent drug and duration of pharmacologic effects. Flurazepam, for example, whose plasma half-life is only 2 to 3 hours, is converted into an active metabolite with a half-life of 50 hours. Hence, administration of flurazepam produces long-lasting effects, despite the fact that within 8 to 12 hours of its administration, flurazepam itself can no longer be detected in the blood.

In patients with liver disease, metabolism of benzodiazepines can decline, thereby prolonging and intensifying responses. Because certain benzodiazepines (oxazepam, temazepam, and lorazepam) undergo very little metabolic alteration, these agents may be preferred for patients with hepatic impairment.

Time Course of Action. Benzodiazepines differ significantly from one another with regard to time course of action. These agents differ in onset of action, duration of action, and tendency to accumulate with repeated dosing.

Because all of the benzodiazepines have essentially equivalent pharmacologic actions, selection among these drugs is based in large part on differences in time course. For example, if a patient needs medication to accelerate falling asleep, a benzodiazepine with a rapid onset of action (e.g., triazolam) would be indicated. However, if medication is needed to prevent waking later in the night, a benzodiazepine with a slower onset (e.g., estazolam) would be preferred. For treatment of anxiety, a drug with an intermediate duration of action is desirable. For treatment of any benzodiazepine-responsive condition in the elderly, a drug such as lorazepam, which is not likely to accumulate with repeated dosing, is generally preferred.

Therapeutic Uses

The benzodiazepines have three principal indications: (1) anxiety, (2) insomnia, and (3) seizure disorders. In addition, these drugs are employed as preoperative medication and in the management of muscle spasm, panic disorder, and withdrawal from alcohol. Although all benzodiazepines share the same pharmacologic properties and, therefore, might be equally effective for all of these applications, not every benzodiazepine is actually employed for all potential uses. The principal factors that determine the actual applications of a particular benzodiazepine are (1) the pharmacokinetic properties of the drug itself, and (2) the research and marketing decisions of pharmaceutical companies. Specific applications of individual benzodiazepines are summarized in Table 27–2.

Anxiety. Benzodiazepines are drugs of first choice for treating anxiety. Although all benzodiazepines have anxiolytic properties, only eight are marketed for this indication (see Table 27–3). Anxiolytic effects result from depressing neurotransmission in the limbic system and cortical areas. Guidelines for managing anxiety with benzodiazepines are presented later in the chapter.

				Table 27–2. Applications of the Benzodiazepines		

	Applications						
Generic Name [Trade Name]	*Anxiety*	*Insomnia*	*Seizures*	*Muscle Spasm, Spasticity*	*Alcohol Withdrawal*	*Induction of Anesthesia*	*Panic Disorder*
Alprazolam [Xanax]	√						√
Chlordiazepoxide [Librium, others]	√				√		
Clonazepam [Klonopin]			√				
Clorazepate [Tranxene, Gen-Xene]	√		√		√		
Diazepam [Valium, others]	√		√	√	√	√	
Estazolam [ProSom]		√					
Flurazepam [Dalmane]		√					
Halazepam [Paxipam]	√						
Lorazepam [Ativan]	√		√		√	√	
Midazolam [Versed]						√*	
Oxazepam [Serax]	√				√		
Prazepam [Centrax]	√						
Quazepam [Doral]		√					
Temazepam [Restoril]		√					
Triazolam [Halcion]		√					

*Midazolam, in conjunction with an opioid analgesic, is also used to produce *conscious sedation,* a semiconscious state suitable for minor surgeries and endoscopic procedures.

Insomnia. Benzodiazepines are drugs of first choice for treating insomnia. These drugs decrease latency time to falling asleep; they reduce awakenings; and they increase total sleeping time. Although all benzodiazepines can relieve insomnia, only five are marketed for this use (see Table 27–4). Management of insomnia with benzodiazepines is discused later in the chapter.

Seizure Disorders. Four benzodiazepines—diazepam, clonazepam, lorazepam, and clorazepate—are employed to treat seizure disorders. This application is discussed in Chapter 22.

Muscle Spasm. One benzodiazepine—diazepam—is used to relieve muscle spasm and spasticity (see Chapter 23). Effects on muscle tone are secondary to actions exerted in the CNS. Diazepam cannot relieve spasm without causing sedation.

Alcohol Withdrawal. Diazepam and other benzodiazepines may be administered to facilitate withdrawal from alcohol (see Chapter 34). These drugs are helpful because cross-dependence with alcohol enables them to suppress symptoms of abstinence in individuals physically dependent on alcohol.

Panic Disorder. Alprazolam [Xanax], in high doses, provides effective treatment of panic disorder. Although several other medications, including imipramine (a tricyclic antidepressant) and phenelzine (a monoamine oxidase–inhibiting antidepressant), are also effective, alprazolam is the only drug actually approved by the FDA for this indication.

Induction of Anesthesia. Three benzodiazepines—diazepam [Valium], lorazepam [Ativan], and midazolam [Versed]—can be given IV for induction of anesthesia. In addition, midazolam, in combination with an opioid analgesic, can be used to produce *conscious sedation*, a semiconscious state suitable for endoscopic procedures and minor surgeries. Benzodiazepines are also used to provide preoperative sedation. All of these uses are discussed in Chapter 30.

Adverse Effects

Benzodiazepines are generally well tolerated, and serious adverse reactions are rare. In contrast to the barbiturates and other general CNS depressants, the benzodiazepines are remarkably safe drugs.

CNS Depression. When taken in sleep-inducing doses, benzodiazepines cause drowsiness, lightheadedness, incoordination, and difficulty in concentrating. When these effects occur at bedtime they are generally inconsequential. However, if sedation and other manifestations of CNS depression persist beyond waking, interference with daytime activities can occur.

Paradoxical Psychologic Effects. When employed to treat anxiety, benzodiazepines sometimes cause paradoxical responses, including insomnia, excitation, euphoria, heightened anxiety, and rage. If these occur, benzodiazepines should be withdrawn.

Anterograde Amnesia. Benzodiazepines can cause anterograde amnesia (impaired recall of events that take place after commencement of treatment). Anterograde amnesia has been especially troublesome with *triazolam* [Halcion]. If patients complain of forgetfulness, the possibility of drug-induced amnesia should be evaluated.

Respiratory Depression. Benzodiazepines are only weak respiratory depressants. Death from overdosage with *oral* benzodiazepines *alone* has never been documented. Hence, in contrast to the barbiturates, benzodiazepines present little risk as vehicles for suicide. It must be emphasized, however, that although respiratory depression with *oral* therapy is rare, benzodiazepines can cause severe respiratory depression when administered *intravenously*. In addition, substantial respiratory depression can result from combining oral benzodiazepines with other CNS depressants (e.g., alcohol, barbiturates, opioids).

Abuse. The abuse potential of the benzodiazepines is lower than that of the barbiturates and most other general CNS depressants. The behavior pattern that constitutes "addiction" is uncommon among patients who take benzodiazepines for therapeutic purposes. When asked about drug-use patterns, individuals who regularly abuse drugs rarely indicate a preference for benzodiazepines over barbiturates. Because their potential for abuse is low, the benzodiazepines are classified under Schedule IV of the Controlled Substances Act. This contrasts with the barbiturates, most of which are classified under Schedule II or III.

Use in Pregnancy and Lactation. Benzodiazepines are highly lipid soluble and can readily cross the placental barrier. Reports based on benzodiazepine use during the first trimester of pregnancy suggest an increased risk of congenital malformations, such as cleft lip, inguinal hernia, and cardiac anomalies. Use near term can cause CNS depression in the neonate. Because they present a risk to the fetus, most benzodiazepines are classified in FDA Pregnancy Category D. Four of these drugs—estazolam, quazepam, temazepam, and triazolam—are classified in Category X. Women of child-bearing age should be warned about the potential for fetal harm and instructed to discontinue benzodiazepines if pregnancy occurs.

Benzodiazepines enter breast milk with ease and may accumulate to toxic levels in the breast-fed infant. Accordingly, these drugs should be avoided by nursing mothers.

Other Adverse Effects. Occasional reactions include weakness, headache, blurred vision, vertigo, nausea, vomiting, epigastric distress, and diarrhea. Neutropenia and jaundice occur rarely.

Drug Interactions

Benzodiazepines undergo very few important interactions with other drugs. Unlike barbiturates, benzodiazepines do not induce hepatic drug-metabolizing enzymes. Hence, benzodiazepines do not accelerate the metabolism of other drugs.

CNS Depressants. The CNS-depressant actions of benzodiazepines will add with those of other CNS depressants (e.g., alcohol, barbiturates, opioids). Hence, although benzodiazepines are very safe when used alone, these drugs can be extremely hazardous in combination with other depressants: *combined overdosage with a benzodiazepine plus another CNS depressants can cause profound respiratory depression, coma, and death. Patients should be warned against use of alcohol and all other CNS depressants.*

Tolerance and Physical Dependence

Tolerance. With prolonged use of benzodiazepines, tolerance develops to some effects—but not to others. No tolerance develops to anxiolytic effects, and tolerance to hypnotic effects is generally low. In contrast, significant tolerance develops to antiseizure effects. Patients tolerant to barbiturates, alcohol, and other general CNS depressants show some cross-tolerance to benzodiazepines.

Physical Dependence. Benzodiazepines can cause physical dependence—but the incidence of *substantial* dependence is low. When benzodiazepines are discontinued following short-term use at therapeutic doses, the resulting withdrawal syndrome is generally mild and often goes unrecognized. Symptoms include anxiety, insomnia, sweating, tremors, and dizziness. Withdrawal from long-term high-dose therapy can elicit more serious reactions, such as panic, paranoia, delirium, hypertension, muscle twitches, and outright convulsions. Symptoms of withdrawal are usually more intense with benzodiazepines that have a short duration of action. With one agent—*alprazolam* [Xanax]—dependence may be a greater problem than with other benzodiazepines. Because the benzodiazepine withdrawal syndrome can resemble an anxiety disorder, care must be taken to differentiate withdrawal from the return of original symptoms.

The intensity of withdrawal symptoms can be minimized by discontinuing treatment gradually. Doses should be gradually tapered over several weeks. Substituting a benzodiazepine with a long half-life for one with a short half-life is also helpful. Patients should be warned against abrupt cessation of treatment. Following discontinuation of treatment, patients should be monitored for 3 weeks for indications of withdrawal or recurrence of original symptoms.

Acute Toxicity

Oral Overdosage. When administered in excessive dosage by mouth, benzodiazepines rarely cause serious toxicity. Symptoms include drowsiness, lethargy, and confusion. Significant cardiovascular and respiratory effects are uncommon. If an individual known to have taken an overdose of benzodiazepines *does* exhibit signs of serious toxicity, it is probable that another drug was taken as well.

Intravenous Toxicity. When injected intravenously, even in therapeutic doses, benzodiazepines can cause severe adverse effects. Life-threatening reactions (e.g., profound hypotension, respiratory arrest, cardiac arrest) occur in about 2% of patients.

General Treatment Measures. Benzodiazepine-induced toxicity is managed in the same fashion as toxicity from barbiturates and other general CNS depressants. Oral benzodiazepines can be removed from the body with gastric lavage followed by ingestion of activated charcoal and a saline cathartic; dialysis may be helpful if symptoms are especially severe. Respiration should be monitored and the airway kept patent. Support of blood pressure with IV fluids and norepinephrine may be required.

Treatment with Flumazenil. Flumazenil [Romazicon] is a competitive benzodiazepine-receptor antagonist. The drug can reverse the *sedative* effects of benzodiazepines, but may not reverse benzodiazepine-induced *respiratory depression*. Flumazenil is approved for treatment of benzodiazepine overdosage and for reversing the effects of benzodiazepines following general anesthesia. The principal adverse effect is precipitation of *convulsions*. This is most likely in patients taking benzodiazepines to treat epilepsy and in patients who are physically dependent on benzodiazepines. Administration of flumazenil is intravenous. Doses are injected slowly (over 30 seconds) and may be repeated every minute as needed. The first dose is 0.2 mg; the second is 0.3 mg; and all subsequent doses are 0.5 mg. Effects of flumazenil fade in about 1 hour; hence, additional dosing may be required.

Preparations, Dosage, and Administration

Preparations and Dosage. Preparations and dosages of the benzodiazepines used for insomnia and anxiety are presented in Tables 27–3 and 27–4. Preparations and dosages of benzodiazepines used to treat other disorders are presented in Chapter 22 (Drugs for Epilepsy), Chapter 23 (Drugs for Muscle Spasm and Spasticity), and Chapter 30 (General Anesthetics).

Routes. All benzodiazepines can be administered orally. In addition, three agents—diazepam, chlordiazepoxide, and lorazepam—may also be administered parenterally (IM and IV). When used for sedation or induction of sleep, benzodiazepines are almost always administered by mouth. Intramuscular and intravenous administration are reserved for acute management of alcohol withdrawal, severe anxiety, status epilepticus, and other emergencies.

Oral. Patients should be advised to take oral benzodiazepines with food if gastric upset occurs. Also, they should be instructed to swallow sustained-release formulations intact, without crushing or chewing. Patients should be warned not to increase the dosage or discontinue therapy without consulting the physician.

For treatment of insomnia, benzodiazepines should be given on an intermittent schedule (e.g., 3 or 4 days a week) in the lowest effective dosage for the shortest duration required. This will minimize physical dependence and associated drug-dependency insomnia.

Intravenous. Intravenous administration is hazardous and must be performed with care. Life-threatening reactions (severe hypotension, respiratory arrest, cardiac arrest) have occurred. In addition, IV administration carries a risk of venous thrombosis, phlebitis, and vascular impairment.

To reduce complications from IV administration, the following precautions should be taken: (1) inject the drug slowly; (2) take care to avoid intra-arterial injection and extravasation; (3) if direct venous injection is impossible, make the injection into infusion tubing as close to the vein as possible; (4) follow the manufacturer's instructions regarding suitable diluents for preparing solutions; and (5) have facilities for resuscitation available.

BARBITURATES

The barbiturates (pronounced bahr-bi-tewr′-ates or bahr-bitch′-oo-rates) have been used since early in the 20th century. These drugs cause relatively nonselective depression of CNS function and are the prototypes of the general CNS depressants. Because they depress multiple aspects of CNS function, barbiturates can be used for daytime sedation, induction of sleep, suppression of seizures,

Table 27–3. Major Drugs for Anxiety

Generic Name	Trade Name	Dosage Forms	Adult Oral Dosage mg/dose	Adult Oral Dosage doses/day	CSA Schedule
Benzodiazepines					
Alprazolam	Xanax	T	0.25–0.5	3	IV
Chlordiazepoxide	Librium, others	C, T, I	5–25	3 or 4	IV
Clorazepate	Tranxene, Gen-Xene	C, T, T-SR	7.5–15	2 to 4*	IV
Diazepam	Valium, others	C-SR, T, L, I	2–10	2 to 4*	IV
Halazepam	Paxipam	T	20–40	3 or 4	IV
Lorazepam	Ativan	T, I	1–3	2 or 3	IV
Oxazepam	Serax	C, T	10–30	3 or 4	IV
Prazepam	Centrax	C, T	10	3†	IV
Nonbenzodiazepine					
Buspirone	BuSpar	T	5–10	3	—

CSA = Controlled Substances Act
Key to dosage forms: C = capsule; C-SR = capsule, sustained-release; I = injection; L = oral liquid; T = tablet; T-SR = tablet, sustained-release
*With the sustained-release formulation, the total daily dose is administered in a single dose.
†May also be administered in a single 20–40 mg dose at bedtime.

and general anesthesia. Barbiturates cause tolerance and dependence, have a high abuse potential, and are subject to multiple drug interactions. Moreover, these drugs are powerful respiratory depressants that can readily prove fatal in overdosage. Because of these undesirable properties, the barbiturates, which were once used widely, have been largely replaced by newer and safer drugs— primarily the benzodiazepines. However, although their use has declined greatly, barbiturates still have important applications (in seizure control and anesthesia). Moreover, barbiturates are valuable from an instructional point of view: by understanding these prototypic agents, we gain an understanding of the general CNS depressants as a group, along with an appreciation as to why these

Table 27–4. Drugs for Insomnia

Generic Name	Trade Name	Dosage Forms	Adult Oral Dose (mg)	CSA Schedule
Benzodiazepines				
Estazolam	ProSom	T	1–2	IV
Flurazepam	Dalmane	C	15–30	IV
Quazepam	Doral	T	7.5–15	IV
Temazepam	Restoril	C	15–30	IV
Triazolam	Halcion	T	0.125–0.5	IV
Barbiturates				
Amobarbital	Amytal	C, T, I	65–200	II
Aprobarbital	Alurate	L	40–160	III
Butabarbital	Butisol, others	C, T, L	50–100	III
Pentobarbital	Nembutal	C, L, I, S	100	II
Phenobarbital	Luminal, others	C, T, L, I	100–320	IV
Secobarbital	Seconal	C, T, RI, I	100	II
Talbutal	Lotusate	T	120	III
Nonbenzodiazepine- Nonbarbiturates				
Chloral hydrate	Noctec, others	C, L, S	500–1000	IV
Ethchlorvynol	Placidyl	C	500–1000	IV
Glutethimide	Doriden	T	250–500	III
Methyprylon	Noludar	C, T	200–400	III
Paraldehyde	Paral	L	4–8 ml	IV
Zolpidem	Ambien	T	10	IV

CSA = Controlled Substances Act
Key to dosage forms: C = capsule; T = tablet; L = oral liquid (includes drops, syrups, and elixirs); I = injection; RI = rectal injection; S = suppository.

Table 27–5. Characteristics of Barbiturate Subgroups

Barbiturate Subgroup	Representative Drug	Lipid Solubility	Time Course Onset (minutes)	Time Course Duration (hours)	Applications
Ultrashort-acting	Thiopental	High	0.5	0.2	Induction of anesthesia; treatment of seizures
Short-to-intermediate-acting	Secobarbital	Moderate	10–15	3–4	Treatment of insomnia
Long-acting	Phenobarbital	Low	60 or less	10–12	Treatment of seizures and insomnia

drugs are used infrequently for anxiety and insomnia.

Classification

The barbiturates can be grouped into three classes based on duration of action: (1) ultrashort-acting agents, (2) short-to-intermediate–acting agents, and (3) long-acting agents. As indicated in Table 27–5, the duration of action of these drugs is inversely related to their lipid solubility. Barbiturates with the highest lipid solubility have the shortest duration of action. Conversely, barbiturates with the lowest lipid solubility have the longest duration.

Duration of action influences the clinical applications of barbiturates. The ultrashort-acting agents (e.g., thiopental) are used for induction of anesthesia. The short-to-intermediate–acting agents (e.g., secobarbital) are used as sedatives and hypnotics. The long-acting agents (e.g., phenobarbital) are used primarily as antiseizure drugs.

Mechanism of Action

Like benzodiazepines, barbiturates bind to the GABA receptor–chloride channel complex (see Fig. 27–1). As a result of binding, these drugs can (1) enhance the inhibitory actions of GABA and (2) directly mimic the actions of GABA. Since barbiturates can directly mimic GABA, there is no ceiling to the degree of CNS depression they can produce. Hence, in contrast to the benzodiazepines, these drugs can readily cause death when taken in overdosage. Although barbiturates can cause general depression of the CNS, they show some selectivity for depressing the *reticular activating system* (RAS), a neuronal network that helps regulate the sleep-wakefulness cycle. By depressing the RAS, barbiturates produce sedation and sleep.

Pharmacologic Effects

CNS Depression. The ability to cause generalized CNS depression underlies the therapeutic effects of the barbiturates as well as many of their adverse effects. As dosage is increased, responses progress from *sedation* to *sleep* to *general anesthesia*.

Most barbiturates can be considered *nonselective* CNS depressants. Exceptions to this rule are phenobarbital and other barbiturates used to control seizures. Seizure control is achieved at doses that have minimal effects on other aspects of CNS function.

Cardiovascular Effects. At hypnotic doses, barbiturates produce modest reductions in blood pressure and heart rate. In contrast, toxic doses can cause profound hypotension and shock. These reactions result from direct depressant effects on the myocardium and vascular smooth muscle.

Induction of Hepatic Drug-Metabolizing Enzymes. Barbiturates stimulate synthesis of hepatic microsomal enzymes, the principal drug-metabolizing enzymes of the liver. As a result, barbiturates can accelerate their own metabolism as well as the metabolism of many other drugs.

Barbiturates stimulate drug metabolism by promoting the synthesis of porphyrin (Fig. 27–2). Porphyrin is then converted into heme, which in turn is converted into cytochrome P-450—a key component of the hepatic drug-metabolizing enzyme system.

Tolerance and Physical Dependence

Tolerance. Tolerance is defined as reduced drug responsiveness that develops over the course of repeated drug use. When barbiturates are taken on a long-term basis, tolerance develops to many—but not all—of their CNS effects. Specifically, tolerance develops to sedative and hypnotic effects and to other effects that underlie barbiturate abuse. However, even with chronic use, *very little tolerance develops to toxic effects*.

In the tolerant user, doses must be increased to elicit the same intensity of response that could formerly be elicited by smaller doses. Hence, individuals who take barbiturates for prolonged periods—be it for therapeutic purposes or for purposes of abuse—require steadily increasing doses to achieve the effects they desire.

It is important to note that *very little tolerance develops to respiratory depression*. Because tolerance to respiratory depression is minimal, and because tolerance does develop to therapeutic effects, with continued treatment, the lethal (respiratory-depressant) dose remains relatively constant while the therapeutic dose climbs higher and higher (Fig. 27–3). As tolerance to therapeutic effects increases, the therapeutic dose grows steadily closer to the lethal dose—a situation that is clearly hazardous.

As a rule, tolerance to one general CNS depressant bestows tolerance to all other general CNS depressants. Hence, there is cross-tolerance among barbiturates, alcohol, benzodiazepines, general anesthetics, chloral hydrate, and a number of other agents. Tolerance to barbiturates and the other general CNS depressants does *not* produce significant cross-tolerance with *opioids* (e.g., morphine).

Physical Dependence. Prolonged administration of barbiturates results in physical dependence—a state in which continued drug use is required to avoid an abstinence (withdrawal) syndrome. Physical dependence is thought to result from adaptive neurochemical changes that occur in response to chronic drug exposure.

Individuals who are physically dependent on barbiturates ex-

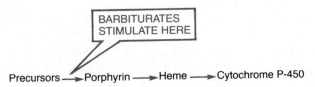

Precursors → Porphyrin → Heme → Cytochrome P-450

BARBITURATES STIMULATE HERE

Figure 27–2. Induction of hepatic microsomal enzymes by barbiturates. By increasing synthesis of porphyrin, barbiturates increase production of cytochrome P-450, a key component of the hepatic drug-metabolizing system.

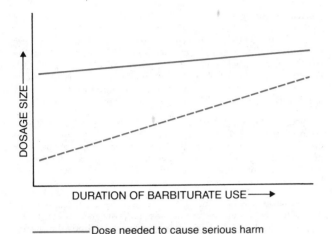

————— Dose needed to cause serious harm

— — — — — Dose needed for desirable effects

Figure 27–3. Development of tolerance to the toxic and subjective effects of barbiturates. With prolonged barbiturate use, tolerance develops. However, less tolerance develops to toxic effects than to desired effects. Consequently, as duration of use increases, the difference between the dose producing desirable effects and the dose producing toxicity becomes progressively smaller, thereby increasing the risk of serious harm.

hibit cross-dependence with other general CNS depressants. Because of cross-dependence, a person physically dependent on barbiturates can prevent development of a withdrawal syndrome by taking any other general CNS depressant (e.g., alcohol, benzodiazepines). As a rule, cross-dependence exists among all of the general CNS depressants. However, there is no significant cross-dependence with opioids.

The general CNS depressant abstinence syndrome can be *severe*. Contrary to popular understanding, abrupt withdrawal from general CNS depressants is more dangerous than withdrawal from opioids. Although withdrawal from opioids is certainly unpleasant, the risk of serious injury is low. In contrast, the abstinence syndrome associated with general CNS depressants can be *fatal*.

The following description illustrates how dangerous withdrawal from general CNS depressants can be. Early reactions include weakness, restlessness, insomnia, hyperthermia, orthostatic hypotension, confusion, and disorientation. By the third day, major convulsive episodes may develop. Approximately 75% of patients experience psychotic delirium (a state similar to alcoholic delirium tremens). In extreme cases, these symptoms may be followed by exhaustion, cardiovascular collapse, and death. The entire abstinence syndrome evolves over approximately 8 days. The intensity of symptoms can be greatly reduced by withdrawing general CNS depressants slowly.

A long-acting barbiturate (e.g., phenobarbital) may be administered to facilitate the withdrawal process. Because of cross-dependence, phenobarbital can substitute for other CNS depressants, and can thereby suppress symptoms of withdrawal. Because of its long half-life, phenobarbital leaves the body slowly, thereby allowing a gradual transition from a drug-dependent state to a drug-free state. When phenobarbital is given to aid withdrawal, its dosage should be reduced gradually over 10 days to 3 weeks.

It is important to note that physical dependence should not be equated with addiction. Addiction is defined as a behavior pattern characterized by (1) compulsive drug use, (2) drug-seeking behavior, and (3) a tendency to relapse following withdrawal. Although physical dependence can contribute to this behavior pattern, physical dependence, by itself, will neither cause nor sustain addictive behavior. The distinction between addiction and physical dependence is discussed at length in Chapter 34 (Drugs of Abuse).

Pharmacokinetics

Lipid solubility has a significant impact on the pharmacokinetic properties of individual barbiturates. As noted earlier, barbiturates of high lipid solubility have a rapid onset and brief duration of action. Onset is rapid because lipid solubility allows these drugs to penetrate the blood-brain barrier with ease, thereby reaching their sites of action quickly. As these drugs undergo uptake by tissues other than the brain, their levels in plasma fall, creating a concentration gradient favoring their movement from the brain back to the blood. Because of this gradient, highly lipid-soluble barbiturates undergo rapid redistribution from the brain back into the blood and then into other tissues. This redistribution terminates their CNS effects.

In comparison to the highly lipid-soluble agents, barbiturates of lower lipid solubility have effects of relatively slow onset but prolonged duration. Onset is delayed because low lipid solubility impedes passage across the blood-brain barrier. Effects are prolonged because their termination is dependent on renal excretion and hepatic metabolism—processes that are slower than simple redistribution of the drug from the brain to other tissues.

With the exception of the highly lipid-soluble agents, all of the barbiturates have long plasma half-lives. These half-lives are so long, in fact, that significant amounts of barbiturate remain in plasma more than 24 hours after giving a single dose. This persistence has two clinical consequences: First, when barbiturates are taken at night to promote sleep, residual drug may cause sedation the following day. Second, since barbiturates are not eliminated entirely in 24 hours, daily administration will cause drug accumulation. As a result, the brain undergoes continuous exposure to progressively higher drug levels—a phenomenon that promotes tolerance.

Therapeutic Uses

Insomnia. By depressing the CNS, barbiturates can promote sleep. However, because they can cause multiple undesired effects, barbiturates have been replaced by benzodiazepines as drugs of first choice for insomnia.

Seizure Disorders. Phenobarbital and certain other barbiturates are employed to treat epilepsy and other seizure disorders (see Chapter 22). These anticonvulsant barbiturates suppress seizures at doses that are essentially nonsedative.

Induction of Anesthesia. Thiopental and other highly lipid-soluble barbiturates are given to induce general anesthesia (see Chapter 30). Unconsciousness develops within seconds of IV injection.

Other Uses. Barbiturates have been used to treat acute manic states and delirium. In children, these drugs can decrease restlessness secondary to colic, pylorospasm, and whooping cough. In addition, they can help reduce anxiety in children prior to minor dental and medical procedures. Excessive excitation from overdosage with CNS stimulants (e.g., amphetamine, theophylline, ephedrine) can be decreased with barbiturates. These drugs can also be employed for emergency treatment of convulsions caused by tetanus, eclampsia, and epilepsy. When administered in anesthetic doses, barbiturates can help reduce mortality from head injury; deep anesthesia reduces the brain's requirements for oxygen and glucose and thereby helps preserve CNS function.

Adverse Effects

Respiratory Depression. Barbiturates reduce ventilation by two mechanisms: (1) depression of brain stem neurogenic respiratory drive, and (2) depression of chemoreceptive mechanisms that control respiratory drive. Doses only three times greater than those needed to induce sleep can cause complete suppression of the neurogenic respiratory drive. With severe overdosage, barbiturates can cause apnea and death.

For most patients, the degree of respiratory depression produced at therapeutic doses is not clinically significant. However, in elderly patients and those with respiratory disease, therapeutic doses can compromise respiration substantially.

Combining a barbiturate with another CNS depressant will intensify respiratory depression.

When barbiturates are employed in anesthetic doses during labor and delivery, respiratory depression may occur in the neonate. The infant should be monitored until respiration is normal.

Suicide. Barbiturates have a low therapeutic index. Accordingly, overdosage can readily result in death. Because of their toxicity, the barbiturates are frequently employed as vehicles for suicide. These drugs should not be dispensed to patients suspected of suicidal tendencies.

Abuse. Barbiturates produce subjective effects that many individuals find desirable. As a result, barbiturates have been popular drugs of abuse. The barbiturates that are most prone to abuse are those in the short-to-intermediate–acting group (e.g., secobarbital). Individual barbiturates within the group are classified under Schedule II or Schedule III of the Controlled Substances Act. These classifications reflect a high potential for abuse. Although barbiturates are frequently abused in nonmedical settings, they are rarely abused during medical use.

Use in Pregnancy. Barbiturates readily cross the placenta and can injure the developing fetus. Women of child-bearing age should be informed about the potential for fetal harm and warned against becoming pregnant. Use of barbiturates during the third trimester may cause drug dependence in the infant.

Exacerbation of Intermittent Porphyria. Barbiturates can intensify attacks of acute intermittent porphyria, a condition brought on by excessive synthesis of porphyrin. Symptoms include nausea, vomiting, abdominal colic, neuromuscular disturbances, and disturbed behavior. Barbiturates exacerbate porphyria by stimulating porphyrin synthesis (see Figure 27–2). Because of their ability to intensify porphyria, barbiturates are *absolutely contraindicated* for individuals with a history of the disorder.

Hangover. Barbiturates have long half-lives and, therefore, can produce residual effects (hangover) when taken to treat insomnia. Hangover can manifest as sedation, impaired judgment, and reduced motor skills. Patients should be forewarned that their ability to perform complex tasks, both manual and intellectual, may be significantly decreased the day after taking a barbiturate to induce sleep.

Paradoxical Excitement. In some patients, especially the elderly and debilitated, barbiturates may cause excitation. The mechanism of this paradoxical response is not known.

Hyperalgesia. Barbiturates can intensify sensitivity to pain. In addition, these drugs may cause pain directly. Treatment has produced muscle pain, joint pain, and pain along nerves.

Drug Interactions

CNS Depressants. Drugs with CNS-depressant properties (e.g., barbiturates, benzodiazepines, alcohol, opioids, antihistamines) intensify each other's effects. If these agents are combined, the degree of CNS depression can be hazardous—perhaps even fatal. Accordingly, patients should be warned emphatically against combining barbiturates with alcohol and other drugs that can depress CNS function.

Interactions Resulting from Induction of Drug-Metabolizing Enzymes. As discussed above, barbiturates stimulate synthesis of hepatic drug-metabolizing enzymes, thereby accelerating metabolism of other drugs. Increased metabolism is of particular concern with *warfarin* (an anticoagulant), *oral contraceptives*, and *phenytoin* (an antiseizure agent). When these drugs are taken concurrently with a barbiturate, their dosages should be increased to account for accelerated degradation.

Following barbiturate withdrawal, rates of drug metabolism gradually decline to baseline values. Several weeks are required for this to occur. Drug dosages that had been increased to account for augmented metabolism must now be reduced to their pre-barbiturate amount.

Acute Toxicity

Acute intoxication with barbiturates is a medical emergency; left untreated, overdosage can be fatal. Poisoning is often the result of attempted suicide, although it can also occur by accident (usually in children and drug abusers). Since acute toxicity from barbiturates and other general CNS depressants is very similar, the discussion below applies to all of these drugs.

Symptoms. Acute barbiturate overdosage produces a classic triad of symptoms: *respiratory depression, coma,* and *pinpoint pupils.* (Pupils may later dilate as hypoxia from respiratory depression sets in.) The three classic symptoms are frequently accompanied by *hypotension* and *hypothermia.* Death is likely to be the result of pulmonary complications and renal failure.

Treatment. Proper management requires an intensive care unit. With vigorous treatment, most patients recover fully.

Treatment has two principal objectives: (1) removal of barbiturate from the body, and (2) maintenance of an adequate oxygen supply to the brain. Oxygenation can be maintained by keeping the airway patent and by administering oxygen.

Several measures can promote barbiturate removal. Unabsorbed drug can be removed from the stomach by gastric lavage and by induction of emesis (e.g., with apomorphine). A saline cathartic can reduce absorption by accelerating drug transit through the intestine. Drug that has been absorbed can be removed rapidly with hemodialysis. (Peritoneal dialysis is significantly slower.) Forced diuresis and alkalinization of urine may facilitate drug removal by the kidneys.

Steps should be taken to prevent hypotension and loss of body heat. Blood pressure can be supported with fluid replacement and dopamine. Body heat can be maintained with blankets and warming devices.

Barbiturate poisoning has no specific antidote. CNS stimulants should definitely *not* be employed. Not only are stimulants ineffective, they are dangerous: use of these drugs to treat barbiturate poisoning has been associated with a significant *increase* in mortality. Naloxone, a drug that can reverse poisoning by opioids, is not effective against poisoning by barbiturates.

Preparations, Dosage, and Administration

Routes. Barbiturates are administered orally, intravenously, intramuscularly, and by rectal suppository.

Oral. Oral administration is employed for daytime sedation and to treat insomnia. Patients should be warned not to increase the dosage or discontinue treatment without consulting the physician. Dosages should be reduced for elderly patients. When terminating therapy, the dosage should be gradually tapered.

Intravenous. Intravenous administration is reserved for general anesthesia and emergency treatment of convulsions. Injections should be made slowly to minimize respiratory depression and hypotension. Blood pressure, pulses, and respiration should be monitored, and facilities for resuscitation should be available. The patient should be under continuous observation. Extravasation may result in local necrosis; hence, care must be taken to insure that extravasation does not occur. Solutions that are cloudy or that contain a precipitate should not be used. Intra-arterial injection should be avoided, since using this route may cause arteriospasm of sufficient duration to cause gangrene.

Intramuscular. Barbiturate solutions are highly alkaline and can cause pain and necrosis when injected IM. Consequently, IM injection is generally avoided. Injection in the vicinity of peripheral nerves can cause irreversible neurologic injury.

Preparations and Dosage. Preparations and dosages for treatment of insomnia are summarized in Table 27–4. Preparations and dosages for treatment of epilepsy are presented in Chapter 22.

NONBENZODIAZEPINE-NONBARBITURATES

BUSPIRONE

Buspirone [BuSpar] is a new and different antianxiety medication. The drug has minimal CNS-depressant actions, and does not enhance the depressant effects of alcohol, barbiturates, and other general CNS depressants. Buspirone is said to reduce anxiety while producing even less sedation than the benzodiazepines. The drug is devoid of hypnotic, muscle relaxant, and anticonvulsant actions.

Mechanism of Action. The mechanism by which buspirone acts has not been established. The drug binds with high affinity to receptors for serotonin and with lower affinity to receptors for dopamine. Buspirone does not bind to receptors for GABA or benzodiazepines.

Pharmacokinetics. Buspirone is well absorbed following oral administration, but undergoes extensive metabolism on its first pass through the liver. Administration with food delays absorption but enhances bioavailability by reducing first-pass metabolism. The drug is excreted in part by the kidneys, primarily as metabolites.

Therapeutic Use. Buspirone is labeled for *short-term* treatment of *anxiety*. However, when taken for as long as 1 year, the drug showed no reduction in antianxiety actions. For treatment of anxiety, the drug appears to be as effective as benzodiazepines. Buspirone lacks sedative effects and is not indicated for insomnia. Use of buspirone is discussed further under *Management of Anxiety* later in the chapter.

Adverse Effects and Interactions. Buspirone is generally well tolerated. The most common reactions are *dizziness, nausea, headache, nervousness, lightheadedness,* and *excitement*. The drug is nonsedative and does not interfere with daytime activities. Furthermore, the drug poses little or no risk of suicide; huge doses (375 mg/day) have been given to healthy volunteers with only moderate effects (nausea, vomiting, dizziness, drowsiness, miosis). Buspirone does not enhance the depressant effects of alcohol, barbiturates, and other general CNS depressants.

Tolerance, Dependence, and Abuse. Buspirone has been used for up to 1 year without evidence of tolerance, physical dependence, or psychologic dependence. No withdrawal symptoms have been observed upon termination of treatment. There is no cross-tolerance between buspirone and benzodiazepines, barbiturates, or other sedative-hypnotics.

To date there is no evidence that buspirone has a liability for abuse. The drug is not regulated under the Controlled Substances Act.

Preparations, Dosage, and Administration. Buspirone [BuSpar] is dispensed in tablets (5 and 10 mg) for oral administration. The usual initial dosage is 5 mg three times a day. Daily dosage may be increased to a maximum of 60 mg.

ZOLPIDEM

Actions and Uses. Zolpidem [Ambien] is a new sedative-hypnotic approved for short-term management of *insomnia*. Although structurally unrelated to the benzodiazepines, zolpidem binds to the GABA receptor–chloride channel complex and shares some properties of the benzodiazepines. Like the benzodiazepines, zolpidem can reduce sleep latency and awakenings and can prolong sleep duration. The drug does not significantly reduce time in REM sleep, and causes little or no rebound insomnia when therapy is discontinued. In contrast to the benzodiazepines, zolpidem lacks anxiolytic, muscle relaxant, and anticonvulsant actions.

Pharmacokinetics. Zolpidem is rapidly absorbed following oral administration. Plasma levels peak in 2 hours. The drug is widely distributed throughout the body, although levels in the brain remain low. Zolpidem is extensively metabolized to inactive compounds that are excreted in the bile, urine, and feces. The drug's half-life is about 2.4 hours.

Adverse Effects. Zolpidem has a side-effect profile like that of the benzodiazepines. *Daytime drowsiness* and *dizziness* are most common, and these occur in only 1% to 2% of patients. At therapeutic doses, zolpidem causes little or no respiratory depression. Safety in pregnancy has not been established.

Tolerance, Dependence, and Abuse. Short-term treatment is not associated with significant tolerance or physical dependence. Withdrawal symptoms are minimal or absent. Similarly, the abuse liability of zolpidem is low. Accordingly, the drug is classified under Schedule IV of the Controlled Substances Act.

Drug Interactions. Like other sedative-hypnotics, zolpidem can intensify the effects of *CNS depressants*. Accordingly, patients should be warned against combining zolpidem with alcohol and all other drugs that can depress CNS function.

Preparations, Dosage, and Administration. Zolpidem [Ambien] is available in 5- and 10-mg tablets for oral use. The usual dosage is 10 mg. The initial dosage should be reduced to 5 mg for elderly and debilitated patients and for those with hepatic insufficiency. Since zolpidem has a rapid onset of action, it should be taken just prior to bedtime to minimize sedation while awake.

MISCELLANEOUS GENERAL CNS DEPRESSANTS

Basic Pharmacologic Profile

The drugs considered in this section have properties very much like those of the barbiturates. All of these agents produce relatively nonselective depression of CNS function.

All of the nonselective CNS depressants are potentially dangerous. These drugs are respiratory depressants and can be lethal in overdosage. Accordingly, these drugs should not be given to patients suspected of suicidal tendencies.

At therapeutic doses, the nonselective CNS depressants can cause substantial drowsiness. Patients should be warned to avoid driving and other hazardous activities.

Concurrent use of these drugs with other CNS depressants (e.g., alcohol, barbiturates, benzodiazepines, opioids, antihistamines) can produce profound depression of CNS function. Accordingly, combinations of CNS depressants should be avoided.

Prolonged use can produce tolerance and physical dependence. Consequently, these agents should be reserved for short-term therapy. In patients who have been treated long-term, termination should be done gradually to minimize the withdrawal reaction.

Many of the nonselective CNS depressants produce subjective effects that individuals prone to drug abuse consider desirable. Because of this abuse potential, agents in this group are classified under Schedule III or IV of the Controlled Substances Act.

In general, acute overdosage resembles poisoning with barbiturates. Characteristic signs are respiratory depression, coma, miosis, and hypotension. Management is the same as with poisoning by barbiturates.

Nonselective CNS depressants should be avoided during pregnancy and lactation. Certain of these agents may cause birth defects if taken during the first trimester. In addition, if these drugs are taken late in pregnancy, the infant may be born drug dependent. The CNS depressants can achieve concentrations in breast milk that are sufficient to cause lethargy in the infant. Nursing mothers should avoid these drugs.

The principal indication for the nonselective CNS depressants is insomnia. Treatment should be short-term. Dosages are summarized in Table 27–4.

Chloral Hydrate

Chloral hydrate [Noctec] is a general CNS depressant with properties similar to those of the barbiturates. Chloral is a prodrug that undergoes rapid conversion to its active form in the liver. The drug's principal application is induction of sleep.

Chloral hydrate is dispensed in capsules, a syrup, and suppositories. Patients should be instructed to swallow the capsules intact, without crushing or chewing. The syrup formulation should be diluted with water, fruit juice, or ginger ale. With oral administration, epigastric distress, nausea, and flatulence are common.

The recommended dosage is 0.5 to 1 gm 30 minutes before bedtime. However, doses in this range are frequently too low to induce sleep. To elicit an adequate response, a dose as large as 2 gm may be needed.

Chloral hydrate is subject to abuse and is classified as a Schedule IV drug. Abuse is similar to that seen in alcoholism. Prolonged consumption of chloral results in substantial tolerance and physical dependence. As a result, chloral addicts may ingest extremely large amounts of the drug. Abrupt withdrawal can cause delirium and seizures. Left untreated, the abstinence syndrome can be fatal.

Glutethimide

Glutethimide [Doriden] is a general CNS depressant with properties similar to those of the barbiturates. In addition, the drug has prominent *anticholinergic* actions. Like the barbiturates, glutethimide can intensify episodes of intermittent porphyria and is contraindicated for patients with this disorder. Acute poisoning produces CNS depression together with anticholinergic responses (e.g., dry mouth, visual disturbance, decreased intestinal motility, atony of the urinary bladder, hyperpyrexia). Glutethimide is a Schedule III drug with an abuse liability like that of the barbiturates.

Glutethimide is indicated for short-term (3 to 7 days) management of insomnia. However, because superior agents are available, and because toxicity can be difficult to manage, it would seem that glutethimide has little to recommend its use. The drug is dispensed in 250- and 500-mg tablets. The usual adult dosage is 250 to 500 mg at bedtime.

Meprobamate

Meprobamate [Miltown, Equanil, others] has pharmacologic properties that lie midway between those of the barbiturates and the benzodiazepines. As a CNS depressant, meprobamate is more selective than the barbiturates but less selective than the benzodiazepines. Meprobamate induces hepatic drug-metabolizing enzymes and can exacerbate intermittent porphyria. Although meprobamate is approved only for treatment of anxiety, the drug is also employed to induce sleep. The usual adult

dosage for anxiety is 1.2 to 1.6 gm/day in three or four divided doses. Meprobamate is classified as a Schedule IV drug.

Paraldehyde

Paraldehyde [Paral] is a CNS depressant with multiple undesirable properties. The drug has a strong odor and unpleasant taste. When administered orally, the drug irritates the throat and stomach; when injected intramuscularly, the drug can produce local necrosis and nerve injury; when injected intravenously, the drug can cause cyanosis, pulmonary edema, hypotension, and venous thrombosis.

Solutions of paraldehyde decompose rapidly to acetic acid. Preparations that smell strongly of acetic acid (i.e., that smell like vinegar) should be discarded. Since decomposition occurs rapidly, paraldehyde in containers that have been open for more than 24 hours should not be used.

Poisoning with paraldehyde is quite different from poisoning with other CNS depressants. In addition to causing respiratory depression and hypotension, paraldehyde causes prominent metabolic acidosis. Symptoms of toxicity include rapid, labored breathing; bleeding gastritis; toxic hepatitis; nephrosis; pulmonary hemorrhage; and edema. An oral dose of 25 ml can be fatal.

The principal indications for paraldehyde are induction of sleep and treatment of alcoholic delirium tremens. The drug is employed almost exclusively in hospitals and institutions. Use by outpatients is rare. Despite its undesirable effects, paraldehyde still has some advocates. Given the availability of clearly superior alternatives, the continued use of this drug is mystifying.

The usual oral dosage for adults is 4 to 8 ml diluted in milk or iced fruit juice to mask the drug's taste. Paraldehyde is a Schedule IV drug and must be dispensed accordingly.

Ethchlorvynol

Ethchlorvynol [Placidyl] is a CNS depressant with a rapid onset and short duration of action. Side effects include dizziness, hypotension, facial numbness, and a mint-like aftertaste. Like the barbiturates, ethchlorvynol can exacerbate acute intermittent porphyria. Ethchlorvynol is classified under Schedule IV and is approved only for short-term management of insomnia. The usual adult dosage is 500 to 1000 mg at bedtime.

Methyprylon

Methyprylon has pharmacologic effects similar to those of the barbiturates. Like the barbiturates, methyprylon can induce hepatic drug-metabolizing enzymes and can exacerbate acute intermittent porphyria. When the drug is administered in therapeutic doses, serious adverse effects are rare. Overdosage causes respiratory depression, hypotension, pulmonary edema, and shock. The only indication for the drug is short-term management of insomnia. The usual adult dosage is 200 to 400 mg before bedtime.

MANAGEMENT OF ANXIETY

Anxiety is a nearly universal experience that often serves an adaptive function. When anxiety is moderate and situationally appropriate, drug therapy may not be needed or even desirable. In contrast, for patients with generalized anxiety disorder, symptoms are prolonged and potentially disabling; hence, anxiolytic therapy is frequently required.

Situational Anxiety versus Generalized Anxiety Disorder

Situational Anxiety. Situational anxiety is a normal response to a stressful situation (e.g., family problems, exams, financial difficulties). Although symptoms may be intense, they are also temporary. If necessary, drugs can be used to provide relief, but treatment should be short-term. Situational anxiety is common among patients with medical illnesses and those anticipating surgery.

Generalized Anxiety Disorder (GAD). The hallmark of GAD is unrealistic or excessive anxiety about two or more life circumstances that lasts for 6 months or longer. Other psychologic manifestations include vigilance, tension, apprehension, poor concentration, and difficulty falling asleep or staying asleep. Somatic manifestations include trembling, muscle tension, restlessness, and signs of autonomic hyperactivity (e.g., palpitations, tachycardia, sweating, clammy hands).

Treatment of GAD consists of psychotherapy and anxiolytic drugs. Psychotherapy provides support and encouragement and can improve coping abilities in anxiety-provoking situations. For some patients this may be all that is needed. However, if symptoms are intensely uncomfortable or disabling, antianxiety drugs are indicated. In most cases, benzodiazepines are preferred. Along with psychotherapy and drugs, the treatment program can include relaxation therapy (meditation, relaxation exercises, biofeedback) to reduce tension.

Drugs Used to Treat Anxiety

Benzodiazepines. Benzodiazepines are drugs of first choice for anxiety. These widely used agents have rendered older anxiolytics obsolete. Since all benzodiazepines have very similar CNS effects, selection among these drugs is largely a matter of physician's preference. Dosages for anxiety are summarized in Table 27–3.

Since the introduction of the benzodiazepines in the 1960's, attitudes toward these drugs have changed. When they first became available, benzodiazepines were used somewhat indiscriminately. In all probability, many people who didn't really need these drugs were receiving them. Because of the freedom with which benzodiazepines had been dispensed, physicians were sometimes accused of poor medical practice. Furthermore, the frequent use of benzodiazepines led to public concerns about "addiction." In response to these developments, two changes took place: (1) physicians restricted their prescribing of benzodiazepines, and (2) patients tended to self-administer less drug than had been prescribed. The unfortunate result is that overtreatment was to some extent replaced with undertreatment.

The current consensus is that the benzodiazepines have a completely legitimate role in the therapy of severe anxiety and that these drugs, like all others, must simply be used with discretion. When they are clearly indicated, benzodiazepines should be prescribed in a sufficient dosage and for a sufficient duration to achieve their objective: relief of symptoms and improvement of overall function. To help insure that benzodiazepines are taken as prescribed, patients should be made to feel that their use of an anxiolytic is appropriate and that they should not be ashamed of their legitimate medical need. Also, patients should be made aware that significant tolerance and physical dependence are unlikely.

It is difficult to predict how long anxiolytic drugs should be taken. To determine the need for continued therapy, patients should be re-evaluated on a regular basis. In some cases, use of an "on-off" dosing schedule may be helpful. In such a regimen, treatment is interrupted periodically (e.g., every 6 to 8 weeks). If anxiety returns, treatment can resume.

Buspirone. Buspirone [BuSpar] is an alternative to the benzodiazepines for treating anxiety. This drug differs from benzodiazepines in four important ways: (1) it does not cause sedation, (2) it has no abuse potential, (3) it does not potentiate other CNS depressants, and (4) its antianxiety effects take a week to begin and several weeks to reach their peak. Because therapeutic effects are delayed, buspirone is not suitable for patients who need immediate relief, nor is it suitable for PRN use. Since buspirone has no abuse potential, the drug may be especially appropriate for patients known to abuse alcohol and other drugs. Because it lacks depressant properties, buspirone is an attractive alternative to benzodiazepines in patients who require long-term therapy but who cannot tolerate benzodiazepine-induced sedation and psychomotor slowing. Buspirone does not display cross-dependence with benzodiazepines. Hence, when patients are switched from benzodiazepines to buspirone, the benzodiazepine should be tapered off prior to initiating buspirone. Patients who have taken benzodiazepines should be told that buspirone will not produce sedation and that its effects will take a week or more to develop; this information will allow expectations to be realistic.

Beta Blockers. Beta-adrenergic blocking agents (e.g., propranolol) can relieve symptoms caused by autonomic hyperactivity (tachycardia, palpitations, tremor, sweating). These drugs may be most valuable as an aid to coping with situational anxiety, such as that experienced by individuals who are overly apprehensive about public speaking.

MANAGEMENT OF INSOMNIA

Sleep Physiology

Sleep is a complex state characterized by a reduced level of consciousness and minimal physical activity. The sleeping state has two primary divisions: *rapid-eye-movement* (REM) sleep and *non-rapid-eye-movement* (NREM) sleep. Sleeping begins with a period of NREM sleep, after which periods of REM sleep and NREM sleep alternate until waking takes place.

REM sleep is the phase during which most recallable dreams occur. A typical night's sleep has four to six REM periods, accounting for approximately 30% of total sleeping time. In males, penile erection is common during REM sleep. This phenomenon is independent of dream content. Except for the benzodiazepines, the drugs used to remedy sleep disorders often reduce the total time spent in REM sleep.

The precise physiologic benefits of sleep have not been established. Some studies suggest that deprivation of REM sleep can produce adverse psychologic reactions; other studies do not support this conclusion. Regardless of the value that specific stages of sleep may or may not have, one thing is clear: when we don't get enough sleep, we tend to be drowsy the next day and less able to function. If fatigue or reduced alertness compromise daytime performance, some form of intervention may be needed.

Causes of Insomnia

Insomnia is defined as an inability to fall asleep or to maintain sleep. About 10% of people in the United States feel they have a significant insomnia problem.

Loss of sleep is often related to medical conditions. Pain keeps people awake. Sleep disturbances are common in patients with psychiatric disorders. Sleep is frequently lost because of concern over impending surgery and other procedures.

At one time or another, nearly everyone suffers from *situational insomnia*. Worry about exams may keep students awake. Job-related pressures may deprive workers of sleep. Unfamiliar surroundings may render sleeping difficult for travelers. Major life stressors (bereavement, divorce, loss of job) frequently disrupt sleep. Other factors, such as uncomfortable bedding, excessive noise, and bright light, can deprive most anyone of sound sleep.

Management Strategy

Treatment is highly dependent on the cause of insomnia. Accordingly, if therapy is to be successful, the underlying reason for sleep loss must be determined. To make this assessment, a thorough history is required.

Nondrug Management. Not everyone with insomnia should be treated with drugs. For some individuals, avoidance of naps and adherence to a regular sleep schedule will be sufficient. For others, decreased consumption of caffeine-containing beverages (e.g., coffee, tea, cola drinks) may be all that is needed. Still others may benefit from restful activity as bedtime approaches. If the history reveals that environmental factors are responsible for lack of sleep, the patient should be advised in ways to correct these factors or to compensate for them. All patients should be counseled about good sleep hygiene (Table 27–6).

Cause-Specific Drug Therapy. When the cause of insomnia is a known medical disorder, hypnotics should not be employed routinely. Rather, medication specific to the primary illness is indicated. For example, if pain is the reason for lack of sleep, analgesics should be prescribed. If insomnia is secondary to major depression, antidepressants are the appropriate treatment. If anxiety is the cause of insomnia, the patient should be given an anxiolytic.

Therapy with Hypnotic Drugs. Hypnotics should be reserved for those patients whose insomnia cannot be managed by other means. If nondrug measures can relieve insomnia, hypnotics should be avoided. Likewise, if insomnia is secondary to an identified and treatable pathology, specific therapies directed at that pathology are clearly preferable to use of hypnotics.

Guidelines for Using Hypnotic Drugs to Treat Insomnia

Drug therapy of insomnia should be short-term. Insomnia is a self-limiting condition and, hence, should not require prolonged treatment. The patient should be reassessed on a regular basis to determine if drug therapy is still needed. If insomnia persists, an underlying pathology may well be the cause. Every effort should be made to diagnose

---

Table 27–6. Measures for Good Sleep Hygiene

1. Establish a regular time to go to bed and a regular time to rise.
2. If you do not fall asleep within 20 to 30 minutes, get up and do something relaxing (e.g., read, listen to music, watch television), and then return to bed when you feel drowsy. Repeat as often as required.
3. Avoid long periods of wakefulness in bed. Don't use your bed for reading or working.
4. Avoid daytime naps.
5. Exercise several days a week, but no later than 3 to 4 hours before bedtime.
6. Create a sleep environment that is comfortable and devoid of loud noises, extreme temperatures, and illuminated clocks.
7. Minimize or eliminate use of alcohol, caffeine, and nicotine.
8. Avoid gastric fullness or hunger at bedtime.
9. Minimize nocturia by minimizing fluid consumption in the evening.

this pathology rather than cover it up with continued use of hypnotics.

Escalation of dosage should be avoided. A need for increased dosage suggests development of tolerance. If hypnotic effects are lost in the course of treatment, it is preferable to interrupt therapy rather than elevate dosage. Interruption will allow tolerance to decline, thereby restoring responsiveness to treatment.

In certain patients, hypnotics must be employed with special caution. Patients who snore heavily and patients with respiratory disorders have reduced respiratory reserve; this low reserve can be further compromised by the respiratory depressant actions of hypnotics. Hypnotic agents are generally contraindicated for use during pregnancy; these drugs have the potential for causing fetal harm, and their use is never an absolute necessity. Except for the benzodiazepines, most hypnotics can be lethal if taken in overdose. Accordingly, these drugs should not be given to individuals suspected of suicidal tendencies.

Patients taking hypnotics should be forewarned that residual CNS depression may be present the following day. Although CNS depression may not be pronounced, it may nonetheless be sufficient to compromise intellectual or physical performance.

When hypnotics are employed, care must be taken to prevent *drug-dependency insomnia*, a condition that can lead to inappropriate prolongation of therapy. Drug-dependency insomnia is a particular problem with the barbiturates, and develops as follows: (1) Insomnia motivates treatment with hypnotics. (2) With continuous drug use, low-level physical dependence develops. (3) Upon cessation of treatment, a mild withdrawal syndrome occurs and disrupts sleep. (4) Failing to recognize that the inability to sleep is a manifestation of drug withdrawal, the patient becomes convinced that insomnia has returned and resumes drug use. (5) Continued drug use leads to heightened physical dependence, making it even more difficult to withdraw medication without producing another episode of drug-dependency insomnia. To minimize drug-dependency insomnia, hypnotics should be employed judiciously. That is, they should be used in the lowest effective dosage for the shortest time required.

Drugs Used to Treat Insomnia

Prescription drugs employed to promote sleep include benzodiazepines, barbiturates, and other general CNS depressants (see Table 27–4). In addition, several over-the-counter sleep aids are available.

The various hypnotic drugs have similarities and differences regarding their effects on sleep. Properties shared by all hypnotics are the ability to accelerate onset of sleep and to maintain sleep. Important differences exist with respect to (1)

suppression of REM sleep, (2) tolerance to hypnotic effects, and (3) tendency to promote rebound insomnia (drug-dependency insomnia).

Benzodiazepines. Benzodiazepines are drugs of first choice for insomnia. These agents are safe, effective, and lack the undesirable properties typical of other hypnotics. Benzodiazepines have a low abuse potential, cause minimal tolerance and physical dependence, present a minimal risk of suicide, and undergo few interactions with other drugs.

Benzodiazepines have multiple desirable effects related to sleep. They decrease the latency to sleep onset; they decrease the number of awakenings; and they increase total sleeping time. In addition, they impart a sense of deep and refreshing sleep. Tolerance to hypnotic actions develops very slowly; benzodiazepines can be taken nightly for several weeks without a noticeable loss in hypnotic effects. Treatment does not significantly reduce the amount of REM sleep, and there is no rebound increase in REM sleep when treatment stops. Furthermore, withdrawal of benzodiazepines is not associated with significant rebound insomnia.

Only five benzodiazepines are marketed specifically for use as hypnotics (see Table 27–4). However, any benzodiazepine with a short-to-intermediate onset could be employed. Two agents—*flurazepam* [Dalmane] and *triazolam* [Halcion]—can be thought of as prototypes of the benzodiazepines used to promote sleep.

The kinetic properties of *triazolam* make this drug especially well suited for treating insomnia. Triazolam is very lipid soluble and, therefore, has a rapid onset of action. In addition, the drug has a short half-life; hence, by morning, plasma drug levels are usually low. As a result, triazolam has little tendency to interfere with daytime function. Curiously, although flurazepam has a very long half-life, this agent, like triazolam, produces minimal daytime sedation.

Barbiturates. The barbiturates are a distant second choice to the benzodiazepines for relieving insomnia. Barbiturates are hazardous and have a high potential for abuse. Tolerance, dependence, and a host of drug interactions further decrease their desirability. Although several barbiturates are approved for insomnia (see Table 27–4), these agents have been largely abandoned in favor of the benzodiazepines.

Several sleep-related effects of the barbiturates differ from those of the benzodiazepines. At the beginning of therapy, barbiturates tend to suppress REM sleep. However, with continued treatment, time spent in REM sleep returns to normal. "Hangover" and residual daytime sedation are relatively common. Tolerance develops rapidly to hypnotic effects; hence, if barbiturates are taken on a routine basis, dosage must be increased periodically to maintain a response. Withdrawal of barbiturates is associated with rebound insomnia and increased REM sleep.

Secobarbital [Seconal], a short-to-intermediate–acting barbiturate, can be considered the prototype of the barbiturates employed to promote sleep. The drug has a rapid onset of action and, therefore, can benefit patients who have difficulty falling asleep. Elimination of secobarbital is relatively rapid. Hence, daytime sedation is less intense than with with long-acting barbiturates.

Other Prescription Sleep Aids. Nonbenzodiazepine-nonbarbiturate hypnotics are listed in Table 27–4. Pharmacologic effects of these drugs are like those of the barbiturates. Benzodiazepines are almost always preferred.

Nonprescription Sleep Aids. Over-the-counter sleep aids (e.g., Compoz, Sominex) contain an *antihistamine* (diphenhydramine, pyrilamine, or doxylamine) as their active ingredient.

Although sedation can be a prominent side effect when antihistamines are taken to treat allergies, relief of insomnia is not always impressive. Antihistamines are less effective than the benzodiazepines, and frequently cause anticholinergic side effects.

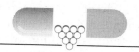

Summary of Major Nursing Implications

BENZODIAZEPINES

The nursing implications summarized here apply to the benzodiazepines as a group and to their use for treating anxiety and insomnia.

 Preadministration Assessment

Therapeutic Goal

Benzodiazepines are used to promote sleep, relieve symptoms of anxiety, suppress seizure disorders (see Chapter 22), relax muscle spasm (see Chapter 23), and ease withdrawal from alcohol (see Chapter 34). They are also used for preanesthetic medication and to induce general anesthesia (see Chapter 30).

Baseline Data

For Insomnia. Determine the nature of the sleep disturbance (prolonged latency, frequent awakenings, early morning awakening) and how long it has lasted. Assess for a possible underlying cause (e.g., medical illness, psychiatric illness, use of caffeine and other stimulants, poor sleep hygiene, major life stressor).

For Anxiety. Determine the nature, duration, and intensity of symptoms. Situational anxiety must be differentiated from generalized anxiety disorder.

Identifying High-Risk Patients

Benzodiazepines are *contraindicated* during *pregnancy* and for patients who experience *sleep apnea.* Use with *caution* in patients with *suicidal tendencies* and a *history of substance abuse.*

 Implementation: Administration

Routes

Oral: *all* benzodiazepines.
IM and IV: *diazepam, chlordiazepoxide,* and *lorazepam.*

Administration

Oral. Advise patients to administer benzodiazepines with food if gastric upset occurs. Instruct patients to swallow sustained-release formulations intact, without crushing or chewing.

Warn patients not to increase the dosage or discontinue treatment without consulting the physician.

To minimize physical dependence when treating insomnia, administer intermittently (three or four nights a week) and use the lowest effective dosage for the shortest duration required.

To minimize the abstinence syndrome, taper the dosage gradually (over several weeks).

Intravenous. Perform IV injections with care. Life-threatening reactions (severe hypotension, respiratory arrest, cardiac arrest) have occurred, along with less serious reactions (venous thrombosis, phlebitis, vascular impairment). To reduce complications, follow these guidelines: (1) make injections slowly; (2) take care to avoid intra-arterial injection and extravasation; (3) if direct venous injection is impossible, inject into infusion tubing as close to the vein as possible; (4) follow the manufacturer's instructions regarding suitable diluents for preparing solutions; and (5) have facilities for resuscitation available.

<table>
<tr><td>✓ **Implementation: Measures to Enhance Therapeutic Effects**</td></tr>
</table>

For Insomnia. Educate patients about good sleep hygiene (see Table 27–6). Reassure patients with situational insomnia that sleep patterns will normalize once the precipitating stressor has been eliminated. Insure that correctable underlying causes of insomnia (psychiatric or medical illness, use of stimulant drugs) are being managed.

For Anxiety. Encourage patients with generalized anxiety disorder to take their medicine as prescribed. Reassure them that significant physical dependence on benzodiazepines is rare. Hence, they should not allow concerns about "addiction" to interfere with compliance.

Ideally, patients will receive psychotherapy, which can provide support, encouragement, and skills for coping with anxiety-provoking situations.

Relaxation therapy (meditation, relaxation exercises, biofeedback) can help reduce tension.

✓ **Ongoing Evaluation and Interventions**

Evaluating Therapeutic Effects

For Insomnia. Insomnia is usually self-limiting. Consequently, drug therapy is usually short-term. Benzodiazepines should be discontinued periodically to determine if they are still required. If insomnia is long-term, make a special effort to identify possible underlying causes (e.g., psychiatric illness, medical illness, use of caffeine and other stimulants).

For Anxiety. For generalized anxiety disorder, benzodiazepines can be discontinued periodically (e.g., every 6 to 8 weeks) to determine if they are still needed.

Minimizing Adverse Effects

CNS Depression. Drowsiness may be present on the day following hypnotic use of benzodiazepines. Warn patients about possible residual CNS depression and advise them to avoid hazardous activities (e.g., driving) if daytime sedation is significant.

Paradoxical Effects. Inform patients about possible paradoxical reactions (rage, excitement, heightened anxiety), and instruct them to notify the physician if these occur. If the reaction is verified, benzodiazepines should be withdrawn.

Physical Dependence. With most benzodiazepines significant physical dependence is rare. However, with one agent—*alprazolam* [Xanax]—substantial dependence has been reported. With all benzodiazepines, development of dependence can be minimized by using the lowest effective dosage for the shortest time necessary and by using intermittent dosing when treating insomnia.

When dependence is mild, withdrawal can elicit insomnia and other symptoms that resemble anxiety. These symptoms must be distinguished from a return of the patient's original anxiety state or sleep disorder. Warn patients about possible drug-dependency insomnia during or after benzodiazepine withdrawal.

When dependence is severe, withdrawal reactions may be serious (panic, paranoia, delirium, hypertension, convulsions). To minimize symptoms, withdraw benzodiazepines slowly (over several weeks). Warn patients against abrupt discontinuation of treatment. After drug cessation, patients should be monitored for 3 weeks for signs of withdrawal or recurrence of original symptoms.

Abuse. The abuse potential of the benzodiazepines is low. However, these drugs *are* abused by some individuals. Be alert to requests for increased dosage, since these may reflect an attempt at abuse. Benzodiazepines are classified under Schedule IV of the Controlled Substances Act and must be dispensed accordingly.

Use in Pregnancy and Lactation. Benzodiazepines may injure the developing fetus, especially during the first trimester. Inform women of childbearing age about the potential for fetal harm and warn them against becoming pregnant. If pregnancy occurs, benzodiazepines should be withdrawn.

Benzodiazepines readily enter breast milk and may accumulate to toxic levels in the breast-fed infant. Warn mothers against breast-feeding.

Minimizing Adverse Interactions

CNS Depressants. Combined overdosage with a benzodiazepine plus another CNS depressant can cause profound respiratory depression, coma, and death. Warn patients against use of alcohol and all other CNS depressants (e.g., opioids, barbiturates, antihistamines).

BARBITURATES

The nursing implications summarized below pertain to the barbiturates as a group. Implications specific to *phenobarbital* in the treatment of epilepsy are summarized in Chapter 22.

✓ Preadministration Assessment

Therapeutic Goal

Barbiturates are used to promote sleep (see Table 27–4), suppress seizures (see Chapter 22), and induce general anesthesia (see Chapter 30).

Baseline Data

For patients with *insomnia*, determine the nature of the sleep disturbance (prolonged latency, frequent awakenings, early morning awakening) and how long it has lasted. Assess for a possible underlying cause (e.g., medical illness, psychiatric illness, use of caffeine and other stimulants, poor sleep hygiene, major life stressor).

Identifying High-Risk Patients

Barbiturates are *contraindicated* for patients with *severe respiratory disease* and *active or latent porphyria*. Also, these drugs should not be dispensed to individuals suspected of *suicidal tendencies* or those with a *history of sedative-hypnotic abuse*. Use with caution in *elderly patients* and those with *respiratory disease*.

**Implementation:
Administration**

Routes

Oral, IV, IM, and rectal.

Administration

Oral. Warn patients not to increase the dosage or discontinue treatment without consulting the physician. Dosages should be reduced for elderly patients.

Intravenous. Make injections slowly to minimize respiratory depression and hypotension. Monitor blood pressure, pulses, and respiration. Have facilities for resuscitation immediately available. Observe the patient continuously. Do not inject solutions that are cloudy or that contain a precipitate. Extravasation may cause local necrosis; take care to insure that extravasation does not occur. Intra-arterial administration may cause gangrene (secondary to arteriospasm) and must be avoided.

Intramuscular. Barbiturate solutions are highly alkaline and can cause pain and necrosis when injected IM. Consequently, IM injection is generally avoided. Avoid injection in the vicinity of peripheral nerves since irreversible nerve damage may result.

 **Ongoing
Evaluation and
Interventions**

Evaluating Therapeutic Effects

Since insomnia is usually self-limiting, drug therapy should be short-term. If insomnia is long-term, make a special effort to identify a possible underlying cause (e.g., psychiatric illness, medical illness, use of caffeine and other stimulants).

Minimizing Adverse Effects

CNS Depression. Inform patients about symptoms of CNS depression (sedation, lethargy, incoordination), and warn them against participation in hazardous activities (e.g., driving, operating machinery). Hospitalized patients may require ambulatory assistance.

Respiratory Depression. Barbiturates are strong respiratory depressants. Use with caution in elderly patients and those with respiratory disease.
When administered in anesthetic doses during labor and delivery, barbiturates can depress respiration in the neonate. Monitor the infant until respiration is normal.

Tolerance. Tolerance develops with prolonged treatment, and cross-tolerance exists with other general CNS depressants, but not with opioids. If tolerance develops, temporary interruption of treatment is preferable to an increase in dosage. Warn patients against escalation of dosage without consulting the physician. To minimize tolerance, employ the lowest effective dosage for the shortest time necessary.

Physical Dependence. Physical dependence develops with prolonged treatment, and cross-dependence exists with other general CNS depressants but not with opioids. The barbiturate abstinence syndrome can be severe, possibly life threatening. Manifestations can be minimized by withdrawing barbiturates slowly. Warn patients against abrupt discontinuation of treatment.

Drug-Dependency Insomnia. When used to treat insomnia, barbiturates may cause drug-dependency insomnia upon cessation of treatment. This must be distinguished from re-emergence of the original sleep disorder. To minimize drug-dependency insomnia, administer barbiturates in the lowest effective dosage for the shortest time necessary.

Abuse. Barbiturates in the short-to-intermediate–acting category (e.g., secobarbital) have a high potential for abuse. Be alert to escalating requests for medication, since these may reflect attempts at abuse. Barbiturates are regulated under the Controlled Substances Act and must be dispensed accordingly.

Suicide. Barbiturates are "drugs of choice" for suicide. Do not dispense these drugs to patients suspected of suicidal tendencies.

Use in Pregnancy. Barbiturates readily cross the placenta and can injure the developing fetus. Inform women of child-bearing age about the potential for fetal harm and warn them against becoming pregnant.

Infants exposed to barbiturates during the third trimester may be born drug dependent; an abstinence syndrome may develop several days after parturition.

Minimizing Adverse Interactions

CNS Depressants. Combined use of barbiturates and other CNS depressants (e.g., benzodiazepines, alcohol, opioids) can cause profound respiratory depression, coma, and death. Warn patients against use of alcohol and all other CNS depressants.

Interactions Secondary to Accelerated Drug Metabolism. Barbiturates induce hepatic drug-metabolizing enzymes, thereby accelerating the degradation of other drugs. Increased metabolism is of particular concern with *warfarin, oral contraceptives,* and *phenytoin.* Advise women taking oral contraceptives to consider an alternative form of birth control.

Management of Toxicity

Overdosage can be life threatening. Manifestations include respiratory depression, coma, pinpoint pupils, and hypotension. Death may result from pulmonary complications or renal failure. Treatment requires an intensive care unit. Principal management objectives are removal of the drug and maintenance of oxygenation. There is no specific antidote to barbiturate poisoning; CNS stimulants should not be employed.

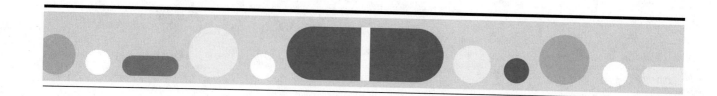

Analgesics

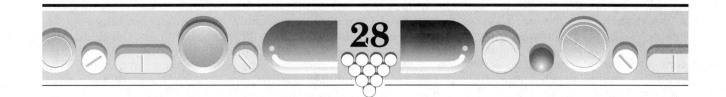

Opioid (Narcotic) Analgesics

Analgesics are drugs that relieve pain without causing loss of consciousness. As a group, the opioids are the most effective analgesics available. The opioid family, whose name derives from opium, includes such widely used agents as morphine, codeine, meperidine [Demerol], and propoxyphene [Darvon].

INTRODUCTION TO THE OPIOIDS

Terminology

Opioid is a general term defined as any drug, natural or synthetic, that has actions similar to those of morphine. The term *opiate* is more specific and applies only to compounds present in opium (e.g., morphine, codeine).

The term *narcotic* has had so many definitions that it can no longer be used with precision. Narcotic has been used to mean analgesic, central nervous system (CNS) depressant, and any drug capable of causing physical dependence. Narcotic has also been employed in a legal context to designate not only the opioids but also such diverse drugs as cocaine, marijuana, and lysergic acid diethylamide (LSD). Because of its more precise definition, *opioid* is clearly preferable to *narcotic* as a label for a discrete family of pharmacologic agents.

Opioid Receptors

The opioids act at multiple receptors both within and outside the CNS. The four most important opioid receptors are designated *mu, kappa, delta,* and *sigma*. Effects mediated by mu receptors include analgesia, respiratory depression, and euphoria. Like mu receptors, kappa and delta receptors also mediate analgesia. Activation of sigma receptors causes psychotomimetic reactions (e.g., hallucinations) and dysphoria. The major functions of mu, kappa, delta, and sigma receptors are summarized in Table 28–1.

Endogenous Opioid Peptides

The body produces three families of peptides that interact with opioid receptors. These peptides are named *enkephalins, endorphins,* and *dynorphins*. Although we know the endogenous opioid peptides serve as neurotransmitters and neurohormones, the precise physiologic role of these compounds is not fully understood. Endogenous opioid peptides are present within and outside the CNS.

Classification of the Opioid Drugs

The opioids are classified on the basis of their actions at opioid receptors. At each receptor type, an opioid can act in one of three ways: as an *agonist, partial agonist,* or *antagonist*. (As discussed in Chapter 6, a partial agonist is a drug that produces low to moderate receptor activation when administered alone, but will block the actions of a full agonist if the two drugs are given concurrently.) Using this basis of classification, the opioids fall into three major groups: (1) pure agonists, (2) mixed-acting agonist-antagonists, and (3) pure antagonists. The actions of drugs in these groups at mu, kappa, and delta receptors are summarized in Table 28–2.

Pure Opioid Agonists. The pure opioid agonists activate mu, kappa, and delta receptors. These drugs have no action at sigma receptors. By

activating mu, kappa, and delta receptors, the pure agonists can produce analgesia, euphoria, sedation, respiratory depression, physical dependence, constipation, and other effects. As indicated in Table 28–3, the pure agonists can be subdivided into two groups: *strong opioid agonists* and *moderate-to-strong opioid agonists*. Morphine is the prototype of the strong agonists. Codeine is the prototype of the moderate-to-strong agonists.

Agonist-Antagonist Opioids. In the United States, five agonist-antagonist opioids are available: pentazocine, nalbuphine, butorphanol, dezocine, and buprenorphine. The actions of these drugs at mu, kappa, and delta receptors are summarized in Table 28–2. When administered alone, the agonist-antagonist opioids produce analgesia. However, if given to a patient taking a pure opioid agonist, these drugs can *antagonize* analgesia caused by the pure agonist.

Pure Opioid Antagonists. The pure opioid antagonists act as antagonists at mu, kappa, and delta receptors. These drugs do not produce analgesia or any of the other effects caused by opioid agonists. The principal use for these agents is reversal of respiratory and CNS depression caused by overdosage with opioid agonists. Naloxone [Narcan] is the prototype of the pure antagonists.

BASIC PHARMACOLOGY OF THE OPIOIDS

MORPHINE

Morphine is the prototype of the strong opioid analgesics and remains the standard by which newer opioids are measured. Morphine has multiple pharmacologic effects, including analgesia, sedation, euphoria, respiratory depression, cough suppression, and suppression of bowel motility. The drug is named after Morpheus, the Greek god of dreams.

Source

Morphine is found in the seed pod of the poppy plant, *Papaver somniferum*. The drug is prepared by extraction from opium, which is the dried juice of the poppy seed pod. In addition to morphine, opium contains two other medicinal compounds: codeine (an analgesic) and papaverine (a smooth muscle relaxant).

Overview of Pharmacologic Actions

Morphine has multiple pharmacologic actions. In addition to relieving pain, the drug causes drowsiness, mental clouding, lowering of anxiety, and a sense of well-being. Through actions in the CNS and periphery, morphine can cause respiratory depression, constipation, urinary retention,

Table 28–1. Responses to Activation of Opioid Receptor Subtypes

Receptor Subtype	Response to Activation
Mu	Analgesia (supraspinal) Respiratory depression Miosis Reduced intestinal motility Euphoria Physical dependence
Kappa	Analgesia (spinal) Respiratory depression* Miosis* Sedation
Delta	Analgesia (spinal)
Sigma	Psychotomimetic effects

*Respiratory depression and miosis caused by kappa activation are less intense than with mu activation.

Table 28–2. Actions of Opioids at Specific Receptors			
	Receptor Type		
Drug	**Mu**	**Kappa**	**Delta**
Pure Agonists			
Morphine, codeine, meperidine, and other morphine-like drugs	Agonist	Agonist	Agonist
Agonist-Antagonists			
Pentazocine*	Antagonist	Agonist	
Nalbuphine	Antagonist	Agonist	
Butorphanol	Antagonist	Agonist	
Dezocine	Antagonist?	Agonist?	
Buprenorphine	Partial agonist	Antagonist	
Pure Antagonists			
Naloxone and naltrexone	Antagonist	Antagonist	Antagonist

*Pentazocine causes psychotomimetic effects through actions at sigma receptors.

orthostatic hypotension, emesis, miosis, cough suppression, and biliary colic. With prolonged treatment, the drug produces tolerance and physical dependence.

Individual effects of morphine may be beneficial, detrimental, or both. For example, analgesia is clearly beneficial, whereas effects such as respiratory depression and urinary retention are clearly detrimental. Certain other effects, such as sedation and reduced bowel motility, may be beneficial *or* detrimental, depending on the circumstances of drug use.

Therapeutic Use: Relief of Pain

The principal indication for morphine is relief of moderate to severe pain. The drug can relieve postoperative pain, chronic pain of cancer, and pain associated with labor and delivery. In addition, morphine is the drug of choice for relieving pain of myocardial infarction (MI) and dyspnea associated with left ventricular failure and pulmonary edema. Morphine may also be administered preoperatively for sedation and reduction of anxiety.

Morphine relieves pain without affecting other senses (e.g., sight, touch, smell, hearing) and without causing loss of consciousness. The drug is more effective against constant, dull pain than against sharp, intermittent pain. However, even sharp pain can be relieved by sufficiently large doses. The ability of morphine to cause mental clouding, sedation, euphoria, and anxiety reduction can contribute to relief of pain.

To understand morphine-induced analgesia, we need to understand pain itself. Pain has two components: *sensation* and *suffering* (emotional reaction to the sensation of pain). Morphine decreases both the sensation of pain as well as the suffering that pain elicits. For some patients, the suffering component may be reduced even though perception of pain remains relatively undiminished. Hence,

morphine may make the patient feel better without actually decreasing pain sensation. Accordingly, patients should not be told that morphine will make their pain go away, because it may not. Rather, patients should be told that morphine will make them feel more comfortable.

The use of morphine and other opioids to relieve pain is discussed in depth later in the chapter under *Clinical Use of Opioids*.

Mechanism of Analgesic Action. Morphine and other opioid agonists are thought to relieve pain by mimicking the actions of endogenous opioid peptides, primarily at mu receptors. This hypothesis is based on the following observations:

1. Opioid peptides and morphine-like drugs both produce analgesia when administered to experimental subjects.
2. Opioid peptides and morphine-like drugs share structural similarities (Fig. 28–1).
3. Opioid peptides and morphine-like drugs bind to the same receptors in the CNS.
4. The receptors to which opioid peptides and morphine-like drugs bind are located in regions of the brain and spinal cord that are associated with perception of pain.
5. Subjects rendered tolerant to analgesia from morphine-like drugs show cross-tolerance to analgesia from opioid peptides.
6. The analgesic effects of opioid peptides and morphine-like drugs can both be blocked by the same antagonist (naloxone).

From these data it is postulated that (1) opioid peptides serve a physiologic role as modulators of pain perception, and that (2) morphine-like drugs produce analgesia by mimicking the actions of endogenous opioid peptides.

Adverse Effects

Respiratory Depression. Respiratory depression is the most serious toxicity of the opioids. At

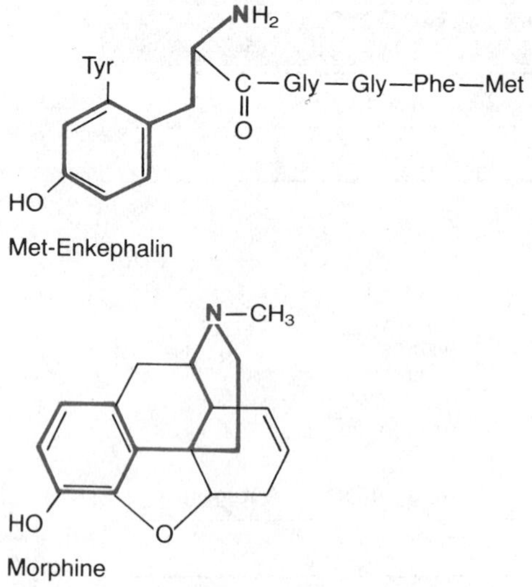

Figure 28–1. Structural similarity between morphine and met-enkephalin. In the morphine structural formula, highlighting indicates the part of the molecule thought responsible for interaction with opioid receptors. In the met-enkephalin structural formula, highlighting indicates the region of structural similarity with morphine.

equianalgesic doses, all of the pure opioid agonists depress respiration to the same degree. Death following overdosage is almost always due to respiratory arrest. Opioids depress respiration primarily through activation of mu receptors, although activation of kappa receptors also contributes. Since the agonist-antagonist opioids (e.g., pentazocine, butorphanol) cause little or no activation of mu receptors (see Table 28–2), respiratory depression with these drugs is much less than with the pure opioid agonists.

The time course of respiratory depression varies with route of administration. Depressant effects begin about 7 minutes after IV injection, 30 minutes after IM injection, and up to 90 minutes after SC injection. With all of these routes, significant depression may persist for 4 to 5 hours. When morphine is administered by spinal injection, onset of respiratory depression may be *delayed for hours*; you should be alert to this possibility.

With prolonged use of opioids, tolerance develops to respiratory depression. Huge doses that would be lethal to nontolerant individuals have been taken by opioid addicts without noticeable effect.

When administered at usual therapeutic doses, opioids rarely cause significant respiratory depression. However, although uncommon, substantial respiratory depression *can* occur. Accordingly, respiratory rate should be determined prior to opioid administration. If the rate is 12 per minute or less, the opioid should be withheld and the physician notified. Certain patients, including the very young, the elderly, and those with respiratory disease (e.g., asthma, emphysema) are especially sensitive to respiratory depression and must be moni-

tored closely. Outpatients should be informed about the risk of respiratory depression and instructed to notify the physician if respiratory distress occurs.

Respiratory depression is increased by concurrent use of other drugs with CNS-depressant actions (e.g., alcohol, barbiturates, benzodiazepines). Accordingly, these drugs should be avoided. Outpatients should be warned against use of alcohol and all other CNS depressants.

Orthostatic Hypotension. Morphine-like drugs lower blood pressure by dilating peripheral arterioles and veins. Vasodilation results primarily from drug-induced release of histamine. Hypotension is mild in the recumbent patient but can be substantial when the patient assumes an erect posture. Patients should be informed about symptoms of hypotension (lightheadedness, dizziness) and instructed to sit or lie down if these occur. Also, patients should be informed that hypotension can be minimized by moving slowly when changing from a supine or seated position to an upright position. Patients should be warned against ambulation if hypotension is significant. Hospitalized patients may require ambulatory assistance. Hypotensive drugs can exacerbate opioid-induced hypotension.

Cough Suppression. Morphine-like drugs act at opioid receptors in the medulla to suppress cough. Suppression of spontaneous cough may lead to accumulation of secretions in the airway. Accordingly, patients should be instructed to actively cough at regular intervals. Lung status should be assessed by auscultation for rales. The ability of opioids to suppress cough is put to clinical use in the form of codeine-based cough remedies.

Constipation. Opioids promote constipation through a combination of effects on the gastrointestinal tract. Through actions exerted in the CNS and locally, these drugs suppress propulsive intestinal contractions, intensify nonpropulsive contractions, increase the tone of the anal sphincter, and inhibit secretion of fluids into the intestinal lumen. Bowel function should be monitored. A diet high in fiber and fluids will minimize disruption of bowel function. A laxative may be needed if constipation cannot be managed with diet alone.

Because of their effects on the intestine, the opioids are highly effective for managing diarrhea. In fact, antidiarrheal use of these drugs preceded their analgesic use by centuries. The effect of opioids on intestinal function is an interesting example of how a drug response can be viewed as detrimental (constipation) or beneficial (relief of diarrhea) depending on who is taking the medication. Opioids employed specifically to treat diarrhea are discussed in Chapter 68.

Urinary Retention. Morphine can cause urinary hesitancy and urinary retention by increasing tone in the sphincter of the bladder. Also, by increasing tone in the detrusor muscle, the drug can elevate pressure within the bladder, causing urinary urgency. In addition to its direct effects on the urinary tract, morphine may interfere with voiding by suppressing awareness of bladder stimuli. Accordingly, patients should be encouraged to void every 4 hours. Urinary hesitancy or retention is especially likely in patients with prostatic hypertrophy.

Urinary retention should be assessed by monitoring intake and output and by palpating the lower abdomen every 4 to 6 hours for bladder distention. If a change in intake-output ratio develops, or if bladder distention is detected, or if the patient reports difficulty in voiding, the physician should be notified. Catheterization may be required.

In addition to causing urinary retention, morphine may decrease urine production. The drug reduces urine formation largely by decreasing renal blood flow, and partly by promoting release of antidiuretic hormone.

Biliary Colic. Morphine can induce spasm of the common bile duct, causing pressure within the biliary tract to rise. Symptoms range from epigastric distress to biliary colic. In patients with preexisting biliary colic, morphine may intensify pain rather than relieve it. Certain opioids (e.g., meperidine) cause less smooth muscle spasm than morphine, and, hence, are less likely to exacerbate biliary colic.

Emesis. Morphine promotes nausea and vomiting through direct stimulation of the chemoreceptor trigger zone (CTZ) of the medulla. These reactions are greatest with the initial dose and diminish with subsequent doses. Nausea and vomiting occur more frequently in ambulatory patients than in those who are stationary, suggesting a vestibular component to these effects. Nausea and vomiting can be reduced by pretreatment with an antiemetic and by having the patient remain still.

Elevation of Intracranial Pressure. Morphine can elevate intracranial pressure (ICP). The mechanism of this effect is indirect: by suppressing respiration, morphine increases the CO_2 content of blood, which dilates the cerebral vasculature, causing ICP to rise. Accordingly, if respiration is maintained at a normal rate, ICP will remain normal as well.

Euphoria/Dysphoria. *Euphoria* is defined as a sense of well-being. Morphine often produces euphoria when administered to patients in pain. Although euphoria can enhance pain relief, it also contributes to the drug's potential for abuse. Euphoria is caused by activation of mu receptors.

In some individuals, morphine causes *dysphoria* (a sense of anxiety and being ill at ease). Dysphoria is uncommon among patients in pain, but

may occur when morphine is taken in the absence of pain.

Sedation. When administered to relieve pain, morphine is likely to cause drowsiness and some mental clouding. Although these effects can complement the drug's analgesic actions, they can also be detrimental. Outpatients should be warned about CNS depression and advised to avoid hazardous activities (e.g., driving) if sedation is significant. Sedation can be minimized by (1) reducing the size of each dose and the dosing interval, (2) using opioids that have short half-lives, and (3) giving small doses of a CNS stimulant (methylphenidate or dextroamphetamine) in the morning and early afternoon.

Miosis. Morphine and other opioids cause pupillary constriction (miosis). In response to toxic doses, the pupil may constrict to "pinpoint" size. Since miosis can impair vision in dim light, room light should be kept bright during waking hours.

Pharmacokinetics

Morphine is administered by several routes: oral, intramuscular, intravenous, subcutaneous, epidural, and intrathecal. Onset of effects is slower with oral administration than with parenteral administration. With four routes—oral, IM, IV, and SC—analgesia persists for 4 to 5 hours. With two routes—epidural and intrathecal—analgesia may persist up to 24 hours.

In order to relieve pain, morphine must cross the blood-brain barrier and enter the CNS. Since the drug is not very lipid soluble, it does not cross the barrier easily. Consequently, only a small fraction of an administered dose reaches sites of analgesic action. Since the blood-brain barrier is not well developed in infants, these patients generally require lower doses than older children and adults.

Morphine is inactivated by hepatic metabolism. When taken by mouth, the drug must pass through the liver on its way to the systemic circulation. Much of an oral dose is inactivated during this first pass through the liver. Consequently, oral doses need to be substantially larger than parenteral doses to produce equivalent analgesic effects. Analgesia and other effects may be intensified and prolonged in patients with liver disease; hence, it may be necessary to reduce the dosage or prolong the dosing interval.

Tolerance and Physical Dependence

With continuous use, morphine can cause tolerance and physical dependence. These phenomena, which are generally inseparable, reflect biochemical adaptations that occur as a compensatory response to prolonged opioid exposure.

Tolerance. Tolerance can be defined as a state in which a large dose is required to produce the same response that could formerly be elicited by a small dose. Alternatively, tolerance can be defined as a condition in which a particular dose produces a smaller response than it could when treatment began.

Tolerance develops to many—but not all—of morphine's actions. With prolonged treatment, tolerance develops to *analgesia, euphoria,* and *sedation.* As a result, with long-term therapy, an increase in dosage may be required to maintain these desirable effects. Fortunately, as tolerance develops to these therapeutic effects, tolerance also develops to *respiratory depression.* As a result, the high doses needed to control pain in the tolerant individual are not associated with increased respiratory depression.

Very little tolerance develops to *constipation* and *miosis.* Even in highly tolerant addicts, constipation remains a chronic problem, and constricted pupils are characteristic.

Cross-tolerance exists among the opioid agonists (e.g., meperidine, methadone, codeine, heroin). Accordingly, individuals tolerant to one of these agents will be tolerant to the others. No cross-tolerance exists between opioids and general CNS depressants (e.g., barbiturates, ethanol, benzodiazepines, general anesthetics).

Physical Dependence. Physical dependence is defined as a state in which an abstinence syndrome will occur if drug use is abruptly discontinued. Opioid dependence results from adaptive biochemical changes that occur in response to the continuous presence of these drugs. Although the exact nature of these changes is unknown, it is clear that once these compensatory changes have taken place, the body requires the continued presence of opioids to function normally. If opioids are withdrawn, an abstinence syndrome will result.

The intensity and duration of the opioid abstinence syndrome depends on the half-life of the drug used and the degree of physical dependence. With opioids that have relatively short half-lives (e.g., morphine) symptoms of abstinence are intense but brief. In contrast, with opioids that have long half-lives (e.g., methadone) symptoms are less intense but more prolonged. With any opioid, the intensity of withdrawal symptoms parallels the degree of physical dependence.

For individuals who are highly dependent, the abstinence syndrome can be extremely unpleasant. Initial reactions include yawning, rhinorrhea, and sweating. Onset occurs about 10 hours after the last dose. These early responses are followed by anorexia, irritability, tremor, and "gooseflesh"—hence, the term "cold turkey." At its peak, the syndrome manifests as violent sneezing, weakness, nausea, vomiting, diarrhea, abdominal cramps, bone and muscle pain, muscle spasm, and kicking movements—hence, "kicking the habit." Adminis-

tration of opioids at any time during withdrawal will rapidly reverse all signs and symptoms. Left untreated, the morphine withdrawal syndrome runs its course in 7 to 10 days. It should be emphasized that although withdrawal from opioids is unpleasant, the syndrome is rarely dangerous. In contrast, withdrawal from general CNS depressants (e.g., barbiturates, alcohol) can be lethal (see Chapter 27).

To minimize the abstinence syndrome, opioids should be withdrawn gradually. When the degree of dependence is moderate, symptoms can be avoided by administering progressively smaller doses over 3 days. When the patient is highly dependent, dosage should be tapered more slowly—over 7 to 10 days. With a proper withdrawal procedure, symptoms of abstinence will resemble those of a mild case of influenza—even when the degree of dependence is high.

It is important to note that physical dependence is rarely a complication when opioids are taken acutely to treat pain. Hospitalized patients receiving morphine 2 to 3 times a day for up to 2 weeks show no significant signs of dependence. If morphine is withheld from these patients, no significant signs of withdrawal can be detected. The issue of physical dependence as a clinical concern is discussed further later in the chapter.

Infants exposed to opioids *in utero* may be born drug dependent. If the infant is not provided with opioids, an abstinence syndrome will occur. Signs of withdrawal include excessive crying, sneezing, tremor, hyperreflexia, fever, and diarrhea. The infant can be weaned from drug dependence by administering dilute opium tincture in progressively smaller doses.

Abuse Liability

Morphine and the other opioids are subject to abuse, largely because of their ability to cause pleasurable experience (e.g., euphoria, sedation, a sensation in the lower abdomen resembling sexual orgasm). Physical dependence contributes to abuse: once dependence exists, the ability of opioids to ward off withdrawal serves to reinforce their desirability in the mind of the abuser.

The abuse liability of the opioids is reflected in their classification under the Controlled Substances Act. (The provisions of this Act are discussed in Chapter 34.) As shown in Table 28–3, morphine and all other strong opioid agonists are classified under Schedule II of the Act. This classification reflects a moderate-to-high abuse liability. The agonist-antagonist opioids have a lower abuse liability and are classified under Schedule IV (pentazocine), Schedule V (buprenorphine), or have no classification at all (dezocine, butorphanol, nalbuphine). Members of the health care team who prescribe, dispense, and administer opioids must

Table 28–3. Opioid Analgesics: Abuse Liability and Maximal Pain Relief

Drug and Category	Controlled Substances Act Schedule	Abuse Liability	Maximal Pain Relief
Strong Opioid Agonists			
Alfentanil	II	High	High
Fentanyl	II	High	High
Hydromorphone	II	High	High
Levorphanol	II	High	High
Meperidine	II	High	High
Methadone	II	High	High
Morphine	II	High	High
Oxymorphone	II	High	High
Sufentanil	II	High	High
Moderate-to-Strong Opioid Agonists			
Codeine	II	Moderate	Moderate-to-high
Hydrocodone	III*	Moderate	Moderate-to-high
Oxycodone	II	Moderate	Moderate-to-high
Propoxyphene	IV	Low	Moderate
Agonist-Antagonist Opioids			
Buprenorphine	V	Low	High
Dezocine	NR	Low	High
Butorphanol	NR	Low	Moderate-to-high
Nalbuphine	NR	Low	Moderate-to-high
Pentazocine	IV	Low	Moderate-to-high

*In the United States, hydrocodone is available only in combination with aspirin or acetaminophen. These combination products are classified under Schedule III.
NR = not regulated under the Controlled Substances Act

adhere to the procedures set forth in the Controlled Substances Act.

Fortunately, abuse is rare when opioids are employed to treat pain. The issue of abuse as a clinical concern is discussed further later in the chapter.

Precautions

Some patients are more likely than others to experience adverse reactions to opioids. Common sense dictates that opioids be used with special caution in these people. Conditions that can predispose patients to adverse reactions are discussed below.

Decreased Respiratory Reserve. Because of its respiratory depressant action, morphine can further compromise respiration in patients with impaired pulmonary function. Accordingly, the drug should be used with caution in patients with asthma, emphysema, kyphoscoliosis, chronic cor pulmonale, and extreme obesity. Caution must also be exercised in patients taking other drugs that can depress respiration (e.g., barbiturates, benzodiazepines, general anesthetics).

Pregnancy. Morphine does not cause birth defects in humans. However, regular use of opioids during pregnancy can cause physical dependence in the fetus. Accordingly, prolonged use by pregnant women should be avoided, if possible.

Labor and Delivery. Use of morphine during delivery can suppress uterine contractions and cause respiratory depression in the neonate. Following delivery, respiration in the neonate should be monitored closely. Respiratory depression can be reversed with naloxone. The use of opioids in obstetrics is discussed further later in the chapter.

Head Injury. In patients with head injury, morphine can exacerbate elevation of intracranial pressure and can complicate diagnosis. Use of opioids in patients with head injury is discussed further later in the chapter.

Other Precautions. *Infants* and *elderly patients* are especially sensitive to the respiratory depressant action of morphine. In patients with *inflammatory bowel disease*, morphine may cause toxic megacolon or paralytic ileus. Since morphine and all other opioids are inactivated by the liver, effects of these agents may be intensified and prolonged in patients with *liver impairment*. Severe hypotension may occur in patients with pre-existing *hypotension* or *reduced blood volume*. In patients with *prostatic hypertrophy*, opioids may cause acute urinary retention; repeated catheterization may be required.

Drug Interactions

The major interactions between morphine and other drugs are summarized in Table 28–4. Some of these interactions are adverse, whereas others are beneficial.

CNS Depressants. All drugs with CNS-depressant actions (e.g., barbiturates, benzodiazepines, alcohol) can intensify sedation and respiratory depression caused by morphine and other opioids. Outpatients should be warned against use of alcohol and all other CNS depressants.

Anticholinergic Drugs. These agents (e.g., antihistamines, tricyclic antidepressants, atropine-like drugs) can exacerbate morphine-induced constipation and urinary retention.

Hypotensive Drugs. Antihypertensive drugs and other drugs that lower blood pressure can exacerbate morphine-induced hypotension.

Monoamine Oxidase (MAO) Inhibitors. The combination of meperidine (a morphine-like drug) with an MAO inhibitor has produced a syndrome characterized by excitation, delirium, hyperpyrexia, convulsions, and severe respiratory depression. Death has occurred. Although this reaction has not been reported with combined use of an MAO inhibitor and morphine, prudence suggests that the combination nonetheless be avoided.

Agonist-Antagonist Opioids. These drugs (e.g., pentazocine, buprenorphine) can precipitate a withdrawal syndrome if administered to an individual who is physically dependent on a pure opioid agonist. The basis of this reaction is considered later in the chapter. Patients taking pure opioid agonists should be weaned from these drugs before treatment with an agonist-antagonist is initiated.

Opioid Antagonists. Opioid antagonists (naloxone, naltrexone) can counteract most actions of morphine and other pure opioid agonists. Opioid antagonists are employed primarily to treat opioid overdosage. The actions and uses of the opioid antagonists are discussed further later in the chapter.

Other Interactions. *Antiemetics* of the phenothiazine type (e.g., promethazine [Phenergan]) may be combined with opioids to reduce nausea and vomiting. *Amphetamines* can enhance opioid-induced analgesia and can help offset sedation.

Toxicity

Clinical Manifestations. Opioid overdosage produces a classic triad of signs: *coma, respiratory depression*, and *pinpoint pupils*. Coma is profound and the patient cannot be aroused. Respiratory rate may be as low as 2 to 4 per minute. Although the pupils are constricted initially, they may dilate as hypoxia sets in secondary to respiratory depression. Hypoxia may cause blood pressure to fall. Prolonged hypoxia may result in shock. When death occurs, respiratory arrest is almost always the immediate cause.

Treatment. Treatment consists primarily of *ventilatory support* and *giving an opioid antagonist*. In most cases, *naloxone* is the antagonist of choice. The pharmacology of naloxone is discussed later in the chapter.

Table 28–4. Interactions of Morphine-Like Drugs with Other Drugs	
Interacting Drugs	**Outcome of the Interaction**
Adverse Interactions	
CNS depressants	Increased respiratory depression and sedation
Barbiturates	
Benzodiazepines	
Alcohol	
General anesthetics	
Antihistamines	
Phenothiazines	
Agonist-antagonist opioids	Precipitation of a withdrawal reaction
Anticholinergic drugs	Increased constipation and urinary retention
Atropine-like drugs	
Antihistamines	
Phenothiazines	
Tricyclic antidepressants	
Hypotensive agents	Increased hypotension
Monoamine oxidase inhibitors	Hyperpyrexic coma
Beneficial Interactions	
Amphetamines	Increased analgesia and decreased sedation
Antiemetics	Suppression of nausea and vomiting
Naloxone	Suppression of symptoms of opioid overdosage

Preparations, Dosage, and Administration

General Guidelines on Dosage and Administration. Dosage must be individualized. High doses are required for patients with a low tolerance to pain or with extremely painful disorders. Patients with sharp, stabbing pain need higher doses than patients with dull pain. Elderly adults generally require lower doses than younger adults. Neonates require relatively low doses because of their poorly developed blood-brain barriers. For all patients, dosage should be reduced as pain subsides. Outpatients should be warned not to increase dosage without consulting the physician.

Before an opioid is administered, respiratory rate, blood pressure, and pulse rate should be determined. The drug should be withheld and the physician notified if respiratory rate is at or below 12 per minute, if blood pressure is significantly below the pretreatment value, or if pulse rate is significantly above or below the pretreatment value.

As a rule, opioids should be administered on a fixed schedule—not on a PRN basis. With a fixed schedule, medication is given before intense pain returns. As a result, the patient is spared needless discomfort; furthermore, anxiety about recurrence of pain is reduced.

Morphine and all other opioid agonists are classified under Schedule II of the Controlled Substances Act, and must be dispensed accordingly.

Preparations. Morphine sulfate is available in six formulations: *standard tablets* (15 and 30 mg); *soluble tablets* (10, 15, and 30 mg); *controlled-release tablets* [MS Contin] (30 mg); *oral solution* [Roxanol] (2, 4, and 20 mg/ml); *rectal suppositories* [RMS] (5, 10, 20, and 30 mg); and solution for injection [Astramorph PF, Duramorph] (concentrations range from 0.5 to 15 mg/ml).

Dosage and Routes of Administration. *Oral.* Oral administration is generally reserved for treating chronic, severe pain, such as that associated with cancer. Because oral morphine undergoes extensive metabolism on its first pass through the liver, oral doses are usually higher than parenteral doses. A typical dosage is 10 to 30 mg repeated every 4 hours as needed. However, oral dosing is highly individualized; hence, some patients may require 75 mg or more. Controlled-release tablets may be administered every 8 to 12 hours. Patient should be instructed to swallow controlled-release tablets intact, without crushing or chewing.

Intramuscular and Subcutaneous. If repeated doses are required, IM injection is preferred, since repeated SC injections can cause local irritation and pain. For adults, dosing is initiated at 5 to 10 mg every 4 hours, and then adjusted up or down based on the patient's response. The usual dosage for children is 0.1 to 0.2 mg/kg repeated every 4 hours as needed.

Intravenous. Intravenous morphine should be injected slowly (over 4 to 5 minutes). Rapid IV injection can cause severe adverse effects (profound hypotension, cardiac arrest, respiratory arrest) and should be avoided. When IV injections are made, an opioid antagonist (e.g., naloxone) and facilities for respiratory support should be available. Injections should be given with the patient lying down to minimize hypotension. The usual dose for adults is 4 to 10 mg (diluted in 4 to 5 ml of water for injection). The usual pediatric dose is 0.05 to 0.1 mg/kg.

Epidural and Intrathecal. When morphine is employed for spinal analgesia, epidural injection is preferred to intrathecal. With either route, onset of analgesia is rapid and the duration prolonged (up to 24 hours). The most troubling side effects of spinal morphine are delayed respiratory depression and delayed cardiac depression. Be alert for possible late reactions. The usual adult epidural dose is 5 mg. Intrathecal doses are much smaller—about one-tenth the epidural dose.

OTHER STRONG OPIOID AGONISTS

In an effort to produce a strong analgesic with a low potential for abuse and respiratory depression, pharmaceutical scientists have created many new opioid analgesics. Unfortunately, none of the newer pure opioid agonists can be considered truly superior to morphine: the newer pure opioids are essentially equal to morphine with respect to analgesic action, abuse liability, and the ability to cause respiratory depression. Also, to varying degrees, all of these drugs can cause sedation, euphoria, constipation, urinary retention, cough suppression, hypotension, and miosis. However, despite their similarities to morphine, the newer drugs do have unique qualities. These special characteristics may render one agent more desirable than another in a particular clinical situation. With all of the newer pure opioid agonists, toxicity can be reversed with an opioid antagonist (e.g., naloxone). Important differences between morphine and the newer strong opioid analgesics are discussed below. Tables 28–5 and 28–6 summarize dosages, routes, and time courses of action for morphine and the newer opioid agonists.

Meperidine

Meperidine [Demerol] shares the major pharmacologic properties of morphine. The drug is employed primarily to relieve pain. For obstetric analgesia, meperidine is preferred to morphine; the drug does not delay or diminish uterine contractions and neonatal respiratory depression is less pronounced.

Meperidine causes less smooth muscle spasm than morphine. As a result, meperidine is less likely to cause constipation, urinary retention, and biliary colic. Meperidine may interact with MAO inhibitors to cause excitation, delirium, hyperpyrexia, and convulsions. Repeated dosing results in accumulation of a toxic metabolite that can cause dysphoria, tremors, myoclonus, and seizures.

Meperidine is available in tablets (50 and 100 mg) and a syrup formulation (10 mg/ml) for oral use, and in solution (50 and 100 mg/ml) for injection (IV, IM, or SC). In addition, the drug is available in single-dose vials, ampuls, and syringes. The usual adult dosage is 50 to 150 mg (IM, SC, or PO) repeated every 3 to 4 hours as needed. The usual dosage for children is 1 to 1.8 mg/kg (IM, SC, or PO) repeated every 3 to 4 hours as needed.

Methadone

Methadone [Dolophine] has pharmacologic properties very similar to those of morphine. The drug is effective orally and has a long duration of action. Repeated dosing can result in accumulation. Methadone is employed to relieve pain and to treat opioid addicts. The use of methadone in drug-abuse treatment programs is discussed in Chapter 34 (Drugs of Abuse).

Methadone is dispensed in standard tablets (5 and 10 mg) and solution (1 and 2 mg/ml) for oral use, and in solution (10 mg/ml) for IM and SC administration. In addition, the drug is available in dispersible 40-mg tablets. This formulation is used

Table 28–5. Clinical Pharmacology of the Pure Opioid Agonists				
		Time Course of Analgesic Effects		
Drug and Route	**Equivalent Dose (mg)***	**Onset (minutes)**	**Peak (minutes)**	**Duration (hours)**
Codeine				
PO	200	30–45	60–120	4
IM	120	10–30	30–60	4
SC	120	10–30	30–60	4
Hydrocodone				
PO	10	10–30	30–60	4–6
Hydromorphone				
PO	7.5	30	90–120	4
IM	1.5	15	30–60	4–5
IV	1.5	10–15	15–30	2–3
SC	1.5	15	30–90	4
Levorphanol				
PO	4	10–60	90–120	4–5
IM	2	—	60	4–5
IV	2	—	Within 20	4–5
SC	2	—	60–90	4–5
Meperidine				
PO	300	15	60–90	2–4
IM	75	10–15	30–50	2–4
IV	75	1	5–7	2–4
SC	75	10–15	30–50	2–4
Methadone				
PO	20	30–60	90–120	4–6†
IM	10	10–20	60–120	4–5†
IV	10	—	15–30	3–4†
Morphine				
PO	60	—	60–120	4–5‡
IM	10	10–30	30–60	4–5
IV	10	—	20	4–5
SC	10	10–30	50–90	4–5
Epidural	10	15–60	—	Up to 24
Intrathecal	10	15–60	—	Up to 24
Oxycodone				
PO	30	—	60	3–4
Oxymorphone				
IM	1	10–15	30–90	3–6
IV	1	5–10	15–30	3–4
SC	1	10–20	—	3–6
Rectal	10	15–30	120	3–6
Propoxyphene				
PO	—§	15–60	120	4–6

*Dose in mg that produces a degree of analgesia equivalent to that produced by a 10-mg intramuscular dose of morphine.
†With repeated doses, methadone's duration of action may increase up to 48 hours.
‡Effects of extended-release tablets may persist for 8 to 12 hours.
§A dose of propoxyphene equivalent to 10 mg of morphine would be too toxic to administer.

only for detoxification and maintenance of opioid addicts. Usual oral analgesic doses for adults range from 2.5 to 20 mg repeated every 3 to 4 hours as needed.

Heroin

Heroin is a strong opioid agonist that is very similar to morphine in structure and actions. Heroin is an effective analgesic and is employed legally in Europe to relieve pain. In the United States, federal legislation prohibits the medical use of this drug. Heroin has been banned from American medicine because of its high abuse liability and because it does not appear to offer any benefits over opioids with a lower abuse potential.

Heroin is preferred to other opioids as a drug of abuse largely because of its pharmacokinetic properties. Heroin has greater lipid solubility than morphine and, therefore, crosses the blood-

brain barrier more readily. As a result, when heroin is injected IV, the drug accumulates in the brain more rapidly and to a higher level than would an equivalent IV dose of morphine. Once in the brain, heroin (diacetylmorphine) is rapidly converted into monoacetyl morphine and then into morphine (Fig. 28–2). It is these metabolites—and not heroin itself—that produce the subjective effects that follow heroin injection. In this regard, heroin can be viewed as a vehicle for facilitating transport of morphine into the brain.

Fentanyl

Fentanyl [Sublimaze, Duragesic] is a strong opioid analgesic with a high milligram potency. The drug is available for parenteral and transdermal administration.

Drug and Route	Equivalent Dose (mg)*	Time Course		
		Onset (minutes)	*Peak (minutes)*	*Duration (hours)*
Alfentanil				
IV	0.3–1	1	2	0.3–0.6
Fentanyl†				
IV	0.1	1–2	3–5	0.5–1
IM	0.1	7–8	20–30	1–2
Sufentanil				
IV	0.02	1–3	20	0.7–2.9

Table 28–6. Clinical Pharmacology of Opioids Used Primarily for General Anesthesia

*Dose in mg that produces a degree of analgesia equivalent to that produced by 10 mg of morphine IM.
†Also given by transdermal patch for prolonged analgesia (see text).

Parenteral. Parenteral fentanyl [Sublimaze] is employed primarily for induction and maintenance of surgical anesthesia. The drug is well suited for these applications because of its rapid onset and relatively short duration of action (see Table 28–6). Most effects are like those of morphine. In addition, fentanyl can cause muscle rigidity, which can interfere with induction of anesthesia. As discussed in Chapter 30 (General Anesthetics), the combination of fentanyl plus droperidol, available commercially as Innovar, is used to produce a state known as "neurolept analgesia."

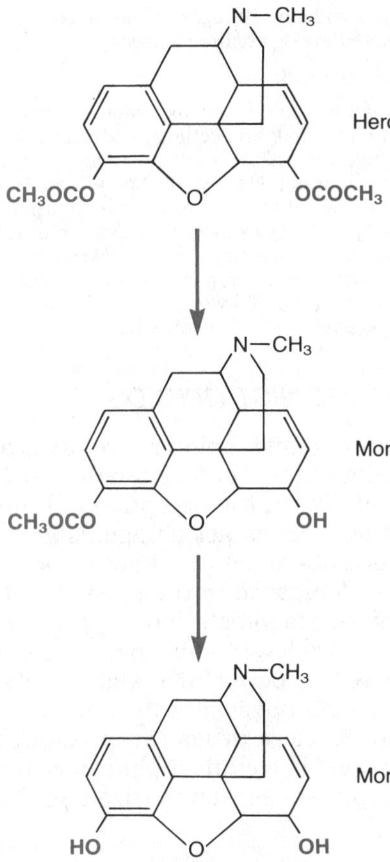

Transdermal. The fentanyl transdermal system [Duragesic] consists of a fentanyl-containing "patch" that is applied to the skin of the upper torso. The drug is slowly released from the patch and absorbed through the skin, reaching effective levels in 24 hours. Levels then remain steady for another 48 hours, after which the patch should be removed and a new patch applied. If a new patch is not applied, effects will nonetheless persist for several hours because of continued absorption of fentanyl that remained in the skin after the old patch was removed. Transdermal fentanyl is indicated for chronic severe pain, such as that associated with cancer. Since onset of analgesia is delayed, fentanyl patches are not well suited for postoperative analgesia.

Transdermal fentanyl has the same adverse effects as other opioids (respiratory depression, sedation, constipation, urinary retention, nausea, and so forth). Adverse effects may persist for hours following patch removal because of continued drug absorption from the skin. Signs of toxicity can be reversed with an opioid antagonist (e.g., naloxone). Used patches should be flushed down the toilet. Unused patches should be stored out of the reach of children.

Fentanyl patches are available in four sizes: proceeding from the smallest to the largest, these deliver fentanyl to the systemic circulation at rates of 25, 50, 75, and 100 μg/hr. If the patient is not already tolerant to opioids, therapy should begin with the smallest patch. If a dosage greater than 100 μg/hr is required, a combination of patches can be applied. Since full analgesic effects can take up to 24 hours to develop, PRN therapy with a short-acting opioid may be required until the patch takes effect. For the majority of patients, patches can be replaced every 72 hours, although some patients may require a new patch every 48 hours. Fentanyl patches are regulated under Schedule II of the Controlled Substances Act.

Alfentanil and Sufentanil

Alfentanil [Alfenta] and sufentanil [Sufenta] are intravenous opioids related to fentanyl. Both drugs are used for induction of anesthesia, for maintenance of anesthesia (in combination with other agents), and as sole anesthetic agents. Pharmacologic effects are like those of morphine. Sufentanil has an especially high milligram potency (about 1000 times that of morphine). As indicated in Table 28–6, both alfentanil and sufentanil have a rapid onset of action. Alfentanil has an unusually brief duration. Both drugs are Schedule II agents.

Hydromorphone, Oxymorphone, and Levorphanol

Basic Pharmacology. All three drugs are strong opioid agonists with pharmacologic actions like those of morphine. All

Figure 28–2. Biotransformation of heroin into morphine. Heroin, as such, is biologically inactive. Once in the body, heroin is converted to monoacetylmorphine (MAM) and then into morphine itself. MAM and morphine are responsible for the effects elicited by injection of heroin.

three are indicated for relief of moderate to severe pain. Dosages and time courses of action are summarized in Table 26–5. Adverse effects include respiratory depression, sedation, cough suppression, constipation, urinary retention, nausea, and vomiting. Toxicity can be reversed with an opioid antagonist (e.g., naloxone). All three drugs are regulated under Schedule II of the Controlled Substances Act.

Preparations, Dosage, and Administration. *Hydromorphone.* Hydromorphone [Dilaudid] is available in oral tablets (1, 2, 3, and 4 mg), rectal suppositories (3 mg), and solution (1, 2, 3, 4, and 10 mg/ml) for IM and SC injection. The usual adult oral dosage is 2 mg every 4 to 6 hours. The adult rectal dosage is 3 mg every 6 to 8 hours. Usual SC and IM dosages are 1 to 4 mg every 4 to 6 hours.

Oxymorphone. Oxymorphone [Numorphan] is available in solution (1 and 1.5 mg/ml) for parenteral administration and in 5-mg rectal suppositories. The initial IV dose is 0.5 mg. Usual SC and IM dosages are 1 to 1.5 mg every 4 to 6 hours as needed. The rectal dosage is 5 mg every 4 to 6 hours.

Levorphanol. Levorphanol [Levo-Dromoran] is available in 2-mg oral tablets and in solution (2 mg/ml) for SC injection. The usual oral or SC dosage for adults is 2 to 3 mg.

MODERATE-TO-STRONG OPIOID AGONISTS

The moderate-to-strong opioid agonists are similar to morphine in most respects. Like morphine, these drugs produce analgesia, sedation, and euphoria. In addition, they can cause respiratory depression, constipation, urinary retention, cough suppression, and miosis. Differences between the moderate-to-strong opioids and morphine are primarily quantitative: the moderate-to-strong opioids produce less analgesia and respiratory depression than morphine and have a somewhat lower potential for abuse. As with morphine, toxicity from the moderate-to-strong agonists can be reversed with naloxone.

Codeine

Actions and Uses. Codeine is indicated for relief of mild to moderate pain. The drug is usually administered by mouth. Maximal analgesic effects are less than with morphine. When taken in its usual analgesic dose (30 mg), codeine produces about as much pain relief as 325 mg of aspirin or 325 mg of acetaminophen.

For analgesic use, codeine is dispensed alone and in combination with a nonopioid analgesic (aspirin or acetaminophen). Since codeine and nonopioid analgesics relieve pain by different mechanisms, the combination of codeine with a nonopioid can produce greater pain relief than either agent alone. Codeine alone is classified under Schedule II of the Controlled Substances Act. The combination preparations are classified under Schedule III. Although codeine is classified along with morphine in Schedule II, codeine's abuse liability appears to be significantly lower than that of morphine.

Codeine is an extremely effective cough suppressant and is widely used for this action. The anti-

tussive dose (10 mg) is lower than analgesic doses. Codeine is dispensed in combination with various agents for suppression of cough. These mixtures are classified under Schedule V.

Preparations, Dosage, and Administration. Codeine is administered orally and parenterally (IV, IM, and SC). For oral therapy, the drug is available in standard and soluble tablets (15, 30, and 60 mg). For parenteral therapy, the drug is dispensed in solution (30 and 60 mg/ml).

The usual analgesic dosage for adults is 15 to 60 mg (PO, IV, IM, or SC) every 3 to 6 hours (to a maximum of 120 mg/24 hr). The usual analgesic dosage for children 1 year and older is 0.5 mg/kg (PO, IM, or SC) every 4 to 6 hours (to a maximum of 60 mg/24 hr).

Propoxyphene

Propoxyphene [Darvon, Dolene] has analgesic effects about equal to those of aspirin. The drug is frequently prescribed in combination with a nonopioid analgesic (aspirin or acetaminophen). These combinations can produce greater pain relief than either propoxyphene or the nonopioid alone. Propoxyphene has a low potential for abuse, primarily because large doses cause toxic psychosis. Furthermore, excessive doses often prove fatal; hence, the drug should not be dispensed to patients with suicidal tendencies. Physical dependence is minimal. Propoxyphene, alone or in combination with a nonopioid analgesic, is classified under Schedule IV of the Controlled Substances Act.

Propoxyphene is available as two salts: propoxyphene hydrochloride and propoxyphene napsylate. Both salts are administered orally. Propoxyphene hydrochloride is dispensed in capsules (32 and 65 mg); the usual adult dosage is 65 mg repeated every 4 hours as needed. The napsylate salt is dispensed in 100-mg tablets and in suspension (10 mg/ml); the usual adult dosage is 100 mg repeated every 4 hours as needed.

Hydrocodone and Oxycodone

Hydrocodone [Vicodin, others] and oxycodone [Roxicodone, Percodan, Percocet] have analgesic actions equivalent to those of codeine. Both drugs are taken orally to relieve pain. The usual dosage for both is 5 mg. Oxycodone is available in 5-mg tablets, in solution (5 and 20 mg/ml), and in combination with aspirin or acetaminophen. Hydrocodone is available only in combination with aspirin or acetaminophen. Oxycodone, alone or combined with aspirin or acetaminophen, is classified under Schedule II. The combination of hydrocodone with aspirin or acetaminophen is classified under Schedule III.

AGONIST-ANTAGONIST OPIOIDS

Five agonist-antagonist opioids are available: pentazocine, nalbuphine, butorphanol, dezocine and buprenorphine. With the exception of buprenorphine, all of these drugs act as agonists at mu receptors and as antagonists at kappa receptors (see Table 28–2). Compared to the pure opioid agonists, the agonist-antagonists have a low potential for abuse, produce less respiratory depression, and generally have less powerful analgesic actions. If given to a patient physically dependent on a pure opioid agonist, these drugs can precipitate a withdrawal reaction. The clinical pharmacology of the agonist-antagonists is summarized in Table 28–7.

Pentazocine

Actions and Uses. Pentazocine [Talwin] was the first agonist-antagonist opioid available and can be considered the prototype for the group. The

Table 28-7. Clinical Pharmacology of Opioid Agonist-Antagonists

Drug and Route	Equivalent Dose (mg)*	Time Course of Analgesic Effects		
		Onset (minutes)	Peak (minutes)	Duration (hours)
Buprenorphine				
IM	0.3	15	60	Up to 6
IV	0.3	<15	<60	Up to 6
Butorphanol				
IM	2-3	10	30-60	3-4
IV	2-3	2-3	30	2-4
Intranasal	2-3	Within 15	60-120	4-5
Dezocine				
IM	10	30	30-150	2-4
IV	10	15	30-150	2-4
Nalbuphine				
IM	10	Within 15	60	3-6
IV	10	2-3	30	3-4
SC	10	Within 15	—	3-6
Pentazocine				
PO	180	15-30	60-90	3†
IM	60	15-20	30-60	2-3†
IV	60	2-3	15-30	2-3†
SC	60	15-20	30-60	2-3†

*Dose in mg that produces a degree of analgesia equivalent to that produced by a 10-mg IM dose of morphine.
†Duration may increase greatly in patients with liver disease.

drug is indicated for mild to moderate pain. Pentazocine is less effective than morphine against severe pain.

As indicated in Table 28-2, pentazocine acts as an *agonist* at kappa and sigma receptors and as an *antagonist* at mu receptors. By activating kappa receptors, the drug produces analgesia, sedation, and respiratory depression. However, unlike the respiratory depression caused by morphine, *respiratory depression caused by pentazocine is limited*: beyond a certain dose, no further depression of respiration occurs. Because it lacks agonist actions at mu receptors, pentazocine produces little or no euphoria. In fact, at supratherapeutic doses, pentazocine produces unpleasant reactions (anxiety, strange thoughts, nightmares, hallucinations). These psychotomimetic effects result from stimulation of sigma receptors. Because of its subjective effects, pentazocine has a low potential for abuse and is classified as a Schedule IV substance.

Adverse effects are generally like those of morphine. However, in contrast to the pure opioid agonists, pentazocine increases cardiac work. Accordingly, a pure agonist (e.g., morphine) is preferred to pentazocine for relieving pain in patients with myocardial infarction.

If administered to a patient who is physically dependent on a pure opioid agonist, pentazocine can precipitate an abstinence syndrome. Recall that mu receptors mediate physical dependence on pure opioid agonists and that pentazocine acts as an antagonist at these receptors. By blocking access of the pure agonist to mu receptors, pentazocine will prevent receptor activation, thereby triggering a withdrawal reaction. Accordingly, *pentazocine and other drugs that block mu receptors should never be administered to a person with physical dependence on a pure opioid agonist.* If a pentazocine-like agent is to be used, the pure opioid agonist must first be withdrawn.

Physical dependence can occur with pentazocine, but symptoms of withdrawal are generally mild (e.g., cramps, fever, anxiety, restlessness). Treatment is rarely required. As with the pure opioid agonists, toxicity from pentazocine can be reversed with naloxone.

Preparations, Dosage, and Administration. For oral therapy pentazocine [Talwin] is dispensed in 50-mg tablets that also contain 0.5 mg of naloxone (to prevent abuse). The usual adult dosage is 50 mg repeated every 3 to 4 hours as needed.

For parenteral therapy, pentazocine is available in solution (30 mg/ml as the lactate salt). Administration is IV, IM, and SC. The usual adult dosage is 30 mg repeated every 3 to 4 hours as needed.

Nalbuphine

Nalbuphine [Nubain] has pharmacologic actions similar to those of pentazocine. The drug is an agonist at kappa receptors and an antagonist at mu receptors. Analgesic effects are somewhat less than those of morphine. Like pentazocine, nalbuphine can cause psychotomimetic reactions. Respiratory depression is limited. With prolonged treatment, physical dependence can develop. Symptoms of abstinence are less intense than with morphine but more intense than with pentazocine. Nalbuphine has a low abuse potential and is not regulated under the Controlled Substances Act. As with the pure opioid agonists, toxicity can be reversed with naloxone. Like pentazocine, nalbuphine will precipitate a withdrawal reaction if administered to an individual who is physically dependent on a pure opioid agonist.

Nalbuphine is dispensed in solution (10 and 20 mg/ml) for IV, IM, and SC injection. The usual adult dosage is 10 mg repeated every 3 to 6 hours as needed.

Butorphanol

Butorphanol [Stadol] has actions similar to those of pentazocine. The drug is an agonist at kappa receptors and an antagonist at mu receptors. Analgesic effects are somewhat less than those of morphine. As with pentazocine, there is a "ceiling" to respiratory depression. The drug can cause psychotomimetic reactions, but these are rare. Butorphanol increases cardiac work and should not be given to patients with myocardial infarction. Physical dependence can occur, but symptoms of withdrawal are relatively mild. The drug may induce a withdrawal reaction in patients physically dependent on a pure opioid agonist. Butorphanol has a low potential for abuse and is not regulated under the Controlled Substances Act. Toxicity can be reversed with naloxone.

Butorphanol is administered parenterally (IM and IV) and by nasal spray. The usual adult IV dosage is 1 mg repeated every 3 to 4 hours as needed. The usual IM dosage is 2 mg every 3 to 4 hours as needed. The usual intranasal dosage is 1 mg (one spray from the metered-dose spray device) repeated in 60 to 90 minutes if needed; the 2-dose sequence may then be repeated every 3 to 4 hours as needed.

Dezocine

Dezocine [Dalgan] is a new opioid agonist-antagonist with analgesic effects equivalent to those of morphine. The drug's adverse effects are like those of the pure opioid agonists, except that there is a ceiling to respiratory depression. Fatal respiratory depression has not been reported. Effects on cardiac performance are modest, but caution should be exercised in patients with coronary artery disease. Dezocine appears to have a low potential for abuse and is not currently regulated under the Controlled Substances Act. The drug is dispensed in solution (5, 10, and 15 mg/ml) for IM and IV administration. The usual IM dosage is 5 to 20 mg repeated every 3 to 6 hours as needed. The usual IV dosage is 2.5 to 10 mg every 2 to 4 hours.

Buprenorphine

Buprenorphine [Buprenex] differs significantly from other opioid agonist-antagonists. The drug is a partial agonist at mu receptors and an antagonist at kappa receptors. Analgesic effects are like those of morphine, but significant tolerance has not been observed. Although buprenorphine can depress respiration, severe respiratory depression has not been reported. Like pentazocine, buprenorphine can precipitate a withdrawal reaction in persons physically dependent on pure opioid agonists. Psychotomimetic reactions can occur but are rare. Physical dependence develops but symptoms of abstinence are delayed; peak responses may not occur until 2 weeks after the last dose was taken. Buprenorphine appears to have a low potential for abuse and is classified as a Schedule V substance.

Although pretreatment with naloxone can prevent toxicity from buprenorphine, naloxone cannot readily reverse toxicity that has already developed. It appears that buprenorphine binds very tightly to its receptors, and cannot be readily displaced by naloxone once it is bound.

Buprenorphine is dispensed in solution (0.3 mg/ml) for administration by IM or slow IV injection. The usual dosage for patients 13 years and older is 0.3 mg repeated every 6 hours as needed.

CLINICAL USE OF OPIOIDS

GENERAL CONSIDERATIONS

Assessment of Pain

To maximize relief, you must first assess the patient's pain. Pain status should be evaluated prior to opioid administration and about 1 hour after. Unfortunately, since pain is a subjective experience affected by multiple factors (e.g., cultural influences, expectations, associated disease), there is no reliable objective method for determining just how much discomfort the patient is under. That is, we cannot measure pain with instruments equivalent to those employed to monitor blood pressure, cardiac performance, and other physiologic parameters. As a result, assessment must ultimately be based on the patient's description of his or her experience. Accordingly, you should ask the patient where the pain is located, what type of pain is present (e.g., dull, sharp, stabbing), how the pain changes with time, what makes the pain better, and what makes the pain worse. In addition, you should assess for psychologic factors that can reduce pain threshold (anxiety, depression, fear, anger).

When attempting to assess pain, keep in mind that what the patient says about his or her pain may not always be the truth. A few patients who are pain free may claim to feel pain so as to receive medication for its euphoriant effects. Conversely, some patients may claim to feel fine even though they are experiencing considerable discomfort. Such patients may misrepresent their experience for any of several reasons: some may fear addiction, some may fear needles, and some may feel a need to be stoic and bear the pain. Patients like these must be listened to with care if their true pain status is to be evaluated and responded to with appropriate measures for relief.

Acute Pain versus Chronic Pain

Opioids are generally reserved for acute pain. With the exception of cancer-caused pain, use of opioids for chronic pain is not usually appropriate. Alternatives to opioids for chronic pain include nonopioid analgesics (acetaminophen and aspirin-like drugs), nerve block, transcutaneous electrical nerve stimulation (TENS), tricyclic antidepressants, and neurosurgery. If disabling pain persists despite these therapies, treatment with an opioid may be indicated.

Dosing Guidelines

Dosage Determination. Dosage of opioid analgesics must be adjusted to accommodate individual variation. "Standard" doses cannot be relied upon as appropriate for all patients. For example, if a "standard" 10-mg dose of morphine were employed for all adults, only about 70% would receive adequate relief; the other 30% would be undertreated. Not all patients have the same tolerance for pain; hence, some will need larger doses than others for the same disorder. Some conditions hurt more than others. For example, patients recovering from open chest surgery are likely to experience greater pain and need larger doses than patients recovering from an appendectomy. Elderly patients metabolize opioids slowly and, therefore, require lower doses than younger adults. Because the blood-brain barrier of newborns is poorly developed, these patients are especially sensitive to opioids; hence, they generally require smaller doses than older infants and young children.

Dosing Schedule. As a rule, *opioids should be administered on a fixed schedule* (e.g., every 4 hours) rather than on a PRN basis. With a fixed schedule, each dose is given before pain returns, thereby sparing the patient needless discomfort. In contrast, when PRN dosing is employed, there can be a long delay between onset of pain and production of relief: each time pain returns, the patient must call the nurse; wait for the nurse to respond; wait for the nurse to evaluate the pain; wait for the nurse to sign out medication; wait for the nurse to prepare and administer the injection; and then wait for the drug to undergo absorption and finally produce analgesia. This delay causes unnecessary discomfort and creates anxiety about pain recurrence. Use of a fixed dosing schedule reduces these problems. As discussed below, allowing the patient to self-administer opioids using a patient-controlled analgesia device can provide even greater protection against pain recurrence than can be achieved by having the nurse administer opioids on a fixed schedule.

Avoiding Withdrawal. When opioids are administered in high doses for 20 days or more, clinically significant physical dependence may develop. Under these conditions, abrupt withdrawal of medication will precipitate an abstinence syndrome. To minimize symptoms of abstinence, opioids should be withdrawn slowly, tapering off the dosage over 3 days. If the degree of dependence is especially high, as can occur in opioid addicts, dosage should be tapered over 7 to 10 days.

PHYSICAL DEPENDENCE, ABUSE, AND ADDICTION AS CLINICAL CONCERNS

Most people in our society, including many health care professionals, harbor strong fears regarding the ability of "narcotics" to cause "addiction." In a clinical setting, such excessive concern is both unwarranted and counterproductive. Because of inappropriate fears, physicians frequently prescribe less pain medication than patients need, and nurses frequently administer less medication than was prescribed. The result, according to one estimate, is that only 25% of patients receive doses of opioids that are sufficient to relieve suffering. One pain specialist described this unacceptable situation as follows: "The excessive and unrealistic concern about the dangers of addiction in the hos-

pitalized medical patient is a significant and potent force for the undertreatment with narcotics."

When treating a patient for pain, you, as a nurse, may have to decide how much opioid to give and when to give it. If you are excessively concerned about the ability of opioids to cause physical dependence and addiction, you will be unable to make a rational decision. Furthermore, in your role as patient advocate, it is your responsibility to intervene and request an increase in dosage if the prescribed dosage has proved inadequate. If you fear that dosage escalation may cause addiction, you are not likely to make such a request.

The object of the following discussion is to dispel excessive concerns about dependence, abuse, and addiction in the medical patient so that these concerns do not result in undermedication and needless suffering.

Definitions

Before we can discuss the clinical implications of physical dependence, abuse, and addiction, we need to define these terms.

Physical Dependence. As discussed previously, physical dependence is a state in which an abstinence syndrome will occur if the dependence-producing drug is abruptly withdrawn. *Physical dependence should NOT be equated with addiction.*

Abuse. Abuse can be broadly defined as drug use that is not socially approved. By this definition, abuse is determined primarily by the reason for drug use and by the setting in which that use occurs—and not by the pharmacologic properties of the drug itself. For example, whereas it is not considered abuse to administer 20 mg of morphine in a hospital to relieve pain, it is considered abuse to administer the same dose of the same drug on the "street" to produce euphoria. The concept of abuse is discussed at length in Chapter 34.

Addiction. For our purposes, the term *addiction* can be defined as a behavior pattern that has three outstanding features: (1) compulsive drug use, (2) preoccupation with securing a drug supply, and (3) a tendency to relapse after withdrawal. Note that by this definition, addiction is not equated with physical dependence. In fact, physical dependence is not even part of the definition. The concept of addiction is discussed further in Chapter 34.

Although physical dependence is not required for addiction to occur, physical dependence *can* contribute to addictive behavior. If an individual has already established a pattern of compulsive drug use, physical dependence can reinforce that pattern. For the individual with a marginal resolve to discontinue opioid use, the desire to avoid symptoms of withdrawal may be sufficient to promote continued drug use. However, in the presence of a strong desire to discontinue opioids, physical dependence, by itself, is insufficient to motivate continued addictive behavior.

Minimizing Fears About Physical Dependence

For the following three reasons, there is little to fear regarding physical dependence upon opioids in the hospitalized patient:

1. Development of significant physical dependence is extremely rare when opioids are given acutely to relieve pain. For most patients, the doses employed and the duration of treatment are insufficient to cause significant dependence.

2. Even when dependence does occur, it is extremely uncommon for patients to develop addictive behavior and continue opioid administration after their pain has subsided. The vast majority of patients who become physically dependent in a clinical setting simply go through gradual withdrawal and never take opioids again. This observation emphasizes the point that physical dependence per se is insufficient to cause addiction.

3. Physical dependence as such is no special problem. As long as the dependent person takes opioids, dependence has no symptoms. Addicts participating in methadone treatment programs can be highly dependent upon methadone, yet they experience no significant ill effects and function normally (as long as they take methadone on a regular schedule). Physical dependence does not prevent methadone-treated addicts from leading productive and fulfilling lives.

From the preceding we can see there is little to fear regarding physical dependence during the therapeutic use of opioids. We can conclude, therefore, that there is no justification for withholding opioids from patients in pain on the basis of concerns about physical dependence.

Minimizing Fears About Addiction

The principal reason for abandoning fears about opioid addiction in patients is simple: *development of addiction to opioids as a result of clinical exposure to these drugs is extremely rare*. Also, as discussed below, if abuse or addiction do occur, it is probable that these behaviors reflect tendencies that existed before the patient entered the hospital, rather than inappropriate medical use of opioids during the hospital stay.

For the purpose of this discussion, the population can be divided into two groups: individuals who are prone to drug abuse and individuals who are not. One source estimates that about 8% of the population is prone to drug abuse, whereas the other 92% is not. Individuals who are prone to drug abuse have a tendency to abuse drugs in the hospital and outside. Nonabusers, on the other hand, will not abuse drugs in a clinical setting or anywhere else. Withholding analgesics from abuse-prone individuals is not going to reverse their tendency to abuse drugs. Conversely, administering opioids to nonabuse-prone persons will not change their personalities and convert them into drug fiends.

If a patient who did not formerly abuse opioids does abuse these drugs following therapeutic exposure, you should not feel responsible for having created an addict. That is, if a patient tries to continue opioid use after leaving the hospital, it is probable that the patient is of the abuse-prone personality type. Therefore, the pattern of abuse that emerged during clinical exposure to opioids was the result of tendencies that were established before the patient ever entered the hospital—and not the consequence of therapy. The only action that might have prevented opioid abuse by such a patient would have been to withhold opioids entirely—an action that would not have been feasible.

Balancing the Need to Provide Pain Relief with the Desire to Minimize Abuse

Although concerns about opioid abuse in the clinical setting are small, they cannot be dismissed entirely. You are still obliged to administer opioids with discretion in an effort to minimize abuse. Some reasonable attempt must be made to determine who is likely to abuse drugs and who is not. As a rule, distinguishing abusers from nonabusers can be done with some confidence. When nonabusers say they need more pain relief, believe them and provide it. In contrast, when an obvious abuser requests more analgesic, some healthy skepticism is in order. When there is doubt as to whether a patient is abuse-prone or not, logic dictates giving the patient the benefit of the doubt and providing the medication. If the patient is an abuser, little harm will result from giving unneeded medication. However, if the patient is a nonabuser, failure to provide medication would prolong suffering for no justifiable reason.

In order to minimize physical dependence and abuse, opioid analgesics should be administered in the lowest effective dosages for the shortest time needed. As pain diminishes, the patient should be switched from an opioid analgesic to a nonopioid analgesic, such as aspirin or acetaminophen.

In summary, when working with opioids, as with any other drugs, you must balance the risks of therapy against the benefits. The risk of addiction from therapeutic use of opioids is real but very small. Consequently, concerns about addiction should play a real but secondary role in making decisions about giving these drugs. Dosages should be sufficient to relieve pain. Suffering because of insufficient dosage is unacceptable. However, it is also unacceptable to promote possible abuse through failure to exercise good judgment.

PATIENT-CONTROLLED ANALGESIA

Patient-controlled analgesia (PCA) is a method of drug delivery that permits the patient to self-administer parenteral (IV, SC, epidural) opioids on an "as-needed" basis. PCA has been employed primarily for relief of pain in postoperative patients. Other candidates include patients experiencing pain caused by cancer, trauma, myocardial infarction, vaso-occlusive sickle cell crisis, and labor. As discussed below, PCA offers several advantages over intramuscular opioids administered by the nurse.

Devices Employed for PCA. PCA has been made possible by the development of reliable PCA devices. A PCA device consists of an electronically controlled infusion pump that can be activated by the patient to deliver a preset bolus dose of an opioid. The opioid is delivered through an indwelling catheter. In addition to providing bolus doses on demand, some PCA devices can deliver a basal infusion of opioid.

An essential feature of all PCA devices is a timing control. This control limits the total dose that can be administered each hour, thereby reducing the risk of overdosage. In addition, the timing control regulates the minimum interval (e.g., 10 minutes) between doses. This interval, referred to as the "lock-out" or "delay" interval, prevents the patient from administering a second dose before the first has had time to produce its full effect.

Drug Selection and Dosage Regulation. The opioids that have been used most extensively for PCA are morphine and meperidine [Demerol]. Other pure opioid agonists (e.g., methadone, hydromorphone, fentanyl) have also been employed, as have agonist-antagonist opioids (e.g., nalbuphine, buprenorphine).

Prior to starting PCA, the postoperative patient should be given an opioid loading dose (e.g., 2 to 10 mg of morphine). Once effective opioid levels have been established with the loading dose, PCA can be initiated, provided the patient has recovered sufficiently from anesthesia. For PCA with morphine, initial bolus doses of 1 mg are typical. The size of the bolus should be increased if analgesia is inadequate, and decreased if excessive sedation occurs. The size of the bolus dose is usually increased during sleeping hours, thereby promoting rest by prolonging the interval between doses.

Comparison of PCA with Traditional Intramuscular Therapy. The objective of therapy with analgesics is to provide comfort while minimizing sedation and other side effects, especially respiratory depression. This objective is best achieved by maintaining plasma levels of opioids that are steady (i.e., that have minimal fluctuations). In this manner, side effects from excessively high levels can be avoided, as can the return of severe pain from low levels.

In the traditional management of postoperative pain, patients are given an IM injection of an opioid every 3 to 4 hours. With this dosing schedule, plasma levels of the opioid can vary widely. Shortly after the injection, plasma levels rise very high, causing excessive sedation and possibly respiratory depression. Late in the dosing interval, pain may return as plasma levels drop to their lowest point.

In contrast to traditional therapy, PCA is ideally suited to maintain steady levels of opioids. This is because PCA relies on small doses given frequently (e.g., 1 mg of morphine every 10 minutes) rather than on large doses given infrequently (e.g., 20 mg of morphine every 3 hours). Maintenance of steady drug levels can be facilitated further if the PCA device is capable of delivering a basal opioid infusion. Because plasma drug levels remain relatively steady, PCA can provide continuous control of pain while avoiding the adverse effects associated with excessive drug levels.

An additional advantage of PCA is rapid relief of pain. Since the patient can self-administer an IV dose of opioid as soon as pain begins to return, there is a minimal delay between detection of pain and restoration of an adequate drug level. With traditional therapy, the patient must wait for the nurse to respond to a request for more drug; this delay can allow pain to become more intense.

Studies indicate that PCA is associated with acceleration of recovery. When compared with patients receiving traditional IM analgesia, postoperative patients receiving PCA show improved early mobilization, greater cooperation during physical therapy, and a shorter hospital stay.

Patient Education. Patient education is essential for successful PCA. Surgical patients should be educated preoperatively. Education should include an explanation of what PCA is along with instruction on how to activate the PCA device (usually by pressing a thumb button on a cord extending from the machine).

Patients should be told not to fear overdosage; the PCA device will not permit self-administration of excessive doses. Patient should be informed that there is a time lag (about 10 minutes) between activation of the device and production of maximal analgesia. To reduce discomfort associated with physical therapy, changing of dressings, ambulation, and other potentially painful activities, patients should be taught to activate the pump prophylactically (e.g., 10 minutes prior to the anticipated activity). Patients should be informed that at night, the PCA device will be adjusted to deliver larger doses than during waking hours; the purpose of this adjustment is to prolong the interval between doses and thereby facilitate sleep.

USE OF OPIOIDS IN SPECIFIC SETTINGS

Postoperative Pain. Opioid analgesics offer several benefits to the postoperative patient. The most obvious is increased comfort through reduction of pain. In addition, by reducing painful sensation, opioids can facilitate early movement and intentional cough. In patients who have undergone thoracic surgery, opioids permit chest movement that would otherwise be too uncomfortable to allow adequate ventilation. By promoting ventilation, opioids can reduce the risk of hypoxia and pneumonitis.

Opioids are not without drawbacks for the postoperative patient. These agents can cause constipation and urinary retention. Suppression of reflex cough can result in respiratory tract complications. In addition, analgesia may delay diagnosis of postoperative complications, since pain will not be present to signal their development.

Obstetric Analgesia. When administered to relieve pain during delivery, opioids may depress fetal respiration and uterine contractions. Since these effects are less likely with *meperidine* than with other strong opioids, meperidine is often the preferred opioid for obstetric use. Dosage should be high enough to reduce maternal discomfort to a tolerable level, but not so high as to cause pronounced respiratory depression in the neonate. Since opioids cross the blood-brain barrier of the infant more readily than that of the mother, doses that have little effect on maternal respiration may nonetheless cause profound respiratory depression in the infant. For meperidine, the usual dosage is 50 to 100 mg every 2 to 3 hours. Administration should be parenteral (IV or IM). Timing of administration is important: if the drug is given too early, it can inhibit or delay the progress of uterine contractions; if given too late, it can cause excessive neonatal sedation and respiratory depression. Following delivery, respiration in the neonate should be monitored closely. Naloxone can reverse respiratory depression and should be on hand.

Head Injury. Opioids must be employed with caution in the patient with head injury. Head injury can cause respiratory depression accompanied by elevation of intracranial pressure; opioids can exacerbate these reactions. In addition, since miosis, mental clouding, and vomiting can be valuable diagnostic signs following head injury, and since opioids can cause these same effects, use of opioids can complicate diagnosis.

Myocardial Infarction. Morphine is the opioid of choice for decreasing pain of myocardial infarction. With careful control of dosage, morphine can reduce discomfort without causing excessive respiratory depression and adverse cardiovascular effects. In addition, by lowering blood pressure, morphine can decrease cardiac work. If excessive hypotension or respiratory depression occur, they can be reversed with naloxone. Since pentazocine and butorphanol increase cardiac work and oxygen demand, these agonist-antagonist opioids should generally be avoided.

Sickle Cell Vaso-occlusive Crisis. Sickle cell disease can produce several types of crises: hemolytic crisis, aplastic crisis, splenic sequestration crisis, and vaso-occlusive crisis. Of these, vaso-occlusive crisis is most common. Vaso-occlusion can cause extreme pain in the affected area (e.g., hands and feet, joints and extremities, abdomen). Acute pain generally lasts for several days, but may then be followed by dull, aching pain that persists for weeks. The mainstays of treatment are hydration and analgesics. Studies have shown that patients generally fail to receive adequate analgesia. If the pain is moderate, a nonopioid analgesic (acetaminophen or a nonsteroidal anti-inflammatory agent) may be sufficient. However, if pain is severe, intensive therapy with an opioid is required. Parenteral (IV or IM) morphine and meperidine have been employed. Patient-controlled analgesia may be especially effective.

Cancer. Treating chronic pain of cancer differs substantially from treating acute pain of other disorders. When treating cancer pain, the objective is to maximize comfort. Psychologic and physical dependence are minimal concerns. Patients should be given as much medication as needed to relieve pain. In the words of one pain specialist, "No patient should wish for death because of the physician's reluctance to use adequate amounts of opioids."

Appropriate management of cancer pain requires appropriate drug selection. Not all patients need a strong opioid. If pain is mild, it can often be relieved with aspirin or another nonopioid analgesic. If pain cannot be relieved with a nonopioid alone, a moderate-to-strong opioid (e.g., codeine) may be added. Only when pain can no longer be controlled with weaker analgesics should a strong opioid be given. Morphine is frequently the drug of choice. Oral therapy is as effective as parenteral therapy and generally preferred. Parenteral opioids should be reserved for patients who cannot take oral drugs because of persistent nausea and vomiting or because of an inability to swallow.

For control of chronic pain, opioids should be given on a fixed schedule (e.g., every 4 hours around the clock) and not on a PRN basis. Use of a fixed schedule insures continuous suppression of pain, thereby sparing the patient discomfort as well as anxiety about pain returning. If breakthrough pain occurs, fixed dosing can be supplemented with PRN dosing.

Over the course of treatment, escalation of opioid dosage may be required. The need for increased dosage may reflect development of tolerance, or it may reflect progression of the disease. Fortunately, tolerance in cancer patients is rarely so great that adequate analgesia can no longer be achieved. Because analgesic needs may increase, patients should be re-evaluated on a regular basis to determine their drug requirements.

A mixture called *Brompton's cocktail*, named after the British hospital in which it was developed, has been advocated for managing cancer pain. A typical cocktail consists of heroin (in variable amounts), 10 mg of cocaine, 2.5 ml of 98% ethanol, 5 ml of syrup, and chloroform water. Controlled studies indicate that oral morphine solution is as effective as Brompton's cocktail and preferred over the cocktail by most patients.

OPIOID ANTAGONISTS

Opioid antagonists are drugs that block the effects of opioid agonists. Two pure antagonists are available: naloxone [Narcan] and naltrexone [Trexan]. Naloxone, the prototype of the opioid antagonists, is employed to treat opioid overdosage, postoperative opioid depression, and opioid-induced neonatal respiratory depression. The only approved application for naltrexone is treatment of opioid addiction.

NALOXONE

Mechanism of Action

Naloxone is a structural analogue of morphine that acts as a competitive antagonist at mu, kappa, and delta opioid receptors. By blocking access of opioid agonists to these receptors, naloxone prevents the agonists from producing effects. Naloxone can reverse most actions of the opioid agonists, including respiratory depression, coma, and analgesia.

Pharmacologic Effects

When administered in the absence of opioids, naloxone has no significant effects. If administered prior to giving an opioid, naloxone will block opioid actions. If administered to a patient who is already receiving opioids, naloxone will reverse analgesia, sedation, euphoria, and respiratory depression. If administered to an individual who is physically dependent on opioids, naloxone will precipitate an immediate withdrawal reaction.

Pharmacokinetics

Naloxone is administered IV, IM, and SC. Following IV injection, effects begin almost immediately, and persist for about 1 hour. Following IM or SC injection, effects begin within 2 to 5 minutes and persist for several hours. Elimination is by hepatic metabolism. Naloxone cannot be used orally because of rapid first-pass inactivation.

Therapeutic Uses

Treatment of Opioid Overdosage. Naloxone is the drug of choice for treating overdosage with pure opioid agonists. The drug reverses respiratory depression, coma, and other signs of opioid toxicity. Naloxone can also reverse toxicity from agonist-antagonist opioids (e.g., pentazocine, nalbuphine). However, the doses required may be higher than those needed to reverse poisoning by pure opioid agonists.

Dosage must be carefully titrated when treating toxicity in opioid addicts. Because the degree of physical dependence in these individuals is likely to be high, if dosage is excessive, naloxone can transform the patient from a state of poisoning to one of acute withdrawal. Accordingly, treatment should be initiated with a series of small doses rather than a single large dose.

In some cases of accidental poisoning, there may be uncertainty as to whether unconsciousness is due to opioid overdosage or to overdosage with a general CNS depressant (e.g., barbiturate, alcohol, benzodiazepine). When uncertainty exists, naloxone is nonetheless indicated. If the cause of poisoning is a barbiturate or another general CNS depressant, naloxone will be of no benefit—but neither will it cause any harm. If a cumulative dose of 10 mg fails to elicit a response, it is unlikely that opioids are involved; hence, other intoxicants should be suspected.

Reversal of Postoperative Opioid Depression. Following surgery, naloxone may be employed to reverse excessive respiratory and CNS depression caused by opioids that had been administered preoperatively or intraoperatively. Dosage should be titrated with care; the objective is to achieve adequate ventilation and alertness without reversing opioid actions to the point of unmasking pain.

Reversal of Neonatal Respiratory Depression. When opioids have been given for analgesia during labor and delivery, respiratory depression in the neonate may occur. If respiratory depression is substantial, naloxone should be administered to restore ventilation.

Preparations, Dosage, and Administration

Preparations and Routes. Naloxone [Narcan] is available in solution (0.4 and 1.0 mg/ml) for IV, IM, and SC injection. A dilute solution (0.02 mg/ml) is available for treating neonates.

Opioid Overdosage. The initial dosage is 0.4 mg for adults and 10 μg/kg for children. The preferred route is IV; IM or SC injection may be employed if IV administration is not possible. Dosing is repeated at 2- to 3-minute intervals until a satisfactory response has been achieved. Additional doses may be needed at 1- to 2-hour intervals for up to 72 hours, depending on the duration of action of the offending opioid.

Postoperative Opioid Depression. Initial therapy for adults consists of 0.1 to 0.2 mg IV repeated every 2 to 3 minutes until an adequate response has been achieved. Additional doses may be required at 1- to 2-hour intervals.

Neonatal Respiratory Depression. The initial dose is 10 μg/kg (IV, IM, or SC). This dose is repeated every 2 to 3 minutes until respiration is satisfactory.

NALTREXONE

Naltrexone [Trexan] is approved only for treating opioid addicts. The purpose of treatment is to prevent euphoria if the addict should take an opioid. Since naltrexone can precipitate a withdrawal reaction in persons who are physically dependent on opioids, candidates for treatment must be detoxified (rendered opioid-free) before naltrexone is given. Although naltrexone can block opioid-induced euphoria, the drug does not prevent craving for opioids. As a result, many addicts fail to comply with the treatment program. Therapy with naltrexone has been considerably less successful than with methadone, a drug that eliminates craving for opioids while blocking euphoria. Naltrexone is dispensed in 50-mg tablets. A typical dosing schedule consists of 100 mg on Monday and Wednesday and 150 mg on Friday. Alternatively, the drug can be administered in daily 50-mg doses.

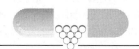

Summary of Major Nursing Implications

PURE OPIOID AGONISTS

Alfentanil	Methadone
Codeine	Morphine
Fentanyl	Oxycodone
Hydrocodone	Oxymorphone
Hydromorphone	Propoxyphene
Levorphanol	Sufentanil
Meperidine	

 Preadministration Assessment

Therapeutic Goal

Relief or prevention of moderate to severe pain while causing minimal respiratory depression, constipation, urinary retention, and other adverse effects.

Baseline Data

Assessment of Pain. Assess pain before administration and 1 hour later Determine the location, time of onset, and quality of pain (e.g., sharp, stabbing, dull). Also, assess for psychologic factors that can lower pain threshold (anxiety, depression, fear, anger). Since pain is subjective and determined by multiple factors (e.g., cultural influences, expectations, associated disease), there is no reliable objective method for determining how much discomfort the patient is experiencing. Ultimately, you must rely on your ability to interpret what patients have to say about their pain. When listening to patients, be aware that a few may claim discomfort when their pain is under control, whereas others may claim to feel fine when they are actually in pain.

Assessment of Vital Signs. Prior to administration, determine respiratory rate, blood pressure, and pulse rate.

Identifying High-Risk Patients

All opioids are *contraindicated* for *premature infants* (both during and after delivery). *Morphine* is contraindicated following *biliary tract surgery*.

Use opioids with *caution* in patients with *head injury, profound CNS depression, coma, respiratory depression, pulmonary disease (e.g., emphysema, asthma), cardiovascular disease, hypotension, reduced blood volume, prostatic hypertrophy, urethral stricture*, and *liver impairment*. Caution is also required when treating *infants, elderly* or *debilitated patients*, and patients receiving *MAO inhibitors, CNS depressants, anticholinergic drugs*, and *hypotensive agents*.

 Implementation: Administration

Routes

Oral, IM, IV, SC, rectal, epidural, intrathecal, and transdermal (fentanyl). Routes for specific opioids are summarized in Tables 28–5 and 28–6.

Dosage

General Guidelines. Adjust dosage to meet individual analgesic needs. Higher doses are required for patients with a low tolerance to pain or with especially painful conditions. Patients with sharp, stabbing pain need higher doses than patients with dull, constant pain. Elderly patients generally require lower doses than younger adults. Neonates require relatively low doses because of their poorly developed blood-brain barriers. For all patients, dosage should be reduced as pain subsides.

Oral doses are larger than parenteral doses. Check to insure that the dose to be administered is appropriate for the intended route.

Tolerance may develop with prolonged treatment, necessitating dosage escalation.

Warn outpatients not to increase dosage without consulting the physician.

Dosage in Patients with Cancer. Cancer is the major disease for which opioids are used chronically. The objective of treatment is to maximize comfort. Physical dependence is a minimal concern. Cancer patients should receive opioids on a fixed schedule around the clock—not on a PRN basis. If breakthrough pain occurs, fixed dosing can be supplemented with PRN dosing. Because of tolerance to opioids or intensification of pain, dosage escalation may eventually be required. Hence, patients should be re-evaluated on a regular basis to determine if pain control is adequate.

Discontinuing Opioids. Although significant dependence in hospitalized patients is rare, it can occur. To minimize symptoms of abstinence, withdraw opioids slowly, tapering the dosage over 3 days. Warn outpatients against abrupt discontinuation of treatment.

Administration

Prior to administration, determine respiratory rate, blood pressure, and pulse rate. Withhold medication and notify the physician if respiratory rate is at or below 12 per minute, if blood pressure is significantly below the pretreatment value, or if the pulse rate is significantly above or below the pretreatment value.

As a rule, opioids should be administered on a fixed schedule and not on a PRN basis. With a fixed schedule, medication is given before intense pain returns, thereby sparing the patient needless discomfort and reducing anxiety about recurrence of pain.

Perform *intravenous* injections slowly (over 4 to 5 minutes). Rapid injection may produce severe adverse effects (profound hypotension, respiratory arrest, cardiac arrest) and should be avoided. When making an IV injection, have an opioid antagonist (e.g., naloxone) and facilities for respiratory support available.

Perform injections (especially IV) with the patient lying down to minimize hypotension.

Opioid agonists are regulated under the Controlled Substances Act and must be dispensed accordingly. All of the pure agonists are Schedule II substances, except for propoxyphene (Schedule IV) and hydrocodone (Schedule III).

Concern for Opioid Abuse as a Factor in Dosage and Administration

Although opioids have a high potential for abuse, abuse is rare in the clinical setting. Consequently, when balancing the risk of abuse against the need to relieve pain, do not give excessive weight to concerns about abuse. The patient must not be allowed to suffer because of your unwarranted fears about abuse and dependence.

Although abuse is rare in the clinical setting, it *can* occur. To keep abuse to a minimum: (1) exercise clinical judgement when interpreting requests for opioid doses that seem excessive, (2) use opioids in the lowest effective doses for the shortest time required, (3) reserve opioid analgesics for patients with moderate to severe pain, and (4) switch to a nonopioid analgesic when the intensity of pain no longer justifies an opioid.

✓ **Implementation: Measures to Enhance Therapeutic Effects**

Responses to analgesics can be reinforced by nondrug measures, such as positioning the patient comfortably, showing concern and interest, and reassuring the patient that the medication will provide relief. Rest, mood elevation, and diversion can raise pain threshold and should be promoted. Conversely, anxiety, depression, fatigue, fear, and anger can lower pain threshold and should be minimized.

Since opioids can relieve the suffering component of pain without necessarily decreasing pain perception, do not tell patients that opioids will make their pain go away. Rather, tell them that their medication will make them more comfortable.

✓ **Ongoing Evaluation and Interventions**

Evaluating Therapeutic Effects

Evaluate for pain control 1 hour after opioid administration. If analgesia is insufficient, consult with the physician about an increase in dosage. Patients taking opioids chronically for suppression of cancer pain should be reevaluated on a regular basis to determine if their dosage is adequate.

Minimizing Adverse Effects

Respiratory Depression. Respiratory depression is the most serious adverse effect of the opioids. Monitor respiration in all patients. If respiratory rate is 12 per minute or less, withhold medication and notify the physician. Warn outpatients about respiratory depression and instruct them to notify the physician if respiratory distress occurs.

Certain patients, including the very young, the elderly, and those with respiratory disease (e.g., asthma, emphysema), are especially sensitive to the respiratory depressant action of opioids and must be monitored closely.

Delayed respiratory depression may develop following spinal administration of *morphine*. Be alert to this possibility.

When employed during labor and delivery, opioids may cause respiratory depression in the *neonate*. Monitor the infant closely. Have naloxone available to reverse opioid toxicity.

Sedation. Inform patients that opioids may cause drowsiness. Warn them against participation in hazardous activities (e.g., driving) if sedation is significant. Sedation can be minimized by (1) using smaller doses given more frequently, (2) using opioids with short half-lives, and (3) giving small doses of a CNS stimulant (methylphenidate or dextroamphetamine) in the morning and early afternoon.

Orthostatic Hypotension. Hypotension results from opioid-induced dilation of arterioles and veins secondary to release of histamine. Monitor blood pressure and pulse rate. Inform patients about symptoms of hypotension (dizziness, lightheadedness) and advise them to sit or lie down if these occur. Inform patients that hypotension can be minimized by moving slowly when assuming an erect posture. Warn patients against ambulation if hypotension is significant. If appropriate, assist hospitalized patients with ambulation.

Constipation. Monitor bowel function and inform the physician if constipation develops. Advise outpatients to increase dietary fiber and fluids. If these measures fail to normalize bowel function, a laxative may be needed.

Urinary Retention. To evaluate urinary retention, monitor intake and output, and palpate the lower abdomen for bladder distention every 4 to 6 hours. If there is a change in intake-output ratio, or if bladder distention is detected, or if the patient reports difficulty in voiding, notify the physician. Catheterization may be required. Interference with voiding is especially likely in patients with prostatic hypertrophy.

Since opioids may suppress awareness of bladder stimuli, encourage patients to void every 4 hours.

Biliary Colic. By constricting the common bile duct, *morphine* can increase pressure within the biliary tract, thereby causing severe pain. Biliary colic is much less likely with *meperidine*.

Emesis. Initial doses of opioids may cause nausea and vomiting. These reactions can be minimized by pretreatment with an antiemetic (e.g., promethazine) and by having the patient remain still. Tolerance to emesis develops quickly.

Cough Suppression. Cough suppression may result in accumulation of secretions in the airway. Instruct patients to cough at regular intervals. Auscultate the lungs for rales.

Miosis. Miosis can impair vision in dim light. Keep hospital room lighting bright during waking hours.

Opioid Dependence in the Neonate. The infant whose mother abused opioids during pregnancy may be born drug dependent. Observe the infant for signs of withdrawal (e.g., excessive crying, sneezing, tremor, hyperreflexia, fever, diarrhea) and notify the physician if these develop (usually within a few days after birth). The infant can be weaned from drug dependence by administering dilute opium tincture in progressively smaller doses.

Minimizing Adverse Interactions

CNS Depressants. Opioids can intensify responses to other CNS depressants (e.g., barbiturates, benzodiazepines, alcohol, antihistamines), thereby presenting a risk of profound sedation and respiratory depression. Warn patients against use of alcohol and other CNS depressants.

Agonist-Antagonist Opioids. These drugs (e.g., pentazocine, nalbuphine) can precipitate an abstinence syndrome if administered to a patient who is physically dependent on a pure opioid agonist. Before administering an agonist-antagonist, make certain that the patient has been withdrawn from opioid agonists.

Anticholinergic Drugs. These agents (e.g., atropine-like drugs, tricyclic antidepressants, phenothiazines) can exacerbate opioid-induced constipation and urinary retention.

Hypotensive Drugs. Antihypertensive agents and other drugs that lower blood pressure can exacerbate opioid-induced orthostatic hypotension.

Opioid Antagonists. Opioid antagonists (naloxone, naltrexone) can precipitate an abstinence syndrome if administered in excessive dosage to a patient who is physically dependent on opioids. To avoid this reaction, carefully titrate the dosage of the antagonist.

AGONIST-ANTAGONIST OPIOIDS

Buprenorphine	Nalbuphine
Butorphanol	Pentazocine
Dezocine	

Except for the differences presented below, the nursing implications for these drugs are much like those of the pure opioid agonists.

Therapeutic Goal

Relief of moderate-to-severe pain.

Routes

Oral, IV, IM, SC, and intranasal (butorphanol). Routes for individual agents are summarized in Table 28–7.

Differences from Pure Opioid Agonists

Maximal pain relief with the agonist-antagonists is generally lower than with pure opioid agonists.

Most agonist-antagonists have a ceiling to respiratory depression, making concerns about insufficient oxygenation low.

Agonist-antagonists cause little euphoria. Hence, abuse liability is low.

Agonist-antagonists increase cardiac work and should not be given to patients with acute myocardial infarction.

Because of their antagonist properties, agonist-antagonists can precipitate an abstinence syndrome in patients physically dependent on opioid agonists. Accordingly, patients must be withdrawn from pure opioid agonists before receiving an agonist-antagonist.

NALOXONE

Therapeutic Goal

Reversal of (1) postoperative opioid depression, (2) neonatal respiratory depression, and (3) overdosage with pure opioid agonists.

Routes

Intravenous, IM, and SC. For initial treatment, administer IV. Once opioid-induced CNS and respiratory depression have been reversed, IM or SC administration may be employed.

Dosage

Titrate dosage carefully. In opioid addicts, excessive doses can transform the patient from a state of opioid poisoning to one of withdrawal. In the postoperative patient, excessive doses can bring on pain by reversing opioid-mediated analgesia.

29

Drugs for Headache

Headache is a common symptom that can be triggered by a variety of stimuli, including stress, fatigue, acute illness, and sensitivity to alcohol. Many people experience mild, episodic headaches that can be relieved with over-the-counter medications (aspirin, acetaminophen, ibuprofen). For these individuals, medical intervention is unnecessary. In contrast, some people experience severe, recurrent, debilitating headaches that are frequently unresponsive to aspirin-like drugs. For these individuals, medical attention is merited. In this chapter, our focus is on these severe forms of headache. Specifically, we will discuss drug therapy of migraine, cluster, and tension-type headaches.

When attempting to treat headache, it is essential to differentiate between headaches that have an identifiable underlying cause (e.g., severe hypertension; hyperthyroidism; tumors; infection; disorders of the eye, ear, nose, sinuses, and throat) and headaches that have no identifiable cause. Obviously, if there is a clear cause of the headache, that cause should be treated directly.

As we consider the drugs for headache, three basic principles should be kept in mind. First, antiheadache drugs may be used in two ways: (1) to abort an ongoing attack, and (2) to prevent attacks from occurring in the first place. Second, not all patients with a particular type of headache respond to the same drugs. Hence, therapy must be individualized. Third, several of the drugs employed to treat severe headaches (ergotamine, pentobarbital, meprobamate, opioids) can cause physical dependence. Accordingly, every effort should be made to keep dependence from developing. If dependence does develop, a withdrawal procedure will be needed.

353

MIGRAINE HEADACHE I: CHARACTERISTICS AND OVERVIEW OF TREATMENT

Characteristics

Migraine headaches are characterized by unilateral, throbbing or nonthrobbing head pain, often associated with nausea, vomiting, diarrhea, photophobia, and irritability. Precipitating factors include anxiety, fatigue, stress, menstruation, alcohol, and tyramine-containing foods. Attacks that are preceded by an aura (typically visual) are termed *classic*, whereas attacks that are not preceded by an aura are termed *common*, the form experienced by most patients. About 60% to 70% of people with migraine are women in their late teens, 20s, or 30s. A family history of the disease is common.

The pathophysiology of migraine is complex and incompletely understood. According to the traditional view, the prodromal aura of classic migraine is caused by constriction of cerebral arteries, whereas the headache itself is caused by subsequent dilation of cerebral and cranial arteries. In support of this view is the observation that the amplitude of arterial pulsations and the intensity of pain decline in parallel in response to drug therapy (ergotamine) and to digital pressure applied to the carotid artery. However, it may be that neurogenic activation of pain fibers, independent of arterial dilatation, is an important contributor to migraine pain.

Overview of Treatment

Drugs for migraine are employed in two ways: (1) to abort an ongoing attack, and (2) to prevent attacks from occurring. The principal drugs used to abort an attack are—in order of increasing effectiveness—*aspirin-like drugs, ergot alkaloids,* and *opioid analgesics.* The principal drugs employed to prevent an attack from occurring are *beta-adrenergic blockers, calcium channel blockers, methysergide,* and *tricyclic antidepressants.*

In addition to drug therapy, nondrug measures should be used. An effort should be made to control or eliminate precipitating factors. Biofeedback and other relaxation techniques can also be helpful.

MIGRAINE HEADACHE II: DRUGS FOR ACUTE THERAPY

The objective of acute therapy is to eliminate headache pain and suppress associated nausea and vomiting. Treatment should commence at the earliest sign of an attack. Because migraine causes gastric stasis, nausea, and vomiting, oral therapy may be ineffective once an attack has begun. Hence, for treatment of an established attack, rectal suppositories or an inhalational preparation may be best.

Drug selection depends on the intensity of the attack. For mild-to-moderate symptoms, an *aspirin-like drug* (aspirin, ibuprofen, acetaminophen) may be sufficient. If this is inadequate, *aspirin combined with codeine* may be tried. If these analgesics prove insufficient, the next attack should be treated with an *ergot alkaloid*—either ergotamine or dihydroergotamine. If these agents fail to relieve pain, an *opioid analgesic* (e.g., meperidine) may be needed. The therapeutic niche of *sumatriptan,* a new drug for migraine, has not been defined.

Metoclopramide may be used as an adjunct to other agents for treating an acute migraine attack. This drug can suppress nausea and vomiting caused by the attack itself and by therapy with ergot alkaloids. In addition, metoclopramide can reverse gastric stasis caused by the attack, thereby facilitating absorption of oral medications. Metoclopramide has no direct effect on migraine pain.

ERGOTAMINE

Mechanism of Antimigraine Action

The actions of ergotamine are complex and the precise mechanism by which the drug stops migraine attacks is not known. Ergotamine can alter transmission at serotonergic (tryptaminergic), dopaminergic, and alpha-adrenergic junctions. In cranial arteries, the drug promotes constriction and reduces the amplitude of pulsations. It can also affect blood flow by depressing the vasomotor center. These vascular effects probably contribute to reduction of migraine pain. In addition, the drug may reduce pain by depressing serotonergic transmission in central pain pathways.

Therapeutic Uses

Ergotamine is the drug of choice for stopping an ongoing migraine attack. It is also used to treat cluster headaches. Because of the risk of dependence (see below), ergotamine should not be taken daily on a long-term basis.

Pharmacokinetics

Administration may be oral, sublingual, rectal, or by inhalation. Bioavailability with oral and sublingual administration is low. Bioavailability with rectal and inhalational administration is higher. Although the half-life of ergotamine is only 2 hours, pharmacologic effects can still be observed 24 hours after administration. The drug is eliminated primarily by hepatic metabolism. Metabolites are excreted in the bile.

Adverse Effects

Ergotamine is well tolerated at usual therapeutic doses. The drug can stimulate the chemoreceptor trigger zone to cause nausea and vomiting in about 10% of those treated. This action can augment nausea and vomiting caused by the migraine itself. Concurrent treatment with metoclopramide or a phenothiazine antiemetic can help suppress these gastrointestinal responses. Other common side effects include weakness in the legs, myalgia, numbness and tingling in fingers and toes, angina-like pain, and tachycardia or bradycardia.

Overdosage

Acute or chronic overdosage can cause serious toxicity (ergotism). Symptoms include the adverse effects seen at therapeutic doses plus signs and symptoms of ischemia caused by constriction of peripheral arteries and arterioles. That is, the extremities become cold, pale, and numb; muscle pain develops; and gangrene may eventually result. Patients should be informed about these signs and symptoms and instructed to report them immediately. The risk of ergotism is highest in patients with sepsis, peripheral vascular disease, and renal or hepatic impairment. Management consists of discontinuing ergotamine, followed by pharmacologic measures to maintain circulation (treatment with anticoagulants, low molecular weight dextran, and/or intravenous nitroprusside as appropriate).

Physical Dependence

Regular daily use of ergotamine, even in moderate doses, can cause physical dependence. The withdrawal syndrome is characterized by headache, nausea, vomiting, and restlessness (i.e., withdrawal resembles a migraine attack). Patients who begin to experience these symptoms are likely to resume taking the drug, thereby perpetuating the cycle of dependence. Hospitalization may be required to break the cycle. To avoid development of dependence, dosage and duration of treatment must be limited (see dosing guidelines below).

Contraindications

Ergotamine is contraindicated for patients with hepatic or renal impairment, sepsis (gangrene has resulted), coronary artery disease, and peripheral vascular disease. In addition, the drug should not be taken during pregnancy (its ability to promote uterine contractions can cause fetal harm or abortion). Ergotamine is classified in FDA Pregnancy Category X: the risk of use by pregnant women clearly outweighs any possible benefits. Warn women of child-bearing age to avoid pregnancy while using this drug.

Preparations, Dosage, and Administration

Ergotamine by itself is available in tablets for sublingual use and in an aerosol for oral inhalation. In addition, ergotamine is dispensed in combination with other drugs for oral and rectal administration.

Sublingual. Ergotamine tartrate [Ergostat] is dispensed in 2-mg tablets for sublingual use. One tablet should be placed under the tongue immediately after onset of aura or headache. If needed, additional tablets can be administered at 30-minute intervals—up to a maximum of 3 tablets/24 hr or 5 tablets/week.

Inhalation. Ergotamine tartrate [Medihaler Ergotamine] is dispensed in an aerosol for oral inhalation. Each inhalation delivers 0.36 mg. One inhalation should be done immediately after onset of aura or headache. If pain is not relieved, additional inhalations can be done at 5-minute intervals—up to a maximum of 6/hr or 15/wk.

Oral. Three oral formulations [Cafergot, Ercaf, Wigraine] contain 1 mg ergotamine tartrate and 100 mg caffeine; a fourth formulation [Cafatine-PB] contains 30 mg pentobarbital and 0.125 mg belladonna alkaloids in addition to the ergotamine and caffeine. The caffeine is present to enhance vasoconstriction and ergotamine absorption. The pentobarbital provides sedation. The belladonna alkaloids suppress emesis. With all four oral formulations, 2 tablets are taken immediately after onset of aura or headache. One additional tablet can be administered every 30 minutes—up to a maximum of 6/attack or 10/wk.

Rectal. Ergotamine is available in three rectal formulations [Cafatine Supps, Cafetrate Supps, Wigraine Supps]. Each contains 2 mg ergotamine tartrate and 100 mg caffeine. No more than 2 suppositories should be administered per attack.

DIHYDROERGOTAMINE

Therapeutic Uses

Dihydroergotamine (IM or IV) is considered the drug of choice for terminating severe, refractory migraine and cluster headaches. Because the drug must be administered parenterally, it is best suited for use in a medical setting (emergency room, physician's office).

Pharmacologic Effects and Contraindications

The actions of dihydroergotamine are similar to those of ergotamine. Like ergotamine, dihydroergotamine alters transmission at serotonergic, dopaminergic, and alpha-adrenergic junctions. In contrast to ergotamine, dihydroergotamine causes minimal peripheral vasoconstriction, little nausea and vomiting, and no physical dependence. However, diarrhea is a prominent side effect. Contraindications are the same as those for ergotamine: coronary artery disease, peripheral vascular disease, sepsis, pregnancy, and hepatic or renal impairment.

Pharmacokinetics

Dihydroergotamine is administered parenterally (IM and IV). Because of extensive first-pass metabolism, the drug is not active orally. Elimination is by hepatic metabolism. An active metabolite (8'-hydroxy-dihydroergotamine) contributes to therapeutic effects. The half-life of dihydroergotamine plus its active metabolite is about 21 hours.

Preparations, Dosage, and Administration

Dihydroergotamine mesylate [D.H.E. 45] is dispensed in solution (1 mg/ml) for IM and IV administration.

Intramuscular. The initial dose is 1 mg immediately after onset of symptoms. Additional 1-mg doses may be given hourly up to a maximum of 3 mg per attack. Dosage should be adjusted early in therapy to determine a minimal effective dose. This dose should be used for subsequent attacks.

Intravenous. One milligram is given initially followed by another mg in 1 hour if needed. Dosage should not exceed 6 mg/wk.

SUMATRIPTAN

Actions and Uses

Sumatriptan [Imitrex] is a promising new drug for migraine. In clinical trials this drug gave complete relief to more than 90% of those treated. Three routes were employed: IV, SC, and PO. Symptoms abated within 10 to 30 minutes after IV administration, within 20 to 60 minutes after SC administration, and within 2 hours after PO administration. Relief was achieved at all stages of the attack. The drug is also active against cluster headaches, although it hasn't been approved for this use.

Sumatriptan is an analogue of serotonin (5-HT), and stimulation of a serotonin receptor subtype (5-HT$_{1D}$) is thought to underlie the drug's antimigraine effects. Observations in support of this hypothesis include (1) sumatriptan binds selectively to 5-HT$_{1D}$ receptors, (2) these receptors are localized on certain cranial blood vessels, and (3) stimulation of these receptors causes the vessels to constrict, a response that could abort a migraine attack. Sumatriptan has no affinity for adrenergic, dopaminergic, or muscarinic receptors. The drug has no analgesic actions in animals and does not affect peripheral blood flow in humans.

Pharmacokinetics

Sumatriptan has very low oral bioavailability and, therefore, is given by injection. Following subcutaneous injection, peak plasma levels are achieved in 5 to 20 minutes. Sumatriptan is converted to inactive metabolites by the liver, and the metabolites are excreted in the urine. The drug's half-life is 2.6 hours.

Adverse Effects

Experience to date indicates that sumatriptan is generally well tolerated. Most side effects have been transient and mild. Reported reactions include *paresthesias* (warmth and tingling), *vertigo, malaise, fatigue, feelings of heaviness,* and *a sense of pressure in the chest.* Transient pain and redness may occur at sites of SC injection.

Angina has occurred with oral and SC administration. Electrocardiographic changes have been observed in patients with coronary artery disease or Prinzmetal's (vasospastic) angina. Sumatriptan is contraindicated for these patients.

Sumatriptan should be avoided during pregnancy. When given daily to pregnant rabbits, the drug is embryolethal at blood levels only three times higher than those achieved with a 6-mg SC injection in humans (which is a typical dose). Accordingly, unless the physician directs otherwise, women should be instructed to avoid the drug if they are pregnant or think they might be, if they are trying to become pregnant, or if they are not using an adequate form of contraception.

Preparations, Dosage, and Administration

Sumatriptan succinate [Imitrex] is available in single-dose vials and prefilled syringes for SC injection. An autoinjector is available for self-administration. The maximum single dose is 6 mg. The maximum that may be given in 24 hours is two 6-mg doses, separated by at least 1 hour. Sumatriptan should be administered no sooner than 24 hours after any ergotamine-containing drug.

MIGRAINE HEADACHE III: PROPHYLACTIC THERAPY

Several drugs, when taken prophylactically, can reduce the frequency and intensity of migraine attacks. Prophylactic therapy is indicated for patients who have not responded adequately to abortive therapy, and for patients whose attacks are especially frequent or severe.

BETA-ADRENERGIC BLOCKING AGENTS

Propranolol is the drug of choice for migraine prophylaxis. This agent can reduce the number and intensity of attacks in about 70% of patients with either common or classic migraine. No loss in benefits has occurred over 1 year of continuous treatment.

Not all beta blockers are active against migraine. Agents with demonstrated efficacy are propranolol, metoprolol, nadolol, and timolol. Agents shown to be ineffective include oxprenolol and pindolol. Because only some beta blockers are effective, whereas all of them are able to block beta-adrenergic receptors, it would appear that a mechanism other than beta blockade is responsible for beneficial effects in migraine.

The basic pharmacology of the beta-adrenergic blocking agents is discussed in Chapter 18.

METHYSERGIDE

Methysergide [Sansert] was the first effective drug for prophylaxis of migraine. This agent is more effective than propranolol, but is also more dangerous. Accordingly, prophylaxis with propranolol is generally preferred. Methysergide is not effective for aborting an ongoing attack. In addition to its utility against migraine, methysergide is a preferred drug for prophylaxis of cluster headaches.

The mechanism by which methysergide provides prophylaxis is not certain. The drug is able to stimulate serotonin receptors in the central nervous system (CNS). Suppression of pain pathways by this mechanism may explain beneficial effects.

Methysergide causes a variety of adverse effects. Fibrotic changes, although rare, are most serious. With long-term therapy, methysergide can cause retroperitoneal, pleuropulmonary, and cardiac fibrosis. Retroperitoneal fibrosis can result in urinary tract obstruction. Pleuropulmonary fibrosis can cause chest pain, dyspnea, and plural effusion. Fibrosis of the aortic and mitral valves can cause murmurs and dyspnea. Fibrotic changes may reverse spontaneously upon cessation of drug use. However, surgical correction may be required. Other adverse effects include vascular insufficiency, CNS reactions (insomnia, altered mood, depersonalization, hallucinations, nightmares), and gastrointestinal disturbances (nausea, vomiting, diarrhea).

The usual adult dosage is 4 to 8 mg daily. Because of its potential for serious toxicity, methysergide should not be taken continuously. Rather, the manufacturer recommends that the drug be discontinued for 3 to 4 weeks every 6 months.

CALCIUM CHANNEL BLOCKERS

Several calcium channel blockers can provide effective prophylaxis of migraine. These include *verapamil, nifedipine, nimodipine,* and *flunarizine* (a drug not yet available in the United States). Curiously, beneficial effects develop slowly, reaching their maximum in 1 to 2 months. Although all of these drugs can relieve vasospasm, it is not clear that vasodilation explains their antimigraine effects. A direct effect on neurons is another possible mechanism.

Except for its cost, *nimodipine* [Nimotop] is especially well suited for migraine prophylaxis. The drug is very lipid soluble and, hence, penetrates the blood-brain barrier with ease. As a result, it can reach effective concentrations in the CNS at relatively low doses, thereby minimizing peripheral vasodilation. Unfortunately, the high price of nimodipine precludes its routine use. The dosage for prophylaxis of migraine is 30 to 60 mg three times a day.

The basic pharmacology of the calcium channel blockers is discussed in Chapter 38.

ANTIDEPRESSANTS

Amitriptyline, a tricyclic antidepressant, provides effective prophylaxis against migraine. In one study, the drug was as effective as methysergide. The mechanism underlying antimigraine actions is not known. Since amitriptyline is effective in patients who are not depressed, it would seem that benefits are *not* dependent on elevation of mood.

Like amitriptyline, *phenelzine*, an MAO inhibitor-type antidepressant, is active against migraine. However, responses are variable, and the drug is potentially much more dangerous than amitriptyline. Accordingly, phenelzine should not be used routinely. Rather, the drug should be reserved for patients who cannot tolerate or who fail to respond to safer drugs.

The basic pharmacology of the antidepressants is discussed in Chapter 25.

CLUSTER HEADACHE

Characteristics

Cluster headaches occur in a series or "cluster" of attacks. Each attack lasts from 15 minutes to 2 hours and is characterized by severe, nonthrobbing, unilateral, oculofrontal or oculotemporal pain. A cluster consists of one or more such attacks every day for 4 to 12 weeks. An attack-free interval of months to years separates each cluster. Although related to migraine, cluster headaches differ in several ways: (1) they are not preceded by an aura, (2) they do not cause nausea and vomiting, (3) they are not associated with a family history of attacks, (4) they are more common in men than women, and (5) the approach to their treatment is different.

Treatment

Primary therapy is directed at preventing attacks. The preferred agent for prophylaxis is *methysergide*. Alternatives include *calcium channel blockers* (e.g., nimodipine), *lithium*, and *glucocorticoids*. When lithium is used, blood levels of the drug must be monitored. Because long-term treatment with glucocorticoids carries a high risk of serious toxicity, use of these drugs should be limited to 3 weeks.

If an attack occurs despite preventative therapy, it can be aborted with an ergot preparation. Because of its rapid action, parenteral dihydroergotamine is preferred. Slower relief can be achieved with an ergotamine-caffeine suppository. Since attacks last less than 2 hours, oral ergotamine, with its slow onset, is less helpful.

An attack may also be terminated by inhalation of 100% oxygen (for 15 minutes or less). This procedure is effective in up to 93% of patients. The mechanism of relief is unknown.

TENSION-TYPE HEADACHES

Characteristics

Tension-type or muscle-contraction headaches are characterized by moderate, generalized (non-localized), nonthrobbing pain associated with scalp formication and a sense of tightness or pressure in the head and neck. Precipitating factors include eye strain, aggravation, frustration, and life's daily stresses. Depressive symptoms (sleep disturbances, including early and frequent awakening) are often present.

Tension-type headaches frequently occur to-gether with migraine. In some patients, migraine headaches experienced early in life are later replaced by an unremitting tension-type headache, a condition referred to as chronic headache syndrome.

Treatment

An acute attack of mild-to-moderate intensity can be relieved with a nonopioid analgesic—acetaminophen or a nonsteroidal anti-inflammatory drug (e.g., aspirin, ibuprofen, naproxen). An analgesic-sedative combination (e.g., aspirin-meprobamate, aspirin-butalbital) may also be used. However, because of their potential for dependence and abuse, these combinations should be reserved for acute therapy of episodic attacks; they are inappropriate for patients with chronic headache syndrome.

If depressive symptoms are present, a tricyclic antidepressant (e.g., amitriptyline) is preferred to analgesics. Administering the antidepressant at bedtime will help relieve depression-related sleep disturbances in addition to relieving headache pain.

For patients with chronic headache syndrome, prophylactic treatment with propranolol plus amitriptyline is helpful. Prophylaxis with a monoamine oxidase inhibitor (e.g., phenelzine) may also be effective.

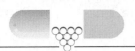

Summary of Major Nursing Implications

ERGOTAMINE

✓ **Preadministration Assessment**

Therapeutic Goal

Termination of migraine or cluster headache.

Baseline Data

Determine the age of onset, frequency, location, intensity, and quality (throbbing or nonthrobbing) of headache as well as the presence or absence of a prodromal aura. Assess for precipitating factors (e.g., stress, anxiety, fatigue) and for a family history of severe headache.

Assess for possible underlying causes of headache (e.g., severe hypertension; hyperthyroidism; infection; tumors; disorders of the eye, ear, nose, sinuses, or throat). If present, these should be treated directly.

Identifying High-Risk Patients

Ergotamine is contraindicated in the presence of *hepatic or renal impairment, sepsis, coronary artery disease, peripheral vascular disease,* and *pregnancy.*

✓ **Implementation: Administration**

Routes

Sublingual, inhalation (ergotamine alone).
Oral, rectal (ergotamine plus caffeine).

Dosage and Administration

Instruct the patient to commence dosing immediately after onset of symptoms.

Ergotamine can cause physical dependence and serious toxicity if taken in excessive dosage. Inform the patient about the risks of dependence and toxicity and the importance of not exceeding the prescribed dosage.

Nausea and vomiting from the headache and from ergotamine itself may prevent complete absorption of oral ergotamine. Concurrent treatment with *metoclopramide* or another antiemetic can minimize these effects.

✓ **Implementation: Measures to Enhance Therapeutic Effects**

Educate the patient in ways to control, avoid, or eliminate precipitating factors (e.g., stress, fatigue, anxiety, menstruation, alcohol, tyramine-containing foods).

Teach the patient biofeedback or another relaxation technique. Advise the patient to rest in a quiet, dark room for 2 to 3 hours after drug administration.

Ongoing Evaluation and Interventions

Evaluating Therapeutic Effects

Determine the size and frequency of doses used and the extent to which therapy has reduced the intensity and duration of attacks.

Minimizing Adverse Effects

Nausea and Vomiting. Minimize these by concurrent therapy with metoclopramide or a phenothiazine-type antiemetic.

Ergotism. Toxicity (ergotism) can result from acute or chronic overdosage. Teach patients the early manifestations of ergotism (muscle pain; paresthesias in fingers and toes; extremities become cold, pale, and numb) and instruct them to report these immediately. To treat: (1) withdraw ergotamine, and (2) administer drugs (anticoagulants, low-molecular-weight dextran, intravenous nitroprusside) as appropriate to maintain circulation.

Physical Dependence. Warn patients not to overuse ergotamine, since overuse can cause physical dependence. Teach patients the signs and symptoms of withdrawal (headache, nausea, vomiting, restlessness) and instruct them to inform the physician if these develop during a drug-free interval. Patients who develop dependence may require hospitalization to bring about withdrawal.

Abortion. Ergotamine is a uterine stimulant that can cause abortion when taken in high doses. Warn women of child-bearing age to avoid pregnancy while using this drug.

Anesthetics

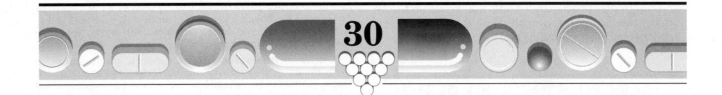

General Anesthetics

*G*eneral anesthetics are drugs that produce unconsciousness and a lack of responsiveness to painful stimuli. These agents can be contrasted with the *local anesthetics*, which do not affect consciousness and reduce sensation only in a limited region of the body. The local anesthetics are discussed in Chapter 31.

General anesthetics can be divided into two groups: (1) inhalation anesthetics, and (2) intravenous anesthetics. The inhalation anesthetics constitute the main focus of this chapter.

When considering the anesthetics, we need to distinguish between the terms *analgesia* and *anesthesia*. Analgesia refers specifically to loss of sensibility to pain. In contrast, anesthesia refers not only to loss of pain but to loss of all other sensations as well (e.g., touch, temperature, taste). Hence, while analgesics (e.g., aspirin, morphine) can selectively reduce pain without affecting other sensory modalities and without reducing consciousness, the general anesthetics have no such selectivity: during general anesthesia, all sensation is lost, and consciousness is lost as well.

The development of general anesthetics has had an incalculable impact on the surgeon's art. The first general anesthetic (ether) was introduced by Dr. William T. Morton in 1846. Prior to this time, surgery was a brutal and exquisitely painful ordeal, undertaken only under the most desperate circumstances. Immobilization of the surgical field was accomplished with the aid of strong men and straps. Survival of the patient was determined by the surgeon's speed—not by his finesse. With the advent of general anesthesia, all of this changed. General anesthesia produced a patient who slept through surgery and experienced no pain. These changes allowed surgeons to develop the lengthy

363

and intricate procedures that are routine today. Such procedures were unthinkable before general anesthetics became available.

BASIC PHARMACOLOGY OF THE INHALATION ANESTHETICS

The information addressed in this section applies to the inhalation anesthetics as a group. We will focus on (1) properties of an ideal anesthetic, (2) pharmacokinetic aspects of inhalation anesthesia, (3) adverse effects of the inhalation anesthetics, and (4) drugs employed as adjuncts to anesthesia.

PROPERTIES OF AN IDEAL INHALATION ANESTHETIC

An ideal inhalation anesthetic would produce unconsciousness, analgesia, muscle relaxation, and amnesia. Furthermore, induction of anesthesia would be brief and pleasant, as would the process of emergence. Depth of anesthesia could be raised or lowered with ease. Adverse effects would be minimal, and the margin of safety would be large. As one might guess, the ideal inhalation anesthetic does not exist: no single agent has all of the properties noted.

BALANCED ANESTHESIA

The term *balanced anesthesia* refers to the use of a combination of drugs to accomplish what usually cannot be achieved using an inhalation anesthetic alone. Put another way, balanced anesthesia is a technique employed to compensate for the lack of an ideal anesthetic. Drugs are combined in balanced anesthesia to insure that induction is smooth and rapid and that analgesia and muscle relaxation are adequate. The agents used most commonly to achieve these goals are (1) short-acting barbiturates (for induction of anesthesia), (2) neuromuscular blocking agents (for muscle relaxation), and (3) opioids and nitrous oxide (for analgesia). The primary benefit of combining drugs to achieve surgical anesthesia is that doing so permits production of full general anesthesia at doses of the inhalation anesthetic that are lower (safer) than those that would be required if surgical anesthesia were attempted using the inhalation anesthetic by itself.

STAGES OF ANESTHESIA

The state of anesthesia has four stages of increasing depth. These stages were first described for patients undergoing anesthesia with ether, an agent whose effects develop slowly. Because modern anesthetics act much more rapidly than ether,

the early stages of anesthesia usually pass so quickly as to be undiscernable. Hence, the stages of anesthesia described below, which are conspicuous during anesthesia with ether, are rarely seen in modern clinical practice.

I. Stage of Analgesia. The initial stage of anesthesia begins with the onset of anesthetic administration and extends until consciousness is lost. Stage I is characterized by analgesia and moderate muscle relaxation. Some major surgeries can be performed at this stage.

II. Stage of Delirium. Stage II begins with loss of consciousness and extends to the onset of the stage of surgical anesthesia. Stage II is characterized by delirious excitement and reflex muscle activity. Respiration is likely to be irregular. Vomiting and urinary or fecal incontinence may occur. Stage II can be troublesome, and anesthesiologists try to hasten passage through this stage.

III. Stage of Surgical Anesthesia. Stage III extends from the end of stage II to the point where spontaneous respiration ceases. Stage III is characterized by deep unconsciousness, varying degrees of respiratory depression, and suppression of certain reflexes. Muscle relaxation is greater than in stages I and II.

Stage III can be subdivided into four planes of increasing depth. As the patient passes through these planes, respiration becomes progressively weaker.

IV. Stage of Medullary Paralysis. Stage IV begins when all spontaneous respiration is lost. Passage into stage IV results from anesthetic overdosage. During this stage, vital signs are dangerously depressed; death results from circulatory collapse.

MOLECULAR MECHANISM OF ACTION

Although several theories have been proposed, the molecular mechanism by which inhalation anesthetics act remains unknown. We do know that general anesthesia results from depression of neuronal activity within the brain and spinal cord. However, we do not know just how this depression is produced.

There is reasonable certainty that general anesthesia is not a receptor-mediated process. General anesthetics come in a wide variety of molecular shapes and sizes. Analysis of these diverse structures does not reveal any relationship between molecular configuration and anesthetic activity. Because of this absence of structure-activity relationships, it is generally assumed that inhalation anesthetics do not produce their effects through interactions with specific neuronal receptors.

If general anesthetics do not act through receptors, how might their effects come about? The available data suggest that inhalation anesthetics act at the level of the neuronal membrane. There is a direct correlation between the potency of an anesthetic and its lipid solubility. That is, the more readily an anesthetic can dissolve in the lipid matrix of neuronal membranes, the more readily that agent can produce anesthesia. By dissolving into neuronal membranes, anesthetics can disrupt membrane structure, thereby suppressing axonal conduction and synaptic transmission. These actions could explain anesthesia. Note that actions at the level of neuronal membranes would predict relatively nonselective interference with all neurons. Experience shows this prediction to be correct.

MINIMUM ALVEOLAR CONCENTRATION

The minimum alveolar concentration, or MAC, is an index of inhalation anesthetic *potency*. The MAC is defined as *the minimum concentration of drug in the alveolar air that will produce immobility in 50% of patients exposed to a painful stimulus.* It should be noted that a *low* MAC indicates *high* anesthetic potency.

From a clinical perspective, knowledge of the MAC of an anesthetic is of great practical value: the MAC tells us approximately how much anesthetic the inspired air must contain to produce anesthesia. A low value for MAC indicates that the inspired air need only contain low concentrations of drug to produce anesthesia. Conversely, when a drug has a high MAC, anesthesia can be achieved only when drug concentration in the inspired air is high. Fortunately, most inhalation anesthetics have very low MACs (Table 30–1), and, therefore, can act at low concentrations. However, one important agent—nitrous oxide—has a MAC that is extremely high. The MAC of nitrous oxide is so high, in fact, that surgical anesthesia cannot be achieved using this drug alone.

PHARMACOKINETICS

Uptake and Distribution

To produce therapeutic effects, an inhalation anesthetic must be present within the central nervous system (CNS) in concentrations sufficient to suppress neuronal excitability. The principal determinants of anesthetic concentration within the CNS are uptake from the lungs and distribution to the CNS and other tissues. The kinetics of anesthetic uptake and distribution are complex and will not be considered in detail.

Uptake. A major determinant of anesthetic uptake is the concentration of anesthetic in the inspired air: the greater the anesthetic concentration, the more rapid uptake will be. Other factors that contribute to anesthetic uptake are pulmonary ventilation, solubility of the anesthetic in blood, and blood flow through the lungs. An increase in any of these factors will increase the rate of uptake.

Distribution. Distribution to specific tissues is determined largely by regional blood flow. Anesthetic levels rise most rapidly in the brain, kidney, heart, and liver—tissues that receive the largest fraction of the cardiac output. Anesthetic levels in these tissues equilibrate with those of the blood within 5 to 15 minutes after the onset of anesthetic administration. In skin and skeletal muscles—tissues with an intermediate blood supply—equilibration occurs more slowly. The most poorly perfused tissues—fat, bone, ligaments, and cartilage—are the last to achieve equilibration with anesthetic levels in the blood.

Metabolism

Inhalation anesthetics undergo very little metabolism. Hence, metabolism does not influence the time course of anesthesia. However, since metabolites are responsible for certain toxicities of inhalation anesthetics (see below), metabolism is nonetheless clinically significant despite its small extent.

Elimination

Inhalation anesthetics are eliminated almost entirely via the lungs; as noted above, hepatic metabolism is a minor contributor to elimination. The same factors that determine anesthetic uptake (pulmonary ventilation, blood flow to the lungs, and anesthetic solubility in blood and tissues) also determine the rate of anesthetic elimination. Since blood flow to the brain is high, anesthetic levels in the brain drop rapidly upon discontinuation of administration. Anesthetic levels in tissues with a lower blood flow decline more slowly. Because levels of anesthetic in the CNS decline more rapidly than levels in other tissues, patients can awaken from anesthesia long before all of the anesthetic has left the body.

Table 30–1. Properties of the Major Inhalation Anesthetics

Drug	MAC* (%)	Analgesic Effect	Effect on Blood Pressure	Effect on Respiration	Muscle Relaxant Effect	Extent of Metabolism	Compatible with Epinephrine
Nitrous oxide	105	+ + + +	→	→	0	0	Yes
Halothane	0.75	+ +	↓	↓ ↓	+	15%	No
Enflurane	1.68	+ +	↓	↓ ↓	+ +	2–5%	Yes†
Isoflurane	1.15	+ +	↓	↓ ↓	+ +	1–2%	Yes
Methoxyflurane	0.16	+ + +	↓	↓ ↓	+	50–70%	—

0 =	No effect	→ =	Little or no change
+ =	Small effect		
+ + =	Moderate effect	↓ =	Moderate decrease
+ + + =	Large effect		
+ + + + =	Very large effect	↓ ↓ =	Large decrease

*Minimal alveolar concentration.
†Enflurane sensitizes the myocardium to catecholamines, but less so than halothane.

ADVERSE EFFECTS

The adverse effects discussed below apply to the inhalation anesthetics as a group. Please note, however, that not all of these effects are seen with every anesthetic agent.

Respiratory and Cardiac Depression. Depression of respiratory and cardiac function is a concern with virtually all inhalation anesthetics. Doses only two to four times greater than those needed for surgical anesthesia are sufficient to depress pulmonary and cardiac function to the point of lethality. To compensate for respiratory depression, almost all patients require mechanical support of ventilation.

Sensitization of the Heart to Catecholamines. Certain inhalation anesthetics can increase the sensitivity of the heart to stimulation by catecholamines (e.g., epinephrine). While in this sensitized state, the heart may develop dysrhythmias in response to catecholamines. Exposure to catecholamines may result from two causes: (1) release of endogenous catecholamines (in response to pain or other stimuli of the sympathetic nervous system), and (2) topical application of catecholamines to control bleeding in the surgical field. Inhalation anesthetics that are especially noted for sensitizing the heart to catecholamines are *halothane* and *methoxyflurane*.

Malignant Hyperthermia. Malignant hyperthermia is a rare and potentially fatal reaction that can be triggered by all inhalation anesthetics. Predisposition to the reaction is genetically based. Malignant hyperthermia is characterized by muscle rigidity and a profound elevation of temperature—sometimes to as high as 43°C. Left untreated, the reaction can rapidly prove fatal. The risk of malignant hyperthermia is greatest when an inhalation anesthetic is used in combination with succinylcholine, a neuromuscular blocker that also can trigger the reaction. Diagnosis and management of malignant hyperthermia are discussed in Chapter 15 (Neuromuscular Blocking Agents).

Aspiration of Gastric Contents. During the state of anesthesia, the reflexes that normally prevent aspiration of gastric contents into the lungs are abolished. Aspiration of gastric fluids can cause bronchospasm and, if bacteria are inhaled, pneumonia. Use of an endotracheal tube isolates the trachea and can thereby prevent these complications.

Toxicity to Operating Room Personnel. Chronic exposure to low levels of anesthetics may have adverse effects on operating room personnel. Suspected reactions include headache, reduced alertness, and possibly spontaneous abortion. The risk of these effects can be reduced by the simple expedient of venting anesthetic gases from the operating room.

Hepatotoxicity. About one patient of each 10,000 receiving inhalation anesthesia develops serious liver dysfunction. At one time, it was thought that halothane was more hepatotoxic than other anesthetics. However, it now appears that all inhalation anesthetics are about equal in their ability to injure the liver.

Renal Toxicity. Renal injury can occur with methoxyflurane. Damage is caused by metabolites of methoxyflurane, and not by the parent compound.

DRUG INTERACTIONS

Several classes of drugs—analgesics, CNS depressants, and CNS stimulants—can influence the amount of anesthetic required to produce anesthesia. Opioid analgesics allow a reduction in anesthetic dosage, since, with this combination, analgesia needn't be produced by the anesthetic alone. Similarly, since CNS depressants (barbiturates, benzodiazepines, alcohol) have additive depressant effects with anesthetics, acute use of these drugs lowers the required dose of anesthetic. Conversely, acute use of CNS stimulants (amphetamines, cocaine) increases the required dose of anesthetic.

ADJUNCTS TO INHALATION ANESTHESIA

Adjuncts to anesthesia are drugs employed to complement the beneficial effects of inhalation anesthetics and to counteract their adverse effects. Some adjunctive agents are administered preoperatively, others are administered intraoperatively, and others postoperatively.

Preanesthetic Medications

Preanesthetic medications are administered for three main purposes: (1) reduction of anxiety, (2) production of perioperative amnesia, and (3) relief of preoperative and postoperative pain. In addition, preanesthetic medications are used prophylactically to suppress adverse responses (excessive salivation, excessive bronchial secretion, coughing, bradycardia, vomiting) to certain anesthetics.

Benzodiazepines. Benzodiazepines (e.g., diazepam) are given preoperatively to reduce anxiety and promote amnesia. The doses employed produce mild sedation with little or no respiratory depression.

Barbiturates. Like the benzodiazepines, barbiturates can relieve anxiety and induce sedation. Respiratory and cardiovascular effects are minimal. Barbiturates with an intermediate duration of action are employed (e.g., pentobarbital, secobarbital).

Opioids. Opioids (e.g., morphine) are administered to relieve preoperative and postoperative pain. These drugs may also benefit the patient by suppressing coughing.

Preanesthetic use of opioids can have adverse effects. Because of their CNS depressant actions, opioids can delay awakening after surgery. Effects on the bowel and urinary tract may result in postoperative constipation and urinary retention. Stimulation of the chemoreceptor trigger zone may induce vomiting. Opioid-induced respiratory depression adds with anesthetic-induced respiratory depression, thereby increasing the risk of postoperative respiratory distress.

Anticholinergic Drugs. Anticholinergic drugs (e.g., atropine) may be given to decrease the risk of bradycardia during surgery. Surgical manipulations can trigger parasympathetic reflexes, which in turn can produce profound vagal slowing of the heart. Pretreatment with a cholinergic antagonist prevents bradycardia from this cause.

At one time, anticholinergic drugs were needed to prevent excessive bronchial secretions associated with anesthesia. Older anesthetic agents (e.g., ether) are highly irritating to the respiratory tract, and can thereby cause profuse bronchial secretions. Cholinergic blockers were given to suppress this response. Since the inhalation anesthetics in use today are nonirritating, bronchial secretions are not increased. Consequently, although anticholinergic agents are still employed as adjuncts to anesthesia, their purpose is no longer to suppress secretion.

Neuromuscular Blocking Agents

Performance of most surgical procedures requires that skeletal muscles be relaxed; neuromuscular blocking agents (e.g., succinylcholine, pancuronium) are given to induce that relaxation. By using neuromuscular blockers, we can reduce the dose of general anesthetic. That is, although it is possible to produce surgical muscle relaxation with an anesthetic alone, the required degree of muscle relaxation can be achieved only with deep anesthesia. When skeletal muscles have been relaxed with a neuromuscular blocker, anesthesia need not be so deep.

Muscle relaxants can have adverse effects. Neuromuscular blocking agents prevent contraction of all skeletal muscles, including the diaphragm and other muscles of respiration. Accordingly, patients require mechanical support of ventilation. Patients recovering from anesthesia may have reduced respiratory capacity due to neuromuscular blockade. Accordingly, respiration must be closely monitored until recovery is complete.

It is important to appreciate that patients under the influence of neuromuscular blocking agents are in a state of total flaccid paralysis. In this condition, a patient could be fully awake while appearing to be asleep. Incidents in which paralyzed patients have been awake during surgery, but unable to communicate their agony, are not unheard of. Because neuromuscular blockade can obscure depth of anesthesia, and because failure to maintain adequate anesthesia can result in true horror, the anesthesiologist must be especially watchful to insure that patients receiving neuromuscular blocking agents also receive adequate amounts of anesthetic.

Postanesthetic Medications

Analgesics. Analgesics are needed to control postoperative pain. If pain is severe, opioids are indicated. For mild pain, aspirin-like drugs may suffice.

Antiemetics. Patients recovering from anesthesia may experience nausea and vomiting. Drugs in the phenothiazine family (e.g., promethazine) have antiemetic properties and are used to reduce nausea and vomiting in postoperative patients.

Muscarinic Agonists. Abdominal distention (from atony of the bowel) and urinary retention are potential postoperative complications. Both conditions can be relieved through stimulation of muscarinic receptors. The muscarinic agonist employed most frequently is bethanechol.

DOSAGE AND ADMINISTRATION

Administration of inhalation anesthetics is performed only by anesthesiologists (physicians) and anesthetists (nurses). Clinicians who lack the training of these specialists have no authority to administer anesthesia. Since knowledge of anesthetic dosage and administration is the responsibility of specialists, and since this text is designed for the beginning student, details regarding dosage and administration will not be presented. The student who desires in-depth information on anesthetic dosage and administration should consult a textbook of anesthesiology.

CLASSIFICATION OF INHALATION ANESTHETICS

Inhalation anesthetics fall into two basic categories: (1) gases, and (2) volatile liquids. The gases, as their name implies, exist in a gaseous state at normal atmospheric pressure. The volatile liquids exist in a liquid state at normal atmospheric pressure, but can be easily volatilized for administration by inhalation.

The anesthetic gases and volatile liquids in current use are listed in Table 30–2. The five volatile

	Anesthetic	
Class	*Generic Name*	*Trade Name*
Volatile liquids	Halothane	Fluothane
	Enflurane	Ethrane
	Isoflurane	Forane
	Methoxyflurane	Penthrane
	Desflurane	Suprane
Gases	Nitrous oxide	
	Cyclopropane*	
	Ethylene*	

*This agent is explosive and used only rarely.

Table 30–2. Classification of the Inhalation Anesthetics

liquids—halothane, enflurane, isoflurane, desflurane, and methoxyflurane—are similar to one another in structure and function. In contrast, the three gases—nitrous oxide, cyclopropane, and ethylene—differ from one another both in structure and pharmacologic properties. Nitrous oxide is the only anesthetic gas that is used extensively.

PROPERTIES OF INDIVIDUAL INHALATION ANESTHETICS

HALOTHANE

Halothane [Fluothane] is the prototype of the current generation of volatile inhalation anesthetics. Halothane was introduced in 1956 and remains the standard against which the newer volatile liquids are compared.

Anesthetic Properties

Halothane is an effective anesthetic. For some procedures, anesthesia may be produced with halothane alone. Other procedures may require a combination of halothane with other drugs.

Potency. Halothane is a high-potency anesthetic. This high potency is reflected in halothane's low MAC (0.75%), which tells us that unconsciousness can be produced when the concentration of halothane in alveolar air is only 0.75%.

Time Course. Induction of anesthesia is smooth and relatively rapid. However, although halothane can act quickly, in actual practice, induction is usually produced with thiopental, a rapid-acting barbiturate. Once the patient is unconscious, depth of anesthesia can be raised or lowered with ease. Patients awaken about 1 hour after ceasing halothane inhalation.

Analgesia. Halothane is only weakly analgesic. Consequently, when this agent is used to provide surgical anesthesia, coadministration of a strong analgesic is usually required. The analgesics most commonly employed are opioids (e.g., morphine) and nitrous oxide.

Muscle Relaxation. Although halothane has muscle-relaxant actions, the degree of relaxation produced is generally inadequate for surgery. Accordingly, concurrent use of a neuromuscular blocking agent (e.g., succinylcholine) is usually required. Although relaxation of *skeletal* muscle is only moderate, halothane does promote significant relaxation of *uterine* muscle. Consequently, when used during parturition, halothane may inhibit uterine contractions, thereby delaying delivery, and possibly increasing postpartum bleeding.

Adverse Effects

Hypotension. Halothane causes a dose-dependent reduction in blood pressure. Doses only twice those needed for surgical anesthesia can produce complete circulatory failure and death.

Halothane promotes hypotension by two mechanisms. First, the drug exerts a direct depressant effect on the myocardium; the resultant decrease in contractility can reduce cardiac output by 20% to 50%. Second, halothane increases vagal tone, thereby slowing heart rate and reducing cardiac output even further.

Respiratory Depression. Halothane produces significant depression of respiration. To insure adequate oxygenation, two measures are employed: (1) mechanical or manual ventilatory support, and (2) enrichment of the inspired gas mixture with additional oxygen.

Sensitization of the Heart to Catecholamines. Halothane sensitizes the heart to catecholamines, thereby increasing the risk of dysrhythmias. Accordingly, caution must be exercised when epinephrine and other catecholamines are employed.

Malignant Hyperthermia. Genetically predisposed patients may experience malignant hyperthermia. Patients with a personal or familial history of malignant hyperthermia should receive halothane only when other options are unavailable.

Other Adverse Effects. Rarely, halothane produces *hepatitis*, sometimes progressing to massive hepatic necrosis and death. Postoperative *nausea* and *vomiting* may occur, but these reactions are less common with halothane than with older anesthetics (e.g., ether). By decreasing blood flow to the kidney, halothane can cause a substantial *decrease in urine formation*.

Elimination

The majority (60% to 80%) of an administered dose is eliminated intact in the exhaled breath.

Hepatic metabolism accounts for a small fraction (about 15%) of elimination.

ISOFLURANE

Isoflurane [Forane] is currently our most widely used inhalation anesthetic. The drug is potent (MAC = 1.15%) and has properties much like those of halothane. Induction of anesthesia is smooth and rapid, depth of anesthesia can be adjusted with speed and ease, and patients emerge from anesthesia rapidly. Like the other volatile-liquid anesthetics, isoflurane causes respiratory depression and hypotension. With isoflurane, hypotension results from vasodilation rather than from reduction of cardiac output. Isoflurane is a more effective muscle relaxant than halothane, but, nonetheless, is usually employed with a neuromuscular blocker. Like halothane, isoflurane suppresses uterine contraction. Only 0.2% of isoflurane undergoes metabolism; the vast majority of the drug is eliminated unchanged in the expired breath.

It is important to note that the cardiac actions of isoflurane differ significantly from those of halothane. Unlike halothane, isoflurane does not cause myocardial depression. Hence, cardiac output is not decreased. Furthermore, isoflurane does not sensitize the myocardium to catecholamines. Hence, patients can be given epinephrine and other catecholamines with little fear of precipitating a dysrhythmia.

ENFLURANE

Enflurane [Ethrane] has pharmacologic properties very similar to those of halothane. Enflurane was introduced in 1973 and still enjoys widespread use.

Comparison of enflurane with halothane reveals important similarities and a few significant differences. Both anesthetics are very potent: the MAC of enflurane is 1.68, compared with 0.75% for halothane. As with halothane, induction of anesthesia is smooth and rapid, and depth of anesthesia can be changed quickly and easily. Like halothane, enflurane produces substantial depression of the respiratory system. Accordingly, patients are likely to require ventilatory support; the concentration of inspired oxygen should be at least 35%. Muscle relaxation induced by enflurane is greater than that induced by halothane. However, despite the ability of enflurane to relax skeletal muscle, neuromuscular blockers are usually employed to permit reduction of enflurane dosage. Like halothane, enflurane can suppress contraction of the uterus, thereby impeding labor. Significantly, sensitization of the myocardium to catecholamines is less with enflurane than with halothane. As a result, patients can be given catecholamines with relative safety. High doses of enflurane can induce seizures, a response not seen with halothane; enflurane should be avoided in patients with a history of seizure disorders. Like halothane, enflurane is eliminated primarily in the exhaled breath as the intact parent compound; about 2% to 5% of an administered dose is eliminated by hepatic metabolism.

METHOXYFLURANE

Methoxyflurane [Penthrane] was introduced in 1960 and belongs to the volatile-liquid class of inhalation anesthetics. Initial use of the drug was widespread. However, the discovery that methoxyflurane can promote severe renal injury caused a sharp decline in its use.

Anesthetic Properties. With a MAC of only 0.16%, methoxyflurane is the most potent of the volatile anesthetics. However, despite this potency, induction of anesthesia is slow. Like the other volatile anesthetics, methoxyflurane causes hypotension and respiratory depression. In contrast to other volatile liquids, methoxyflurane produces excellent analgesia, and does not inhibit uterine contraction.

Metabolism and Renal Toxicity. Methoxyflurane undergoes more extensive metabolism than any other inhalation anesthetic. Between 50% and 70% of the drug is converted to metabolites. Of the metabolites produced, fluoride is the most important. When present in sufficient concentration, fluoride acts directly on renal tubules to cause injury. If renal injury is extensive, death can result. In order to cause renal toxicity, fluoride must achieve blood levels of 40 μM or more. To produce fluoride levels of this magnitude, methoxyflurane must be administered in large amounts. Low-dose, short-term use will not generate enough fluoride to injure the kidneys.

Therapeutic Use. Because of its ability to promote renal injury, methoxyflurane is not used extensively. The principal application of the drug is production of analgesia during labor. Methoxyflurane is acceptable for this application because the doses required are small—so small that there is no risk of generating fluoride in amounts sufficient to injure the kidneys. Methoxyflurane is preferable to the other volatile anesthetics for use during labor because it does not suppress uterine contractions.

DESFLURANE

Desflurane [Suprane] is a new volatile anesthetic nearly identical in structure to isoflurane. Induction occurs more rapidly than with any other volatile anesthetic; depth of anesthesia can be changed quickly; and recovery occurs about 5 minutes after ceasing inhalation. Desflurane is indicated for *maintenance* of anesthesia in adults and children and for *induction* of anesthesia in adults. The drug is not approved for induction in infants and children because of a high incidence of respiratory difficulties (laryngospasm, apnea, increased secretions), which are due to the drug's pungency. Like isoflurane, desflurane can cause respiratory depression and hypotension secondary to vasodilation. Postoperative nausea and vomiting are possible. Malignant hypertension has occurred in experimental animals. Desflurane undergoes even less metabolism than isoflurane; hence, the risk of postoperative organ injury is probably low.

NITROUS OXIDE

Nitrous oxide, also known as "laughing gas," differs from the volatile-liquid anesthetics in its pharmacologic properties and applications. With respect to pharmacologic properties, nitrous oxide differs from other inhalation anesthetics in two important ways: (1) whereas other inhalation agents have high *anesthetic* potency, the *anesthetic* potency of nitrous oxide is very *low*, and (2) whereas other inhalation agents lack *analgesic* potency, the *analgesic* potency of nitrous oxide is very *high*. These properties have given nitrous oxide a unique pattern of use: because of its low anesthetic potency, nitrous oxide is never employed as a primary anesthetic agent; however, because of its high analgesic potency, nitrous oxide is employed with great regularity as an adjuvant to provide supplemental analgesia for other inhalation agents.

Because nitrous oxide has such low anesthetic potency, *it is virtually impossible to produce surgical anesthesia employing nitrous oxide alone.* The low anesthetic potency of nitrous oxide is reflected in the drug's extremely high MAC, which is greater than 100%. A MAC of this value tells us that even if it were possible to administer 100% nitrous oxide (i.e., inspired gas that contains only nitrous oxide and no oxygen), this concentration of nitrous oxide would still be insufficient to produce surgical anesthesia. Since practical considerations (i.e., the need to administer at least 30% oxygen) limit the maximum usable concentration of nitrous oxide to 70%, and since much higher concentrations are needed to approach production of surgical anesthesia, it is clear that full anesthesia cannot be achieved with nitrous oxide by itself.

Despite its low anesthetic potency, nitrous oxide may well be our most widely used inhalation agent; *almost all patients undergoing general anesthesia receive nitrous oxide to supplement the analgesic effects of the primary anesthetic.* As indicated in Table 30–1, the analgesic effects of nitrous oxide are substantially greater than those of the other inhalation agents. Reflecting the drug's analgesic potency is the fact that inhalation of 20% nitrous oxide can produce pain relief equivalent to that of morphine. The advantage of providing analgesia with nitrous oxide, rather than relying entirely on the primary anesthetic for pain relief, is that the use of nitrous oxide allows the dosage of the primary anesthetic to be significantly decreased—usually by 50% or more. This reduction in dosage results in decreased respiratory and cardiovascular depression, and also leads to faster emergence. When employed in combination with other inhalation anesthetics, nitrous oxide is administered at a concentration of 70%.

When administered at therapeutic concentrations, nitrous oxide has practically no adverse effects. The drug is not toxic to the CNS, nor does it cause cardiovascular or respiratory depression. Furthermore, it is unlikely to precipitate malignant hyperthermia.

In certain settings, nitrous oxide can be used alone. When administered by itself, nitrous oxide is employed for *analgesia*—not *anesthesia.* Nitrous oxide alone is used for analgesia in dentistry and during delivery.

OBSOLETE INHALATION ANESTHETICS

Several once-popular anesthetics are now obsolete. These agents include *ethylene, cyclopropane, diethyl ether* (ether), *vinyl ether,* and *ethyl chloride.* Use of these agents has declined for two reasons: (1) all of these compounds are *explosive,* and (2) these drugs offer no advantages over newer, less hazardous anesthetics.

INTRAVENOUS ANESTHETICS

Intravenous anesthetics may be used alone or to supplement the effects of inhalation agents. When combined with inhalation anesthetics, intravenous agents offer two potential benefits: (1) they permit dosage of the inhalation agent to be reduced, and (2) they produce effects that cannot be achieved with an inhalation agent alone. Several of the drug families discussed in this section (opioids, barbiturates, benzodiazepines) have been considered at length in previous chapters. Accordingly, discussion here is limited to their use in anesthesia.

SHORT-ACTING BARBITURATES (THIOBARBITURATES)

Short-acting barbiturates, administered intravenously, are employed for *induction of anesthesia.* Three agents are available: (1) *thiopental sodium* [Pentothal], (2) *methohexital sodium* [Brevital], and (3) *thiamylal sodium* [Surital]. Almost every time an inhalation anesthetic is used, one of the short-acting barbiturates is administered first for induction.

Thiopental. Thiopental [Pentothal] was the first short-acting barbiturate to be introduced and is the prototype for the group. This drug acts rapidly to produce unconsciousness. Analgesic and muscle-relaxant effects are weak.

Thiopental has a rapid onset and short duration of action. Unconsciousness occurs within 10 to 20 seconds after IV injection. If administration of thiopental is not followed by inhalation anesthesia, the patient will wake up in approximately 10 minutes.

The time course of thiopental-induced anesthesia is determined by the drug's pattern of distribution. Thiopental is highly lipid soluble and, therefore, enters the brain rapidly to begin its effects. Anesthesia is terminated as thiopental undergoes redistribution from the brain and blood to other tissues. Practically no metabolism of the drug takes place between the time of administration and the time of awakening.

Like most of the inhalation anesthetics, thiopental causes cardiovascular and respiratory depression. If administered too rapidly, the drug may cause apnea.

BENZODIAZEPINES

When administered in large doses, benzodiazepines produce unconsciousness and amnesia. Because of this ability, intravenous benzodiazepines are occasionally given to induce anesthesia; however, the short-acting barbiturates are generally preferred for this application. Three benzodiazepines—diazepam, lorazepam, and midazolam—are administered intravenously for induction. Diazepam is the prototype for the group. The basic pharmacology of the benzodiazepines is discussed in Chapter 27.

Diazepam. Induction with IV diazepam [Valium] is slower than with barbiturates; unconsciousness develops in about 1 minute. Diazepam is not analgesic and causes very little muscle relaxation. Intravenous diazepam usually produces only moderate cardiovascular and respiratory depression; however, respiratory depression is occasionally severe. Accordingly, whenever diazepam is administered intravenously, facilities for support of respiration must be immediately available.

Midazolam. Intravenous midazolam [Versed] may be used for *induction of anesthesia* and to produce *conscious sedation*. When used for induction, midazolam is given by itself. Unconsciousness develops in 80 seconds.

Conscious sedation can be produced by combining midazolam with an opioid analgesic (e.g., morphine). The state is characterized by sedation, analgesia, amnesia, and an absence of anxiety. The patient is unperturbed and passive, but responsive to commands, such as "open your eyes." Conscious sedation persists for an hour or so and is suitable for minor surgeries and endoscopic procedures.

Midazolam can cause dangerous cardiorespiratory effects, including respiratory depression and respiratory and cardiac arrest. Accordingly, the drug should be used only in settings that permit constant monitoring of cardiac and respiratory status. Facilities for resuscitation must be immediately available. The risk of adverse effects can be minimized by injecting midazolam slowly (over 2 or more minutes) and by waiting another 2 or more minutes for full effects to develop before giving additional doses.

PROPOFOL

Propofol [Diprivan] is a new intravenous sedative-hypnotic used for induction and maintenance of anesthesia. Like thiopental, propofol has a rapid onset and short duration of action. Unconsciousness develops within 60 seconds and lasts for 3 to 5 minutes. As with thiopental, redistribution from the brain to other tissues explains the speed of awakening. Although its effects are brief, propofol persists in the body with a half-life of 3 to 5 hours.

Propofol can cause respiratory depression (including apnea), cardiac depression, hypotension, and pain at the site of injection. Because of the risk of cardiovascular depression, the drug should be used with caution in elderly patients, hypovolemic patients, and patients with compromised myocardial function. Pain at the injection site can be minimized by using a large vein and mixing propofol with a small amount of lidocaine (a local anesthetic) just prior to injection.

ETOMIDATE

Etomidate [Amidate] is a potent hypnotic agent used for induction of surgical anesthesia. Unconsciousness develops rapidly and lasts for 5 minutes. The drug has no analgesic actions. Adverse effects associated with single injections include transient apnea, venous pain at the injection site, and suppression of plasma cortisol levels for 6 to 8 hours. Repeated administration can cause hypotension, oliguria, electrolyte disturbances, and a high incidence (50%) of postoperative nausea and vomiting.

KETAMINE

Anesthetic Effects. Ketamine [Ketalar] produces a state known as *dissociative anesthesia*, in which the patient feels dissociated from his or her environment. In addition, the drug causes sedation, immobility, analgesia, and amnesia; responsiveness to pain is lost. Induction is rapid, and emergence begins within 10 to 15 minutes. Full recovery, however, may take several hours.

Adverse Psychologic Reactions. During recovery from ketamine, unpleasant psychologic reactions may occur. Possible reactions include hallucinations, disturbing dreams, and delirium. In some cases, these reactions recur days and even weeks after ketamine had been used. To minimize adverse psychologic effects, the patient should be kept in a soothing, stimulus-free environment until recovery is complete. Premedication with diazepam or midazolam reduces the risk of adverse reactions. Psychologic reactions are *least* likely in children under the age of 15 and in adults over the age of 65.

Therapeutic Uses. Ketamine is especially valuable for producing anesthesia in young children for minor surgical and diagnostic procedures; the drug is frequently used to facilitate changing of burn dressings. Because of its potential for adverse psychologic effects, ketamine should be avoided in patients with a history of psychiatric illness.

NEUROLEPTIC-OPIOID COMBINATION: DROPERIDOL PLUS FENTANYL

A unique state, known as *neurolept analgesia*, can be produced with a combination of fentanyl, a potent opioid, plus droperidol, a neuroleptic (antipsychotic) agent. The combination of fentanyl plus droperidol is available premixed under the trade name *Innovar*.

Neurolept analgesia is characterized by quiescence, indifference to surroundings, and insensitivity to pain; the patient appears to be asleep but is not (i.e., complete loss of consciousness does not occur). In large part, neurolept analgesia is similar to the dissociative anesthesia produced by ketamine. Neurolept analgesia is employed for diagnostic and minor surgical procedures (e.g., bronchoscopy, repeated changing of burn dressings).

Adverse effects include hypotension and respiratory depression. Respiratory depression can be severe and may persist for several hours. Respiratory assistance is likely to be required.

For some procedures, the combination of fentanyl plus droperidol is supplemented with nitrous oxide. The state produced by this three-drug regimen is called *neurolept anesthesia*. Neurolept anesthesia produces more analgesia and a greater reduction of consciousness than occurs with neurolept analgesia. Neurolept anesthesia can be used for major surgical procedures.

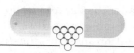

Summary of Major Nursing Implications

ALL GENERAL ANESTHETICS

Nursing management of the patient receiving general anesthesia is almost exclusively preoperative and postoperative. (Intraoperative management is the responsibility of anesthesiologists and anesthetists.) Accordingly, our summary of anesthesia-related nursing implications is divided into two sections: (1) implications that pertain to the preoperative patient, and (2) implications that pertain to the postoperative patient. Intraoperative implications are not considered.

It should be noted that the nursing implications summarized here are restricted to those that are directly related to anesthesia; nursing implications regarding the overall management of the surgical patient (i.e., implications unrelated to anesthesia) are not presented. (Overall nursing management of the surgical patient is discussed fully—and appropriately—in medical-surgical texts.)

Nursing implications for drugs employed as adjuncts to anesthesia (barbiturates, benzodiazepines, anticholinergic agents, opioids, neuromuscular blocking agents) have been summarized in previous chapters. Only those implications that apply specifically to the adjunctive use of these agents are addressed here.

 Preoperative Patients: Counseling Assessment, and Medication

Counseling

Anxiety is common among patients anticipating surgery; the patient may fear the surgery itself, or may be concerned about the possibility of waking up or experiencing pain during the procedure. Since excessive anxiety can disrupt the smoothness of the surgical course (in addition to being distressing to the patient), you should attempt to dispel preoperative fears. To some extent, fear can be allayed by reassuring the patient that anesthesia will keep him or her asleep for the entire procedure, will prevent pain, and will create amnesia about the experience.

Assessment

Medication History. The patient may be taking drugs that can affect responses to anesthetics. Drugs that act on the respiratory and cardiovascular systems are of particular concern. To decrease the risk of adverse interactions, obtain a thorough history of drug use. All drugs—prescription medications, over-the-counter preparations, and illicit agents—should be considered.

Respiratory and Cardiovascular Function. Most general anesthetics produce cardiovascular and respiratory depression. In order to evaluate the effects of anesthesia, baseline values for blood pressure, heart rate, and respiration are required. Also, any disease of the cardiovascular and respiratory systems should be noted.

Preoperative Medication

Preoperative medications (e.g., benzodiazepines, opioids, anticholinergic agents) are employed to (1) calm the patient, (2) provide analgesia, and (3) counteract adverse effects of general anesthetics. As a rule, the nurse is responsible for administering these drugs. Since preoperative medication can have a significant impact on the overall response to anesthesia, it is important that these drugs be administered at an appropriate time—typically 30 to 60 minutes before surgery. Because preoperative medication may produce drowsiness or reduce blood pressure, the patient should remain in bed. A calm environment will complement the effect of sedatives.

✓ **Postoperative Patients: Ongoing Evaluation and Interventions**

When receiving a patient for postoperative care, you should know all of the drugs the patient has received (anesthetics and adjunctive medications). With this information, you will be able to anticipate the time course of emergence from anesthesia as well as potential drug-related postoperative complications.

Evaluations and Interventions That Pertain to Specific Organ Systems

Cardiovascular and Respiratory Systems. Anesthetics depress cardiovascular and respiratory function. Monitor vital signs until they return to normal. Determine blood pressure, pulse rate, and respiration immediately upon receipt of the patient, and repeat monitoring at brief intervals until recovery is complete. During the recovery period, observe the patient for respiratory and cardiovascular distress. Be alert for (1) reductions in blood pressure, (2) altered cardiac rhythm, and (3) shallow, slow, or noisy breathing. Have facilities for respiratory support available.

Central Nervous System. Return of CNS function is gradual, and precautions must be taken until recovery is complete. When appropriate, employ side rails or straps to avoid accidental falls. Assist ambulation until the patient is able to stand steadily. During the early stage of emergence, the patient may be able to hear, although he or she may appear unconscious; exercise discretion in conversation.

Gastrointestinal Tract. Bowel function may be compromised by the surgery itself or by the drugs employed as adjuncts to anesthesia (e.g., opioids, anticholinergics). Constipation or atony of the bowel may occur. Monitor bowel function. A muscarinic agonist (e.g., bethanechol) may be needed to restore peristalsis.

Nausea and vomiting are potential postanesthetic reactions. To reduce the risk of aspiration, position the patient with his or her head to the side. Have equipment for suctioning available. Antiemetic medication may be needed.

Urinary Tract. Anesthetics and their adjuncts can disrupt urinary tract function. Anesthetics can decrease urine production by reducing renal blood flow; opioids and anticholinergic drugs can cause urinary retention. Monitor urine output. If the patient fails to void, notify the physician. Catheterization or medication (e.g., bethanechol) may be required.

Management of Postoperative Pain

As anesthesia wears off, the patient may experience postoperative pain. An opioid may be required. Since respiratory depression from opioids will add to residual respiratory depression from anesthesia, use opioids with caution; balance the need to relieve pain against the need to maintain ventilation.

Implications for Ketamine

Adverse psychologic reactions can develop as the patient emerges from ketamine-induced anesthesia. To minimize these reactions, provide the patient with a calm and stimulus-free environment until recovery is complete.

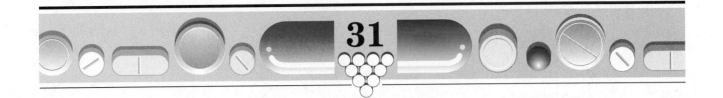

Local Anesthetics

Local anesthetics are drugs that block conduction of nerve impulses along axons. Conduction blockade occurs only in those neurons located near the site of anesthetic administration. The great advantage of local anesthesia, as compared with inhalation anesthesia, is that sensation can be suppressed without causing generalized depression of the entire nervous system. Hence, local anesthetics allow performance of medical and surgical procedures with much less risk than that associated with general anesthetics.

We will begin our study of local anesthetics by considering the pharmacology of the local anesthetics as a group. After that, we will discuss three prototypic agents: procaine, lidocaine, and cocaine. We will finish the chapter by discussing specific routes of anesthetic administration.

BASIC PHARMACOLOGY OF THE LOCAL ANESTHETICS

CLASSIFICATION

Most local anesthetics fall into one of two groups: *esters* or *amides*. The ester-type anesthetics, represented by *procaine* [Novocain], are drugs that contain an ester linkage in their structure. The amide-type agents, represented by *lidocaine* [Xylocaine], contain an amide linkage. Structural formulas for these two drugs are shown in Figure 31–1. As we will discuss in detail later, the ester-type agents and amide-type agents differ in two important ways: (1) method of inactivation, and (2) relative ability to promote allergic re-

ESTER-TYPE LOCAL ANESTHETICS

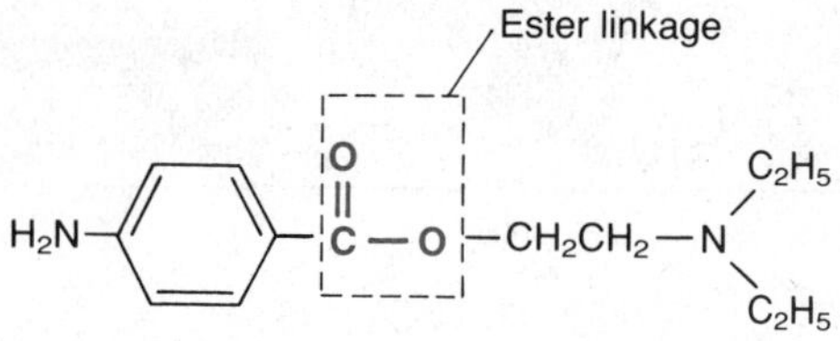

Procaine

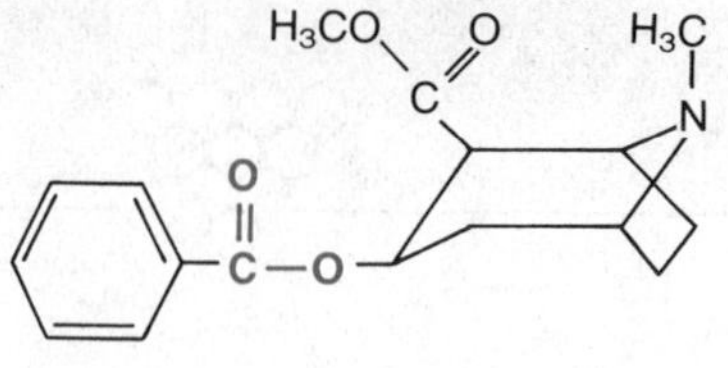

Cocaine

Figure 31–1. Structural formulas of representative local anesthetics.

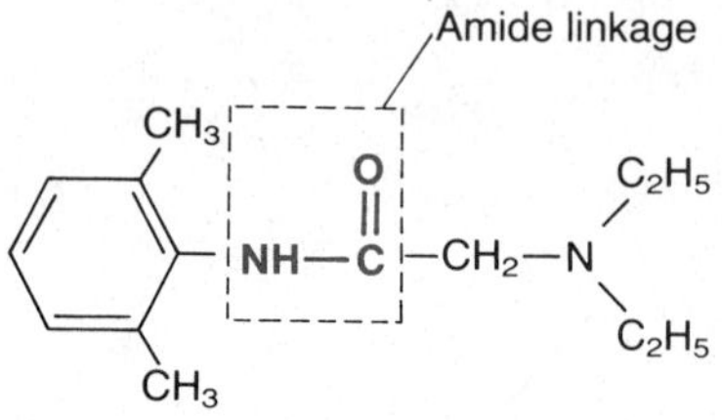

AMIDE-TYPE LOCAL ANESTHETICS

Lidocaine

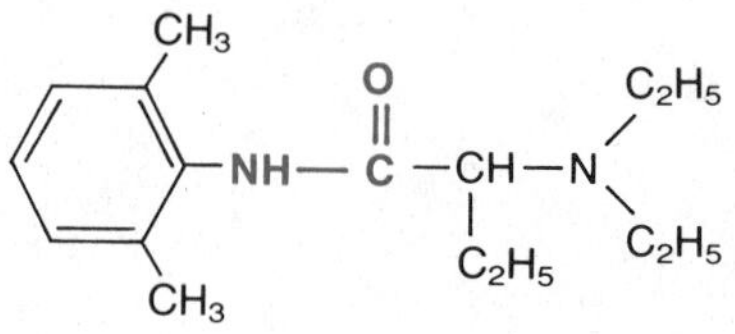

Etidocaine

sponses. Characteristic properties of the esters and amides are summarized in Table 31–1.

MECHANISM OF ACTION

Local anesthetics stop axonal conduction by *blocking sodium channels* in the axonal membrane. Recall that propagation of an action potential requires that sodium ions move from outside the axon to the inside. This influx takes place through sodium channels. Hence, by blocking axonal sodium channels, local anesthetics prevent sodium entry, and thereby bring conduction to a halt.

Table 31–1. Contrasts Between Ester and Amide Local Anesthetics

	Ester-type Anesthetics	Amide-type Anesthetics
Characteristic chemistry	Ester bond	Amide bond
Representative agent	Procaine	Lidocaine
Incidence of allergic reactions	Low	Very low
Method of metabolism	Plasma esterases	Hepatic enzymes

SELECTIVITY OF ANESTHETIC EFFECTS

Local anesthetics are nonselective modifiers of neuronal function. That is, these drugs will block the propagation of action potentials in all neurons to which they have access. The only way that we can achieve selectivity is through delivery of the anesthetic to a limited area.

Although local anesthetics can block traffic in all neurons, anesthesia develops faster in some neurons than in others. Specifically, small, nonmyelinated neurons undergo blockade more rapidly than large, myelinated neurons. Because neurons develop conduction blockade at different rates, there is a temporal sequence in which sensations are lost: pain perception is the first sensation to diminish—followed in order by perception of cold, warmth, touch, and deep pressure.

It should be noted that the effects of local anesthetics are not limited to sensory nerves; these drugs also block impulse conduction in motor nerves.

TIME COURSE OF LOCAL ANESTHESIA

Under ideal conditions, local anesthesia would begin promptly and would persist for a time neither longer nor shorter than needed. Unfortu-

Table 31-2. Local Anesthetics Used Topically: Trade Names, Indications, and Time Course of Action

	Generic Name	Trade Name	Indications		Time Course of Action*	
			Skin	Mucous Membranes	Peak Effect (minutes)	Duration (minutes)
Amides	Dibucaine†	Nupercainal	✓		<15	180–240
	Lidocaine†	Xylocaine, Solarcaine	✓	✓	2–5	30–60
Esters	Benzocaine	Many names	✓	✓	1	30–60
	Butamben	Butesin	✓		—	—
	Cocaine			✓	2–5	30–120
	Tetracaine†	Pontocaine	✓	✓	3–8	30–60
Others	Dyclonine	Dyclone		✓	<10	<60
	Pramoxine	Tronothane, others	✓		3–5	—

*Based primarily on application to mucous membranes.
†Also administered by injection.

nately, although onset of anesthesia is usually rapid (see Tables 31–2 and 31–3), duration of anesthesia is often nonideal: in some cases, anesthesia persists longer than necessary; in others, repeated administration is needed to maintain anesthesia of sufficient duration.

Onset of local anesthesia is determined largely by the molecular properties of the anesthetic. Before anesthesia can occur, the anesthetic must diffuse from its site of administration to its sites of action within the axonal membrane; anesthesia will be delayed until this movement has occurred. The ability of an anesthetic to penetrate the axonal membrane is determined by three properties: *molecular size, lipid solubility*, and *degree of ionization at tissue pH*. Anesthetics of small size, high lipid solubility, and low ionization cross the axonal membrane relatively rapidly. In contrast, anesthetics of large size, low lipid solubility, and high ionization cross more slowly. Those agents that penetrate the axon most rapidly will have the fastest onset of action.

Termination of local anesthesia occurs as molecules of anesthetic diffuse out of nerves and are carried away in the blood. The same factors that determine onset of anesthesia (molecular size, lipid solubility, degree of ionization) also help determine duration. In addition, *regional blood flow* is an important determinant of how long anesthesia will last. In those areas where blood flow is high, anesthetic will be carried away quickly, and, hence, effects will terminate with relative haste. In regions where blood flow is low, anesthesia will be more prolonged.

Table 31-3. Injectable Local Anesthetics: Trade Names and Time Course of Action

	Generic Name	Trade Name	Time Course of Action*	
			Onset (minutes)	Duration (hours)
Esters	Procaine	Novocain	2–5	0.25–0.5
	Chloroprocaine	Nesacaine	6–12	0.25–0.5
	Tetracaine†	Pontocaine	≤15	2–3
Amides	Lidocaine†	Xylocaine, others	0.5–1	0.5–1
	Prilocaine	Citanest	1–2	0.5–1.5
	Mepivacaine	Carbocaine, Isocaine, Polocaine	3–5	0.75–1.5
	Bupivacaine	Marcaine, Sensorcaine	5	2–4
	Etidocaine	Duranest	3–5	2–3

*Values are for *infiltration* anesthesia in the absence of epinephrine (epinephrine prolongs duration two- to three-fold).
†Also administered topically.

USE WITH VASOCONSTRICTORS

Local anesthetics are frequently administered in combination with a vasoconstrictor (usually epinephrine). The function of the vasoconstrictor is to decrease blood flow to the site.

Concurrent use of a vasoconstrictor offers several benefits. (1) By decreasing local blood flow, the vasoconstrictor will delay absorption of anesthetic into the systemic circulation, thereby prolonging anesthesia. (2) By delaying absorption, the vasoconstrictor allows the use of anesthetic in doses that are significantly smaller than those that would be required if regional blood flow were normal. (3) By permitting a reduction in anesthetic dosage, the vasoconstrictor decreases the risk of systemic toxicity. (4) By slowing anesthetic absorption, the vasoconstrictor helps establish a favorable balance between the rate of entry of anesthetic into the general circulation and the capacity of the body to convert the anesthetic to inactive metabolites.

It should be noted that absorption of the vasoconstrictor into the blood can result in systemic toxicity (e.g., palpitations, tachycardia, nervousness, hypertension). If adrenergic stimulation from absorption of epinephrine is excessive, symptoms can be controlled with alpha- and beta-adrenergic antagonists.

FATE IN THE BODY

Absorption and Distribution. Although administered for local effects, local anesthetics do get absorbed into the bloodstream and distributed to all parts of the body. The rate of absorption is determined in large part by blood flow to the area of administration.

Metabolism. The process by which a particular local anesthetic is metabolized depends on the category (ester or amide) to which it belongs. *Ester-type* local anesthetics are broken down in the *blood* by enzymes known as *esterases*. In contrast, metabolism of the *amide-type* agents takes place in the *liver*. For both types of drugs, metabolism results in inactivation.

The balance between rate of absorption and rate of metabolism is of clinical significance. If a local anesthetic is absorbed more slowly than it is metabolized, plasma drug levels will remain low and systemic reactions will be minimal. However, if absorption occurs too swiftly, absorption will outpace metabolism, plasma drug levels will rise, and the risk of systemic toxicity will increase.

ADVERSE EFFECTS

Adverse effects can occur locally or distant from the site of administration. Systemic effects are most common.

Central Nervous System. When absorbed in sufficient amounts, local anesthetics cause central nervous system (CNS) excitation followed by depression. During the excitatory phase, convulsions may occur. These can be controlled with intravenous diazepam or, if necessary, a neuromuscular blocking agent (e.g., succinylcholine). Depressant effects range from drowsiness to unconsciousness; death can occur from depression of respiration. If respiratory depression is prominent, mechanical ventilation with oxygen is indicated.

Cardiovascular System. Systemic absorption of local anesthetics can cause vasodilation and cardiac suppression. Local anesthetics can decrease excitability in the myocardium and in the conducting system, thereby causing *bradycardia, A-V heart block, reduced contractile force*, and sometimes *cardiac arrest*. The combination of vasodilation and cardiac suppression can produce *hypotension*.

Allergic Reactions. A variety of hypersensitivity reactions, ranging from allergic dermatitis to anaphylaxis, have occurred in response to local anesthetics. These reactions, which are relatively uncommon, are much more likely with the *ester-type* anesthetics (e.g., procaine) than with the amides. Patients allergic to one ester-type anesthetic are likely to be allergic to all other ester-type agents. Fortunately, cross-hypersensitivity between the esters and amides has not been observed. Hence, the amides can be used when allergies contraindicate use of ester-type anesthetics.

Use in Labor and Delivery. Local anesthetics can depress uterine contractility and decrease maternal expulsion effort. Both actions can prolong labor. Also, local anesthetics can cross the placenta, causing bradycardia and CNS depression in the neonate.

PROPERTIES OF INDIVIDUAL LOCAL ANESTHETICS

PROCAINE

Procaine [Novocain] was synthesized in 1905 and is the prototype of the ester-type local anesthetics. The drug is ineffective topically and, hence, must be administered by injection. Administration in combination with epinephrine delays absorption. Procaine is readily absorbed, but systemic toxicity is rare; plasma esterases rapidly convert the drug to inactive, nontoxic products. Being an ester-type anesthetic, procaine is more likely to cause allergic responses than are the amide-type anesthetics. Individuals allergic to procaine are likely to be allergic to all other ester-type anesthetics—but not to the amides.

For many years, procaine was the local anesthetic most preferred for use by injection. However, with the development of newer agents, use of procaine has sharply declined. Once popular in dentistry, procaine is rarely employed in this setting today.

Preparations. Procaine hydrochloride [Novocain] is available in solution (1%, 2%, and 10%) for administration by injection. Dilution is required for use by some routes. Epinephrine (at a final concentration of 1:100,000 or 1:200,000) may be combined with procaine to delay absorption.

LIDOCAINE

Lidocaine was introduced in 1948 and is the prototype of the amide-type agents. One of today's most widely used local anesthetics, lidocaine can be administered topically and by injection. Anesthesia from lidocaine is more rapid, more intense, and of longer duration than that produced by an equal dose of procaine. Effects can be prolonged by coadministration with epinephrine. Allergic reactions are rare; individuals allergic to ester-type anesthetics are not cross-allergic to lidocaine. If plasma levels of lidocaine climb too high, CNS and cardiovascular toxicity can result. Inactivation is by hepatic metabolism.

In addition to its use in local anesthesia, lidocaine is used to treat dysrhythmias (see Chapter 44). Control of dysrhythmias results from suppression of cardiac excitability.

Preparations. Lidocaine hydrochloride [Xylocaine, others] is dispensed in several formulations (cream, ointment, jelly, solution, aerosol) for topical administration. Lidocaine for injection is available in concentrations ranging from 0.5% to 20%; some preparations contain epinephrine (1:50,000, 1:100,000, or 1:200,000).

COCAINE

Cocaine was the first local anesthetic discovered. Clinical use was initiated in 1884 by Sigmund Freud and Karl Koller. Freud described the physiologic effects of cocaine, while Koller focused on the drug's anesthetic actions. As can be seen from its structure (Fig. 31–1), cocaine is an ester-type anesthetic. In addition to causing local anesthesia, cocaine has pronounced effects on the CNS and structures regulated by sympathetic nerves. Autonomic and CNS effects are due in large part to the drug's ability to block uptake of norepinephrine by adrenergic neurons.

Anesthetic Use. Cocaine is an excellent local anesthetic. Administration is topical. The drug is employed for anesthesia of the ear, nose, and throat. Anesthesia has a rapid onset and persists for about an hour. Unlike other local anesthetics, cocaine causes intense vasoconstriction. Accordingly, the drug should not given in combination with epinephrine or other vasoconstrictors. Despite its ability to constrict blood vessels, cocaine is readily absorbed following application to mucous membranes; significant effects on the brain and heart can result. The drug is inactivated by plasma esterases and by enzymes in the liver.

Central Nervous System Effects. Cocaine produces generalized CNS stimulation. Moderate doses cause euphoria, loquaciousness, reduced fatigue, and increased sociability and alertness. Excessive doses can cause seizures. Excitation is followed by CNS depression; respiratory arrest and death can result.

Although cocaine does not seem to cause substantial physical dependence, psychologic dependence can be profound. The drug is subject to widespread abuse and is classified under Schedule II of the Controlled Substances Act. Cocaine abuse is discussed in Chapter 34.

Cardiovascular Effects. Cocaine stimulates the heart and causes vasoconstriction. These effects result from (1) central stimulation of the sympathetic nervous system, and (2) blockade of norepinephrine uptake in the periphery. Stimulation of the heart can produce tachycardia and potentially fatal dysrhythmias. Hypertension can result from vasoconstriction. Cocaine presents an especially serious risk to individuals with cardiovascular disease (e.g., hypertension, angina pectoris).

When used for local anesthesia, cocaine should not be combined with epinephrine, since the combination would increase the risk of cardiovascular toxicity. Furthermore, since a vasoconstrictor will not significantly retard cocaine absorption, the combination would be irrational in addition to dangerous.

Preparations and Administration. Cocaine hydrochloride is available in soluble tablets (135 mg), as a powder (5 and 25 gm), and in solution (40 and 100 mg/ml). Administration is topical. For application to the ear, nose, or throat, a 4% solution is usually employed. The drug must be dispensed in accord with provisions of the Controlled Substances Act.

OTHER LOCAL ANESTHETICS

In addition to the drugs discussed above, several other local anesthetics are available. These agents differ from one another with respect to indications, routes of administration, mode of elimination, time course of action, and toxicity.

The local anesthetics can be grouped according to those that are administered topically and those that are administered by injection. (Very few agents are administered by both routes, largely because the drugs that are suitable for topical application are usually too toxic for parenteral use.) Table 31–2 lists the topically administered local anesthetics along with trade names and time courses of action. Table 31–3 presents equivalent information for the injectable agents.

CLINICAL USE OF LOCAL ANESTHETICS

GENERAL PRECAUTIONS

When local anesthetics are administered parenterally, the following precautions apply. Severe reactions can occur with inadvertent injection into arter4ies and veins. To avoid intravascular injection, aspirate prior to injection. Because serious systemic reactions may occur, parenteral local anesthetics should be given only when equipment for resuscitation is immediately available. Following an injection, the patient should be monitored periodically for cardiovascular status, respiratory function, and state of consciousness. To reduce the risk of toxicity, local anesthetics should be administered in the lowest effective dosage.

TECHNIQUES EMPLOYED TO PRODUCE LOCAL ANESTHESIA

Local anesthetics may be employed in two basic ways: *topically* (for surface anesthesia) and *by injection*. Injection is used to produce infiltration anesthesia, nerve-block anesthesia, intravenous regional anesthesia, epidural anesthesia, and spinal anesthesia. The type of anesthesia produced is determined by the site of injection. The characteristics of surface anesthesia and the various types of anesthesia that result from injection are discussed below. It should be noted that injection of local anesthetics requires special skills. Hence, administration is usually performed by an anesthesiologist.

Surface Anesthesia

Surface anesthesia is produced by applying a local anesthetic to the skin or mucous membranes. The agents employed most commonly are *lidocaine, tetracaine,* and *cocaine.*

Systemic Toxicity. Topical anesthetics can be absorbed in amounts sufficient to produce systemic toxicity. Cardiovascular and CNS reactions are of principal concern. Since the extent of absorption is proportional to the surface area over which the anesthetic is applied, the risk of toxicity is greatest when a large surface area is involved. Also, since absorption occurs more readily through mucous membranes than through the skin, anesthetics applied to mucous membranes are more likely to produce systemic toxicity. If the skin is abraded or otherwise injured, anesthetic absorption will be increased, as will the risk of toxicity.

Therapeutic Uses. Local anesthetics are applied to the *skin* to relieve pain, itching, and soreness of various causes, including infection, thermal burns, sunburn, diaper rash, wounds, bruises, abrasions, plant poisoning, and insect bites. Application may be made to *mucous membranes* of the nose, mouth, pharynx, larynx, trachea, bronchi, vagina, and urethra. In addition, local anesthetics may be used to relieve discomfort associated with hemorrhoids, anal fissures, and pruritus ani.

Infiltration Anesthesia

Infiltration anesthesia is achieved by injecting a local anesthetic directly into the immediate area of surgery or manipulation. Anesthesia can be prolonged by combining the anesthetic with epinephrine. However, epinephrine should not be used in areas supplied by end arteries (toes, fingers, nose, ears, penis), since restriction of blood flow at these sites may cause gangrene. The agents given most frequently for infiltration anesthesia are *procaine, lidocaine,* and *bupivacaine.*

Nerve Block Anesthesia

Nerve block anesthesia is achieved by injecting a local anesthetic into or near the nerves that *supply* the surgical field, but at a site *distant* from the field. An advantage of this technique is that anesthesia can be produced using doses that are smaller than those needed for infiltration anesthesia. Drugs employed for nerve block anesthesia include *procaine, chlorprocaine, lidocaine, mepivacaine,* and *prilocaine.*

Intravenous Regional Anesthesia

Intravenous regional anesthesia is employed to anesthetize the limbs. Anesthesia is produced by injection into a distal vein of an arm or leg. Prior to anesthetic administration, blood must be removed from the vein (usually by application of an Esmarch bandage), and a tourniquet must be applied to the limb (proximal to the site of anesthetic injection) to prevent anesthetic from entering the general circulation. Following injection, the anesthetic diffuses from the vasculature and becomes evenly distributed to all areas of the occluded limb. Safe administration requires that the tourniquet produce complete blockade of arterial flow throughout the procedure. When the tourniquet is loosened at the end of surgery, about 15% to 30% of administered anesthetic is released into the systemic circulation. *Prilocaine* and *lidocaine* are the preferred agents for intravenous regional anesthesia.

Epidural Anesthesia

Epidural anesthesia is achieved by injecting a local anesthetic into the epidural space (i.e., within the spinal column but outside the dura mater). Diffusion of anesthetic across the dura into the subarachnoid space produces anesthesia of nerve roots and of the spinal cord itself. Diffusion through intervertebral foramina blocks nerves located in the paravertebral region. With epidural administration, anesthetic can reach the systemic circulation in significant amounts. As a result, when the technique is used during delivery, neonatal depression may result. *Lidocaine* and *bupivacaine* are popular drugs for epidural anesthesia. Because of the risk of cardiac arrest, the 0.75% solution of bupivacaine should not be used for epidural anesthesia in obstetric patients.

Spinal (Subarachnoid) Anesthesia

Technique. Spinal anesthesia is produced by injecting local anesthetic into the subarachnoid space. Injection is made in the lumbar region below the termination of the cord. Spread of anesthetic within the subarachnoid space determines the level of anesthesia achieved. Movement of anesthetic within the subarachnoid space is determined by two factors: (1) the density of the anesthetic solution, and (2) the position in which the patient is lying. Anesthetics employed most commonly are *lidocaine* and *tetracaine.*

Adverse Effects. The most significant adverse effect of spinal anesthesia is *hypotension.* Blood pressure is reduced by venous dilation occurring secondary to blockade of sympathetic nerves. (Loss of venous tone decreases the return of blood to the heart, causing a reduction in cardiac output and a corresponding fall in blood pressure.) Loss of venous tone can be compensated for by placing the patient in a 10- to 15-degree head-down position, which will promote venous return to the heart. If blood pressure cannot be restored through head-down positioning alone, drugs may be indicated; ephedrine and mephentermine have been employed to promote vasoconstriction and enhance cardiac performance.

Autonomic blockade may disrupt function of the intestinal and urinary tracts, causing fecal incontinence, urinary incontinence, or urinary retention. The physician should be notified if the patient fails to void within 8 hours of the end of surgery.

Spinal anesthesia frequently causes headache. These "spinal" headaches are posture dependent and can be relieved by having the patient assume a supine position.

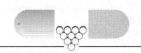

Summary of Major Nursing Implications

INJECTED LOCAL ANESTHETICS

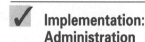

✓ Preadministration Assessment

Therapeutic Goal

Production of local anesthesia for surgical, dental, and obstetric procedures.

Identifying High-Risk Patients

Ester-type local anesthetics are *contraindicated* for patients with a *history of serious allergic reactions to these drugs.*

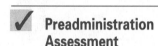

✓ Implementation: Administration

Preparation of the Patient

The nurse may be responsible for preparing the patient to receive an injectable local anesthetic. Preparation includes cleansing the injection site, shaving the site when indicated, and placing the patient in a position appropriate for receipt of the injection. Children, elderly patients, and patients who are uncooperative may require restraint prior to injection by some routes.

Administration

Injection of local anesthetics is performed by clinicians with special training in their use (physicians, dentists, nurse anesthetists).

✓ Ongoing Evaluation and Interventions

Minimizing Adverse Effects

Systemic Reactions. Absorption into the general circulation can cause systemic toxicity. Effects on the CNS and heart are of greatest concern. CNS toxicity manifests as a brief period of excitement, possibly including convulsions, followed by CNS depression, which can result in respiratory depression. Cardiotoxicity can manifest as bradycardia, A-V heart block, and cardiac arrest. Monitor blood pressure, pulse, respiratory rate, and state of consciousness. Have facilities for cardiopulmonary resuscitation available. Manage convulsions with IV diazepam or a neuromuscular blocking agent.

Allergic Reactions. Severe allergic reactions are rare, but can occur. These are most likely with ester-type anesthetics. Avoid ester-type agents in patients with a history of allergy to these drugs.

Labor and Delivery. Use of local anesthetics during delivery can cause bradycardia and CNS depression in the newborn. Monitor cardiac status.

Self-Inflicted Injury. Since anesthetics eliminate pain, and since pain warns us about injury, the patient recovering from anesthesia must be protected from inadvertent harm until anesthesia wears off. Caution the patient against activities that might result in unintentional harm. Position the patient comfortably.

Spinal Headache and Urinary Retention. Patients recovering from spinal anesthesia may experience headache and urinary retention. Headache is posture-dependent and can be minimized by having the patient remain supine for about 12 hours. Notify the physician if the patient fails to void within 8 hours.

TOPICAL LOCAL ANESTHETICS

Preadministration Assessment

Therapeutic Goal

Reduction of discomfort associated with local disorders of the skin and mucous membranes.

Identifying High-Risk Patients

Ester-type local anesthetics are *contraindicated* for patients with a *history of serious allergic reactions to these drugs.*

Implementation: Administration

Routes

Topical application to skin and mucous membranes.

Administration

Apply in the lowest effective dosage to the smallest area required. If possible, avoid application to skin that is abraded or otherwise injured.

Ongoing Evaluation and Interventions

Minimizing Adverse Effects

Systemic Toxicity. Absorption into the general circulation can cause systemic toxicity. Effects on the heart (bradycardia, A-V heart block, cardiac arrest) and CNS (excitation, possibly including convulsions, followed by depression) are of greatest concern. Monitor blood pressure, pulse, respiratory rate, and state of consciousness. Have facilities for cardiopulmonary resuscitation available.

The risk of systemic toxicity is determined by the extent of absorption. To minimize absorption, apply topical anesthetics to the smallest surface area needed, and, when possible, avoid application to injured skin.

Allergic Reactions. Severe allergic reactions are rare but can occur; these are most likely with ester-type anesthetics. Avoid ester-type agents in patients with a history of allergy to these drugs.

Other Central Nervous System Drugs

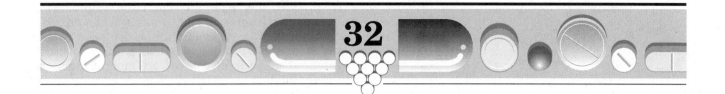

Central Nervous System Stimulants

Central nervous system (CNS) stimulants increase the activity of CNS neurons. This increase can be produced in either of two ways: (1) enhancement of excitation, or (2) suppression of inhibition. Most CNS stimulants work by the first mechanism. In sufficient dosage, all of the CNS stimulants can cause convulsions.

Clinical applications of the CNS stimulants are limited. Currently, these drugs have two principal indications: (1) attention-deficit hyperactivity disorder in children, and (2) narcolepsy. In addition, CNS stimulants can be used to treat obesity. At one time, CNS stimulants were administered to counteract poisoning by CNS depressants; however, this use has been discredited.

It is important to note that CNS stimulants are not equivalent to antidepressants. The antidepressants act selectively to alter mood, and, hence, can relieve depression while leaving other CNS functions unaffected. In contrast, CNS stimulants cannot elevate mood without producing generalized excitation. Accordingly, the role of CNS stimulants in treating depression is minor.

Our principal focus in this chapter is on two groups of drugs: *methylxanthines* (e.g., caffeine) and *amphetamines*. These agents are by far the most widely used CNS stimulants.

METHYLXANTHINES

The methylxanthines are derivatives of xanthine (pronounced "zan'theen"), hence the family name.

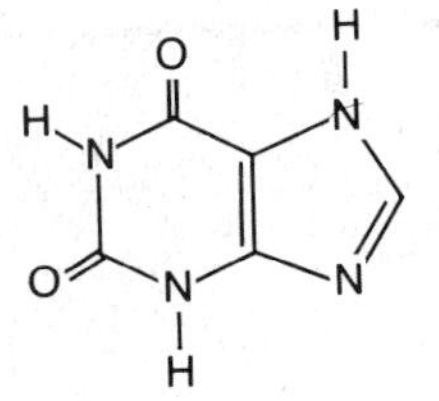

Figure 32–1. Structural formulas of the methylxanthines.

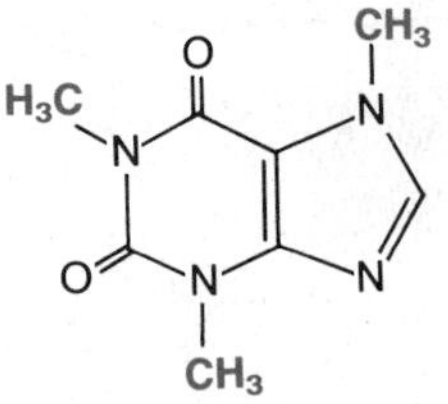

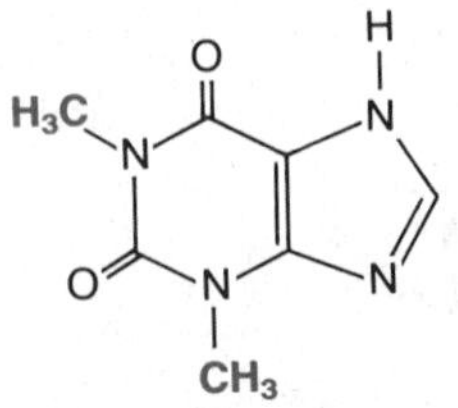

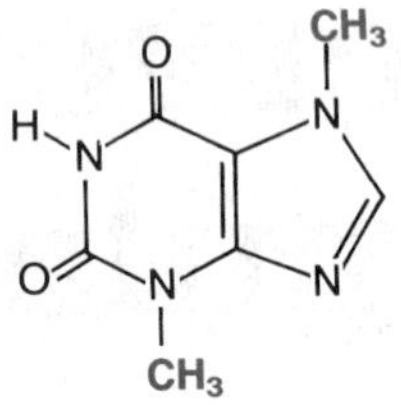

As indicated in Figure 32–1, these compounds consist of a xanthine nucleus to which one or more methyl groups have been attached. Caffeine, the most familiar member of the family, will serve as our prototype.

CAFFEINE

Caffeine is consumed worldwide for its stimulant effects. In the United States, per capita consumption is about 200 mg per day–mostly in the form of coffee. Although clinical applications of caffeine are few, caffeine remains of interest because of its widespread ingestion for nonmedical purposes.

Dietary Sources

Caffeine is present in chocolate and in beverages prepared from various natural products. Common dietary sources are coffee, tea, and cola drinks. The caffeine in cola drinks derives partly from the cola nut and partly from caffeine added by the manufacturer. Caffeine is also present in many noncola soft drinks. The caffeine content of chocolate and caffeine-containing beverages is indicated in Table 32–1.

Mechanism of Action

Several mechanisms of action have been proposed for caffeine and the other methylxanthines. These are (1) enhancement of calcium permeability in the sarcoplasmic reticulum, (2) reversible blockade of adenosine receptors, and (3) inhibition of cyclic nucleotide phosphodiesterase, resulting in accumulation of cyclic adenosine monophosphate (cyclic AMP).

Pharmacologic Effects

Central Nervous System. In low doses, caffeine decreases drowsiness and fatigue, and increases the capacity for prolonged intellectual exertion. With increasing dosage, caffeine produces nervousness, insomnia, and tremors. When administered in very large amounts, the drug can cause convulsions. Despite popular belief, there is little evidence that caffeine can restore mental function in individuals intoxicated with alcohol.

Heart. High doses of caffeine stimulate the heart. When caffeine-containing beverages are consumed in excessive quantities, dysrhythmias may result.

Blood Vessels. Caffeine affects blood vessels in the periphery differently from those in the CNS. In the *periphery*, caffeine promotes *vasodilation*, whereas in the *CNS*, caffeine promotes *vasoconstriction*. The ability of caffeine to constrict cerebral blood vessels is thought to underlie the drug's ability to relieve certain types of headache.

Bronchi. Caffeine and other methylxanthines cause relaxation of bronchial smooth muscle, and thereby promote bronchodilation. Theophylline is an especially effective bronchodilator and, because of this action, is widely prescribed to treat asthma.

Kidney. Caffeine is a diuretic. The mechanism underlying increased urine formation is not fully understood.

Reproduction. When applied to cells in culture, caffeine can cause chromosomal damage and mutations. However, the concentrations of caffeine required to elicit these responses are much greater than those that can be achieved in the body by drinking caffeine-containing beverages. Although there has been concern that ingestion of caffeine by pregnant women might cause fetal harm, studies have failed to demonstrate an association between caffeine consumption and birth defects. Nonetheless, the drug has caused birth defects in animals. Accordingly, it would seem prudent to minimize ingestion of caffeine during pregnancy.

Table 32–1. Dietary Caffeine	
Source	**Caffeine Content**
Coffee: Regular	
Brewed	40–180 mg/cup
Instant	30–120 mg/cup
Coffee: Decaffeinated	
Brewed	2–5 mg/cup
Instant	1–5 mg/cup
Tea	
Brewed	20–110 mg/cup
Instant	25–50 mg/cup
Cola drinks	40–60 mg/12 oz
Cocoa	2–50 mg/cup
Chocolate milk	2–7 mg/5 oz
Milk chocolate	1–15 mg/oz
Baker's chocolate	25–35 mg/oz

Pharmacokinetics

Caffeine is readily absorbed from the gastrointestinal (GI) tract and achieves peak plasma levels within 1 hour. Plasma half-life ranges from 3 to 7 hours. Elimination is by hepatic metabolism.

Therapeutic Uses

Promoting Wakefulness. Caffeine is used primarily as an aid to staying awake. The drug is marketed in various over-the-counter preparations [NōDōz, Vivarin, others] for this purpose. Of course, individuals desiring increased alertness needn't take a pill to obtain their caffeine; they can get just as much caffeine by drinking coffee or some other caffeine-containing beverage.

Other Applications. Intravenous caffeine can help relieve headache induced by spinal puncture. The drug is used orally to enhance analgesia induced by opioids and non-narcotic agents (e.g., aspirin). Caffeine has been administered on an investigational basis to treat neonatal apnea.

Acute Toxicity

Caffeine poisoning is characterized by intensification of the responses seen at low doses. Stimulation of the CNS results in excitement, restlessness, and insomnia; if the dosage is sufficiently high, convulsions may occur. Tachycardia and respiratory stimulation are likely. Sensory phenomena (ringing in the ears, flashing lights) are common. Death from caffeine overdose is rare. When fatalities have occurred, between 5 and 10 gm have been ingested.

Preparations, Dosage, and Administration

Oral. Oral caffeine is dispensed in tablets (100, 150, and 200 mg) and timed-release capsules (200 mg). The usual dosage is 100 to 200 mg every 3 to 4 hours as needed.

Parenteral. Caffeine plus sodium benzoate is dispensed as an injection (250 mg/ml in 2-ml ampuls) for IV and IM administration. The usual adult dose (IM or IV) is 500 mg. The dose for infants and children is 8 mg/kg.

THEOPHYLLINE

Theophylline is similar to caffeine in most of its pharmacologic actions. Like caffeine, theophylline is an effective CNS stimulant. In contrast to caffeine, theophylline has important applications in the treatment of asthma; benefits derive from the drug's ability to promote bronchodilation. Antiasthmatic applications of theophylline are discussed in Chapter 64.

THEOBROMINE

Theobromine is a methylxanthine that occurs naturally in the seeds of *Theobroma cocao*, from which cocoa and chocolate are made. The caffeine content of these seeds is relatively low. Although there are similarities between theobromine and caffeine, these compounds do differ. The most distinct difference is that caffeine is a CNS stimulant, whereas theobromine is not. Accordingly, any CNS excitation produced by ingestion of cocoa and chocolate derives from their caffeine content and not from theobromine.

AMPHETAMINES

The amphetamine family consists of amphetamine, dextroamphetamine, and methamphetamine. All are powerful CNS stimulants. In addition to their central actions, amphetamines have significant actions in the periphery—actions that can cause cardiac stimulation and vasoconstriction. The amphetamines have a high potential for abuse. As a result, therapeutic applications are limited.

Chemistry

Dextroamphetamine and Levamphetamine. The amphetamines are molecules that contain an asymmetric carbon atom. Because of that asymmetric carbon, amphetamines can exist as mirror images of each other. Such compounds are termed optical isomers or enantiomers. Dextroamphetamine and levamphetamine, whose structures are shown in Figure 32–2, illustrate the mirror-image concept. As can be seen, dextroamphetamine and levamphetamine both contain the same atomic components—but those components are arranged differently around the asymmetric carbon. Because of this structural difference, these compounds have distinctly different pharmacologic properties. Dextroamphetamine is more selective than levoamphetamine for causing CNS stimulation and, hence, produces fewer peripheral side effects.

Amphetamine. The term *amphetamine* refers not to a single compound but rather to a 50:50 mixture of two enantiomers: dextroamphetamine and levamphetamine. (In chemistry, we refer to such equimolar mixtures of enantiomers as being racemic.)

Mechanism of Action

The amphetamines produce their effects by promoting the release of biogenic amines (dopamine, serotonin, norepinephrine) from neurons. Amphetamines promote transmitter release in the CNS and in the periphery. Many of the effects of the amphetamines are due to the release of norepinephrine. However, release of dopamine and serotonin is also important.

Pharmacologic Effects

Central Nervous System. The amphetamines have prominent effects on mood and arousal. At usual doses, these drugs increase wakefulness and alertness, reduce fatigue, elevate mood, and augment self-confidence and initiative. Euphoria, talkativeness, and increased motor activity are likely.

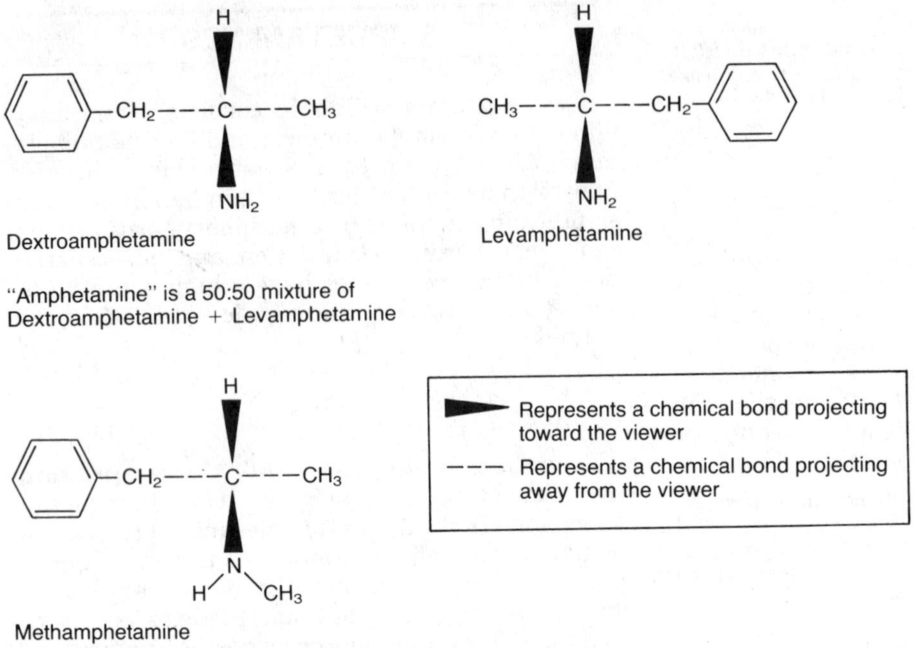

Dextroamphetamine

Levamphetamine

"Amphetamine" is a 50:50 mixture of
Dextroamphetamine + Levamphetamine

Methamphetamine

◀ Represents a chemical bond projecting
toward the viewer

--- Represents a chemical bond projecting
away from the viewer

Figure 32–2. Structural formulas of the amphetamines. "Amphetamine" is a 50:50 mixture of dextroamphetamine plus levamphetamine. Note that dextroamphetamine and levamphetamine are simply mirror images of each other. Both compounds contain the same atomic components.

Task performance that had been reduced by fatigue or boredom improves.

In addition to psychic stimulation, the amphetamines have several other CNS effects. Stimulation of the medullary respiratory center increases respiration. Effects on the hypothalamic feeding center depress appetite. By a mechanism that is not understood, amphetamines can enhance the analgesic effects of morphine and other opioids.

Cardiovascular System. Cardiovascular effects occur secondary to release of norepinephrine from sympathetic nerves. Norepinephrine acts in the heart to increase atrioventricular (A-V) conduction, heart rate, and force of contraction. Excessive cardiac stimulation can produce dysrhythmias. In blood vessels, norepinephrine promotes constriction. Excessive vasoconstriction can produce hypertension.

Tolerance

With regular amphetamine use, tolerance develops to elevation of mood, suppression of appetite, and stimulation of the heart and blood vessels. In highly tolerant users, doses up to 1000 mg (IV) every few *hours* may be required to maintain euphoric effects. This compares with *daily* doses of 5 to 30 mg for nontolerant individuals.

Physical Dependence

Chronic use of amphetamines produces physical dependence. If amphetamines are abruptly withdrawn after prolonged use, an abstinence syndrome will result. Symptoms of withdrawal include exhaustion, depression, prolonged sleep,

excessive eating, and a craving for more drug. Sleep patterns may take months to normalize.

Abuse

Because of their ability to produce euphoria (extreme mood elevation), amphetamines have a high potential for abuse; psychologic dependence can occur. By way of comparison, the psychologic effects of amphetamine are practically indistinguishable from those of cocaine. Because of their abuse potential, amphetamines are classified under Schedule II of the Controlled Substances Act and must be dispensed accordingly. Whenever amphetamines are used therapeutically, their potential for abuse must be weighed against any benefits they may have to offer.

Adverse Effects

Psychosis. Excessive amphetamine usage produces a state of paranoid psychosis, characterized by hallucinations and paranoid delusions (suspiciousness, feelings of being watched). Amphetamine-induced psychosis looks very much like schizophrenia. Symptoms are thought to result from release of dopamine. Consistent with this hypothesis is the observation that symptoms can be alleviated with dopamine-receptor blocking agents (e.g., haloperidol). Left untreated, amphetamine-induced psychosis usually resolves spontaneously within a week.

In some individuals, amphetamine use can unmask latent schizophrenia. For these individuals, symptoms of psychosis will not clear spontaneously. Psychiatric care is likely to be needed.

CNS Stimulation. Stimulation of the CNS can cause *insomnia, restlessness,* and *extreme loquaciousness.* These effects can occur at therapeutic doses.

Cardiovascular Effects. Stimulation of the heart and blood vessels can result in *dysrhythmias, anginal pain,* and *hypertension.* Accordingly, amphetamines must be employed with extreme caution in patients with cardiovascular disease.

Acute Toxicity

Symptoms. Overdosage produces dizziness, confusion, hallucinations, paranoid delusions, palpitations, dysrhythmias, and hypertension. Death is rare. Fatal overdosage is associated with convulsions, coma, and cerebral hemorrhage.

Treatment. Hallucinations can be controlled with chlorpromazine (an antipsychotic drug). An alpha-adrenergic blocker (e.g., phentolamine) can reduce hypertension by promoting vasodilation. Because of its ability to block alpha receptors, chlorpromazine will contribute to lowering of blood pressure. Seizures can be managed with diazepam. Acidification of the urine will accelerate amphetamine excretion.

Therapeutic Uses

Narcolepsy. Narcolepsy is a disorder characterized by daytime somnolence and uncontrollable attacks of sleep. By stimulating the CNS, amphetamines can promote arousal and thereby alleviate these symptoms.

Attention-Deficit Hyperactivity Disorder (ADHD). ADHD is a childhood condition characterized by inattentiveness, impulsiveness, and hyperactivity. Symptoms include failure to complete tasks, difficulty concentrating on schoolwork, switching excessively from one activity to another, excessive calling out in class, difficulty awaiting one's turn in group activities, excessive running about, and excessive movement during sleep. Onset of symptoms occurs between 3 and 7 years of age. Symptoms must be present for 6 months to make a diagnosis. Since other disorders (especially anxiety and depression) may cause similar symptoms, diagnosis of ADHD must be done with care. Former names for ADHD—*hyperkinetic syndrome* and *minimal brain dysfunction*—are misleading and should be abandoned.

Children with ADHD respond dramatically to amphetamine therapy. The amphetamines increase attention span and goal-oriented behavior while decreasing impulsiveness, distractibility, hyperactivity, and restlessness. Overall behavior becomes more tolerable to parents and teachers. Tests of cognitive function (memory, reading, arithmetic) often improve significantly. The calming effect of amphetamines on children is paradoxical and not understood. In addition to drug therapy, treatment should involve behavior modification for the child and counseling for parents and teachers.

The decisions to commence and continue drug therapy are difficult to make and depend in part on cultural expectations. Drugs are not indicated if symptoms are mild. Furthermore, when drugs *are* employed, they should be interrupted periodically to assess the need for their continuation. Many children can reduce or eliminate drug use on weekends and holidays—and in no case should treatment continue for more than 1 school year without interruption. The summer school break is often a good opportunity for a prolonged drug holiday, with treatment resuming, if indicated, after school recommences.

The principal adverse effects of treatment are *insomnia* and *suppression of growth.* Insomnia results from CNS stimulation and can be minimized by taking the last dose of the day no later than 6 hours before bedtime. Growth suppression occurs secondary to appetite suppression. Growth rate should be monitored. Once treatment ceases, a rebound increase in growth usually takes place. Other adverse effects include *headache* and *abdominal pain,* which occur in 10% of those treated, and lethargy and listlessness, which can occur when dosage is excessive.

In addition to amphetamines, two other stimulants—*methylphenidate* [Ritalin] and *pemoline* [Cylert]—are used to treat ADHD. The pharmacology of these drugs is discussed later in the chapter. Of the agents available to treat ADHD, methylphenidate and dextroamphetamine are preferred.

Obesity. Because of their ability to suppress appetite, the amphetamines have been employed as adjunctive aids in programs for weight loss. However, because of their high abuse potential, and because they offer no advantages over less dangerous drugs, amphetamines are not generally recommended for weight reduction. (In some states, the use of amphetamines for weight reduction is prohibited.) When deciding to employ amphetamines to promote weight loss, the risks of abuse must be carefully weighed against the potential benefits. Prescriptions for weight control should be short-term. Amphetamines should not be provided when overeating is the result of psychologic factors, since amphetamines are ineffective under these conditions.

Preparations, Dosage, and Administration

Amphetamines are available in a variety of formulations (standard tablets, long-acting tablets, standard capsules, sustained-release capsules, elixir) for oral use. Formulations and dosages for specific applications are summarized in Table 32–2. Amphetamines are not approved for IV administration. Amphetamines for IV use are available only through illegal sources. Amphetamines are regulated under Schedule II of the Controlled Substances Act and must be dispensed accordingly.

METHYLPHENIDATE

Although methylphenidate [Ritalin] is structurally dissimilar from the amphetamines, the phar-

Generic Name	Trade Name	Dosage Forms	Daily Dosage Range (mg)		
			ADHD	*Obesity*	*Narcolepsy*
Amphetamine sulfate	—	T	2.5–40	5–30	5–60
Dextroamphetamine sulfate	Dexedrine, others	T, E, SRC	2.5–40	5–30	5–60
Methamphetamine hydrochloride	Desoxyn	T, LAT	5–25	10–15	—
Amphetamine complex*	Biphetamine	C	12.5–40	12.5–20	—
Methylphenidate	Ritalin	T, LAT	10–60	—	10–60

*Amphetamine complex is a resin complex containing equimolar amounts of amphetamine and dextroamphetamine.
C = capsule, SRC = sustained-release capsule, T = tablet, LAT = long-acting tablet, E = elixir, ADHD = attention-deficit hyperactivity disorder in children.

macologic effects of methylphenidate and the amphetamines are nearly identical. Consequently, methylphenidate can be considered an amphetamine in all but structure and name. The mechanism of action, adverse effects, and abuse liability of methylphenidate are the same as those of the amphetamines. Methylphenidate has two indications: (1) narcolepsy, and (2) attention-deficit hyperactivity disorder (ADHD) in children. Like the amphetamines, methylphenidate is administered orally. Preparations and dosages are listed in Table 32–2. Methylphenidate is classified under Schedule II of the Controlled Substances Act and must be dispensed accordingly. Guidelines for treatment of ADHD are presented in the discussion of amphetamines.

MISCELLANEOUS CNS STIMULANTS

PEMOLINE

Actions, Uses, and Adverse Effects. Pemoline is a CNS stimulant with effects much like those of the amphetamines. The drug differs from the amphetamines primarily in that it causes less cardiac stimulation and vasoconstriction. The only approved indication for pemoline is attention-deficit hyperactivity disorder. The drug has been used investigationally in narcolepsy but is not approved for this application. Adverse effects are like those of other CNS stimulants. In addition, pemoline is suspected of being hepatotoxic. Hence, patients should undergo periodic tests of liver function. The abuse potential of pemoline is less than that of the amphetamines and methylphenidate. As a result, pemoline is classified under Schedule IV of the Controlled Substances Act, whereas the amphetamines and methylphenidate are classified under Schedule II.

Preparations, Dosage, and Administration. Pemoline [Cylert] is dispensed in standard tablets (18.75, 37.5, and 75 mg) and in chewable tablets (37.5 mg) for oral use. Initial dosage for treatment of attention-deficit hyperactivity disorder is 37.5 mg/day administered as a single dose in the morning. The maximum maintenance dosage is 112.5 mg daily.

STRYCHNINE

Strychnine was introduced in the 16th century as a rat poison. At one time, the drug was also employed therapeutically. Although strychnine is no longer used as a medicine, it remains a source of accidental poisoning and is of interest for that reason.

Strychnine is a powerful convulsant that stimulates the CNS at all levels. The drug produces stimulation by blocking receptors for glycine, an inhibitory neurotransmitter.

Strychnine Poisoning

Causes. A common cause of strychnine poisoning is ingestion of strychnine-based rodenticides by children. Poisoning also occurs through the use of "street drugs" to which strychnine has been added. (Since strychnine does not enhance the effects of illicit drugs, the practice of mixing this agent with street drugs is not only dangerous, it is also devoid of any pharmacologic rationale.) The lethal dose in children is about 15 mg. Doses between 50 and 100 mg are lethal in adults.

Symptoms. The first manifestation of strychnine poisoning is stiffness in the muscles of the face and neck. This response is followed by a generalized increase in reflex excitability. During the early stages of poisoning, the victim is fully conscious. As poisoning progresses, convulsions occur. Strychnine-induced convulsions are characterized by tonic contraction of all voluntary muscles; contraction of the diaphragm, abdominal muscles, and thoracic muscles stops respiration. Convulsive episodes alternate with periods of depression until the victim dies or until the poisoning is successfully treated. Few patients survive beyond the fifth convulsive episode; some are killed by the first. Death is from respiratory arrest.

Treatment. Management is directed primarily at control of convulsions and support of respiration. Intravenous diazepam is the treatment of choice to suppress convulsions. In cases of severe poisoning, general anesthesia or neuromuscular blockade may be needed to eliminate convulsive activity. If anticonvulsant therapy fails to permit adequate breathing, mechanical support of respiration is indicated.

DOXAPRAM

Doxapram [Dopram] stimulates the CNS at all levels. The drug is employed clinically for its ability to stimulate respiration. However, since the doses required to increase respiration are close to those that can produce generalized CNS stimulation and convulsions, doxapram must be used with great care. Furthermore, although doxapram is labeled for treatment of general CNS depressant poisoning, its use for this purpose should be discontinued. Experience has shown that respiratory depression from CNS depressant poisoning can be managed more safely and effectively with mechanical support of ventilation than with pharmacologic stimulation of respiration.

ANOREXIANTS (NONAMPHETAMINES)

Anorexiants are drugs that suppress appetite. These agents are intended for use in the context of a comprehensive weight reduction program—one that includes exercise, behavior modification, and a strict, low-calorie diet. Anorexiants are not indicated as the sole means of controlling caloric intake. These drugs are recommended for short-term use only.

Several types of drugs can suppress appetite. Nonamphetamine anorexiants are discussed in this section. Use of amphetamines to control appetite is discussed above.

Prescription Agents

The nonamphetamine anorexiants that require a prescription are listed in Table 32–3. None of these drugs is more effective than the amphetamines at suppressing appetite. However, the abuse potential and adverse effects of the nonamphetamine anorexiants are generally less than those of the amphetamines.

With the exception of fenfluramine (see below), all of the drugs in Table 32–3 are CNS stimulants. Consequently, these drugs, like the amphetamines, can increase alertness, decrease fatigue, and induce nervousness and insomnia. Because of their potential to interfere with sleep, anorexiants should be administered no later than 4 o'clock in the afternoon. Upon discontinuation of treatment, fatigue and depression may replace CNS stimulation.

Like the amphetamines, most of the nonamphetamine anorexiants have effects in the periphery as well as in the CNS. Peripheral effects of greatest significance are tachycardia, anginal pain, and hypertension. Accordingly, the anorexiants should be used with caution in patients with cardiovascular disease.

Although the abuse potential of the nonamphetamine anorexiants is generally lower than that of the amphetamines, abuse of any of these agents can occur. As shown in Table 32–3, classification of these drugs under the Controlled Substances Act ranges from Schedule II to Schedule IV—indicating that some anorexiants have a greater abuse potential than others. To reduce abuse, an attempt should be made to identify abuse-prone patients prior to treatment.

Tolerance is common and may be seen in 6 to 12 weeks. Tolerance to the anorexiant effects of one agent produces cross-tolerance to the others. If tolerance develops, the appropriate response is to discontinue the drug rather than increase the dosage.

Anorexiants are not recommended for use during pregnancy for two reasons. First, these drugs are not very effective during pregnancy; hence there is little point in taking them. Second, *in utero* exposure to anorexiants poses an increased risk of cleft palate and congenital heart defects.

Fenfluramine. Fenfluramine [Pondimin] is unique among the prescription anorexiant drugs. Unlike the other anorexiants, fenfluramine is a CNS *depressant*, promoting sedation and drowsiness rather than excitation and insomnia. Fenfluramine should not be combined with other CNS depressants, since excessive CNS depression may result. Because of its depressant properties, fenfluramine is useful for treating obesity in patients for whom excitation must be avoided. Fenfluramine has a low abuse potential and is classified under Schedule IV of the Controlled Substances Act.

Nonprescription Agents

Phenylpropanolamine. Phenylpropanolamine is a sympathomimetic drug similar to ephedrine. This agent stimulates adrenergic receptors directly and also promotes norepinephrine release. These actions result in cardiac stimulation and vasoconstriction. The most common indication for the drug is nasal congestion.

In addition to its use as a decongestant, phenylpropanolamine is the active ingredient in various over-the-counter weight-loss aids. The abuse potential of this drug appears to be very low. However, phenylpropanolamine is not without adverse effects, excessive elevation of blood pressure being of particular concern. Although phenylpropanolamine is currently available without prescription, some authorities believe that this drug should be more tightly regulated.

Benzocaine. Benzocaine is a local anesthetic that is also marketed as an aid to weight reduction. The drug is administered in the form of candy or chewing gum. In theory, benzocaine reduces food consumption by decreasing the ability to taste. However, there is no convincing evidence that benzocaine is effective in facilitating weight loss.

COCAINE

Cocaine is a powerful CNS stimulant with a high potential for abuse. The only clinical application of this drug—local anesthesia—is discussed in Chapter 31. The basic pharmacology of cocaine as well as cocaine abuse is discussed in Chapter 34.

Generic Name	Trade Name	Dosage Forms	Usual Adult Dosage*	CSA Schedule
Benzphetamine	Didrex	T	25–50 mg 1–3 times/day	III
Diethylpropion	Tenuate, Tepanil	T, LAT	25 mg 3 times/day	IV
Fenfluramine	Pondimin	T	20 mg 3 times/day	IV
Mazindol	Mazanor, Sanorex	T	1 mg 3 times/day	IV
Phendimetrazine	Many names	T, C, SRC	35 mg 2–3 times/day	III
Phenmetrazine	Preludin	LAT	25 mg 2–3 times/day	II
Phentermine	Many names	T, C	8 mg 3 times/day	IV

Table 32–3. Anorexiants Available by Prescription

*Dosage is for tablet formulation.
C = capsule, T = tablet, LAT = long-acting tablet, SRC = sustained-release capsule.
CSA = Controlled Substances Act.

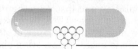

Summary of Major Nursing Implications

AMPHETAMINES AND METHYLPHENIDATE

Preadministration Assessment

Therapeutic Goal

Amphetamines and methylphenidate: Reduction of symptoms in children with attention-deficit hyperactivity disorder (ADHD). Reduction of sleep attacks in patients with narcolepsy.

Amphetamines only: Facilitation of weight loss in conjunction with a comprehensive weight loss program.

Baseline Data

Children with ADHD. Document the degree of inattentiveness, impulsivity, hyperactivity, and other symptoms of ADHD. Symptoms must be present for at least 6 months to allow a diagnosis of ADHD. Obtain baseline values of height and weight.

Narcolepsy. Document the frequency and circumstances of sleep attacks.

Identifying High-Risk Patients

Amphetamines are *contraindicated* for patients with *symptomatic cardiovascular disease, advanced arteriosclerosis, hypertension, hyperthyroidism, agitated states*, and a *history of drug abuse* and in those who have taken *monoamine oxidase (MAO) inhibitors* within the previous 2 weeks.

Implementation: Administration

Route

Oral.

Administration

Instruct the patient to swallow sustained-release and long-acting tablets intact, without crushing or chewing.

Children with ADHD should take the last dose of the day at least 6 hours before bedtime.

Amphetamines and methylphenidate are classified under Schedule II of the Controlled Substances Act and must be dispensed accordingly.

Implementation: Measures to Enhance Therapeutic Effects

Children with ADHD

In addition to drug therapy, treatment should include behavior modification for the child and counseling for parents and teachers.

Ongoing Evaluation and Interventions

Evaluating Therapeutic Effects

Children with ADHD. Monitor for reductions in symptoms (impulsiveness, hyperactivity, inattentiveness) and for improvement in cognitive function. Periodic drug holidays are required to determine if therapy is still needed. Continuous treatment for longer than 1 school year should not be done.

Minimizing Adverse Effects

Excessive CNS Stimulation. Amphetamines and methylphenidate can cause restlessness and insomnia. Advise patients to use the smallest dose required and to avoid dosing late in the day. Advise patients to minimize or eliminate dietary caffeine (e.g., coffee, tea, caffeine-containing soft drinks).

Cardiovascular Effects. Warn patients about cardiovascular responses (palpitations, hypertension, angina, dysrhythmias) and instruct them to notify the physician if these develop.

Psychosis. Amphetamines can induce a state of paranoid psychosis. If psychosis develops, therapy should be discontinued. For most individuals, symptoms resolve within a week. For some patients, drug-induced psychosis may represent unmasking of latent schizophrenia; these patients will require psychiatric care.

Withdrawal Reactions. Abrupt discontinuation can produce extreme fatigue and depression. To minimize these responses, withdraw amphetamines and methylphenidate gradually.

Minimizing Abuse

If the medical history reveals that the patient is prone to drug abuse, monitor use of amphetamines and methylphenidate closely.

Avoid routine use of amphetamines for weight loss.

CAFFEINE

General Considerations

Caffeine is administered to promote wakefulness. Warn patients against habitual caffeine use to compensate for chronic lack of sleep. Advise patients to consult the physician if fatigue is persistent or recurrent.

Minimizing Adverse Effects

Cardiovascular Effects. Inform patients about cardiovascular responses to caffeine (palpitations, rapid pulse, dizziness) and instruct them to discontinue caffeine if these occur.

Excessive CNS Stimulation. Warn patients that overdosage can cause convulsions. Advise them to take no more caffeine than is needed.

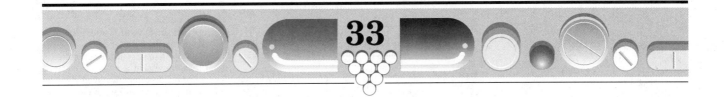

Aliphatic Alcohols: Ethanol and Methanol

There are two aliphatic alcohols of pharmacologic interest: ethanol and methanol. Ethanol, the inebriant in alcoholic beverages, will be the principal focus of this chapter. Methanol is included because of its capacity for toxicity; methanol has no recreational or therapeutic uses. In addition to ethanol and methanol, we will discuss disulfiram [Antabuse], a drug used in the treatment of alcoholism.

ETHANOL

Ethanol (ethyl alcohol) is more commonly known simply as *alcohol*. We will refer to ethanol by its common name in this chapter. The structural formula of alcohol is shown in Figure 33–1.

Although alcohol does have some therapeutic applications, alcohol is of primary interest because of its nonmedical use. In our society, alcohol is the only psychoactive drug with which self-induced intoxication is considered socially acceptable. Two of three American adults drink alcohol, and at least 12% of these drink heavily. Excessive use of alcohol is a major public health problem. Chronic alcohol abuse is costly in terms of damaged health, disrupted families, and lost productivity.

In this chapter, we will limit consideration to the pharmacologic consequences of alcohol ingestion.

399

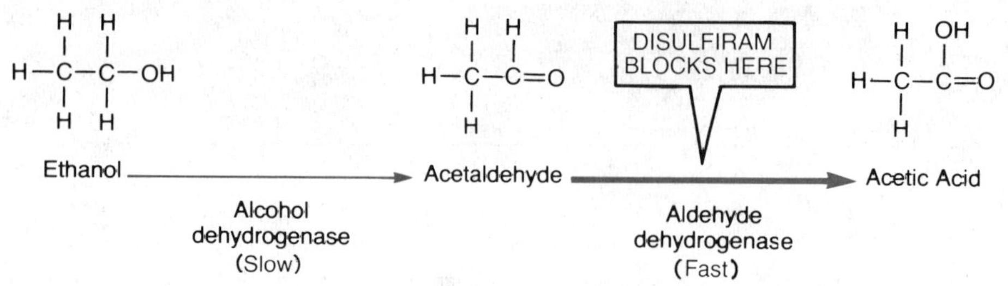

Figure 33–1. Ethanol metabolism and the effect of disulfiram. Conversion of ethanol into acetaldehyde takes place slowly (at a rate of about 15 ml/hr). Consumption of more than 15 ml/hr will cause ethanol to accumulate. Effects of disulfiram result from accumulation of acetaldehyde secondary to inhibition of aldehyde dehydrogenase.

In discussing the pharmacology of alcohol we will consider the effects of both moderate and excessive consumption. Alcohol abuse is addressed in Chapter 34.

Central Nervous System Effects

Acute Effects. Alcohol is a central nervous system (CNS) depressant. Like the barbiturates, alcohol causes general (relatively nonselective) depression of CNS function. Alcohol appears to affect the nervous system primarily by enhancing the actions of gamma-aminobutyric acid (GABA), an inhibitory neurotransmitter.

The effects of alcohol on the CNS are dose dependent. When dosage is low, the higher brain centers (cortical areas) are primarily affected. As dosage is increased, more primitive brain areas (e.g., medulla) become depressed. With depression of cortical function, thought processes and learned behaviors are altered, inhibitions are released, and self-restraint is replaced by increased sociability and expansiveness. Cortical depression also results in significant impairment of motor function. As CNS depression deepens, reflexes diminish greatly and consciousness becomes impaired. At very high doses, alcohol produces a state of general anesthesia. (Alcohol is not actually used for anesthesia because anesthetic doses are very close to being lethal.) Table 33–1 summarizes the effects of alcohol as a function of blood alcohol level and indicates the brain areas involved.

Chronic Effects. When consumed chronically and in excess, alcohol can produce severe neurologic and psychiatric disorders. Injury to the CNS is caused by the direct actions of alcohol and by the nutritional deficiencies frequently suffered by chronic heavy drinkers.

Two neuropsychiatric syndromes commonly seen in alcoholics are *Wernicke's encephalopathy* and *Korsakoff's psychosis*. Both disorders are caused by thiamine deficiency, which results from poor diet and alcohol-induced suppression of thiamine absorption. Wernicke's encephalopathy is characterized by confusion, nystagmus, and abnormal ocular movements. This syndrome is readily reversible with thiamine. Korsakoff's psychosis is characterized by polyneuropathy, inability to convert short-term memory to long-term memory, and confabulation. Korsakoff's psychosis is not reversible.

Perhaps the most dramatic effect of long-term excessive alcohol consumption is enlargement of the cerebral ventricles, presumably in response to atrophy of the cerebrum itself. These gross anatomic changes are associated with impairment of intellectual function and memory. With cessation of drinking, ventricular enlargement and cognitive deficits reverse (partially) in some individuals, but not in all.

Other Pharmacologic Effects

Cardiovascular System. When alcohol is consumed acutely and in moderate doses, cardiovas-

Table 33–1. Central Nervous System Responses at Various Blood Alcohol Levels

Blood Alcohol Level (%)	Pharmacologic Response	Brain Area Affected
0.50	Peripheral collapse	Medulla
0.45	Respiratory depression	
0.40	Stupor, coma	Diencephalon
0.35	Apathy, inertia	
0.30	Altered equilibrium	Cerebellum
	Double vision	Occipital lobe
0.25	Altered perception	
0.20	↓ Motor skills	Parietal lobe
	Slurred speech	
0.15	Tremors	
	Ataxia	
0.10	↓ Attention	Frontal lobe
	Loquaciousness	
	Altered judgment	
0.05	Increased confidence	
	Euphoria, ↓ inhibitions	

cular effects are minor, the most prominent effect being *dilation of cutaneous blood vessels*—an action that increases blood flow to the skin. By increasing blood flow to the body surface, alcohol imparts a sensation of warmth, while at the same time promoting heat loss. Hence, despite images of Saint Bernards with little barrels of whiskey about their necks, alcohol may do more harm than good for the individual stranded in the snow and suffering from hypothermia. Acute alcohol consumption also produces a modest rise in blood pressure.

Although the cardiovascular effects of moderate alcohol consumption are unremarkable, chronic and excessive alcohol consumption is clearly harmful. Abuse of alcohol results in *direct damage to the myocardium*, thereby increasing the risk of heart failure. Some investigators believe that alcohol may be the major cause of cardiomyopathy in the Western world.

Not all of the cardiovascular effects of alcohol are deleterious: there is clear evidence that people who drink *moderately* (1 to 3 drinks/day) experience less coronary artery disease (CAD) than abstainers. It is important to note, however, that with *heavy* drinking (5 or more drinks/day) the risk of CAD is greatly increased. Recent evidence suggests that moderate alcohol intake reduces CAD in large part by raising levels of HDL-cholesterol. (As discussed in Chapter 45, HDL-cholesterol protects against CAD, whereas LDL-cholesterol promotes it.)

Respiration. Like all other CNS depressants, alcohol depresses respiration. Respiratory depression from moderate drinking is negligible. However, when consumed in excessive amounts, alcohol can cause death by respiratory arrest. The respiratory depressant effects of alcohol are potentiated by other CNS depressants (e.g., benzodiazepines, opioids, barbiturates).

Stomach. Immoderate use of alcohol can cause *erosive gastritis*. About one third of alcoholics have this disorder. Alcohol causes gastritis by two mechanisms. First, alcohol stimulates secretion of gastric acid. Second, when present in high concentrations, alcohol can injure the gastric mucosa directly.

Liver. Acute use of alcohol causes reversible accumulation of fat and protein in the liver. However, when alcohol consumption is chronic, accumulation of fat and protein eventually leads to *cirrhosis*—a condition characterized by proliferation of fibrous tissue and destruction of liver parenchymal cells. Although various factors can cause cirrhosis, alcohol abuse is unquestionably the major cause of *fatal* cirrhosis.

Kidney. Alcohol is a diuretic. The drug promotes urine formation by inhibiting the release of antidiuretic hormone (ADH) from the pituitary. Since ADH acts on the kidney to promote water reabsorption, thereby decreasing urine formation, a reduction in circulating ADH will increase urine formation.

Sexual Function. Alcohol has both psychologic and physiologic effects related to human sexual behavior. Although alcohol is not exactly an aphrodisiac, the ability of alcohol to release people from their inhibitions has been known to inspire sexual activity. Ironically, the physiologic effects of alcohol may frustrate attempts at consummating the sexual activity that the psychologic effects of alcohol helped bring about: objective measurements in males and females show that alcohol significantly decreases our physiologic capacity for sexual responsiveness.

The opposing psychologic and physiologic effects of alcohol on sexual function were noted long ago by no less an authority than William Shakespeare. In *Macbeth* (Act 2, Scene 2) Macduff inquires of a porter "What . . . does drink especially provoke?" To which the porter replies,

> . . . *Lechery, sir, it provokes, and unprovokes; it provokes the desire, but it takes away the performance.*

In males, long-term use of alcohol may promote *feminization*. Symptoms include testicular atrophy, impotence, sterility, and breast enlargement.

Impact on Longevity. The effects of alcohol on life span depend on the amount of alcohol consumed. Heavy drinkers have a higher mortality rate than the population at large. Causes of increased mortality include cirrhosis, respiratory disease, and cancer. The risk of death associated with alcohol abuse increases markedly in individuals who consume six or more drinks per day. Interestingly, people who consume *moderate* amounts of alcohol live *longer* than those who abstain. This increase in longevity results from alcohol's ability to suppress development of coronary atherosclerosis.

Pharmacokinetics

Absorption. Alcohol is absorbed from the stomach and small intestine. About 20% of ingested alcohol is absorbed from the stomach. Gastric absorption is relatively slow and is delayed even further by the presence of food. Milk is especially effective at retarding absorption. Absorption from the small intestine is rapid and largely independent of the presence of food; about 80% of ingested alcohol is absorbed from this site. Because most alcohol is absorbed from the small intestine, gastric emptying time (the time required for the contents of the stomach to be released into small intestine) is a major determinant of individual variation in alcohol absorption.

Distribution. Alcohol is distributed to all tissues and body fluids. The drug crosses the blood-brain barrier with ease, allowing alcohol in the brain to equilibrate rapidly with alcohol in the blood. Alcohol also crosses the placenta and can affect the developing fetus.

Metabolism. Alcohol is metabolized in the liver. The metabolic pathway is shown in Figure 33–1. As depicted, the process begins with the conversion of alcohol to acetaldehyde. This reaction is *slow* and puts a limit on the rate at which alcohol can be inactivated. Once formed, acetaldehyde undergoes *rapid* conversion to acetic acid. Through a series of reactions, acetic acid is then used to synthesize cholesterol, fatty acids, and other compounds.

The kinetics of alcohol metabolism differ from those of most other drugs. With most drugs, as plasma drug levels rise, the amount of drug metabolized per unit time increases. This is not true for alcohol: as the alcohol content of blood increases, there is no change in the speed of alcohol breakdown. That is, alcohol is metabolized at a *constant rate*—regardless of how much alcohol is in the body. The average rate at which individuals can metabolize alcohol is about *15 ml per hour*.

There is some variation among individuals in their capacity for alcohol metabolism. Since metabolism of alcohol is generally proportional to body weight, large people usually metabolize alcohol more rapidly than small people. Also, because alcohol, like the barbiturates, can stimulate hepatic drug metabolism, individuals who consume alcohol chronically in large amounts can usually metabolize the drug faster than people who drink moderately.

Because alcohol is metabolized at a slow and constant rate, there is a limit to how much alcohol one can consume without having the drug accumulate in the body. For practical purposes, that limit is about *one drink per hour*. Consumption of more than one drink per hour—be that drink beer, wine, straight whiskey, or a cocktail—will result in alcohol buildup.

The information in Table 33–2 helps explain why we are unable to metabolize more than one drink's worth of alcohol per hour. As the table indicates, beer, wine, and whiskey differ from one another with respect to alcohol concentration and usual serving size. However, despite these differences, it turns out that *the average can of beer, the average glass of wine, and the average shot of whiskey all contain the same amount of alcohol, namely, 18 ml*. Since the liver can metabolize about 15 ml of alcohol per hour, and since the average alcoholic drink contains 18 ml of alcohol, one drink contains just about the amount of alcohol that the liver can comfortably process. Consumption of more than one drink per hour will overwhelm the capacity of the liver for alcohol metabolism, and, therefore, will cause alcohol to accumulate.

Table 33–2. Alcohol Content of Beer, Wine, and Whiskey

	Wine	Beer	Whiskey
Usual serving	1 glass	1 can or bottle	1 shot
Serving size	150 ml (5 ounces)	360 ml (12 ounces)	45 ml (1.5 ounces)
Alcohol concentration	12%[a]	5%[c]	40%[e]
Alcohol per serving	18 ml[b]	18 ml[d]	18 ml[f]

[a]The alcohol content of wine varies from 8% to 20%; typical table wines contain 12%.
[b]The alcohol in a 5-ounce glass of wine varies from 12 ml to 30 ml, depending on the alcohol concentration in the wine. Wine with 12% alcohol has 18 ml alcohol per 5-ounce glass.
[c]The alcohol content of beer varies: 5% alcohol is typical of American premium beers; cheaper American beers and light beers have less alcohol (2.4% to 5%); and imported beers may have more alcohol (6%). Beer sold in Europe may have 7% to 8% alcohol.
[d]The alcohol in a 12-ounce can of beer varies from 9 ml to 29 ml, depending on the alcohol concentration in the beer. Beer with 5% alcohol has 18 ml per 12-ounce can.
[e]Whiskeys and other distilled spirits (e.g., rum, vodka, gin) are usually 80 proof (40% alcohol) but may also be 100 proof (50% alcohol).
[f]The alcohol in a 1.5-ounce shot of whiskey can be either 18 ml or 22.5 ml, depending on the proof of the whiskey. Eighty-proof whiskey has 18 ml alcohol per 1.5-ounce serving.

Blood Levels of Alcohol. Since alcohol in the brain rapidly equilibrates with alcohol in the blood, blood levels of alcohol are predictive of CNS effects. The behavioral effects associated with specific blood levels of alcohol are summarized in Table 33–1. The earliest effects (euphoria, reduced inhibitions, increased confidence) are seen when blood alcohol content is about 0.05%. As blood alcohol rises, intoxication becomes more intense. When blood alcohol exceeds 0.4%, there is a substantial risk of respiratory depression, peripheral collapse, and death.

It must be noted that not all people with the same blood level of alcohol will be affected to the same extent. There is individual variability in responsiveness to alcohol just as with all other drugs. Variability in alcohol responsiveness is illustrated in Figure 33–2. As the figure shows, a blood alcohol level of 0.1% will produce intoxication in 50% of the population. However, although the average person will be intoxicated with 0.1% blood alcohol, this relationship does not hold for everyone. For example, as can be seen from Figure 33–2, 10% of the population will be intoxicated when their blood level of alcohol is only 0.03%. At the other extreme, some individuals can have 0.3% alcohol in their blood and still be relatively sober.

Tolerance

Chronic consumption of alcohol produces tolerance. As a result, in order to alter consciousness,

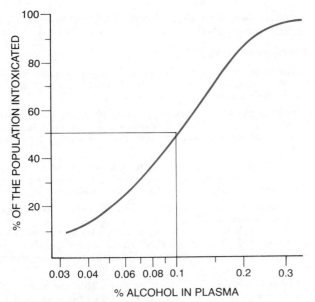

Figure 33–2. Individual variation in alcohol responsiveness. This graph shows the percentage of the population that will be intoxicated at particular blood levels of alcohol. As indicated, 50% of the population will be intoxicated at a blood alcohol level of 0.1% (100 mg/100 ml)—the level that constitutes statutory intoxication in most states.

people who drink on a regular basis require larger amounts of alcohol than people who drink only on occasion. Tolerance to alcohol confers cross-tolerance to general anesthetics, barbiturates, and other general CNS depressants. However, no cross-tolerance develops to opioids. Tolerance subsides within a few weeks following cessation of alcohol use.

Although tolerance develops to many of the effects of alcohol, *very little tolerance develops to respiratory depression.* Consequently, the lethal dose of alcohol for chronic, heavy drinkers is not much greater than the lethal dose for nondrinkers. Alcoholics may tolerate blood alcohol levels as high as 0.4% (four times the amount normally defined by law as intoxicating) with no marked reduction in consciousness; however, if blood levels rise only slightly above this level, death may result.

Physical Dependence

Chronic use of alcohol produces physical dependence. If alcohol is withdrawn abruptly, an abstinence syndrome will result. The intensity of the abstinence syndrome is proportional to the degree of physical dependence. Individuals who are physically dependent on alcohol show cross-dependence with other general CNS depressants (e.g., barbiturates, chloral hydrate, benzodiazepines) but not with opioids. The alcohol withdrawal syndrome and its management are discussed in detail later in the chapter.

Drug Interactions

CNS Depressants. The CNS effects of alcohol are additive with the effects of other CNS depressants (e.g., barbiturates, benzodiazepines, opioids). Consumption of alcohol with other CNS depressants will intensify the psychologic and physiologic manifestations of CNS depression. Combining alcohol with other CNS depressants greatly increases the risk of death from respiratory depression.

Aspirin-like Drugs. Like alcohol, the aspirin-like drugs can injure the gastrointestinal mucosa. The combined effects of alcohol and aspirin-like drugs can result in significant gastric bleeding.

Disulfiram. The combination of alcohol with disulfiram [Antabuse] can cause a variety of adverse effects, some of which are extremely hazardous. These effects, and the use of disulfiram in the treatment of alcoholism, are discussed later in the chapter.

Vasodilators. The vasodilating effects of alcohol are additive with those of other drugs that promote vasodilation (e.g., nitroglycerin, hydralazine). The combination of alcohol with other vasodilating agents can cause significant hypotension.

Use in Pregnancy and Lactation

Pregnancy. Consumption of alcohol during pregnancy can cause *fetal alcohol syndrome* (FAS). This syndrome is seen in one out of three children born to alcoholic mothers. Children with FAS are characterized by mild-to-moderate mental retardation, slow growth rate, craniofacial malformations, and limb abnormalities. Also, resistance to infection is greatly reduced (apparently secondary to immune system derangement).

In addition to FAS, alcohol use during pregnancy can result in *stillbirth, spontaneous abortion, low birth weight,* and *mental retardation.* (Alcohol may be the greatest teratogenic cause of mental deficiency in the Western world.) Neonates whose mothers consumed large amounts of alcohol during pregnancy may be born with *physical dependence* on alcohol. These infants will need to undergo withdrawal therapy.

From the above, it is clear that pregnancy is a contraindication to use of alcohol. Mild FAS has been caused by consuming as little as 30 ml of alcohol per day. Drinking 30 ml of alcohol twice weekly is associated with an increase in second trimester spontaneous abortion. Although there may be some small amount of alcohol that can be consumed safely during pregnancy, we do not know what that amount is. Consequently, in the interests of fetal health, pregnant women should be advised to avoid alcohol entirely.

Lactation. Unless alcohol consumption is extremely heavy, alcohol in breast milk is not likely to reach levels that can affect the nursing infant. (Alcohol does enter breast milk, but significant amounts will not be present until maternal blood levels of alcohol reach 0.3%—a level associated with gross intoxication.) Use of alcohol during lactation may inhibit the milk-ejection reflex.

Acute Overdosage

Acute overdosage with alcohol produces vomiting, coma, pronounced hypotension, and respiratory depression. The combination of vomiting and unconsciousness can result in aspiration, which in turn can result in pulmonary obstruction and pneumonia. Alcohol-induced hypotension results from a direct effect on peripheral blood vessels, and cannot be corrected with vasoconstrictors (e.g., epinephrine). Hypotension can lead to renal failure (secondary to compromised renal blood flow) and to cardiovascular shock, which is a common cause of alcohol-related death. Although death can also result from respiratory depression, this is not the usual cause.

Since the symptoms of acute alcohol poisoning can mimic symptoms of other pathologies (e.g., diabetic coma, skull fracture), a definitive diagnosis may not be possible without measuring alcohol in the blood, urine, or expired air. The smell of "alcohol" on the breath is not a reliable means of diagnosis, since the breath odors we associate with alcohol consumption are due to impurities in alcoholic beverages—and not to alcohol itself. Hence, these odors may or may not be present.

Alcohol poisoning is treated like poisoning with all other general CNS depressants. Details of management are discussed in Chapter 27. Alcohol can be removed from the body by gastric lavage and dialysis. Stimulants (e.g., caffeine, pentylenetetrazol) should not be administered.

Summary of Precautions and Contraindications

Alcohol can injure the gastrointestinal mucosa and should not be consumed by persons with *peptic ulcer disease*. Alcohol is harmful to the liver and should not be used by individuals with *liver disease*. Alcohol should be avoided during *pregnancy* because of the risk of fetal alcohol syndrome, mental retardation, reduced birth weight, stillbirth, and spontaneous abortion.

Alcohol must be used with caution by patients with *epilepsy*. During alcohol use, the CNS is depressed. When alcohol consumption ceases, the CNS undergoes rebound excitation, and this excitation can precipitate seizures.

Alcohol can cause serious adverse effects if combined with *CNS depressants, aspirin-like drugs,*

vasodilators, and *disulfiram*. These combinations should be avoided.

Therapeutic Uses

Although our emphasis has been on the nonmedical use of alcohol, it should be remembered that alcohol does have therapeutic applications.

Topical. Alcohol applied to the skin can promote cooling in febrile patients. Topical alcohol is also a popular skin disinfectant. In addition, alcohol application can help prevent decubitus ulcers.

Oral. Because of its ability to promote gastric secretion, alcohol can serve as an aid to digestion in bedridden patients. Oral alcohol is frequently used as self-medication for insomnia.

Intravenous. Solutions of alcohol (5% or 10%) in 5% dextrose are administered by slow IV infusion to provide calories and fluid replacement. Intravenous alcohol is also used to treat poisoning by methanol (see below). At one time, IV alcohol was employed to delay preterm labor; this application is essentially obsolete.

Local Injection. Injection of alcohol within the vicinity of nerves produces nerve block. This technique can be used to relieve pain of trigeminal neuralgia, inoperable carcinoma, and other causes.

DRUGS EMPLOYED IN THE TREATMENT OF ALCOHOLISM

Alcoholism can be defined (simplistically) as chronic ingestion of excessive amounts of alcohol. With the exception of cigarette smoking, alcoholism is the largest drug-related public health problem in the United States. The cost of alcoholism both in dollars and quality of life is beyond measurement.

The consequences of alcohol abuse are numerous. Alcoholism produces psychologic derangements, including anxiety, depression, and suicidal ideation. Malnutrition, secondary to inadequate diet and malabsorption, is common. Poor work performance and disruption of family life reflect the social deterioration suffered by alcoholics. Lastly, chronic alcohol abuse is harmful to the body, resulting in liver disease, cardiomyopathy, and brain damage—not to mention injury from automotive and other types of accidents.

When treating alcoholism, the principal objective is to modify patterns of drinking (i.e., to reduce or completely eliminate alcohol consumption). In addition, alcoholics often need therapy for malnutrition. Drugs employed to attain these objectives are discussed below.

DRUGS USED TO FACILITATE WITHDRAWAL

As stated previously, chronic use of alcohol produces physical dependence, and abrupt withdrawal will produce an abstinence syndrome. When the degree of physical dependence is low, withdrawal symptoms are mild (disturbed sleep, weakness, nausea, anxiety, mild tremors) and last for less than a day. In contrast, the withdrawal syndrome experienced by individuals highly dependent upon alcohol is severe. Symptoms begin 12 to 72 hours after the last drink and continue for 5 to 7 days. Early manifestations include cramps, vomiting, hallucinations, and intense tremors; heart rate, blood pressure, and temperature may rise; and tonic-clonic seizures may develop. As the syndrome progresses, disorientation and loss of insight occur. A few alcoholics (less than 1%) experience *delirium tremens* (severe persecutory hallucinations). These hallucinations can be so vivid and lifelike that alcoholics often cannot distinguish them from reality. In extreme cases, alcohol withdrawal can result in cardiovascular collapse and death.

Management of withdrawal depends on the degree of alcohol dependence. When dependence is mild, withdrawal can be accomplished on an outpatient basis and without the use of drugs. However, when dependence is great, withdrawal carries a risk of death. In this case, hospitalization and drug therapy are indicated.

The objective of drug therapy is to suppress symptoms of abstinence. In theory, any drug that has cross-dependence with alcohol (i.e., any of the general CNS depressants) should be effective. However, in actual practice, the *benzodiazepines*, especially *chlordiazepoxide* [Librium] and *diazepam* [Valium], have been the drugs of choice. Use of *atenolol* (a beta-adrenergic blocking agent) in conjunction with benzodiazepines appears promising. Combined therapy with atenolol may permit use of lower benzodiazepine doses and may accelerate improvement in vital signs. When drugs are employed to treat withdrawal, initial doses should be sufficient to suppress severe symptoms. Doses are then decreased gradually until drugs are no longer needed.

DISULFIRAM

Therapeutic Use. Disulfiram [Antabuse] is taken by alcoholics to help them refrain from drinking. This drug discourages drinking by causing severe adverse effects if alcohol is ingested. Disulfiram has no applications outside the treatment of alcoholism.

Mechanism of Action. As indicated in Figure 33–1, disulfiram acts by disrupting alcohol metabolism. Specifically, disulfiram causes *irreversible inhibition of aldehyde dehydrogenase*, the enzyme that converts acetaldehyde to acetic acid. As a result, if alcohol is ingested, *acetaldehyde* will accumulate to toxic levels, producing unpleasant and potentially dangerous effects.

Pharmacologic Effects. The constellation of adverse effects caused by alcohol plus disulfiram is referred to as the *acetaldehyde syndrome*. This syndrome can be very dangerous—even fatal. In its "mild" form, the syndrome manifests as nausea, copious vomiting, flushing, palpitations, headache, sweating, thirst, chest pain, weakness, blurred vision, and hypotension; blood pressure may ultimately decline to shock levels. This reaction, which may last from 30 minutes to several hours, can be brought on by consuming as little as 7 ml of alcohol.

In its more severe manifestations, the acetaldehyde syndrome is life-threatening. Potential reactions include marked respiratory depression, cardiovascular collapse, cardiac dysrhythmias, myocardial infarction, acute congestive heart failure, convulsions, and death. Clearly, the acetaldehyde syndrome is not simply unpleasant; this syndrome can be extremely hazardous and must be avoided.

In the absence of alcohol, disulfiram rarely causes significant effects. Drowsiness and skin eruptions may occur during initial drug use. These responses diminish with time.

Patient Selection. Because of the severity of the acetaldehyde syndrome, candidates for therapy must be carefully chosen. Alcoholics who lack the determination to stop drinking should not be given disulfiram. In other words, disulfiram must not be administered to those alcoholics who are likely to attempt drinking while undergoing treatment.

Patient Education. Patient education is an extremely important component of disulfiram therapy. Patients must be thoroughly informed about the potential hazards of treatment. That is, they must be made aware that consumption of any alcohol while taking disulfiram may produce a severe, potentially fatal, reaction. Patients must be warned to avoid all forms of alcohol, including alcohol found in sauces and cough syrups, and alcohol applied to the skin in after-shave lotions, colognes, and liniments. Patients should be made aware that the effects of disulfiram will persist for about 2 weeks after the last dose is taken; alcohol must not be consumed until this interval is over. Individuals using disulfiram should be encouraged to carry identification indicating their status.

Preparations, Dosage, and Administration. Disulfiram [Antabuse] is dispensed in tablets (250 and 500 mg) for oral use. At least 12 hours must elapse between the patient's last drink and initiation of treatment. The initial dosage is 500 mg once daily for 1 to 2 weeks. Maintenance dosages range from 125 to 500 mg a day, usually taken as a single dose in the morning. Therapy may last for months or even years.

OTHER DRUGS USED IN THE TREATMENT OF ALCOHOLISM

Malnutrition is a common problem in the chronic alcoholic. Poor nutrition results from two factors: (1) poor diet, and (2) malabsorption of nutrients and vitamins. Malabsorption is caused by alcohol-induced damage to the gastrointestinal mu-

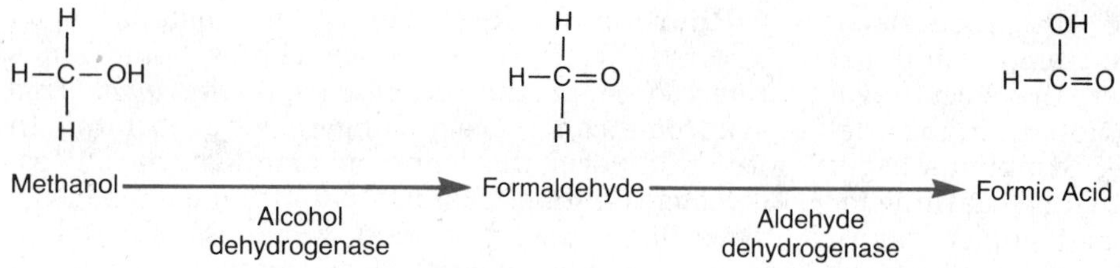

Figure 33-3. Metabolism of methanol. Toxicity associated with methanol results from production of toxic metabolites: formaldehyde and formic acid.

cosa. Poor diet is due in part to the fact that alcoholics can meet up to 50% of their caloric needs with alcohol, and, therefore, consumption of foods with greater nutritional value tends to be subnormal. Because of their poor nutritional state, alcoholics are in need of fat, protein, and vitamins. The B vitamins (thiamine, folic acid, cyanocobalamin) are especially needed. To correct nutritional deficiencies, a program of dietary modification and vitamin supplements should be implemented.

Alcoholics frequently require fluid replacement therapy and antibiotics. Fluids are needed to replace fluids lost because of gastritis or because of vomiting associated with withdrawal. Antibiotics may be needed to manage pneumonitis, a common complication of alcoholism.

METHANOL

Methanol, also known as *methyl alcohol* or *wood alcohol*, is of purely toxicologic interest; the drug has no therapeutic applications. Methanol poisoning produces multiple symptoms, including headache, severe abdominal pain, back pain, labored breathing, and blurred vision. Coma may develop rapidly. Death, preceded by blindness, results from respiratory arrest. As little as 4 ml of methanol can cause blindness. Eighty to 150 ml is usually fatal.

The adverse effects of methanol ingestion are caused by products of methanol metabolism and not by methanol itself. As indicated in Figure 33-3, metabolism of methanol produces *formaldehyde* and *formic acid*, the immediate causes of toxicity. Formic acid produces *severe acidosis*. Formaldehyde, in the presence of acidosis, causes *blindness*. Because methanol must be metabolized before toxicity results, signs of poisoning may not appear until 8 to 36 hours after drug ingestion.

The key to treatment is reversal of acidosis, which can be accomplished by infusing alkali (e.g., bicarbonate). The more rapidly pH is returned to normal, the better the chances of preventing blindness.

Methanol poisoning is also treated by administering *ethanol*. Benefits derive from preventing the conversion of methanol to its toxic metabolites. Alcohol blocks the formation of these metabolites by competing with methanol for alcohol dehydrogenase, the enzyme that converts methanol into formaldehyde.

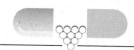

Summary of Major Nursing Implications

DISULFIRAM

Preadministration Assessment

Therapeutic Goal

Facilitation of abstinence from alcohol.

Patient Selection

Candidates for therapy must be chosen carefully. Disulfiram must not be given to alcoholics who are likely to attempt drinking while taking this drug.

Identifying High-Risk Patients

Disulfiram is *contraindicated* for *patients suspected of being incapable of abstinence from alcohol,* for patients with *myocardial disease, coronary occlusion, or psychosis,* and for patients who have recently received *alcohol, metronidazole, paraldehyde,* or *alcohol-containing medications* (e.g., cough syrups, tonics).

Implementation: Administration

Route

Oral.

Administration

Instruct the patient not to administer the first dose until at least 12 hours after his or her last drink.

Dosing is done once daily and may continue for months or even years. Tablets may be crushed or mixed with liquid.

Implementation: Measures to Enhance Therapeutic Effects

Patient education is essential for safety. Inform patients about the potential hazards of treatment, and warn them to avoid all forms of alcohol, including alcohol in vinegar, sauces, and cough syrups, and alcohol applied to the skin in after-shave lotions, colognes, and liniments. Inform patients that the effects of disulfiram will persist for about 2 weeks after the last dose and that alcohol must not be consumed during this interval. Encourage patients to carry identification to alert emergency health care personnel to their condition.

34

Drugs of Abuse

From the dawn of civilization mind-altering drugs have held a fascination for mankind. Throughout history, people have taken drugs to elevate mood, release inhibitions, distort perceptions, induce hallucinations, and modify thinking. The majority of those who use mind-altering drugs restrict usage to socially approved patterns. However, some individuals self-administer drugs to excess. Excessive drug use is our concern in this chapter.

Drug abuse confronts the clinician in a variety of ways, making knowledge of abuse a necessity. Important areas in which expertise on drug abuse may be applied include (1) diagnosis and treatment of acute toxicity, (2) diagnosis and treatment of secondary medical complications of drug abuse, (3) facilitating drug withdrawal in the physically dependent user, and (4) educating and counseling drug abusers.

We will approach drug abuse in two stages. First, we will discuss general issues regarding drug abuse. Second, we will discuss the pharmacology of specific abused agents. Topics addressed in the general discussion include (1) definitions of abuse, addiction, and psychoactive substance dependence; (2) factors contributing to abuse; (3) methods for modifying drug-using behavior; and (4) the Controlled Substances Act. As we discuss specific agents, we will focus on (1) patterns of use, (2) subjective and behavioral effects, (3) physiologic effects, (4) tolerance and dependence, (5) withdrawal techniques, and (6) manifestations and management of toxicity.

GENERAL CONSIDERATIONS ON DRUG ABUSE

DEFINITIONS: DRUG ABUSE, ADDICTION, PSYCHOACTIVE SUBSTANCE DEPENDENCE

Drug Abuse

Drug abuse can be defined as *using a drug in a fashion inconsistent with social norms and with the intent of altering one's psychologic state.* Traditionally, the term abuse also implies drug usage that is harmful to the individual or society. As we shall see, although we can give abuse a general definition, deciding whether a particular instance of drug use constitutes "abuse" is often difficult.

Whether or not drug use is considered abuse depends, in part, on the purpose for which a drug is taken. Not everyone who takes large doses of psychoactive agents is an abuser. For example, we do not consider it abuse to take opioids in large doses on a long-term basis to relieve pain caused by cancer. However, we do consider it abusive for an otherwise healthy individual to take those same opioids in the same doses for the purpose of producing euphoria.

When we speak of drug abuse, we should be aware that abuse can have different degrees of severity. Some people, for example, use opioids (e.g., heroin) only occasionally, whereas heroin use by others is habitual and compulsive. Although both patterns of drug use are socially condemned, and therefore constitute abuse, there is an obvious quantitative difference between taking heroin once or twice and using the drug compulsively.

Note that by the definition given above, *drug abuse is a culturally defined concept.* Because abuse is culturally defined, and because societies differ from one another and are changeable, there can be wide variations in what is labeled abuse. *What is defined as abuse can vary from one culture to another.* For example, in the United States, moderate consumption of alcohol is not usually considered abuse. In contrast, any ingestion of alcohol would be considered abuse in some Moslem societies. Furthermore, *what is defined as abuse can vary from one time to another within the same culture.* For example, when a few Americans first began to experiment with LSD and other psychedelic drugs, these agents were legal and their use was not generally disapproved. However, as use of psychedelics became widespread, our societal posture changed and legislation was passed to make the manufacture, sale, and use of these drugs illegal.

Within the United States there is divergence of opinion about what constitutes drug abuse. For example, some people would consider *any* use of marijuana to be drug abuse, whereas others would call smoking marijuana abusive only if it were done *habitually.* Similarly, although many Americans do not seem to consider cigarette smoking to be drug abuse (even though the practice is compulsive and clearly harmful to the individual and society), there are others who believe very firmly that cigarette smoking constitutes a blatant form of drug abuse.

As we can see, distinguishing between culturally acceptable drug use and drug use that is to be called abuse is more in the realm of social science than pharmacology. Accordingly, since this is a pharmacology text and not a sociology text, we will not attempt to define just what patterns of drug use do or do not constitute abuse. Instead, we will focus on the pharmacologic properties of abused drugs—leaving distinctions about what is and is not abuse to sociologists and legislators. Fortunately, we *can* identify the drugs that tend to be abused and discuss their pharmacology without having to resolve all arguments about what patterns of use should or should not be considered abusive.

Addiction

For our purposes, we will define addiction as a *behavior pattern* that has three outstanding features: (1) *compulsive drug use,* (2) *preoccupation with securing a drug supply,* and (3) *a tendency to relapse following withdrawal.* To illustrate this definition, let's consider the cigarette smoker. Smokers typify addicts in that smokers carry out all three behaviors that constitute our criteria for addiction. First, smokers are highly compulsive about using their drug. Second, smokers will do almost anything, from rummaging through ashtrays to braving severe weather, in order to provide an uninterrupted drug supply. Third, smokers who have stopped for a time have a very high rate of relapse. Clearly, the cigarette smoker provides an excellent example of a drug addict within the definition given.

Please note that by our definition, *addiction is not equated with physical dependence: being physically dependent is not the same as being addicted.* Many people are physically dependent upon drugs but would not be considered addicts according to our definition. These people are not considered addicts because they do not demonstrate the behavior pattern that constitutes addiction. Patients with terminal cancer, for example, are often physically dependent on opioids; however, since these people do not take opioids compulsively, their drug use does not meet our criteria for addiction. Similarly, some degree of physical dependence occurs in all individuals who take barbiturates to control epilepsy; despite their physical dependence, epileptics do not carry out stereotypic addictive behavior and, therefore, cannot be considered addicted under our definition.

Having stressed that physical dependence and addiction are different from each other, we must note that these two phenomena are not entirely unrelated. As discussed below, although physical dependence is not the same as addiction, physical dependence often contributes to addictive behavior.

Psychoactive Substance Dependence

Psychoactive substance dependence is a syndrome described in the American Psychiatric Association's *Diagnostic and Statistical Manual of Mental Disorders*, 3rd edition, revised (DSM-III-R). According to the DSM-III-R, a diagnosis of psychoactive substance dependence can be made if at least three of the following symptoms have been present for at least 1 month, or have occurred repeatedly over a longer time:

1. Takes substance in larger amounts or for longer times than intended.
2. Persistently desires to reduce or eliminate drug use, or fails in actual efforts to reduce or eliminate drug use.
3. Spends a great deal of time acquiring or using the substance, or recovering from its effects.
4. Intoxication or withdrawal frequently interferes with occupational or family obligations, or with the safe performance of hazardous activities (e.g., driving).
5. Reduces or gives up important social, occupational, or recreational activities in order to acquire or use the substance.
6. Continues substance use despite awareness of adverse psychologic, physiologic, or social consequences.
7. Is markedly tolerant to the substance.
8. Has experienced characteristic withdrawal symptoms.
9. Often takes the substance to avoid or relieve symptoms of withdrawal.

As defined in the DSM-III-R, psychoactive substance dependence may be *mild*, *moderate*, or *severe*. The syndrome is considered *mild* if occupational, social, and interpersonal impairment is mild and there are few (or no) symptoms in excess of the three required for a diagnosis. The syndrome is considered *severe* if occupational, social, and interpersonal impairment is severe, and there are many symptoms in excess of the three required for a diagnosis. The syndrome is considered *moderate* if functional impairment and symptoms are intermediate between those of mild dependence and severe dependence. *Addiction*, as defined above, can be considered a severe case of psychoactive substance dependence.

Please note that psychoactive substance dependence is a clinical syndrome and should not be equated with *physical dependence* (see below). Furthermore, although physical dependence, as manifested by withdrawal symptoms, is one of the possible diagnostic criteria for psychoactive substance dependence, it need not be present to make a diagnosis.

FACTORS CONTRIBUTING TO DRUG ABUSE

Drug abuse is the end result of a progressive involvement with drugs. Taking psychoactive drugs is usually initiated out of curiosity. From this initial involvement, the user can progress to occasional use. Occasional use can then evolve into compulsive use. Factors that play a role in the progression from experimental use to compulsive use are discussed below.

Reinforcing Properties of Drugs. Although there are several reasons for *initiating* drug use (e.g., curiosity, peer pressure), individuals would not *continue* drug use unless drugs gave them desirable feelings or experiences that they otherwise would not have. By making people feel "good," drugs reinforce the reasons for their use. Conversely, if drugs did not give people experiences that they found desirable, the reasons for initiating drug use would not be reinforced, and drug use would stop.

Reinforcement by drugs can occur in two ways. First, drugs can give the individual an experience that is pleasurable. Cocaine, for example, produces a state of euphoria. Second, drugs can reduce the intensity of unpleasant experience. For example, drugs can reduce anxiety and stress.

The reinforcing properties of drugs can be clearly demonstrated in experiments with animals. In the laboratory, animals will *self-administer* most of the drugs that are abused by humans (e.g., opioids, barbiturates, alcohol, cocaine, amphetamines, phencyclidine, nicotine, caffeine). When these drugs are made freely available, animals develop patterns of drug use that are similar to those of humans. Animals will self-administer these drugs (except for nicotine and caffeine) in preference to eating, drinking, or sexual activity. If permitted, these animals often die from lack of food and fluid. These observations strongly suggest that pre-existing psychopathology is not necessary for drug abuse to take place. Rather, these studies suggest that drug abuse results, in large part, from the reinforcing properties of drugs themselves.

Physical Dependence. Physical dependence is defined as *a state in which an abstinence syndrome will occur if drug use is discontinued.* The degree of physical dependence is determined largely by dosage size and duration of drug use. Physical dependence is greatest in those who use large doses for a prolonged period. The more physically dependent a person is, the more intense the withdrawal syndrome will be. Substantial physical dependence develops to the opioids (e.g., morphine, heroin) and to central nervous system (CNS) depressants (e.g., barbiturates, alcohol). Physical dependence tends to be less prominent with other abused drugs (e.g., psychostimulants, psychedelics, marijuana).

Physical dependence can contribute to compulsive drug use. Once dependence has developed, the desire to avoid withdrawal becomes a motivator for continued drug administration. Furthermore, if the drug is administered after the onset of withdrawal, its ability to alleviate the discomfort of withdrawal can reinforce its desirability. It must be noted, however, that although physical dependence plays a role in the abuse of drugs, physical dependence should not be viewed as the primary cause of addictive behavior. Rather, physical dependence is just one of several factors that can contribute to the development and continuation of compulsive use.

Psychologic Dependence. Psychologic dependence can be defined as *an intense subjective need for a drug.* Individuals who are psychologically dependent feel very strongly that their sense of well-being is dependent upon continued drug use; a sense of "craving" is felt when the drug is unavailable. There is no question that psychologic dependence can be a major factor in addictive behavior. For example, it is psychologic dependence—and not physical dependence—that plays the principal role in causing renewed use of opioids by addicts who had previously gone through withdrawal.

Social Factors. Social factors can play an important role in the development of drug abuse. The desire for social status and approval is a common reason for initiating drug use. Also, since initial drug experiences are frequently unpleasant, the desire for social approval can be one of the most compelling reasons for repeating drug use after the initial exposure. For example, most people do not especially enjoy their first cigarette; if it were not for peer pressure, many people would quit before reaching the point where they began to experience smoking as pleasurable. Similarly, initial use of heroin, with its accompanying nausea and vomiting, is often deemed unpleasant; peer pressure is a common reason for maintaining heroin use long enough to develop tolerance to these undesirable effects.

Drug Availability. Drug availability is clearly a factor in the development and maintenance of abuse. Drug abuse can flourish only in those environments where drugs can be readily obtained. In contrast, where procurement of drugs is difficult, drug abuse is minimal. The ready availability of drugs in hospitals and clinics is a major reason for the unusually high incidence of addiction seen among pharmacists, nurses, and physicians. It is the desire to reduce drug abuse through reducing drug availability that provides much of the rationale for law enforcement efforts directed against the manufacture and distribution of illicit drugs.

Vulnerability of the Individual. Some individuals are more prone to becoming drug abusers than others. By way of illustration, let's consider three individuals from the same social setting who have equal access to the same psychoactive drug. The first person experiments with the drug briefly and never uses it again. The second person progresses from experimentation to occasional drug use. The third goes on to take the drug compulsively. Since social factors, drug availability, and the properties of the drug itself were the same for all three individuals, these factors cannot explain the three different patterns of drug use that developed. We must conclude, therefore, that these three patterns developed because of differences in the users themselves: one individual was not prone to drug abuse, one had only moderate tendencies toward abuse, and the third was highly vulnerable to becoming an abuser.

Several psychologic factors have been associated with tendencies toward drug abuse. Drug abusers are frequently individuals who are impulsive, have a low tolerance for frustration, and are rebellious against social norms. Other psychologic factors that seem to predispose individuals to abusing drugs include depressive disorders, anxiety disorders, and antisocial personality. It is also clear that individuals who abuse one type of drug are likely to abuse other drugs.

There is speculation that some instances of drug abuse may actually be attempts at self-medication to relieve emotional discomfort. For example, some people may use alcohol and other depressants as a means of controlling severe anxiety. Although their drug use may appear excessive, it may be no more than is needed to prevent feelings that are deemed intolerable.

Genetics may also contribute to drug abuse. Vulnerability to alcoholism, for example, may be the result of an inherited predisposition.

APPROACHES TO MODIFYING DRUG-USING BEHAVIOR

In the treatment of drug abuse, the *ideal* goal is *complete cessation* of drug use. However, total abstinence is not the only outcome that can be considered successful. Treatment that changes drug use from compulsive to moderate will allow an increase in productivity, better physical health, and a decrease in socially unacceptable behavior. Clearly, this outcome is beneficial both to the individual and to society—even though some degree of drug use continues. It must be noted, however, that in the treatment of some forms of abuse, nothing short of total abstinence can be considered a true success. Experience has shown that abusers of *cigarettes, alcohol,* and *opioids* are rarely capable of sustained moderation. Hence, for many of these individuals, abstinence must be complete if there is to be any hope of avoiding a return to compulsive drug use.

Multiple techniques are employed in efforts to modify drug-using behavior. Techniques that have shown some degree of success include (1) therapy directed at resolving emotional problems that underlie drug use, (2) substitution of alternative rewards for the rewards of drug use, (3) threats and external pressure to discourage drug use, and (4) use of pharmacologic agents to modify the effects of abused drugs. It is not uncommon for a treatment program to incorporate two or more of these behavior modification methods. It is worth noting that at least two approaches to reducing drug abuse have *not* met with much success. These are (1) *prolonged* hospitalization, and (2) traditional individual psychotherapy in the absence of other forms of treatment.

Of the pharmacologic aids for modifying drug-using behavior, *disulfiram* [Antabuse] and *naltrexone* [Trexan] have proved most beneficial—and even these drugs are not employed widely. Disulfiram helps the alcoholic avoid drinking (see Chapter 29). Naltrexone, an opioid antagonist, is employed to treat opioid abuse (see below).

THE CONTROLLED SUBSTANCES ACT

The *Comprehensive Drug Abuse Prevention and Control Act of 1970,* known informally as the *Controlled Substances Act,* is the principal federal legislation addressing drug abuse. One objective of the Act is to reduce the chances that drugs originating from legitimate sources will become available to drug abusers. To accomplish this goal, the Act sets forth regulations for the handling of controlled substances by manufacturers, distributors, pharmacists, nurses, and physicians. Enforcement of the Act is the responsibility of the *Drug Enforcement Administration (DEA),* an arm of the United States Department of Justice.

Record Keeping. In order to keep track of controlled substances that originate from legitimate sources, a written record must be made of all transactions involving these agents. Every time a controlled substance is purchased or dispensed, the transfer must be recorded. Physicians, pharmacists, and hospitals must keep a current inventory of all controlled substances in stock. This inventory must be reported to the DEA every 2 years. Although not specifically obliged to do so by the Act, many hospitals require that floor stocks of controlled substances be counted at the beginning and end of each nursing shift.

Drug Enforcement Administration Schedules. Each drug preparation regulated under the Controlled Substances Act has been assigned to one of five categories: Schedule I, II, III, IV, or V. Drugs in Schedule I have a high potential for abuse and have no approved medical uses in the United States. In contrast, drugs in Schedules II through V all have approved applications. Assignment of drugs to Schedules II through V is based on their abuse potential and their potential for causing physical or psychologic dependence. Drugs in Schedule II have the highest potential for abuse and dependence. Drugs in the remaining schedules have decreasing abuse and dependence liabilities. Table 34–1 lists the primary drugs that belong to each of the five DEA Schedules.

Scheduling of drugs under the Controlled Substances Act undergoes periodic re-evaluation. With increased understanding of the abuse and dependence liabilities of a drug, the DEA may choose to reassign that drug to a different Schedule.

Prescriptions. The Controlled Substances Act places restrictions on prescribing drugs in Schedules II through V. (Drugs in Schedule I have no approved uses and, therefore, are not prescribed at all.) Only those physicians who have registered with the DEA are authorized to prescribe controlled drugs. Regulations on prescribing controlled substances are summarized below.

Schedule II. All prescriptions for Schedule II drugs must be typed or filled out in ink or indelible pencil and signed by the prescribing physician. Oral prescriptions may be made, but only in emergencies, and a written prescription must follow within 72 hours. Prescriptions of Schedule II drugs cannot be refilled. Hence, a new prescription must be written if continued therapy is needed.

Schedules III and IV. Prescriptions for drugs in Schedules III and IV may be oral or written. If authorized by the physician, these prescriptions may be refilled up to five times. Refills must be made within 6 months of the original order. If additional medication is needed beyond the amount provided for in the original prescription, a new prescription must be written.

Schedule V. The same regulations for prescribing drugs in Schedules III and IV apply to drugs in Schedule V. In addition, Schedule V drugs may be dispensed *without* a prescription provided the following conditions are met: (1) the drug is dispensed by a pharmacist, (2) the amount dispensed is very limited, (3) the recipient is at least 18 years old and can prove it, (4) the pharmacist writes and initials a record indicating the date, the name and amount of the drug, and the name and address of the recipient, and (5) state and local laws do not prohibit dispensing Schedule V drugs without a prescription.

Labeling. When drugs in Schedules II, III, and IV are dispensed, their containers must bear this label: *Caution—Federal law prohibits the transfer*

Table 34–1. Drug Classification Under the Controlled Substances Act

Schedule I Drugs	Schedule II Drugs	Schedule III Drugs	Schedule IV Drugs	Schedule V Drugs
Opioids Acetylmethadol Heroin Normethadone Many others	*Opioids* Alfentanil Codeine Fentanyl Hydromorphone Levorphanol Meperidine Methadone Morphine Opium tincture Oxycodone Oxymorphone Sufentanil	*Opioids* Hydrocodone syrup Paregoric	*Opioids* Pentazocine Propoxyphene	*Opioids* Buprenorphine Diphenoxylate plus atropine
Psychedelics Bufotenin Diethyltryptamine Dimethyltryptamine Ibogaine *d*-Lysergic acid diethylamide (LSD) Mescaline 3,4-Methylenedioxy- methamphetamine (MDMA) Psilocin Psilocybin	*Psychostimulants* Amphetamine Cocaine Dextroamphetamine Methamphetamine Methylphenidate Phenmetrazine	*Stimulants* Benzphetamine Phendimetrazine	*Stimulants* Diethylpropion Fenfluramine Mazindol Pemoline Phentermine	
Cannabis Derivatives Hashish Marijuana	*Barbiturates* Amobarbital Pentobarbital Secobarbital	*Barbiturates* Aprobarbital Butabarbital Metharbital Talbutal Thiamylal Thiopental	*Barbiturates* Mephobarbital Methohexital Phenobarbital	
Others Methaqualone Phencyclidine	*Cannabinoids* Dronabinol (THC) Nabilone	*Miscellaneous* *Depressants* Glutethimide Methyprylon	*Benzodiazepines* Alprazolam Chlordiazepoxide Clonazepam Clorazepate Diazepam Estazolam Flurazepam Halazepam Lorazepam Midazolam Oxazepam Prazepam Quazepam Temazepam Triazolam	
		Anabolic Steroids Fluoxymesterone Methyltestosterone Nandrolone Oxandrolone Stanozolol Testosterone	*Miscellaneous* *Depressants* Chloral hydrate Ethchlorvynol Ethinamate Meprobamate Paraldehyde	

of this drug to any person other than the patient for whom it was prescribed. The label must also indicate whether the drug belongs to Schedule II, III, or IV. The symbols C-II, C-III, and C-IV are used to indicate the Schedule.

State Laws. All states have their own laws regulating drugs of abuse. In many cases, the provisions of the state law are more stringent than those of the federal law. As a rule, whenever there is a difference between state and federal laws, the more severe of the two takes precedence.

PROPERTIES OF ABUSED DRUGS

In this section we will discuss the pharmacologic properties of specific drugs of abuse. As indicated in Table 34–2, these agents fall into six major pharmacologic categories: (1) opioids, (2) psychostimulants, (3) depressants, (4) psychedelics, (5) anabolic steroids, and (6) miscellaneous drugs of abuse. The basic pharmacology of many of the con-

trolled substances has been presented in previous chapters; hence, their discussion here will be brief. Agents that have *not* been addressed previously (e.g., marijuana, LSD) are discussed in greater depth. Structural formulas of representative controlled substances are shown in Figure 34–1. Street names for some abused drugs are summarized in Table 34–3.

OPIOIDS

The opioids (e.g., morphine, heroin) are major drugs of abuse. This fact is underscored by the classification of most opioids as Schedule II substances. The basic pharmacology of the opioids is discussed in Chapter 28.

Patterns of Use

Opioid abuse is encountered in all segments of American society. Formerly, opioid use was limited almost exclusively to lower socioeconomic groups

Table 34–2. Pharmacologic Categorization of Abused Drugs	
Category	**Examples**
Opioids	Heroin Morphine Meperidine Hydromorphone
Psychostimulants	Cocaine Dextroamphetamine Methamphetamine Methylphenidate
Depressants: *Barbiturates*	Amobarbital Secobarbital Pentobarbital Phenobarbital
Depressants: *Benzodiazepines*	Diazepam Chlordiazepoxide Lorazepam
Depressants: *Miscellaneous*	Alcohol Methaqualone Chloral hydrate Meprobamate
Psychedelics	LSD Mescaline Psilocybin Dimethyltryptamine
Anabolic Steroids	Nandrolone Oxandrolone Testosterone
Miscellaneous	Marijuana Phencyclidine Nicotine Caffeine Nitrous oxide Amyl nitrite

residing in cities. However, opioids are now used by people outside cities and by people of means—although the urban poor still constitute the majority of abusers.

For most abusers, initial exposure to opioids occurs management in a medical setting. The overwhelming majority of individuals who go on to abuse opioids began their drug use illicitly. Only an exceedingly small percentage of those exposed to opioids therapeutically develop a pattern of compulsive drug use.

Opioid abuse by health care providers deserves special attention. It is well established that physicians, nurses, and pharmacists, as a group, abuse opioids to a greater extent than all other groups with similar educational backgrounds. The vulnerability of health care professionals to opioid abuse is primarily the result of easy drug access.

Subjective and Behavioral Effects

Moments after IV injection, heroin produces a sensation in the lower abdomen similar to sexual orgasm. This initial reaction, known as a "rush" or

"kick," persists for about 45 seconds. After this, the user experiences a prolonged sense of euphoria (well-being); there is a feeling that "all is well with the world." It is for these extended effects, rather than the initial rush, that most opioid abuse occurs.

It is interesting to note that when individuals first use opioids, nausea and vomiting are prominent, and an overall sense of *dysphoria* may be felt. In many cases, were it not for peer pressure, individuals would not continue opioid use long enough to allow these unpleasant reactions to be replaced by a more agreeable experience.

Preferred Drugs and Routes of Administration

Among street users, *heroin* is the opioid of choice. This agent is easy to procure and is taken by about 90% of opioid abusers. The popularity of heroin is related to its high lipid solubility, which allows the drug to readily cross the blood-brain barrier, and thereby produce initial effects that are both immediate and intense. It is this combination of speed and intensity that sets heroin apart from other opioids, and makes it such a desirable drug.

It should be noted that when heroin is administered orally or subcutaneously, as opposed to intravenously, the drug's effects cannot be distinguished from those of morphine and other opioids. This observation is not surprising when we realize that once in the brain, heroin is rapidly converted into morphine, the active form through which heroin produces its effects.

Nurses and physicians who abuse opioids often select *meperidine* [Demerol] as their drug of choice. This agent has distinct advantages for these particular users. First, unlike heroin, meperidine is highly effective when administered orally; hence, meperidine abuse need not be associated with tell-tale signs of repeated injections. Second, meperidine produces less pupillary constriction than other opioids, thereby minimizing awkward questions about miosis. Lastly, meperidine has minimal effects on smooth muscle function; hence, constipation and urinary retention are less than with other opioid preparations.

Tolerance and Physical Dependence

Tolerance. With prolonged opioid use, tolerance develops to many—but not all—opioid effects. Effects to which tolerance *does* develop include euphoria, respiratory depression, and nausea. In contrast, little or no tolerance develops to constipation and miosis. Because tolerance to respiratory depression develops in parallel with tolerance to euphoria, respiratory depression is not increased as higher doses are taken to produce desired subjective effects. Persons tolerant to one opioid are cross-tolerant to other opioids. However, there is

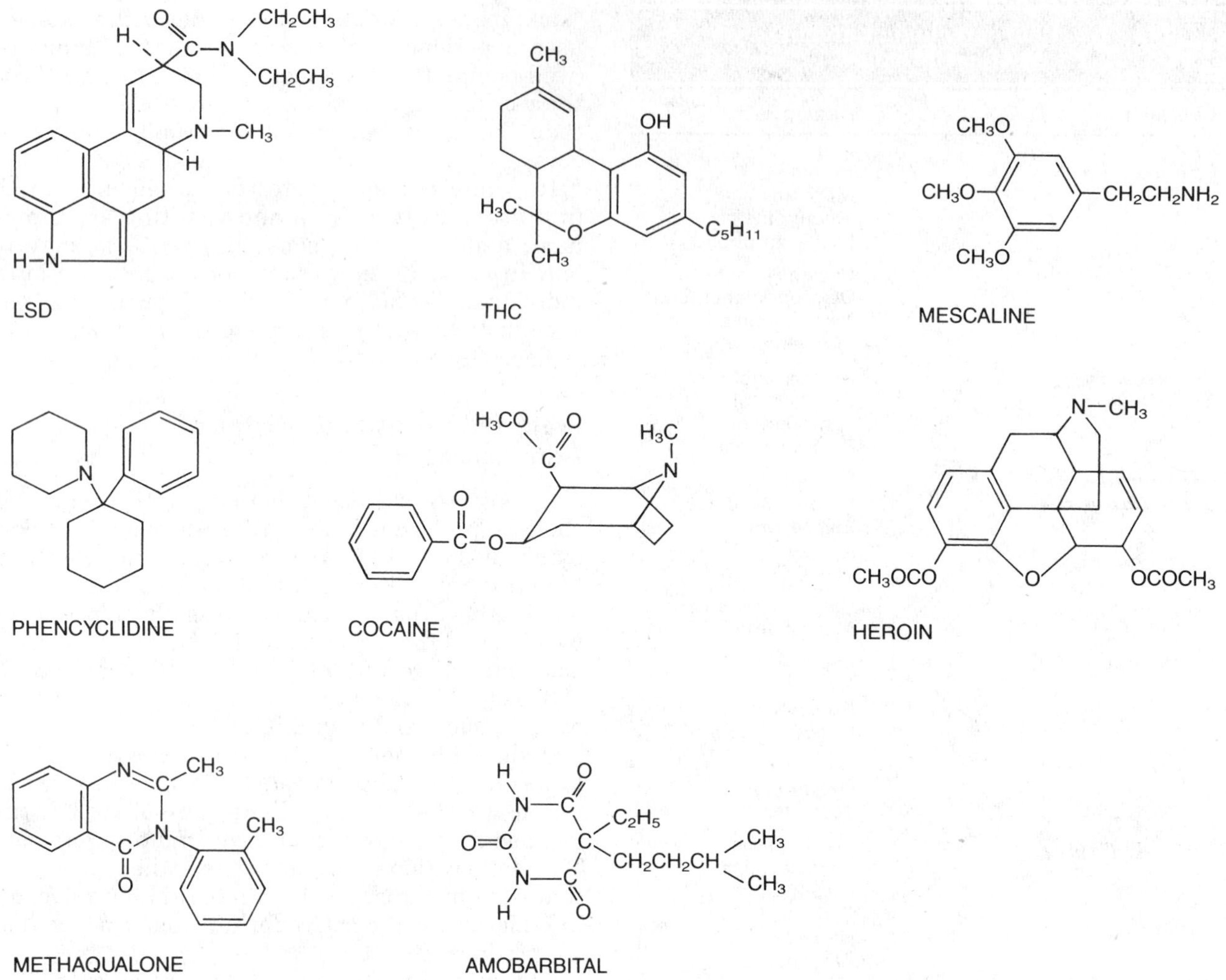

Figure 34–1. Structural formulas of representative drugs of abuse. (LSD = *d*-lysergic acid diethylamide; THC = tetrahydrocannabinol)

no cross-tolerance between opioids and general CNS depressants (e.g., barbiturates, benzodiazepines, alcohol).

Physical Dependence. Long-term opioid use produces substantial physical dependence. The abstinence syndrome resulting from opioid withdrawal is described in Chapter 28. It is important to note that although the opioid withdrawal syndrome can be extremely unpleasant, it is rarely dangerous.

Following the acute abstinence syndrome, which takes about 10 days to run its course, opioid addicts may experience a milder but protracted phase of withdrawal. This second phase, which may persist for months, is characterized by insomnia, irritability, and fatigue. Gastrointestinal hyperactivity and premature ejaculation may also be problems.

Treatment of Acute Toxicity

Treatment of acute opioid toxicity is discussed at length in Chapter 28 and will only be summarized here. Overdosage produces a classic triad of symptoms: *respiratory depression, coma,* and *pinpoint pupils. Naloxone,* an opioid antagonist, is the treatment of choice. This agent rapidly reverses all signs of opioid poisoning. However, dosage must be titrated carefully, since, if too much naloxone is given, the addict will swing from a state of intoxication to one of withdrawal. Because of its short half-life, naloxone must be re-administered every few hours until opioid concentrations have dropped to nontoxic levels—a process that sometimes takes days. Failure to repeat naloxone dosing may result in the death of a patient who had earlier been rendered symptom free.

Withdrawal Techniques

Persons who are physically dependent on opioids will experience unpleasant symptoms if drug use is abruptly discontinued. Techniques for minimizing discomfort are discussed below.

Table 34–3. Street Names for Abused Drugs	
Drug	**Street Names**
Psychedelics	
d-Lysergic acid diethylamide	LSD, LSD-25, acid, blotter, microdot
Dimethyltryptamine	DMT, businessman's trip
Mescaline	Peyote, cactus buttons
3,4-Methylenedioxy- methamphetamine	MDMA, ecstasy, XTC
2,5-Dimethoxy-4- methylamphetamine	DOM, STP
Psilocybin	Magic mushrooms
Psilocin	Magic mushrooms
Psychostimulants	
Amphetamine	Bennies, hearts, whites, cartwheels
Dextroamphetamine	Dexies, oranges, footballs
Methamphetamine	Speed, bombita, crank, crystal meth, ice
Biphetamine	Black beauties
Cocaine	Coke, crack, snow, blow, freebase, pasta, bazooka
General CNS Depressants	
Pentobarbital	Yellow jackets
Secobarbital	Red devils
Miscellaneous Agents	
Phencyclidine	PCP, angel dust, dummy dust, hog, peacepill, rocket fuel, sheets
Marijuana	Pot, grass, reefer, weed, Panama red, Acapulco gold, many others

Use of Methadone. Methadone, an oral opioid with a long duration of action, is the agent most commonly employed for easing opioid withdrawal. The first step in methadone-aided withdrawal is to substitute methadone for the opioid upon which the addict is dependent. Because opioids display cross-dependence with one another, methadone will prevent an abstinence syndrome. Once the subject has been stabilized on methadone, withdrawal is accomplished by administering methadone in gradually smaller doses. The resultant abstinence syndrome is mild, with symptoms resembling those of moderate influenza. The entire process of methadone substitution and withdrawal takes about 10 days to complete.

When substituting methadone for another opioid, suppression of the abstinence syndrome requires that methadone dosage be closely matched to the existing degree of physical dependence. Hence, to insure that methadone dosing is adequate, the extent of physical dependence must be assessed. This can be accomplished by taking a history on the extent of drug use and by clinical observation of the patient. Of these two approaches, observation of the patient is the more reliable. Estimates of drug use based on patient histories may be unreliable for the following reasons: (1) street users don't know the purity of the drugs they have taken, (2) claims of drug use may be inflated in hopes of receiving larger doses of methadone, and (3) addicts from the ranks of the health care professions may report minimal con-

sumption to downplay the extent of abuse. Because information from addicts is not likely to permit accurate assessment of dependence, it is essential to observe the patient to make certain that the methadone dosage is sufficient to suppress withdrawal.

Use of methadone for *maintenance therapy* and *suppressive therapy* is discussed separately below.

Use of Clonidine. Clonidine is a centrally acting alpha$_2$-adrenergic agonist. When administered to an individual who is physically dependent on opioids, clonidine can suppress some—but not all—symptoms of abstinence. Clonidine is most effective against symptoms related to autonomic hyperactivity (nausea, vomiting, diarrhea). Modest relief is provided from muscle aches, restlessness, anxiety, and insomnia. Opioid craving is not diminished.

Use of Opioid Antagonists. Once a patient has withdrawn from opioids, remaining drug free can be very difficult. Use of opioid antagonists is one means of discouraging renewed abuse. Opioid antagonists can decrease abuse by blocking euphoria and all other opioid effects. By preventing pleasurable effects, opioid antagonists eliminate the reinforcing properties of drug use. When the former addict learns that opioid administration will not produce desired responses, drug-using behavior will cease.

Of the opioid antagonists available, *naltrexone* is the agent best suited for treating opioid abuse.

Naltrexone is desirable because it is orally usable and because its long half-life permits alternate-day dosing. In contrast to naltrexone, naloxone has low oral efficacy and a half-life that is so short that multiple daily doses would be needed. These properties make naloxone impractical for deterring opioid abuse.

Methadone for Maintenance and Suppressive Therapy

In addition to its role in facilitating opioid withdrawal, methadone can be used for *maintenance therapy* and *suppressive therapy*. These therapies are employed to modify drug-using behavior in the addict who is not yet a candidate for withdrawal.

Maintenance Therapy. Methadone maintenance consists of transferring the addict from the abused opioid to oral methadone. By taking methadone, the addict avoids withdrawal and the need to procure illegal drugs. Methadone maintenance is most effective when done in conjunction with nondrug measures directed at altering patterns of drug use.

Suppressive Therapy. The objective of suppressive therapy is to prevent the reinforcing effects of opioid-induced euphoria. Suppression is achieved by giving the addict progressively larger doses of methadone until a very high daily dose (120 mg) is reached. Building up to this dose creates a high degree of tolerance. Hence, no subjective effects are experienced from the methadone itself. Since cross-tolerance exists between opioids, once the patient is tolerant to methadone, taking street drugs, even in high doses, cannot produce significant psychologic effects. As a result, individuals made tolerant to opioids with methadone will not experience the reinforcing effects of illicit drugs.

Use of methadone to treat opioid addicts is restricted to agencies approved by the FDA and state authorities. These restrictions on the nonanalgesic use of methadone are needed to control methadone abuse, since the drug has about the same abuse liability as morphine and other strong opioids.

Sequelae of Compulsive Opioid Use

Surprisingly, chronic opioid use has very few direct detrimental effects. Addicts in treatment programs have been maintained on high doses of methadone for years with no significant impairment of health. Furthermore, individuals on methadone maintenance can be successful socially and at work. It appears, then, that opioid use is not necessarily associated with poor health, lack of productivity, or inadequate social interaction.

Although opioids have few *direct* ill effects, there *are* many *indirect* hazards. These indirect risks stem largely from the lifestyle of the opioid user and from the impurities common to street drugs. Infections secondary to sharing nonsterile needles occur frequently. The infections that opioid abusers acquire include septicemia, subcutaneous ulcers, hepatitis, and HIV infection. Foreign-body emboli have resulted from impurities in opioid preparations. Opioid users suffer an unusually high death rate. Some deaths reflect the violent nature of the subculture in which opioid use often takes place. Many other deaths result from accidental overdosage.

GENERAL CNS DEPRESSANTS

The family of CNS depressants consists of barbiturates, benzodiazepines, alcohol, and a variety of other agents. With the exception of the benzodiazepines, all of these drugs are more alike than different. The benzodiazepines have properties that set them apart. The basic pharmacology of the CNS depressants is discussed in Chapters 27 and 33. A brief overview of these agents is given below.

Barbiturates

The barbiturates embody all of the properties that typify the general CNS depressants and can be considered the prototypes of the group. Depressant effects are dose dependent and range from mild sedation to sleep to coma to death. With prolonged use, barbiturates produce tolerance and physical dependence.

The abuse liability of the barbiturates stems from their ability to produce subjective effects similar to those of alcohol. The barbiturates with the highest potential for abuse are those with a short-to-intermediate duration of action. These agents (amobarbital, pentobarbital, secobarbital) are classified as Schedule II substances. Other barbiturates appear under Schedules III and IV (see Table 34–1). Despite legal restrictions, barbiturates are available cheaply and in abundance.

Tolerance. With regular use of barbiturates, tolerance develops to some effects but not to others. Tolerance to *subjective* effects is significant. As a result, progressively larger doses are needed to produce desired psychologic responses. Unfortunately, very little tolerance develops to *respiratory depression*. Consequently, as barbiturate use continues, the dose needed to produce subjective effects becomes closer and closer to the dose that can cause fatal respiratory depression. (This contrasts to the pattern seen with opioids, in which tolerance to subjective effects and respiratory depression develops in parallel.) Individuals who are tolerant to barbiturates show cross-tolerance to other CNS depressants (e.g., alcohol, benzodiazepines, general anesthetics). However, little or no cross-tolerance develops to opioids.

Physical Dependence and Withdrawal Techniques. Chronic barbiturate use can produce substantial physical dependence. Cross-dependence exists between barbiturates and other CNS depressants, but not with opioids. When physical dependence is great, the associated abstinence syndrome can be severe—sometimes even fatal (see Chapter 27). In contrast, the opioid abstinence syndrome, although unpleasant, is rarely life threatening.

One technique for easing barbiturate withdrawal employs phenobarbital, a barbiturate with a long duration of action. Because of cross-dependence, substitution of phenobarbital for the abused barbiturate suppresses symptoms of abstinence. Once the patient has been stabilized on phenobarbital, the dosage is gradually tapered off, thereby minimizing symptoms of abstinence.

Acute Toxicity. Overdosage with barbiturates produces a triad of symptoms: *respiratory depression*, *coma*, and *pinpoint pupils*. These are the same symptoms that accompany opioid poisoning. Treatment is directed at maintaining respiration and removing the drug from the body. Details are given in Chapter 27. Barbiturate overdosage has no specific antidote. Naloxone, which reverses poisoning by opioids, is not effective against poisoning by barbiturates.

Benzodiazepines

Benzodiazepines differ significantly from barbiturates. Benzodiazepines are much safer than the barbiturates, and overdosage with *oral* benzodiazepines *alone* is rarely lethal. However, the risk of death is greatly increased when oral benzodiazepines are combined with other CNS depressants (e.g., alcohol, barbiturates), or when benzodiazepines are administered *intravenously*. If severe overdosage occurs, signs and symptoms can be reversed with *flumazenil*, a benzodiazepine antagonist. In contrast to barbiturates, benzodiazepines do not produce significant tolerance when taken repeatedly. Furthermore, when benzodiazepines are taken in therapeutic doses, physical dependence is usually mild. However, substantial dependence can develop with prolonged, high-dose administration. When physical dependence is present, the abstinence syndrome can be minimized by withdrawing benzodiazepines slowly. The abuse liability of the benzodiazepines is much lower than that of the barbiturates. As a result, benzodiazepines are classified as Schedule IV agents. Benzodiazepines are discussed at length in Chapter 27.

Alcohol

The basic pharmacology of alcohol is discussed at length in Chapter 33. Emphasis here is on alcohol abuse.

Abuse of alcohol is second only to cigarette smoking as America's most serious drug problem. Alcoholism damages the physical and mental health of the abuser and is extremely costly to society. Reasons for alcohol use vary. Some people seek euphoria and release of emotions, others want relief from anxiety or depression, and, for many people, genetic factors are thought to underlie excessive alcohol use.

Alcoholism can be defined as a chronic primary disorder characterized by impaired control over drinking, preoccupation with the drug alcohol, use of alcohol despite awareness of adverse consequences, and distortions in thinking, especially as evidenced by denial of a drinking problem. The development and manifestations of alcoholism are influenced by genetic, psychosocial, and environmental factors. The disease is often progressive and fatal. In the United States, about 8% of adults are alcoholics.

Abuse of alcohol can produce a variety of adverse effects. Pathologies related to alcoholism include neurologic injury, cardiomyopathy, cirrhosis of the liver, erosive gastritis, respiratory disease, and nutritional deficiencies. Alcohol abuse during pregnancy can result in stillbirth, spontaneous abortion, low birth weight, mental retardation, and fetal alcohol syndrome. As a group, alcoholics have a higher death rate than nonalcoholics. Interestingly, although *heavy* alcohol use is clearly detrimental, individuals who consume alcohol *moderately* tend to live somewhat longer than total abstainers.

Chronic alcohol consumption produces substantial tolerance. Tolerance is both pharmacokinetic (accelerated alcohol metabolism) and pharmacodynamic. Pharmacodynamic tolerance is evidenced by an increase in the blood alcohol level required to produce intoxication. Alcoholics may tolerate blood alcohol levels of 200 to 400 mg/dl—2 to 4 times the level that defines legal intoxication in most states—with no marked reduction in consciousness. It should be noted, however, that very little tolerance develops to respiratory depression. Hence, as the alcoholic consumes increasing amounts in an effort to produce desired psychologic effects, the risk of death from respiratory arrest gets increasingly high. Cross-tolerance exists with general anesthetics and other CNS depressants, but not with opioids.

Physical dependence develops with chronic alcohol use. There is cross-dependence with other CNS depressants, but not with opioids. The alcohol withdrawal syndrome, which can be severe, is described in Chapter 33. Withdrawal symptoms can be eased with a *benzodiazepine* (usually *chlordiazepoxide*), since cross-dependence allows the benzodiazepine to suppress symptoms. Once the patient has been stabilized with chlordiazepoxide, this drug can be gradually withdrawn, thereby minimizing symptoms of abstinence. *Atenolol* (a beta-adrenergic blocking agent) may be a useful adjunct to chlordiazepoxide during the withdrawal process.

Once withdrawal has been accomplished, continued abstention can be facilitated with *disulfiram* [Antabuse]. This drug discourages alcohol consumption by causing an intense adverse reaction if *any* alcohol is consumed. In some cases, this reaction has been fatal. Accordingly, only those alcoholics who are judged capable of *complete* abstinence are appropriate candidates for disulfiram therapy. The pharmacology and clinical use of disulfiram are discussed at length in Chapter 33.

Other Depressants

In addition to barbiturates, benzodiazepines, and alcohol, other CNS depressants (e.g., paraldehyde, meprobamate, methaqualone, chloral hydrate) are subject to abuse. As discussed in Chapter 27, the pharmacologic properties of these drugs are similar to those of the barbiturates.

Methaqualone. Methaqualone is unique among the CNS depressants and requires special comment. Until recently, methaqualone [Quaalude] was available legally for use as a sedative. However, because of its high abuse potential and the availability of superior alternatives (benzodiazepines), methaqualone has been withdrawn from the market. This drug differs from other depressants in that overdosage is not characterized by obvious signs of CNS depression. Rather, poisoning can produce restlessness, hypertonia, and convulsions.

PSYCHOSTIMULANTS: AMPHETAMINES AND COCAINE

In this section, we will focus on those CNS stimulants that have a high potential for abuse: amphetamines, cocaine, and related substances. Because of their considerable abuse liability, these drugs are classified as Schedule II agents. In addition to stimulating the CNS, the amphetamines and cocaine can stimulate the heart, blood vessels, and other structures under sympathetic control. Because of these peripheral actions, these agents are also referred to as *sympathomimetics*.

Stimulants that are *not* addressed in this chapter are ones whose abuse potential is moderate-to-low or nonexistent. Agents in this group include Schedule III stimulants (e.g., benzphetamine), Schedule IV stimulants (e.g., diethylpropion), and stimulants that are not regulated at all (e.g., caffeine). The pharmacology of some of these drugs is discussed in Chapter 32.

Amphetamines

The amphetamines are the prototypes of the psychostimulants. The basic pharmacology of these agents is summarized below and discussed at length in Chapter 32.

Forms and Routes. The amphetamine family includes dextroamphetamine, methamphetamine, and amphetamine (a racemic mixture of dextroamphetamine and levamphetamine). When taken for purposes of abuse, amphetamines are usually administered orally or IV. In addition, a form of dextroamphetamine known as "ice" or "crystal meth" can be smoked. The only legal route of administration for amphetamines is oral.

Subjective and Behavioral Effects. Amphetamines produce arousal and elevation of mood. Euphoria is likely and talkativeness is prominent. A sense of increased physical strength and mental capacity occurs. Self-confidence rises. The amphetamine user feels little or no need for food and sleep. Orgasm is delayed, intensified, and more pleasurable.

Adverse CNS Effects. Amphetamines can produce a psychotic state characterized by hallucinations and paranoid ideation. This condition closely resembles paranoid schizophrenia. Psychosis can be triggered by a single amphetamine dose—but occurs most commonly in the context of long-term abuse. Amphetamine-induced psychosis usually resolves spontaneously following drug withdrawal. If needed, an antipsychotic agent (e.g., haloperidol) can be given to suppress symptoms.

Adverse Cardiovascular Effects. Because of their sympathomimetic actions, amphetamines can cause vasoconstriction and excessive stimulation of the heart. These actions can lead to hypertension, angina pectoris, and dysrhythmias. Vasoconstriction can be relieved with an alpha-adrenergic blocker (e.g., phentolamine). Cardiac stimulation can be reduced with a beta blocker (e.g., labetalol).

Tolerance, Dependence, and Withdrawal. Prolonged amphetamine use results in tolerance to mood elevation, appetite suppression, and cardiovascular effects. Although physical dependence is only moderate, psychologic dependence can be intense. Amphetamine withdrawal can produce dysphoria and a strong sense of craving. Other symptoms include fatigue, prolonged sleep, excessive eating, and depression. Depression can persist for months and is a common reason for resuming amphetamine use.

Cocaine

Cocaine is a stimulant with CNS effects similar to those of the amphetamines. In addition to its CNS actions, cocaine can produce local anesthesia (see Chapter 31) as well as vasoconstriction and cardiac stimulation. In recent years, use of a form of cocaine known as "crack" has reached epidemic proportions, especially among adolescents. Crack is extremely addictive, and the risk of lethal overdosage is high.

Formulations. Cocaine is available in two forms: *cocaine hydrochloride* and *cocaine base* (alkaloidal cocaine, freebase cocaine, "crack"). Cocaine base is heat stabile, whereas cocaine hydrochloride is not. Cocaine hydrochloride is available as a white powder that is frequently diluted ("cut") before sale. Cocaine base is sold in the form of crystals ("rocks") that consist of nearly pure cocaine. Cocaine base is widely known by the street name of "crack," a term inspired by the sound that the crystals make when they are heated.

Routes of Administration. Cocaine *hydrochloride* is usually administered *intranasally*. The drug is "snorted" (inhaled into the nose) and absorbed across the nasal mucosa into the bloodstream. In addition to intranasal administration, cocaine hydrochloride is often injected IV. The hydrochloride form cannot be smoked because of its instability at high temperatures.

Cocaine *base* is administered by *smoking*, a process referred to as "freebasing." Smoking delivers large amounts of cocaine to the lungs, and absorption is very rapid. Subjective and physiologic effects are equivalent to those elicited by IV injection.

Subjective Effects, Patterns of Use, and Addiction. The psychologic effects of cocaine appear to result from activation of dopamine receptors secondary to cocaine-induced blockade of dopamine reuptake. At usual doses, cocaine produces euphoria similar that produced by amphetamine. In a laboratory setting, individuals familiar with the effects of cocaine are unable to distinguish between cocaine and amphetamine. Interestingly, lidocaine (a local anesthetic similar to cocaine) produces subjective effects that are indistinguishable from those of cocaine (when both drugs are administered intranasally).

As with many other psychoactive drugs, the intensity of subjective responses depends on the rate at which plasma drug levels rise. Since cocaine levels rise relatively slowly with intranasal administration, this route produces responses of low intensity. In contrast, since intravenous administration and smoking cause nearly instantaneous elevations of plasma drug levels, these routes produce responses that are very intense.

When crack cocaine is smoked, desirable subjective effects begin to fade within minutes, and are often replaced by dysphoria. In an attempt to avoid dysphoria and regain euphoria, the cocaine user may administer repeated doses of the drug at short intervals. This pattern of use can rapidly lead to addiction.

Acute Toxicity. Overdosage is frequent and deaths have occurred. Mild overdosage produces agitation, dizziness, tremor, and blurred vision.

Severe overdosage can produce hyperpyrexia, convulsions, ventricular dysrhythmias, and hemorrhagic stroke. Angina pectoris and myocardial infarction may develop secondary to coronary artery spasm. Psychologic manifestations of overdosage include severe anxiety, paranoid ideation, and hallucinations (visual, auditory, or tactile).

Although there is no specific antidote to cocaine toxicity, most symptoms can be controlled with drugs. Paranoia may respond to *haloperidol*. Intravenous *diazepam* can reduce anxiety and suppress seizures. *Antidysrhythmic drugs* should be used to normalize cardiac rhythm. Severe hypertension can be corrected with oral *nifedipine* or intravenous *nitroprusside, phentolamine,* or *labetalol*. Hyperthermia should be reduced with external cooling.

Chronic Toxicity. When administered intranasally on a long-term basis, cocaine can cause atrophy of the nasal mucosa and loss of sense of smell. In extreme cases, necrosis and perforation of the nasal septum have occurred. Nasal pathology results from local ischemia secondary to chronic, cocaine-induced vasoconstriction. Injury to the lungs can occur from smoking cocaine base.

Toxicity from Use During Pregnancy and Lactation. Cocaine is highly lipid soluble and can readily cross the placenta, allowing the drug to accumulate in the fetal circulation. Use of cocaine during pregnancy has been associated with spontaneous abortion, premature delivery, and retardation of intrauterine growth. In addition, congenital abnormalities (e.g., cardiac anomalies, skull malformations) have been reported. Neonates exposed to cocaine during gestation have displayed signs of CNS irritability (increased muscle tone, tremor, electroencephalogram [EEG] abnormalities) that in some cases have persisted for months. Cerebral infarction has occurred in newborns whose mothers took cocaine just prior to labor. Maternal use of cocaine can produce intoxication in the breast-fed infant.

Tolerance, Dependence, and Withdrawal. In striking contrast to amphetamine use, cocaine use does not produce tolerance to elevation of mood. In fact, it appears that as cocaine use continues, sensitivity to subjective effects increases rather than decreases.

Physical dependence on cocaine is similar to dependence on amphetamines. Withdrawal can produce dysphoria, craving, fatigue, severe depression, and prolonged sleep. Depression and inability to experience pleasure may last for days or even weeks. Drugs used to suppress cocaine craving include *desipramine* (a tricyclic antidepressant), *amantadine,* and *bromocriptine,* all of which promote activation of dopamine receptors.

Addiction to crack cocaine can be very difficult to treat. The crack addict is typically unresponsive to persuasion and traditional psychotherapeutic techniques. If treatment on an outpatient basis is ineffective, admission to a treatment facility that prevents all access to cocaine may be helpful.

MARIJUANA AND RELATED PREPARATIONS

Cannabis sativa, the Source of Marijuana

The source of marijuana is *Cannabis sativa*, the Indian hemp plant—an unusual plant in that it has separate male and female forms. Psychoactive compounds are present in all parts of the male and female plants. However, the greatest concentration of psychoactive substances is found in the flowering tops of the females.

The two most common *Cannabis* derivatives are *marijuana* and *hashish*. Marijuana is a preparation consisting of leaves and flowers of male and female plants. Alternative names for marijuana include *grass, weed, pot*, and *dope*. The terms *joint* and *reefer* apply to marijuana cigarettes. Hashish is a dried preparation of the resinous exudate from female flowers. Hashish is considerably more potent than marijuana.

Patterns of Use

In the United States, marijuana is by far the most commonly used illicit drug. Marijuana is used by people in all levels of society, and by people in rural areas and in cities. During the 1960's and early 1970's, use of marijuana increased sharply. However, between 1978 and 1988, reported use among high school seniors declined by about 50%. Millions of Americans use marijuana occasionally. A small percentage smoke the drug daily.

Psychoactive Component

The major psychoactive substance in *Cannabis sativa* is *delta-9-tetrahydrocannabinol (THC)*, an oily chemical with high lipid solubility. The structure of THC appears in Figure 34–1.

The THC content of *Cannabis* preparations is variable. The highest concentrations are found in the flowers of the female plant. The lowest concentrations are in the seeds. Depending on growing conditions and the strain of the plant, THC in marijuana preparations may range from 1% to 11%.

Mechanism of Action

THC has several possible mechanisms. Perhaps the most important of these is activation of specific cannabinoid receptors found in various brain regions. The endogenous ligand for these receptors appears to be *anandamide*, a derivative of arachidonic acid unique to the brain. Other proposed mechanisms are (1) activation of phospholipase A_2 in the brain, resulting in increased production of prostaglandin E_2, and (2) augmentation of neuronal membrane fluidity through interaction with membrane lipids.

Pharmacokinetics

Administration by Smoking. When marijuana or hashish is smoked, about 60% of the THC content is absorbed. Absorption from the lungs is rapid. Subjective effects begin in minutes and peak in 20 to 30 minutes. Effects from a single marijuana cigarette may persist 2 to 3 hours. Termination of effects results from metabolic conversion of THC to inactive products.

Oral Administration. When marijuana or hashish is taken orally, practically all of the THC undergoes absorption. However, the majority of absorbed THC is metabolically inactivated on its first pass through the liver. Hence only 6% to 20% of absorbed drug actually reaches the general circulation. Because of this extensive first-pass metabolism, oral doses must be 3 to 10 times greater than smoked doses to produce equivalent effects. With oral administration, effects are delayed and prolonged; responses begin 30 to 50 minutes after drug ingestion and persist for up to 12 hours.

Behavioral and Subjective Effects

Marijuana produces three principal subjective effects: *euphoria, sedation*, and *hallucinations*. This set of responses is unique to marijuana; no other psychoactive drug produces all three. Because of this singular pattern of effects, marijuana is in a class by itself.

Effects of Low-to-Moderate Doses. Responses to low doses of THC are variable and depend on several factors, including dosage size, route of administration, setting of drug use, and expectations and previous experience of the user. The following effects are common: (1) euphoria and relaxation, (2) gaiety and a heightened sense of the humorous, (3) increased sensitivity to visual and auditory stimuli, (4) enhanced sense of touch, taste, and smell, (5) increased appetite and ability to appreciate the flavor of food, and (6) distortion of time perception such that short spans seem much longer than they actually are. In addition to these effects, which might be considered pleasurable (or at least innocuous), moderate doses can produce undesirable responses. These include (1) impairment of short-term memory, (2) decreased capacity to perform multistep tasks, (3) impairment of driving skills (which can be substantially worsened by concurrent use of alcohol), (4) temporal disintegration (inability to distinguish between past, present, and future), (5) depersonalization (a sense of strangeness about the self), (6) decreased ability to perceive the emotions of others, and (7) reduced interpersonal interaction.

High-Dose Effects. In high doses, marijuana can have serious adverse psychologic effects. The user may experience hallucinations, delusions, and feelings of paranoia. Euphoria may be replaced by intense anxiety. And a dissociative state in which the user feels "outside of himself or herself" may occur. In extremely high doses, marijuana can produce a state resembling toxic psychosis, which may persist for weeks. Because of the widespread use of marijuana, psychiatric emergencies caused by the drug are not uncommon.

Not everyone is equally vulnerable to the adverse psychologic effects of marijuana. Some individuals experience ill effects only at extremely high doses. In contrast, others routinely experience adverse effects at moderate doses. Schizophrenics are at unusually high risk for adverse reactions. In the stabilized schizophrenic, marijuana can precipitate an acute psychotic episode.

Effects of Chronic Use. Chronic, excessive use of marijuana has been associated with a behavioral phenomenon known as the *amotivational syndrome*. This syndrome is characterized by apathy, dullness, poor grooming, reduced interest in achievement, and disinterest in the pursuit of conventional goals. The precise relationship between marijuana and development of the syndrome is not known, nor is it certain what other factors, in addition to marijuana, may contribute. Available data do not suggest that the amotivational syndrome is due to organic brain damage.

Physiologic Effects

Cardiovascular Effects. Marijuana produces a dose-related increase in heart rate. Increases of 20 to 50 beats/min are typical. However, rates up to 140 beats/min are not uncommon. Pretreatment with propranolol will prevent marijuana-induced tachycardia, but will not block the drug's subjective effects. Marijuana causes orthostatic hypotension and pronounced reddening of the conjunctivae. These responses apparently result from vasodilation.

Respiratory Effects. When used *acutely*, marijuana produces *bronchodilation*. However, when smoked *chronically*, the drug causes airway *constriction*. In addition, chronic use is closely associated with development of bronchitis, sinusitis, and asthma. Lung cancer is another possible outcome. Experiments in animals have shown that tar from marijuana smoke is a more potent carcinogen than tar from cigarettes.

Effects on Reproduction. Studies in animals have shown multiple effects on reproduction. In males, marijuana decreases spermatogenesis and testosterone levels. In females, the drug reduces levels of follicle stimulating hormone, luteinizing hormone, and prolactin. In some species, marijuana has caused birth defects. However, teratogenesis has not been proved in humans.

Tolerance and Dependence

When taken in extremely high doses, marijuana can produce tolerance and physical dependence. Neither effect, however, is remarkable. Some tolerance develops to the cardiovascular, perceptual, and motor effects of marijuana. Little or no tolerance develops to subjective effects.

To demonstrate physical dependence on marijuana, the drug must be given in exceptionally high doses—and even then the degree of dependence is only moderate. Symptoms brought on by abrupt discontinuation of high-dose marijuana include irritability, restlessness, nervousness, insomnia, reduced appetite, and weight loss. Tremor, hyperthermia, and chills may also occur. Symptoms subside in 4 to 5 days. When marijuana use has been moderate, no symptoms of withdrawal are noted.

Therapeutic Uses

Suppression of Emesis. Intense nausea and vomiting are common side effects of cancer chemotherapy. In certain patients these responses can be suppressed more effectively with cannabinoids than with traditional antiemetics (e.g., prochlorperazine, metoclopramide). Two cannabinoid preparations are available: *dronabinol* (THC) and *nabilone* (a synthetic derivative of dronabinol). Dosage forms and dosages are presented in Chapter 68.

Appetite Stimulation. Dronabinol (THC) was recently approved for stimulating appetite in patients with AIDS. The goal of treatment is to decrease anorexia, thereby preventing or reversing weight loss.

Comparison of Marijuana with Alcohol

In several important ways, responses to marijuana and alcohol are quite different. Whereas increased hostility and aggression are common sequelae of alcohol consumption, aggressive behavior is rare among marijuana users. Although loss of judgment and control can occur with either drug, such losses are much greater with alcohol. For the marijuana user, increased appetite and food intake are typical. In contrast, the heavy drinker often suffers from nutritional deficiencies. Lastly, whereas marijuana can cause toxic psychosis, dissociative phenomena, and paranoia, these severe adverse psychologic reactions rarely occur with alcohol.

PSYCHEDELICS

The psychedelics are a fascinating drug family for which LSD can be considered the prototype. Other family members include mescaline, dimethyltryptamine (DMT), and psilocin. The psychedelics are so named because of their ability to produce what has been termed a *psychedelic state*. Individuals in this state show an increased awareness of sensory stimuli, and are likely to perceive the world around them as beautiful and harmonious; the normally insignificant may assume exceptional meaning; the "self" may seem split into an "observer" and a "doer"; and boundaries between "self" and "nonself" may fade, producing a sense of unity with the cosmos.

Psychedelic drugs are often referred to as *hallucinogens* or *psychotomimetics*. These names reflect the ability of these agents to produce hallucinations as well as mental states that in many ways resemble psychosis.

It is important to note that although psychedelic drugs are able to cause hallucinations and psychotic-like states, these responses are not the most characteristic effects of these drugs. The characteristic that truly distinguishes the psychedelics from other agents is *their ability to bring on the same types of alterations in thought, perception, and feeling that otherwise occur only in dreams*. In essence, the psychedelics seem able to activate mechanisms for dreaming without causing unconsciousness.

d-Lysergic Acid Diethylamide (LSD)

History. The first person to experience LSD was a Swiss chemist named Albert Hofman. In 1943, 5 years after LSD was first synthesized, Hofman accidentally ingested a minute amount of the drug. The result was a dream-like state accompanied by perceptual distortions and vivid hallucinations. The high potency and unusual actions of LSD led to speculation that the drug might provide a model for studying psychosis. Unfortunately, that speculation did not prove correct: extensive research revealed that the effects of LSD could not be equated with idiopathic psychosis. With the realization that LSD did not produce a "model psychosis," medical interest in the drug declined. Not everyone, however, lost interest in the effects of LSD on the human psyche; during the decade of the 1960's, nonmedical experimentation with the drug flourished. This widespread use of LSD caused substantial societal concern, and, by 1970, LSD had been classified as a Schedule I substance. Despite regu-

latory efforts, street use of LSD continues, although to a lesser extent than during 1960's.

Patterns of Use. The pattern of use for LSD is unique. In contrast to most abused substances, LSD is rarely taken repetitively on a long-term basis. For the typical user, intervals of days to months separate individual LSD experiences. The drug is taken primarily by college students and the economically well off. LSD is not popular among the urban poor. Use of LSD peaked in the late 1960's and has since declined.

Mechanism of Action. LSD acts at multiple sites in the brain and spinal cord. Effects are thought to result from activation of serotonin$_2$ receptors at these sites.

Pharmacokinetics. LSD is usually administered orally but can also be injected or smoked. With oral administration, initial effects can be felt in minutes. Over the next few hours, responses become progressively more intense. About 12 hours after LSD ingestion, responses begin to subside. Interestingly, the plasma half-life of LSD is only about 3 hours. Hence, plasma levels of the drug begin to fall long before subjective effects begin their decline.

Subjective and Behavioral Effects. Responses to LSD can be diverse, complex, and changeable. The drug can alter thinking, feeling, perception, sense of self, and sense of relationship to the environment and other people. LSD-induced experiences may be sublime or they may be terrifying. Just what will be experienced during any particular "trip" cannot be predicted.

Perceptual alterations can be dramatic. Colors may appear iridescent or glowing, kaleidoscopic images may appear, and vivid hallucinations may occur. Sensory experiences may merge so that colors seem to be heard and sounds seem to be visible. Afterimages may occur, causing current perceptions to overlap with preceding perceptions. The LSD user may feel a sense of wonderment and awe at the beauty of commonplace things.

LSD can have profound effects on affect. Emotions may range from elation, good humor, and euphoria to sadness, dysphoria, and fear. The intensity of emotion may be overwhelming.

Thoughts may turn inward. Attitudes may be reevaluated, and old values assigned new priorities. A sense of new and important insight may be felt. However, despite the intensity of these experiences, enduring changes in beliefs, behavior, and personality are rare.

Physiologic Effects. LSD produces few physiologic effects. Activation of the sympathetic nervous system can produce tachycardia, elevation of blood pressure, mydriasis, piloerection, and hyperthermia. Neuromuscular effects (tremor, incoordination, hyperreflexia, muscular weakness) may also occur.

Tolerance and Dependence. Tolerance to LSD develops rapidly. Substantial tolerance can be seen after just three or four daily doses. Tolerance to subjective and behavioral effects develops to a greater extent than to cardiovascular effects. Cross-tolerance exists with LSD, mescaline, and psilocybin, but not with DMT. Since DMT is similar to LSD, the absence of cross-tolerance is surprising. There is no cross-tolerance with amphetamines or THC. Upon cessation of LSD use, tolerance fades rapidly. Abrupt withdrawal of LSD is not associated with an abstinence syndrome. Hence, there is no evidence for physical dependence.

Toxicity. Toxic reactions to LSD are primarily psychologic. The drug has never been a direct cause of death, although fatalities have occurred from accidents and suicides.

Acute panic reactions are relatively common and may be associated with a fear of disintegration of the self. Such "bad trips" can usually be managed by a process of "talking down" (providing emotional support and reassurance in a nonthreatening environment). Panic episodes can also be managed with an *antianxiety agent* (e.g., diazepam). *Phenothiazines* (e.g., chlorpromazine) can antagonize the effects of LSD, but are rarely needed.

About 15% of LSD users experience "flashbacks"—recurrences of LSD experiences long after drug use has ceased. Flashbacks may be precipitated by several causes, including marijuana use, fatigue, and anxiety. Surprisingly, phenothiazines exacerbate flashbacks rather than provide relief.

In addition to panic reactions and flashbacks, LSD can cause other adverse psychologic effects. Depressive episodes, dissociative reactions, and distortions of body image may occur. When an LSD experience has been intensely terrifying, the user may be left with persistent residual fear. The drug may also cause prolonged psychotic reactions. In contrast to acute effects, which differ substantially from symptoms of schizophrenia, prolonged psychotic reactions mimic schizophrenia faithfully.

Therapeutic Uses. LSD has no recognized therapeutic applications. The drug has been evaluated for possible use in treating alcoholism, opioid addiction, and psychiatric disorders. In addition, LSD has been studied as a possible means of promoting psychologic well-being in patients with terminal cancer. However, for all of these potential uses, LSD proved either ineffective or impractical.

3,4-Methylenedioxy-methamphetamine (MDMA)

Use of MDMA ("ecstasy") came to prominence in the mid-1980's, especially among college students. Although originally unregulated, the drug was soon classified as a Schedule I substance. MDMA has mixed properties of a psychedelic drug and a psychostimulant. Low doses produce LSD-like psychedelic effects, and higher doses produce amphetamine-like stimulant effects. Moderate doses appear to facilitate interpersonal relationships: users report a sense of closeness with others, lowering of defenses, reduced anxiety, enhanced communication, and increased sociability. Because of these favorable psychologic effects, MDMA was used briefly in psychotherapy. Unfortunately, the drug can cause serious adverse effects. When administered to rats and monkeys in doses only 2 to 4 times greater than those that produce hallucinations in humans, MDMA can cause irreversible destruction of serotonergic neurons, resulting in passivity and insomnia. We do not know if MDMA is neurotoxic in humans. Other adverse effects include tingling and cold sensations as well as neurologic effects (spasmodic jerking, jaw clenching, and teeth grinding).

Mescaline, Psilocybin, Psilocin, and Dimethyltryptamine

In addition to LSD, the family of psychedelic drugs includes mescaline, psilocin, psilocybin, dimethyltryptamine (DMT), and several related compounds (see Table 34–1). Some psychedelics are synthetic and some are naturally occurring. DMT and LSD represent the synthetic compounds. Mescaline, a constituent of the peyote cactus, and psilocin, a constituent of "magic mushrooms," represent the compounds found in nature.

The subjective and behavioral effects of the miscellaneous psychedelic drugs are similar to those of LSD. Like LSD, these drugs can elicit modes of thought, perception, and feeling that are normally restricted to dreams. In addition, these drugs can cause hallucinations and can induce mental states that resemble psychosis.

The miscellaneous psychedelics differ from LSD with respect to potency and time course of action. LSD is the most potent of the psychedelics, producing its full spectrum of effects at doses as low as 0.5 μg/kg. Psilocin and psilocybin are 100 times less potent than LSD, and mescaline is 4000 times less potent than LSD. Whereas LSD has effects that are prolonged (responses only begin to decline after 12 hours), the effects of mescaline and DMT are much shorter: responses to mescaline usually terminate within 8 to 12 hours, and responses to DMT terminate within 1 to 2 hours.

PHENCYCLIDINE

Phencyclidine ("PCP," "angel dust," "peace pill") was originally developed as an anesthetic for animals. The drug was tried briefly as a general anesthetic for humans, but was withdrawn because it produced severe emergence delirium. Although rejected for therapeutic use, phencyclidine has become widely used as a drug of abuse. Use has grown in large part because the drug can be synthesized easily by the amateur chemist, making it cheap and abundant. The popularity of phencyclidine is disturbing in that the drug causes a high incidence of severe adverse effects—effects that make it one of the most dangerous drugs of abuse.

Chemistry and Pharmacokinetics

Chemistry. Phencyclidine is a weak organic base with high lipid solubility. The drug is chemically related to ketamine, an unusual general anesthetic (see Chapter 30). The structural formula of phencyclidine appears in Figure 34–1.

Pharmacokinetics. Phencyclidine can be administered orally, intranasally, intravenously, and by smoking. For administration by smoking, the drug is usually sprinkled on plant matter (e.g., oregano, parsley, tobacco, marijuana). Because of its high lipid solubility, phencyclidine is readily absorbed from all sites.

Once absorbed, phencyclidine undergoes substantial gastroenteric recirculation. Because it is a base, phencyclidine in the blood can be drawn into the acidic environment of the stomach (by the pH-partitioning effect); from the stomach, the drug reenters the intestine, from which it then is reabsorbed into the blood. This cycling from the blood to the gastrointestinal tract and back to the blood prolongs the drug's sojourn in the body. Elimination occurs eventually through a combination of hepatic metabolism and renal excretion.

Mechanism of Action

The mechanism by which phencyclidine affects the CNS is not known with certainty. There is good evidence suggesting that the drug *does* act at specific receptors. However, the exact nature of those receptors is unknown. Available data indicate that phencyclidine does not act through neuronal systems that employ dopamine, norepinephrine, or serotonin as their transmitters.

Subjective and Behavioral Effects

Phencyclidine produces a unique set of effects. Responses include CNS depression, CNS excitation, analgesia, and hallucinations. This response profile is not seen with any other drug of abuse. Because of its singular range of effects, phencyclidine is in a class by itself.

Effects of Low-to-Moderate Doses. At low doses, phencyclidine produces effects like those of alcohol. Low-dose intoxication is characterized by euphoria, release of inhibitions, and emotional lability. Nystagmus, slurred speech, and motor incoordination may also occur.

As dosage is increased, the clinical picture becomes more variable and complex. Symptoms include excitation, disorientation, anxiety, disorganized thoughts, altered body image, and reduced perception of tactile and painful stimuli. Mood may be volatile and hostile. Bizarre behavior may develop. Heart rate and blood pressure are elevated.

High-Dose (Toxic) Effects. High doses of phencyclidine can cause severe adverse physiologic and psychologic effects. Death may result from a variety of causes.

Psychologic effects include confusional states, combativeness, hallucinations, and psychosis. The psychosis closely resembles schizophrenia and may persist for weeks. Individuals with pre-existing psychoses are especially vulnerable to psychotogenic effects. Attempts at suicide may be made.

The physiologic effects of high-dose phencyclidine are varied. Motor effects range from muscular rigidity to convulsions. Cardiovascular effects include severe hypertension, tachycardia, and cardiac arrest. Respiratory depression is likely. At very high doses, phencyclidine can produce analgesia, anesthesia, and even coma. Other effects include hypersalivation, sweating, and fever.

Treatment of toxicity is primarily supportive. In addition, attempts may be made to hasten exit of the drug from the body. Psychotic reactions are best managed by isolating the patient from external stimuli. "Talking down" is not effective, and antipsychotic drugs are of limited help. Physical restraint may be needed to prevent self-inflicted harm and to protect others from assault. If respiration is depressed, mechanical support of ventilation may be needed. Severe hypertension can be managed with a *vasodilator* (e.g., diazoxide). Seizures can be controlled with *IV diazepam. Haloperidol* can suppress symptoms of psychosis. If fever is high, external cooling can help lower temperature.

Elimination of phencyclidine can be accelerated in two ways: continuous gastric lavage, and acidification of the urine (e.g., with ammonium chloride). Continuous lavage is effective because of the gastroenteric recirculation that the drug undergoes. Acidification of urine promotes phencyclidine excretion by reducing tubular reabsorption of this weak base. The combination of continuous gastric lavage plus acidification of the urine reduces the plasma half-life of phencyclidine from 3 days down to 1 day.

INHALANTS

The inhalants are a diverse group of drugs that have only one characteristic in common—administration by inhalation. These drugs can be divided into three major classes: (1) anesthetics, (2) vasodilators, and (3) organic solvents.

Anesthetics

Provided that dosage is modest, anesthetics produce subjective effects that are similar to those of alcohol (euphoria, exhilaration, loss of inhibitions). The anesthetics that have seen the most widespread nonmedical use are *nitrous oxide* ("laughing gas") and *ether*. One reason for the popularity of these drugs is ease of administration: neither agent requires exotic equipment to be used. For nitrous oxide, ready availability also promotes use: small cylinders of the drug, marketed for aerating whipped cream, can be purchased without restriction.

Vasodilators

The abuse potential of vasodilators is due mostly to a reputed ability of these drugs to prolong and intensify sexual orgasm. Production of lightheadedness and euphoria may also contribute to abuse. Two vasodilators—*amyl nitrite* and *isobutyl nitrite*—have been extensively abused. Of these, only amyl nitrite is used medically (to treat angina pectoris). Effects begin seconds after inhalation and fade rapidly. Primary side effects are pulsatile headache and orthostatic hypotension. Preparations of amyl nitrite are known on the street as "poppers" or "snappers." These terms reflect the fact that amyl nitrite is packaged in glass ampules that make a popping sound when snapped open to allow inhalation of their contents.

Organic Solvents

A wide assortment of solvents have been inhaled to induce intoxication. These compounds include gasoline, lighter fluid, paint thinner, nail-polish remover, benzene, acetone, toluene, chloroform, and model-airplane glue. The principal users of these agents are children and the very poor—people who, because of age or insufficient funds, lack access to more conventional drugs of abuse.

The organic solvents depress CNS function. In low amounts, these agents produce effects somewhat like those of alcohol (exhilaration, impaired judgment, altered perception of reality). When inhaled to excess, solvents can produce coma and death.

Multiple serious toxicities are associated with inhalation of solvents. Gasoline can cause lead poisoning; chloroform is toxic to the heart, liver, and kidneys; and toluene can cause severe brain damage and bone marrow depression. Many solvents can damage the heart; fatal dysrhythmias have occurred secondary to drug-induced heart block.

TOBACCO

Tobacco smoking is the largest preventable cause of death in the United States. Of the three modes in which tobacco is smoked (cigarettes, cigars, pipes), cigarettes produce the greatest mortality. In the discussion below, we will consider tobacco smoke in its entirety, rather than focussing on nicotine alone. The pharmacology of nicotine is discussed at length in Chapter 14 and will only be summarized here.

CNS Effects. Smoking cigarettes has a mild stimulant effect and produces an alerting pattern on the EEG. Smoking facilitates memory while decreasing irritability, aggressiveness, and appetite. At least some of these CNS effects are due to the nicotine content of tobacco.

Chronic Toxicity from Smoking. Adverse effects of chronic tobacco smoking range from vascular diseases (coronary artery disease, cerebrovascular disease, peripheral vascular disease); to chronic lung disease; to cancers of the larynx, esophagus, oral cavity, lung, bladder, and pancreas. Smoking during pregnancy carries an increased risk of low birth weight, spontaneous abortion, perinatal mortality, and sudden infant death. Quantitatively, cardiovascular disease is the greatest danger of smoking.

Fortunately, many adverse effects of smoking are reversible. Within 5 to 10 years after smoking has ceased, the risks of smoking-related disease for the ex-smoker are only slightly higher than the risks for the person who has never smoked.

Harmful Components of Tobacco Smoke. Cigarette smoke contains a large assortment of hazardous substances, including carbon monoxide, hydrogen cyanide, ammonia, nitrosamines, nicotine, and tar. (Tar is composed of a variety of polycyclic hydrocarbons, some of which are proven carcinogens.) The components of smoke that are considered most dangerous are carbon monoxide, nicotine, and tar.

Tolerance and Dependence. Tolerance develops to some effects of tobacco but not to others. Tolerance develops to nausea and dizziness, which frequently occur in the unseasoned smoker. However, no tolerance develops to the cardiovascular effects of smoking; even veteran smokers continue to experience an increase in heart rate and blood pressure whenever they smoke.

Chronic cigarette smoking produces physical dependence. Within 24 hours after smoking has stopped, an abstinence syndrome begins. The tobacco abstinence syndrome is characterized by irritability, anxiety, restlessness, reduced ability to concentrate, increased appetite, insomnia, and a craving for cigarettes. Symptoms may persist for weeks or months. Women report more discomfort than men. Experience has shown that abrupt discontinuation of smoking is preferable to gradual reduction; all that gradual reduction seems to do is prolong suffering.

Nicotine gum and *nicotine patches* (see Chapter 14) are available to facilitate withdrawal. These products reduce some signs of abstinence but not others, indicating that lack of nicotine is not the only factor contributing to the tobacco abstinence syndrome. When used as part of a quit-smoking program, these nicotine products can be a significant help. Individuals who benefit most are those with the highest degree of physical dependence. Unfortunately, long-term success rates have not been impressive.

ANABOLIC STEROIDS

Many athletes take anabolic steroids (androgens) in an effort to enhance athletic performance. *Perceived* benefits include increased muscle mass and strength, accelerated healing after muscle injury, heightened aggressiveness, and increased energy. Because of the massive doses that are often employed, the risk of adverse effects is substantial. With long-term use of steroids, an addiction syndrome develops. Because of their abuse potential, most androgens are now classified as Schedule III drugs (see Table 34–1). The basic pharmacology of androgens and their abuse by athletes are discussed at length in Chapter 54.

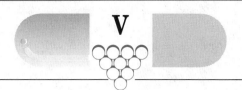

V

Drugs That Affect Fluid and Electrolyte Balance

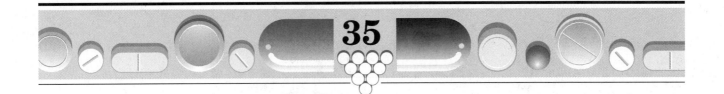

Diuretics

D iuretics are drugs that increase the output of urine. These agents have two major applications: (1) treatment of hypertension, and (2) mobilization of edematous fluid (associated with heart failure, cirrhosis, and kidney disease). In addition, because of their ability to maintain urine flow, diuretics are used to prevent renal failure.

REVIEW OF RENAL ANATOMY AND PHYSIOLOGY

Understanding the diuretic drugs requires a basic knowledge of the anatomy and physiology of the kidney. Accordingly, we will review these topics before discussing the diuretics themselves.

ANATOMY

The basic functional unit of the kidney is the *nephron*. As indicated in Figure 35–1, the nephron has four functionally distinct regions: (1) the *glomerulus,* (2) the *proximal convoluted tubule,* (3) the *loop of Henle,* and (4) the *distal convoluted tubule.* All nephrons are oriented within the kidney such that the upper portion of Henle's loop is located within the renal *cortex* and the lower end of the loop descends toward the renal *medulla.* Without this orientation the kidney would be unable to produce concentrated urine.

In addition to the nephrons, the *collecting ducts* (the tubules into which the nephrons pour their contents) play a critical role in kidney function. As

431

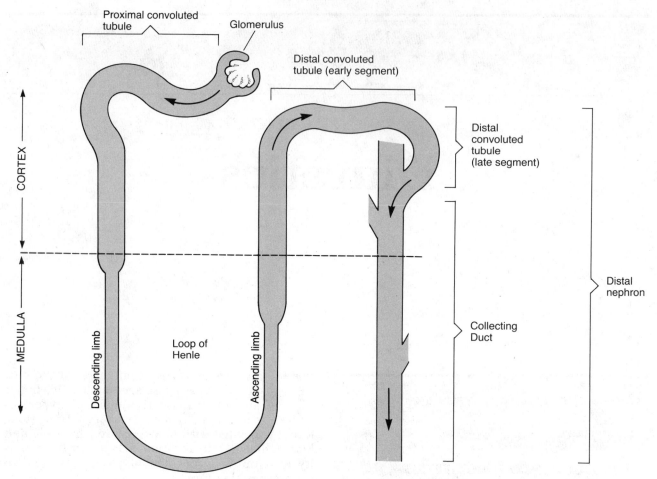

Figure 35–1. Schematic representation of a nephron and collecting duct.

suggested by Figure 35–1, the final segment of the distal convoluted tubule plus the collecting duct into which it empties can be considered a single functional unit: *the distal nephron.*

PHYSIOLOGY

Overview of Kidney Functions

The kidney serves three basic functions: (1) cleansing of extracellular fluid (ECF) and maintenance of ECF volume and composition, (2) maintenance of acid-base balance, and (3) excretion of metabolic wastes and foreign substances (e.g., drugs, toxins). Of these three functions, maintenance of ECF volume and composition is the one most affected by diuretics.

The Three Basic Renal Processes

The effects of the kidney on ECF are the net result of three basic processes: (1) *filtration,* (2) *reabsorption,* and (3) *active secretion.* We should note that in order to cleanse the entire ECF, huge volumes of plasma must be filtered. Furthermore,

in order to maintain homeostasis, practically everything that has been filtered must be reabsorbed—leaving behind only a small volume of urine for excretion.

Filtration. Filtration occurs at the *glomerulus* and is the first step in urine formation. Virtually all small molecules (electrolytes, amino acids, glucose, drugs, metabolic wastes) present in plasma undergo filtration, whereas cells and large molecules (lipids, proteins) remain behind in the blood. The most prevalent constituents of the filtrate are sodium ions and chloride ions. Bicarbonate ions and potassium ions are also present, but in smaller amounts.

The filtration capacity of the kidney is huge. Each minute the kidney produces 125 ml of filtrate, which adds up to 180 L/day. Since the total volume of ECF is only 12.5 L, the kidney can process the equivalent of all the ECF in the body every 100 minutes. Hence, the ECF undergoes complete cleansing many times each day.

Please note that filtration is a *nonselective* process and, therefore, cannot regulate the composition of urine. Reabsorption and secretion, processes that display a significant degree of selectivity, are the primary determinants of what the urine ultimately contains—and of these two processes, reabsorption is by far the more important.

Reabsorption. Greater than 99% of the water, electrolytes, and nutrients that are filtered at the glomerulus undergo reabsorption. This reabsorption conserves valuable constituents of the filtrate while allowing wastes to be excreted. Reabsorption of solutes (e.g., electrolytes, amino acids, glucose) takes place by way of *active transport*. Water then follows passively along the osmotic gradient created by solute reuptake. Specific sites along the nephron at which reabsorption takes place are discussed below. It is primarily through interference with reabsorption that diuretics produce their effects.

Active Tubular Secretion. The kidney has two kinds of "pumps" for active secretion. These pumps transport compounds from the plasma into the lumen of the nephron. One kind of pump is selective for *organic acids*, and the other transports *organic bases*. Together, these pumps can promote the excretion of a wide assortment of molecules, including metabolic wastes, drugs, and toxins. The pumps for active secretion are located in the *proximal convoluted tubule*.

Processes of Reabsorption That Occur at Specific Sites Along the Nephron

Since most diuretics act by disrupting solute reabsorption, to understand the diuretics, we must first understand the major processes by which the nephron reabsorbs filtered solutes. Since sodium and chloride ions are the predominant solutes in the filtrate, it is the reabsorption of these ions that is of greatest interest. As we discuss reabsorption, numeric values will be given for the percentage of solute reabsorbed at specific sites along the nephron; bear in mind that these values are only approximations. Figure 35–2 provides a summary of the sites of sodium and chloride reabsorption, indicating the amount of reabsorption that occurs at each site.

Proximal Convoluted Tubule. The proximal convoluted tubule (PCT) has a high reabsorptive capacity. As indicated in Figure 35–2, *a large frac-*

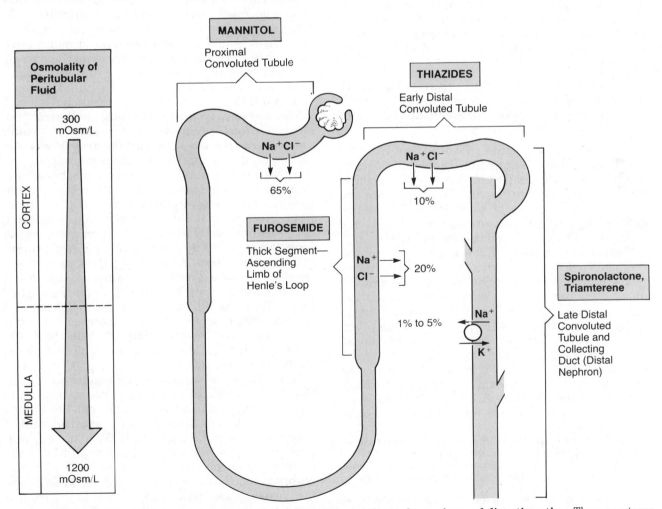

Figure 35–2. Schematic diagram of a nephron showing sites of sodium absorption and diuretic action. The percentages indicate how much of the filtered sodium and chloride is reabsorbed at each site.

tion (about 65%) *of filtered sodium and chloride is reabsorbed at the PCT.* In addition, essentially all of the bicarbonate and potassium in the filtrate is reabsorbed here. As sodium, chloride, and other solutes are actively reabsorbed, water follows passively. Since solutes and water are reabsorbed to an equal extent, the tubular urine remains isotonic (i.e., its tonicity is 300 mOsm/L). By the time the filtrate leaves the PCT, sodium and chloride are the only solutes that remain in significant amounts.

Loop of Henle. The *descending limb* of the loop of Henle is freely permeable to water. Hence, as tubular urine moves down the loop and passes through the hypertonic environment of the renal medulla, water is drawn from the loop into the interstitial space. This process decreases the volume of the tubular urine and causes the urine to become concentrated (tonicity is increased to about 1200 mOsm/L).

Within the thick segment of the *ascending limb* of the loop of Henle, *about 20% of filtered sodium and chloride is reabsorbed* (see Fig. 35–2). Since, unlike the descending limb, the ascending limb is not permeable to water, water must remain in the loop as reabsorption of sodium and chloride takes place. This process causes the tonicity of the tubular urine to return to that of the original filtrate (300 mOsm/L).

Distal Convoluted Tubule (Early Segment). *About 10% of filtered sodium and chloride is reabsorbed in the early segment of the distal convoluted tubule.* Water follows passively.

Late Distal Convoluted Tubule and Collecting Duct (Distal Nephron). The distal nephron is the site of two important processes. The first involves the exchange of sodium for potassium and is under the influence of aldosterone. The second determines the final concentration of the urine and is regulated by antidiuretic hormone (ADH).

Sodium-Potassium Exchange. Aldosterone, the principal mineralocorticoid of the adrenal cortex, stimulates reabsorption of sodium from the distal nephron. At the same time, aldosterone causes potassium to be secreted. Although not directly coupled, these two processes—sodium retention and potassium excretion—can be envisioned as an exchange mechanism. This exchange is shown schematically in Figure 35–2. Aldosterone promotes sodium-potassium exchange by stimulating cells of the distal nephron to synthesize more of the pumps responsible for sodium and potassium transport.

Regulation of Urine Concentration by Antidiuretic Hormone. Although of great physiologic significance, the effects of ADH have little to do with the actions of diuretics. Hence, discussion of this physiologically important topic is presented in small type.

Antidiuretic hormone acts on the collecting duct to regulate conservation of water. To understand the effects of ADH, we need to know four facts:

1. In the absence of ADH, the collecting duct is impermeable to water.
2. The collecting duct is oriented such that it begins in the cortex of the kidney and then passes down through the hypertonic renal medulla (see Fig. 35–2).
3. Tubular urine entering the collecting duct is isotonic (i.e., 300 mOsm/L).
4. Antidiuretic hormone acts on the collecting duct to increase its permeability to water.

By rendering the collecting duct permeable to water, ADH allows water to be drawn from the duct as it passes through the hypertonic renal medulla. Because of this reabsorption of water, urine that entered the duct in a relatively dilute state becomes concentrated and reduced in volume.

In the absence of ADH, water cannot be reabsorbed in the collecting duct. As a result, large volumes of dilute urine are produced. The clinical syndrome resulting from ADH deficiency is known as *diabetes insipidus.*

INTRODUCTION TO THE DIURETICS

HOW DIURETICS WORK

Most diuretics share the same basic mechanism of action: blockade of sodium and chloride reabsorption. By blocking the reabsorption of these prominent solutes, diuretics create osmotic pressure within the nephron that prevents the passive reabsorption of water. Hence, diuretics cause water and solutes to be retained within the nephron, and thereby promote their excretion.

The increase in urine flow that a diuretic produces is directly related to the amount of sodium and chloride reabsorption that the drug blocks. Accordingly, drugs that block solute reabsorption to the greatest degree will produce the most profound diuresis. Since the amount of solute in the nephron becomes progressively smaller as filtrate flows from the proximal tubule to the collecting duct, *drugs whose site of action is early in the nephron have the opportunity to block the greatest amount solute reabsorption. Accordingly, these agents produce the greatest diuresis.* Conversely, since most of the filtered solute has already been reabsorbed by the time the filtrate reaches the distal parts of the nephron, diuretics that act at these distal sites have very little reabsorption available to block. Consequently, distally acting agents produce relatively scant diuresis.

It is instructive to look at the quantitative relationship between blockade of solute reabsorption and production of diuresis. Recall that the kidney produces 180 L of filtrate a day, practically all of which normally is reabsorbed. With filtrate production at this volume, a diuretic will increase daily urine output by 1.8 L for each 1% of solute reabsorption that is blocked. A 3% blockade of solute reabsorption will produce 5.4 L of urine a day—a rate of fluid loss that would reduce body weight by 12 pounds in 24 hours. Clearly, with only a small blockade of reabsorption, diuretics can produce a profound effect on the fluid and electrolyte composition of the body.

ADVERSE IMPACT ON EXTRACELLULAR FLUID

In order to promote excretion of water, diuretics must compromise the normal operation of the kidney. By doing so, diuretic drugs can cause *hypovolemia* (from excessive fluid loss), *acid-base imbalance,* and *disturbance of electrolyte levels.* These adverse effects can be minimized by using short-acting diuretics and by timing drug administration such that the kidney is allowed to operate in a drug-free manner between periods of diuresis. Both measures will give the kidney periodic opportunities to readjust the ECF so as to compensate for any undesired alterations produced under the influence of diuretics.

CLASSIFICATION OF DIURETICS

There are four major categories of diuretic drugs: (1) *high-ceiling (loop) diuretics* (e.g., furosemide), (2) *thiazide diuretics* (e.g., hydrochlorothiazide), (3) *osmotic diuretics* (e.g., mannitol), and (4) *potassium-sparing diuretics.* The last group, the potassium-sparing agents, can be subdivided into aldosterone antagonists (e.g., spironolactone) and nonaldosterone antagonists (e.g., triamterene).

In addition to the four major categories of diuretics, there is a fifth group: the *carbonic anhydrase inhibitors.* Although the carbonic anhydrase inhibitors are classified as diuretics, these drugs are employed primarily to lower intraocular pressure, and not to increase urine production. Consequently, the carbonic anhydrase inhibitors are discussed in Chapter 69 (Drugs for Disorders of the Eye).

HIGH-CEILING (LOOP) DIURETICS

The high-ceiling agents are the most effective diuretics available. These drugs produce greater loss of fluid and electrolytes than any other diuretics. Because their site of action is in the loop of Henle, the high-ceiling agents are also known as *loop diuretics.*

FUROSEMIDE

Furosemide [Lasix] is the most frequently prescribed loop diuretic and will serve as our prototype for the family.

Mechanism of Action

Furosemide acts in the thick segment of the ascending limb of Henle's loop to block reabsorption of sodium and chloride (see Fig. 35–2). By blocking solute reabsorption, furosemide prevents passive reabsorption of water. Since a substantial amount (20%) of filtered NaCl is normally reabsorbed in the loop of Henle, interference with reabsorption can produce profound diuresis.

Pharmacokinetics

Furosemide can be administered orally and intravenously. With oral administration, diuresis begins in 60 minutes and persists for 8 hours. Oral therapy is used when rapid onset of effects is not required. Effects of intravenous furosemide begin within 5 minutes and last for 2 hours. Intravenous therapy is used in critical situations (e.g., pulmonary edema) that demand immediate mobilization of fluid. Furosemide undergoes hepatic metabolism followed by renal excretion.

Therapeutic Uses

Furosemide is a powerful drug that is generally reserved for situations that require rapid or massive mobilization of fluid. This drug should be avoided when less efficacious diuretics (thiazides) will suffice. Conditions that justify use of furosemide include (1) *pulmonary edema associated with congestive heart failure,* (2) *edema of hepatic, cardiac, or renal origin that has been unresponsive to less efficacious diuretics,* and (3) *hypertension that cannot be controlled with other diuretics.* Furosemide is especially useful in patients with severe renal impairment, since, unlike the thiazides (see below), this drug can promote diuresis even when renal blood flow and glomerular filtration rate are low. If treatment with furosemide alone is insufficient, a thiazide diuretic may be added to the regimen. There is no benefit to combining furosemide with another high-ceiling agent.

Adverse Effects

Dehydration. Because of its high diuretic capacity, furosemide can mobilize enough fluid to cause severe dehydration. Signs of developing dehydration include dry mouth, unusual thirst, and oliguria (scanty urine output). Impending dehydration can also be anticipated from excessive loss of weight. If dehydration occurs, furosemide should be withheld.

Dehydration can promote thrombosis and embolism. Symptoms include headache and pain in the chest, calves, or pelvis. The physician should be notified if these develop.

The risk of dehydration and its sequelae can be minimized by initiating therapy with low doses, adjusting the dosage carefully, monitoring weight loss every day, and administering furosemide on an intermittent schedule.

Hypotension. Furosemide can cause a substantial drop in blood pressure. The mechanism of this effect is not fully understood, although loss of volume is certainly a contributing factor. Signs of hypotension include dizziness, lightheadedness, and fainting. If blood pressure falls precipitously, furosemide should be discontinued. Because of the risk of hypotension, blood pressure should be monitored on a routine basis.

Outpatients should be taught to self-monitor their blood pressure and instructed to notify the physician if it drops substantially. Also, patients should be informed about symptoms of postural hypotension (dizziness, lightheadedness) and advised to sit or lie down if these occur. Patients should be taught that postural hypotension can be minimized by moving slowly when changing from a seated or supine position to an upright position.

Electrolyte Imbalance. Furosemide can produce excessive loss of electrolytes, especially sodium, chloride, and potassium. Sodium and chloride are lost because their reabsorption is blocked in the loop of Henle; potassium is lost through increased secretion in the distal nephron. Loss of these electrolytes can cause muscle fatigue, cramps, and dysrhythmias. As discussed below under *Drug Interactions*, loss of potassium is of special concern for patients taking digoxin, a drug used to treat heart failure. Electrolyte imbalance can be minimized by monitoring electrolyte status and by administering furosemide on an intermittent schedule. Additional measures may be required to maintain potassium at acceptable levels; these include consumption of potassium-rich foods (e.g., citrus fruits, potatoes, bananas) and treatment with a potassium-sparing diuretic or potassium supplements.

Ototoxicity. Rarely, loop diuretics cause hearing impairment. With furosemide, deafness has been transient. With ethacrynic acid (another loop diuretic), irreversible hearing loss has occurred. The ability to impair hearing is unique to the high-ceiling agents; diuretics in other classes are not ototoxic. Because of the risk of hearing loss, caution should be exercised when high-ceiling diuretics are used in combination with other ototoxic drugs (e.g., aminoglycoside antibiotics).

Hyperglycemia. Elevation of plasma glucose levels is a potential, albeit uncommon, complication of furosemide therapy. Hyperglycemia appears to result from inhibition of insulin release. Increased glycogenolysis and decreased glycogen synthesis may also contribute. When furosemide is taken by a diabetic, the patient should be especially diligent about monitoring blood glucose content.

Hyperuricemia. Elevation of plasma uric acid content is a frequent side effect of treatment. For most patients, furosemide-induced hyperuricemia is asymptomatic. However, for patients predisposed to gout, elevation of uric acid levels may precipitate a gouty attack. Patients should be informed about symptoms of gout (tenderness or swelling in joints) and instructed to notify the physician if these develop.

Use in Pregnancy. When administered to pregnant laboratory animals, high-ceiling diuretics have caused maternal death, abortion, fetal resorption, and other adverse effects. There are no definitive studies on the effects of loop diuretics during human pregnancy. However, given the toxicity displayed in animals, prudence dictates that pregnant women use these drugs only if absolutely required.

Drug Interactions

Digoxin. Digoxin is used to treat congestive heart failure (see Chapter 42) and cardiac dysrhythmias (see Chapter 44). In the presence of low potassium levels, the risk of serious digoxin toxicity (ventricular dysrhythmias) is greatly increased. Since high-ceiling diuretics promote potassium loss, use of these drugs in combination with digoxin can increase the risk of dysrhythmias. This interaction is unfortunate in that most patients who take digoxin for heart failure must also take a diuretic as part of their therapy. To reduce the chances of digoxin toxicity, potassium levels should be monitored routinely, and, when indicated, potassium supplements or a potassium-sparing diuretic should be given.

Lithium. Lithium is used to treat manic-depressive illness (see Chapter 26). In the presence of low sodium levels, excretion of lithium is reduced. By lowering sodium levels, furosemide can cause lithium to accumulate to toxic levels. Accordingly, lithium levels should be monitored, and, if they climb too high, lithium dosage should be reduced.

Ototoxic Drugs. The risk of furosemide-induced hearing loss is increased by concurrent use of other ototoxic drugs (e.g., aminoglycoside antibiotics). Accordingly, combined use of these drugs should be avoided.

Potassium-Sparing Diuretics. The potassium-sparing diuretics (e.g., spironolactone, triamterene) can help counterbalance the potassium-wasting effects of furosemide, thereby reducing the risk of hypokalemia.

Antihypertensive Agents. The hypotensive effects of furosemide add with those of other hypotensive drugs. To avoid excessive reductions in blood pressure, patients may need to reduce or eliminate use of hypotensive medications.

Preparations, Dosage, and Administration

Oral. Furosemide [Lasix] is available in tablets (20, 40, and 80 mg) and in solution (10 mg/ml and 40 mg/5 ml) for oral use. The initial dosage for adults is 20 to 80 mg/day as a single dose. The maximum daily dosage is 600 mg. Twice-daily dosing (8 AM and 2 AM) is common. Administration late in the day produces nocturia and should be avoided.

Parenteral. Furosemide is available as an injection (10 mg/ml) for IV and IM administration. The usual parenteral dose for adults is 20 to 40 mg, repeated in 1 or 2 hours if needed. Intravenous administration should be done slowly (over 1 to 2 minutes). For high-dose therapy, furosemide can be administered by continuous infusion at a rate of 4 mg/min or slower.

ETHACRYNIC ACID AND BUMETANIDE

Ethacrynic acid [Edecrin] and bumetanide [Bumex] have pharmacologic properties very similar to those of furosemide. All of these drugs share the same mechanism of action, therapeutic uses, and adverse effects. Dosages and time courses of action are summarized in Table 35–1.

THIAZIDES AND RELATED DIURETICS

The thiazide diuretics (also known as benzothiadiazides) have effects similar to those of the loop diuretics. Like the loop diuretics, thiazides increase renal excretion of sodium, chloride, potassium, and water. In addition, thiazides elevate plasma levels of uric acid and glucose. The principal difference between the thiazides and the high-ceiling diuretics is that the maximum diuresis produced by the thiazides is considerably lower than the maximum diuresis produced by the high-ceiling agents.

HYDROCHLOROTHIAZIDE

Hydrochlorothiazide is the most widely used thiazide diuretic and will serve as our prototype for the family. Because of its use in hypertension, a very common disorder, hydrochlorothiazide is one of the most widely used of all prescription drugs.

Mechanism of Action

Hydrochlorothiazide promotes urine production by blocking the reabsorption of sodium and chloride in the *early segment of the distal convoluted tubule* (see Fig. 35–2). Retention of sodium and chloride in the nephron causes water to be retained as well, thereby producing an increased flow of urine. Since only 10% of filtered sodium and chloride is normally reabsorbed at the site where thiazides act, the maximum urine flow that these drugs can produce is low relative to the maximum flow that the high-ceiling diuretics produce.

The ability of thiazides to promote diuresis is dependent on adequate kidney function. These drugs are ineffective when glomerular filtration rate (GFR) is low (less than 15 to 20 ml/min). Hence, in contrast to the high-ceiling agents, thiazides cannot be used to promote fluid loss in patients with severe renal impairment.

Pharmacokinetics

Diuresis begins about 2 hours after oral administration. Effects peak within 4 to 6 hours, and may persist for up to 12 hours. Most of the drug is excreted unchanged in the urine.

Therapeutic Uses

Essential Hypertension. The primary indication for hydrochlorothiazide is hypertension, a condition for which thiazides are often drugs of first choice. For many hypertensive patients, blood pressure can be controlled with a thiazide alone,

Drug	Route	Onset	Duration	Usual Adult Dosage
Furosemide [Lasix]	Oral	Within 60 min	6–8 hr	20 to 80 mg on 2 to 4 consecutive days each week
	IV	Within 5 min	2 hr	20 to 40 mg, repeated in 1 to 2 hours if needed
Ethacrynic acid [Edecrin]	Oral	Within 30 min	6–8 hr	50 to 100 mg daily or on alternate days
	IV	Within 5 min	2 hr	50 mg or 0.5 to 1 mg/kg
Bumetanide [Bumex]	Oral	30–60 min	4–6 hr	0.5 to 2 mg on alternate days
	IV	Within min	0.5–1 hr	0.5 to 1 mg, repeated in 2 to 3 hours if needed

Table 35–1. High-Ceiling (Loop) Diuretics: Routes, Dosages, and Time Course — Time Course of Events

although many other patients require multiple-drug therapy. The role of thiazides in hypertension is discussed in Chapter 40.

Edema. Thiazides are preferred drugs for mobilizing *edema associated with mild-to-moderate congestive heart failure.* These drugs are also given to mobilize *edema associated with hepatic or renal disease.*

Diabetes Insipidus. Diabetes insipidus is a rare condition characterized by excessive production of urine. In these patients, thiazides *reduce* urine production by 30% to 50%. The mechanism of this paradoxical effect is unknown.

Adverse Effects

The adverse effects of the thiazide diuretics are similar to those of the high-ceiling agents. In fact, with the exception that thiazides lack ototoxic actions, the adverse effects of the thiazides and loop diuretics are nearly identical.

Alteration of Extracellular Fluid Composition. Loss of sodium, chloride, and water can lead to *electrolyte imbalance* and *dehydration.* It should be noted, however, that since the diuresis produced by thiazides is moderate, these drugs have less of an impact on ECF than the loop diuretics. To evaluate fluid and electrolyte status, electrolyte levels should be determined periodically, and the patient should be weighed on a regular basis.

Hypokalemia. Like the high-ceiling diuretics, the thiazides can cause hypokalemia from excessive potassium excretion. As noted previously, potassium loss is of particular concern for patients taking *digoxin.* Potassium levels should be measured periodically, and, if serum potassium falls below 3.5 mEq/L, treatment with potassium supplements or a potassium-sparing diuretic should be instituted. Hypokalemia can be minimized by eating potassium-rich foods (e.g., citrus fruits, bananas).

Hyperglycemia. Like the loop diuretics, the thiazides can elevate plasma levels of glucose. Significant hyperglycemia develops only in diabetics, and these patients should be especially diligent about monitoring blood glucose. To maintain normal glucose levels, the diabetic may require larger doses of a hypoglycemic drug (insulin or an oral hypoglycemic agent).

Hyperuricemia. The thiazides, like the loop diuretics, can cause retention of uric acid, thereby elevating plasma uric acid levels. Although hyperuricemia is usually asymptomatic, it may precipitate gouty arthritis in patients with a history of the disorder. Plasma levels of uric acid should be measured periodically.

Use in Pregnancy and Lactation. The thiazides have direct and indirect effects on the developing fetus. By reducing blood volume, thiazides can decrease placental perfusion, and may thereby compromise fetal nutrition and growth. Furthermore, thiazides can cross the placental barrier to produce fetal harm directly; potential effects include electrolyte imbalance, hypoglycemia, jaundice, and hemolytic anemia. Because of the potential for fetal harm, *thiazides should not be used routinely during pregnancy.* Edema of pregnancy is not an indication for diuretic therapy—except when unusually severe. In contrast, edema from pathologic causes (e.g., heart failure, cirrhosis) does constitute a legitimate indication for thiazide use.

Thiazides enter breast milk and can be hazardous to the nursing infant. Women who are taking thiazides should be cautioned against breast-feeding.

Drug Interactions

The important drug interactions of the thiazides are nearly identical to those of the loop diuretics. By promoting potassium loss, thiazides can increase the risk of toxicity from *digoxin.* By counterbalancing the potassium-wasting effects of the thiazides, the *potassium-sparing diuretics* can help prevent hypokalemia. By lowering blood pressure, thiazides will augment the effects of other *antihypertensive drugs.* By promoting sodium loss, thiazides can reduce renal excretion of *lithium,* thereby causing the drug to accumulate, possibly to toxic levels. In contrast to the loop diuretics, the thiazides can be combined with *ototoxic agents* without an increased risk of hearing loss.

Preparations, Dosage, and Administration

Hydrochlorothiazide [HydroDIURIL, others] is dispensed in tablets (25, 50, and 100 mg) and solution (10 and 100 mg/ml) for oral administration. Like practically all other thiazides, hydrochlorothiazide is administered only by mouth. The usual adult dosage is 25 to 50 mg once or twice daily. To minimize nocturia, the drug should not be administered late in the day. To minimize electrolyte imbalance, the drug should be administered on an intermittent basis (e.g., every other day). In addition to being marketed alone, hydrochlorothiazide is available in fixed-dose combinations with potassium-sparing diuretics; trade names are Dyazide, Moduretic, Aldactazide, Maxzide, and Spirozide.

OTHER THIAZIDE-TYPE DIURETICS

In addition to hydrochlorothiazide, 12 other thiazides (and related drugs) are approved for use in the United States (Table 35–2). All have pharmacologic properties similar to those of hydrochlorothiazide. With the exception of chlorothiazide, these drugs are administered only by mouth. (Chlorothiazide can be administered IV as well as orally.) Although the thiazides differ from one another in milligram potency (see Table 35–2), at therapeutically equivalent doses, all can elicit the same degree of diuresis. Although most have the same onset of action (1 to 2 hours after administration), these drugs differ significantly with respect to duration of action. As with hydrochlorothiazide, disturbance of electrolyte balance can be minimized through alternate-day dosing. Nocturia can be minimized by avoiding dosing in the late afternoon.

Table 35–2 lists four drugs—chlorthalidone, indapamide, metolazone, and quinethazone—that are not true thiazides. How-

Table 35–2. Thiazides and Related Diuretics: Dosages and Time Course of Effects

Generic Name	Trade Name	Time Course of Effects		Optimal Oral Adult Dosage (mg/day)
		Onset (hours)	Duration (hours)	
Thiazides				
Chlorothiazide	Diuril, Diurigen	1–2	6–12	500–2000
Hydrochlorothiazide	Esidrix, Oretic, HydroDIURIL, others	2	6–12	25–100
Bendroflumethiazide	Naturetin	2	6–12	2.5–15
Benzthiazide	Exna	2	6–12	50–200
Hydroflumethiazide	Diucardin, Saluron	2	6–12	25–200
Methyclothiazide	Aquatensen, Enduron	2	24	2.5–10
Polythiazide	Renese	2	24–48	1–4
Trichlormethiazide	Metahydrin, Naqua Diurese	2	24	1–4
Related Drugs				
Chlorthalidone	Hygroton, Thalitone	2	24–72	25–200
Indapamide	Lozol	1–2	up to 36	2.5–5
Metolazone	Zaroxolyn, Mykrox	1	12–24	2.5–20
Quinethazone	Hydromox	2	18–24	50–100

ever, these agents *are* very similar to the thiazides both in structure and function; hence their inclusion in the group.

POTASSIUM-SPARING DIURETICS

The potassium-sparing diuretics can elicit two potentially useful responses. First, these drugs produce a modest increase in urine production. Second, these drugs produce a substantial *decrease in potassium excretion*. Because their diuretic effects are limited, the potassium-sparing drugs are rarely employed to promote diuresis. However, because of their marked ability to decrease potassium excretion, these drugs are used with great regularity to counteract potassium loss caused by the loop diuretics and thiazides.

There are two subcategories of potassium-sparing diuretics: (1) aldosterone antagonists and (2) nonaldosterone antagonists. Only one aldosterone antagonist—spironolactone—is approved for use in the United States. Two nonaldosterone antagonists—triamterene and amiloride—are currently employed.

SPIRONOLACTONE

Mechanism of Action

Spironolactone [Aldactone] blocks the actions of aldosterone in the distal nephron. Since aldosterone acts to promote sodium uptake in exchange for potassium secretion (see Fig. 35–2), inhibition of aldosterone by spironolactone will have the op-

posite effect: *retention of potassium and increased excretion of sodium.* The diuresis caused by spironolactone is scanty because most of the filtered sodium load has already been absorbed by the time the filtrate reaches the distal nephron. (Recall that the degree of diuresis a drug produces is directly proportional to the amount of sodium reuptake that the drug blocks.)

As indicated in Table 35–3, the effects of spironolactone are delayed, taking up to 48 hours to develop. To understand this delay, recall that aldosterone acts by stimulating cells of the distal nephron to synthesize the proteins required for sodium and potassium transport. By preventing aldosterone's action, spironolactone blocks the synthesis of new proteins, but does not stop existing transport proteins from doing their job. Hence, the effects of spironolactone are not visible until the existing proteins complete their normal life cycle—a process that takes a day or two to run its course.

Therapeutic Uses

Spironolactone is indicated primarily for patients with *hypertension* and *edema*. Although it can be employed alone, the drug is used most frequently in combination with a thiazide or loop diuretic. The purpose of spironolactone in these combinations is to counteract the potassium-wasting effects of the more powerful diuretics. Spironolactone also makes a small contribution to diuresis. In addition to its use in hypertension and edema, spironolactone can be given to block the effects of aldosterone in patients with *primary hyperaldosteronism.*

Table 35–3. Potassium-Sparing Diuretics: Names, Dosages, and Time Course of Effects

Generic Name	Trade Name	Time Course of Effects		Usual Adult Dosage (mg/day)
		Onset (hours)	*Duration (hours)*	
Spironolactone	Aldactone	24–48	48–72	25–400
Triamterene	Dyrenium	2–4	12–16	200–300
Amiloride	Midamor	2	24	5–20

Adverse Effects

Hyperkalemia. The potassium-sparing effects of spironolactone can result in hyperkalemia, a condition that can produce fatal dysrhythmias. Although hyperkalemia is most likely when spironolactone is used alone, this condition can also develop when spironolactone is used in conjunction with potassium-wasting agents (thiazides and high-ceiling diuretics). Because of the risk of hyperkalemia, *spironolactone must never be combined with potassium supplements or with another potassium-sparing diuretic*. If hyperkalemia develops, spironolactone should be discontinued and potassium intake restricted; injection of insulin will help lower potassium levels by promoting uptake of potassium into cells.

Endocrine Effects. Spironolactone is a steroid derivative with a structure similar to that of the steroid hormones (e.g., progesterone, estradiol, testosterone). As a result, spironolactone can cause a variety of endocrine effects, including *gynecomastia, menstrual irregularities, impotence, hirsutism,* and *deepening of the voice*.

Preparations, Dosage, and Administration

Spironolactone [Aldactone] is dispensed in tablets (25, 50, and 100 mg) for oral administration. The usual adult dosage is 25 to 100 mg a day. Spironolactone is also marketed in fixed-dose combinations with hydrochlorothiazide; trade names are Aldactazide and Spirozide.

TRIAMTERENE

Mechanism of Action

Like spironolactone, triamterene disrupts sodium-potassium exchange in the distal nephron. However, in contrast to spironolactone, which reduces ion transport indirectly through blockade of aldosterone, triamterene is a *direct inhibitor* of the exchange mechanism itself. The net effect of this inhibition is a decrease in sodium reuptake and a reduction in potassium secretion. Hence, sodium excretion is increased, while potassium is conserved. Because it inhibits ion transport directly, triamterene acts much more quickly than spironolactone. As indicated in Table 35–3, initial responses develop in hours, as compared with days for spironolactone. Like spironolactone, triamterene is unable to cause more than a scant diuresis.

Therapeutic Uses

Triamterene can be used alone or in combination with other diuretics to treat *hypertension* and *edema*. When used alone, triamterene produces mild diuresis. When combined with other diuretics (e.g., furosemide, hydrochlorothiazide), triamterene augments diuresis and helps counteract the potassium-wasting effects of the more powerful diuretic drugs. It is the latter effect for which triamterene is principally employed.

Adverse Effects

Hyperkalemia. Excessive potassium accumulation is the drug's most significant adverse effect. Hyperkalemia is most likely when triamterene is used alone, but can also occur when the drug is combined with thiazides or high-ceiling agents. Triamterene should never be used in conjunction with another potassium-sparing diuretic or with potassium supplements.

Other Adverse Effects. Relatively common side effects include *nausea, vomiting, leg cramps,* and *dizziness. Blood dyscrasias* occur rarely.

Preparations, Dosage, and Administration

Triamterene [Dyrenium] is available in 50- and 100-mg capsules for oral use. The usual initial dosage is 100 mg twice a day. The maximum daily dosage is 300 mg. Triamterene is also marketed in fixed-dose combinations with hydrochlorothiazide under the trade names Dyazide and Maxzide.

AMILORIDE

Pharmacologic Properties. Amiloride has actions similar to those of triamterene. Both drugs inhibit potassium loss by direct blockade of sodium-potassium exchange in the distal nephron. Also, both drugs produce only modest diuresis. Although it can be employed alone as a diuretic, amiloride is used primarily to counteract potassium loss caused by more powerful diuretics (thiazides, high-ceiling agents). The major adverse effect of amiloride is hyperkalemia. Accordingly, concurrent use of other potassium-sparing diuretics or potassium supplements must be avoided.

Preparations, Dosage, and Administration. Amiloride [Midamor] is dispensed in 5-mg tablets for oral use. Dosing is begun at 5 mg a day and may be increased to a maximum of 20 mg. Amiloride is available in a fixed-dose combination with hydrochlorothiazide under the trade name Moduretic.

OSMOTIC DIURETICS

Four compounds—mannitol, urea, glycerin, and isosorbide—are classified as osmotic diuretics. However, of the four, only mannitol is used for its diuretic actions. The osmotic agents differ from other diuretics both in mechanism of action and clinical applications.

MANNITOL

Mannitol [Osmitrol] is a simple six-carbon sugar that possesses the four properties characteristic of an osmotic diuretic:

1. The drug is freely filtered at the glomerulus.
2. It undergoes minimal reabsorption.
3. It is not metabolized to a significant degree.
4. It is pharmacologically inert (i.e., it has no direct effects on the biochemistry or physiology of cells).

Mechanism of Diuretic Action

Mannitol promotes diuresis by creating an osmotic force within the lumen of the nephron. Unlike other solutes, mannitol undergoes minimal reabsorption after filtration. As a result, most of the drug remains within the nephron, creating an osmotic force that inhibits passive reabsorption of water. Hence, urine flow increases. The degree of diuresis produced is directly related to the concentration of mannitol in the filtrate; the more mannitol present, the greater the diuresis. Mannitol has no significant effect on the excretion of potassium and other electrolytes.

Pharmacokinetics

Mannitol does not diffuse across the gastrointestinal epithelium and cannot be transported by the uptake systems that absorb dietary sugars. Accordingly, in order to reach the circulation, the drug must be given parenterally. Following IV injection, mannitol distributes freely to extracellular water. Diuresis begins in 30 to 60 minutes and persists for 6 to 8 hours. Most of the drug is excreted intact in the urine.

Adverse Effects

Edema. Mannitol can leave the vascular system at all capillary beds except those of the brain. When the drug exits capillaries it draws water along, causing edema. Mannitol must be used with extreme caution in patients with heart disease, since it may precipitate congestive heart failure (CHF) and fulminating pulmonary edema in these patients. If signs of pulmonary congestion or CHF develop, use of the drug must cease immediately. Mannitol must also be discontinued if patients with heart failure or pulmonary edema develop renal failure, since the resultant drug accumulation would increase the risk of cardiac or pulmonary injury.

Other Adverse Effects. Common responses include *headache, nausea,* and *vomiting. Fluid and electrolyte imbalance* may also occur.

Therapeutic Uses

Prophylaxis of Renal Failure. Under certain conditions (e.g., dehydration, severe hypotension, hypovolemic shock), blood flow to the kidney is decreased, causing a great reduction in filtrate volume. When the volume of filtrate is this low, the transport mechanisms of the nephron are able to reabsorb virtually all of the sodium and chloride present, causing complete reabsorption of water as well. As a result, urine production ceases, and kidney failure follows. The risk of renal failure can be reduced with mannitol. Since filtered mannitol is not reabsorbed—even when filtrate volume is small—filtered mannitol will remain in the nephron, drawing water along with it. Hence, mannitol can preserve urine flow and may thereby prevent renal failure. Thiazides and loop diuretics are not as effective for this application because, under conditions of low filtrate production, there is such an excess of reabsorptive capacity (relative to the amount of filtrate) that these drugs are unable to produce sufficient blockade of reabsorption to promote diuresis.

Reduction of Intracranial Pressure. Intracranial pressure (ICP) that has been elevated by cerebral edema can be reduced with mannitol. The drug lowers ICP because its presence in the cerebral vasculature creates an osmotic force that draws edematous fluid out of the brain. There is no risk of increasing cerebral edema because mannitol cannot exit the capillary beds of the brain.

Reduction of Intraocular Pressure. Mannitol and other osmotic agents can lower intraocular pressure (IOP). Mannitol reduces IOP by rendering the plasma hyperosmotic with respect to intraocular fluids, thereby creating an osmotic force that draws ocular fluid into the blood. Use of mannitol to lower IOP is reserved for patients who have not responded to more conventional treatment.

Preparations, Dosage, and Administration

Mannitol [Osmitrol] is administered by IV infusion. Solutions for IV use range in concentration from 5% to 25%. Dosing is complex and varies with the objectives of therapy (prevention of renal failure, lowering of ICP, lowering of IOP). The usual adult dosage for prevention of renal failure is 50 to 100 gm over 24 hours. The rate of infusion should be set to elicit a urine flow of at least 30 to 50 ml/hr. It should be noted that mannitol may crystallize out of solution if exposed to low temperature. Accordingly, preparations should be observed for crystals prior to use. Preparations that contain crystals should be warmed (to redissolve the mannitol) and then cooled to body temperature for administration. A filter needle is employed to withdraw mannitol from the vial, and an in-line filter is used to prevent any crystals that may be present from entering the circulation. If urine flow declines to a very low rate or ceases entirely, the infusion should be stopped.

UREA, GLYCERIN, AND ISOSORBIDE

In addition to mannitol, three other drugs—urea, glycerin, and isosorbide—are classified as osmotic diuretics. Like mannitol, these agents are freely filtered at the glomerulus and undergo limited reabsorption. It is these properties that promote osmotic diuresis. It must be noted, however, that although urea, glycerin, and isosorbide can produce diuresis, none of these drugs is actually used for this purpose. Application of these agents is limited to reducing intraocular and intracranial pressure. Urea [Ureaphil] is administered intravenously. Glycerin [Osmoglyn] and isosorbide [Ismotic] are administered orally.

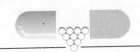

Summary of Major Nursing Implications

HIGH-CEILING (LOOP) DIURETICS

Furosemide

Ethacrynic Acid

Bumetanide

 Preadministration Assessment

Therapeutic Goal

High-ceiling diuretics are indicated for patients with (1) pulmonary edema associated with congestive heart failure; (2) edema of hepatic, cardiac, or renal origin that has been unresponsive to less effective diuretics; and (3) hypertension that cannot be controlled with thiazide and potassium-sparing diuretics.

Baseline Data

For all patients, obtain baseline values for weight, blood pressure (sitting and supine), pulse, respiration, and electrolytes (sodium, potassium, chloride). For patients with edema, record sites and extent of edema. For patients with ascites, measure abdominal girth.

Identifying High-Risk Patients

Use with *caution* in patients with *cardiovascular disease, renal impairment, diabetes mellitus,* or a *history of gout* and in patients taking *digoxin, lithium, ototoxic drugs,* or *antihypertensive drugs.*

 Implementation: Administration

Routes

Furosemide and bumetanide: Oral, IV, IM.
Ethacrynic acid: Oral, IV.

Administration

Oral. Dosing may be done once daily, twice daily, or on alternate days. Instruct patients who are using once-a-day or alternate-day dosing to take their medication in the morning. Instruct patients using twice-a-day dosing to take their medication at 8 AM and 2 PM (to minimize nocturia).

Advise patients to administer *furosemide* with food if GI upset occurs.

Parenteral. Administer IV injections slowly (over 1 to 2 minutes). For high-dose therapy, administer by continuous infusion. Discard discolored solutions.

Promoting Compliance

Increased frequency of urination is inconvenient and can discourage compliance. To promote compliance, forewarn patients that treatment will increase urine volume and frequency of voiding, and inform them that these effects will subside 6 to 8 hours after dosing. Inform patients that nighttime diuresis can be minimized by avoiding dosing late in the day.

 Ongoing Evaluation and Interventions

Evaluating Therapeutic Effects

Monitor blood pressure and pulse rate, weigh the patient daily, and evaluate for decreased edema.

Monitor intake and output. Notify the physician if oliguria (urine output less than 25 ml/hr) or anuria (no urine output) develops.

Instruct outpatients to weigh themselves daily, preferably in the morning before eating, and to maintain a weight record.

Minimizing Adverse Effects

Dehydration. Excessive fluid loss can cause dehydration. Signs include dry mouth, unusual thirst, and oliguria. Withhold the drug if these appear.

Dehydration can promote thromboembolism. Monitor the patient for symptoms (headache; pain in the chest, calves, or pelvis), and notify the physician if these develop.

The risk of dehydration and its sequelae can be minimized by (1) initiating therapy with low doses, (2) adjusting the dosage carefully, (3) monitoring weight loss daily, and (4) using an intermittent dosing schedule.

Hypotension. Monitor blood pressure, and, if it falls precipitously, withhold medication and notify the physician.

Teach outpatients to self-monitor blood pressure, and instruct them to notify the physician if pressure drops substantially.

Inform patients about signs of postural hypotension (dizziness, lightheadedness), and advise them to sit or lie down if these occur. Inform patients that postural hypotension can be minimized by moving slowly when changing from a seated or supine position to an upright position.

Electrolyte Imbalance. High-ceiling diuretics can produce excessive loss of sodium, potassium, and chloride. Signs of electrolyte imbalance include muscle fatigue, cramps, and dysrhythmias. Electrolyte imbalance can be minimized by intermittent dosing and regular monitoring of urinary and plasma electrolytes. If electrolyte imbalance is severe, diuretic dosage should be reduced or treatment should be interrupted.

Potassium loss is a special problem: if serum potassium falls below 3.5 mEq/L, fatal dysrhythmias may result. The risk of hypokalemia can be reduced by consumption of potassium-rich foods (e.g., bananas, citrus fruits, potatoes) and by use of potassium supplements *or* a potassium-sparing diuretic.

Ototoxicity. Rarely, high-ceiling diuretics cause hearing loss. Inform patients about possible hearing loss, and instruct them to notify the physician if a hearing deficit develops. Exercise caution when high-ceiling diuretics are used concurrently with other ototoxic drugs (e.g., aminoglycosides).

Hyperglycemia. High-ceiling diuretics may elevate blood glucose levels in diabetics. Advise diabetic patients to be especially diligent about monitoring blood glucose.

Hyperuricemia. High-ceiling diuretics frequently cause *asymptomatic* hyperuricemia, although gout-prone patients may experience a *gouty attack*. Inform patients about signs of gout (tenderness or swelling in joints), and instruct them to notify the physician if these occur.

Minimizing Adverse Interactions

Digoxin. By lowering potassium levels, high-ceiling diuretics increase the risk of fatal dysrhythmias from digoxin. Serum potassium levels must be monitored and maintained above 3.5 mEq/L.

Lithium. High-ceiling diuretics can suppress lithium excretion, thereby causing the drug to accumulate, possibly to toxic levels. Plasma lithium content should be monitored routinely. If drug levels become elevated, lithium dosage should be reduced.

Ototoxic Drugs. The risk of hearing loss from high-ceiling diuretics is increased in the presence of other ototoxic drugs (e.g., aminoglycosides). Exercise caution when such combinations are employed.

Antihypertensive Agents. The hypotensive effects of high-ceiling diuretics add with those of other antihypertensive drugs. To avoid an excessive drop in blood pressure, dosages of other antihypertensive drugs may need to be reduced.

THIAZIDE DIURETICS

Thiazide diuretics have actions very similar to those of the high-ceiling diuretics. Hence, nursing implications for the thiazides are nearly identical to those of the high-ceiling agents.

Preadministration Assessment

Therapeutic Goal

Thiazide diuretics are used to treat *hypertension* and *edema*.

Baseline Data

For all patients, obtain baseline values for weight, blood pressure (sitting and supine), pulse, respiration, and electrolytes (sodium, potassium, chloride). For patients with edema, record sites and extent of edema.

Identifying High-Risk Patients

Use with *caution* in patients with *cardiovascular disease, renal impairment, diabetes mellitus,* or a *history of gout* and in patients taking *digoxin, lithium,* or *antihypertensive drugs.*

Implementation: Administration

Routes

Oral: all thiazide-type diuretics.
Intravenous: chlorothiazide.

Administration

Dosing may be done once daily, twice daily, or on alternate days. When once-a-day dosing is employed, instruct patients to take their medicine early in the day to minimize nocturia. When twice-a-day dosing is employed, instruct patients to take their medicine at 8 AM and 2 PM.

Advise patients to administer thiazides with or after meals if GI upset occurs.

Promoting Compliance

See implications for *High-Ceiling Diuretics.*

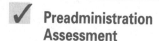

Evaluating Therapeutic Effects

See implications for *High-Ceiling Diuretics.*

Minimizing Adverse Effects

Like the high-ceiling diuretics, thiazides can cause *dehydration, electrolyte imbalance (including hypokalemia), hypotension, hyperglycemia,* and *hyperuricemia.* For implications regarding these effects, see implications for *High-Ceiling Diuretics.*

Thiazides can cause fetal harm and can enter breast milk. These drugs should be avoided during pregnancy unless absolutely required. Caution women not to breast-feed.

Minimizing Adverse Interactions

Like high-ceiling diuretics, thiazides can interact adversely with *digoxin, lithium,* and *antihypertensive drugs.* For nursing implications regarding these interactions, see implications for *High-Ceiling Diuretics.*

POTASSIUM-SPARING DIURETICS

Spironolactone

Triamterene

Amiloride

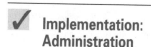

Therapeutic Goal

Potassium-sparing diuretics are given primarily to counterbalance the potassium-losing effects of thiazides and high-ceiling diuretics.

Baseline Data

Obtain baseline values for serum potassium content.

Identifying High-Risk Patients

Potassium-sparing diuretics are *contraindicated* for patients with *hyperkalemia* and for *patients taking potassium supplements or another potassium-sparing diuretic.*

Route

Oral.

Administration

Advise patients to take these drugs with or after meals if GI upset occurs.

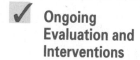

Evaluating Therapeutic Effects

Monitor serum potassium levels on a regular basis. The objective is to maintain serum potassium levels between 3.5 and 5 mEq/L.

Minimizing Adverse Effects

Hyperkalemia. Hyperkalemia is the principal adverse effect. Unless clearly indicated, potassium supplements should be avoided. Instruct patients to restrict intake of potassium-rich foods (e.g., citrus fruits, bananas). If serum potassium levels rise above 5 mEq/L, or if signs of hyperkalemia develop (e.g., abnormal cardiac rhythm), withhold medication and notify the physician. Insulin can be given to drive potassium levels down.

Endocrine Effects. *Spironolactone* may cause *menstrual irregularities* and *impotence.* Inform patients about these effects, and instruct them to notify the physician if they occur.

Minimizing Adverse Interactions

Use of a potassium-sparing diuretic with *potassium supplements* or with *another potassium-sparing diuretic* can cause hyperkalemia. These combinations should be avoided.

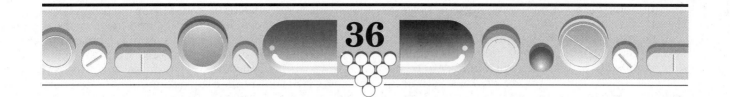

Agents Affecting the Volume and Ion Content of Body Fluids

The drugs discussed in this chapter are used to correct disturbances in the volume and ionic composition of body fluids. Three groups of agents are considered: (1) drugs used to correct disorders of fluid volume and osmolality, (2) drugs used to correct disturbances of hydrogen ion concentration (acid-base status), and (3) drugs used to correct electrolyte imbalances.

DISORDERS OF FLUID VOLUME AND OSMOLALITY

Good health requires that both the volume and osmolality of extracellular and intracellular fluids remain within a normal range. If a substantial alteration in either the volume or osmolality of these fluids develops, significant harm can result.

Maintenance of fluid volume and osmolality is primarily the job of the kidneys, and, even under adverse conditions, renal mechanisms usually succeed in keeping the volume and composition of body fluids within acceptable limits. However, circumstances can arise in which the regulatory powers of the kidneys are exceeded. When this occurs,

447

disruption of fluid volume, osmolality, or both can result.

Abnormal states of hydration can be divided into two major categories: *volume contraction* and *volume expansion*. Volume contraction is defined as a decrease in total body water, whereas volume expansion is an increase in total body water. States of volume contraction and volume expansion have three subclassifications based on alterations in extracellular fluid osmolality. For volume contraction, the three subcategories are *isotonic* contraction, *hypertonic* contraction, and *hypotonic* contraction. The states of volume expansion may also be subclassified as either *isotonic, hypertonic,* or *hypotonic*. Descriptions and causes of these abnormal states are discussed below.

In the clinical setting, changes in osmolality are described in terms of the sodium content of plasma. Sodium is used as the reference for classification because this ion is the principal extracellular solute. (Plasma sodium content ranges from 135 to 145 mEq/L.) In most cases, the total osmolality of plasma is equal to approximately twice the osmolality of sodium. That is, total plasma osmolality usually ranges from 280 to 300 mOsm/kg water.

VOLUME CONTRACTION

Isotonic Contraction

Definition and Causes. Isotonic contraction is defined as volume contraction in which *sodium and water are lost in isotonic proportions*. Hence, although there is a decrease in the total volume of extracellular fluid, there is no change in osmolality. Causes of isotonic contraction include vomiting, diarrhea, kidney disease, and misuse of diuretics. Isotonic contraction is characteristic of cholera, an infection that produces vomiting and severe diarrhea.

Treatment. Lost volume should be replaced with fluids that are isotonic to plasma. This can be accomplished by infusion of isotonic (0.9%) sodium chloride in sterile water, a solution in which both sodium and chloride are present at a concentration of 145 mEq/L. Volume should be replenished slowly so as to avoid pulmonary edema.

Hypertonic Contraction

Definition and Causes. Hypertonic contraction is defined as volume contraction in which *loss of water exceeds loss of sodium*. Hence, there is a reduction in extracellular fluid volume coupled with an increase in osmolality. Because of extracellular hypertonicity, water is drawn out of cells, thereby producing intracellular dehydration and partial compensation for lost extracellular volume.

Causes of hypertonic contraction include excessive sweating, osmotic diuresis, and feeding of excessively concentrated foods to infants. Hypertonic contraction may also develop secondary to extensive burns or disorders of the central nervous system (CNS) that render the patient unable to report sensations of thirst.

Treatment. Volume replacement in hypertonic contraction should be performed with hypotonic fluids (e.g., 0.11% sodium chloride) or fluids containing no solutes at all. Initial therapy may consist simply of oral administration of water. Alternatively, 5% dextrose can be infused intravenously; since dextrose is rapidly metabolized to carbon dioxide and water, dextrose solutions can be looked upon as the osmotic equivalent of water alone. Volume replenishment should be done in stages. About 50% of the estimated loss should be replaced during the first few hours of treatment. The remainder should be replenished over 1 to 2 days.

Hypotonic Contraction

Definition and Causes. Hypotonic contraction is defined as volume contraction in which *loss of sodium exceeds loss of water*. Hence, both the volume and the osmolality of extracellular fluid are reduced. Since intracellular osmolality now exceeds the osmolality of extracellular fluid, extracellular volume becomes diminished further by movement of water into cells.

The principal cause of hypotonic contraction is excessive loss of sodium through the kidneys. This may occur because of diuretic therapy, chronic renal insufficiency, or lack of aldosterone (the adrenocortical hormone that promotes renal retention of sodium).

Treatment. If hyponatremia is mild and if renal function is adequate, hypotonic contraction can be corrected by infusion of *isotonic* sodium chloride solution for injection; plasma tonicity will be adjusted by the kidneys. However, if the sodium loss is severe, a *hypertonic* (e.g., 3%) solution of sodium chloride should be infused. Administration should continue until plasma sodium concentration has been raised to about 130 mEq/L. Patients should be monitored for signs of fluid overload (distention of neck veins, peripheral or pulmonary edema). When hypotonic contraction is due to low levels of aldosterone, patients should receive hormone replacement therapy along with intravenous infusion of isotonic sodium chloride.

VOLUME EXPANSION

Volume expansion is defined as an increase in the total volume of body fluid. As with volume contraction, volume expansion may be isotonic, hypertonic, or hypotonic. Volume expansion may result from an overdose with therapeutic fluids (e.g., sodium chloride infusion) or may be associated with disease states (e.g., congestive heart failure, nephrotic syndrome, cirrhosis of the liver with ascites). The principal drugs employed to correct volume expansion are diuretics and the agents used to treat heart failure. These drugs are discussed in Chapters 35 and 42, respectively.

ACID-BASE DISTURBANCES

Maintenance of acid-base balance is a complex process, the full discussion of which is beyond the scope of this text. Hence, consideration here is condensed.

Acid-base status is regulated by multiple systems. The most important of these are (1) the bicarbonate–carbonic acid buffer system, (2) the respiratory system, and (3) the kidneys. The respiratory system influences pH through control of CO_2 exhalation. Since CO_2 represents volatile carbonic acid, exhalation of CO_2 tends to elevate pH (reduce acidity), whereas CO_2 retention (secondary to respiratory depression) tends to lower pH. The kidneys influence pH through regulation of bicarbonate excretion. By retaining bicarbonate, the kidneys can raise pH. Conversely, by increasing the excretion of bicarbonate, the kidneys can compensate for alkalosis.

There are four principal types of acid-base imbalance: (1) respiratory alkalosis, (2) respiratory acidosis, (3) metabolic alkalosis, and (4) metabolic acidosis. The causes and treatments of these states are discussed below.

Respiratory Alkalosis

Causes. Respiratory alkalosis is produced by hyperventilation. Deep and rapid breathing increases loss of CO_2, which in turn lowers the pCO_2 of blood and increases the pH. Mild hyperventilation may result from a number of causes, including hypoxia, pulmonary disease, and drugs (especially aspirin and other salicylates). Severe hyperventilation can be caused by injury to the CNS and by hysteria.

Treatment. Management of respiratory alkalosis is dictated by the severity of pH elevation. When alkalosis is mild, no specific treatment is indicated. The severe respiratory alkalosis produced by hysteria can be controlled by having the patient rebreathe his or her CO_2-laden expired breath. This can be accomplished by holding a paper bag over the nose and mouth. A similar effect can be achieved by having the patient inhale a gas mixture containing 5% CO_2. A sedative (e.g., diazepam) can help suppress the hysteria.

Respiratory Acidosis

Causes. Respiratory acidosis results from retention of CO_2 secondary to hypoventilation. Reduced exhalation of CO_2 raises plasma pCO_2, which in turn causes plasma pH to fall. Primary causes of impaired ventilation are (1) depression of the medullary respiratory center, and (2) pathologic changes in the lungs. With time, the kidneys compensate for respiratory acidosis by excreting less bicarbonate.

Treatment. Primary treatment of respiratory acidosis is directed at correcting the respiratory impairment. The patient may also need oxygen and ventilatory assistance. Infusion of *sodium bicarbonate* solution is indicated if acidosis is severe.

Metabolic Acidosis

Causes. Principal causes of metabolic acidosis are chronic renal failure, loss of bicarbonate during severe diarrhea, and metabolic disorders that result in overproduction of lactic acid (lactic acidosis) or ketoacids (ketoacidosis). Metabolic acidosis may also result from poisoning by methanol and certain medications (e.g., aspirin and other salicylates).

Treatment. Treatment of metabolic acidosis consists of efforts to correct the underlying cause, and, if the acidosis is severe, administration of an alkalinizing salt (e.g., sodium bicarbonate, sodium citrate, sodium lactate).

When an alkalinizing salt is indicated, *sodium bicarbonate* is generally preferred. Administration may be oral or intravenous. If acidosis is mild, oral administration is preferred. Intravenous infusion is usually reserved for severe reductions of pH. When sodium bicarbonate is given IV in the treatment of acute, severe acidosis, caution must be exercised to avoid excessive elevation of plasma pH, since rapid conversion from acidosis to alkalosis can be hazardous. Also, because of the sodium content of sodium bicarbonate, care should be taken to avoid hypernatremia.

Metabolic Alkalosis

Causes. Metabolic alkalosis is characterized by increases in both the pH and bicarbonate content of plasma. Causes include excessive loss of gastric acid (through vomiting or suctioning) and administration of alkalinizing salts (e.g., sodium bicarbonate). The body compensates for metabolic alkalosis by (1) hypoventilation (causing retention of CO_2), (2) increased renal excretion of bicarbonate, and (3) accumulation of organic acids.

Treatment. In most cases, metabolic alkalosis can be corrected by infusing a solution of sodium chloride plus potassium chloride. This facilitates renal excretion of bicarbonate, and thereby promotes normalization of plasma pH. When alkalosis is severe, direct correction of pH is indicated. This can be accomplished by infusing dilute (0.1 N) *hydrochloric acid* through a central venous catheter or by administering an acid-forming salt, such as *ammonium chloride*. Ammonium chloride must not be given to patients with liver failure, since the drug is likely to cause hepatic encephalopathy in these patients.

POTASSIUM IMBALANCES

Potassium is the most abundant *intracellular* cation, having a concentration within cells of about 150 mEq/L. In contrast, *extracellular* concentrations are low (4 to 5 mEq/L). Potassium plays a major role in the conduction of nerve impulses and in maintaining the electrical excitability of muscle. Potassium also helps regulate acid-base balance.

REGULATION OF POTASSIUM LEVELS

Serum levels of potassium are regulated primarily by the kidneys. Under steady-state conditions, urinary output of potassium equals intake. Renal excretion of potassium is increased by aldosterone, an adrenal steroid that promotes conservation of sodium while increasing potassium loss. Potassium excretion is also increased by most diuretics. Potassium-sparing diuretics (e.g., spironolactone) are the exception to this rule.

Potassium levels are influenced by extracellular pH. In the presence of extracellular *alkalosis*, potassium uptake by cells is *enhanced*, causing a *reduction* in extracellular potassium levels. Conversely, extracellular *acidosis* promotes the *exit* of potassium from cells, thereby causing extracellular *hyperkalemia*.

Insulin has a profound effect on potassium: in high doses, insulin stimulates potassium uptake by cells. This ability has been exploited to treat hyperkalemia.

HYPOKALEMIA

Causes and Consequences

Hypokalemia is defined as a deficiency of potassium in the blood. By definition, hypokalemia exists when serum potassium levels fall below 3.5 mEq/L. The most common cause of hypokalemia is treatment with thiazide or loop diuretics (see Chapter 35). Other causes include insufficient potassium intake; alkalosis and excessive insulin (both of which decrease extracellular potassium levels by driving potassium into cells); increased

renal excretion of potassium (e.g., as caused by aldosterone); and potassium loss associated with vomiting, diarrhea, and abuse of laxatives. Hypokalemia may also occur because of excessive loss of potassium in sweat. As a rule, potassium depletion is accompanied by loss of chloride. Insufficiency of both ions produces *hypokalemic alkalosis*.

Hypokalemia has adverse effects on skeletal muscle, smooth muscle, and the heart. Symptoms associated with hypokalemia include weakness or paralysis of skeletal muscle, abnormalities in cardiac impulse conduction, and intestinal dilatation and ileus. In patients taking digoxin (a cardiac drug), concurrent hypokalemia is the principal cause of digoxin toxicity.

Prevention and Treatment

Potassium depletion is treated with a potassium salt. Potassium salts may also be used for *prophylaxis* against insufficiency. For either treatment or prophylaxis, the salt that is generally preferred is *potassium chloride*. The chloride salt of potassium is preferred because chloride deficiency frequently coexists with deficiency of potassium. Other salts (e.g., potassium gluconate, potassium citrate) are also available.

Potassium chloride may be administered orally or IV. Oral administration is preferred for prophylaxis and for treatment of mild deficiency. The intravenous route is employed for severe deficiency and for patients who cannot take potassium orally.

Oral Potassium Chloride. *Uses, Dosage, and Preparations.* Oral potassium chloride may be used for both prevention and treatment of potassium deficiency. Doses for prophylaxis range from 16 to 24 mEq per day. Doses for correction of deficiency range from 40 to 100 mEq per day.

Oral potassium chloride is available in solution and in solid formulations (powder, standard tablets, effervescent tablets, enteric-coated tablets, wax-matrix tablets, microencapsulated particles in capsules). The solution is preferred.

Adverse Effects. Potassium chloride *irritates the gastrointestinal tract*, frequently causing abdominal discomfort, nausea, vomiting, and diarrhea. Solid forms of potassium chloride (tablets, capsules) can produce high local concentrations of potassium, resulting in severe intestinal injury (ulcerative lesions, bleeding, perforation); death has occurred. These severe effects are less likely with wax-matrix tablets and with capsules that contain microencapsulated particles than with other solid formulations. To minimize gastrointestinal effects, oral potassium chloride should be taken with meals or with a full glass of water. If symptoms of irritation occur, administration should be discontinued. Rarely, oral potassium chloride produces *hyperkalemia*. This dangerous development is much more likely with intravenous therapy.

Intravenous Potassium Chloride. Intravenous potassium chloride is indicated for prevention and treatment of hypokalemia. Intravenous solutions must be diluted (preferably to 40 mEq/L or less) and infused slowly (generally no faster than 10 mEq/hr in adults).

The principal complication of IV therapy is *hyperkalemia*, a condition that can prove fatal. To reduce the risk of hyperkalemia, serum potassium levels should be measured prior to starting the infusion and periodically throughout the treatment interval. In addition, renal function should be assessed before and during treatment to insure adequate output of urine. If renal failure develops, the infusion should be stopped immediately. Changes in the electrocardiogram (EKG) can provide an early indication that potassium toxicity is developing. Symptoms and treatment of hyperkalemia are discussed in the section that follows.

Contraindications to Potassium Use. Potassium should be avoided under conditions that predispose patients to hyperkalemia (e.g., severe renal impairment, use of potassium-sparing diuretics, hypoaldosteronism). Potassium must also be avoided when hyperkalemia already exists.

HYPERKALEMIA

Causes and Consequences

Causes. Hyperkalemia (excessive elevation of serum potassium content) can result from a number of causes. These include severe tissue trauma, untreated Addison's disease, acute acidosis (which draws potassium out of cells), misuse of potassium-sparing diuretics, and overdosage with intravenous potassium.

Consequences. The most serious consequence of hyperkalemia is disruption of the electrical activity of the heart. Because hyperkalemia alters the generation and conduction of cardiac impulses, alterations in the EKG and in cardiac rhythm are usually the earliest signs that potassium levels are climbing dangerously high. With mild elevation of serum potassium (5 to 7 mEq/L), the T wave heightens and the PR interval becomes prolonged. When serum potassium reaches 8 to 9 mEq/L, cardiac arrest occurs, possibly preceded by ventricular tachycardia or fibrillation.

Effects of hyperkalemia are not limited to the heart. Elevation of serum potassium may cause confusion, anxiety, dyspnea, weakness or heaviness of the legs, and numbness or tingling of the hands, feet, and lips.

Treatment

Treatment is begun by withholding any foods and medicines that contain potassium. After this,

management consists of measures that (1) counteract potassium-induced cardiotoxicity, and (2) lower extracellular levels of potassium. Specific steps include (1) infusion of a *calcium salt* (e.g., calcium gluconate) to offset effects of hyperkalemia on the heart; (2) infusion of *glucose* and *insulin* to promote uptake of potassium by cells and thereby decrease extracellular potassium levels; and (3) if acidosis is present (which is likely), infusion of *sodium bicarbonate* in order to move pH toward alkalinity, and thereby increase cellular uptake of potassium. If the preceding measures prove inadequate, steps can be taken to remove potassium. These include (1) oral or rectal administration of *sodium polystyrene sulfonate*, an exchange resin that absorbs potassium, and (2) peritoneal or extracorporeal dialysis.

MAGNESIUM IMBALANCES

Magnesium is required for the activity of many enzymes and for binding of messenger RNA to ribosomes. In addition, magnesium helps regulate neurochemical transmission and the excitability of muscle. The concentration of magnesium within cells is about 40 mEq/L, much higher than its concentration outside cells (about 2 mEq/L).

HYPOMAGNESEMIA

Causes and Consequences

Low levels of magnesium may result from a variety of causes, including diarrhea, hemodialysis, kidney disease, and prolonged intravenous feeding with magnesium-free solutions. Hypomagnesemia may also be seen in chronic alcoholics and in people with diabetes mellitus or pancreatitis. Frequently, patients with magnesium deficiency also present with hypocalcemia and hypokalemia.

Prominent symptoms of hypomagnesemia involve cardiac and skeletal muscle. In the presence of low levels of magnesium, release of acetylcholine at the neuromuscular junction is enhanced. This can increase muscle excitability to the point of tetany. Hypomagnesemia also increases excitability of neurons within the CNS, causing disorientation, psychoses, and seizures.

In the kidneys, hypomagnesemia may lead to nephrocalcinosis (formation of miniscule calcium stones within nephrons). Renal injury occurs when the stones become large enough to block the flow of tubular urine.

Prevention and Treatment

Frank hypomagnesemia is treated with parenteral magnesium sulfate. For prophylaxis against magnesium deficiency, an oral preparation (magnesium gluconate, magnesium hydroxide) may be used.

Magnesium Gluconate and Magnesium Hydroxide. Tablets of magnesium gluconate or magnesium hydroxide may be taken as supplements to dietary magnesium to help prevent development of hypomagnesemia. Milk of magnesia (a liquid formulation of magnesium hydroxide) may also be used for prophylaxis. With any of these oral magnesium preparations, excessive doses may cause diarrhea. The adult and pediatric dosage for prevention of deficiency is 5 mg/kg/day.

Magnesium Sulfate. *Uses, Administration, and Dosage.* Magnesium sulfate (IM or IV) is the preferred treatment for severe hypomagnesemia. The IM dosage is 0.5 to 1 gm four times a day. For IV therapy, a 10% solution can be used; the infusion rate is 1.5 ml/min or less.

Adverse Effects. Excessive levels of magnesium cause *neuromuscular blockade.* Paralysis of the respiratory muscles is of particular concern. By suppressing neuromuscular transmission, magnesium excess can intensify the effects of neuromuscular blocking agents (e.g., tubocurarine, succinylcholine). Hence, caution must be exercised in patients receiving these drugs. The neuromuscular blocking actions of magnesium can be counteracted with calcium. Accordingly, when parenteral magnesium is being employed, an injectable form of calcium (e.g., calcium gluconate) should be immediately available.

In the heart, excessive levels of magnesium can suppress impulse conduction through the A-V node. Accordingly, magnesium sulfate is contraindicated for patients with A-V heart block.

To minimize the risk of toxicity, serum content of magnesium should be monitored. Respiratory paralysis occurs at concentrations of 12 to 15 mEq/L. When magnesium levels exceed 25 mEq/L, cardiac arrest may take place.

HYPERMAGNESEMIA

Toxic elevation of magnesium levels is most common in patients with renal insufficiency, especially when magnesium-containing antacids or cathartics are being used. Symptoms of mild intoxication include muscle weakness (resulting from inhibition of acetylcholine release), hypotension, sedation, and EKG changes. As noted above, respiratory paralysis is likely when plasma levels reach 12 to 15 mEq/L. At higher concentrations of magnesium, there is a risk of cardiac arrest. Muscle weakness and paralysis can be counteracted with an intravenous calcium preparation.

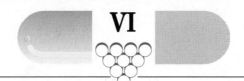

Cardiovascular Drugs

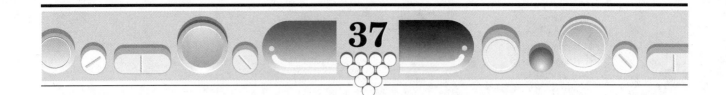

Angiotensin-Converting Enzyme Inhibitors

Angiotensin-converting enzyme (ACE) inhibitors are important drugs for treating hypertension and congestive heart failure. The primary effects of these drugs — vasodilation and reduction of blood volume — result from inhibiting ACE, a key component of the renin-angiotensin-aldosterone system (RAAS). Accordingly, before discussing the pharmacology of the ACE inhibitors, we will review the physiology of ACE and the RAAS.

PHYSIOLOGY OF THE RENIN-ANGIOTENSIN-ALDOSTERONE SYSTEM

The RAAS plays an important role in regulating blood pressure, blood volume, and fluid and electrolyte balance. The system exerts its effects through the actions of angiotensin II and aldosterone. The major components of the system are depicted in Figure 37–1.

TYPES OF ANGIOTENSIN

Before discussing the physiology of the RAAS, we need to introduce the angiotensin family: an-

455

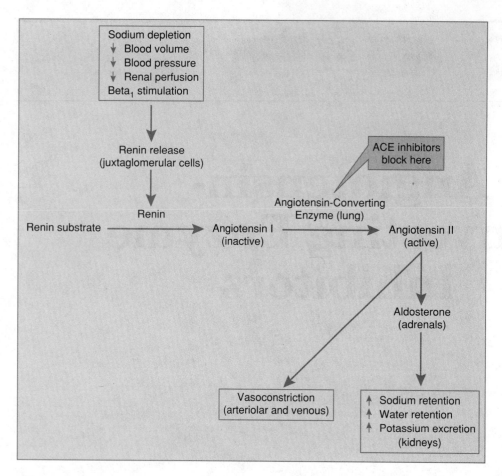

Figure 37–1. Components of the renin-angiotensin-aldosterone system.

giotensin I, angiotensin II, and angiotensin III. All three compounds are small polypeptides. Angiotensin I is the precursor of angiotensin II (see Fig. 37–1) and has very little biologic activity. In contrast, the biologic activity of angiotensin II is extremely high. Angiotensin III is formed by the degradation of angiotensin II, and has only moderate biologic activity.

ACTIONS OF ANGIOTENSIN II

The most prominent actions of angiotensin II are vasoconstriction and promotion of aldosterone release. Both actions result in elevation of blood pressure.

Vasoconstriction. Angiotensin II is an extremely potent vasoconstrictor. This agent acts directly on vascular smooth muscle to cause contraction. Vasoconstriction is most prominent in arterioles, although venous contraction occurs as well. As a result of angiotensin-induced vasoconstriction, blood pressure is elevated.

Release of Aldosterone. Angiotensin II acts directly on the adrenal cortex to promote synthesis and secretion of aldosterone. Aldosterone, in turn, acts on the kidney to cause retention of sodium

and excretion of potassium and hydrogen. Because water is retained along with sodium, aldosterone increases plasma volume, and thereby increases blood pressure. The adrenal cortex is highly sensitive to angiotensin. As a result, angiotensin can stimulate aldosterone release even when angiotensin levels are too low to induce vasoconstriction. Aldosterone secretion is enhanced when sodium levels are low and when potassium levels are high.

FORMATION OF ANGIOTENSIN II

As indicated in Figure 37–1, there are two reactions in the formation of angiotensin II. Both reactions take place within the vascular system. In the first reaction, angiotensin I is formed from renin substrate, which is also known as *angiotensinogen*. The enzyme that catalyzes this reaction is *renin* (pronounced "ree′nin"). Renin is produced by the kidney and is the rate-limiting enzyme in angiotensin II formation. In step two, angiotensin I is converted into angiotensin II. The enzyme responsible for this reaction is *angiotensin-converting enzyme* (ACE). ACE is located on the luminal surface of all blood vessels. The vasculature of the lungs is especially rich in the enzyme. Since ACE is present in abundance, conversion of angiotensin

I to angiotensin II occurs almost instantaneously after angiotensin I is formed.

REGULATION OF RENIN RELEASE

Renin is produced by juxtaglomerular cells of the kidney and undergoes controlled secretion into the bloodstream. As noted above, renin is the rate-limiting element in angiotensin II formation. Since renin must be released into the blood to produce its effects, the rate of renin release determines the rate at which angiotensin II is formed.

As indicated in Figure 37–1, release of renin is triggered by multiple factors. Release *increases* in response to a *decline* in blood pressure, blood volume, plasma sodium content, or renal perfusion pressure. Reduced renal perfusion pressure is an especially important stimulant of renin release and can occur in response to (1) stenosis of the renal arteries, (2) reduced systemic blood pressure, and (3) reduced plasma volume (brought on by dehydration, hemorrhage, or chronic sodium depletion). For the most part, these factors increase renin release through effects exerted locally within the kidney. However, some of these factors may also promote renin release through activation of the sympathetic nervous system. Sympathetic nerves increase secretion of renin by causing stimulation of beta$_1$-adrenergic receptors on juxtaglomerular cells.

Release of renin is *suppressed* by factors opposite to those that cause release. That is, renin secretion is inhibited by elevation of blood pressure, elevation of blood volume, and elevation of plasma sodium content. Hence, as blood pressure, blood volume, and plasma sodium content increase in response to renin release, further release of renin is suppressed. In this regard we can view release of renin as being regulated by a classic negative feedback loop.

THE ROLE OF THE RENIN-ANGIOTENSIN-ALDOSTERONE SYSTEM IN REGULATING BLOOD PRESSURE

Since a decline in blood pressure stimulates renin release (and angiotensin II formation), whereas factors that increase blood pressure suppress renin release, it is clear that the RAAS is poised to participate in the regulation of intravascular pressure. However, although this system does indeed contribute to blood pressure control, its role in the *normovolemic, sodium-replete* individual is only modest. In contrast, the system can be a major factor in maintaining blood pressure in the presence of *hemorrhage, dehydration,* or *sodium depletion.*

The role of the RAAS in hypertension is undergoing re-evaluation. Initially, it was thought that excess activity of the system was a causative factor in only two relatively rare forms of hypertension: (1) malignant hypertension, and (2) hypertension occurring secondary to renal arterial stenosis. For the most prevalent form of hypertension (essential hypertension), it was thought that the RAAS was not a significant contributing factor. The basis of this belief was simple: most people with hypertension have normal levels of plasma renin activity. However, despite this apparent normalcy of the RAAS, *drugs that block the formation of angiotensin II were found capable of lowering blood pressure in a broad spectrum of hypertensive states.* This discovery came as a major surprise. Given the clinical efficacy of drugs that block angiotensin II production, it appears that the role of the RAAS in causing hypertension is much greater than originally suspected.

ANGIOTENSIN-CONVERTING ENZYME INHIBITORS

The ACE inhibitors were developed in the late 1970's. Since the introduction of captopril, the first of these drugs, six more ACE inhibitors have become available. For all of these agents, beneficial effects result from suppressing angiotensin II formation. The principal indications for these drugs are hypertension and congestive heart failure. Their most prominent adverse effects are hypotension and persistent cough.

CAPTOPRIL

Captopril [Capoten] was the first ACE inhibitor to be widely employed and will serve as our prototype for the family. The drug is administered orally to treat hypertension and congestive heart failure. The most common adverse effects of concern are hypotension, hyperkalemia, and cough.

Pharmacologic Effects

The pharmacologic effects of captopril result from inhibition of ACE. By inhibiting ACE, the drug prevents conversion of angiotensin I, a compound with minimal biologic activity, into angiotensin II, a potent vasoconstrictor and stimulant of aldosterone release. The major response to reduced angiotensin II production is *vasodilation*, primarily in arterioles and to a lesser degree in veins. Reduced aldosterone release (secondary to reduced angiotensin II production) promotes renal retention of potassium and increased excretion of sodium and water.

Pharmacokinetics

Captopril is rapidly absorbed following oral administration. The extent of absorption is about 70%. Absorption can be reduced significantly by food. Accordingly, captopril should be administered at least 1 hour before meals. Elimination is rapid: the plasma half-life of the drug is less than 2 hours. Approximately 50% of each dose is excreted unchanged in the urine. As a result, renal impairment prolongs the drug's half-life; this can cause significant drug accumulation if the dosage is not reduced.

Therapeutic Uses

Hypertension. Captopril has broad applications in hypertension. The drug is especially effective against malignant hypertension and hypertension secondary to renal arterial stenosis. Captopril is also useful against essential hypertension of mild to moderate intensity. In this disorder, maximal benefits may take several weeks to develop.

The mechanism by which captopril lowers blood pressure in essential hypertension is only partially understood. *Initial* responses are proportional to angiotensin II levels and are clearly related to reduced formation of this compound. However, with *prolonged* therapy, blood pressure often undergoes an additional decline. During this second phase, there is no correspondence between reductions in blood pressure and reductions in angiotensin II levels. Hence, the mechanism underlying the long-term antihypertensive effects of captopril remains to be established.

Captopril offers several advantages over many other antihypertensive drugs. In contrast to the sympatholytic agents, captopril does not interfere with cardiovascular reflexes. Hence, exercise capacity is not impaired and orthostatic hypotension is minimal. In addition, captopril can be used safely in patients with bronchial asthma, a condition that precludes the use of beta$_2$-adrenergic antagonists. Captopril does not promote hypokalemia, hyperuricemia, or hyperglycemia—side effects seen with thiazide diuretics. Lastly, captopril does not induce lethargy, weakness, or sexual dysfunction—responses that are common with older antihypertensive agents.

Congestive Heart Failure. Captopril produces multiple benefits in congestive heart failure (CHF). By lowering arteriolar tone, captopril improves regional blood flow and, by reducing cardiac afterload, increases cardiac output. By causing venous dilation, the drug reduces pulmonary congestion and peripheral edema. By dilating blood vessels in the kidney, the drug increases renal blood flow, thereby promoting excretion of sodium and water. This loss of fluid has two beneficial effects: (1) it helps reduce edema, and (2) by lowering blood volume, it decreases venous return to the heart, thereby reducing right-heart size.

Adverse Effects

Captopril is generally well tolerated. In a group of patients receiving high-dose therapy (about 350 mg/day), less than 12% discontinued treatment because of intolerable reactions. The incidence of adverse effects can be minimized by using low doses (less than 150 mg/day).

First-Dose Hypotension. A precipitous drop in blood pressure may occur following the first dose of captopril and other ACE inhibitors. This reaction is caused by widespread vasodilation secondary to abrupt lowering of angiotensin II levels. First-dose hypotension is most likely in patients with severe hypertension, in patients taking diuretics, and in patients who are sodium depleted or volume depleted. To minimize the first-dose effect, initial doses should be low. Also, diuretics should be temporarily discontinued, starting 2 to 3 days before initiating captopril therapy. Blood pressure should be monitored for several hours following the first captopril dose. If hypotension develops, the patient should assume a supine position. If necessary, blood pressure can be raised with an infusion of normal saline.

Cough. Persistent, dry, irritating, nonproductive cough can develop with captopril and other ACE inhibitors. This reaction occurs in 1% to 12% of those treated, and is the most common reason for discontinuing therapy. Cough is more troublesome when the patient is supine, and occurs more frequently in women than men.

Hyperkalemia. Inhibition of aldosterone release (secondary to inhibition of angiotensin II production) can cause potassium retention by the kidney. As a rule, significant potassium accumulation is limited to patients taking potassium supplements or a potassium-sparing diuretic. For most other patients, hyperkalemia is rare. Patients should be instructed to avoid potassium supplements and potassium-containing salt substitutes unless they are prescribed by the physician.

Renal Failure. ACE inhibitors can cause severe renal insufficiency in patients with renal artery stenosis. In the presence of renal artery stenosis, the kidneys release large amounts of renin. The resulting high levels of angiotensin II serve to maintain glomerular filtration by two mechanisms: (1) elevation of blood pressure, and (2) constriction of efferent glomerular arterioles. When ACE is inhibited in these patients, causing angiotensin II levels to fall, the mechanisms that had been maintaining glomerular filtration fail, causing urine production to drop precipitously. Not surprisingly, *ACE inhibitors are contraindicated for patients with renal artery stenosis.*

Fetal Injury. Use of ACE inhibitors during the *second* and *third* trimesters of pregnancy can injure the developing fetus. Specific effects include hypotension, hyperkalemia, skull hypoplasia, anuria, renal failure (reversible and irreversible), and death. Women who become pregnant while using ACE inhibitors should discontinue treatment as soon as possible. Infants who have been exposed to ACE inhibitors during the second or third trimester should be closely monitored for hypotension, oliguria, and hyperkalemia. Exposure to ACE inhibitors during the *first* trimester is not associated with fetal injury; pregnant women who have taken ACE inhibitors during the first trimester should be told this.

Angioedema. Angioedema is a rare and potentially fatal reaction. Symptoms, which result from increased capillary permeability, include giant wheals and edema of the tongue, glottis, and pharynx. Severe reactions should be treated with subcutaneous epinephrine. If angioedema develops, captopril should be discontinued and never used again.

Dysgeusia and Rash. Dysgeusia (impaired or distorted sense of taste) and rash are common. Rashes (macropapular, morbilliform, others) develop in up to 10% of those treated. The incidence of dysgeusia is about 4%. For some patients, dysgeusia may result in anorexia and weight loss. If these complications arise, captopril should be withdrawn. Both reactions resolve following cessation of treatment. At one time, researchers thought that rash and dysgeusia were related to the sulfhydral group in the captopril molecule. However, this appears to be untrue, since ACE inhibitors that lack a sulfhydral group also cause these reactions.

Neutropenia. Neutropenia, with its associated risk of infection, is a rare but serious complication of therapy. Neutropenia is most likely in patients with renal impairment and in those with collagen vascular diseases (e.g., systemic lupus erythematosus, scleroderma). These patients should be followed closely. Fortunately, neutropenia is reversible if detected early. To promote early detection, a white blood cell count with differential should be obtained every 2 weeks during the first 3 months of therapy and periodically thereafter. If neutropenia develops, captopril should be withdrawn immediately; neutrophil counts should normalize in approximately 2 weeks. In the absence of early detection, neutropenia may progress to fatal agranulocytosis. Patients should be informed about early signs of infection (e.g., fever, sore throat) and instructed to report these immediately.

Other Adverse Effects. Captopril can cause a variety of *gastrointestinal disturbances* (e.g., nausea, vomiting, diarrhea, abdominal pain). *Proteinuria* has occurred, most often in patients with pre-existing renal disease. *Neurologic effects* include headache, dizziness, fatigue, paresthesias, and insomnia.

Drug Interactions

Diuretics. Diuretics may intensify first-dose hypotension. To prevent this interaction, diuretics should be withdrawn 2 to 3 days prior to initiating treatment with captopril. Diuretic therapy can be resumed later if needed.

Antihypertensive Agents. The hypotensive effects of captopril are often additive with those of other antihypertensive drugs (e.g., diuretics, sym-patholytics, vasodilators, calcium channel blockers). When captopril is added to an antihypertensive regimen, dosages of other drugs may require reduction.

Drugs That Raise Potassium Levels. Captopril increases the risk of hyperkalemia caused by *potassium supplements* and *potassium-sparing diuretics.* The risk of hyperkalemia is increased because, by suppressing aldosterone secretion, captopril can reduce excretion of potassium. To minimize the risk of hyperkalemia, potassium supplements and potassium-sparing diuretics should be employed only when clearly indicated.

Lithium. ACE inhibitors can increase serum lithium levels, causing toxicity. Lithium levels should be monitored frequently.

Preparations, Dosage, and Administration

Preparations. Captopril [Capoten] is dispensed in tablets (12.5, 25, 50, and 100 mg) for oral use. Also, the drug is available in a fixed-dose combination formulation with hydrochlorothiazide under the trade name Capozide.

Dosage and Administration. Captopril should be taken 1 hour before meals. Dosage must be individualized. The usual starting dosage for adults is 25 mg three times a day. For patients at high risk of first-dose hypotension, a smaller initial dosage should be employed (e.g., 6.25 mg three times a day). To achieve an optimum response, the dosage is gradually increased (to a maximum of 450 mg/day). Dosage must be lowered in patients with renal disease.

ENALAPRIL

Enalapril [Vasotec] is a prodrug that must be converted into its active form (enalaprilat) by the liver. Enalaprilat is a potent inhibitor of ACE.

Actions and Uses. Enalapril has pharmacologic actions and therapeutic uses like those of captopril. Approved indications are hypertension and congestive heart failure.

Pharmacokinetics. Enalapril is rapidly absorbed from the gastrointestinal (GI) tract, even in the presence of food. The extent of absorption is about 60%. Conversion to enalaprilat takes several hours. As a result, peak effects are delayed. Enalaprilat has a plasma half-life of 11 hours, considerably longer than that of captopril. Hence, unlike captopril, which must be administered two or three times a day, enalapril can be administered once a day. Renal insufficiency delays excretion of enalapril, and can thereby promote drug accumulation. To avoid accumulation, dosage should be reduced in the presence of kidney disease.

Adverse Effects and Interactions. Enalapril is generally well tolerated. Like captopril, enalapril can cause first-dose hypotension, persistent cough, hyperkalemia, angioedema, and renal failure (in patients with renal artery stenosis). Common but less serious reactions include headache

Table 37–1. ACE Inhibitors: Uses and Dosages

Generic Name [Trade Name]	Approved Uses		Dosage for Hypertension
	HTN	CHF	
Benazepril [Lotensin]	√		Initial: 10 mg once a day Usual: 20–40 mg 1 or 2 times/day Maximum: 80 mg/day In renal impairment: reduce dosage
Captopril [Capoten]	√	√	Initial: 25 mg 2 or 3 times/day Usual: 25–150 mg 2 or 3 times/day Maximum: 450 mg/day In renal impairment: reduce dosage
Enalapril [Vasotec]	√	√	Initial: 5 mg once a day Usual: 10–40 mg once or divided Maximum: 40 mg/day In renal impairment: reduce dosage
Fosinopril [Monopril]	√		Initial: 10 mg once a day Usual: 20–40 mg 1 or 2 times/day Maximum: 80 mg/day In renal impairment: no change in dosage
Lisinopril [Prinivil] [Zestril]	√		Initial: 10 mg once a day Usual: 20–40 mg once a day Maximum: 80 mg/day In renal impairment: reduce dosage
Quinapril [Accupril]	√		Initial: 10 mg once a day Usual: 20–80 mg once or divided Maximum: 80 mg/day In renal impairment: reduce dosage
Ramipril [Altace]	√		Initial: 2.5 mg once a day Usual: 5–10 mg 1 or 2 times/day Maximum: 20 mg/day In renal impairment: reduce dosage

HTN = hypertension, CHF = congestive heart failure

(5%), dizziness (5%), and fatigue (3%). Neutropenia and proteinurea have been reported. Rash and dysgeusia occur, but less frequently than with captopril. Like captopril, enalapril has important interactions with diuretics, antihypertensive agents, potassium supplements, potassium-sparing diuretics, and lithium.

Preparations, Dosage, and Administration. *Oral.* Enalapril maleate [Vasotec] is available in tablets (2.5, 5, 10, and 20 mg) for oral use. In contrast to captopril, enalapril may be administered with meals. The initial daily dosage is 2.5 mg for patients taking diuretics and for patients with kidney disease. An initial dosage of 5 mg/day is appropriate for most other patients. Maintenance dosages range from 10 to 40 mg/day.

Intravenous. The active form of enalapril (enalaprilat) [Vasotec I.V.] is available in solution (1.25 mg/ml) for intravenous administration. The initial dose is 1.25 mg administered over 5 minutes. Doses may be increased up to 5 mg, and may be repeated every 6 hours for up to 48 hours.

NEWER ACE INHIBITORS: BENAZEPRIL, FOSINOPRIL, LISINOPRIL, QUINAPRIL, AND RAMIPRIL

In addition to captopril and enalapril, five other ACE inhibitors are approved for use in the United States. All are similar to captopril. Their trade names, uses, and dosages are summarized in Table 37-1.

Basic Pharmacology. The newer ACE inhibitors have the same mechanism of action as captopril (inhibition of angiotensin-converting enzyme) and they all produce similar pharmacologic effects. All are approved for hypertension. However, in contrast to captopril and enalapril, none is approved for CHF. All share the same major adverse effects: persistent cough, first-dose hypotension, hyperkalemia, angioedema, and renal failure (if given to patients with renal artery stenosis). Furthermore, they all have important interactions with the same drugs: diuretics, antihypertensive agents, potassium supplements, potassium-sparing diuretics, and lithium. Except for lisinopril, all are prodrugs that undergo conversion to their active forms in the small intestine and liver.

Dosage and Administration. Like captopril, all of the newer ACE inhibitors are administered orally. However, they all differ from captopril in that (1) they can be administered with food, and (2) they have prolonged half-lives and, therefore, can be administered once daily. Dosages for hypertension are summarized in Table 37-1. With the exception of fosinopril, all of these drugs require a reduction in dosage for patients with renal insufficiency.

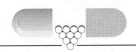

Summary of Major Nursing Implications

ANGIOTENSIN-CONVERTING ENZYME INHIBITORS

Benazepril	Lisinopril
Captopril	Quinapril
Enalapril	Ramipril
Fosinopril	

Unless indicated otherwise, the implications summarized below pertain to all of the ACE inhibitors.

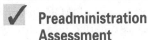

Preadministration Assessment

Therapeutic Goal

Reduction of blood pressure in patients with hypertension (all ACE inhibitors).

Hemodynamic improvement in patients with congestive heart failure *(captopril, enalapril)*.

Baseline Data

Determine blood pressure and obtain white blood cell count and differential.

Identifying High-Risk Patients

ACE inhibitors are *contraindicated* during the *second and third trimesters of pregnancy* and for patients with *renal artery stenosis* or a *history of hypersensitivity reactions* (e.g., angioedema) *to ACE inhibitors.* Exercise *caution* in patients with *salt or volume depletion, renal impairment,* or *collagen disease,* and in those taking *potassium supplements, potassium-sparing diuretics,* or *lithium.*

Implementation: Administration

Routes

Oral: all ACE inhibitors.
Intravenous: *enalaprilat* only.

Dosage and Administration

Begin therapy with low doses and then gradually increase the dosage.
Instruct patients to administer *captopril* 1 hour before meals.

Ongoing Evaluation and Interventions

Monitoring Summary

Monitor blood pressure closely for 2 hours after the first dose, and periodically thereafter. Obtain a white blood cell count and differential every 2 weeks for the first 3 months of therapy and periodically thereafter.

Evaluating Therapeutic Effects

Hypertension. Monitor for lowering of blood pressure. The usual target pressure is systolic/diastolic of 140/90 mm Hg.

Congestive Heart Failure. Monitor for lessening of signs and symptoms (e.g., dyspnea, cyanosis, jugular vein distention, edema).

Minimizing Adverse Effects

First-Dose Hypotension. Severe hypotension can occur with the first dose. Minimize with low initial doses and by withdrawing diuretics 1 week before treatment. Monitor blood pressure for 2 hours following the first dose. Instruct patients to lie down if hypotension develops. If necessary, infuse normal saline to restore pressure.

Cough. Warn patients about the possibility of persistent, dry, irritating, nonproductive cough. Instruct them to consult the physician if cough is bothersome. Therapy may need to be discontinued.

Hyperkalemia. ACE inhibitors may increase potassium levels. Instruct patients to avoid potassium supplements, potassium-containing salt substitutes, and potassium-sparing diuretics unless they are prescribed by the physician.

Fetal Injury. Warn women of child-bearing age that use of ACE inhibitors during the *second* and *third* trimester of pregnancy can cause fetal injury (hypotension, hyperkalemia, skull hypoplasia, anuria, reversible and irreversible renal failure, death). If the patient becomes pregnant, withdraw ACE inhibitors as soon as possible. Closely monitor infants who have been exposed to ACE inhibitors during the second or third trimester for hypotension, oliguria, and hyperkalemia. Reassure women who took ACE inhibitors during the *first* trimester that this does *not* represent a risk to the fetus.

Angioedema. This is a rare and potentially fatal reaction whose symptoms include giant wheals and edema of the tongue, glottis, and pharynx. If angioedema occurs, discontinue the ACE inhibitor and never use it again. Treat severe reactions with subcutaneous epinephrine.

Renal Failure. Renal failure is a risk for patients with renal artery stenosis. ACE inhibitors are contraindicated for these people.

Rash and Dysgeusia (mainly with *captopril*). Minimize these reactions by avoiding high doses. Instruct patients to notify the physician if rash or dysgeusia persist. If dysgeusia results in anorexia and weight loss, withdraw the drug. Rash and dysgeusia resolve with cessation of treatment.

Neutropenia (mainly with *captopril*). Neutropenia poses a high risk of infection. Inform patients about early signs of infection (fever, sore throat, mouth sores) and instruct them to notify the physician if these occur. Obtain white blood cell counts and differential every 2 weeks during the first 3 months of therapy and periodically thereafter. If neutropenia develops, withdraw the drug immediately; neutrophil counts should normalize in approximately 2 weeks. Neutropenia is most likely in patients with renal impairment and collagen vascular diseases (e.g., systemic lupus erythematosus, scleroderma); monitor these patients closely.

Minimizing Adverse Interactions

Diuretics. Diuretics may intensify first-dose hypotension. Withdraw diuretics 1 week prior to beginning an ACE inhibitor. Diuretics may be resumed later if needed.

Antihypertensive Agents. The effects of ACE inhibitors are additive with those of other antihypertensive drugs (e.g., diuretics, sympatholytics, vasodilators, calcium channel blockers). When an ACE inhibitor is added to an antihypertensive regimen, dosages of the other drugs may require reduction.

Drugs That Elevate Potassium Levels. ACE inhibitors increase the risk of hyperkalemia associated with *potassium supplements* and *potassium-sparing diuretics*. This risk can be minimized by avoiding potassium supplements and potassium-sparing diuretics except when they are clearly indicated.

Lithium. ACE inhibitors can increase serum levels of lithium, causing toxicity. Monitor lithium levels frequently.

Calcium Channel Blockers

C alcium channel blockers are drugs that prevent calcium ions from entering cells. These drugs have their greatest effects on the heart and blood vessels. Over the last decade, the calcium channel blockers have assumed a prominent role in the treatment of hypertension and angina pectoris. In addition, some of these drugs are used to treat cardiac dysrhythmias. Alternative names for the calcium channel blockers are *calcium antagonists* and *slow channel blockers*.

CALCIUM CHANNELS: PHYSIOLOGIC FUNCTIONS AND CONSEQUENCES OF BLOCKADE

Calcium channels are specialized pores in the cytoplasmic membrane that regulate the entry of calcium ions into cells. Calcium entry plays a critical role in the function of vascular smooth muscle and the heart.

Vascular Smooth Muscle

The role of calcium channels in vascular smooth muscle (VSM) is to regulate contraction. When a muscle action potential travels down the surface of a smooth muscle cell, calcium channels are caused to open and calcium ions flow inward, thereby initiating the contractile process. If calcium channels

465

are blocked, contraction will be prevented, and vasodilation will result.

At therapeutic doses, calcium channel blockers act selectively on *peripheral arterioles* and *arteries and arterioles of the heart*. These drugs have no significant effect on veins.

Heart

Myocardium. In cardiac muscle, calcium entry promotes contraction. Hence, calcium influx has a positive inotropic effect (increased force of contraction). If calcium channels in atrial and ventricular muscle are blocked, contractile force will diminish.

Sinoauricular Node. Pacemaker activity of the sinoauricular (S-A) node is regulated by calcium influx. When calcium channels are open, spontaneous discharge of the S-A node increases. Conversely, when calcium channels close, pacemaker activity declines. Hence, the effect of calcium channel blockade is to reduce heart rate.

Atrioventricular Node. Impulses that originate in the S-A must pass through the atrioventricular (A-V) node on their way to the ventricles. Regulation of A-V conduction plays a critical role in coordinating contraction of the ventricles with contraction of the atria.

The excitability of A-V nodal cells is regulated by calcium entry. When calcium channels are open, calcium entry increases, and cells of the A-V node discharge more readily. Conversely, when calcium channels are closed, discharge of A-V nodal cells is suppressed. Hence, the effect of calcium channel blockade is to decrease velocity of conduction through the A-V node.

CLASSIFICATION OF CALCIUM CHANNEL BLOCKERS

The calcium channel blockers can be grouped on the basis of their chemical structures and their prominent pharmacologic effects.

Chemical Classification

The calcium channel blockers used in the United States belong to three chemical families. The largest family is the *dihydropyridines*, for which *nifedipine* is the prototype. This family name is encountered frequently and is worth remembering. The other two families consist of orphans: *verapamil* is the only *phenylakylamine*, and *diltiazem* is the only *benzothiazepine*. The drug names are important; the family names are not.

Pharmacodynamic Classification

The calcium channel blockers can be placed into two pharmacodynamic groups: (1) agents that act on VSM *and* the heart, and (2) agents that act mainly on VSM. Individual calcium channel blockers differ with respect to their abilities to block calcium channels in the heart and VSM. These differences are based on structural differences among the drugs and on structural differences among calcium channels. All of the calcium channel blockers are able to block calcium channels in VSM. However, at usual therapeutic doses, only two agents—verapamil and diltiazem—produce significant blockade of calcium channels in the heart. As a result, verapamil and diltiazem have clinically significant effects on the heart *and* VSM, whereas all of the other calcium channel blockers (which happen to be dihydropyridines) act almost exclusively on VSM. Because of these pharmacodynamic differences, verapamil and diltiazem can be used to treat cardiac dysrhythmias in addition to hypertension and angina pectoris. In contrast, major applications of the dihydropyridines are limited to hypertension and angina.

AGENTS THAT ACT ON VASCULAR SMOOTH MUSCLE AND THE HEART

VERAPAMIL

Verapamil [Calan, Isoptin, Verelan] blocks calcium channels in blood vessels and in the heart. Major indications for the drug are angina pectoris, essential hypertension, and cardiac dysrhythmias. Verapamil was the first calcium channel blocker available and will serve as our prototype for the group.

Hemodynamic Effects

The overall hemodynamic response to verapamil is the net result of (1) direct effects on the heart and blood vessels, and (2) reflex responses.

Direct Effects. By blocking calcium channels in the heart and blood vessels, verapamil has five direct effects: (1) blockade at peripheral arterioles causes dilation, and thereby reduces arterial pressure; (2) blockade at arteries and arterioles of the heart increases coronary perfusion; (3) blockade at the S-A node reduces heart rate; (4) blockade at the A-V node decreases A-V nodal conduction; and (5) blockade in the myocardium decreases force of contraction. Of the effects on the heart, reduced A-V conduction is the most important.

Indirect (Reflex) Effects. Verapamil-induced lowering of blood pressure activates the baroreceptor reflex, causing increased firing of sympathetic nerves to the heart. Norepinephrine released from these nerves acts to increase heart rate, A-V conduction, and force of contraction. However, since these same three parameters are suppressed by the direct actions of verapamil, the direct and indirect effects tend to negate each other.

Net Effect. Since the direct effects of verapamil on the heart are counterbalanced by indirect effects, the drug has little or no net effect on cardiac performance: for most patients, heart rate, A-V conduction, and contractility are not noticeably altered. Consequently, the overall cardiovascular effect of verapamil is simply vasodilation accompanied by reduced arterial pressure and increased coronary perfusion.

Pharmacokinetics

Verapamil may be administered orally and intravenously. The drug is well absorbed following oral administration, but undergoes extensive metabolism on its first pass through the liver. Consequently, only about 20% of an oral dose reaches the systemic circulation. Effects begin in 30 minutes and peak within 5 hours. Elimination is primarily by hepatic metabolism. Because the drug is eliminated by the liver, doses must be reduced substantially in patients with liver dysfunction.

Therapeutic Uses

Angina Pectoris. Verapamil is used widely to treat angina pectoris. The drug is approved for both vasospastic angina and effort-induced angina. Benefits in both types of angina derive from vasodilation. The role of verapamil in antianginal therapy is discussed further in Chapter 41.

Essential Hypertension. Verapamil is a first-line drug for treatment of chronic hypertension. The drug lowers blood pressure by promoting dilation of arterioles. The role of verapamil and other calcium channel blockers in hypertension is discussed in Chapter 40.

Cardiac Dysrhythmias. Verapamil is used to slow ventricular rate in patients with atrial flutter, atrial fibrillation, and paroxysmal supraventricular tachycardia. Benefits derive from the drug's ability to suppress impulse conduction through the A-V node, thereby preventing the ventricles from being driven at an excessive rate. Antidysrhythmic applications are discussed in Chapter 44.

Migraine. Verapamil has been used on an investigational basis to relieve migraine headache. This application is discussed in Chapter 29.

Adverse Effects

Common Effects. Verapamil is generally well tolerated. *Constipation* occurs frequently and is the most common cause of complaints. This prob-

lem, which can be especially severe in the elderly, can be minimized by increasing dietary fluids and fiber. Other common effects—*dizziness, facial flushing, headache,* and *edema of the ankles and feet*—occur secondary to vasodilation. *Gingival hyperplasia* (overgrowth of gum tissue) may also develop.

Cardiac Effects. Blockade of calcium channels in the heart can compromise cardiac function. In the S-A node, calcium channel blockade can cause bradycardia; in the A-V node, blockade can cause partial or complete A-V block; in the myocardium, blockade can decrease contractility. When the heart is healthy, these effects are minimal. However, in patients with certain cardiac diseases, verapamil can seriously exacerbate dysfunction. Accordingly, the drug must be used with special caution in patients with cardiac failure, and must not be used at all in patients with sick sinus syndrome or second-degree or third-degree A-V block.

Drug Interactions

Digoxin. Like verapamil, digoxin suppresses impulse conduction through the A-V node. Accordingly, when these drugs are used concurrently, the risk of A-V block is increased. Patients receiving the combination should be monitored closely.

With long-term use, verapamil increases plasma levels of digoxin by 50% to 70%. Digoxin dosage should be reduced to prevent toxicity.

Beta-Adrenergic Blocking Agents. Drugs that block beta$_1$ receptors in the heart have the same cardiac effects as verapamil: decreased heart rate, decreased A-V conduction, and decreased contractility. Hence, when a beta blocker and verapamil are used concurrently, there is a risk of excessive cardiosuppression. To minimize this risk, beta blockers and *intravenous* verapamil should be administered several hours apart from each other.

Toxicity

Clinical Manifestations. Overdosage can produce severe hypotension and cardiotoxicity (bradycardia, A-V block, ventricular tachydysrhythmias).

Treatment. *General Measures.* Verapamil can be removed from the gastrointestinal tract with an emetic or with gastric lavage followed by a cathartic. Intravenous calcium gluconate can counteract vasodilation and the drug's negative inotropic effects, but will not reverse A-V block.

Hypotension. Hypotension can be treated with intravenous *norepinephrine,* which promotes vasoconstriction (by activating alpha$_1$ receptors on blood vessels) and increases cardiac output (by activating beta$_1$ receptors in the heart). Placing the patient in Trendelenburg's position (inclined with the head down) and administering IV fluids may also be helpful.

Bradycardia and A-V Block. Bradycardia and A-V block can be treated with isoproterenol (a beta-adrenergic agonist) and with atropine (an anticholinergic drug that will block parasympathetic influences on the heart). If pharmacologic measures are inadequate, electronic pacing may be required.

Ventricular Tachydysrhythmias. The preferred treatment for ventricular dysrhythmias is DC cardioversion. Antidysrhythmic drugs (procainamide, lidocaine) may also be tried.

Preparations, Dosage, and Administration

Oral. Verapamil is available in regular tablets (40, 80, and 120 mg) as Calan and Isoptin; in sustained-release tablets (120, 180, and 240 mg) as Calan SR and Isoptin SR; and in sustained-release capsules (180 and 240 mg) as Verelan. The sustained-release formulations are approved only for essential hypertension. Instruct patients to swallow sustained-release formulations intact, without crushing or chewing.

The usual initial dosage for *angina pectoris* is 80 to 120 mg three times a day. The usual initial dosage for *essential hypertension* is 80 mg three times a day (using standard tablets) or 240 mg of a sustained release formulation (administered once a day in the morning with food). Dosages should be reduced for elderly patients and for patients with advanced renal or liver disease. Dosages for dysrhythmias are presented in Chapter 44.

Intravenous. Intravenous verapamil [Isoptin] is used to treat cardiac dysrhythmias. Since IV verapamil can cause severe adverse cardiovascular effects, blood pressure and the electrocardiogram (EKG) should be monitored, and equipment for resuscitation should be immediately available. Intravenous dosages for dysrhythmias are presented in Chapter 44.

DILTIAZEM

Like verapamil, diltiazem [Cardizem, Dilacor] blocks calcium channels in the heart and blood vessels. As a result, the actions and applications of these drugs are very similar.

Hemodynamic Effects. Diltiazem has the same effects on cardiovascular function as verapamil: both drugs lower blood pressure through arteriolar dilation and both have little net effect on the heart, since their direct suppressant actions are balanced by reflex cardiac stimulation.

Therapeutic Uses. Like verapamil, diltiazem is used to treat angina pectoris, essential hypertension, and cardiac dysrhythmias (atrial flutter, atrial fibrillation, paroxysmal supraventricular tachycardia).

Pharmacokinetics. Oral diltiazem is well absorbed and then extensively metabolized on its first pass through the liver. As a result, bioavailability is only about 50%. Effects begin rapidly (within a few minutes) and peak within half an hour. The drug undergoes nearly complete metabolism prior to elimination in the urine and feces.

Adverse Effects. The adverse effects of diltiazem are like those of verapamil, except that diltiazem causes less constipation. The most common effects are dizziness, flushing, headache, and edema of the ankles and feet. Like verapamil, diltiazem can exacerbate cardiac dysfunction in patients with bradycardia, sick-sinus syndrome, second- or third-degree A-V block, or congestive heart failure.

Drug Interactions. Like verapamil, diltiazem can exacerbate digoxin-induced suppression of A-V conduction, and can intensify the cardiosuppressant effects of beta blockers. Patients receiving diltiazem concurrently with digoxin or a beta blocker should be monitored closely for cardiac status.

Preparations, Dosage, and Administration. *Oral* diltiazem is available in standard tablets (30, 60, 90, and 120 mg) as Cardizem and in sustained-release capsules (60, 90, 120, 180, and 240 mg) as Cardizem SR, Cardizem CD, and Dilacor XR. The drug is also available in solution (5 mg/ml) for *parenteral* administration. The usual initial dosage for *hypertension* is 180 mg once a day with Cardizem CD or 60 to 120 mg twice a day with Cardizem SR or Dilacor XR. *Angina pectoris* can be treated with standard tablets (30 mg qid initially and 60 mg qid for maintenance).

DIHYDROPYRIDINES: AGENTS THAT ACT MAINLY ON VASCULAR SMOOTH MUSCLE

All of the drugs discussed in this section belong to the *dihydropyridine* family. At therapeutic doses, these drugs produce significant blockade of calcium channels in blood vessels and minimal blockade of calcium channels in the heart. The dihydropyridines are similar to verapamil in some respects, but quite different in others.

NIFEDIPINE

Nifedipine [Adalat, Procardia] was the first dihydropyridine available and will serve as our prototype for the family. Like verapamil, nifedipine blocks calcium channels in VSM and thereby promotes vasodilation. However, in contrast to verapamil, nifedipine produces very little blockade of calcium channels in the heart. As a result, nifedipine cannot be used to treat dysrhythmias, does not cause adverse cardiac effects, and is less likely than verapamil to exacerbate pre-existing cardiac disorders. Nifedipine also differs from verapamil in that nifedipine is more likely to cause reflex tachycardia. Contrasts between nifedipine and verapamil are summarized in Table 38–1.

Hemodynamic Effects

Direct Effects. The direct effects of nifedipine on the cardiovascular system are limited to blockade of calcium channels in vascular smooth muscle. Blockade of calcium channels in peripheral arterioles causes vasodilation, and thereby lowers arterial pressure. Blockade of calcium channels in arteries and arterioles of the heart increases coronary perfusion. Since nifedipine does not block cardiac calcium channels at usual therapeutic doses, the drug causes minimal reductions in automaticity, A-V conduction, and contractile force.

Indirect (Reflex) Effects. By lowering blood pressure, nifedipine activates the baroreceptor reflex, thereby causing sympathetic stimulation of the heart. Since nifedipine has minimal direct cardiosuppressant actions, cardiac stimulation is unopposed; hence, heart rate and contractile force increase.

Net Effect. The overall hemodynamic response to nifedipine is simply the sum of its direct effect (vasodilation) and indirect effect (reflex cardiac stimulation). Hence, nifedipine (1) lowers blood pressure, (2) increases heart rate, and (3) increases contractile force.

Pharmacokinetics

Nifedipine is well absorbed following oral administration, but undergoes extensive first-pass metabolism. As a result, only about 50% of an oral dose reaches the systemic circulation. Effects begin within 30 minutes and peak in 1 to 3 hours. The drug is fully metabolized prior to excretion in the urine.

Table 38–1. Comparisons and Contrasts Between Verapamil and Nifedipine

	Drug	
Property	Verapamil	Nifedipine
Direct Effects on the Heart and Blood Vessels		
Arteriolar dilation	Yes	Yes
Effects on the heart		
↓ Automaticity	Yes	No
↓ A–V conduction	Yes	No
↓ Contractility	Yes	No
Indications		
Hypertension	Yes	Yes
Angina pectoris	Yes	Yes
Dysrhythmias	Yes	No
Adverse Effects		
Exacerbation of A–V block Sick–sinus syndrome Congestive heart failure	Yes	No
Constipation	Yes	No
Reflex tachycardia	No	Yes
Edema (ankles and feet)	Yes	Yes
Flushing	Yes	Yes
Headache	Yes	Yes
Dizziness	Yes	Yes
Drug Interactions		
Exacerbates A–V block caused by digoxin	Yes	No
Augments cardiosuppressant effects of beta blockers	Yes	No

Therapeutic Uses

Angina Pectoris. Nifedipine is indicated for vasospastic angina and angina of effort. The drug is usually combined with a beta blocker to prevent reflex stimulation of the heart, which could intensify anginal pain. The role of nifedipine in angina is discussed further in Chapter 41.

Hypertension. Nifedipine is used widely to treat *essential hypertension* and *hypertensive emergencies*. For therapy of essential hypertension, only the sustained-release formulation is approved. The use of nifedipine in hypertensive emergencies is discussed in Chapter 40.

Migraine. Nifedipine has been used on an investigational basis to relieve migraine headache. This application is discussed in Chapter 29.

Adverse Effects

Some adverse effects of nifedipine are like those of verapamil, whereas others are quite different. Like verapamil, nifedipine can cause *flushing, dizziness, headache, peripheral edema,* and *gingival hyperplasia*. In contrast to verapamil, nifedipine

does *not* cause much constipation. Also, since nifedipine causes minimal blockade of calcium channels in the heart, the drug is not likely to exacerbate A-V block, congestive heart failure, bradycardia, or sick-sinus syndrome. Accordingly, nifedipine is preferred to verapamil for patients with these disorders.

A response that occurs with nifedipine that does not occur with verapamil is *reflex tachycardia*. This response is problematic in that it increases cardiac oxygen demand, and can thereby increase pain in patients with angina. To prevent reflex tachycardia, nifedipine can be combined with a beta-adrenergic blocker (e.g., propranolol).

Drug Interactions

Beta-Adrenergic Blockers. Beta blockers are combined with nifedipine to prevent reflex tachycardia. It is important to note that whereas beta blockers can *decrease* the adverse cardiac effects of *nifedipine*, they can *intensify* the adverse cardiac effects of *verapamil* and *diltiazem*.

Toxicity

When taken in excessive dosage, nifedipine loses its selectivity. Hence, toxic doses affect the heart in addition to blood vessels. Consequently, the manifestations and treatment of nifedipine overdosage are the same as those described above for verapamil.

Preparations, Dosage, and Administration

Nifedipine is available in capsules (10 and 20 mg) as Adalat and Procardia and in sustained-release tablets (30, 60, and 90 mg) as Procardia XL. Instruct patients to swallow sustained-release tablets whole, without crushing or chewing.

For treatment of *angina pectoris*, the usual initial dosage is 10 mg three times a day. The usual maintenance dosage is 10 to 20 mg three times a day. The maximum recommended dosage is 180 mg/day.

For *essential hypertension*, only the sustained-release tablets are approved. The usual initial dosage is 30 mg once a day.

OTHER DIHYDROPYRIDINES

All of these drugs are similar to nifedipine, the prototype of the dihydropyridines. Like nifedipine, these drugs produce greater blockade of calcium channels in VSM than in the heart.

Nicardipine. At therapeutic doses, nicardipine [Cardene, Cardene SR] produces selective blockade of calcium channels in blood vessels, and has minimal direct effects on the heart. The drug is indicated for essential hypertension and for effort-induced angina pectoris. The most common adverse effects are flushing, headache, asthenia (weakness), dizziness, palpitations, and edema of the ankles and feet. Gingival hyperplasia (overgrowth of gum tissue) has been reported. Like nifedipine, this drug can be combined safely with a beta-adrenergic blocker to promote therapeutic effects and suppress reflex tachycardia. Nicardipine is available in standard capsules (20 and 30 mg) and sustained-release capsules (30, 45, and 60 mg) for oral use. The usual initial dosage for angina pectoris is 20 mg tid using the standard capsules. The usual initial dosage for essential hypertension is 20 mg tid (using standard capsules) or 30 mg bid (using sustained-release capsules).

Amlodipine. At therapeutic doses, amlodipine [Norvasc] produces "selective" blockade of calcium channels in blood vessels, having minimal direct effects on the heart. Approved indications are essential hypertension and angina pectoris (effort-induced and vasospastic). Amlodipine is administered orally and absorbed slowly; peak plasma levels develop in 6 to 12 hours. The drug has a long half-life (30 to 50 hours) and, therefore, is effective with once-a-day dosing. The principal adverse effects are peripheral and facial edema. Flushing, dizziness, and headache may also occur. In contrast to other dihydropyridines, amlodipine causes little reflex tachycardia. The usual initial dosage for hypertension and angina pectoris is 5 mg once a day.

Isradipine. Like nifedipine, isradipine [DynaCirc] produces relatively selective blockade of calcium channels in blood vessels. In the United States, the drug is approved only for hypertension. Isradipine is rapidly absorbed following oral administration, but undergoes extensive metabolism on its first pass through the liver. The drug and its metabolites are excreted in the urine. The most common side effects are facial flushing (11%), headache (14%), dizziness (7%), and ankle edema (7%). In contrast to nifedipine, isradipine causes minimal reflex tachycardia. The drug is available in 2.5- and 5-mg capsules. The usual antihypertensive dosage is 2.5 to 5 mg twice a day.

Felodipine. Felodipine [Plendil] produces "selective" blockade of calcium channels in blood vessels. In the United States, the drug is approved only for essential hypertension. Felodipine is well absorbed following oral administration, but undergoes extensive first-pass metabolism. As a result, bioavailability is only 20%. Plasma levels peak in 2.5 to 5 hours and then decay with a half-life of 24 hours. Because of this prolonged half-life, felodipine is effective with once-a-day dosing. Characteristic adverse effects are reflex tachycardia, peripheral edema, headache, facial flushing, and dizziness. Gingival hyperplasia has been reported. Felodipine is dispensed in 5- and 10-mg extended-release tablets. The usual dosage for hypertension is 5 to 10 mg once a day.

Nimodipine. Nimodipine [Nimotop] produces selective blockade of calcium channels in *cerebral blood vessels*. The drug's only approved application is prophylaxis of neurologic injury following rupture of an intracranial aneurysm. Benefits derive from preventing the cerebral arterial spasm that follows subarachnoid hemorrhage (SAH) and can result in ischemic neurologic injury. Dosing (60 mg every 4 hours) should begin within 96 hours of SAH and should continue for 21 days. As discussed in Chapter 29, nimodipine may also be useful against migraine.

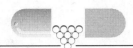

Summary of Major Nursing Implications

VERAPAMIL AND DILTIAZEM

**Preadministration
Assessment**

Therapeutic Goal

Verapamil and diltiazem are indicated for *hypertension, angina pectoris,* and *cardiac dysrhythmias.*

Baseline Data

For *all patients,* determine blood pressure and pulse rate, and obtain laboratory evaluations of liver and kidney function. For patients with *angina pectoris,* obtain baseline data on the frequency and severity of anginal attacks. For baseline data relevant to *hypertension,* refer to Chapter 40.

Identifying High-Risk Patients

Verapamil and diltiazem are *contraindicated* for patients with *severe hypotension, sick-sinus syndrome* (in the absence of electronic pacing), and *second- or third-degree A-V block.* Use with *caution* in patients with *congestive heart failure* or *liver dysfunction* and in patients *taking digoxin* or *beta-adrenergic blocking agents.*

**Implementation:
Administration**

Routes

Oral, intravenous.

Administration

Oral. *Verapamil* and *diltiazem* may be used for angina pectoris and essential hypertension. *Verapamil* may be used with digoxin to control ventricular rate in patients with atrial fibrillation and atrial flutter.

Sustained-release formulations are reserved for essential hypertension. Instruct patients to swallow sustained-release formulation whole, without crushing or chewing.

Prior to administration, measure blood pressure and pulse rate. If hypotension or bradycardia is detected, withhold medication and notify the physician.

Intravenous. Intravenous therapy is used for cardiac dysrhythmias. Perform injections slowly (over 2 to 3 minutes). Monitor the EKG for A-V block, sudden reduction in heart rate, and prolongation of the P-R or Q-T interval. Have facilities for cardioversion and cardiac pacing immediately available.

**Ongoing
Evaluation and
Interventions**

Evaluating Therapeutic Effects

Angina Pectoris. Keep an ongoing record of anginal attacks, noting the time and intensity of each attack and the likely precipitating event. Teach outpatients to chart the time, intensity, and circumstances of their attacks.

Essential Hypertension. Monitor blood pressure periodically. The goal is to reduce systolic/diastolic pressure to 140/90 mm Hg. Teach patients to self-monitor their blood pressure and to maintain a blood pressure record.

Minimizing Adverse Effects

Cardiosuppression. Verapamil and diltiazem can cause bradycardia, A-V block, and congestive heart failure. Inform patients about manifestations of cardiac effects (e.g., slow heart beat, shortness of breath, weight gain) and instruct them to notify the physician if these occur. If cardiac impairment is severe, drug use should be discontinued.

Peripheral Edema. Inform patients about signs of edema (swelling in ankles or feet) and instruct them to notify the physician if these occur. If necessary, edema can be reduced with a diuretic.

Constipation. This response occurs primarily with *verapamil*. Constipation can be minimized by increasing dietary fluids and fiber.

Minimizing Adverse Interactions

Digoxin. The combination of digoxin with verapamil or diltiazem increases the risk of partial or complete A-V block. Monitor for indications of impaired A-V conduction.

Verapamil (and possibly diltiazem) can increase plasma levels of digoxin. Digoxin dosage should be reduced.

Beta-Adrenergic Blocking Agents. Concurrent use of a beta blocker with verapamil or diltiazem can cause bradycardia, A-V block, or congestive heart failure. Monitor the patient closely for cardiac suppression. Administer *intravenous verapamil* and beta blockers several hours apart from each other.

Managing Acute Toxicity

Remove unabsorbed drug with an emetic or with gastric lavage followed by a cathartic. Give intravenous calcium to help counteract excessive vasodilation and reduced myocardial contractility.

To raise blood pressure, give intravenous norepinephrine. Intravenous fluids and placing the patient in Trendelenburg's position can also help.

Bradycardia and A-V block can be reversed with isoproterenol and atropine. If these drugs are inadequate, electronic pacing may be required.

Ventricular tachydysrhythmias can be treated with DC cardioversion. Antidysrhythmic drugs (lidocaine or procainamide) may also be used.

DIHYDROPYRIDINES

Amlodipine	Nifedipine
Isradipine	Nicardipine
Felodipine	Nimodipine

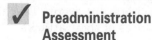
✓ **Preadministration Assessment**

Therapeutic Goal

Amlodipine, nifedipine, and *nicardipine* are approved for *essential hypertension* and *angina pectoris. Isradipine* and *felodipine* are approved for *hypertension* only.

Baseline Data

See implications for verapamil and diltiazem

Identifying High-Risk Patients

Use bipyridines with *caution* in patients with *hypotension, sick-sinus syndrome* (in the absence of electronic pacing), *angina pectoris* (because of reflex tachycardia), *congestive heart failure,* and *second- or third-degree A-V block.*

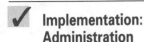

Route

All bipyridines are given orally.

Administration

Instruct patients to swallow sustained-release formulations whole, without crushing or chewing.

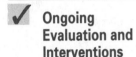

Evaluating Therapeutic Effects

See implications for verapamil and diltiazem.

Minimizing Adverse Effects

Reflex Tachycardia. Reflex tachycardia can be suppressed with a beta blocker.

Peripheral Edema. Inform patients about signs of edema (swelling in ankles or feet) and instruct them to notify the physician if these occur. If necessary, edema can be reduced with a diuretic.

Managing Acute Toxicity

See implications for verapamil and diltiazem.

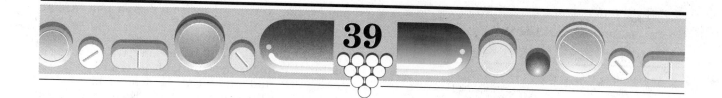

Vasodilators

Vasodilation can be produced with a wide variety of drugs. The major classes of vasodilators along with representative agents are shown in Table 39–1. Some of these drugs act primarily on arterioles, some act primarily on veins, and some dilate both types of vessel. The vasodilators are widely used, having indications that range from hypertension to angina pectoris to heart failure. Many of the vasodilators have been discussed in previous chapters. Four agents—hydralazine, minoxidil, diazoxide, and nitroprusside—are introduced here.

In approaching the vasodilators, we will begin by considering concepts that apply to the vasodilators as a group. We will then discuss the pharmacology of individual agents.

BASIC CONCEPTS IN VASODILATOR PHARMACOLOGY

SELECTIVITY OF VASODILATORY EFFECTS

It is important to appreciate that vasodilators differ from one another with respect to the types of blood vessels they affect. Some agents (e.g., hydralazine) produce selective dilation of arterioles. Others (e.g., nitroglycerin) produce selective dilation of veins. And still others (e.g., prazosin) exert approximately equal effects on arterioles and veins. The selectivity of the major vasodilators is summarized in Table 39–2.

The selectivity of a vasodilator determines its hemodynamic effects. For example, dilators of *re-*

Table 39–1. Types of Vasodilators

Category	Examples
Angiotensin-Converting Enzyme Inhibitors	Captopril Enalapril Lisinopril
Organic Nitrates	Nitroglycerin Isosorbide dinitrate
Calcium Channel Blockers	Verapamil Nifedipine Diltiazem
Sympatholytics Alpha–adrenergic blockers	Phentolamine Prazosin Terazosin
Ganglionic blockers	Mecamylamine Trimethaphan
Adrenergic neuron blockers	Reserpine Guanethidine
Centrally acting agents	Clonidine Methyldopa
Other Important Vasodilators	Hydralazine Minoxidil Nitroprusside Diazoxide

sistance vessels (arterioles) cause a decrease in cardiac *afterload* (the force against which the heart must work to pump blood). By decreasing afterload, arteriolar dilators reduce cardiac work while at the same time causing cardiac output and tissue perfusion to increase. In contrast, dilators of *capacitance vessels* (veins) cause a reduction in cardiac *preload* (the force with which blood is returned to the heart). By decreasing preload, venous dilators cause a decrease in cardiac filling

Table 39–2. Vasodilator Selectivity

Vasodilator	Site of Vasodilation	
	Arterioles	*Veins*
Diazoxide	+	
Hydralazine	+	
Minoxidil	+	
Diltiazem	+	
Nifedipine	+	
Verapamil	+	
Prazosin	+	+
Terazosin	+	+
Phentolamine	+	+
Nitroprusside	+	+
Captopril	+	+
Enalapril	+	+
Lisinopril	+	+
Nitroglycerin		+
Isosorbide dinitrate		+

and cardiac work, along with a decrease in cardiac output and tissue perfusion.

Because hemodynamic responses to arteriolar and venous dilation differ, the selectivity of a vasodilator is a major determinant of its effects, both therapeutic and undesired. Undesired effects related to selective dilation of arterioles and veins are discussed below. Therapeutic implications of selective dilation are discussed in Chapters 40, 41, and 42—the chapters in which the primary uses of the vasodilators are presented.

OVERVIEW OF THERAPEUTIC USES

The vasodilators, as a group, have a broad spectrum of applications. Principal indications are *essential hypertension, hypertensive crisis, angina pectoris,* and *congestive heart failure.* Additional indications include *pheochromocytoma, peripheral vascular disease,* and *production of controlled hypotension during surgery.* The specific applications of any particular agent are determined by its pharmacologic profile. Important facets of that profile are route of administration, site of vasodilation (arterioles, veins, or both), and intensity and duration of effects.

ADVERSE EFFECTS RELATED TO VASODILATION

Postural Hypotension

Postural (orthostatic) hypotension is defined as a fall in blood pressure brought on by moving from a supine or seated position to an upright position. The underlying cause of orthostatic hypotension is relaxation of smooth muscle in *veins.* Because of venous relaxation, gravity causes blood to "pool" within veins, thereby decreasing venous return to the heart. This reduction in venous return causes a decrease in cardiac output and a corresponding drop in blood pressure. Hypotension from venous dilation is minimal in recumbent subjects because gravity has only a small effect on venous return when we are lying down.

Patients receiving vasodilators should be informed about symptoms of hypotension (lightheadedness, dizziness) and advised to sit or lie down if these occur, since failure to do so may result in fainting. In addition, patients should be informed that they can minimize hypotension by avoiding abrupt transitions from a supine or seated position to an upright position.

Reflex Tachycardia

Reflex tachycardia results from dilation of *arterioles;* venous dilation is not a significant factor. The mechanism of reflex tachycardia is as follows:

(1) arteriolar dilation causes a decrease in arterial pressure; (2) baroreceptors in the aortic arch and carotid sinus sense the vasomotor center of the medulla; and (3) in an attempt to bring blood pressure back up, the medulla sends impulses along sympathetic nerves instructing the heart to beat faster.

Reflex tachycardia is undesirable for two reasons. First, tachycardia counteracts the hypotensive effects of arteriolar dilation, thereby negating the therapeutic response for which the drug was given. Second, reflex tachycardia can put an unacceptable burden on the heart.

To help prevent vasodilator-induced reflex tachycardia, patients can be pretreated with a beta-adrenergic blocking agent (e.g., propranolol), which will block sympathetic stimulation of the heart.

Expansion of Blood Volume

Prolonged use of *arteriolar* dilators can cause an increase in blood volume (secondary to chronic reduction of blood pressure). This increase in blood volume represents an attempt by the body to restore blood pressure to pretreatment levels.

Blood volume is increased by two mechanisms. First, reduced blood pressure triggers secretion of aldosterone by the adrenal glands. Aldosterone then acts on the kidney to promote retention of sodium and water, thereby increasing blood volume. The second mechanism also involves the kidney: by reducing arterial pressure, vasodilators decrease renal blood flow and glomerular filtration rate; because filtrate volume is decreased, the kidney is able to reabsorb an increased amount of sodium and water, which causes blood volume to expand.

Increased plasma volume can negate the beneficial effects of vasodilator therapy. For example, if plasma volume increases during the treatment of hypertension, blood pressure will rise, and the benefits of therapy will be cancelled. To prevent the kidney from neutralizing the beneficial effects of arteriolar dilation, patients often receive concurrent therapy with a diuretic, which will prevent fluid retention and volume expansion.

PHARMACOLOGY OF INDIVIDUAL VASODILATORS

Our focus in this section is on four drugs: hydralazine, minoxidil, diazoxide, and sodium nitroprusside. All of the other vasodilators are discussed at length in other chapters; hence, their discussion here is brief.

HYDRALAZINE

Cardiovascular Effects

Hydralazine [Alazine, Apresoline] causes selective dilation of arterioles. The drug has little or no effect on veins. Arteriolar dilation results from a direct action on vascular smooth muscle; the precise mechanism is not known. In response to arteriolar dilation, peripheral resistance and arterial blood pressure fall. In addition, heart rate and myocardial contractility increase, largely by reflex mechanisms. Since hydralazine acts selectively on arterioles, postural hypotension is minimal.

Pharmacokinetics

Absorption and Time Course of Action. Hydralazine is readily absorbed following oral administration. Effects are apparent within 45 minutes and persist for 6 hours or more. When the drug is given parenterally, effects begin rapidly (within 10 minutes) and last for 2 to 4 hours.

Metabolism. Hydralazine is inactivated by a metabolic process known as *acetylation*. The ability to acetylate hydralazine and other drugs is genetically determined. Some people are rapid acetylators, whereas others are slow acetylators. The distinction between rapid and slow acetylators can be clinically significant, in that individuals who acetylate hydralazine slowly are likely to have higher blood levels of the drug. These high drug levels can result in excessive vasodilation and other adverse effects. To avoid undesired drug accumulation, the dosage of hydralazine for slow acetylators should be reduced.

Adverse Effects

Reflex Tachycardia. By lowering arterial blood pressure, hydralazine can trigger reflex stimulation of the heart, thereby causing cardiac work and myocardial oxygen demand to increase. Because hydralazine-induced reflex tachycardia is frequently severe, the drug is almost always used in combination with a beta-adrenergic blocking agent. In fact, the only patients who are not given a beta blocker are those who have heart failure. (Beta blockers are not used during heart failure because they would further decrease cardiac output.)

Increased Blood Volume. Hydralazine-induced hypotension can cause sodium and water retention and a corresponding increase in blood volume. Expansion of blood volume can be prevented with a diuretic.

Systemic Lupus Erythematosus–like Syndrome. Hydralazine can cause an acute rheumatoid syndrome that closely resembles systemic lupus erythematosus (SLE). This syndrome is characterized by muscle pain, joint pain, fever, nephritis, pericarditis, and the presence of antinuclear antibodies. The syndrome occurs most frequently in slow acetylators, and is rare when hydralazine dosage is kept below 200 mg per day. If an SLE-like reaction occurs, hydralazine should be discontinued. Symptoms are usually reversible, but may take 6 or more months to subside. In some cases, rheumatoid symptoms persist for years.

Other Adverse Effects. Common responses include *headache, dizziness, weakness,* and *fatigue.* These reactions are related to hydralazine-induced hypotension.

Drug Interactions

Hydralazine is combined with *beta-adrenergic blockers* to protect against reflex tachycardia, and with *diuretics* to prevent sodium and water retention and expansion of blood volume. Drugs that lower blood pressure will intensify hypotensive responses to hydralazine. Accordingly, if hydralazine is used with other *antihypertensive agents,* care must be taken to avoid excessive hypotension.

Therapeutic Uses

Essential Hypertension. Oral hydralazine can be used to lower blood pressure in patients with essential hypertension. The regimen almost always includes a beta blocker, and may also include a diuretic. Although commonly employed in the past, hydralazine has been largely replaced by newer antihypertensive agents (see Chapter 40).

Hypertensive Crisis. Parenteral hydralazine is used to lower blood pressure rapidly in severe hypertensive episodes. The drug should be administered in small, incremental doses. If dosage is excessive, severe hypotension may replace the hypertension. Treatment of hypertensive emergencies is discussed further in Chapter 40.

Congestive Heart Failure. As discussed in Chapter 42, hydralazine can be used on a short-term basis to reduce afterload in patients with congestive heart failure. With prolonged therapy, tolerance to hydralazine develops.

Preparations, Dosage, and Administration

Preparations. Hydralazine [Alazine, Apresoline] is dispensed in tablets (10, 25, 50, and 100 mg) for oral use and as an injection (20 mg/ml in 1-ml ampuls) for parenteral administration. Hydralazine is also available in fixed-dose combinations with hydrochlorothiazide, a diuretic.

Oral Therapy. Dosage should be small initially (10 mg four times a day) and then gradually increased. Rapid increases may produce excessive hypotension. Usual maintenance dosages for adults range from 25 to 100 mg two times a day. Daily doses greater than 200 mg are associated with an increased incidence of adverse effects and should be avoided.

Parenteral Therapy. Parenteral administration (IV and IM) is reserved for hypertensive crises. The usual dose is 20 to 40 mg, repeated as needed. Blood pressure should be monitored frequently to minimize excessive hypotension. In most cases, patients can be switched from hydralazine injections to oral therapy within 48 hours.

MINOXIDIL

Minoxidil [Loniten, Minodyl] produces more intense vasodilation than hydralazine, but also causes more severe adverse reactions. Because it is both very effective and very hazardous, minoxidil is reserved for patients with severe hypertension that has been refractory to less dangerous drugs.

Cardiovascular Effects

Like hydralazine, minoxidil produces selective dilation of *arterioles.* Little or no venous dilation occurs. Arteriolar dilation decreases peripheral resistance and arterial blood pressure. In response to the reduction in blood pressure, reflex mechanisms cause an increase in heart rate and myocardial contractility. These responses can increase cardiac oxygen demand, and can thereby exacerbate angina pectoris.

Vasodilation results from a direct action on vascular smooth muscle (VSM). In order to relax VSM, minoxidil must first be metabolized to minoxidil sulfate. This metabolite then causes potassium channels in VSM to open. The resultant efflux of potassium hyperpolarizes VSM cells, thereby reducing their ability to contract.

Pharmacokinetics

Minoxidil is rapidly and completely absorbed following oral administration. Vasodilation is maximal within 2 to 3 hours and then gradually declines. Residual effects may persist for 2 days or more. Minoxidil is extensively metabolized; metabolites and parent drug are eliminated in the urine.

Adverse Effects

Reflex Tachycardia. Blood pressure reduction triggers reflex tachycardia. Tachycardia is a serious side effect and can be minimized by concurrent use of a beta blocker.

Sodium and Water Retention. Fluid retention is both common and serious. Volume expansion may be so severe as to cause cardiac decompensation. Management of fluid retention requires a high-ceiling diuretic (e.g., furosemide) used alone or in combination with a thiazide diuretic. If diuretics are inadequate, dialysis must be employed, or minoxidil must be withdrawn.

Hypertrichosis. About 80% of patients taking minoxidil for 4 weeks or more develop hypertrichosis (excessive growth of hair). Hair growth begins on the face and later develops on the arms, legs, and back. Hypertrichosis is presumed to result from increased cutaneous blood flow secondary to vasodilation. Direct effects on hair follicles may also be involved. Overgrowth of hair is a cosmetic problem and can be controlled by shaving or using a depilatory. However, many patients (primarily women) find hypertrichosis both unmanageable and intolerable and refuse to continue treatment.

Pericardial Effusion. Rarely, minoxidil-induced fluid retention results in pericardial effusion (fluid accumulation beneath the pericardium). In most cases, pericardial effusion is asymptomatic. However, in some cases, fluid accumulation becomes so great as to cause cardiac tamponade (compression of the heart with a resultant decrease in cardiac performance). If tamponade occurs, it must be treated by pericardiocentesis or by surgical drainage.

Other Adverse Effects. Minoxidil may cause *nausea, headache, fatigue, breast tenderness, glucose intolerance, thrombocytopenia,* and *skin reactions* (rashes, Stevens-Johnson syndrome). In addition, the drug has caused *hemorrhagic cardiac lesions* in experimental animals.

Therapeutic Uses

The only cardiovascular indication for minoxidil is *severe hypertension.* Because of its serious adverse effects, minoxidil is reserved for patients who have failed to respond to safer drugs. To minimize adverse cardiovascular responses (reflex tachycardia, expansion of blood volume, pericardial effusion), minoxidil should be used with a beta blocker and intensive diuretic therapy.

Topical minoxidil [Rogaine] is used to promote hair growth in balding men (see Chapter 70).

Preparations, Dosage, and Administration

Minoxidil [Loniten, Minodyl] is dispensed in 2.5- and 10-mg tablets for oral administration. The initial dosage is 5 mg once a day; the maximum dosage is 100 mg/day. The usual adult dosage is 10 to 40 mg/day administered in single or divided doses. When a rapid response is needed, a loading dose of 5 to 20 mg is given followed by doses of 2.5 to 10 mg every 4 hours.

DIAZOXIDE

Diazoxide [Hyperstat IV] is a close relative of the thiazide diuretics, but is devoid of diuretic actions. The drug is used primarily for hypertensive emergencies.

Cardiovascular Effects

Like hydralazine and minoxidil, diazoxide produces selective dilation of *arterioles;* the drug has no significant effect on veins. Intravenous diazoxide causes a rapid drop in diastolic and systolic pressure. Reduced arterial pressure triggers reflex tachycardia along with an increase in myocardial contractility; these effects combine to increase cardiac output. Arteriolar dilation also promotes substantial salt and water retention.

Vasodilation results from a direct effect on vascular smooth muscle (VSM). Diazoxide activates potassium channels in VSM, which results in hyperpolarization and a reduced ability to contract.

Pharmacokinetics

Diazoxide is administered intravenously, either as a bolus injection or by infusion. Bolus injection is generally preferred. Effects begin within minutes and may persist for hours. Most of the drug is eliminated unchanged in the urine.

Adverse Effects

Reflex Tachycardia. Reflex tachycardia occurs in response to lowering of blood pressure. If necessary, this reaction can be blunted with a beta blocker.

Salt and Water Retention. Diazoxide causes substantial retention of salt and water. This response is due largely to a reduction in glomerular filtration rate. If fluid retention is severe, edema and even congestive heart failure can result. Expansion of blood volume and edema can be prevented with a diuretic; a high-ceiling agent (e.g., furosemide) is preferred.

Hyperglycemia. Like the thiazide diuretics, diazoxide can suppress release of insulin, and can thereby cause blood glucose to rise. For most patients, the degree of hyperglycemia is insignificant. However, for patients with diabetes, hyperglycemia may be substantial. Blood glucose should be monitored daily in diabetic patients, and, if hyperglycemia develops, insulin dosage should be increased.

Hyperuricemia. Like the thiazide diuretics, diazoxide can decrease renal excretion of uric acid, thereby raising uric acid levels in blood. For most patients, hyperuricemia is asymptomatic. However, in gout-prone individuals, retention of uric acid may result in a gouty attack.

Other Adverse Effects. Diazoxide may cause *gastrointestinal effects* (nausea, vomiting, anorexia), *headache, flushing, hypotension,* and *temporary interruption of labor.* Rapid injection of large doses may produce *severe hypotension, anginal symptoms,* and *myocardial infarction.*

Drug Interactions

Diuretics. *High-ceiling diuretics* are used to counteract diazoxide-induced retention of salt and water. Since *thiazide diuretics* might potentiate the hyperglycemic and hyperuricemic effects of diazoxide, these diuretics should be avoided.

Antihypertensive Drugs. With the exception of high-ceiling diuretics, antihypertensive drugs should not be used routinely in combination with diazoxide. The concurrent use of diazoxide with other hypotensive agents may cause excessive lowering of blood pressure.

Therapeutic Uses

Parenteral diazoxide is reserved for acute treatment of hypertensive emergencies (e.g., malignant hypertension, hypertensive encephalopathy). Therapy with oral antihypertensive agents should be instituted as soon as possible. In most cases, diazoxide can be discontinued within 4 to 5 days.

Preparations, Dosage, and Administration

Diazoxide [Hyperstat IV] is dispensed as an injection (15 mg/ml) for IV administration. Until recently, it was common practice to administer diazoxide as a single, large (300 mg) IV bolus. This practice is no longer recommended. Currently, it is considered safer and more effective to use a series of "minibolus" injections, rather than one large injection. Accordingly, treatment should begin with a dose of 1 to 3 mg/kg injected by rapid (30 seconds or less) IV push. Dosing is then repeated every 5 to 15 minutes until the desired reduction in blood pressure has been achieved. Once hypertension has been controlled, injections can be made every 4 to 24 hours. Blood pressure should be monitored closely until an acceptable and stable level has been produced; hourly monitoring should be performed thereafter. The patient should remain recumbent for at least 30 minutes after diazoxide injection. After 4 or 5 days of treatment, the patient can usually be switched to oral antihypertensive therapy.

SODIUM NITROPRUSSIDE

Sodium nitroprusside [Nipride, Nitropress] is a potent and efficacious vasodilator. It is also the fastest acting antihypertensive agent available. Because of these qualities, nitroprusside is a drug of choice for treating hypertensive emergencies.

Cardiovascular Effects

In contrast to hydralazine, minoxidil, and diazoxide, nitroprusside causes *venous* dilation in addition to *arteriolar* dilation. Curiously, although nitroprusside is an effective arteriolar dilator, reflex tachycardia is minimal. Administration is by IV infusion, and onset of effects is immediate. By adjusting the infusion rate, blood pressure can be depressed to almost any level desired. When the infusion is stopped, blood pressure returns to pretreatment levels in minutes. Nitroprusside can trigger retention of sodium and water; furosemide can help offset this effect.

Mechanism of Action

Once in the body, nitroprusside breaks down to release *nitric oxide*, which then activates *guanylate cyclase*, an enzyme present in vascular smooth muscle. Guanylate cyclase catalyzes the production of *cyclic GMP*, which, through a series of reactions, causes vasodilation. This mechanism is similar to that of nitroglycerin.

Metabolism

As shown in Figure 39–1, nitroprusside contains five *cyanide* groups, which are split free in the first step of nitroprusside metabolism. The reaction that frees the cyanide is very rapid and takes place within red blood cells. Once freed, the cyanide groups are rapidly converted to *thiocyanate* in the liver; *thiosulfate* is a required co-factor for this reaction. Thiocyanate is eliminated by the kidneys over several days.

Adverse Effects

Excessive Hypotension. If administered too rapidly, nitroprusside can cause a precipitous fall in blood pressure, resulting in headache, palpitations, nausea, vomiting, and sweating. Blood pressure should be monitored continuously.

Cyanide Poisoning. On rare occasions, nitroprusside therapy has resulted in the accumulation of lethal amounts of cyanide. Cyanide buildup is most likely in patients with liver disease and in those with low stores of thiosulfate, the co-factor needed for cyanide detoxification. The chances of cyanide poisoning can be minimized by avoiding prolonged infusion in patients with liver disease and by co-administration of thiosulfate. If cyanide toxicity occurs, nitroprusside should be discontinued.

Thiocyanate Toxicity. When nitroprusside is given for several days, thiocyanate (a metabolite of nitroprusside) may accumulate. Although much less hazardous than cyanide, thiocyanate can also cause adverse effects. These effects, which involve the central nervous system, include disorientation, psychotic behavior, and delirium. To minimize toxicity, patients receiving nitroprusside for more than 3 days should be monitored for plasma levels of thiocyanate. These levels should not be allowed to exceed 0.1 mg/ml.

Therapeutic Uses

Hypertensive Emergencies. Nitroprusside is used to produce rapid lowering of blood pressure in hypertensive emergencies. Oral antihypertensive medication should be initiated at the same time that blood pressure is being reduced with nitroprusside. During nitroprusside treatment, furosemide may be needed to prevent excessive retention of fluid.

Other Uses. Nitroprusside is approved for production of controlled hypotension during surgery (to reduce bleeding in the surgical field). In addition, the drug has been employed on an investigational basis to treat severe, refractory congestive heart failure and myocardial infarction.

Preparations, Dosage, and Administration

Sodium nitroprusside [Nipride, Nitropress] is dispensed in powdered form (50 mg) to be dissolved and diluted for IV infu-

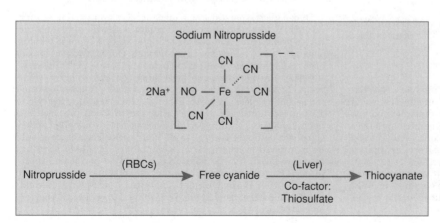

Figure 39–1. Structure and metabolism of sodium nitroprusside. Note the five cyanide groups in nitroprusside and their liberation by metabolism. (RBCs = red blood cells)

sion. Fresh solutions may have a faint brown coloration; solutions that are deeply colored (blue, green, dark red) should be discarded. Solutions of nitroprusside can be degraded by light and should be protected with an opaque material.

Blood pressure can be adjusted to practically any level by increasing or decreasing the rate of infusion. The initial infusion rate is 0.3 μg/kg/min. The maximal rate is 10 μg/kg/min. If infusion at the maximal rate for 10 minutes fails to produce an adequate drop in blood pressure, administration should be discontinued. During the infusion, blood pressure should be monitored continuously, either with an arterial line or an electronic monitoring device. No other drugs should be mixed with the infusion solution.

ANGIOTENSIN-CONVERTING ENZYME INHIBITORS

Inhibitors of angiotensin-converting enzyme (ACE) promote vasodilation by preventing the conversion of angiotensin I (a weak vasoconstrictor) into angiotensin II (an extremely powerful vasoconstrictor). The primary indication for ACE inhibitors is essential hypertension. These drugs can also benefit patients with congestive heart failure. The basic pharmacology of the ACE inhibitors is presented in Chapter 37. The use of these drugs to treat hypertension and heart failure is discussed in Chapters 40 and 42, respectively.

ORGANIC NITRATES

The organic nitrates (e.g., nitroglycerin, isosorbide dinitrate) produce selective dilation of veins; dilation of arterioles is minimal. The primary indication for these drugs is angina pectoris. Nitroglycerin is also given to treat congestive heart failure and myocardial infarction, and to provide controlled hypotension during surgery. The pharmacology of the organic nitrates is discussed in Chapter 41.

CALCIUM CHANNEL BLOCKERS

The calcium channel blockers (e.g., verapamil, nifedipine) produce vasodilation by preventing calcium entry into vascular smooth muscle. At therapeutic doses, these drugs produce se-lective dilation of arterioles; very little venous dilation occurs. The vasodilating ability of these drugs is exploited in the treatment of essential hypertension and angina pectoris. The calcium channel blockers are the subject of Chapter 38.

SYMPATHOLYTICS

Sympatholytics are drugs that promote vasodilation by preventing the sympathetic nervous system from causing vasoconstriction. Some of these drugs act by direct blockade of adrenergic receptors on blood vessels. Others act on sympathetic ganglia, adrenergic neurons, or within the central nervous system.

Alpha-Adrenergic Blocking Agents. The alpha blockers promote vasodilation by preventing stimulation of alpha-adrenergic receptors on veins and arterioles. In their capacity as vasodilators, these drugs have multiple therapeutic applications, including essential hypertension, peripheral vascular disease, and pheochromocytoma. The alpha blockers are discussed in Chapter 18.

Ganglionic Blocking Agents. The ganglionic blocking agents interrupt impulse transmission through all ganglia of the autonomic nervous system. By doing so, these drugs prevent sympathetic stimulation of arterioles and veins. Ganglionic blockers are used to treat hypertensive emergencies and severe cases of essential hypertension. In addition, these drugs are given to produce hypotension during surgery. The ganglionic blockers are discussed in Chapter 14.

Adrenergic Neuron Blocking Agents. Adrenergic neuron blockers act within terminals of adrenergic neurons to cause a reduction in norepinephrine release. By decreasing the release of norepinephrine from sympathetic nerves that control vasomotor tone, these drugs promote vasodilation. Their principal indication is essential hypertension. The adrenergic neuron blockers are discussed in Chapter 19.

Centrally Acting Agents. The centrally acting sympatholytics act within the central nervous system to inhibit outflow of impulses along sympathetic nerves. These agents are used primarily in the treatment of hypertension. Their pharmacology is discussed in Chapter 19.

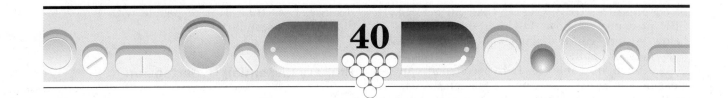

Drug Therapy of Hypertension

HYPERTENSION: DEFINITION, TYPES, AND CONSEQUENCES
Definition and Diagnosis
Types of Hypertension
Consequences of Hypertension

OBJECTIVES OF ANTIHYPERTENSIVE THERAPY

MANAGEMENT OF HYPERTENSION I: LIFESTYLE CHANGES

MANAGEMENT OF HYPERTENSION II: PHARMACOLOGIC THERAPY
Review of Blood Pressure Control
Antihypertensive Mechanisms: Sites of Drug Action and Effects Produced
The Antihypertensive Drugs
Fundamentals of Antihypertensive Therapy
Individualizing Therapy
Minimizing Adverse Effects
Promoting Compliance

DRUGS FOR HYPERTENSIVE EMERGENCIES

Hypertension (elevated blood pressure) is a common, chronic disorder that affects about 50 million Americans. Left untreated, hypertension can lead to heart disease, kidney disease, blindness, and stroke. Conversely, a treatment program of lifestyle changes and drug therapy can reduce both blood pressure and the risk of long-term complications.

Unfortunately, drug therapy does not cure hypertension, it only reduces symptoms. Accordingly, for most patients, treatment must continue lifelong. As a result, noncompliance can be a significant problem.

Many different drugs are used to treat hypertension. All of these have been introduced in previous chapters. Hence, in this chapter, rather than struggling with a huge array of new drugs, we will simply be discussing the antihypertensive applications of drugs with which we are already familiar.

In approaching our study of antihypertensive therapy, we will begin by discussing the nature of hypertension and nondrug methods of treatment. Following that we will discuss drug therapy of chronic hypertension. We will complete the chapter by discussing drugs used for hypertensive emergencies.

HYPERTENSION: DEFINITION, TYPES, AND CONSEQUENCES

DEFINITION AND DIAGNOSIS

Hypertension is defined as systolic blood pressure (SBP) greater than 140 mm Hg or diastolic

483

blood pressure (DBP) greater than 90 mg Hg. If SBP pressure is above 140 mm Hg and DBP is below 90 mm Hg, a diagnosis of *isolated systolic hypertension* applies.

As shown in Table 40–1, hypertension can be classified as Stage 1, 2, 3, or 4, based on the degree of blood pressure elevation. This new classification scheme was introduced in the fifth report of the Joint National Committee (JNC) on Detection, Evaluation, and Treatment of Hypertension (1993). When SBP and DBP fall into different categories, classification is based on the *higher* category. For example, an individual with SBP/DBP of 185/105 mm Hg would be diagnosed as having Stage 3 hypertension, and an individual with SBP/DBP of 185/85 would be diagnosed as having Stage 3 isolated systolic hypertension.

Diagnosis of hypertension should not be based on a single blood pressure determination. Rather, if an initial screening shows that blood pressure is elevated (but does not represent an immediate danger), it should be measured again on two subsequent visits 1 week to several weeks later. At each visit, two measurements should be made and averaged. If these readings confirm that SBP is indeed greater than 140 mm Hg or DBP is greater than 90 mm Hg, a diagnosis of hypertension can be made.

TYPES OF HYPERTENSION

There are two broad categories of hypertension: *primary hypertension* and *secondary hypertension*. As indicated in Table 40–2, primary hypertension is by far the most common form of hypertensive disease. Less than 10% of people with hypertension have a secondary form.

Primary (Essential) Hypertension

Primary hypertension is defined as hypertension that has no identifiable cause. A diagnosis of primary hypertension is made by ruling out probable specific causes of blood pressure elevation. Primary hypertension is a chronic, progressive disorder. In the absence of treatment, patients will experience a continuous, gradual rise in blood pressure over the remainder of their lives.

In the United States, primary hypertension affects about 20% of adults aged 25 to 74. Some people are more likely to experience hypertension than others: older people experience more hypertension than younger people, African Americans experience more hypertension than white Americans, postmenopausal women experience more hypertension than premenopausal women, and obese people experience more hypertension than people of normal weight.

Although the cause of primary hypertension is unknown, the condition *can* be successfully treated. It should be understood, however, that treatment is not curative: drugs can lower blood pressure, but they do not eliminate the underlying pathology. Consequently, treatment usually must continue lifelong.

Primary hypertension is also referred to as *essential hypertension*. This alternative name preceded the term primary hypertension and reflects our ignorance about the cause of the disease. Historically, it had been noted that as people grew older, their blood pressure rose. Why older people

Table 40–1. Classification of Blood Pressure for Adults Age 18 Years and Older		
Category*	Systolic (mm Hg)	Diastolic (mm Hg)
Normal†	<130	<85
High Normal	130–139	85–89
Hypertension‡		
STAGE 1 (mild)	140–159	90–99
STAGE 2 (moderate)	160–179	100–109
STAGE 3 (severe)	180–209	110–119
STAGE 4 (very severe)	≥210	≥120

*When systolic and diastolic pressures fall into different categories, the *higher* category should be selected to classify the individual's blood pressure status. For instance, 130/85 mm Hg should be classified as high normal, and 180/120 mm Hg should be classified as Stage 4 hypertension.

†Optimal blood pressure with respect to cardiovascular risk is SBP <120 mm Hg and DBP <80 mm Hg. However, unusually low readings should be evaluated for clinical significance.

‡Based on the average of two or more readings taken at each of two or more visits following an initial screening. Isolated systolic hypertension (ISH) is defined as SBP ≥140 mm Hg and DBP <90 mm Hg and staged appropriately (e.g., 170/85 mm Hg is defined as Stage 2 ISH).

Data from the fifth report of the Joint National Committee on Detection, Evaluation, and Treatment of High Blood Pressure, 1993.

Table 40–2. Types of Hypertension and Their Frequency	
Type of Hypertension	Frequency (%)
Primary (Essential) Hypertension	92
Secondary Hypertension	
Chronic renal disease	4
Renovascular disease	2
Coarctation	0.3
Primary aldosteronism	0.2
Cushing's syndrome	0.1
Pheochromocytoma	0.1
Oral contraceptive-induced	1

had elevated blood pressure was (and remains) unknown. One hypothesis noted that as people aged, their vascular systems offered greater resistance to blood flow. In order to move blood against this increased resistance, a compensatory increase in blood pressure was required. Therefore, the hypertension that occurred with age was seen as being "essential" for providing adequate perfusion of tissues—hence, the term *essential hypertension*. Over time, the term essential hypertension came to be applied to all cases of hypertension for which an underlying cause could not be identified.

Secondary Hypertension

Secondary hypertension is defined as an elevation of blood pressure occurring in response to an identified primary cause. The most common causes are listed in Table 40–2.

Because secondary hypertension is due to identified causes, it may be possible to treat that cause directly, rather than relying on drugs to provide symptomatic relief. As a result, some individuals with secondary hypertension can actually be cured. For example, if hypertension occurs secondary to pheochromocytoma (a catecholamine-secreting tumor), surgical removal of the tumor may produce permanent cure. When cure is not possible, secondary hypertension can be managed with the same drugs used to lower blood pressure in primary hypertension.

CONSEQUENCES OF HYPERTENSION

Chronic hypertension is associated with increased morbidity and mortality. Left untreated, chronically elevated blood pressure can lead to *heart disease* (left ventricular hypertrophy, myocardial infarction, angina pectoris), *kidney disease*, *blindness*, and *stroke*. The degree of injury is di-

rectly related to the degree of blood pressure elevation: the higher the pressure, the greater the injury. In addition, certain risk factors (e.g., obesity, sedentary lifestyle) can intensify injury. Deaths related to chronic hypertension result largely from cerebral hemorrhage, congestive heart failure, renal failure, and myocardial infarction.

Unfortunately, despite its potential for serious harm, hypertension usually remains asymptomatic until long after injury has begun to occur. That is, hypertension can exist for years before overt pathology is evident. Because injury occurs slowly and progressively, and because hypertension rarely causes noticeable discomfort, many people with this disease are unaware of its presence. Furthermore, many other people, even though diagnosed as hypertensive, may forgo therapy because hypertension doesn't make them feel bad.

OBJECTIVES OF ANTIHYPERTENSIVE THERAPY

Treatment of hypertension has two objectives: (1) reduction of SBP/DBP to 140/90 mm Hg, and (2) prevention of long-term complications. Furthermore, these goals should be achieved without decreasing quality of life with the drugs used for treatment. Extensive clinical trials have demonstrated unequivocally that when the blood pressure of hypertensive individuals is lowered, morbidity is decreased and life is prolonged. Antihypertensive therapy decreases the risk of heart disease, kidney disease, blindness, and stroke.

MANAGEMENT OF HYPERTENSION I: LIFESTYLE CHANGES

Lifestyle changes (previously termed nonpharmacologic therapy) can decrease blood pressure in many people with hypertension. These changes are useful by themselves and, when implemented in conjunction with drug therapy, can reduce the number of required drugs and their dosages.

Weight Reduction. There is a direct relationship between obesity and elevation of blood pressure. Clinical studies indicate that weight loss can reduce blood pressure in 60% to 80% of overweight hypertensive individuals. Consequently, a restricted-calorie diet is recommended for all patients whose weight exceeds 110% of ideal. The diet should be low in saturated fats, and total dietary fat should not exceed 30% of caloric intake.

Sodium Restriction. Epidemiologic studies indicate that increased dietary sodium chloride (salt) is associated with elevated blood pressure. Furthermore, clinical trials have shown that reduction of dietary sodium can lower blood pressure. Also, salt restriction can enhance the hypotensive effects of drugs. Accordingly, it is recommended that all people with hypertension consume no more than 6 gm of sodium chloride (2.3 gm of sodium) a day. To facilitate salt restriction, patients should be given information on the salt content of foods.

Alcohol Restriction. Excessive alcohol consumption can raise blood pressure and create resistance to antihypertensive drugs. Accordingly, patients should be counseled to limit alcohol intake to 1 ounce a day. One ounce of ethanol is equivalent to about two mixed drinks, two glasses of wine, or two cans of beer.

Exercise. Regular aerobic exercise (e.g., jogging, walking, swimming, bicycling) can reduce blood pressure by about 10 mm Hg, even in the absence of weight reduction. Patients with a sedentary lifestyle should be encouraged to develop an appropriate exercise program. An activity as simple as brisk walking for 30 to 45 minutes three to five times a week can be beneficial.

Smoking Cessation. Although not directly related to hypertension, smoking is a major risk factor for cardiovascular disease and should be avoided. Furthermore, smoking may impair the ability of antihypertensive drugs to protect against cardiovascular disease. All patients who smoke should be forcefully encouraged to quit.

MANAGEMENT OF HYPERTENSION II: PHARMACOLOGIC THERAPY

Drug therapy is indicated if blood pressure is still excessive 3 to 6 months after implementation of lifestyle changes. The decision to use drugs should be the result of collaboration between clinician and patient. A wide range of antihypertensive drugs is available, permitting versatility in the regimen. Consequently, for the majority of patients, it should be possible to establish a treatment program that is effective and yet devoid of objectionable side effects. After 12 months of successful therapy, an attempt should be made to reduce the number of drugs taken and their dosages.

REVIEW OF BLOOD PRESSURE CONTROL

Before discussing the antihypertensive drugs, it will be helpful to review the major mechanisms by which blood pressure is controlled. This information will enable us to better understand the mechanisms by which drugs bring blood pressure down to an acceptable level.

Principal Determinants of Blood Pressure

The principal determinants of blood pressure are summarized in Figure 40–1. As indicated, arterial pressure is the product of cardiac output and peripheral resistance. An increase in either factor will increase blood pressure.

As shown in the figure, cardiac output is influenced by four factors: (1) heart rate, (2) myocardial contractility (force of contraction), (3) blood volume, and (4) venous return of blood to the heart. An increase in any of these factors will increase cardiac output, thereby causing blood pressure to rise. Conversely, by reducing these factors, we can cause blood pressure to fall. Drugs that affect these factors are (1) beta blockers, which decrease heart rate and contractile force, (2) diuretics, which decrease blood volume, and (3) venodilators, which reduce venous return.

Peripheral vascular resistance is regulated by arteriolar constriction. Accordingly, we can reduce blood pressure with drugs that promote arteriolar dilation.

Systems That Help Regulate Blood Pressure

Having established that blood pressure is determined by heart rate, myocardial contractility, blood volume, venous return, and arteriolar constriction, we will now examine how these factors are regulated. Two regulatory systems are of particular significance: (1) the sympathetic nervous system, and (2) the renin-angiotensin-aldosterone system.

Sympathetic Control of Blood Pressure. The sympathetic nervous system employs a reflex circuit—*the baroreceptor reflex*—to keep blood pressure at a preset level. This circuit operates as follows: (1) Baroreceptors in the aortic arch and carotid sinus sense the status of blood pressure and relay this information to the brainstem. (2) When blood is perceived as being too low, the brainstem sends impulses along sympathetic nerves to stimulate the heart and blood vessels. (3) Blood pressure is then elevated by (a) stimulation of beta$_1$ receptors in the heart, resulting in increased cardiac output, and (b) stimulation of vascular alpha$_1$ receptors, resulting in vasoconstriction. (4) When blood pressure has been reduced to an acceptable level, sympathetic stimulation of the heart and vascular smooth muscle subsides.

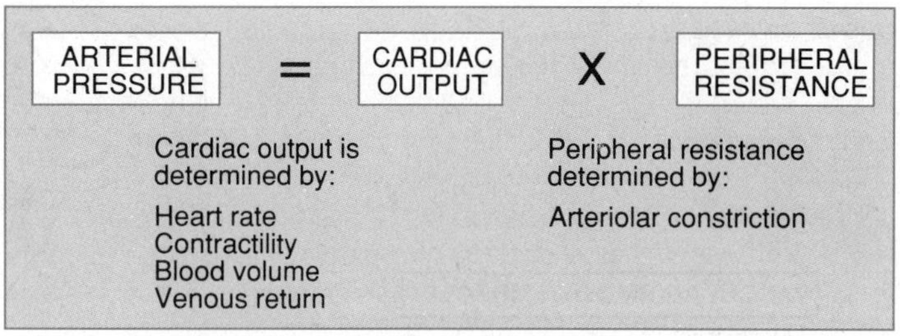

Figure 40-1. Primary determinants of arterial blood pressure.

The baroreceptor reflex frequently opposes our attempts to reduce blood pressure with drugs. Opposition occurs because the "set point" of the baroreceptors tends to be abnormally high in people with hypertension. That is, the baroreceptors are set to perceive excessively high blood pressure as being "normal" (i.e., appropriate). As a result, the system operates to maintain blood pressure at pathologic levels. Consequently, when we attempt to lower blood pressure using drugs, the reduced (healthier) pressure is interpreted by the baroreceptors as being below what it should be, and, in response, signals are sent out along sympathetic nerves to "correct" the reduction. These signals produce reflex tachycardia and vasoconstriction—responses that can counteract the hypotensive effects of drugs. Clearly, if treatment is to succeed, the regimen must compensate for the resistance offered by the baroreceptor reflex. Inclusion of a beta blocker, which will block reflex tachycardia, can be an effective method of compensation. Fortunately, when blood pressure has been suppressed with drugs for an extended period, the baroreceptors become reset at a lower level. Consequently, as therapy proceeds, sympathetic reflexes offer progressively less resistance to the hypotensive effects of medication.

Renin-Angiotensin-Aldosterone System. The renin-angiotensin-aldosterone system (RAAS) can elevate blood pressure, thereby negating the hypotensive effects of our drugs. The RAAS is discussed at length in Chapter 37 and will be reviewed briefly here.

How does the RAAS elevate blood pressure? The process begins with the release of renin from juxtaglomerular cells of the kidney. These cells release renin in response to several factors: reduced renal blood flow, reduced blood volume, reduced blood pressure, and stimulation of beta$_1$-adrenergic receptors on the cell surface. Following its release, renin promotes the conversion of angiotensinogen into angiotensin I, a weak vasoconstrictor. After this, angiotensin-converting enzyme (ACE) acts on angiotensin I to form angiotensin II, a compound that causes intense constriction of arterioles and veins, thereby elevating blood pressure. In addition, angiotensin II causes release of aldosterone (from the adrenal cortex), which acts on the kidneys to promote retention of sodium and water.

The resultant increase in blood volume contributes to increased arterial pressure.

Since drug-induced reductions in blood pressure can activate the RAAS, this system can counteract the effects we are trying to achieve. We have two methods available to cope with this problem. First, we can suppress renin release with beta blockers. Second, we can prevent the conversion of angiotensin I into angiotensin II with an ACE inhibitor.

ANTIHYPERTENSIVE MECHANISMS: SITES OF DRUG ACTION AND EFFECTS PRODUCED

As discussed above, drugs can lower blood pressure by reducing heart rate, myocardial contractility, blood volume, venous return, and the tone of arteriolar smooth muscle. In this section we will survey the principal mechanisms by which drugs produce these effects.

The major mechanisms for lowering blood pressure are summarized in Figure 40-2 and Table 40-3. The figure indicates the nine principal sites at which antihypertensive drugs act. The table summarizes the effects brought about by drug actions exerted at these sites. The sites of drug action and the resultant effects are described briefly below. Sites numbered 1 through 9 below correspond with sites 1 through 9 in the figure and table.

1. Central Nervous System. Antihypertensive drugs acting in the brainstem suppress sympathetic outflow to the heart and blood vessels, resulting in decreased heart rate, decreased myocardial contractility, and vasodilation. Vasodilation contributes most to reductions in blood pressure. Dilation of arterioles reduces blood pressure by decreasing vascular resistance. Dilation of veins decreases blood pressure by decreasing venous return to the heart.

2. Sympathetic Ganglia. Ganglionic blockade reduces sympathetic stimulation of the heart and blood vessels. Antihypertensive effects result primarily from dilation of arterioles and veins. Ganglionic blocking agents produce such a profound reduction in blood pressure that they are employed only for hypertensive emergencies.

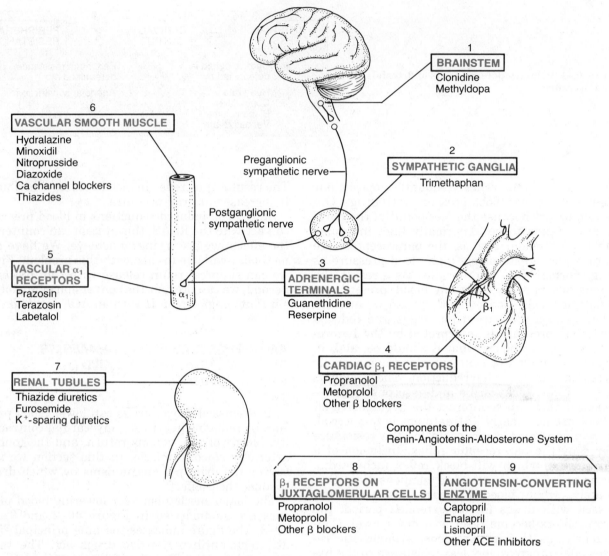

Figure 40–2. Sites of action of antihypertensive drugs. Note that some antihypertensive agents act at more than one site: beta blockers act at sites 4 and 8, and thiazides act at sites 6 and 7. The hemodynamic consequences of drug actions at the sites depicted are summarized in Table 40–3.

3. Terminals of Adrenergic Nerves. Antihypertensive agents acting at adrenergic nerve terminals decrease the release of norepinephrine, resulting in decreased sympathetic stimulation of the heart and blood vessels.

4. Beta₁-Adrenergic Receptors on the Heart. Blockade of cardiac beta₁ receptors prevents sympathetic stimulation of the heart. As a result, heart rate and myocardial contractility decline.

5. Alpha₁-Adrenergic Receptors on Blood Vessels. Blockade of vascular alpha₁ receptors promotes dilation of arterioles and veins. Arteriolar dilation reduces peripheral resistance. Venous dilation reduces venous return of blood to the heart.

6. Vascular Smooth Muscle. Several antihypertensive drugs (Fig. 40–2) act directly on vascular smooth muscle to cause relaxation. Two of

these agents—sodium nitroprusside and diazoxide—are used only for hypertensive emergencies. The rest are employed to treat essential hypertension.

7. Renal Tubules. Diuretics act on renal tubules to promote salt and water excretion. As a result, blood volume declines, causing blood pressure to fall.

8. Beta₁ Receptors on Juxtaglomerular Cells. Blockade of beta₁ receptors on juxtaglomerular cells suppresses release of renin. The resultant decrease in angiotensin II levels has two effects: (1) vasodilation, and (2) suppression of aldosterone-mediated volume expansion.

9. Angiotensin-Converting Enzyme. Inhibitors of angiotensin-converting enzyme suppress formation of angiotensin II. This results in (1) vasodilation, and (2) suppression of aldosterone-mediated volume expansion.

Table 40–3. Summary of Antihypertensive Effects Elicited by Drug Actions at Specific Sites

Site of Drug Action*	Representative Drug	Drug Effects
1. Brainstem	Clonidine	Suppression of sympathetic outflow decreases sympathetic stimulation of the heart and blood vessels.
2. Sympathetic ganglia	Trimethaphan	Ganglionic blockade reduces sympathetic stimulation of the heart and blood vessels.
3. Adrenergic nerve terminals	Guanethidine	Reduced norepinephrine release decreases sympathetic stimulation of the heart and blood vessels.
4. Cardiac beta$_1$ receptors	Propranolol	Beta$_1$ blockade decreases heart rate and myocardial contractility.
5. Vascular alpha$_1$ receptors	Prazosin	Alpha$_1$ blockade causes vasodilation.
6. Vascular smooth muscle	Hydralazine	Relaxation of vascular smooth muscle causes vasodilation.
7. Renal tubules	Chlorothiazide	Promotion of diuresis results in decreased blood volume.
8. Beta$_1$ receptors on juxtaglomerular cells	Propranolol	Beta$_1$ blockade suppresses renin release, resulting in (1) vasodilation secondary to reduced production of angiotensin II, and (2) prevention of aldosterone-mediated volume expansion.
9. Angiotensin–converting enzyme (ACE)	Captopril	Inhibition of ACE decreases formation of angiotensin II and thereby prevents (1) vasoconstriction, and (2) aldosterone-mediated volume expansion.

*Sites 1 through 9 in this table correspond to sites 1 through 9 in Figure 40–20.

THE ANTIHYPERTENSIVE DRUGS

In this section we will consider the principal drugs employed to treat *chronic* hypertension. Drugs used in *hypertensive emergencies* are considered later in the chapter.

The antihypertensive drugs and their classes are summarized in Table 40–4. All of these drugs have been discussed in previous chapters. Accordingly, discussion here is limited to their use in hypertension. Of primary interest are mechanisms of antihypertensive action and major adverse effects.

Diuretics

Diuretics are a mainstay of antihypertensive therapy. These drugs reduce blood pressure when used alone and they can enhance the effects of other hypotensive drugs. The basic pharmacology of the diuretics is discussed in Chapter 35.

Thiazide Diuretics. The thiazide diuretics (e.g., hydrochlorothiazide) are the most commonly used antihypertensive drugs. Thiazides reduce blood pressure by two mechanisms: reduction of blood volume and reduction of arterial resistance. Reduced blood volume is responsible for initial antihypertensive effects. Reduced vascular resistance develops over time and is responsible for long-term antihypertensive effects. The mechanism by which thiazides reduce vascular resistance has not been established.

The principal adverse effect of thiazides is *hypokalemia*. This effect can be minimized by consuming potassium-rich foods (e.g., bananas, citrus fruits) and by using potassium supplements or a potassium-sparing diuretic. Other side effects include *hyperglycemia*, *hyperuricemia*, and *excessive fluid loss*.

High-Ceiling (Loop) Diuretics. High-ceiling diuretics (e.g., furosemide) produce much greater diuresis than the thiazides. For most individuals with essential hypertension, the amount of fluid loss that loop diuretics can produce is greater than is needed or desirable. Consequently, loop diuretics are not used routinely. Rather, they are reserved for those few patients who need greater diuresis than can be achieved with thiazides.

Like the thiazides, the loop diuretics lower blood pressure by reducing blood volume. However, in contrast to the thiazides, the loop diuretics do not promote vasodilation.

Adverse effects are like those of the thiazides: *excessive fluid loss*, *hypokalemia*, *hyperglycemia*, and *hyperuricemia*.

Potassium-Sparing Diuretics. The degree of diuresis induced by the potassium-sparing agents (e.g., spironolactone) is small. Consequently, these drugs are not very effective as hypotensive agents. However, because of their ability to conserve potassium, these drugs can play an important role in an antihypertensive regimen. That role is to balance potassium loss caused by thiazides or loop diuretics. The most significant adverse effect of the potassium-sparing agents is *hyperkalemia*. Because of the risk of hyperkalemia, potassium-sparing diuretics must not be used in combination with potassium supplements or with ACE inhibitors, which also pose a risk of hyperkalemia.

	Table 40–4. Drugs for Chronic Hypertension		
Diuretics	**Sympatholytics**	**Others**
Thiazides and Related Diuretics	***Beta Blockers***	***ACE Inhibitors***
Bendroflumethiazide	Acebutolol	Benazepril
Benzthiazide	Atenolol	Captopril
Chlorothiazide	Betaxolol	Enalapril
Cyclothiazide	Bisoprolol	Fosinopril
Hydrochlorothiazide	Metoprolol	Lisinopril
Hydroflumethiazide	Nadolol	Quinapril
Indapamide	Penbutolol	Ramipril
Methyclothiazide	Pindolol	
Metolazone	Propranolol	***Calcium Channel Blockers***
Polythiazide	Timolol	Amlodipine
Quinethazone		Diltiazem
Trichlormethiazide	***Alpha₁ Blockers***	Felodipine
	Doxazosin	Isradipine
Loop Diuretics	Prazosin	Nicardipine
Furosemide	Terazosin	Verapamil
Ethacrynic acid		
Bumetanide	***Combined Alpha₁ and Beta Blocker***	***Direct-Acting Vasodilators***
	Labetalol	Hydralazine
Potassium-Sparing Diuretics		Minoxidil
Spironolactone	***Centrally Acting Agents***	
Triamterene	Clonidine	
Amiloride	Methyldopa	
	Adrenergic Neuron Blockers	
	Guanethidine	
	Reserpine	

Sympatholytics (Adrenergic Antagonists)

Sympatholytic drugs suppress the influence of the sympathetic nervous system on the heart, blood vessels, and other structures. These drugs are used widely in the treatment of hypertension.

As indicated in Table 40–4, there are five subcategories of sympatholytic drugs: (1) beta-adrenergic blockers, (2) centrally acting agents, (3) adrenergic neuron blockers, (4) alpha₁-adrenergic blockers, and (5) a category that contains only one agent, labetalol, which blocks alpha₁- and beta-adrenergic receptors.

Beta-Adrenergic Blockers. The beta blockers (e.g., propranolol, metoprolol) are among the most widely used antihypertensive drugs. However, despite their efficacy and frequent use, the exact mechanism by which these drugs reduce blood pressure is somewhat uncertain.

The beta blockers have at least three useful actions in hypertension. First, blockade of cardiac beta₁ receptors decreases heart rate and contractility, thereby decreasing cardiac output. Second, beta blockers can suppress reflex tachycardia caused by vasodilators in the regimen. Third, blockade of beta₁ receptors on juxtaglomerular cells of the kidney reduces release of renin, thereby reducing angiotensin II–mediated vasoconstriction and aldosterone-mediated volume expansion.

Beta blockers can produce a variety of adverse effects. Blockade of cardiac beta₁ receptors can produce *bradycardia, decreased atrioventricular (A-V) conduction,* and *reduction of contractility.* Consequently, beta blockers should not be used by patients with sick-sinus syndrome, congestive heart failure, or second- or third-degree A-V block. Blockade of beta₂ receptors in the lung can promote *bronchoconstriction.* Accordingly, beta blockers should be avoided by patients with asthma. If an asthmatic individual absolutely must use a beta blocker, a beta₁-selective agent (e.g., metoprolol) should be employed. Beta blockers can mask signs of hypoglycemia and, therefore, must be used with caution in patients with *diabetes.* Through actions exerted in the central nervous system, beta blockers can cause *insomnia, depression, bizarre dreams,* and *sexual dysfunction.*

The basic pharmacology of the beta blockers is discussed in Chapter 18.

Centrally Acting Agents: Clonidine and Methyldopa. Clonidine and methyldopa act within the brainstem to suppress sympathetic outflow to the heart and blood vessels. The mechanisms by which these agents reduce sympathetic outflow are discussed in Chapter 19. Both clonidine and methyldopa can cause *drying of the mouth, drowsiness,* and *sexual dysfunction.* In addition, clonidine can cause *severe rebound hypertension* if treatment is abruptly discontinued. Additional adverse effects of methyldopa include *hemolytic anemia* (accompanied by a positive direct Coombs' test) and *liver disorders*.

Adrenergic Neuron Blockers: Guanethidine and Reserpine. Guanethidine and reserpine decrease blood pressure through actions exerted within the terminals of postganglionic sympathetic neurons. Guanethidine inhibits release of norepinephrine, whereas reserpine causes norepinephrine depletion. Both actions result in decreased sympathetic stimulation of the heart and blood vessels.

The major adverse effect of guanethidine is *severe orthostatic hypotension* resulting from decreased sympathetic tone to veins. Because of the risk of postural hypotension, guanethidine is a last-choice agent for chronic hypertension.

The major adverse effect of reserpine is *depression*. Accordingly, reserpine is absolutely contraindicated for patients with a history of depressive illness.

The basic pharmacology of reserpine and guanethidine is discussed in Chapter 19.

Alpha₁-Adrenergic Blockers. The alpha₁ blockers (e.g., prazosin, terazosin) prevent stimulation of alpha₁ receptors on arterioles and veins, thereby preventing sympathetically mediated vasoconstriction. The resultant vasodilation reduces both peripheral resistance and venous return to the heart.

The most disturbing side effect of alpha blockers is *orthostatic hypotension*. Hypotension can be especially severe with the initial dose. Significant hypotension continues with subsequent doses but is less profound.

The basic pharmacology of the alpha blockers is discussed in Chapter 18.

Alpha₁-Adrenergic and Beta-Adrenergic Blocker: Labetalol. Labetalol is unusual in that it can block alpha₁ receptors as well as beta receptors. Lowering of blood pressure results from a combination of actions: (1) alpha₁ blockade promotes dilation of arterioles and veins, (2) blockade of cardiac beta₁ receptors reduces heart rate and contractility, and (3) blockade of beta₁ receptors on juxtaglomerular cells suppresses release of renin. Like other nonselective beta blockers, labetalol can exacerbate bradycardia, A-V heart block, congestive heart failure, and asthma. Blockade of venous alpha₁ receptors can produce postural hypotension.

Direct-Acting Vasodilators: Hydralazine and Minoxidil

Hydralazine and minoxidil reduce blood pressure by promoting dilation of *arterioles*. Neither drug causes significant dilation of veins. Because venous dilation is minimal, these agents produce very little orthostatic hypotension. With both

drugs, lowering of blood pressure may be followed by reflex tachycardia, renin release, and fluid retention. Reflex tachycardia and release of renin can be prevented with a beta blocker. Fluid retention can be prevented with a diuretic.

The most disturbing adverse effect of *hydralazine* is a syndrome resembling *systemic lupus erythematosus* (SLE). Fortunately, this reaction is rare when the drug is used at recommended doses. If an SLE-like reaction occurs, hydralazine should be withdrawn. Hydralazine is considered a third-choice drug for chronic hypertension.

Minoxidil is substantially more toxic than hydralazine. By causing fluid retention, minoxidil can promote *pericardial effusion* (accumulation of fluid beneath the myocardium) that, in some cases, may progress to *cardiac tamponade* (compression of the heart). A less serious effect is *hypertrichosis* (excessive hair growth). Because of its capacity for significant harm, minoxidil is not used routinely in chronic hypertension. Instead, minoxidil is reserved for patients with severe hypertension who have not responded to less dangerous drugs.

The basic pharmacology of hydralazine and minoxidil is discussed in Chapter 39.

Calcium Channel Blockers

The calcium channel blockers used most frequently are verapamil, diltiazem, and nifedipine. Discussion here is limited to these drugs. All three agents reduce blood pressure by causing dilation of *arterioles*.

Like other vasodilators, calcium channel blockers can cause *reflex tachycardia*. This reaction is greatest with nifedipine and minimal with verapamil and diltiazem. Reflex tachycardia is low with verapamil and diltiazem because these drugs have direct suppressant effects on the heart. Since nifedipine does not block cardiac calcium channels, reflex tachycardia with this drug can be substantial.

Because of their ability to compromise cardiac performance, verapamil and diltiazem must be used cautiously in patients with bradycardia, congestive heart failure, or A-V heart block. These precautions do not apply to nifedipine.

The basic pharmacology of the calcium channel blockers is discussed in Chapter 38.

Angiotensin-Converting Enzyme Inhibitors

The ACE inhibitors used most frequently in hypertension are captopril and enalapril. Our discussion will be limited to these two drugs. Both agents lower blood pressure by preventing the conversion of angiotensin I into angiotensin II, thereby preventing angiotensin II–mediated vasoconstriction and aldosterone-mediated volume expansion. Principal adverse effects are *persistent cough, first-dose hypotension*, and *hyperkalemia* (secondary to suppression of aldosterone release). Because of the risk of hyperkalemia, these drugs must not be used in combination with potassium supplements or potassium-sparing diuretics. ACE inhibitors can cause fetal harm during the second and third trimesters of pregnancy, and, therefore, must not be given to pregnant women. These are the only antihypertensive drugs that are specifically contraindicated for use during pregnancy. The basic pharmacology of the ACE inhibitors is discussed in Chapter 37.

FUNDAMENTALS OF ANTIHYPERTENSIVE THERAPY

The Basic Strategy

The basic approach to treating hypertension is outlined in Figure 40–3. As shown, lifestyle changes should be tried first. If these fail to produce an adequate response, they should be continued and drug therapy should be started. Treatment should begin with a single drug, usually a diuretic or a beta blocker. If the initial drug fails to produce an adequate response, another drug may be added or substituted. However, before another drug is considered, possible reasons for failure with the initial drug should be assessed. These reasons include poor compliance, excessive salt intake, and the presence of secondary hypertension. If treatment with two drugs is unsuccessful, a third may be added.

Guidelines for Drug Selection

As indicated in Table 40–5, the antihypertensive drugs can be placed in two major therapeutic groups: (1) drugs for initial therapy, and (2) supplemental drugs. For initial therapy, a *diuretic* or a *beta blocker* is generally preferred. This preference is based on long-term controlled trials that show conclusively that beta blockers and diuretics can reduce morbidity and mortality in hypertensive patients. The alternative drugs for initial therapy—*ACE inhibitors, calcium channel blockers, alpha$_1$-adrenergic blockers, and labetalol*—are equally effective in reducing blood pressure. However, because these drugs have not been used in

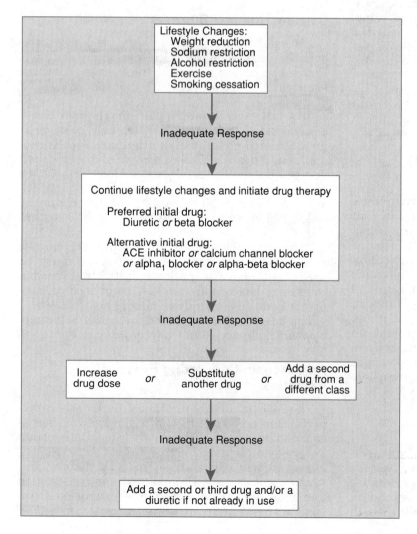

Figure 40–3. Algorithm for treating hypertension.

Drugs for Initial Therapy

Preferred Agents*	Alternatives†
Beta blockers	ACE inhibitors
Diuretics	Alpha₁ blockers
	Alpha-beta blocker
	Calcium channel blockers

Supplemental Drugs
Centrally acting sympatholytics
Adrenergic neuron blockers
Direct-acting vasodilators

*Diuretics and beta blockers are preferred because these drugs have a demonstrated ability to reduce morbidity and mortality.

†Although these drugs can reduce blood pressure, we do not yet know if they can reduce morbidity and mortality.

Based on recommendations in the fifth report of the Joint National Committee on Detection, Evaluation, and Treatment of High Blood Pressure, 1993.

long-term controlled trials, we do not yet know if they can reduce morbidity and mortality. Hence, it is recommended that they be reserved for special indications and for patients who have not responded to beta blockers and diuretics. The drugs classified as supplemental—*centrally acting sympatholytics, adrenergic neuron blockers, and direct-acting vasodilators*—are associated with a high incidence of undesirable effects. Hence, these drugs are not well suited for initial monotherapy.

An important guideline for drug selection is that each drug in the regimen belong to a different class. That is, each drug should have a different mechanism of action. In accord with this guideline, it would be appropriate to combine a beta blocker, a diuretic, and a vasodilator, since each of these drugs lowers blood pressure by a different mechanism. In contrast, it would be inappropriate to combine two thiazide diuretics or two beta blockers or two vasodilators.

To insure maximum benefits with minimum harm, it is essential that treatment be tailored to the individual patient. This important topic is addressed below under *Individualizing Therapy*.

Benefits of Multidrug Therapy

Treatment with multiple drugs can offer significant benefits. First, by employing drugs that have different mechanisms of action, we can increase our chances of success: attacking blood pressure control at several sites is more likely to be effective than an attack that centers on just one site. Second, when drugs are used in combination, each agent can be administered in a lower dosage than would be possible if that drug were used alone; as a result, both the frequency and the intensity of side effects are reduced. Third, when proper combinations are selected, one agent can offset the adverse effects of another. For example, if a vasodilator is used alone, reflex tachycardia is likely. However, if a vasodilator is combined with a beta blocker, reflex tachycardia will be minimal.

Dosing

For each drug in the regimen, *dosage should be low initially and then gradually increased*. There are several reasons for this approach. First, for most people with chronic hypertension, the disease poses no immediate threat to well-being. Hence, there is no need to lower blood pressure rapidly using large doses. Second, when blood pressure is reduced slowly, baroreceptors gradually reset to the new, lower pressure. Therefore, when dosage is increased gradually, sympathetic reflexes will offer less resistance to the hypotensive effects of therapy. Third, since there is no need to drop blood pressure rapidly, and since higher doses carry a higher risk of adverse effects, use of high initial doses would needlessly increase the risk of unpleasant responses.

Step-Down Therapy

After blood pressure has been controlled for at least 1 year, an attempt should be made to reduce dosages and the number of drugs taken. Of course, lifestyle modifications should be continued. When reductions are made slowly and progressively, many patients are able to maintain blood pressure control with less medication—and some can be maintained with no drugs at all. If drugs are discontinued, regular follow-up is essential, since blood pressure will usually return to hypertensive levels—although it may take years to do so.

INDIVIDUALIZING THERAPY

Treating Patients with Co-existing Diseases

Antihypertensive drugs that can exacerbate co-existing disorders must be avoided. In our discussion of specific antihypertensive drugs, we noted that certain agents can aggravate certain disease states. We saw, for example, that reserpine can intensify depression, and that beta blockers can exacerbate congestive heart failure, A-V heart block, and asthma. Other conditions that can be aggravated by antihypertensive drugs are presented in Table 40–6. To help avoid drug-disease mismatches, the medical history should identify all co-existing pathophysiology. With this information, the physician will be able to choose drugs that are least likely to make co-existing disorders worse.

Table 40–6. Pathophysiologic Conditions that Require Cautious Use or Complete Avoidance of Certain Antihypertensive Drugs

Pathophysiologic Condition	Drugs to Be Avoided or Used with Caution	Reason for Concern
Cardiovascular		
Congestive heart failure	Beta blockers Labetalol Verapamil Diltiazem	These drugs act on the heart to decrease myocardial contractility and can thereby further reduce cardiac output.
A-V heart block	Beta blockers Labetalol Verapamil Diltiazem	These drugs act on the heart to suppress A-V conduction and can thereby intensify A-V block.
Coronary artery disease	Guanethidine Hydralazine	Reflex tachycardia induced by these drugs can precipitate an anginal attack.
Post myocardial infarction	Guanethidine Hydralazine	Reflex tachycardia induced by these drugs can increase cardiac work and oxygen demand.
Other		
Renal insufficiency	K^+-sparing diuretics K^+ supplements	Use of these agents can lead to dangerous accumulations of potassium.
Asthma	Beta blockers Labetalol	$Beta_2$ blockade promotes bronchoconstriction.
Depression	Reserpine	Reserpine causes depression.
Diabetes mellitus	Thiazides Furosemide Beta blockers	Thiazides and furosemide promote hyperglycemia; beta blockers suppress glycogenolysis and can mask signs of hypoglycemia.
Gout	Thiazides Furosemide	These diuretics promote hyperuricemia.
Hyperkalemia	K^+-sparing diuretics ACE inhibitors	These drugs cause potassium accumulation.
Hypokalemia	Thiazides Furosemide	These diuretics promote potassium loss.
Collagen diseases	Hydralazine	Hydralazine can precipitate a lupus erythematosus–like syndrome.
Liver disease	Methyldopa	Methyldopa is hepatotoxic.
Pre-eclampsia	ACE inhibitors	These drugs can injure the fetus.

Treating Patients in Special Populations

African Americans. Hypertension is the major health problem of African-American adults. Hypertension develops earlier in blacks than in whites, has a significantly higher incidence, and is likely to be more severe. As a result, African Americans face a greater risk of heart disease, end-stage renal disease, and stroke. Available data indicate that blacks and whites respond equally to treatment—although not always to the same drugs. Controlled trials have shown that *diuretics* can decrease morbidity and mortality in blacks. Accordingly, these agents are drugs of first choice. Monotherapy with *calcium channel blockers, alpha₁ blockers,* and *labetalol* are equally effective in blacks and whites. In contrast, *beta blockers* and *ACE inhibitors* are less effective in blacks than in whites. Because African Americans have a high incidence of salt sensitivity, obesity, and cigarette use, lifestyle changes are especially important for people in this group.

Children. The incidence of secondary hypertension in children is much higher than in adults. Accordingly, efforts to diagnose and treat an underlying cause should be especially diligent. For children with primary hypertension, treatment is the same as for adults.

The Elderly. The incidence of hypertension in people over the age of 60 is approximately 65%, and the prevalence of isolated systolic hypertension is greater than in younger adults. In clinical trials, treatment has reduced the incidence of stroke by 36% and myocardial infarction by 27%. Although all antihypertensive drugs are effective in older adults, only the *beta blockers* and *diuretics* have been shown in controlled trials to reduce morbidity and mortality. Hence, these drugs are often preferred. Since cardiovascular reflexes are blunted in the elderly, treatment carries a significant risk of orthostatic hypotension. Accordingly, initial doses should be lower than for younger adults. Furthermore, drugs that are especially likely to cause orthostatic hypotension (e.g., guanethidine, alpha blockers, labetalol) should be used with caution.

Treating Hypertension During Pregnancy

When treating hypertension associated with pregnancy, it is essential to distinguish between chronic hypertension and pre-eclampsia, since chronic hypertension is relatively benign, whereas pre-eclampsia can lead to life-threatening complications for the mother and fetus.

Chronic Hypertension. Chronic hypertension is defined as hypertension that was present prior to pregnancy or that developed before the 20th week of gestation. Since elevated maternal blood pressure is not a direct threat to the fetus, the goal of treatment is to minimize the risk of hypertension to the mother while avoiding drug-induced harm to the fetus. With the exception of the ACE inhibitors, antihypertensive drugs that were being taken before pregnancy can be continued. *ACE inhibitors are contraindicated* because of their potential for fetal harm. When drug therapy is initiated during pregnancy, *methyldopa* is recommended, since this drug has been evaluated most extensively. Regardless of the drugs employed, treatment should not be too aggressive, since an excessive drop in blood pressure could compromise uteroplacental blood flow.

Pre-eclampsia. Pre-eclampsia is a pregnancy-specific condition characterized by hypertension in association with proteinuria, edema, or both. Liver dysfunction and coagulation abnormalities may also be present. The disorder may progress rapidly to eclampsia (pre-eclampsia plus convulsions). Treatment of pre-eclampsia consists of hospitalization, reduction of blood pressure, and prophylaxis of threatened seizures. The preferred drug for lowering blood pressure is *methyldopa*. Alternatives include *hydralazine* and *calcium channel blockers. ACE inhibitors can cause fetal harm and are contraindicated.* If pre-eclampsia progresses to eclampsia, immediate delivery or abortion is required. Recent evidence indicates that pre-eclampsia can be prevented by prophylaxis with low-dose aspirin (60 to 100 mg/day).

MINIMIZING ADVERSE EFFECTS

Antihypertensive drugs can produce many unwanted effects, including hypotension, sedation,

and disruption of sexual function. (Although not stressed previously, practically all antihypertensive drugs can interfere with sexual feelings or performance.)

The fundamental strategy for decreasing side effects is to tailor the regimen to the sensitivities of the patient. Simply put, if one drug causes effects that are objectionable, a more acceptable drug should be substituted. The best way to identify unacceptable responses is to encourage the patient to report them.

Adverse effects caused by exacerbation of co-existing diseases are both predictable and avoidable. By taking a thorough medical history, we can greatly reduce the chances of an inappropriate drug-disease match.

Use of high initial doses and rapid dosage escalation can increase the incidence and severity of adverse effects. Accordingly, doses should be low initially and then gradually increased. Remember, there is usually no need to reduce blood pressure rapidly. Hence, it makes no sense to give large initial doses that can produce a rapid fall in blood pressure but that also produce intense undesired responses.

PROMOTING COMPLIANCE

The major cause of treatment failure in patients with chronic hypertension is lack of adherence to the therapeutic regimen. In this section we will consider the causes of noncompliance and then discuss some solutions.

Why Compliance Can Be Difficult to Achieve

Much of the difficulty in promoting compliance stems from the nature of hypertension itself. Hypertension is a *chronic, slowly progressing* disease that, through much of its course, is *devoid of overt symptoms.* Because symptoms are absent, it can be difficult to convince patients that they are ill and need treatment. In addition, since there are no symptoms to relieve, drugs cannot produce an obvious therapeutic response. In the absence of such a response, it can be difficult for patients to believe that their medication is doing anything useful.

Because hypertension progresses very slowly, the disease tends to encourage procrastination. For most people, the adverse effects of hypertension will not become manifest for many years. Realizing this, patients may reason (incorrectly) that they can postpone therapy without significantly increasing their risk.

The negative aspects of treatment also contribute to noncompliance. Antihypertensive regimens can be complex and expensive. In addition, treatment must continue lifelong. Lastly, antihypertensive drugs can cause a number of adverse effects, ranging from sedation to hypotension to disruption of sexual function. It is difficult to convince people who are feeling good to start taking drugs that may make them feel worse. Some people may decide that exposing themselves to the negative effects of therapy today is paying too high a price to avoid the adverse consequences of hypertension at some indefinite time in the future.

Ways to Promote Compliance

Patient Education. Compliance requires motivation, and patient education can help provide it. Patients should be taught about the consequences of hypertension and the benefits of treatment. Because hypertension does not cause discomfort, it may not be clear to patients that their condition is indeed serious. Patients must be made to understand that, left untreated, hypertension can cause heart disease, kidney disease, blindness, and stroke. In addition, patients should appreciate that with proper therapy the risks of these long-term complications can be minimized, resulting in a longer and healthier life. Lastly, patients must understand that drugs do not cure hypertension—they only control symptoms. Hence, for treatment to be effective, medication must usually be taken lifelong.

Self-Monitoring. Patients should be taught the goal of treatment (reduction of SBP/DBP to 140/90 mm Hg) and they should be taught to monitor and record their blood pressure daily. This will increase patient involvement and will provide positive feedback that can help promote compliance.

Minimize Side Effects. Common sense dictates that if we expect patients to comply with long-term treatment, we must keep undesired effects to a minimum. As discussed above, adverse effects can be minimized by (1) encouraging patients to report side effects, (2) discontinuing objectionable drugs and substituting more acceptable ones, (3) avoiding drugs that can exacerbate coexisting pathology, and (4) using doses that are low initially and then gradually increased.

Establish a Collaborative Relationship. The patient who feels like a collaborative partner in the treatment program is more likely to comply than is the patient who feels that treatment is being imposed. Collaboration allows the patient to help set treatment goals, help create the treatment program, and participate in evaluating progress. In addition, a collaborative relationship facilitates communication about side effects. This is especially important with respect to drug-induced sexual dysfunction, which patients may be reluctant to discuss.

Simplify the Regimen. Antihypertensive regimens may consist of several drugs taken multiple times a day. Such complex regimens are a deterrent to compliance. Therefore, in order to promote compliance, steps should be taken to make the dosing schedule as simple as possible. Once an effective regimen has been established, an attempt should be made to switch to once-a-day or twice-a-day dosing. If an appropriate combination product is available (e.g., a fixed-dose combination of a thiazide diuretic plus a potassium-sparing diuretic), the combination product may be substituted for its components.

Other Measures. Compliance can be promoted by giving positive reinforcement when therapeutic goals are achieved. Involvement of family members in the program can be helpful. Also, compliance can be promoted by scheduling office visits at convenient times, and by following up on patients whose appointments are missed. For many patients, antihypertensive therapy represents a significant economic burden; devising a regimen that is effective and yet keeps costs low will certainly encourage compliance.

DRUGS FOR HYPERTENSIVE EMERGENCIES

A hypertensive emergency exists when diastolic pressure exceeds 120 mm Hg. The severity of the emergency is determined by the likelihood of organ damage. When excessive blood pressure is associated with papilledema (edema of the retina), intracranial hemorrhage, myocardial infarction, or acute congestive heart failure, a severe emergency exists and blood pressure must be lowered rapidly (within 1 hour). If severe hypertension is present but does not yet pose an immediate threat of organ damage, it is preferable to reduce blood pressure more slowly (over 24 to 48 hours). (Rapid reductions in blood pressure can cause cerebral ischemia, myocardial infarction, and renal failure. Hence, pressure should be reduced gradually whenever possible.)

The major drugs used for hypertensive emergencies are discussed below. All reduce blood pressure by causing vasodilation. With the exception of nifedipine, all are administered intravenously.

Nifedipine. Oral nifedipine [Adalat, Procardia] is the preferred therapy for most hypertensive emergencies. This calcium channel blocker lowers blood pressure by dilating arterioles. In patients with severe hypertension, nifedipine produces a 20% reduction in both systolic and diastolic pressure within 20 to 30 minutes. "Overshoot" (excessive lowering of pressure) is rare. The dosage is 5 to 20 mg repeated every 4 to 6 hours. To insure a rapid response, patients should be instructed to bite the nifedipine capsule and swallow its contents. The basic pharmacology of nifedipine is discussed in Chapter 38.

Sodium Nitroprusside. When acute, severe hypertension demands a rapid but controlled reduction in pressure, intravenous nitroprusside [Nipride, Nitropress] is usually the drug of first choice. Nitroprusside is a direct-acting vasodilator that relaxes smooth muscle of arterioles and veins. Effects begin in seconds and then fade rapidly when administration ceases. Nitroprusside is administered by continuous IV infusion using a pump to control the rate of flow. The usual infusion rate is 0.5 to 8 μg/kg/min. To avoid overshoot, continuous monitoring of blood pressure is required. Because nitroprusside has an extremely short duration of action, overshoot can be corrected quickly by reducing the rate of the infusion. Prolonged infusion (longer than 72 hours) can produce toxic accumulation of thiocyanate and should be avoided. The basic pharmacology of nitroprusside is discussed in Chapter 39.

Labetalol. Labetalol [Trandate, Normodyne] blocks alpha- and beta-adrenergic receptors. Blood pressure is reduced by arteriolar dilation secondary to alpha blockade. Beta blockade prevents reflex tachycardia in response to reduced arterial pressure; hence, the drug is probably safe for patients with angina pectoris and myocardial infarction. Beta blockade can aggravate bronchial asthma, congestive heart failure, A-V heart block, cardiogenic shock, and bradycardia. Accordingly, labetalol should not be given to patients with these disorders. Administration is by slow IV injection.

Diazoxide. Diazoxide [Hyperstat IV] causes selective dilation of arterioles. Effects begin within minutes and may persist for hours. The drug can be administered by IV bolus or by slow IV infusion (over 15 to 30 minutes). Diazoxide can produce reflex tachycardia and should be avoided in patients with angina. Reflex tachycardia can be reduced with a beta blocker. Fluid retention may occur and can be controlled with a diuretic. Hyperglycemia may be a complication for patients with diabetes. The basic pharmacology of diazoxide is discussed in Chapter 39.

Trimethaphan. Trimethaphan [Arfonad] is a ganglionic blocking agent that dilates arterioles and veins. Effects begin and end within minutes. Like nitroprusside, trimethaphan must be administered by continuous IV infusion, using a pump to control the rate of flow. Continuous monitoring of blood pressure is required. Prominent side effects (dry mouth, blurred vision, urinary retention, paresis of the bowel) result from parasympathetic blockade. The basic pharmacology of trimethaphan is discussed in Chapter 14.

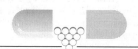

Summary of Major Nursing Implications

ANTIHYPERTENSIVE DRUGS

✔ **Preadministration Assessment**

Therapeutic Goal

The objective of antihypertensive therapy is to reduce SBP/DBP to 140/90 mm Hg, to prevent the long-term sequelae of hypertension (heart disease, kidney disease, blindness, stroke), and to minimize drug affects that can reduce quality of life.

Baseline Data

The following tests should be done in all hypertensive patients: blood pressure; electrocardiogram; complete urinalysis; hemoglobin and hematocrit; and blood levels of sodium, potassium, calcium, creatinine, glucose, uric acid, triglycerides, and cholesterol (total and HDL-cholesterol).

Identifying High-Risk Patients

When taking the patient history, attempt to identify drugs that can raise blood pressure or that can interfere with the effects of antihypertensive drugs. Some drugs of concern are listed below under *Minimizing Adverse Interactions*.

The patient history should identify co-existing pathologies that either contraindicate use of specific agents (e.g., congestive heart failure contraindicates use of beta blockers) or that require drugs to be used with special caution (e.g., thiazide diuretics must be used with caution in patients with gout or diabetes). For risk factors that pertain to specific antihypertensive drugs, refer to the chapters in which those drugs are discussed.

✔ **Implementation: Administration**

Routes

All drugs used in chronic hypertension can be administered orally. None are administered by injection.

Dosage

To minimize adverse effects, dosages should be low initially and then gradually increased. It is counterproductive to employ high initial dosages that produce a rapid fall in pressure but that also produce intense undesired responses that can discourage compliance. After 12 months of successful treatment, an attempt should be made to reduce dosages to their lowest effective level.

Simplifying the Regimen

An antihypertensive regimen can consist of several drugs taken multiple times a day. Once an effective regimen has been established, attempt to switch to once-a-day or twice-a-day dosing. If an appropriate combination product is available (e.g., a fixed-dose combination of a thiazide diuretic plus a potassium-sparing diuretic), substitute the combination product for its components.

Implementation: Measures to Enhance Therapeutic Effects

Lifestyle Changes

Lifestyle changes can lower blood pressure. These should be tried for 3 to 6 months before implementing drug therapy, and should be continued if drug therapy is nonetheless required.

Weight Reduction. Help overweight patients develop a restricted-calorie diet. The diet should be low in saturated fats, and total fat content should not exceed 30% of caloric intake. Target weight is 110% of ideal weight or less.

Sodium Restriction. Encourage patients to consume no more than 6 gm of salt (2.3 gm of sodium) daily and provide them with information on the salt content of foods.

Alcohol Restriction. Encourage patients who drink alcohol to limit consumption to 1 ounce a day. One ounce of ethanol is equivalent to about two mixed drinks, two glasses of wine, or two cans of beer.

Exercise. Encourage patients who have a sedentary lifestyle to establish a regular program of aerobic exercise (e.g., walking, jogging, swimming, bicycling).

Smoking Reduction or Cessation. Strongly encourage patients to quit smoking.

Promoting Compliance

Noncompliance is the major cause of treatment failure. Compliance can be difficult to achieve for the following reasons: hypertension is devoid of overt symptoms; drugs do not make people feel better and may make them feel worse; regimens can be complex and expensive; complications of hypertension take years to develop, thereby providing a misguided rationale for postponing treatment; and treatment is usually lifelong. Measures to promote compliance are summarized below.

Provide Patient Education. Educate patients about the long-term consequences of hypertension and the ability of lifestyle changes and drug therapy to decrease morbidity and prolong life. Inform patients that drugs do not cure hypertension and, therefore, must usually be taken lifelong.

Encourage Self-Monitoring. Make sure that patients know the treatment goal (reduction of SBP/DBP to 140/90 mm Hg) and teach them to monitor and chart their own blood pressure. This will increase patient involvement and help them see the benefits of therapy.

Minimize Side Effects. Adverse drug effects are an obvious deterrent to compliance. Measures to reduce undesired effects are discussed below, under *Minimizing Adverse Effects.*

Establish a Collaborative Relationship. Encourage patients to be active partners in setting treatment goals, creating a treatment program, and evaluating progress.

Simplify the Regimen. Simplification measures are discussed above, under *Simplifying the Regimen.*

Other Measures. Additional measures to promote compliance include providing positive reinforcement when treatment goals are achieved, involving family members in the treatment program, scheduling office visits at convenient times, following up on patients who miss an appointment, and devising a program that is effective but keeps costs low.

 Ongoing Evaluation and Interventions

Evaluating Treatment

Monitor blood pressure periodically. The goal is to reduce SBP/DBP to 140/90 mm Hg. Teach patients to self-monitor their blood pressure and to maintain a blood pressure record.

Minimizing Adverse Effects

General Considerations. The fundamental strategy for decreasing adverse effects is to tailor the regimen to the sensitivities of the patient. If a drug causes objectionable effects, a more acceptable drug should be substituted.

Inform patients about the potential side effects of treatment and encourage them to report objectionable responses.

Avoid drugs that can exacerbate co-existing pathology. For example, do not give beta blockers to patients who have congestive heart failure, A-V heart block, or asthma. A list of pathologies and drugs to avoid is given in Table 40–6.

Initiate therapy with low doses and increase them gradually.

Adverse Effects of Specific Drugs. For measures to minimize adverse effects of specific antihypertensive drugs (e.g., beta blockers, diuretics, ACE inhibitors) refer to the chapters in which those drugs are discussed.

Minimizing Adverse Interactions

When taking the patient history, identify drugs that can raise blood pressure or interfere with the effects of antihypertensive drugs. Drugs of concern include oral contraceptives, nasal decongestants and other cold remedies, nonsteroidal anti-inflammatory drugs, glucocorticoids, appetite suppressants, tricyclic antidepressants, monoamine oxidase inhibitors, cyclosporine, erythropoietin, and alcohol (in large quantities).

Antihypertensive regimens frequently contain two or more drugs, thereby posing a potential risk of adverse interactions (e.g., ACE inhibitors can increase the risk of hyperkalemia caused by potassium-sparing diuretics). For interactions that pertain to specific antihypertensive drugs, refer to the chapters in which those drugs are discussed.

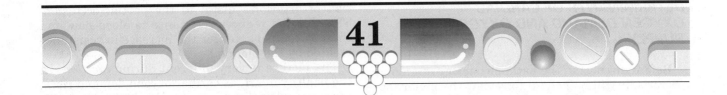

Drug Therapy of Angina Pectoris

Angina pectoris is defined as sudden pain beneath the sternum, often radiating to the left shoulder and arm. Anginal pain is precipitated when the oxygen supply to the heart is insufficient to meet oxygen demand. Most often, anginal pain occurs secondary to atherosclerosis of the coronary arteries. Hence, angina should be seen as a symptom of a disease and not as a disease in its own right.

Three drug families are used to treat angina. These are the *organic nitrates* (e.g., nitroglycerin), the *beta blockers* (e.g., propranolol), and the *calcium channel blockers* (e.g., verapamil). Our principal focus will be on the organic nitrates. The beta blockers and the calcium channel blockers are discussed at length in other chapters; hence, consideration here is limited to their use in angina pectoris.

ANGINA PECTORIS: PATHOPHYSIOLOGY AND TREATMENT STRATEGY

Angina pectoris has two major forms: (1) classic angina (exertional or effort-induced angina) and (2) variant angina (Prinzmetal's or vasospastic angina). Of the two conditions, classic angina is the more common.

501

DETERMINANTS OF CARDIAC OXYGEN DEMAND AND OXYGEN SUPPLY

Before discussing the pathophysiology of angina pectoris, it will be helpful to review the major factors that determine cardiac oxygen demand and oxygen supply.

Oxygen Demand. The principal determinants of cardiac oxygen demand are *heart rate, myocardial contractility*, and, most importantly, *intramyocardial wall tension*. Wall tension is determined by two factors: (1) systemic arterial resistance (cardiac afterload), and (2) the degree of ventricular diastolic dilation, which is determined by ventricular filling pressure (cardiac preload). From the preceding, we can see that cardiac oxygen demand is determined by four major factors: (1) heart rate, (2) contractility, (3) afterload, and (4) preload. Drugs that reduce these factors will reduce oxygen demand.

Oxygen Supply. Cardiac oxygen supply is determined by myocardial blood flow. Under resting conditions, the heart extracts nearly all of the oxygen delivered to it by the coronary vessels. Hence, the only way to accommodate an increase in oxygen demand is to increase blood flow. When oxygen demand increases, coronary arterioles dilate, and the resultant decrease in vascular resistance allows blood flow to increase. During exertion, coronary blood flow increases to four to five times the flow rate at rest.

CLASSIC ANGINA PECTORIS (EXERTIONAL ANGINA)

Pathophysiology. Classic angina pectoris is triggered most often by an increase in physical activity. Emotional excitement, large meals, and cold exposure may also precipitate an attack. Because classic angina usually occurs in response to strain, this condition is known alternatively as *exertional angina* or *angina of effort*.

The underlying cause of exertional angina is *coronary artery disease* (CAD), a condition characterized by deposition of fatty plaque on the arterial wall. If an artery is only partially occluded by plaque, blood flow will be reduced and angina pectoris will result. However, if complete vessel blockage occurs, blood flow will stop and myocardial infarction (heart attack) will result.

The impact of CAD on the balance between myocardial oxygen demand and oxygen supply is illustrated in Figure 41–1. As the figure depicts, in both the healthy heart and the heart with CAD, oxygen supply and oxygen demand are in balance when the subject is *at rest*. (In the presence of CAD, resting oxygen demand is met through dila-

tion of arterioles distal to the partial occlusion. This dilation reduces resistance to blood flow and thereby compensates for the increase in resistance created by the plaque.)

The picture is very different during *exertion*. In the healthy heart, as cardiac oxygen demand rises, coronary arterioles dilate, causing blood flow to increase. This increase keeps oxygen supply in balance with oxygen demand. In people with CAD, arterioles in the affected region are already fully dilated at rest. Hence, when exertion occurs, there is no way to increase blood flow to compensate for the increase in oxygen demand. The resultant imbalance between oxygen supply and oxygen demand is the cause of anginal pain.

Treatment Strategy. The goal of therapy is to reduce the intensity and frequency of anginal attacks. Because anginal pain results from an imbalance between oxygen supply and oxygen demand, logic dictates two possible remedies: (1) we might increase cardiac oxygen supply, or (2) we might decrease oxygen demand. Since the underlying cause of classic angina is occlusion of the coronary arteries, there is little we can do to increase cardiac oxygen supply. Hence, the first remedy is not a real option. Consequently, the principal way that we can relieve the pain of classic angina is to *decrease cardiac oxygen demand*. As discussed above, we can reduce oxygen demand with drugs that decrease heart rate, contractility, afterload, or preload.

Overview of Therapeutic Agents. Classic angina can be treated with three types of drugs: *organic nitrates, beta blockers*, and *calcium channel blockers*. All of these agents relieve the pain of classic angina primarily by decreasing cardiac oxygen demand. It should be noted that these drugs only provide symptomatic relief; they do not affect the underlying pathology (CAD).

Nondrug Therapy. Patients should attempt to avoid factors that can precipitate angina. These include overexertion, heavy meals, emotional stress, and exposure to cold.

Risk factors for classic angina should be corrected. Important among these are smoking, obesity, hypertension, hyperlipidemia, and a sedentary lifestyle. Patients should be strongly encouraged to quit smoking. Overweight patients should be given a restricted-calorie diet; the diet should be low in saturated fats, and total fat content should not exceed 30% of caloric intake. The target weight is 110% of ideal or less. Patients with a sedentary lifestyle should be encouraged to establish a regular program of aerobic exercise (e.g., walking, jogging, swimming, bicycling). Hypertension and hyperlipidemia are major risk factors and should be treated. These disorders are discussed in Chapters 40 and 45.

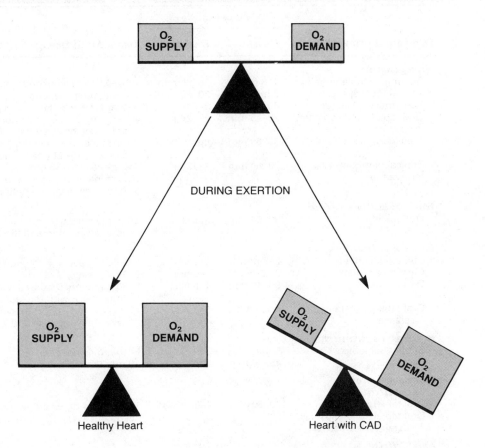

DURING REST
Healthy Heart and Heart with CAD

DURING EXERTION

Healthy Heart   Heart with CAD

Figure 41–1. Effect of exertion on the balance between oxygen supply and oxygen demand in the healthy heart and the heart with coronary artery disease (CAD). In the *healthy heart,* O_2 supply and O_2 demand are always in balance; during exertion, coronary arteries dilate, producing an increase in blood flow to meet the increase in O_2 demand. In the *heart with CAD,* O_2 supply and demand are in balance only during rest. During exertion, dilation of coronary arteries cannot compensate for the increase in O_2 demand, and an imbalance results.

VARIANT ANGINA PECTORIS (PRINZMETAL'S ANGINA, VASOSPASTIC ANGINA)

Pathophysiology. Variant angina pectoris is caused by *coronary artery spasm,* which restricts blood flow to the myocardium. Hence, as in classic angina, pain is secondary to insufficient oxygenation of the heart. In contrast to classic angina, whose symptoms occur primarily at times of exertion, variant angina can cause pain at any time, even during rest and sleep. Frequently, variant angina occurs in conjunction with classic angina. Alternative names for variant angina are *vasospastic angina* and *Prinzmetal's angina.*

Treatment Strategy. The goal of therapy is to reduce the incidence and severity of attacks. In contrast to classic angina, which is treated primarily by reducing oxygen demand, variant angina is treated by *increasing cardiac oxygen supply.* This makes sense since the pain is caused by a reduction in oxygen supply, rather than by an increase in demand. Oxygen supply is increased with vasodilators, which prevent or relieve coronary artery spasm.

Overview of Therapeutic Agents. Vasospastic angina is treated with two groups of drugs: *calcium channel blockers* and *organic nitrates.* Both drug classes act by relaxing coronary artery spasm. *Beta blockers,* which are effective in classic angina, are *not* effective against variant angina. As with classic angina, therapy is symptomatic only; drugs do not alter the underlying pathology.

ORGANIC NITRATES

The organic nitrates are the oldest and most frequently used antianginal drugs. These agents relieve angina by causing vasodilation. Nitroglycerin, the most familiar organic nitrate, will serve as our prototype for the family. A complete listing of organic nitrates appears in Table 41–1.

NITROGLYCERIN

Nitroglycerin has been used to treat angina since 1879. This drug is effective, fast acting, and inexpensive. Despite the development of newer an-

Table 41–1. Organic Nitrates: Formulations, Dosages, and Time Course			
Drug and Formulation	**Time Course**		**Usual Adult Dosage and Comments**
	Onset	*Duration*	
Nitroglycerin			
Sublingual tablets	1–3 min	30–60 min	0.15–0.6 mg as needed
Translingual spray	2 min	30–60 min	0.4–0.8 mg as needed
Transmucosal tablets	3 min	3–5 hr	1–2 mg every 3–8 hr
Oral tablets and capsules, sustained-release	20–45 min	8–12 hr	2.5–6.5 mg 3 or 4 times daily; to avoid tolerance, administer only once or twice daily. Do not crush or chew
Transdermal systems	30–60 min	up to 24 hr	1 patch a day; to avoid tolerance, remove after 12–14 hr, allowing 10–12 patch-free hr each day
Topical ointment	20–60 min	2–12 hr	1–2 inches (15–30 mg) every 4–8 hr
Intravenous	1–2 min	3–5 min	5 μg/min initially, then increased gradually as needed. Tolerance develops with prolonged continuous infusion
Isosorbide Mononitrate			
Oral tablets	30–60 min	hours	20 mg twice daily; to avoid tolerance, take the 1st dose upon awakening and the 2nd dose 7 hr later
Isosorbide Dinitrate			
Sublingual tablets	2–5 min	1–3 hr	2.5–10 mg every 4–6 hr; do not crush or chew
Chewable tablets	2–5 min	1–3 hr	5–10 mg every 2–3 hr
Oral tablets	20–40 min	4–6 hr	5–30 mg every 6 hr; to avoid tolerance, take only 2 or 3 times daily, with the last dose no later than 7 PM
Oral tablets, sustained release	up to 4 hrs	6–8 hrs	40 mg every 6–12 hr; to avoid tolerance, take only once or twice daily (at 8 AM and 2 PM)
Erythrityl Tetranitrate			
Sublingual tablets	5 min	3 hr	5–10 mg as needed
Oral tablets	15–30 min	6 hr	10 mg 3 times a day
Pentaerythritol Tetranitrate			
Oral tablets	20–60 min	4–5 hr	10–40 mg 4 times a day
Oral tablets and capsules, sustained release	30 min	up to 12 hr	30–80 mg every 12 hr; do not crush or chew
Amyl Nitrite			
Inhalant	30 sec	3–5 min	0.18 or 0.3 ml

tianginal agents, nitroglycerin remains the drug of choice for relieving acute anginal attacks.

Vasodilator Actions

Nitroglycerin acts directly on vascular smooth muscle (VSM) to promote vasodilation. At usual therapeutic doses, the drug acts primarily on *veins*; dilation of arterioles is only modest.

The biochemical events that lead to vasodilation are outlined in Figure 41–2. The process begins with uptake of nitrate by VSM, followed by conversion of nitrate to its active form: *nitric oxide*. As indicated, this conversion requires the presence of *sulfhydryl groups*. Nitric oxide activates guanylate cyclase, an enzyme that catalyzes the formation of cyclic GMP. Through a series of reactions, cyclic GMP decreases intracellular calcium levels. Since calcium is required for VSM contraction, the reduction in calcium results in vasodilation. For our purposes, the most important aspect of this sequence is the conversion of nitrate to its active form (nitric oxide) in the presence of a sulfhydryl source.

Mechanism of Antianginal Effects

Classic Angina. Nitroglycerin decreases the pain of exertional angina *primarily by decreasing cardiac oxygen demand*. Oxygen demand is decreased as follows: by dilating veins, nitroglycerin decreases venous return to the heart, and thereby decreases ventricular filling; the resultant decrease in wall tension decreases oxygen demand.

In patients with classic angina, nitroglycerin does not appear to increase blood flow to ischemic areas of the heart. This statement is based on two observations. First, nitroglycerin does not dilate atherosclerotic coronary arteries. Second, when nitroglycerin is injected directly into coronary arteries during an anginal attack, the drug does not relieve pain. Both observations suggest that the antianginal effects of nitroglycerin result from effects on peripheral blood vessels—and not from effects on coronary blood flow.

Variant Angina. In patients with variant angina, nitroglycerin acts by relaxing or preventing spasm in coronary arteries. Hence, the drug *increases oxygen supply* rather than decreasing oxygen demand.

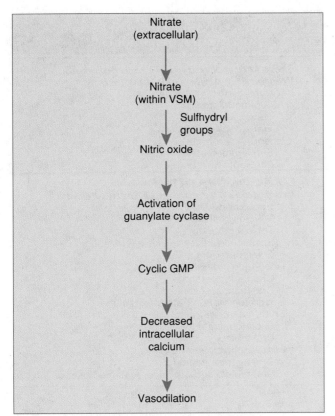

Figure 41–2. Biochemistry of nitrate-induced vasodilation. Note that sulfhydryl groups are needed to catalyze the conversion of nitrate to its active form, nitric oxide. If sulfhydryl groups are depleted from vascular smooth muscle (VSM), tolerance to nitrates will occur.

Pharmacokinetics

Absorption. Nitroglycerin is *highly lipid soluble* and crosses membranes with ease. Because of this property, nitroglycerin can be administered by uncommon routes (sublingual, buccal, transdermal) as well as by more conventional routes (oral, intravenous).

Metabolism. Nitroglycerin undergoes *rapid inactivation* by hepatic enzymes. As a result, the drug has a plasma half-life of only 5 to 7 minutes. When nitroglycerin is administered orally, most of each dose is destroyed on its first pass through the liver.

Adverse Effects

Nitroglycerin is generally well tolerated. Principal adverse effects—headache, hypotension, and tachycardia—occur secondary to vasodilation.

Headache. Initial therapy can produce severe headache. This response diminishes over the first few weeks of treatment. In the meantime, headache can be reduced with aspirin, acetaminophen, or another mild analgesic.

Orthostatic Hypotension. Relaxation of venous smooth muscle causes blood to pool in veins when the patient assumes an erect posture. This pooling decreases venous return to the heart, which reduces cardiac output, causing blood pressure to fall. Symptoms of orthostatic hypotension include lightheadedness and dizziness. Patients should be instructed to sit or lie down if these occur. Lying with the feet elevated promotes venous return, and can thereby help restore blood pressure.

Reflex Tachycardia. Although nitroglycerin acts primarily on veins, the drug can also dilate arterioles, causing arterial pressure to fall. By lowering blood pressure, nitroglycerin can activate the baroreceptor reflex, causing sympathetic stimulation of the heart. The resultant increase in heart rate increases cardiac oxygen demand, and can thereby negate the benefits of therapy. Pretreatment with a beta-adrenergic blocking agent or with verapamil (a calcium channel blocker that directly affects the heart) can prevent sympathetic cardiac stimulation.

Drug Interactions

Hypotensive Drugs. Nitroglycerin can intensify the effects of other hypotensive agents. Consequently, care should be exercised when nitroglycerin is used concurrently with beta blockers, calcium channel blockers, diuretics, and all other drugs that can lower blood pressure. Also, patients should be advised to avoid alcohol.

Beta Blockers, Verapamil, and Diltiazem. These drugs can suppress nitroglycerin-induced tachycardia. Beta blockers do so by preventing sympathetic activation of $beta_1$-adrenergic receptors on the heart. Verapamil and diltiazem prevent tachycardia through direct suppression of pacemaker activity in the sinoauricular (S-A) node.

Tolerance

Tolerance to nitroglycerin-induced vasodilation can develop rapidly (over the course of a single day). The mechanism underlying tolerance is depletion of sulfhydryl groups in VSM; in the absence of sulfhydryl groups, nitroglycerin and other nitrates cannot be converted to their active form, nitric oxide. Patients who develop tolerance to nitroglycerin display cross-tolerance to the other nitrates and vice versa. Development of tolerance is most likely with high-dose therapy and with uninterrupted therapy. To prevent tolerance, nitroglycerin and other nitrates should be used in the lowest effective dosages, and long-acting preparations (e.g., nitroglycerin transdermal patches) should be used on an intermittent schedule that allows at least 8 drug-free hours every day. If tolerance develops, it can be reversed by withholding nitrates until the sulfhydryl content of VSM has been replenished.

Preparations and Routes of Administration

Nitroglycerin is available in an assortment of formulations for administration by a variety of routes (see Table 41–1). This proliferation of dosage forms reflects efforts to delay hepatic metabolism, and thereby prolong therapeutic effects. Trade names are summarized in Table 41–2.

All nitroglycerin preparations produce qualitatively similar responses; differences relate only to time course of action. With some preparations, effects begin rapidly and then fade within 30 to 60 minutes. With others, effects begin slowly but persist for hours. With one preparation (transmucosal tablets), effects begin rapidly and then persist.

Applications of specific preparations are based on their time course of action. Preparations with a *rapid onset* are employed to *terminate an ongoing anginal attack*. When used for this purpose, rapid-acting preparations are administered as soon as

Table 41–3. Applications of Organic Nitrate Preparations

Short-Acting Nitrates for Prophylaxis and Treatment of Acute Angina Pectoris
Nitroglycerin
  Sublingual tablets
  Translingual spray
  Transmucosal tablets*
Isosorbide dinitrate
  Sublingual tablets
  Chewable tablets

Long-Acting Nitrates for Sustained Prophylaxis (Prevention) of Angina Pectoris†
Nitroglycerin
  Transdermal patches
  Topical ointment
  Sustained-release capsules and tablets
  Transmucosal tablets*
Isosorbide dinitrate
  Oral tablets, standard
  Oral tablets, sustained-release
Isosorbide mononitrate (oral tablets)
Erythrityl tetranitrate
  Sublingual tablets
  Oral tablets
Pentaerythritol tetranitrate
  Oral tablets, standard
  Oral tablets and capsules, sustained-release

*Used for acute therapy *and* sustained prophylaxis.
†All of these pose a risk of tolerance.

Table 41–2. Trade Names for Organic Nitrates

Generic Name	Trade Name(s)
Nitroglycerin	
Sublingual tablets	Nitrostat
Translingual spray	Nitrolingual
Transmucosal tablets	Nitrogard
Oral tablets, SR	Nitrong
Oral capsules, SR	Nitro-Bid Plateau Caps, Nitroglyn, Nitrocine Timecaps
Transdermal systems	Deponit, Minitran, Nitrodisc, Nitro-Dur, Nitrocine, Transderm-Nitro
Topical ointment	Nitro-Bid, Nitrol
Intravenous	Nitro-Bid IV, Tridil
Isosorbide Mononitrate	
Oral tablets	ISMO
Isosorbide Dinitrate	
Sublingual tablets	Isordil, Sorbitrate
Chewable tablets	Sorbitrate
Oral tablets	Isordil Titradose, Sorbitrate
Oral tablets, SR	Dilatrate S-R, Iso-Bid, Isordil Tembids, Isotrate Timecelles, Sorbitrate SA
Erythrityl Tetranitrate	
Sublingual tablets	Cardilate
Oral tablets	Cardilate
Pentaerythritol Tetranitrate	
Oral tablets	Pentylan, Peritrate
Oral tablets, SR	Peritrate SA
Oral capsules, SR	Duotrate, Duotrate 45
Amyl Nitrite	
Inhalant	Generic only

SR = sustained release

pain begins. Rapid-acting preparations can also be used for *prophylaxis of angina*. For this purpose, these preparations are taken just prior to anticipated exertion. *Long-acting preparations* are used to provide *sustained protection* against anginal attacks. To provide protection, these preparations are administered on a fixed schedule (but one that permits at least 8 drug-free hours each day). Applications of specific preparations are summarized in Table 41–3.

Sublingual Tablets. When administered sublingually (beneath the tongue), nitroglycerin is absorbed directly through the oral mucosa and into the bloodstream. Hence, unlike orally administered drugs, which must pass through the liver on their way to the systemic circulation, sublingual nitroglycerin bypasses the liver, and thereby temporarily avoids metabolism. Because the liver is bypassed, sublingual doses can be low (between 0.15 and 0.6 mg). These doses are about 10 times lower than those required when nitroglycerin is taken orally.

Effects of sublingual nitroglycerin begin rapidly—in 1 to 3 minutes—and persist for up to 1 hour. Because sublingual administration works fast, this route is ideal for (1) termination of an ongoing anginal attack, and (2) short-term prophylaxis when exertion is anticipated.

To terminate an acute anginal attack, sublingual nitroglycerin should be administered as soon as pain begins. Administration should not be delayed until the pain has become severe. If 1 tablet is insufficient, 1 or 2 additional tablets should be taken at 5-minute intervals. If pain persists, the patient should contact a physician or report to an emergency facility, since anginal pain that is unresponsive to nitroglycerin may indicate myocardial infarction.

Sublingual administration is unfamiliar to most patients. Accordingly, education about this route should be provided. The patient should be instructed to place the tablet under the tongue and leave it there while it dissolves. Nitroglycerin tablets formulated for sublingual use are ineffective if swallowed.

Nitroglycerin tablets are chemically unstable and can lose effectiveness over time. Shelf life can be prolonged by storing tablets in a tightly closed, dark container. Under these conditions, tablets should remain effective for at least 6 months after the container is first opened. As a rule, nitroglycerin tablets should be discarded after this time. Patients should be instructed to write the date of opening on the container and to discard unused tablets 6 months later.

Translingual Spray. Nitroglycerin can be delivered to the oral mucosa using a metered-dose spray device. Each activation delivers a 0.4-mg dose. Indications for nitroglycerin spray are the same as those for sublingual tablets: (1) suppression of an acute anginal attack, and (2) prophylaxis of angina when exertion is anticipated. As with sublingual tablets, no more than three doses should be administered within a 15-minute interval. Patients should be instructed not to inhale the spray.

Transmucosal (Buccal) Tablets. Administration of transmucosal nitroglycerin tablets consists of placing the tablet between the upper lip and the gum, or in the buccal area between the cheek and the gum. The tablet will adhere to the oral mucosa and slowly dissolve over 3 to 5 hours. As the tablet dissolves, nitroglycerin is absorbed directly through the oral mucosa and into the bloodstream, thereby bypassing the liver. Like sublingual nitroglycerin, transmucosal nitroglycerin has a rapid onset of action. Hence, transmucosal administration can be used to terminate an ongoing anginal attack, and to provide short-term prophylaxis prior to exertion. In addition, since the effects of transmucosal nitroglycerin are prolonged, this formulation can be used for sustained prophylaxis. Patients should be instructed not to chew or swallow these tablets.

Sustained-Release Oral Tablets and Capsules. Sustained-release oral formulations are intended for long-term prophylaxis only; these formulations cannot act quickly enough to terminate an ongoing anginal attack. Sustained-release tablets and capsules contain a large dose of nitroglycerin that is slowly absorbed across the gastrointestinal wall. In theory, doses are large enough so that amounts of nitroglycerin sufficient to produce a therapeutic response will survive passage through the liver. Because they produce sustained blood levels of nitroglycerin, these formulations can cause tolerance. To reduce the risk of tolerance, these products should be taken only once or twice daily. Patients should be instructed to swallow sustained-release formulations intact.

Topical Ointment. Topical nitroglycerin ointment is used for sustained protection against anginal attacks. The ointment is applied to the skin of the chest, back, abdomen, or anterior thigh. (Since nitroglycerin acts primarily by dilating *peripheral* veins, there is no mechanistic advantage to applying topical nitroglycerin directly over the heart.) Following topical application, nitroglycerin is absorbed through the skin and then into the bloodstream. Effects begin within 20 to 60 minutes and may persist for up to 12 hours.

Nitroglycerin ointment (2%) is dispensed from a tube, and the length of the ribbon squeezed from the tube determines the dosage. (One inch contains about 15 mg of nitroglycerin.) The usual adult dosage is 1 to 2 inches applied every 4 to 8 hours. The ointment should be spread over a 6-inch by 6-inch area and then covered with a plastic wrap. Sites of application should be rotated to minimize irritation of the skin. As with other long-acting formulations, uninterrupted use can cause tolerance.

Transdermal Delivery Systems. Transdermal delivery systems for nitroglycerin, which look somewhat like adhesive bandages, contain a reservoir from which nitroglycerin is slowly released. Following its release, the drug is absorbed through the skin and then into the bloodstream. The rate of release is constant for any particular transdermal patch and, depending upon the system used, can range from 0.1 to 0.6 mg/hour. Effects begin within 30 to 60 minutes and persist as long as the patch remains in place (up to 14 hours). Transdermal patches are applied once daily to a hairless area of skin. The site should be rotated to avoid local irritation.

Tolerance develops if the patches are used continuously (24 hours a day every day). Accordingly, a daily "patch-free" interval of 10 to 12 hours is recommended. This can be accomplished by applying a new patch each morning, leaving it in place for 12 to 14 hours, and then removing it in the evening.

Intravenous Infusion. Intravenous nitroglycerin is employed only rarely to treat angina pectoris. When used for angina, IV nitroglycerin is limited to patients who have failed to respond to other medications. Additional uses of IV nitroglycerin include treatment of congestive heart failure associated with acute myocardial infarction, treatment of perioperative hypertension, and production of controlled hypotension for surgery.

Intravenous nitroglycerin has a very short duration of action; hence, continuous infusion is required. The rate is 5 μg/minute initially and then increased gradually until an adequate response has been achieved. Heart rate and blood pressure must be monitored continuously.

Stock solutions of nitroglycerin must be diluted for intravenous therapy. Since ampules of nitroglycerin prepared by different manufacturers can differ both in volume and nitroglycerin concentration, the label must be read carefully when dilutions are made.

Administration should be performed using a *glass* IV bottle and the administration set provided by the manufacturer. Nitroglycerin absorbs into standard polyvinyl chloride tubing; hence, this tubing should be avoided.

Discontinuing Nitroglycerin

Long-acting preparations (transdermal patches, topical ointment, sustained-release oral tablets or capsules) should be discontinued slowly. If these preparations are withdrawn abruptly, vasospasm may result.

Summary of Therapeutic Uses

Acute Therapy of Angina. For acute treatment of angina pectoris, nitroglycerin is administered in sublingual tablets, transmucosal tablets, and a translingual spray. All three dosage forms can be used to abort an ongoing anginal attack and to provide prophylaxis in anticipation of exertion.

Sustained Therapy of Angina. For sustained prophylaxis against angina, nitroglycerin is administered in the following formulations: topical ointment, transdermal patches, transmucosal tablets, or sustained-release oral tablets or capsules.

Intravenous Therapy. Intravenous nitroglycerin is indicated for perioperative control of blood pressure, production of controlled hypotension during surgery, and treatment of congestive heart failure associated with acute myocardial infarction. In addition, IV nitroglycerin is used to treat angina pectoris when symptoms cannot be controlled with preferred medications.

OTHER ORGANIC NITRATES

Isosorbide Dinitrate, Isosorbide Mononitrate, Erythrityl Tetranitrate, Pentaerythritol Tetranitrate

All of these nitrates have pharmacologic actions identical to those of nitroglycerin. All are used to treat angina pectoris. Pharmacologic differences among these drugs relate to routes of administration and time course of action (see Table 41–1). These differences determine whether a particular drug or do-

sage form will be used for acute therapy, sustained prophylaxis, or both (see Table 41–3). As with nitroglycerin, tolerance can develop to long-acting preparations. To avoid tolerance, long-acting preparations should be used on an intermittent schedule—one that allows at least 8 drug-free hours a day.

AMYL NITRITE

Amyl nitrite is an ultrashort-acting agent used to treat acute episodes of angina pectoris. The drug's mechanism of action is the same as that of nitroglycerin. Amyl nitrite is a volatile liquid that is dispensed in glass ampuls. For administration, an ampul is crushed, allowing the volatile compound to be inhaled. Effects begin within 30 seconds and terminate in 3 to 5 minutes. Amyl nitrite is highly flammable and should not be used near flame. The drug is reputed to intensify sexual orgasm and has been abused for that purpose (see Chapter 34).

BETA-ADRENERGIC BLOCKING AGENTS

Beta-adrenergic blocking agents (e.g., propranolol, metoprolol) are important drugs for treating *classic angina pectoris*, but are *not* effective against vasospastic angina. When administered on a fixed dosing schedule, beta blockers can provide sustained protection against effort-induced anginal pain. Exercise tolerance is increased and the frequency and intensity of attacks are lowered. All of the beta blockers appear equally effective.

Beta blockers reduce anginal pain by *decreasing cardiac oxygen demand*. This is accomplished primarily through blockade of beta$_1$ receptors in the heart, which decreases heart rate and contractility. Beta blockers can reduce oxygen demand further by causing a modest reduction in arterial pressure (afterload). In patients taking vasodilators (e.g., nitroglycerin), beta blockers provide the additional benefit of blunting reflex tachycardia.

For treatment of classic angina, dosage should be low initially and then gradually increased. The dosing goal is to lower resting heart rate to 50 to 60 beats/min, and limit exertional heart rate to about 100 beats/min. Beta blockers should not be withdrawn abruptly, since doing so can increase the incidence and intensity of anginal attacks, and may even precipitate myocardial infarction.

Beta blockers can produce a variety of adverse effects. Blockade of cardiac beta$_1$ receptors can produce *bradycardia, decreased atrioventricular (A-V) conduction*, and *reduction of contractility*. Consequently, beta blockers should not be used by patients with sick-sinus syndrome, congestive heart failure, or second- or third-degree A-V block. Blockade of beta$_2$ receptors in the lung can promote *bronchoconstriction*. Accordingly, beta blockers should be avoided by patients with asthma. If an asthmatic individual absolutely must use a beta blocker, a beta$_1$-selective agent (e.g., metoprolol) should be employed. Beta blockers can mask signs of hypoglycemia and, therefore, must be used with caution in patients with *diabetes*. Through effects on the central nervous system, these drugs can cause *insomnia*, *depression*, *bizarre dreams*, and *sexual dysfunction*.

The basic pharmacology of the beta blockers is discussed in Chapter 18.

CALCIUM CHANNEL BLOCKING AGENTS

The calcium channel blockers used most frequently are *verapamil*, *diltiazem*, and *nifedipine*. Accordingly, our discussion will focus on these three drugs. *All three* agents can block calcium channels in *vascular smooth muscle*, primarily in arterioles. The result is arteriolar dilation and reduction of peripheral resistance (afterload). In addition, *verapamil* and *diltiazem* can block calcium channels in the *heart*, and can thereby decrease heart rate, A-V conduction, and contractility.

Calcium channel blockers are used to treat both classic angina and variant angina. In *variant angina*, these drugs promote relaxation of coronary artery spasm, thereby *increasing cardiac oxygen supply*. In *classic angina*, these drugs promote relaxation of peripheral arterioles; the resultant decrease in afterload *reduces cardiac oxygen demand*. Verapamil and diltiazem can produce modest additional reductions in oxygen demand by suppressing heart rate and contractility.

The major adverse effects of the calcium channel blockade are cardiovascular. Dilation of peripheral arterioles lowers blood pressure, and can thereby induce *reflex tachycardia*. This reaction is greatest with nifedipine and minimal with verapamil and diltiazem. Because of their suppressant effects on the heart, verapamil and diltiazem must be used cautiously in patients taking beta blockers and in patients with bradycardia, congestive heart failure, or A-V heart block. These precautions do not apply to nifedipine.

The basic pharmacology of the calcium channel blockers is discussed in Chapter 38.

INVASIVE PROCEDURES USED TO TREAT ANGINA

CORONARY ARTERY BYPASS GRAFTING

Coronary artery bypass grafting (CABG) is a surgical procedure used to increase blood flow to ischemic areas of the heart. In this procedure, one end of a segment of healthy blood vessel is grafted onto the aorta, and the other end is connected to the diseased coronary artery at a point distal to the region of atherosclerotic plaque. Hence, the graft constitutes a shunt whereby blood flow can bypass the occluded section of a diseased coronary vessel. Following surgery, most patients remain in the hospital for a week, and then recuperate for another 6 weeks at home. The cost of a bypass operation is about $30,000. Once considered exotic, coronary bypass surgery has become commonplace; more than 200,000 Americans undergo the procedure annually.

Although the effects of bypass surgery can be dramatic, they can also be short-lived: only 65% of grafts remain patent after 5 to 11 years. Patency can be prolonged by antiplatelet therapy (daily low-dose aspirin) and by reducing risk factors for angina.

The great frequency with which bypass surgery is performed suggests that the procedure may not always be employed judiciously. It seems very likely that many of the individuals who receive bypass grafts could be treated just as effectively with drugs—an alternative that is safer and much less expensive. Accordingly, it has been recommended that bypass surgery be reserved for those patients who have severe angina and who have been refractory to drug therapy; in addition, patients should be good candidates for surgery.

PERCUTANEOUS TRANSLUMINAL CORONARY ANGIOPLASTY

Percutaneous transluminal coronary angioplasty (PTCA) is an alternative to CABG for treatment of classic angina pectoris. In PTCA, a miniature catheter containing a deflated balloon is inserted into the femoral artery, threaded up into the aorta, and then manipulated into the occluded coronary artery. The balloon is then inflated, thereby flattening the obstruction and allowing blood to flow. Unfortunately, re-occlusion occurs in about one third of patients within 6 to 8 months, necessitating a repeat of the procedure. As with CABG, PTCA should be reserved for patients who have not responded to drug therapy of angina.

PTCA offers three major advantages over bypass surgery. First, PTCA does not require general anesthesia. Second, recovery from PTCA occurs quickly, allowing most patients to return to work within 1 to 2 days. Third, the cost of PTCA is about $15,000—roughly half the cost of a bypass operation.

SUMMARY OF THERAPEUTIC MEASURES

In the preceding sections, we have discussed three drug families and two invasive procedures that can be used to treat angina pectoris. In this section, we consider guidelines for implementing these therapeutic modalities. It should be noted that these guidelines are general and intended only to provide a basic understanding as to when a specific modality might be employed.

CLASSIC ANGINA PECTORIS

Treatment of angina can be approached in a stepwise fashion (Table 41–4). Progression from one step to the next is based on the frequency and intensity of attacks and on the patient's response to therapy. Some patients can be treated with a single drug, some require two or three drugs; and some may require surgical intervention.

Step 1. If anginal attacks are infrequent (no more than one a day), then PRN therapy with sublingual nitroglycerin or another fast-acting nitrate is often sufficient. Likewise, if attacks occur predictably with exertion, taking a fast-acting nitrate 5 minutes before the anticipated activity may be all that is needed.

Step 2. When anginal episodes occur more than once a day, a drug that can provide sustained prophylaxis should be added to the regimen. Usually, a beta blocker is chosen. In fact, in the absence of specific contraindications (asthma, bradycardia, congestive heart failure, A-V heart block), a trial with a beta blocker is recommended for all patients who have frequent anginal attacks. To be effective, the drug must be taken on a fixed schedule. Therapy with a fast-acting nitrate should continue on a PRN basis. In addition to providing prophylaxis, the beta blocker will suppress nitrate-induced reflex tachycardia.

Calcium channel blockers are an alternative to beta blockers for sustained prophylaxis. Since calcium channel blockers do not promote bronchocon-

striction, they are preferred to beta blockers for patients with asthma. Nifedipine, which lacks cardiosuppressant effects, is safer than beta blockers for patients with bradycardia, A-V heart block, or congestive heart failure. This is not true of verapamil and diltiazem—calcium channel blockers that, like beta blockers, can suppress cardiac function. When used for prophylaxis of angina, calcium channel blockers must be taken on a regular schedule. A fast-acting nitrate should be used as needed to supplement antianginal effects.

Long-acting nitrate preparations (e.g., transdermal nitroglycerin) can also be used for sustained prophylaxis. However, because tolerance can develop quickly, these preparations would seem less well suited than beta blockers or calcium channel blockers for continuous protection against angina.

Step 3. Patients who do not respond to two drugs (a nitrate plus either a beta blocker or a calcium channel blocker) should receive a trial with three drugs: a nitrate, a beta blocker, and a calcium channel blocker (usually nifedipine). The benefit of taking three drugs is that oxygen demand is reduced by multiple mechanisms: nitrates reduce preload (by dilating veins); calcium channel blockers reduce afterload (by dilating arterioles); and beta blockers reduce heart rate and contractility. It should be noted that when a calcium channel blocker is to be combined with a beta blocker, *nifedipine* is preferred to verapamil and diltiazem. Nifedipine is preferred because it does not directly affect the heart and, therefore, will not intensify the cardiosuppressant effects of beta blockade.

Step 4. If the combination of a nitrate, a beta blocker, and a calcium channel blocker fails to provide relief from angina, CABG or PTCA may be indicated. Note that invasive procedures should be considered only after more conservative treatment has been attempted.

Reduction of Risk Factors. At all stages, the treatment program should reduce anginal risk factors: obese patients should lose weight, smokers should quit, sedentary patients should get aerobic exercise, and patients with hypertension or hyperlipidemia should receive appropriate therapy.

VARIANT ANGINA PECTORIS

Treatment of vasospastic angina can proceed in three steps. For initial therapy, either a calcium channel blocker or a nitrate is selected. If either drug alone is inadequate, then combined therapy with a calcium channel blocker *plus* a nitrate should be tried. If this combination fails to control anginal attacks, CABG may be indicated.

Table 41–4. Stepwise Therapy of Classic Angina Pectoris

Step 1: Nitrates

Step 2: Nitrates + beta blocker *or*
Nitrates + calcium channel blocker

Step 3: Nitrates + beta blocker + calcium channel blocker

Step 4: CABG *or* PTCA

At all stages, the treatment program should encourage reduction of angina risk factors: obese patients should lose weight, smokers should quit, sedentary patients should get aerobic exercise, and patients with hypertension or hyperlipidemia should receive appropriate therapy.

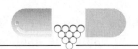

Summary of Major Nursing Implications

NITROGLYCERIN

**Preadministration
Assessment**

Therapeutic Goal

Reduction of the frequency and intensity of anginal attacks.

Baseline Data

Obtain baseline data on the frequency and intensity of anginal attacks, the location of anginal pain, and the factors that precipitate attacks.

The patient interview and physical examination should identify risk factors for angina pectoris, including treatable contributing pathophysiologic conditions (e.g., hypertension, hyperlipidemia).

Identifying High-Risk Patients

Use with *caution* in *hypotensive patients* and patients taking *drugs that can lower blood pressure, including alcohol and antihypertensive medications.*

**Implementation:
Administration**

Routes and Administration

Sublingual. Use: prophylaxis or termination of an acute anginal attack.

Instruct patients to place the tablet under the tongue and leave it there until fully dissolved; the tablet should not be swallowed.

Inform patients that if 1 tablet fails to relieve pain, 1 or 2 additional tablets should be taken at 5-minute intervals. Instruct patients to seek medical help immediately if pain is not relieved within 15 minutes.

Instruct patients to store tablets in a dark, tightly closed bottle that contains no other medications. Instruct patients to write the date of opening on the bottle and to discard unused medication after 6 months.

Translingual Spray. Use: prophylaxis or termination of an acute anginal attack.

Instruct patients to direct the spray against the oral mucosa. Warn patients against inhaling the spray.

Transmucosal (Buccal) Tablets. Uses: (1) prophylaxis or termination of an acute anginal attack, and (2) sustained prophylaxis.

Instruct patients to place the transmucosal tablet between the upper lip and the gum or in the buccal area between the cheek and the gum. Inform patients that the tablet will adhere to the oral mucosa and slowly dissolve over 3 to 5 hours. To achieve sustained prophylaxis, a tablet should be administered every 3 to 8 hours.

Sustained-Release Oral Tablets and Capsules. Use: sustained protection against anginal attacks.

To avoid tolerance, administer only once or twice daily.

Instruct patients to swallow these preparations intact, without chewing or crushing.

Topical Ointment. Use: sustained protection against anginal attacks.

Before applying a new dose, remove ointment remaining from the previous dose.

Technique of administration: (1) squeeze a ribbon of ointment of prescribed length onto the applicator paper provided; (2) using the applicator paper, spread the ointment over a 6-inch by 6-inch area (application may be made to the chest, back, abdomen, upper arm, or anterior thigh); and (3) cover the ointment with plastic wrap. Avoid touching the ointment.

Rotate the application site to minimize local irritation.

Transdermal Delivery Systems. Use: sustained protection against anginal attacks.

Instruct patients to apply transdermal patches to a hairless area of skin, using a new patch and a different site each day.

Instruct patients to remove the patch after 12 to 14 hours, allowing 10 to 12 "patch-free" hours each day. This practice will prevent tolerance.

Intravenous. Uses: (1) angina pectoris refractory to more conventional therapy, (2) perioperative control of blood pressure, (3) production of controlled hypotension during surgery, and (4) congestive heart failure associated with acute myocardial infarction.

Perform IV administration using a glass IV bottle and the administration set provided by the manufacturer; avoid standard IV tubing. Dilute stock solutions before use.

Administer by continuous infusion. The rate is slow initially (5 μg/min) and then gradually increased until an adequate response is achieved.

Monitor cardiovascular status constantly.

Terminating Therapy

Warn patients against abrupt withdrawal of long-acting preparations (transdermal systems, topical ointment, sustained-release tablets and capsules).

Implementation: Measures to Enhance Therapeutic Effects

Reducing Risk Factors

Precipitating Factors. Advise patients to avoid activities that are likely to elicit an anginal attack (e.g., overexertion, heavy meals, emotional stress, cold exposure).

Weight Reduction. Help overweight patients develop a restricted-calorie diet. The diet should be low in saturated fats, and total fat content should not exceed 30% of caloric intake. Target weight is 110% of ideal or less.

Exercise. Encourage patients who have a sedentary lifestyle to establish a regular program of aerobic exercise (e.g., walking, jogging, swimming, bicycling).

Smoking Cessation. Strongly encourage patients to quit smoking.

Contributing Disease States. Insure that patients with contributing pathology (especially hypertension or hypercholesterolemia) are receiving appropriate treatment.

Ongoing Evaluation and Interventions

Evaluating Therapeutic Effects

Have the patient keep a record of the frequency and intensity of anginal attacks, the location of anginal pain, and the factors that precipitate attacks.

Minimizing Adverse Effects

Headache. Inform patients that headache will diminish with continued drug use. Advise patients that headache can be relieved with aspirin, acetaminophen, or another mild analgesic.

Orthostatic Hypotension. Inform patients about symptoms of hypotension (e.g., dizziness, lightheadedness) and advise them to sit or lie down if these occur. Inform patients that hypotension can be minimized by moving slowly when changing from a sitting or supine position to an upright posture.

Reflex Tachycardia. This reaction can be suppressed by concurrent treatment with a *beta blocker, verapamil,* or *diltiazem.*

Minimizing Adverse Interactions

Hypotensive Agents. Nitroglycerin can interact with other hypotensive drugs to produce excessive lowering of blood pressure. Advise patients to avoid *alcohol.* Exercise caution when nitroglycerin is used in combination with *beta blockers, calcium channel blockers, diuretics,* and *all other drugs that can lower blood pressure.*

ISOSORBIDE MONONITRATE, ISOSORBIDE DINITRATE, ERYTHRITYL TETRANITRATE, PENTAERYTHRITOL TETRANITRATE

All four drugs have pharmacologic actions identical to those of nitroglycerin. Differences relate only to specific applications (see Table 41–3) and to dosage forms, routes of administration, and time course of action (see Table 41–2). Hence, the implications presented for nitroglycerin apply to these drugs as well.

Drug Therapy of Congestive Heart Failure

Congestive heart failure (CHF) is a syndrome characterized by reduced cardiac output. CHF is a common disorder that affects about 1% of the American population. The principal drugs employed for treatment are *diuretics*, *vasodilators*, and *inotropic agents*. Most of this chapter is dedicated to drugs known as cardiac glycosides (e.g., digoxin), the inotropic drugs encountered most frequently. Diuretics and vasodilators are discussed at length in other chapters; hence, their consideration here is brief. Before discussing the cardiac glycosides we will (1) review the factors that determine cardiac output, (2) discuss the pathophysiology of CHF, and (3) establish an overview of CHF therapy.

FACTORS THAT DETERMINE CARDIAC OUTPUT

Before discussing CHF and its treatment, it will be helpful to review the major factors that determine cardiac output.

The basic equation for cardiac output is

$$CO = HR \times SV$$

where CO is cardiac output, HR is heart rate, and SV is stroke volume. Clearly, factors that alter heart rate or stroke volume will alter cardiac output.

Heart rate is controlled by the autonomic nervous system. Rate is increased by the sympathetic branch acting through beta$_1$-adrenergic receptors in the sinoauricular (S-A) node. Rate is decreased by the parasympathetic branch acting through muscarinic receptors in the S-A node.

Stroke volume is determined largely by three factors: (1) myocardial contractility, (2) cardiac afterload, and (3) cardiac preload. *Myocardial contractility* is defined as the force with which the ventricles contract. Contractility can be increased by the sympathetic nervous system acting through beta$_1$-adrenergic receptors in the myocardium. More importantly, contractility is increased by cardiac dilatation, in accordance with the Frank-Starling relationship (see below).

Cardiac *afterload* is defined as the force against which the heart must work to pump blood. Afterload is determined by arteriolar resistance. Accordingly, when arterioles constrict, afterload is increased and cardiac output declines. Conversely, when arterioles dilate, afterload is reduced and cardiac output increases.

Cardiac *preload* is defined as ventricular filling pressure, or the force with which blood is returned to the heart. Preload is determined by blood volume and venous contraction; an increase in either will cause preload to increase. Increased preload results in increased ventricular filling, which, because of the Frank-Starling relationship (see below), increases stroke volume and cardiac output.

The *Frank-Starling relationship* between ventricular diameter and contractile force is depicted in Figure 42–1. As the curves indicate, contractile force (which determines stroke volume) increases with an increase in ventricular diameter. This means that *as ventricular filling increases, the force of contraction will increase as well*. Because of this relationship, the healthy heart is able to precisely match its output to the volume of blood delivered by the veins: if venous return increases, cardiac output increases correspondingly; conversely, if venous return declines, cardiac output declines to the same extent. Hence, *under normal physiologic conditions, venous return is the principal determinant of stroke volume and cardiac output*.

Why does contractile force change as a function of ventricular diameter? Recall that muscle contraction results from the interaction of two proteins: actin and myosin. As the heart stretches in response to increased ventricular filling, actin and myosin are brought into a more optimal alignment with each other, which allows them to interact with greater force.

RELATIONSHIP OF VENTRICULAR
FIBER LENGTH TO CONTRACTILE FORCE

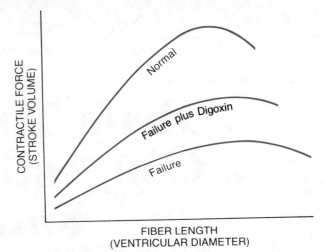

Figure 42–1. Relationship of ventricular diameter to contractile force. In the normal heart and the failing heart, increased fiber length produces increased contractile force. However, for any given fiber length, contractile force in the failing heart is much less than in the healthy heart. By increasing cardiac contractility, digoxin shifts the relationship between fiber length and stroke volume in the failing heart toward that in the normal heart.

PATHOPHYSIOLOGY OF CONGESTIVE HEART FAILURE

CHF is a pathophysiologic state characterized by an inability of the heart to pump sufficient blood to meet the metabolic needs of tissues. CHF is a not a specific disease. Rather, it is a clinical syndrome that can be precipitated by multiple factors, including hypertension, valvular heart disease, coronary artery disease, myocardial infarction, dysrhythmias, and aging of the heart muscle. Early symptoms include fatigue and shortness of breath. As cardiac performance deteriorates further, blood backs up behind the failing ventricles, causing venous distention, peripheral edema, and pulmonary congestion (edema)—hence, the term *congestive*. Heart failure is extremely common, affecting about 3 million people in the United States alone. For most patients, CHF is a chronic disorder that requires continuous treatment with drugs.

Primary Pathology of CHF

The primary defect in CHF is a reduction in ventricular contractility. This decrease in contractile force is responsible for the reduction in cardiac output that characterizes CHF. The cellular changes that underlie reduced contractility are not known.

Physiologic Adaptations to Reduced Cardiac Output

In response to reductions in the pumping ability of the heart, the body undergoes several adaptive changes. Some of these help improve tissue perfusion, whereas others compound existing problems.

Cardiac Dilatation. Dilatation of the heart is characteristic of CHF. Cardiac dilatation results from a combination of increased preload (see below) and reduced contractile force. Reduced contractility lowers the amount of blood ejected during systole, causing end-systolic volume to rise. The increase in preload increases diastolic filling, which causes the heart to expand even further.

Because of the Frank-Starling mechanism discussed above, the increase in heart size that occurs during CHF helps improve cardiac output. That is, as the heart fails and its volume expands, contractility increases, causing a corresponding increase in stroke volume. However, it must be noted that the maximal contractile force that can be developed by the failing heart is considerably lower than the maximal force of the healthy heart. This limitation is reflected in the Frank-Starling curve for the failing heart shown in Figure 42–1.

If cardiac dilatation is insufficient to maintain cardiac output, other factors come into play. As discussed below, these are not always beneficial.

Increased Sympathetic Tone. Heart failure causes arterial pressure to fall. In response, baroreceptor reflexes increase sympathetic output to the heart, veins, and arterioles; at the same time, parasympathetic effects on the heart are reduced. The consequences of increased sympathetic tone are summarized below.

1. *Increased heart rate.* Acceleration of heart rate increases cardiac output, thereby helping improve tissue perfusion. However, if heart rate increases too much, there will be insufficient time for ventricular filling, and cardiac output will fall.
2. *Increased contractility.* Increased myocardial contractility has the obvious benefit of increasing cardiac output. The only detriment is an increase in cardiac oxygen demand.
3. *Increased venous tone.* Elevation of venous tone increases cardiac preload, and thereby increases ventricular filling. Because of the Frank-Starling relationship, increased filling increases stroke volume. Unfortunately, if preload is excessive, blood will back up behind the failing ventricles, thereby aggravating pulmonary and peripheral edema. Furthermore, excessive preload can dilate the heart so much that stroke volume will begin to decline (see Fig. 42–1).
4. *Increased arteriolar tone.* Elevation of arteriolar tone increases arterial pressure, thereby increasing perfusion of vital organs. Unfortu-

nately, increased arterial pressure also means that the heart must pump against greater resistance. Since cardiac reserve is minimal in CHF, the heart may be unable to meet this challenge, and cardiac output may decline.

Water Retention and Increased Blood Volume. Water retention results from two mechanisms. (1) Reduced cardiac output causes a reduction in renal blood flow (RBF), which, in turn, decreases glomerular filtration rate. As a result, urine production is decreased and water is retained. This retention of fluid increases blood volume. (2) Water retention also occurs because of activation of the renin-angiotensin-aldosterone system (see below).

As with other adaptive responses to CHF, increased blood volume can be both beneficial and harmful. Increased blood volume will increase preload, thereby increasing ventricular filling and stroke volume. However, as noted above, if preload is too high, edema of the lungs and periphery may result.

Activation of the Renin-Angiotensin-Aldosterone System. Several factors, including reduced arterial pressure and reduced renal blood flow, promote release of *renin* from the kidney. Renin then accelerates production of *angiotensin II*, which acts directly to cause *constriction of arterioles and veins*, thereby increasing preload and afterload. In addition, angiotensin II causes release of *aldosterone* (from the adrenal cortex), which acts on the kidneys to promote *retention of sodium and water*. As discussed above, all of these effects (increased preload, increased afterload, and retention of sodium and water with resultant increased blood volume) can be both beneficial and detrimental. (The renin-angiotensin-aldosterone system is discussed in depth in Chapter 37.)

The Vicious Cycle of "Compensatory" Physiologic Responses

As discussed above, reduced cardiac output leads to four compensatory responses: (1) cardiac dilatation, (2) activation of the sympathetic nervous system, (3) retention of water with expansion of blood volume, and (4) activation of the renin-angiotensin-aldosterone system. Although these responses represent the body's attempt to compensate for reduced cardiac output, they can actually make matters worse: if increases in heart rate, preload, and afterload are excessive, they will reduce cardiac output rather than increase it. Hence, as depicted in Figure 42–2, the "compensatory" responses can create a self-sustaining cycle of maladaptation that further impairs cardiac output and tissue perfusion. Drug therapy attacks this cycle at several points, causing it to cease.

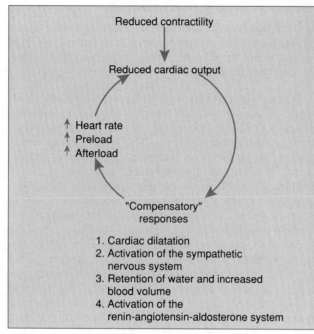

Reduced contractility

Reduced cardiac output

↑ Heart rate
↑ Preload
↑ Afterload

"Compensatory"
responses

1. Cardiac dilatation
2. Activation of the sympathetic
   nervous system
3. Retention of water and increased
   blood volume
4. Activation of the
   renin-angiotensin-aldosterone system

Figure 42–2. The vicious cycle of maladaptive compensatory responses to a failing heart.

Signs and Symptoms of CHF

The prominent signs and symptoms of CHF are a direct consequence of the pathophysiology described above. Decreased tissue perfusion results in reduced exercise tolerance, fatigue, and shortness of breath; shortness of breath may also stem from pulmonary edema. Increased sympathetic tone produces tachycardia. Increased preload and reduced systolic ejection result in cardiomegaly (increased heart size). The combination of increased venous tone plus increased blood volume helps cause pulmonary edema, peripheral edema, hepatomegaly (increased liver size), and distention of the jugular veins. Weight gain results from fluid retention.

TREATMENT GOALS AND STRATEGIES

Therapy of CHF has three major goals: (1) relief of pulmonary and peripheral congestive symptoms, (2) improvement of functional capacity and quality of life, and (3) prolongation of life expectancy. To achieve these goals, three strategies are employed. The first is treatment of correctable underlying causes of CHF, such as hypertension, dysrhythmias, and aortic stenosis. The second is implementation of nondrug measures, specifically, restriction of salt intake and physical activities. Third, if the first two strategies prove insufficient, drug therapy should be employed.

OVERVIEW OF DRUGS USED TO TREAT CHF

Congestive heart failure is treated with three classes of drugs: (1) diuretics, (2) vasodilators, and (3) inotropic agents. The role of these drugs in CHF is discussed below.

DIURETICS

Diuretics are first-line drugs for all patients with CHF. By reducing blood volume, these drugs can decrease preload, afterload, pulmonary edema, peripheral edema, and cardiac distention. It is important to note, however, that excessive diuresis is hazardous and must be avoided: if blood volume drops too low, cardiac output and blood pressure may fall precipitously, thereby further compromising tissue perfusion. The basic pharmacology of the diuretics is discussed in Chapter 35. The role of diuretics in CHF is summarized below.

Thiazide Diuretics. The thiazide diuretics (e.g., hydrochlorothiazide) produce moderate diuresis. These oral agents are used for long-term therapy of chronic CHF when edema is not too great. Since thiazides are ineffective when glomerular filtration rate (GFR) is low, these drugs cannot be used if cardiac output is greatly reduced. The principal adverse effect of the thiazides is *hypokalemia*, which increases the risk of digoxin-induced dysrhythmias (see below).

High-Ceiling (Loop) Diuretics. The loop diuretics (e.g., furosemide) produce profound diuresis. In contrast to the thiazides, these drugs can promote fluid loss even when GFR is low. Hence, loop diuretics are preferred to thiazides when cardiac output is greatly reduced. Administration is oral and intravenous. Because they can mobilize large volumes of water, and because they work when GFR is low, loop diuretics are drugs of choice for patients with severe CHF. Like the thiazides, these drugs can cause *hypokalemia*, thereby increasing the risk of digoxin toxicity. In addition, loop diuretics can cause *severe hypotension* secondary to excessive volume reduction.

Potassium-Sparing Diuretics. In contrast to the thiazides and loop diuretics, the potassium-sparing diuretics (e.g., spironolactone) promote only scant diuresis. In patients with CHF, these drugs are employed to counteract potassium loss caused by thiazide and loop diuretics, thereby lowering the risk of digoxin-induced dysrhythmias. Not surprisingly, the principal adverse effect of the potassium-sparing drugs is *hyperkalemia*. These drugs should not be used in combination with angiotensin-converting enzyme inhibitors, which also promote retention of potassium, and would thereby greatly increase the risk of hyperkalemia.

VASODILATORS

Vasodilators are important drugs for treating CHF. As discussed below, these drugs differ from one another with respect to route of administration (oral versus intravenous) and site action (arterioles, veins, or both). Route of administration determines whether a drug will be used acutely or long term. Site of action determines the specific hemodynamic benefits the drug will have in CHF.

Drugs that dilate *veins* increase venous capacitance and thereby decrease cardiac *preload*. By decreasing preload, venodilators can reduce cardiac distention as well as pulmonary and peripheral edema.

Drugs that dilate *arterioles* have three beneficial effects. (1) Arteriolar dilation reduces cardiac *afterload*, thereby allowing stroke volume and cardiac output to increase. (2) By increasing cardiac output and dilating arterioles in the kidney, these drugs increase renal perfusion, thereby promoting loss of fluid. (3) In skeletal muscle, arteriolar dilation increases local perfusion.

Intravenous Agents for Acute Care

Nitroglycerin. Intravenous nitroglycerin is a powerful *venodilator* that produces a dramatic reduction in preload. The drug's effects have been described as being equivalent to "pharmacologic phlebotomy." In CHF, nitroglycerin is used to relieve acute severe pulmonary edema. Principal adverse effects are *hypotension* and resultant *reflex tachycardia*. The basic pharmacology of nitroglycerin is discussed in Chapter 41.

Sodium Nitroprusside. This drug acts rapidly to dilate *arterioles and veins*. Arteriolar dilation reduces afterload and thereby increases cardiac output. Venodilation reduces preload and thereby decreases pulmonary and peripheral congestion. The drug is indicated for short-term therapy of severe refractory CHF. The principal adverse effect is *profound hypotension*. Blood pressure must be monitored continuously. The basic pharmacology of nitroprusside is discussed in Chapter 39.

Oral Agents for Long-Term Therapy

Angiotensin-Converting Enzyme (ACE) Inhibitors. ACE inhibitors (e.g., captopril, enalapril) are the most frequently used vasodilators for long-term therapy of CHF. By suppressing production of angiotensin II, these drugs promote *dilation of arterioles and veins* and *decrease release of aldosterone*. Arteriolar dilation improves regional blood flow and, by reducing afterload, increases stroke volume and cardiac output. Venous dilation reduces preload, and thereby reduces pulmonary congestion, peripheral edema, and cardiac dilatation. By dilating renal blood vessels, ACE inhibitors improve renal blood flow, thereby enhancing excretion of sodium and water. Suppression of aldosterone release further enhances excretion of sodium, while at the same time causing retention of potassium. From the foregoing, we can see that giving an ACE inhibitor is much like giving three different drugs: an arteriolar dilator, a venodilator, and a diuretic. The principal adverse effects of the ACE inhibitors are *hypotension* (secondary to arteriolar dilation), *hyperkalemia* (secondary to decreased aldosterone release), and *cough* (the mechanism of which is unknown). Because of their ability to elevate potassium levels, ACE inhibitors should not be used in combination with potassium supplements or potassium-sparing diuretics; hyperkalemia could result. The basic pharmacology of the ACE inhibitors is discussed in Chapter 37.

Isosorbide Dinitrate. This drug belongs to the same family as nitroglycerin. Like nitroglycerin, isosorbide dinitrate (ISDN) causes selective dilation of veins. In patients with severe refractory CHF, the drug can reduce congestive symptoms and improve exercise capacity. Principal adverse effects are *orthostatic hypotension* and *reflex tachycardia*. The basic pharmacology of ISDN is discussed in Chapter 41.

Hydralazine. Hydralazine causes selective dilation of arterioles. By doing so, the drug can improve cardiac output and renal blood flow. For treatment of CHF, hydralazine is always used in combination with ISDN, since the drug is relatively ineffective by itself. With continued use for 4 to 6 weeks, tolerance develops to hydralazine's effects, thereby greatly limiting its utility. The basic pharmacology of hydralazine is discussed in Chapter 39.

INOTROPIC AGENTS

Inotropic agents are drugs that increase myocardial contractility. These agents are given to improve performance of the failing heart. Three types of inotropic drugs are available: *cardiac glycosides, sympathomimetics*, and *phosphodiesterase (PDE) inhibitors*. The sympathomimetics and PDE inhibitors currently available can be administered only by intravenous infusion. Accordingly, their use is restricted to acute care of the hospitalized patient. At this time, the cardiac glycosides are the only inotropic agents that can be used orally. Hence, these are the only inotropics suited for long-term CHF treatment.

Cardiac Glycosides

The cardiac glycosides (e.g., digoxin) are the oldest and most frequently prescribed inotropic drugs. These agents are used widely for long-term therapy of chronic CHF, but should not be used for acute heart failure. The pharmacology of the cardiac glycosides is discussed at length later in the chapter.

Sympathomimetic Drugs: Dopamine and Dobutamine

The basic pharmacology of dopamine and dobutamine is presented in Chapter 17. Discussion here is limited to the use of these drugs in CHF.

Dopamine. Dopamine is a catecholamine that can activate (1) beta$_1$-adrenergic receptors in the heart, (2) dopamine receptors in the kidney, and (3) at high doses, alpha$_1$-adrenergic receptors in blood vessels. Activation of beta$_1$ receptors increases myocardial contractility, thereby improving cardiac performance. Beta$_1$ activation can also increase heart rate, creating a risk of tachycardia. Activation of dopamine receptors dilates renal blood vessels, thereby increasing renal blood flow and urine output. Activation of alpha$_1$ receptors increases vascular resistance (afterload), which can further compromise cardiac output. Dopamine is administered by continuous infusion, and constant monitoring of blood pressure, the electrocardiogram (EKG), and urine output are required. The drug is employed as a short-term rescue measure for patients with severe, acute cardiac failure.

Dobutamine. Dobutamine is a synthetic catecholamine that causes selective activation of beta$_1$-adrenergic receptors. By doing so, the drug can increase myocardial contractility, thereby improving cardiac performance. In contrast to dopamine, dobutamine does not activate alpha$_1$ receptors and, therefore, does not increase vascular resistance. As a result, the drug is generally preferred to dopamine for short-term treatment of acute CHF. Administration is by continuous infusion.

Phosphodiesterase Inhibitors

Amrinone. Amrinone [Inocor] increases myocardial contractility and promotes vasodilation. Both effects result from intracellular accumulation of cyclic AMP (cAMP) secondary to inhibition of phosphodiesterase III, the enzyme that normally degrades cAMP. Comparative studies indicate that improvements in cardiac function elicited by amrinone are superior to those elicited by dopamine or dobutamine. Like dopamine and dobutamine, amrinone is administered by intravenous infusion and, therefore, is not suitable for outpatient use. Amrinone is indicated for short-term (2- to 3-day) treatment of CHF in patients who have not responded to digoxin, diuretics, and vasodilators. The drug should be protected from light and should not be mixed with glucose-containing solutions. Constant monitoring is required. The initial dose is 0.75 mg/kg (IV) administered over 2 to 3 minutes. The maintenance infusion is 5 to 10 μg/kg/min.

Milrinone. Like amrinone, milrinone [Primacor] inhibits phosphodiesterase III. The resultant increase in intracellular cAMP increases myocardial contractility and promotes vasodilation. The drug is administered by IV infusion and is indicated only for short-term therapy of severe CHF. Dosing is complex.

Vesnarinone. Vesnarinone is an investigational drug under study for treatment of heart failure. Like amrinone and milrinone, vesnarinone inhibits phosphodiesterase III, and thereby increases myocardial contractility and relaxes vascular smooth muscle. In addition, by affecting sodium and potassium channels, the drug prolongs the action potential duration and slows heart rate, thereby decreasing the risk of dysrhythmias.

Clinical effects are highly dose dependent. When administered in *high* doses (120 mg/day), vesnarinone produces a fivefold *increase* in mortality, which is greater than the increase in mortality reported for any other inotropic drug. In striking contrast, when given in *low* doses (60 mg/day), vesnarinone decreases mortality by 62%, which is two to four times greater than the decrease in mortality reported for any other drug used for heart failure. Because the toxic dose (120 mg/day) is only twice the beneficial dose (60 mg/day), vesnarinone clearly has a very narrow margin of safety.

The mechanism underlying reduced mortality is not known. The low doses that are responsible for reduced mortality produce no significant hemodynamic change. Hence, it would appear that reduced mortality cannot be explained by an increase in contractility.

The major adverse effect of vesnarinone is reversible neutropenia, which occurs in 2.5% of patients. Neutrophil counts must be monitored.

DRUG SELECTION IN CHRONIC CHF

The choice of drugs for treating chronic CHF has undergone significant change in recent years. The role of the cardiac glycosides—agents with serious toxicities—has diminished. Traditionally, practically all patients were given a cardiac glycoside. However, it is now clear that not everyone needs one of these drugs. Patients with mild to moderate CHF may respond adequately to nondrug measures (rest and restriction of sodium intake). If these measures are inadequate, drugs are indicated. Treatment can begin with a two-drug regimen: a diuretic combined with either digoxin or an ACE inhibitor. If more intensive therapy is needed, we can treat the patient with three drugs: a diuretic, digoxin, and an ACE inhibitor.

CARDIAC (DIGITALIS) GLYCOSIDES

The cardiac glycosides are naturally occurring compounds that have profound effects on the heart. These drugs alter both the mechanical and the electrical components of cardiac function. These actions have made the glycosides important medications for treating CHF and cardiac dysrhythmias. Because they are prepared by extraction from *Digitalis purpura* (purple foxglove) and *Digitalis lanata* (white foxglove), the cardiac glycosides are also known as *digitalis glycosides*.

The cardiac glycosides are one of our most widely used groups of prescription drugs. They are also among the most dangerous. The frequent use of these drugs is attributable to their ability to improve cardiac performance in patients with CHF. The high incidence of toxicity results from their propensity to cause dysrhythmias—at doses that are very close to therapeutic. There is no question that the cardiac glycosides are a mixed blessing, having the potential for life-saving benefits as well as life-threatening harm. Accordingly, it is essential that we use these drugs with respect, caution, and skill.

In the United States, only three cardiac glycosides are available: digoxin, digitoxin, and deslanoside. Of these, digoxin is by far the most widely prescribed.

DIGOXIN

Digoxin [Lanoxin, Lanoxicaps] is the most widely used cardiac glycoside. In fact, of all medicines employed in the United States, digoxin is one of the 10 most frequently prescribed. The principal indication for digoxin is CHF. In addition, the drug is used to treat dysrhythmias (see Chapter 44).

Chemistry

As shown in Figure 42–3, digoxin consists of three components: (1) a steroid nucleus, (2) a lactone ring, and (3) three molecules of digitoxose (a sugar). It is because of the sugars that digoxin is known as a *glycoside*. The region of the molecule composed of the steroid nucleus plus the lactone ring (i.e., the region without the sugar molecules) is responsible for the pharmacologic effects of digoxin. The sugars serve only to increase solubility.

Mechanical Effects on the Heart

Digoxin exerts a *positive inotropic* action on the heart. That is, the drug *increases the force of ventricular contraction*, and thereby increases cardiac output.

Mechanism of Inotropic Action. Digoxin increases myocardial contractility by inhibiting an enzyme known as *sodium, potassium-ATPase* (Na^+,K^+-ATPase). By way of an indirect process (see below), inhibition of Na^+,K^+-ATPase promotes *calcium accumulation* within cardiac cells. It is this increase in intracellular calcium that is responsible for increased contractile force. Calcium augments force of contraction by facilitating the interaction of myocardial contractile proteins (actin and myosin).

To understand how inhibition of Na^+,K^+-ATPase causes intracellular calcium to rise, we must first understand the normal role of Na^+,K^+-ATPase in the cardiac cell. That role is illustrated in Figure 42–4. As indicated, when an action potential passes along the cardiac cell membrane (sarcolemma), Na^+ ions and Ca^{++} ions enter the cell, and K^+ ions exit. Once the action potential has passed, these ion fluxes must be reversed so that the original ionic composition of the cell can be restored. Na^+,K^+-ATPase is critical to this restorative process. As shown in the figure, Na^+,K^+-ATPase acts as a "pump" to draw extracellular K^+ ions into the cell, while simultaneously extruding intracellular Na^+. The energy required for pumping Na^+ and K^+ is provided by the breakdown of ATP—hence, the name Na^+,K^+-ATPase. To complete the normalization of cellular ionic composition, Ca^{++} ions must leave the cell. Extrusion of Ca^{++} is accomplished through an exchange process in which extracellular Na^+ ions are taken into the cell while Ca^{++} ions exit. This exchange of Na^+ for Ca^{++} is a passive (energy-independent) process.

We can now answer the question, how does the ability of digoxin to inhibit Na^+,K^+-ATPase produce an increase in intracellular Ca^{++} levels? By inhibiting Na^+,K^+-ATPase, digoxin prevents the cardiac cell from restoring its proper ionic composition following the passage of an action potential. Inhibition of Na^+,K^+-ATPase blocks uptake of K^+ and extrusion of Na^+. Hence, with each successive action potential, intracellular K^+ levels decline while levels of Na^+ within the cell rise. It is this rise in Na^+ that leads to the rise in intracellular Ca^{++}. In the presence of excess intracellular Na^+, further Na^+ entry is suppressed. Since Na^+ entry is suppressed, the passive exchange of Ca^{++} for Na^+ cannot take place; hence, Ca^{++} accumulates within the cell.

Relationship of Potassium to Inotropic Action. Potassium ions compete with digoxin for binding to Na^+,K^+- ATPase. This competition is of great clinical significance. Because potassium competes with digoxin, when potassium levels are low, binding of digoxin to Na^+,K^+-ATPase will increase. This increase can produce excessive inhibition of Na^+,K^+-ATPase with resultant toxicity. Conversely, when levels of potassium are high, inhibition of Na^+,K^+-ATPase by digoxin is reduced, causing a reduction in the therapeutic response. Because increases in potassium can impair therapeutic responses, whereas decreases in potassium can cause toxicity, it is imperative that potassium levels be kept within the normal physiologic range (3.5 to 5 mEq/L).

Beneficial Effects in CHF

Increased Cardiac Output. The primary effect of digoxin is to increase myocardial contractility, which in turn causes an increase in cardiac output. As shown in Figure 42–1, by increasing contractility, digoxin shifts the relationship of fiber length to stroke volume in the failing heart toward that in the healthy heart. Consequently, at any given heart size, the stroke volume of the failing heart increases, causing cardiac output to rise.

Consequences of Increased Cardiac Output. As a result of increased cardiac output, three major secondary responses occur: (1) sympathetic tone declines, (2) urine production increases, and (3) renin release declines. These responses can lead to reversal of virtually all signs and symptoms of CHF.

Decreased Sympathetic Tone. By increasing contractile force and cardiac output, digoxin increases arterial blood pressure. In response, sympathetic nerve traffic to the heart and blood vessels is reduced via the baroreceptor reflex. (Recall that a compensatory *increase* in sympathetic tone had taken place because of CHF.)

The decrease in sympathetic tone has several beneficial effects. First, heart rate is reduced, thereby allowing more complete ventricular filling. Second, afterload is reduced (because of reduced arteriolar constriction), thereby allowing more complete ventricular emptying. Third, preload is reduced (because of reduced venous constriction),

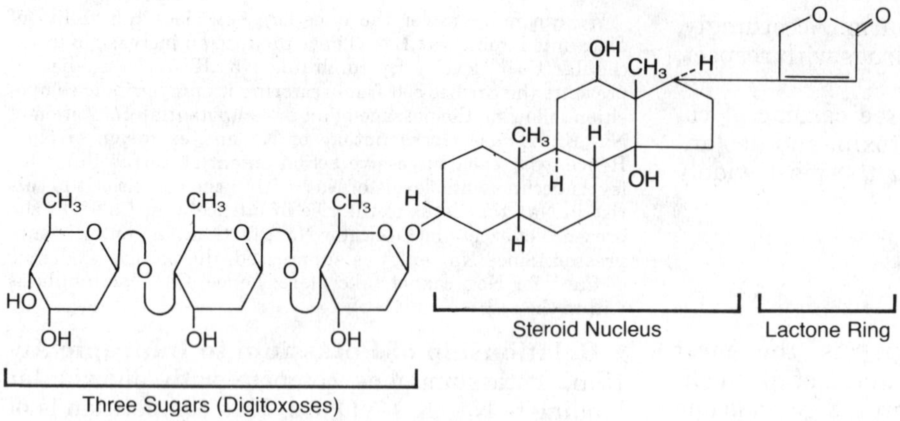

Figure 42–3. Structure of digoxin.

Three Sugars (Digitoxoses)

Steroid Nucleus

Lactone Ring

thereby reducing cardiac distention, pulmonary congestion, and peripheral edema.

Increased Urine Production. The increase in cardiac output increases renal blood flow, and thereby increases production of urine. This loss of water reduces blood volume, which in turn reduces cardiac distention, pulmonary congestion, and peripheral edema.

Decreased Renin Release. As arterial pressure rises, release of renin declines, causing levels of aldosterone and angiotensin II to decline as well. The decrease in angiotensin II decreases vasoconstriction, thereby further reducing afterload and preload. The decrease in aldosterone reduces retention of sodium and water, which reduces blood volume, which in turn further reduces preload.

Summary of Effects in CHF. In summary, we can see that through direct and indirect mechanisms, digoxin has the potential to correct all of the overt manifestations of heart failure: cardiac output improves, heart rate decreases, heart size declines, constriction of arterioles and veins decreases, water retention reverses, blood volume declines, peripheral and pulmonary edema decrease, and weight is lost (because of water loss). In addition, exercise tolerance improves and fatigue is reduced. Given this impressive spectrum of responses, in combination with the prevalence of heart disease, we can appreciate why digoxin is widely prescribed. There is, however, one important caveat to keep in mind: *the efficacy of digoxin in CHF depends on cardiac reserve—if the heart is too sick, the drug will not be able to help very much.*

Evaluating Digoxin Therapy of CHF

When attempting to assess the effectiveness of digoxin, we must rely on secondary responses (e.g., increased urine production, weight loss, decreased edema, decreased jugular distention) as indices of beneficial drug action. We are obliged to rely on these secondary effects because we cannot directly measure the primary actions of digoxin (increased contractility and increased cardiac output).

Unfortunately, although information on secondary responses is clearly valuable, that value is limited. Information on secondary responses can only provide a general notion as to whether or not improvement has taken place. Accordingly, secondary responses do not offer a precise therapeutic endpoint. That is, secondary responses can only tell us if we're moving in the right direction; they cannot tell us when (or if) we have reached our

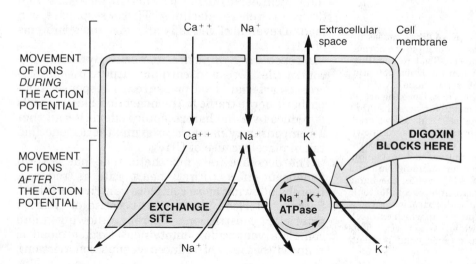

Figure 42–4. Ion fluxes across the cardiac cell membrane. During the action potential, Na⁺ and Ca⁺⁺ enter the cardiac cell and K⁺ exits. Following the action potential, Na⁺, K⁺-ATPase pumps Na⁺ out of the cell and takes up K⁺. Ca⁺⁺ leaves the cell in exchange for the uptake of Na⁺. By inhibiting Na⁺,K⁺-ATPase, digoxin prevents the extrusion of Na⁺, causing Na⁺ to accumulate inside the cell. The resulting buildup of intracellular Na⁺ suppresses the Na⁺-Ca⁺⁺ exchange process, thereby causing intracellular levels of Ca⁺⁺ to rise.

therapeutic goal (maximal improvement of cardiac performance). This leaves us in the uncomfortable position of being unable to know with certainty just how beneficial treatment has been.

Electrical Effects on the Heart

The effects of digoxin on the electrical activity of the heart are of therapeutic and toxicologic importance. It is because of its electrical effects that digoxin is useful for treating dysrhythmias (see Chapter 44). Ironically, these same electrical effects are responsible for *causing* dysrhythmias—the most serious toxicity of digoxin.

The electrical effects of digoxin can be bewildering in their complexity. Through a combination of actions, digoxin can alter the electrical activity of noncontractile tissue (S-A node, A-V node, Purkinje fibers) as well as the activity of ventricular muscle. In these various tissues, digoxin can alter automaticity, refractoriness, and impulse conduction. Whether these parameters are increased or decreased depends on cardiac status, digoxin dosage, and the particular tissue examined.

Although the electrical effects of digoxin are many and varied, only a few are clinically significant. These are discussed below.

Mechanisms for Altering Electrical Activity of the Heart. Digoxin alters the electrical properties of the heart by two basic mechanisms: (1) *inhibition of* Na^+, K^+-*ATPase* and (2) *enhancement of vagal influences on the heart*. By inhibiting Na^+,K^+-ATPase, digoxin alters the distribution of ions (Na^+, K^+, Ca^{++}) across cardiac cell membranes. This change in ion distribution can alter the electrical responsiveness of the cells involved. Since *hypokalemia* intensifies inhibition of Na^+,K^+-ATPase, hypokalemia will intensify alterations in cardiac electrical properties.

Digoxin acts in two ways to enhance vagal effects on the heart. First, the drug acts in the central nervous system to increase the firing rate of vagal fibers that innervate the heart. Second, digoxin increases the responsiveness of the S-A node to acetylcholine (the neurotransmitter released by the vagus). The net result of these vagotonic effects is (1) decreased automaticity of the S-A node, and (2) decreased conduction through the A-V node.

Effects on Specific Regions of the Heart. In the *S-A node*, digoxin *decreases automaticity* (by the vagotonic mechanisms just mentioned). In the *A-V node*, digoxin *decreases conduction velocity* and *prolongs the effective refractory period*; these effects, which can promote varying degrees of A-V heart block, result primarily from the drug's vagotonic actions. In *Purkinje fibers*, digoxin-induced inhibition of Na^+,K^+-ATPase results in *increased automaticity*; this increase can generate ectopic foci that, in turn, can cause ventricular dysrhythmias. In the *ventricular myocardium*, digoxin acts to *shorten the effective refractory period* and (possibly) to *increase automaticity*.

Cardiotoxicity: Production of Cardiac Dysrhythmias

Production of dysrhythmias is the most serious adverse effect of digoxin. The drug causes dysrhythmias by altering the electrical properties of the heart.

Because serious dysrhythmias are a potential consequence of therapy, all patients should be evaluated frequently for changes in heart rate and rhythm. If significant changes occur, digoxin should be withheld and the physician consulted. Outpatients should be taught to monitor their pulses and instructed to report any significant changes in rate or regularity.

Types of Digoxin-Induced Dysrhythmias. Digoxin can mimic practically all types of dysrhythmias. A-V block with escape beats is among the most common. Ventricular flutter and ventricular fibrillation are the most dangerous.

Mechanism of Ventricular Dysrhythmia Generation. Digoxin-induced *ventricular* dysrhythmias result from a combination of three factors: (1) suppression of A-V conduction, (2) increased automaticity of Purkinje fibers, and (3) shortening of the effective refractory period in ventricular muscle. Increased Purkinje fiber automaticity and shortening of the effective refractory period of the ventricular myocardium predispose the ventricles to development of ectopic beats. The reduction in A-V conduction facilitates expression of ectopic ventricular activity: by preventing atrial impulses from reaching the ventricles, A-V block allows potential beats of ventricular origin to become manifest.

**Predisposing Factors. *Hypokalemia. The most common cause of dysrhythmias in patients receiving digoxin is hypokalemia secondary to the use of diuretics.* Less common causes of hypokalemia include vomiting and diarrhea. Hypokalemia promotes dysrhythmias by increasing digoxin-induced inhibition of Na^+,K^+-ATPase, which, in turn, leads to increased automaticity of Purkinje fibers. Because low potassium can precipitate dysrhythmias, *it is imperative that serum potassium levels be kept within a normal range.* If diuretic therapy causes potassium levels to fall, a potassium-sparing diuretic (e.g., spironolactone) can be added to the regimen to correct the problem. Potassium supplements may also be used. Patients should be taught to recognize symptoms of hypokalemia (e.g., muscle weakness) and instructed to notify the physician if these develop.

Elevated Digoxin Levels. *Digoxin has a narrow therapeutic range: drug levels only slightly higher than therapeutic greatly increase the risk of toxicity.* Possible causes of excessive digoxin levels include (1) intentional or accidental overdosage, (2) increased digoxin absorption, and (3) decreased digoxin elimination.

If plasma digoxin levels are monitored and kept within the therapeutic range, the chances of a dysrhythmia will be reduced. However, it is important to note that careful control over drug levels will not eliminate the risk entirely. As discussed above, there is only a loose relationship between digoxin levels and clinical effects. As a result, some patients may experience dysrhythmias even when drug levels are well within what is normally considered the therapeutic range.

Heart Disease. The ability of digoxin to cause dysrhythmias is greatly increased by the presence of heart disease. Doses of digoxin that have no adverse effects on healthy volunteers can precipitate serious dysrhythmias in patients with CHF. The probability and severity of a dysrhythmia are directly related to the severity of the underlying disease. Since heart disease is the reason for taking digoxin, it should be no surprise that people taking the drug are at risk of dysrhythmias.

Diagnosis of Cardiotoxicity. Diagnosis of digoxin-induced dysrhythmias is not a simple matter. Much of the difficulty stems from the fact that the failing heart is prone to developing dysrhythmias spontaneously. Hence, when a dysrhythmia occurs, we cannot simply assume that digoxin is the cause; the possibility that the dysrhythmia is the direct result of heart disease must also be evaluated. Compounding diagnostic difficulties is the poor correlation between plasma digoxin levels and dysrhythmia onset. Because of this loose correspondence, the presence of an apparently excessive digoxin level does not necessarily indicate that digoxin is responsible for the problem. Laboratory data required for diagnosis include digoxin levels, serum electrolytes, and an EKG. Ultimately, diagnosis is based on experience and clinical judgment. Resolution of the dysrhythmia following digoxin withdrawal confirms the diagnosis.

Management of Digoxin-Induced Dysrhythmias. When accurately diagnosed and properly treated, digoxin-induced dysrhythmias can almost always be controlled. Basic management measures are as follows:

1. *Withdraw digoxin and potassium-wasting diuretics.* For many patients, no additional treatment will be needed. To help insure that medication is stopped, a written order to withhold digoxin should be made.
2. *Monitor serum potassium.* If the potassium level is low or nearly normal, potassium (IV or PO) should be administered. Potassium will displace digoxin from Na^+,K^+-ATPase and will thereby help reverse toxicity. However, if potassium levels are *high* or if *A-V block is present*, no more potassium should be given. Under these conditions, more potassium may cause complete A-V block.
3. Some patients may require an antidysrhythmic drug. *Phenytoin* and *lidocaine* are most effective. Quinidine, another antidysrhythmic drug, can cause plasma levels of digoxin to rise. Accordingly, quinidine should not be used.
4. Patients who develop bradycardia or A-V block can be treated with atropine. (Atropine helps by blocking the vagal influences that underlie bradycardia and A-V block.) Alternatively, electronic pacing may be employed.
5. When overdosage is especially severe, digoxin levels can be lowered using *Fab antibody fragments* [Digibind]. These fragments, which are administered intravenously, bind to digoxin and thereby prevent it from acting. *Cholestyramine* and *activated charcoal*, agents that also bind digoxin, can be administered orally to suppress absorption of digoxin from the gastrointestinal tract.

It should be noted that attempts to treat digoxin-induced dysrhythmias with electrical countershock can be extremely hazardous: countershock may convert a relatively benign dysrhythmia into ventricular fibrillation. If countershock must be employed, very low current should be used.

Noncardiac Adverse Effects

Digoxin's principal noncardiac toxicities concern the gastrointestinal (GI) system and the central nervous system (CNS). Since adverse effects on these systems frequently precede development of dysrhythmias, symptoms involving the GI tract and CNS can provide advance warning of more serious toxicity. Accordingly, patients should be taught to recognize these effects and instructed to notify the physician if they occur.

Gastrointestinal Tract. *Anorexia, nausea,* and *vomiting* are the most common GI effects of digoxin. These responses result primarily from stimulation of the chemoreceptor trigger zone of the medulla. Digoxin rarely causes diarrhea.

Central Nervous System. *Fatigue* is the most frequent CNS effect. *Visual disturbances* (e.g., blurred vision, yellow tinge to vision, appearance of halos around dark objects) are also relatively common.

Reducing the Risk of Toxicity

Patient education can help reduce the incidence of toxicity. Patients should be warned about digoxin-induced dysrhythmias and should be instructed to take their medication exactly as prescribed. In addition, they should be informed about symptoms of developing toxicity (altered heart rate or rhythm, visual or gastrointestinal disturbances) and instructed to notify the physician if these develop. If a potassium supplement or potassium-sparing diuretic is part of the regimen, it should be taken exactly as prescribed.

Drug Interactions

Diuretics. *Thiazides* and *loop diuretics* promote loss of potassium, thereby increasing the risk of digoxin-induced dysrhythmias. Accordingly, when digoxin and these diuretics are used concurrently, serum potassium levels must be monitored and maintained within a normal range (3.5 to 5 mEq/L). If hypokalemia develops, potassium levels can be restored with potassium supplements, a potassium-sparing diuretic, or both.

Insulin. Insulin promotes potassium uptake by cells. This action can produce hypokalemia, and can thereby precipitate digoxin toxicity. Consequently, insulin must be used with caution.

Sympathomimetics. Sympathomimetic drugs (e.g., dopamine, dobutamine) act on the heart to increase the rate and force of contraction. The increase in contractile force can add to the positive inotropic effects of digoxin. These complementary actions can be beneficial. In contrast, the ability of sympathomimetics to increase heart rate may be detrimental: a higher heart rate can increase the risk of a tachydysrhythmia.

Quinidine. Quinidine is an antidysrhythmic drug that can cause plasma levels of digoxin to rise. Quinidine increases digoxin levels by (1) displacing digoxin from tissue binding sites, and (2) reducing the renal excretion of digoxin. By elevating levels of free digoxin, quinidine can promote digoxin toxicity. Accordingly, concurrent use of quinidine and digoxin should be avoided.

Verapamil. Verapamil, a calcium-channel blocker, can significantly increase plasma levels of digoxin. If the combination is employed, digoxin dosage must be reduced.

Other Interactions. Various drugs can lower plasma levels of digoxin, apparently by decreasing digoxin absorption. Agents reported to reduce digoxin levels include *antacids, oral aminoglycoside antibiotics* (e.g., kanamycin, neomycin), *kaolin-pectin antidiarrheal suspensions*, and certain combinations of anticancer drugs.

Pharmacokinetics

Absorption. Absorption of oral digoxin can be variable, ranging from 55% to 90%. The extent of absorption is lowest and most variable with digoxin *tablets*. Absorption from digoxin *capsules* [Lanoxicaps] is more complete and less variable. However, although digoxin capsules permit excellent absorption, they do have a drawback: they are much more expensive than the tablets. Hence, it may be preferable to reserve the capsules for patients in whom stable drug levels cannot be achieved with tablets.

Until recently, there was considerable variability in the absorption of digoxin from tablets prepared by different manufacturers. This variability resulted from differences in the rate and extent of tablet dissolution. Because of this variable bioavailability, it had been recommended that patients not switch between different digoxin brands.

Today, bioavailability of digoxin in tablets produced by different companies is fairly uniform, making brands of digoxin more interchangeable than they had been. However, given the narrow therapeutic range of the drug, some authorities still recommend that patients not switch between brands of digoxin tablets—even when prescriptions are written generically—except with the approval and supervision of the physician.

Distribution. Digoxin undergoes wide distribution throughout the body and crosses the placenta. High levels are achieved in cardiac and skeletal muscle, owing largely to binding to Na^+,K^+-ATPase. About 23% of digoxin in plasma is bound to proteins (mainly albumin).

Elimination. Digoxin is eliminated primarily by *renal excretion*. Hepatic metabolism is minimal. Because digoxin is eliminated by the kidneys, *alterations in renal function can have a significant impact on digoxin blood levels: if kidney function declines, digoxin may accumulate to levels that are toxic.* Accordingly, dosage must be reduced in patients with renal impairment. Because digoxin is not metabolized to any significant extent, changes in liver function do not affect plasma digoxin content.

Half-life and Time to Plateau. The half-life of digoxin is about 1.5 days. Hence, in the absence of a loading dose, about 6 days (4 half-lives) are required for plateau levels to be achieved. When use of the drug is discontinued, another 6 days are required for body stores to be eliminated.

Single-Dose Time Course. Effects of a single dose of digoxin begin 30 minutes to 2 hours after oral administration and peak within 4 to 6 hours. Effects of intravenous digoxin begin rapidly (within 5 to 30 minutes), and peak in 1 to 4 hours.

A Note on Plasma Digoxin Levels. Most hospitals are equipped to measure plasma levels of digoxin. Knowledge of these levels can be useful for (1) establishing dosage, (2) monitoring compliance, (3) diagnosing toxicity, and (4) determining the cause of therapeutic failure. For digoxin, the usual therapeutic range is 0.5 to 2.0 ng/ml. Levels above 2.5 ng/ml are toxic.

Although knowledge of digoxin plasma levels can aid the clinician, it must be understood that the extent of this aid is limited. The correlation between plasma levels of digoxin and clinical effects—both therapeutic and adverse—is not very tight: drug levels that are safe and effective for patient A may be subtherapeutic for patient B and toxic for patient C. Because of interpatient variability, knowledge of digoxin levels does not permit precise predictions of therapeutic effects or toxicity. Hence, information regarding drug levels must not be relied upon too heavily. Rather, this information should be seen as but one factor among several to be considered when evaluating clinical responses.

Preparations, Dosage, and Administration

Preparations. Digoxin [Lanoxin] is available in tablets (0.125, 0.25, and 0.5 mg), as a pediatric elixir (0.05 mg/ml), and as an injection (0.1 and 0.25 mg/ml). Digoxin is also available in capsules (0.05, 0.1, and 0.2 mg) under the trade name Lanoxicaps.

Administration. Digoxin can be administered *orally* and *intravenously*. *Intramuscular* administration causes severe pain and tissue damage and should be avoided. Prior to administration, the rate and regularity of the heart beat should be determined. If heart rate is less than 60 beats per minute or if a change in rhythm is detected, digoxin should be withheld and the physician notified. When digoxin is given IV, cardiac status should be monitored continuously for 1 to 2 hours.

Dosage Determination in CHF. For several reasons, establishing a safe and effective dosage is difficult. First, since digoxin has a narrow therapeutic range, the dosing target is small, making it difficult to hit. Second, as discussed above, when treating CHF with digoxin, we lack a clear-cut therapeutic endpoint. Without such an endpoint, we cannot determine with certainty if the dosage is greater or smaller than required. Third, monitoring digoxin plasma levels is only moderately helpful. Because of substantial interpatient variability, drug levels that may be safe and effective in one patient may be ineffective or toxic in another. Hence, we cannot rely heavily on the concept of "standard therapeutic plasma levels" when attempting to establish digoxin dosage. Ultimately, determining the most desirable dosage must be based on careful observation of the patient; signs of beneficial and adverse responses must be monitored and the dosage adjusted accordingly.

Digitalization. When maximal effects must be achieved rapidly, a loading dose is required. (As noted above, 6 days are needed for plasma drug levels to reach plateau if no loading dose is employed.) By convention, the process of using a loading dose to achieve high levels of digoxin quickly is termed *digitalization*. Digitalization can be accomplished with an initial oral dose of 0.5 to 0.75 mg followed by doses of 0.25 to 0.5 mg at intervals of 6 to 8 hours until digitalization is complete (usually with a total dose of 0.75 to 1.25 mg).

Maintenance Doses. After initial digitalization, a transition to smaller doses is required for maintenance therapy. When this transition is made, it is imperative that a new medication order be written for the lower dosage to avoid inadvertent continued administration of the large digitalizing doses.

The dosing objective in maintenance therapy is to establish doses that are high enough to be effective but not so high as to cause toxicity. As discussed above, *dosing is highly individualized and based largely on clinical observation.* Because digoxin is eliminated by the kidneys, *maintenance doses must be reduced if renal function declines.* Maintenance dosages for adults usually range from 0.125 to 0.5 mg daily.

DIGITOXIN

Digitoxin [Crystodigin] is similar to digoxin in most respects. These drugs have the same mechanism of action (inhibition of Na^+, K^+-ATPase), the same applications (treatment of CHF and dysrhythmias), and they produce the same toxicities (cardiac dysrhythmias). The principal differences between these drugs are pharmacokinetic. The most outstanding property of digitoxin is its prolonged half-life—a characteristic that makes management of toxicity very difficult. Accordingly, digitoxin is used much less frequently than digoxin.

Contrasts with Digoxin

The major differences between digitoxin and digoxin concern pharmacokinetics, especially absorption, route of elimination, and plasma half-life. Pharmacokinetic contrasts between these drugs are summarized in Table 42–1.

Absorption. Digitoxin is highly lipid soluble. As a result, the drug undergoes "complete" (90% to 100%) absorption following oral administration. In contrast, absorption of digoxin is both incomplete and variable.

Elimination. Unlike digoxin, which is eliminated by the kidneys, digitoxin is eliminated by the *liver*. The capacity of the liver to metabolize digitoxin is large—so large, in fact, that

Table 42–1. Pharmacokinetic Properties of Digoxin and Digitoxin

Pharmacokinetic Property	Cardiac Glycoside	
	Digoxin	*Digitoxin*
Absorption		
Tablets	55–90%	90–100%
Elixir	75–85%	
Capsules	90–100%	
Plasma Protein Binding	23%	95%
Route of Elimination	Renal	Hepatic
Plasma Half-Life		
Normal renal function	1.5 days	1 wk
Severe renal impairment	5 days	1 wk
Single-Dose Time Course		
Onset (oral)	1.5–6 hr	3–4 hr
Peak (oral)	4–6 hr	6–12 hr
Time to Plateau*	6–7 days	4–5 wk
Plasma Drug Levels†		
Therapeutic	0.5–2.0 ng/ml	14–26 ng/ml
Toxic	>2.5 ng/ml	>35 ng/ml

*In the absence of a loading dose.
†There is significant individual variation in responses to digoxin and digitoxin. Levels that are safe and effective for patient A may be subtherapeutic for patient B and toxic for patient C.

inactivation of digitoxin continues at a high rate even in the presence of liver disease. Hence, a decline in liver function rarely necessitates a reduction in dosage.

Half-Life and Time to Plateau. The half-life of digitoxin is about 7 days—considerably longer than the 1.5-day half-life of digoxin. Because of its prolonged half-life, digitoxin requires about 4 weeks to reach plateau (in the absence of a loading dose). More importantly, the drug's long half-life dictates that, in the event of toxicity, plasma levels will take a long time to decline to ones that are safe. This slow decline makes management of digitoxin overdosage very difficult.

Plasma Drug Levels. As indicated in Table 42–1, the usual therapeutic range for *total* plasma digoxin is 14 to 26 ng/ml. Toxicity occurs at levels above 35 ng/ml. These levels are much higher than those for digoxin. This is because digitoxin is highly bound to plasma proteins. As a result, plasma levels of digitoxin must be higher than those of digoxin in order to produce equivalent concentrations of *free* drug—the form that is responsible for therapeutic and toxic effects.

Therapeutic Use

For most patients with CHF, digoxin is preferred to digitoxin. This preference is based on the relatively short half-life of di-goxin, a property that allows digoxin levels to be reduced more quickly in the event of toxicity. However, although digoxin is usually preferred, when there is a need for plasma drug levels to be very stable, digitoxin—with its prolonged half-life and reliable absorption—might be superior. Similarly, when compliance is a problem, maintenance of therapeutic drug levels can be achieved best with digitoxin: if a dose is missed, the long half-life of digitoxin will prevent plasma drug levels from declining significantly during the extended interval between doses. If kidney function is poor, elimination of digoxin will be delayed, possibly resulting in drug accumulation; hence, in patients with renal impairment, digitoxin may be preferred.

Preparations, Dosage, and Administration

Preparations. Digitoxin [Crystodigin] is dispensed in tablets (0.05, 0.1, 0.15, and 0.2 mg) for oral use.

Dosing. As with digoxin, dosing is highly individualized. If plateau drug levels must be achieved quickly, an initial series of digitalizing doses is required. For rapid digitalization in adults, an initial oral dose of 0.8 mg is followed by two or three doses of 0.2 mg at 6- to 8-hour intervals. Maintenance dosages for adults range from 0.05 to 0.3 mg/day.

Summary of Major Nursing Implications

DIGOXIN

Preadministration Assessment

Therapeutic Goal

Digoxin is used to treat *congestive heart failure* and certain *cardiac dysrhythmias.* Be sure to confirm which disorder the drug is being used for.

Baseline Data

Assess for signs and symptoms of CHF, including fatigue, weakness, cough, shortness of breath, cyanosis, tachycardia, cardiomegaly, hepatomegaly, jugular distention, edema, and weight gain.

The physician may order an EKG plus laboratory data on serum electrolytes, kidney function, and liver function.

Identifying High-Risk Patients

Digoxin is *contraindicated* for patients experiencing *ventricular fibrillation*, *ventricular tachycardia*, or *digoxin toxicity.* Exercise caution in the presence of conditions that can predispose the patient to serious adverse responses to digoxin; these include *hypokalemia*, *partial A-V block*, *advanced heart failure*, and *renal impairment.*

Implementation: Administration

Routes

Oral, slow IV injection.

Administration

Oral. Determine heart rate and regularity prior to administration. If heart rate is less than 60 beats per minute or if a change in rhythm is detected, withhold digoxin and notify the physician.

Since digoxin has a long half-life, an initial series of large doses may be ordered to establish therapeutic drug levels quickly. Following this initial digitalization, smaller doses are used for maintenance. When the dosage is changed to the smaller amounts employed for maintenance, it is imperative that the medication order used during digitalization be replaced with an order for the smaller dosage.

Warn patients not to "double up" on doses in attempts to compensate for missed doses.

Intravenous. Monitor cardiac status closely for 1 to 2 hours following IV injection.

Promoting Compliance

Since digoxin has a narrow therapeutic range, rigid adherence to the prescribed dosage is essential. Inform patients that failure to take digoxin exactly as prescribed may lead to toxicity or therapeutic failure. Warn patients against switching between brands or formulations of digoxin, since variations in bioavailability may lead to altered responses. If poor compliance is suspected, serum drug levels may help in assessing the extent of noncompliance.

Advise patients to reduce intake of salt and to minimize strenuous activity. Advise obese patients to adopt a reduced-calorie diet. Precipitating factors for CHF (e.g., hypertension, valvular heart disease) should be corrected.

Evaluating Therapeutic Effects

Monitor for improvements in signs and symptoms of CHF (e.g., increased urine output, weight loss, reduction in edema, increased exercise capacity, decreased jugular distention, reduced heart size, and slowing of heart rate).

Plasma drug levels can help determine the cause of therapeutic failure. The therapeutic range for digoxin is 0.5 to 2 ng/ml.

Minimizing Adverse Effects

Cardiotoxicity. Dysrhythmias are the most serious adverse effect of digoxin.

Monitor hospitalized patients for alterations in heart rate or rhythm, and withhold digoxin if significant changes develop.

Inform outpatients about the danger of dysrhythmias. Teach them to monitor their pulses for rate and rhythm, and instruct them to notify the physician if significant changes occur. Provide patient with an EKG rhythm strip; this can be used by physicians unfamiliar with the patient (e.g., when the patient is traveling) to verify suspected changes in rhythm.

Hypokalemia—usually diuretic-induced—is the most frequent underlying cause of digoxin-induced dysrhythmias. Monitor serum potassium concentrations. If hypokalemia develops, potassium levels can be raised with potassium supplements, with a potassium-sparing diuretic, or both. Teach patients to recognize early signs of hypokalemia (e.g., muscle weakness) and instruct them to notify the physician if these develop. Severe vomiting and diarrhea can increase potassium loss; exercise caution if these events occur.

To treat digoxin-induced dysrhythmias: (1) withdraw digoxin and diuretics (make sure that a written order for digoxin withdrawal is made), (2) administer potassium (unless potassium levels are above normal or A-V block is present), (3) administer an antidysrhythmic drug (phenytoin or lidocaine, but not quinidine) if indicated, (4) manage bradycardia with atropine or electrical pacing, and (5) treat with Fab fragments if toxicity is life-threatening. Electrical countershock is generally avoided, since ventricular fibrillation may result.

Noncardiac Effects. Nausea, vomiting, diarrhea, fatigue, and visual disturbances (blurred or yellow vision) frequently foreshadow more serious toxicity (dysrhythmias) and should be reported immediately. Inform patients about these early indications of toxicity, and instruct them to notify the physician if they develop.

Minimizing Adverse Interactions

Diuretics. Thiazide diuretics and loop diuretics increase the risk of dysrhythmias by promoting potassium loss. Monitor potassium levels. If hypokalemia develops, it should be corrected with potassium supplements, a potassium-sparing diuretic, or both.

Insulin. Insulin can cause hypokalemia by promoting uptake of potassium by cells. Use insulin with caution.

Implementation: Measures to Enhance Therapeutic Effects

Ongoing Evaluation and Interventions

Sympathomimetic Agents. Sympathomimetic drugs (e.g., dopamine, dobutamine) stimulate the heart, thereby increasing the risk of tachydysrhythmias and ectopic pacemaker activity. When sympathomimetics are combined with digoxin, monitor closely for dysrhythmias.

Quinidine. Quinidine can elevate plasma levels of digoxin. If quinidine is employed concurrently with digoxin, digoxin dosage must be reduced. Do not use quinidine to treat digoxin-induced dysrhythmias.

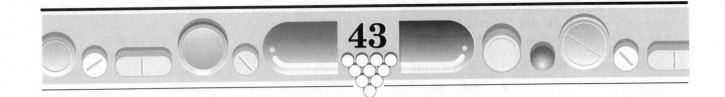
Management of Myocardial Infarction

Myocardial infarction (MI) is defined as necrosis of the myocardium resulting from acute occlusion of a coronary artery. In the United States, MI strikes about 1.5 million people each year and is the most common cause of death. Risk factors include advanced age, a family history of MI, sedentary lifestyle, obesity, high serum cholesterol, hypertension, smoking, and diabetes. The objectives of this chapter are to describe the pathophysiology of MI and to discuss interventions that can help reduce morbidity and mortality.

PATHOPHYSIOLOGY OF MYOCARDIAL INFARCTION

Myocardial infarction occurs when blood flow to a region of the myocardium (heart muscle) is stopped because of platelet plugging and thrombus formation in a coronary artery—almost always at a site of a fissured or ruptured atherosclerotic plaque. Myocardial injury is ultimately the result of an imbalance between oxygen demand and oxygen supply.

In response to local ischemia (insufficient oxygen), a dramatic redistribution of ions takes place. Hydrogen ions accumulate in the myocardium, and

531

calcium ions become sequestered in mitochondria. The resultant acidosis and functional calcium deficiency alter the distensibility of cardiac muscle. Sodium ions accumulate in myocardial cells and promote edema. Potassium ions are lost from myocardial cells, thereby setting the stage for dysrhythmias.

Local metabolic changes begin rapidly following coronary artery occlusion. Within seconds, metabolism shifts from aerobic to anaerobic. High energy stores of ATP and creatine phosphate become depleted. As a result, contraction ceases in the affected region.

If blood flow is not restored, cell death occurs within 2 to 6 hours. Clear indices of cell death—myocyte disruption, coagulative necrosis, elevation of serum enzymes–are present by 24 hours. By 4 days, monocyte infiltration and removal of dead myocytes weaken the infarcted area, making it vulnerable to expansion and rupture. Healing begins in 10 to 12 days with deposition of collagen, and is usually complete with dense scar formation in 4 to 6 weeks.

The degree of residual cardiac dysfunction depends on how much of the myocardium was damaged. With infarction of 10% of left ventricular (LV) mass, the ejection fraction will be reduced. With 25% LV infarction, dilatation and congestive heart failure occur. With 40% LV infarction, cardiogenic shock and death are likely.

CLINICAL DIAGNOSIS OF MYOCARDIAL INFARCTION

Myocardial infarction is diagnosed by the presence of chest pain, EKG changes, and elevated serum levels of myocardial enzymes. Other symptoms include sweating, weakness, and a sense of impending doom. About 20% of people with MI experience no symptoms.

Chest Pain. Patients undergoing acute MI typically experience severe substernal pressure that they characterize as unbearable crushing or constricting pain. The pain often radiates down the arms and up to the jaw. Acute MI can be differentiated from angina pectoris in that pain caused by MI lasts longer (20 to 30 minutes) and is not relieved by nitroglycerin. Some patients confuse the pain of MI with indigestion.

EKG Changes. Myocardial infarction often produces characteristic changes in the EKG (Fig. 43–1). These changes occur because conduction of electrical impulses through the heart becomes altered in the region of myocardial injury and cell death. Elevation of the ST segment occurs almost immediately in response to acute ischemia. Following a period of ST elevation, a prominent Q wave (>0.04 second duration) develops in the majority of patients. (Q waves are small or absent in the normal EKG.) Over time, the ST segment returns to baseline, after which a symmetrical inverted T wave appears. This T wave inversion may resolve within weeks to months. Q waves may resolve over a period of years.

Elevation of Serum Myocardial Enzymes. Enzymes present in myocardial cells are released into the blood as a result of cardiac injury. For diagnosis of infarction, the best enzyme to measure is the MB isozyme of creatine kinase. This form of creatine kinase is found primarily in the heart, and not in skeletal muscle. Hence, an increase in serum levels of the MB isozyme is a certain marker for cardiac injury. Following an acute MI, serum levels of the MB isozyme peak after 24 hours, and then return to baseline values in 36 to 72 hours.

For patients who have normal levels of the MB isozyme, but for whom infarction is nonetheless suspected, serum levels of lactate dehydrogenase may be measured. These levels begin to rise 1 to 2 days after infarction, peak in 3 to 5 days, and then remain above normal for another 7 to 10 days.

ACUTE MANAGEMENT OF MYOCARDIAL INFARCTION

The acute phase of management refers to the interval between the onset of symptoms and discharge from the hospital (usually in 6 to 10 days). The goal of therapy is to bring cardiac oxygen supply back in balance with oxygen demand. This can be accomplished by (1) restoring blood flow to the myocardium, and (2) reducing myocardial oxygen demand. The first few hours of treatment are the most critical.

Management of acute MI should take place in a cardiac care unit. Standard treatment consists of bed rest (for the first days), supplemental oxygen, opioids (e.g., morphine), antianxiety agents (e.g., diazepam), and heparin.

The major threats to life during acute MI are ventricular dysrhythmias, cardiogenic shock, and congestive heart failure. These complications must be treated as they arise.

REPERFUSION THERAPY: THROMBOLYTIC AND NONDRUG THERAPY

The goal of reperfusion therapy is to restore blood flow through the blocked coronary artery. Reperfusion therapy is the most effective way to preserve myocardial function and limit infarct size. Reperfusion can be accomplished with drugs (thrombolytic agents) and by nondrug measures

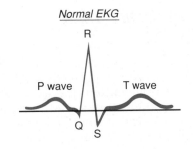

Normal EKG

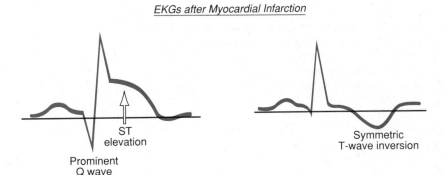

Figure 43–1. EKG changes associated with myocardial infarction.

EKGs after Myocardial Infarction

(percutaneous transluminal coronary angioplasty, coronary artery bypass grafting). Of these options, thrombolytic therapy is preferred. However, if thrombolytic therapy is contraindicated, the nondrug methods may be an option.

Thrombolytic Therapy

Thrombolytic drugs dissolve clots. They accomplish this by converting plasminogen into plasmin, a proteolytic enzyme that digests the fibrin meshwork that holds clots together. At this time, four fibrinolytic drugs are available: *streptokinase, urokinase, alteplase,* and *anistreplase.* The basic pharmacology of these drugs is presented in Chapter 46. Discussion here is limited to their use in MI.

Thrombolytic therapy is now standard treatment for early MI. When thrombolytics are given soon enough, the occluded artery can be opened in 80% of patients. Clinical trials have shown that timely therapy improves ventricular function, limits infarct size, and reduces mortality. Restoration of blood flow reduces or eliminates chest pain, and often reduces ST elevation as well. To be effective, treatment should be initiated within 4 to 6 hours of the onset of symptoms—and preferably sooner. Current guidelines restrict thrombolytic therapy to patients younger than 76 and to those whose ischemic pain began no more than 4 to 6 hours before treatment is to begin. Under typical conditions, all of the available thrombolytics are equally beneficial. However, under *ideal* conditions, alteplase may be superior (see discussion of the GUSTO trial in Chapter 46).

To prevent re-occlusion, which occurs in 10% to 20% of patients, *heparin* and *aspirin* are used as adjuncts to thrombolytic therapy. Heparin (IV) should be initiated no later than 90 minutes after thrombolysis and continued for 5 days. The drug is most critical during the first 24 hours following thrombolytic therapy. Low-dose aspirin (160 mg per day) helps prevent re-occlusion by suppressing platelet aggregation. Therapy should begin immediately after onset of MI symptoms.

Nondrug Methods of Reperfusion

Percutaneous Transluminal Coronary Angioplasty (PTCA). PTCA is a mechanical technique for recanalizing an occluded coronary artery. In this procedure, a catheter containing a deflated balloon is worked into the affected artery, after which the balloon is inflated. This opens the vessel and allows blood to flow. PTCA can be used as primary therapy for acute MI, or as secondary therapy when thrombolysis has failed. When PTCA is used as primary therapy, the success rate is about equal to that of thrombolysis. At this time, it is not known which procedure—PTCA or thrombolysis—provides the best long-term reduction in morbidity and mortality. The rate of re-occlusion after PTCA is about 30% within 6 to 8 months.

Coronary Artery Bypass Graft (CABG). A CABG may be needed to treat acute or recurrent MI. Candidates include patients for whom thrombolysis was unsuccessful and for whom PTCA is contraindicated or has failed to recanalize the occluded artery. Although a CABG may be done as primary therapy for MI, the procedure is clearly impractical for *routine* use.

DRUG THERAPY (OTHER THAN THROMBOLYTICS)

Morphine. Intravenous morphine controls the pain of MI and also provides hemodynamic benefits. By promoting venodilation, the drug reduces cardiac preload. By promoting modest arterial dilation, morphine may cause some reduction in afterload. The combined reductions in preload and afterload lower cardiac oxygen demand, thereby helping preserve the ischemic myocardium.

Beta-Adrenergic Blocking Agents. When given to patients undergoing acute MI, beta-adrenergic blocking agents (e.g., metoprolol) can reduce cardiac pain, infarct size, and mortality. As an MI evolves, traffic along sympathetic nerves to the heart increases greatly, as does the number of beta receptors on the heart. As a result, heart rate and force of contraction rise substantially, thereby increasing cardiac oxygen demand. By preventing beta receptor activation, beta blockers lower heart rate and contractility, and thereby reduce oxygen demand. Furthermore, by prolonging diastolic filling time, these drugs increase coronary blood flow and oxygen supply. Presumably, clinical benefits derive at least in part from the reduction in oxygen demand and the increase in oxygen supply. Beta blockers are contraindicated for patients with overt heart failure, pronounced bradycardia, hypotension, and heart block greater than first degree. The basic pharmacology of the beta blockers is discussed in Chapter 18.

Nitrates. Intravenous nitroglycerin and nitroprusside can reduce infarct size and mortality. Both drugs are vasodilators. Clinical benefits result from reduced oxygen demand (secondary to reduced preload and afterload) and perhaps from increased collateral blood flow in the ischemic region of the heart.

COMPLICATIONS OF ACUTE MYOCARDIAL INFARCTION AND THEIR MANAGEMENT

Myocardial infarction predisposes the heart and vascular system to serious complications. Among the most severe are ventricular dysrhythmias, cardiogenic shock, and congestive heart failure.

Ventricular Dysrhythmias. These develop frequently and are the major cause of death following MI. Sudden death from dysrhythmias occurs in 15% of patients during the first hour. Ultimately, ventricular dysrhythmias cause 60% of infarction-related deaths. Lidocaine has been used widely for prophylaxis of life-threatening dysrhythmias. However, there is no evidence that this practice reduces mortality. Programmed ventricular stimulation with guided antidysrhythmic therapy may be lifesaving for some patients.

Cardiogenic Shock. Shock results from greatly reduced tissue perfusion secondary to impaired cardiac function. Shock develops in 7% to 15% of patients during the first few days after MI and has a mortality rate of up to 90%. Patients at highest risk are those with large infarcts, a previous infarct, a low ejection fraction (less than 35%), diabetes, and advanced age. Drug therapy includes inotropic agents (e.g., dopamine, dobutamine) to increase cardiac output and vasodilators (nitroglycerin, nitroprusside) to improve tissue perfusion and reduce cardiac work and oxygen demand. Unfortunately, although these drugs can improve hemodynamic status, they do not seem to reduce mortality. Restoration of cardiac perfusion with PTCA or CABG may be of value.

Congestive Heart Failure (CHF). CHF secondary to acute MI can be treated with a combination of drugs. A diuretic (e.g., furosemide) is given to decrease preload and pulmonary congestion. Inotropic agents (e.g., digoxin) increase cardiac output by enhancing contractility. Vasodilators improve hemodynamic status by reducing preload and/or afterload. Angiotensin-converting enzyme (ACE) inhibitors, which reduce both preload and afterload, can be especially helpful.

Cardiac Rupture. Weakening of the myocardium predisposes the heart wall to rupture. Following rupture, shock and circulatory collapse develop rapidly. Death is often immediate. Fortunately, cardiac rupture is rare (less than 2% incidence). Patients at highest risk are those with a large anterior infarction. Cardiac rupture is most likely within the first days after MI. Early treatment with vasodilators and beta-adrenergic blocking agents may reduce the risk of wall rupture.

Arterial Embolism and Deep Venous Thrombosis. Arterial embolism occurs when a thrombus in the heart breaks free and becomes lodged in a systemic artery. The incidence of embolism is 2% to 6%. Deep venous thrombosis of the legs develops in 17% to 38% of patients, usually within a few days of the MI. The incidence of embolism and thrombosis can be reduced with heparin (IV or SC). Treatment should begin soon (within 12 to 18 hours) after the onset of MI symptoms and should continue for 10 days.

Pericarditis. About 10% of patients with acute MI develop pericarditis, usually within 2 to 4 days. This inflammation develops in response to transmural necrosis. Symptoms can be reduced with aspirin, an anti-inflammatory drug.

LONG-TERM MANAGEMENT AFTER MYOCARDIAL INFARCTION

As a rule, patients who survive the acute phase of MI can be discharged from the hospital after 6 to 10 days. However, these patients are still at risk of reinfarction (5% to 15% incidence within the first year) and other complications, (e.g., dysrhythmias, congestive heart failure). Accordingly, long-term preventive treatment is indicated. Drug therapy and nondrug methods are employed.

DRUG THERAPY

Aspirin and Oral Anticoagulants. Aspirin inhibits platelet aggregation, thereby reducing the risk of reinfarction and stroke. The drug is clearly effective in post MI patients and now constitutes standard therapy. Treatment is initiated immediately after onset of symptoms and continues for at least several years. Low-dose therapy (160 mg per day) suppresses platelet aggregation while causing minimal side effects.

Oral anticoagulants (e.g., warfarin) reduce the incidence of reinfarction, stroke, and mortality. Duration of treatment is 3 to 6 months. Candidates for therapy include patients with left ventricular thrombus, threatened thrombus, atrial fibrillation, and those with a history of emboli. When oral anticoagulants are used, it may be appropriate to postpone therapy with aspirin.

Beta-Adrenergic Blocking Agents. Clinical studies indicate that these drugs help reduce mortality following MI. Treatment has been continued for up to 6 years.

Angiotensin-Converting Enzyme Inhibitors. ACE inhibitors promote vasodilation. In post MI patients, these drugs can improve exercise tolerance, reduce ventricular enlargement, and prevent further ventricular dilatation. Their impact on mortality is not known.

Antidysrhythmic Agents. Premature ventricular complexes in the post MI patient are considered predictors of sudden death from ventricular dysrhythmias. Unfortunately, attempts to prevent dysrhythmias by giving antidysrhythmic drugs prophylactically have failed to reduce mortality. Worse yet, attempted prophylaxis of ventricular dysrhythmias with two drugs—encainide and flecainide—has actually *increased* mortality. Similarly, when quinidine was employed to prevent supraventricular dysrhythmias, it too increased mortality. Therefore, since prophylaxis with antidysrhythmic drugs has not reduced mortality—and may in fact increase mortality—antidysrhythmic drugs should be withheld until a dysrhythmia actually occurs.

NONDRUG THERAPY

Reduction of risk factors for MI can increase long-term survival. Patients who smoke must be discouraged from doing so. Patients with high serum cholesterol should be given an appropriate dietary plan and, if necessary, treated with lipid-lowering drugs. Diabetes and hypertension increase the risk of mortality and must be controlled.

Exercise training can be valuable for two reasons: (1) it reduces complications associated with prolonged bed rest, and (2) it accelerates return to an optimal level of functioning. Although exercise is safe for most patients, there is concern about cardiac risk and impairment of infarct healing in patients whose infarct is large.

Psychologic reactions to MI are common and can impede recovery. These reactions include anxiety, denial, and depression with associated social and sexual dysfunction. The clinician should be alert to these reactions and make counseling available when appropriate.

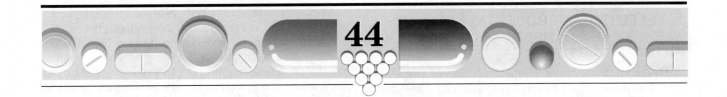

Antidysrhythmic Drugs

A dysrhythmia is defined as an abnormality in the rhythm of the heart beat. In their mildest forms, dysrhythmias have only modest effects on cardiac output. However, in their most severe forms, dysrhythmias can so disable the heart that no blood is pumped at all. Because of their ability to compromise cardiac function, dysrhythmias are associated with a high degree of morbidity and mortality.

There are two basic types of dysrhythmias: *tachydysrhythmias* (dysrhythmias in which heart rate is increased) and *bradydysrhythmias* (dysrhythmias in which heart rate is slowed). In this chapter, we will only consider the tachydysrhythmias. This is by far the largest group of dysrhythmias and the group that responds best to drugs. We will not discuss the bradydysrhythmias as they are few in number and are commonly treated with electronic pacing. When drugs are indicated, atropine (see Chapter 13) and isoproterenol (see Chapter 17) are usually the agents of choice.

It is important to appreciate that virtually all of the drugs used to *treat* dysrhythmias can also *cause* dysrhythmias. These drugs can create new dysrhythmias and worsen existing ones. Accordingly, antidysrhythmic drugs should be employed only when the benefits of treatment clearly outweigh the risks.

A note on terminology: dysrhythmias are also known as *arrhythmias*. Since the term *arrhythmia* denotes an *absence* of cardiac rhythm whereas *dysrhythmia* denotes *abnormal* rhythm, dysrhythmia would seem to be the more appropriate term.

ELECTRICAL PROPERTIES OF THE HEART

Dysrhythmias result from alteration of the electrical impulses that regulate cardiac rhythm—and antidysrhythmic drugs produce rhythm control by correcting or compensating for these alterations. Accordingly, if we want to understand the generation of dysrhythmias as well as the drugs used to treat them, we must first understand the electrical properties of the heart. To establish that understanding, we will review the following: (1) timing and pathways of impulse conduction, (2) cardiac action potentials, and (3) basic elements of the electrocardiogram.

IMPULSE CONDUCTION: PATHWAYS AND TIMING

For the heart to pump effectively, contraction of the the atria and ventricles must be coordinated. Coordination is achieved through precise timing and routing of impulse conduction. In the healthy heart, impulses originate in the S-A node, spread rapidly through the atria, pass slowly through the A-V node, and then spread rapidly through the ventricles via the His-Purkinje system (Fig. 44–1). Details of conduction are discussed below.

Sinoauricular (S-A) Node. Under normal circumstances, the S-A node serves as the pacemaker for the heart. Pacemaker activity results from spontaneous phase-4 depolarization (see below). Since sinus node cells usually discharge at a rate higher than that of other cells that display automaticity, the S-A node normally dominates all other potential pacemakers.

After the S-A node discharges, impulses spread rapidly through the atria along the *internodal pathways*. This rapid conduction allows the atria to contract in unison.

Atrioventricular (A-V) Node. Impulses originating in the atria must travel through the A-V node in order to reach the ventricles. In the healthy heart, impulses arriving at the A-V node are *delayed* before going on to produce ventricular excitation. This delay at the A-V node provides time for blood to fill the ventricles prior to ventricular contraction.

His-Purkinje System. The fibers of the His-Purkinje system consist of specialized conducting tissue. The function of these fibers is to conduct electrical excitation very rapidly to all parts of the ventricles. Stimulation of the His-Purkinje system is caused by impulses leaving the A-V node. These impulses are conducted rapidly down the bundle of His, enter the right and left bundle branches, and then distribute to the many fine branches of the Purkinje fibers (see Fig. 44–1). Because impulses travel quickly through this system, all regions of the ventricles are stimulated simultaneously, producing synchronized ventricular contraction with resultant forceful ejection of blood.

CARDIAC ACTION POTENTIALS

Cardiac cells, like neurons, can initiate and conduct action potentials—self-propagating waves of depolarization followed by repolarization.

In the heart, two kinds of action potentials occur: *fast potentials* and *slow potentials*. These potentials differ from each other with respect to the mechanisms by which they are generated, the kinds of cells in which they occur, and the drugs to which they respond.

Profiles of fast and slow potentials are depicted in Figure 44–2. Please note that action potentials in this figure represent the electrical activity of *single cardiac cells*. Such single-cell recordings, which are made using experimental preparations, should not be confused with the electrocardiogram, which is made using surface electrodes, and reflects the electrical activity of the *entire heart*.

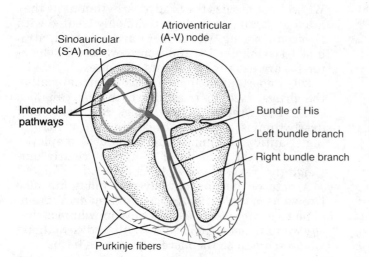

Figure 44–1. Impulse conduction pathways.

A **Myocardium and His-Purkinje System**

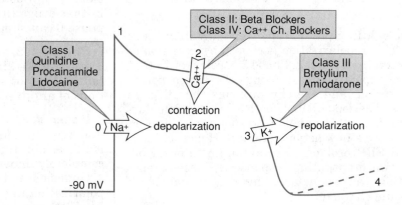
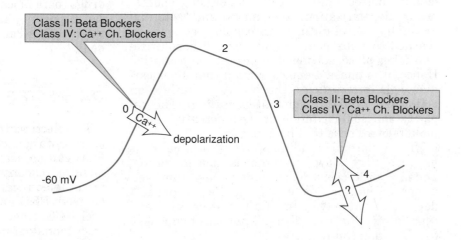

Figure 44–2. Ion fluxes during cardiac action potentials and effects of antidysrhythmic drugs.

A, Fast potential of the His-Purkinje system and atrial and ventricular myocardium. Blockade of sodium influx by Class I drugs slows conduction in the His-Purkinje system. Blockade of calcium influx by beta blockers and calcium channel blockers decreases contractility. Blockade of potassium efflux by Class III drugs delays repolarization and thereby prolongs the effective refractory period.

B, Slow potential of the sinoauricular (S-A) node and atrioventricular (A-V) node. Blockade of calcium influx by beta blockers and calcium channel blockers slows A-V conduction. These same drugs decrease S-A nodal automaticity (phase 4 depolarization); the ionic basis of this effect is not known.

B **S-A Node and A-V Node**

Fast Potentials

Fast potentials occur in fibers of the *His-Purkinje system* and in *atrial and ventricular muscle*. These responses serve to conduct electrical impulses rapidly throughout the heart.

Cardiac action potentials are generated by the movement of ions into and out of cells. These ion fluxes take place by way of specific channels in the cell membrane. In the resting cardiac cell, negatively charged ions cover the inner surface of the cell membrane while positively charged ions cover the external surface. Because of this separation of charge, the cell membrane is said to be *polarized*. Under proper conditions, channels in the cell membrane open, allowing positively charged ions to rush in. This influx eliminates the charge difference across the cell membrane; hence, the cell is said to *depolarize*. Following depolarization, positively charged ions are extruded from the cell, causing the cell to return to its original polarized state.

As indicated in panel A of Figure 44–2, fast po-

tentials have five distinct phases, labeled 0, 1, 2, 3, and 4. As we discuss each phase, we will focus on its ionic basis and its relationship to the actions of antidysrhythmic drugs.

Phase 0. In phase 0, the cell undergoes *rapid depolarization* in response to *influx of sodium ions*. Phase 0 is important in that the speed of phase-0 depolarization determines the velocity of impulse conduction. Drugs that decrease the rate of phase-0 depolarization (by blocking sodium channels) will slow impulse conduction though the His-Purkinje system and myocardium.

Phase 1. During phase 1, rapid (but partial) repolarization takes place. Phase 1 has no relevance to antidysrhythmic drugs.

Phase 2. Phase 2 consists of a prolonged plateau in which the membrane potential remains relatively stable. During this phase, *calcium* enters the cell and promotes contraction of atrial and ventricular muscle. Drugs that reduce calcium entry during phase 2 do *not* influence *cardiac rhythm*.

However, since calcium influx is required for contraction, these drugs *can reduce* myocardial *contractility*.

Phase 3. In phase 3, rapid repolarization takes place. This repolarization is caused by *extrusion of potassium* from the cell. Phase 3 is relevant in that delay of repolarization prolongs the action potential duration, and thereby prolongs the effective refractory period (ERP). (The ERP is the time during which a cell is unable to respond to excitation and initiate a new action potential. Hence, extending the ERP prolongs the minimum interval between two propagating responses.) Phase-3 repolarization can be delayed by drugs that block potassium channels.

Phase 4. During phase 4, two types of electrical activity are possible: (1) the membrane potential may remain *stable* (solid line in Fig. 44–2A), or (2) the membrane may undergo *spontaneous depolarization* (dotted line). In cells undergoing spontaneous depolarization, the membrane potential gradually rises until a threshold potential is reached. At this point, rapid phase-0 depolarization takes place, setting off a new action potential. Hence, it is phase-4 depolarization that gives cardiac cells *automaticity* (the ability to initiate an action potential through self-excitation). The capacity for self-excitation makes potential pacemakers of all cells that have it.

Under normal conditions, His-Purkinje cells undergo very slow spontaneous depolarization, and myocardial cells do not undergo any. However, under pathologic conditions, significant phase-4 depolarization may occur in all of these cells, and especially in Purkinje fibers. When this happens, a dysrhythmia can result.

Slow Potentials

Slow potentials occur in cells in the *S-A node* and *A-V node*. The profile of a slow potential is depicted in Figure 44–2B. Like fast potentials, slow potentials are generated by ion fluxes.

From a physiologic and pharmacologic perspective, slow potentials have three features of special significance: (1) phase-0 depolarization is slow and mediated by calcium influx, (2) these potentials conduct slowly, and (3) spontaneous phase-4 depolarization in the S-A node normally determines heart rate.

Phase 0. Phase 0 (depolarization phase) of slow potentials differs significantly from phase 0 of fast potentials. As we can see from Figure 44–2, whereas phase 0 of fast potentials is caused by an *inward rush of sodium*, phase 0 of slow potentials is caused by *slow influx of calcium*. Because calcium influx is slow, the rate of depolarization is slow; and because depolarization is slow, these potentials conduct slowly. This explains why impulse

conduction through the A-V node is delayed. Phase 0 of the slow potential is of therapeutic significance in that drugs that suppress calcium influx during phase 0 can suppress A-V conduction.

Phases 1, 2, and 3. Slow potentials lack a phase 1 (see Fig 44–2B). Phases 2 and 3 of the slow potential are not significant with respect to the actions of antidysrhythmic drugs.

Phase 4. Cells of the S-A node and A-V node undergo spontaneous phase-4 depolarization. The ionic basis of this phenomenon is complex and incompletely understood.

Under normal conditions, the rate of phase-4 depolarization in cells of the S-A node is faster than in all other cells of the heart. As a result, the S-A discharges first and determines heart rate. Hence, the S-A node is referred to as the cardiac *pacemaker*.

As indicated in Figure 44–2B, two classes of drugs (beta blockers and calcium channel blockers) can suppress phase-4 depolarization. By doing so, these agents can decrease automaticity in the S-A node.

THE ELECTROCARDIOGRAM

The electrocardiogram (EKG) provides a graphic representation of cardiac electrical activity. The EKG can be used to identify dysrhythmias and to monitor responses to therapy. (Note: In referring to the electrocardiogram, two abbreviations may be used: EKG and ECG. Many people prefer EKG over ECG, since ECG sounds much like EEG [electroencephalogram] when spoken aloud.)

The major components of an EKG are illustrated in Figure 44–3. As we can see, three features are especially prominent: the *P wave*, the *QRS complex*, and the *T wave*. The P wave is caused by *depolarization in the atria*. Hence, the P wave cor-

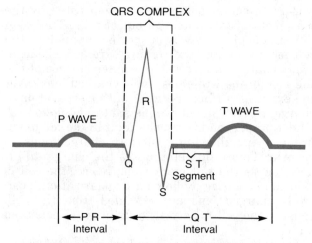

Figure 44–3. The electrocardiogram.

responds to atrial contraction. The QRS complex is caused by *depolarization of the ventricles*. Hence, the QRS complex corresponds to ventricular contraction. If conduction through the ventricles is slowed, the QRS complex will widen. The T wave is caused by *repolarization of the ventricles*. Hence, this wave is not associated with overt physical activity of the heart.

In addition to the features just described, the EKG has three other components of interest: the *PR interval*, the *QT interval*, and the *ST segment*. The PR interval is defined as the time between the onset of the P wave and the onset of the QRS complex. Lengthening of this interval indicates a delay in conduction through the A-V node. Several drugs increase the PR interval. The QT interval is defined as the time between the onset of the QRS complex and the completion of the T wave. This interval is prolonged by drugs that delay ventricular repolarization. The ST segment is the portion of the EKG that lies between the end of the QRS complex and the beginning of the T wave. Digoxin depresses the ST segment.

GENERATION OF DYSRHYTHMIAS

Dysrhythmias arise from two fundamental causes: *disturbances of impulse formation* (automaticity) and *disturbances of impulse conduction*. One or both of these disturbances underlie all dysrhythmias. Factors that may lead to altered automaticity or conduction include hypoxia, electrolyte imbalance, cardiac surgery, reduced coronary blood flow, myocardial infarction, and all of the antidysrhythmic drugs.

Disturbances of Automaticity

Disturbances of automaticity can occur in any area of the heart. Cells normally capable of automaticity (cells of the S-A node, A-V node, and His-Purkinje system) can produce dysrhythmias if their normal rate of discharge changes. In addition, dysrhythmias may be produced if tissues that do not normally express automaticity (atrial and ventricular muscle) develop spontaneous phase-4 depolarization.

Altered automaticity in the S-A node can produce tachycardia or bradycardia. Excessive discharge of sympathetic neurons that innervate the S-A node can augment automaticity to such a degree that *sinus tachycardia* results. Excessive vagal (parasympathetic) discharge can suppress automaticity to such a degree that *sinus bradycardia* results.

Increased automaticity of Purkinje fibers is a common cause of dysrhythmias. The increase can be brought about by injury or by excessive stimulation of Purkinje fibers by the sympathetic ner-

vous system. If Purkinje fibers begin to discharge faster than the S-A node, they will escape control by the S-A node and potentially serious dysrhythmias may result.

Under special conditions, automaticity may develop in cells of atrial and ventricular muscle. Dysrhythmias will result if these cells begin to fire faster than the S-A node.

Disturbances of Conduction

A-V Block. Impaired conduction through the A-V node produces varying degrees of A-V block. If impulse conduction is delayed (but not prevented entirely), the block is termed *first degree*. If some impulses pass through the node but others do not, the block is termed *second degree*. If all traffic through the A-V node stops, the block is termed *third degree*.

Recirculating Activation (Reentry). Recirculating activation, also referred to as *reentry*, is a generalized mechanism by which dysrhythmias can be produced. Reentry causes dysrhythmias by establishing a localized, self-sustaining circuit capable of repetitive cardiac stimulation. Reentry results from a unique form of conduction disturbance. The mechanism of reentrant activation and the effects of drugs on this process are described below.

The mechanism for establishing a reentrant circuit is depicted in Figure 44–4, panels A and B. In the figure, the inverted Y-shaped structure represents a branched Purkinje fiber terminating on a strip of ventricular muscle; the muscle appears as a horizontal bar. Normal impulse conduction is shown in Figure 44–4A. As indicated by the arrows, impulses travel down both branches of the Purkinje fiber to cause excitation of the muscle at two separate locations. Impulses created within the muscle travel in both directions (to the right and to the left) away from their sites of origin. Those impulses that are moving toward each other meet at a point midway between the two branches of the Purkinje fiber. Since the muscle in the wake of both impulses is in a refractory state, neither impulse can proceed further, and both impulses come to a stop.

Figure 44–4B depicts a reentrant circuit. The shaded area in branch 1 of the Purkinje fiber represents a region of *one-way* conduction block. This region prevents conduction of impulses downward (toward the muscle) but does not prevent impulses from traveling upward. (Impulses can travel back up the block because impulses in *muscle* are very strong and, therefore, are able to pass the block, whereas impulses in the Purkinje fiber are weaker and unable to pass.) A region of one-way block is essential for reentrant activation.

How does one-way block lead to reentrant activation? As an impulse travels down the Purkinje fiber, it is stopped in branch 1 but continues unimpeded in branch 2. Upon reaching the tip of branch 2, the impulse stimulates the muscle. As described above, the impulse in the muscle travels to the right and to the left away from its site of origin. However, in this new situation, as the impulse travels toward the impaired branch of the Purkinje fiber, it meets no impulse coming from the other direction; hence, the impulse continues on, resulting in the stimulation of the terminal end of branch 1. This stimulation causes an impulse to travel backward up the Purkinje fiber. Since blockade of conduction is unidirectional, the impulse passes through the region of block and then back down into branch 2, causing reentrant activation of this branch. Under proper conditions,

A   Normal Conduction

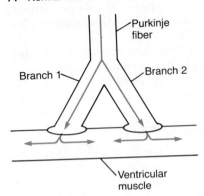

B   Reentrant Activation

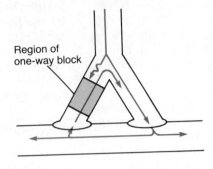

Figure 44–4. Reentrant activation: mechanism and drug effects. *A,* In normal conduction, impulses from the branched Purkinje fiber stimulate the strip of ventricular muscle in two places. Within the muscle, waves of excitation spread from both points of excitation, meet between the Purkinje fibers, and cease further travel. *B,* In the presence of one-way block, the strip of muscle is excited at only one location. Impulses spreading from this area meet no impulses coming from the left and can therefore travel far enough to stimulate branch 1 of the Purkinje fiber. This stimulation passes back up the fiber, past the region of one-way block, and then stimulates branch 2, causing reentrant activation. *C,* Elimination of reentry by a drug that improves conduction in the sick branch of the Purkinje fiber. *D,* Elimination of reentry by a drug that further suppresses conduction in the sick branch, thereby converting one-way block into two-way block.

C   Drug Effect I

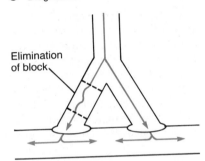

D   Drug Effect II

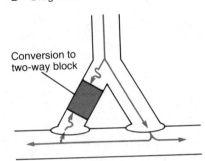

the impulse will continue to cycle indefinitely, resulting in re-petitive ectopic beats.

There are two mechanisms by which drugs can abolish a reentrant dysrhythmia. First, drugs can improve conduction in the sick branch of the Purkinje fiber, and can thereby eliminate the one-way block (Fig. 44–4C). Alternatively, drugs can suppress conduction in the sick branch, and thereby convert unidirectional block into two-way block (Fig. 44–4D).

CLASSIFICATION OF ANTIDYSRHYTHMIC DRUGS

The antidysrhythmic drugs fall into five groups (Table 44–1). As indicated in the table, there are four major classes of antidysrhythmic drugs (Classes I, II, III, and IV) and a fifth group that includes adenosine and digoxin. Membership in Classes I through IV relates to drug effects on ion movements during slow and fast potentials (see Fig. 44–2).

Class I: Sodium Channel Blockers. Class I drugs produce blockade of cardiac sodium channels (see Fig. 44–2). By doing so, these drugs slow the rate of impulse conduction in the atria, ventricles, and His-Purkinje system. Class I constitutes the largest group of antidysrhythmic drugs.

Class II: Beta Blockers. Class II consists of beta-adrenergic blocking agents. As suggested by Figure 44–2, these drugs reduce calcium entry (during fast and slow potentials) and they depress phase-4 depolarization (in slow potentials only). Beta blockers have three prominent effects on the heart: in the S-A node they reduce automaticity; in the A-V node they slow conduction velocity; and in the atria and ventricles they reduce contractility. Cardiac effects of the beta blockers are nearly identical to those of the calcium channel blockers.

Class III: Drugs That Delay Repolarization. Class III drugs produce blockade of potassium channels (Fig. 44–2A), and thereby delay repolarization of fast potentials. By delaying repolarization, these drugs prolong both the action potential duration and the effective refractory period.

Class IV: Calcium Channel Blockers. Only one calcium channel blocker—verapamil—is approved for antidysrhythmic use. As indicated in Figure 44–2, calcium channel blockade has the same impact on cardiac action potentials as beta blockade. As a result, verapamil and the beta blockers have nearly identical effects on cardiac function—namely, reduction of automaticity in the S-A node, delay of conduction through the A-V node, and reduction of myocardial contractility.

Table 44-1. Classes of Antidysrhythmic Drugs

Class I: Sodium Channel Blockers

Class IA
Quinidine [Quinidex, others]
Procainamide [Pronestyl, others]
Disopyramide [Norpace]

Class IB
Lidocaine [Xylocaine]
Phenytoin [Dilantin]
Mexiletine [Mexitil]
Tocainide [Tonocard]

Class IC
Flecainide [Tambocor]
Propafenone [Rhythmol]

Other Class I
Moricizine [Ethmozine]

Class II: Beta Blockers
Propranolol [Inderal]
Acebutolol [Sectral]
Esmolol [Brevibloc]

Class III: Drugs That Delay Repolarization
Amiodarone [Cordarone]
Betylium [Bretylol]
Sotalol [Betapace]

Class IV: Calcium Channel Blockers
Verapamil [Isoptin, Calan, Verelan]

Other Antidysrhythmic Drugs
Adenosine [Adenocard]
Digoxin [Lanoxin, Lanoxicaps]

Antidysrhythmic effects derive from suppressing A-V nodal conduction.

Other Antidysrhythmic Drugs. *Digoxin* and *adenosine* do not fit into any of the four major classes of antidysrhythmic drugs. Both of these agents decrease conduction through the A-V node and reduce automaticity in the S-A node.

PRODYSRHYTHMIC EFFECTS OF ANTIDYSRHYTHMIC DRUGS

Virtually all of the drugs used to treat dysrhythmias have prodysrhythmic (proarrhythmic) effects. That is, *all of these drugs can worsen existing dysrhythmias and generate new ones*. This ability was documented dramatically in the CAST study (Cardiac Arrhythmia Suppression Trial) in which use of Class IC drugs (encainide and flecainide) to prevent dysrhythmias after myocardial infarction actually *doubled* the mortality rate. Because of their prodysrhythmic actions, antidysrhythmic drugs should be used only when dysrhythmias are symptomatically significant, and then only when the potential benefits of treatment clearly outweigh the risks. Applying this guideline, it would be inappropriate to give antidysrhythmic drugs to a patient with nonsustained ventricular tachycardia, since this dysrhythmia does not significantly reduce car-

diac output. Conversely, when a patient is facing death from ventricular fibrillation, any therapy that might work must be tried; the risk of prodysrhythmic effects is clearly outweighed by the potential benefits of stopping the fibrillation. Regardless of the particular circumstances of drug use, all patients must be followed closely.

OVERVIEW OF COMMON DYSRHYTHMIAS AND THEIR TREATMENT

The common dysrhythmias can be divided into two major groups: *supraventricular dysrhythmias* and *ventricular dysrhythmias*. In general, ventricular dysrhythmias are more dangerous than supraventricular dysrhythmias. With either type, intervention is required only if the dysrhythmia interferes with effective ventricular pumping. Treatment usually proceeds in two phases: (1) *termination* of the dysrhythmia (with electrical countershock, drugs, or both), followed by (2) *long-term suppression* with drugs.

Therapy of the common dysrhythmias is summarized in Table 44–2. As indicated, drugs are not always the preferred treatment. In fact, drugs constitute the first line of treatment for only two of the common dysrhythmias: ventricular premature beats and digoxin-induced ventricular dysrhythmias. For several dysrhythmias, DC cardioversion (electrical countershock) is the preferred therapy. In one case (supraventricular tachycardia), maneuvers that increase vagal tone are the treatment of choice.

It is important to appreciate that drug therapy of dysrhythmias is highly empirical (i.e., based largely on the response of the patient and not on scientific principles). In practice, this means that even after a dysrhythmia has been identified, we cannot predict with certainty just which drugs will be effective. Frequently, trials with several drugs are required before control of rhythm is achieved. In the discussion below, only first-choice drugs are considered.

SUPRAVENTRICULAR DYSRHYTHMIAS

Supraventricular dysrhythmias are dysrhythmias that arise in areas of the heart above the ventricles (atria, S-A node, A-V node). Supraventricular dysrhythmias per se are not especially harmful. This is because dysrhythmic activity within the atria does not significantly reduce cardiac output (except in patients with valvular disorders and heart failure). Supraventricular *tachy*dysrhythmias *can* be dangerous, however, in that

	Acute Treatment		
Type of Dysrhythmia	*Preferred*	*Alternatives*	**Long-Term Suppression**
Supraventricular			

Supraventricular tachycardia	Vagotonic maneuvers	To terminate:
		  Beta blocker (II)
		  Verapamil (IV)
		  Digoxin
		  Adenosine
			Quinidine (IA)
			Procainamide IA)
			Other drugs

Atrial flutter and atrial fibrillation	Cardioversion	To slow ventricular response:
		  Beta-blocker (II)
		  Verapamil (IV)
		  Digoxin
			Quinidine (IA)*
			Procainamide (IA)
			Other drugs

Ventricular			
Sustained ventricular tachycardia	Cardioversion	Lidocaine (IB) Procainamide (IA) Bretylium (III)	Quinidine (IA) Procainamide (IA) Other drugs
Ventricular fibrillation	Cardioversion	Lidocaine (IB)† Procainamide (IA)† Bretylium (III)†	Amiodarone (III)
Ventricular premature beats	Asymptomatic patients need no treatment	Beta-blocker (II)‡	
Digoxin-induced ventricular dysrhythmias	Lidocaine (IB)	Phenytoin (IB)	

Table 44–2. Treatment of Common Dysrhythmias

*Quinidine may *increase* mortality in these patients.
†Cardioversion is the treatment of choice. Drugs are given to prevent recurrence.
‡Beta blockers are used only if the dysrhythmia is symptomatic.

atrial impulses are likely to traverse the A-V node, resulting in excitation of the ventricles. If the atria drive the ventricles at an excessive rate, diastolic filling will be incomplete and cardiac output will decline. Hence, when treating supraventricular dysrhythmias, the objective is frequently one of *blocking impulse conduction through the A-V node* and *not* elimination of the dysrhythmia itself. Of course, if treatment did abolish the dysrhythmia, this outcome would not be undesirable. As indicated in Table 44–2, acute treatment of supraventricular dysrhythmias is accomplished with vagotonic maneuvers, DC cardioversion, and certain drugs: Class II, Class IV, adenosine, and digoxin.

Supraventricular Tachycardia. Supraventricular tachycardia (SVT) is caused by a rapidly firing ectopic focus located in the atria or in the A-V node. Heart rate is increased to 150 to 250 beats per minute. SVT is best treated by maneuvers that increase vagal tone, such as carotid sinus massage or the Valsalva maneuver. If vagal maneuvers are ineffective, intravenous adenosine or verapamil should be given. If these drugs fail, others may be tried (see Table 44–2). Once the dysrhythmia has been controlled, long-term prophylaxis with quinidine may prevent its recurrence.

Atrial Flutter. Atrial flutter is caused by an ectopic atrial focus discharging at a rate of 250 to 350 times a minute. Ventricular rate is considera-

bly slower than this, however, because the A-V node is unable to transmit impulses at such a high rate. Typically, one atrial impulse out of three manages to reach the ventricles. The treatment of choice is DC cardioversion, which almost always converts atrial flutter to normal sinus rhythm. If cardioversion is ineffective, drugs may be employed; the objective is to decrease the number of atrial impulses that pass to the ventricles. The drug of choice for atrial flutter is digoxin. Verapamil or a beta blocker may also be effective. Long-term therapy with quinidine has been used to prevent the dysrhythmia from recurring. However, recent analysis of older data indicates that quinidine can actually *increase* mortality in these patients. It is not known whether other drugs used for prophylaxis pose a similar danger.

Atrial Fibrillation. Atrial fibrillation is caused by multiple atrial ectopic foci firing in random order; each focus stimulates only a small area of atrial muscle. This chaotic excitation produces a highly irregular atrial rhythm. Depending upon the extent of impulse transmission through the A-V node, ventricular rate may be rapid or nearly normal. Treatment is the same as for atrial flutter. Cardioversion is the preferred therapy. If cardioversion is ineffective, digoxin can be used to reduce the number of atrial impulses reaching the ventricles. Long-term quinidine therapy may prevent the dysrhythmia from recurring, but may also *increase* the risk of mortality.

VENTRICULAR DYSRHYTHMIAS

In contrast to atrial dysrhythmias, which are generally benign, ventricular dysrhythmias can cause significant disruption of cardiac pumping. Accordingly, the usual objective is to abolish the dysrhythmia. Cardioversion is often the treatment of choice. When antidysrhythmic drugs are indicated, Classes I and III are usually employed.

Sustained Ventricular Tachycardia. Ventricular tachycardia arises from a single, rapidly firing ventricular ectopic focus. The focus drives the ventricles at a rate of 150 to 250 beats per minute. Since the ventricles cannot pump effectively at these rates, immediate treatment is required. Cardioversion is the treatment of choice. If cardioversion fails to normalize rhythm, lidocaine should be administered. If lidocaine is also ineffective, bretylium or procainamide should be tried. As indicated in Table 44–2, quinidine, procainamide, and other drugs can be employed for long-term suppression.

Ventricular Fibrillation. Ventricular fibrillation is a life-threatening emergency and requires immediate treatment. This dysrhythmia results from the asynchronous discharge of multiple ventricular ectopic foci. Because many different foci are firing, and because each focus initiates contraction in its immediate vicinity, localized twitching takes place all over the ventricles, making coordinated ventricular contraction impossible. As a result, the pumping action of the heart stops. In the absence of blood flow, the patient becomes unconscious and cyanotic. If heartbeat is not restored rapidly, death soon follows. Electrical countershock (cardioversion) is applied to eliminate fibrillation and restore cardiac function. If necessary, lidocaine can be used to enhance the effects of cardioversion. Procainamide and bretylium may also be helpful. Amiodarone can be used for long-term suppression.

Ventricular Premature Beats. Ventricular premature beats (VPBs) are beats that occur before they should in the cardiac cycle. These beats are caused by ectopic ventricular foci. VPBs may arise from a single ectopic focus or from several foci. In the absence of additional signs of heart disease, VPBs are benign and not usually treated. However, in the presence of acute myocardial infarction, VPBs may predispose the patient to ventricular fibrillation. In this case, therapy is required. A beta blocker is the agent of choice. Because VPBs are associated with a premature QRS complex on the EKG, this dysrhythmia is also known as *premature ventricular complexes.*

Digoxin-Induced Ventricular Dysrhythmias. Digoxin toxicity can mimic practically all types of dysrhythmias. Varying degrees of A-V block are among the most common. Ventricular flutter and ventricular fibrillation are the most dangerous. Digoxin causes dysrhythmias by increasing automaticity in the atria, ventricles, and His-Purkinje system, and by decreasing conduction through the A-V node.

With accurate diagnosis and proper treatment, digoxin-induced dysrhythmias can almost always be controlled. Treatment is discussed at length in Chapter 42. If antidysrhythmic drugs are required, lidocaine and phenytoin are the agents of choice. In patients with digoxin toxicity, cardioversion may bring on ventricular fibrillation. Accordingly, this procedure should be used only when absolutely required.

CLASS I: SODIUM CHANNEL BLOCKERS

Class I antidysrhythmic drugs produce blockade of cardiac sodium channels. By doing so, these drugs decrease conduction velocity in the atria, ventricles, and His-Purkinje system.

There are three subgroups of Class I agents. Drugs in all three groups block sodium channels. In addition, Class IA agents delay repolarization, whereas Class IB agents accelerate repolarization. Class IC agents have pronounced prodysrhythmic actions.

The Class I drugs are similar in action and structure to the local anesthetics. In fact, one of these drugs—lidocaine—has both local anesthetic and antidysrhythmic applications. Because of their relationship to the local anesthetics, Class I agents are sometimes referred to as *local anesthetic antidysrhythmic agents.*

Some important properties of the Class I drugs and other antidysrhythmics are summarized in Table 44–3.

CLASS IA AGENTS

Quinidine

Quinidine is the oldest and most thoroughly studied of the Class IA drugs. Accordingly, quinidine will serve as our prototype for the group. Quinidine is the most frequently used oral antidysrhythmic agent.

Chemistry and Source. Quinidine is similar to quinine in structure and actions. The natural source of both drugs is the bark of the South American cinchona tree. Accordingly, these agents are referred to as *cinchona alkaloids.* Like quinine,

Drug	**Usual Route**	**Effects on the EKG**	**Antidysrhythmic Applications**

Table 44–3. Properties of Antidysrhythmic Drugs

Drug	Usual Route	Effects on the EKG	Antidysrhythmic Applications
Class IA			
Quinidine	PO	Widens QRS, prolongs QT	Broad spectrum: used for long-term suppression of ventricular and supraventricular dysrhythmias
Procainamide	PO	Widens QRS, prolongs QT	Broad spectrum: similar to quinidine, but toxicity makes it less desirable for long-term use
Disopyramide	PO	Widens QRS, prolongs QT	Ventricular dysrhythmias
Class IB			
Lidocaine	IV	No significant change	Ventricular dysrhythmias
Mexiletine	PO	No significant change	Ventricular dysrhythmias
Tocainide	PO	No significant change	Life-threatening ventricular dysrhythmias
Phenytoin	PO	No significant change	Digoxin-induced ventricular dysrhythmias
Class IC			
Flecainide	PO	Widens QRS, prolongs PR	Life-threatening ventricular dysrhythmias
Propafenone	PO	Widens QRS, prolongs PR	Life-threatening ventricular dysrhythmias
Other Class I			
Moricizine	PO	Widens QRS, prolongs PR	Life-threatening ventricular dysrhythmias
Class II			
Propranolol	PO	Prolongs PR, bradycardia	Dysrhythmias caused by excessive sympathetic activity; control of ventricular rate in patients with supraventricular tachydysrhythmias
Acebutolol	PO	Prolongs PR, bradycardia	Premature ventricular beats
Esmolol	IV	Prolongs PR, bradycardia	Control of ventricular rate in patients with supraventricular tachydysrhythmias
Class III			
Amiodarone	PO	Widens QRS, prolongs PR and QT	Life-threatening ventricular dysrhythmias
Bretylium	IV	Prolongs QT	Life-threatening ventricular dysrhythmias
Sotalol	IV	Prolongs PR and QT	Life-threatening ventricular dysrhythmias
Class IV			
Verapamil	PO	Prolongs PR	Control of ventricular rate in patients with supraventricular tachydysrhythmias
Others			
Adenosine	IV	Prolongs PR	Termination of paroxysmal supraventricular tachycardia
Digoxin	PO	Prolongs PR, depresses ST	Control of ventricular rate in patients with supraventricular tachydysrhythmias

quinidine has antimalarial and antipyretic properties.

Effects on the Heart. By blocking sodium channels, quinidine *slows impulse conduction* in the atria, ventricles, and His-Purkinje system. In addition, the drug *delays repolarization* at these sites. Both actions contribute to suppression of dysrhythmias.

Quinidine is strongly *anticholinergic* (atropine-like) and blocks vagal input to the heart. The resultant *increase* in S-A nodal automaticity and A-V conduction can drive the ventricles at an excessive rate. To prevent excessive ventricular stimulation, patients are usually pretreated with digoxin, verapamil, or a beta blocker, all of which suppress A-V conduction.

Effects on the EKG. Quinidine has two pronounced effects on the EKG. The drug *widens the QRS complex* (by slowing depolarization of the ventricles) and *prolongs the QT interval* (by delaying ventricular repolarization).

Therapeutic Uses. Quinidine is a *broad spectrum* drug that is active against *supraventricular and ventricular dysrhythmias*. The drug's principal indication is long-term suppression of dysrhythmias, including supraventricular tachycardia, atrial flutter, atrial fibrillation, and sustained ventricular tachycardia. To prevent quinidine from increasing ventricular rate, patients are usually pretreated with an A-V nodal blocking agent (digoxin, verapamil, beta blocker). A recent analysis of older studies indicates that quinidine may actually *in-*

crease mortality in patients with *atrial flutter and atrial fibrillation*.

Pharmacokinetics. Quinidine is rapidly absorbed following oral administration. Peak responses to quinidine *sulfate* develop in 30 to 90 minutes; responses to quinidine *gluconate* develop more slowly, peaking after 3 to 4 hours. Elimination is by hepatic metabolism, and patients with liver dysfunction may require a reduction in dosage. Therapeutic plasma levels are 2 to 5 μg/ml.

Adverse Effects. *Diarrhea.* Diarrhea and other gastrointestinal symptoms develop in about 33% of patients. These reactions can be immediate and intense, and frequently force discontinuation of treatment. Gastric upset can be reduced by administering quinidine with food.

Cinchonism. Cinchonism is characterized by tinnitus (ringing in the ears), headache, nausea, vertigo, and disturbed vision. These symptoms can develop with just one quinidine dose.

Cardiotoxicity. At high concentrations, quinidine can cause severe cardiotoxicity (sinus arrest, A-V block, ventricular tachydysrhythmias, asystole). These reactions occur secondary to increased automaticity of Purkinje fibers and reduced conduction throughout all regions of the heart.

As cardiotoxicity develops, the EKG will change. Important danger signals are *widening of the QRS complex* (by 50% or more) and excessive *prolongation of the QT interval*. The physician should be notified immediately if these changes occur.

Arterial Embolism. Embolism is a potential complication of treating atrial fibrillation. During atrial fibrillation, thrombi may form in the atria. When sinus rhythm is restored, these thrombi may be dislodged and cause embolism. To reduce the risk of embolism, anticoagulants can be given for 1 to 2 weeks prior to quinidine. Signs of embolism (e.g., sudden chest pain, dyspnea) should be reported immediately.

Other Adverse Effects. Quinidine can cause alpha-adrenergic blockade, resulting in vasodilation and subsequent *hypotension*. This reaction is much more serious with intravenous therapy than with oral therapy. Rarely, quinidine has caused *hypersensitivity reactions*, including fever, anaphylactic reactions, and thrombocytopenia.

Drug Interactions. *Digoxin.* Quinidine can double digoxin levels. The increase is caused by displacing digoxin from plasma albumin and by decreasing digoxin elimination. When these drugs are used concurrently, digoxin dosage must be reduced. Also, patients should be monitored closely for digoxin toxicity (dysrhythmias). Because of its interaction with digoxin, quinidine is a last-choice drug for treating digoxin-induced dysrhythmias.

Other Interactions. Because of its anticholinergic actions, quinidine can intensify the effects of other *atropine-like drugs*; one possible result is excessive tachycardia. *Phenobarbital, phenytoin,* and *other drugs that induce hepatic drug metabolism* can shorten the half-life of quinidine by as much as 50%. Quinidine can intensify the effects of *warfarin* by a mechanism that is not known.

Preparations, Dosage, and Administration. *Preparations.* Quinidine is available as three salts: *quinidine sulfate, quinidine gluconate,* and *quinidine polygalacturonate*. Because these salts have different molecular weights, equal doses of these preparations (on a milligram basis) do not provide equal amounts of quinidine. A 200-mg dose of quinidine sulfate is equivalent to 275 mg of either quinidine gluconate or quinidine polygalacturonate. *Quinidine sulfate* [Quinora, Quinidex Extentabs] is dispensed in standard tablets (200 and 300 mg) and sustained-release tablets (300 mg). *Quinidine gluconate* [Quinalan, Quinaglute Dura-Tabs] is available in sustained-release tablets (324 mg) and as an injection (80 mg/ml). *Quinidine polygalacturonate* [Cardioquin] is available in 275-mg tablets.

Dosage. The usual dosage of *quinidine sulfate* is 200 to 400 mg every 4 to 6 hours. The usual dosage of *quinidine gluconate* is 324 to 648 mg every 8 to 12 hours. Dosage is adjusted to produce plasma quinidine levels between 2 and 5 μg/ml.

Administration. Quinidine is almost always administered by mouth. If time permits, a small test dose (200 mg PO or IM) should be given prior to the full therapeutic dose in order to assess for hypersensitivity. Intramuscular administration is painful and produces erratic absorption. Intravenous injection carries a great risk of adverse cardiovascular reactions; hence, continuous cardiovascular monitoring is required.

Procainamide

Procainamide [Pronestyl, Procan SR] is similar to quinidine in actions and applications. Like quinidine, procainamide is active against a broad spectrum of dysrhythmias. Unfortunately, serious side effects frequently limit the drug's use.

Effects on the Heart and EKG. Like quinidine, procainamide blocks cardiac sodium channels, thereby decreasing conduction velocity in the atria, ventricles, and His-Purkinje system. Also, the drug delays repolarization. In contrast to quinidine, procainamide is only weakly anticholinergic. Hence, procainamide is not likely to increase ventricular rate. Effects on the EKG are the same as those of quinidine: widening of the QRS complex and prolongation of the QT interval.

Therapeutic Uses. Procainamide is effective against a broad spectrum of atrial and ventricular dysrhythmias. Like quinidine, the drug can be used for long-term suppression. However, since prolonged therapy is often associated with serious adverse effects (see below), procainamide is less desirable than quinidine for long-term use. In contrast to quinidine, procainamide can be used to *terminate* ventricular tachycardia and ventricular fibrillation.

Pharmacokinetics. Routes are oral, IV, and IM. Peak plasma levels develop 1 hour after oral administration. Procainamide has a short half-life and requires more frequent dosing than quinidine.

Elimination is by hepatic metabolism and renal excretion. The major metabolite—N-acetylprocainamide (NAPA)—has antidysrhythmic properties of its own. NAPA is excreted by the kidneys and can accumulate to toxic levels in patients with renal dysfunction.

Adverse Effects. *Systemic Lupus Erythematosus–like Syndrome.* Prolonged treatment with procainamide is associated with severe immunologic reactions. Within a year, about 70% of patients develop antinuclear antibodies (ANA)—antibodies directed against the patient's own nucleic acids. If procainamide is continued, between 20% and 30% of patients with ANA will go on to develop symptoms resembling those of systemic lupus erythematosus (SLE). These symptoms include pain and inflammation of the joints, pericarditis, fever, and hepatomegaly. When procainamide is withdrawn, symptoms usually slowly subside. If the patient has a life-threatening dysrhythmia for which no alternative drug is available, procainamide can be continued and the symptoms of SLE can be controlled with a nonsteroidal anti-inflammatory agent (e.g., aspirin) or a glucocorticoid. All patients taking procainamide chronically should be tested for ANA. If the ANA titer rises, discontinuation of treatment should be considered.

Blood Dyscrasias. About 0.5% of patients develop blood dyscrasias, including *neutropenia, thrombocytopenia,* and *agranulocytosis.* Fatalities have occurred. These reactions usually develop during the first 12 weeks of treatment. Complete blood counts should be obtained weekly during this time and periodically thereafter. Also, complete blood counts should be obtained promptly at the first sign of infection, bruising, or bleeding. If blood counts indicate bone marrow suppression, procainamide should be withdrawn. Hematologic status usually returns to baseline within 1 month.

Cardiotoxicity. Procainamide has cardiotoxic actions like those of quinidine. Danger signs are QRS widening (>50%) and excessive prolongation of the QT interval. If these develop, the drug should be withheld and the physician informed.

Other Adverse Effects. Like quinidine, procainamide can cause *gastrointestinal symptoms* and *hypotension.* However, these are much less prominent than with quinidine. Procainamide is a derivative of procaine (a local anesthetic) and patients with a history of *procaine allergy* are at high risk of having an allergic response to procainamide. As with quinidine, *arterial embolism* may occur during treatment of atrial fibrillation.

Preparations, Dosage, and Administration. Oral. Procainamide [Pronestyl, Procan SR] is available in tablets and capsules (250, 375, and 500 mg) and sustained-release tablets (250, 500, 750, and 1000 mg). The usual maintenance dosage is 50 mg/kg/day in divided doses. Standard tablets and capsules are administered every 3 to 4 hours and sustained-release tablets every 6 hours. Dosage is adjusted to maintain plasma drug levels between 4 and 10 µg/ml.

Parenteral. Procainamide injection (100 and 500 mg/ml) is available for IM and IV administration. Intramuscular injection is made deep into the gluteal muscle; dosage is 0.5 to 1.0 gm repeated every 4 to 8 hours.

Intravenous infusion may be performed at an initial rate of 20 mg/min (maximal loading dose is 500 to 600 mg). After the loading period, an infusion rate of 2 to 6 mg/min should be employed. Once the dysrhythmia has been controlled, the patient should be switched to oral procainamide. Three hours should elapse between terminating the infusion and the first oral dose.

Disopyramide

Disopyramide is a Class I drug with actions like those of quinidine. However, because of prominent side effects, indications for disopyramide are limited.

Effects on the Heart and EKG. Cardiac effects are similar to those of quinidine. By blocking sodium channels, disopyramide decreases conduction velocity in the atria, ventricles, and His-Purkinje system. In addition, the drug delays repolarization. Anticholinergic actions are greater than those of quinidine. In contrast to quinidine, disopyramide causes a pronounced *reduction in contractility.* Like quinidine, disopyramide causes widening of the QRS complex and prolongation of the Q-T interval.

Adverse Effects. *Anticholinergic responses* are most common. These include dry mouth, blurred vision, constipation, and urinary hesitancy or retention. Urinary retention frequently requires discontinuation of treatment.

Because of its negative inotropic effects, disopyramide can cause *severe hypotension* (secondary to reduced cardiac output) and can *exacerbate congestive heart failure* (CHF). The drug should not be administered to patients with CHF or to patients taking beta blockers. Whenever disopyramide is used, pressor drugs should be immediately available.

Therapeutic Uses. Disopyramide is indicated only for ventricular dysrhythmias (VPBs, ventricular tachycardia, ventricular fibrillation). The drug is reserved for patients who cannot tolerate safer medications (e.g., quinidine, procainamide).

Preparations, Dosage, and Administration. Disopyramide [Norpace] is available in standard and extended-release capsules (100 and 150 mg). An initial loading dose (200 to 300 mg) is followed by maintenance doses (100 to 200 mg) every 6 hours.

CLASS IB AGENTS

As a group, Class IB agents differ from quinidine and the other Class IA agents in two respects: (1) whereas Class IA agents *delay* repolarization, Class IB agents *accelerate* repolarization, and (2) Class IB agents have little or no effect on the EKG.

Lidocaine

Lidocaine [Xylocaine], an intravenous agent, is used only against ventricular dysrhythmias. In addition to its antidysrhythmic applications, lidocaine is employed as a local anesthetic (see Chapter 31).

Effects on the Heart and EKG. Lidocaine has three significant effects on the heart. (1) Like other Class I drugs, lidocaine blocks cardiac sodium channels and thereby *slows conduction* in the atria, ventricles, and His-Purkinje system. (2) The drug *reduces automaticity* in the ventricles and His-Purkinje system by a mechanism that is not understood. (3) Lidocaine *accelerates repolarization* (shortens action potential duration and the ERP). In contrast to quinidine and procainamide, lidocaine is devoid of anticholinergic properties. Also, lidocaine has no significant impact on the EKG: a small reduction in the QT interval may occur, but there is no widening of the QRS complex.

Pharmacokinetics. Lidocaine undergoes rapid metabolism by the liver. If the drug were administered orally, most of each dose would be inactivated on its first pass through the liver. For this reason, administration is by intravenous infusion.

Because lidocaine is rapidly degraded, plasma drug levels can be easily controlled: if drug levels climb too high, the infusion can be slowed and the liver will quickly remove excess drug from the circulation. The therapeutic range for lidocaine is 1.5 to 5 µg/ml.

Antidysrhythmic Use. Antidysrhythmic use of lidocaine is limited to short-term therapy of *ventricular* dysrhythmias. Because its levels can be easily controlled, lidocaine is the drug of choice for several ventricular dysrhythmias, including those associated with myocardial infarction, cardiac surgery, and digoxin toxicity. Lidocaine is not active against supraventricular dysrhythmias.

Adverse Effects. Lidocaine is generally well tolerated. However, adverse central nervous system (CNS) effects can occur. High therapeutic doses can cause *drowsiness, confusion,* and *paresthesias.* Toxic doses may produce *convulsions* and *respiratory arrest.* Consequently, whenever lidocaine is used, equipment for resuscitation must be available. Convulsions can be managed with diazepam or phenytoin.

Preparations, Dosage, and Administration. Administration is parenteral only. The usual route is intravenous. Intramuscular injection can be used in emergencies. Blood pressure and the EKG should be monitored for signs of toxicity.

Intravenous. Lidocaine [Xylocaine] preparations intended for intravenous administration are clearly labeled as such. These contain no preservatives or catecholamines. (Lidocaine used for local anesthesia frequently contains epinephrine.) *Preparations that contain epinephrine or another catecholamine must never be administered intravenously, since doing so can cause severe hypertension and life-threatening dysrhythmias.*

Intravenous therapy is initiated with a loading dose followed by continuous infusion for maintenance. The usual loading dose is 50 to 100 mg (1 mg/kg) administered at a rate of 25 to 50 mg/min. An infusion rate of 1 to 4 mg/min is used for maintenance; the rate is adjusted on the basis of cardiac response. Intravenous lidocaine should be discontinued as soon as is possible, usually within 24 hours. Lidocaine for IV administration is dispensed in concentrated and dilute formulations. The concentrated forms must be diluted with 5% dextrose in water.

To avoid toxicity, the dosage should be reduced in patients with impaired hepatic function or impaired hepatic blood flow (e.g., elderly patients, patients with cirrhosis, shock, or CHF).

Intramuscular. Lidocaine is dispensed in an automatic injection device [Lido-Pen Auto-Injector] for IM administration. A dose of 300 mg is injected into the deltoid muscle. This dose can be repeated in 60 to 90 minutes if necessary. The patient should be switched to IV lidocaine as soon as is possible.

Phenytoin

Phenytoin [Dilantin] is an antiseizure drug that is also used to treat digoxin-induced dysrhythmias. The basic pharmacology of phenytoin is presented in Chapter 22 (Drugs for Epilepsy). Discussion here is limited to antidysrhythmic applications.

Effects on the Heart and EKG. Like lidocaine, phenytoin reduces automaticity (especially in the ventricles), and has little or no effect on the EKG. In contrast to lidocaine (and practically all other antidysrhythmic agents), phenytoin *increases* A-V nodal conduction.

Pharmacokinetics. Phenytoin has two unfortunate kinetic properties. First, metabolism of the drug is subject to wide interpatient variation. Second, doses only slightly greater than therapeutic are likely to cause toxicity. Because of these characteristics, maintenance of therapeutic plasma levels (5 to 20 µg/ml) is difficult.

Adverse Effects and Interactions. The most common adverse reactions are *sedation, ataxia,* and *nystagmus.* With too rapid intravenous administration, phenytoin can cause *hypotension, dysrhythmias,* and *cardiac arrest. Gingival hyperplasia* is a frequent complication of long-term treatment. Phenytoin is subject to a large number of undesirable drug interactions (see Chapter 22).

Antidysrhythmic Applications. Phenytoin is a second-choice drug after lidocaine for treating digoxin-induced dysrhythmias. The ability of phenytoin to increase A-V nodal conduction can help counteract the reduction in A-V conduction caused by digoxin intoxication. Phenytoin should not be used to treat atrial fibrillation or atrial flutter, since enhanced A-V conduction could increase the number of atrial impulses reaching the ventricles, thereby driving the ventricles at an excessive rate.

Dosage and Administration. Phenytoin [Dilantin] is administered orally and intravenously. For oral therapy, a loading dose (14 mg/kg) is followed by daily maintenance doses (200 to 400 mg).

Intravenous administration is reserved for severe, acute dysrhythmias. Blood pressure and the EKG must be monitored continuously. Phenytoin is not soluble in water and must be diluted in the medium supplied by the manufacturer. This medium is highly alkaline (pH 12) and will cause phlebitis if given by continuous infusion. Consequently, administration is by intermittent injections. Intravenous injections must be performed slowly (50 mg/min or less), since rapid injection can cause cardiovascular collapse. Treatment is begun with a series of loading doses (50 to 100 mg every 5 minutes until the dysrhythmia has been controlled or until toxicity appears). Maintenance dosages range from 200 to 400 mg/day.

Mexiletine

Mexiletine [Mexitil] is an oral congener of lidocaine used to treat symptomatic ventricular dysrhythmias. Principal indications are VPBs and sustained ventricular tachycardia. Like lidocaine, mexiletine does not alter the EKG. The drug is eliminated by hepatic metabolism; hence, effects may be prolonged in patients with liver disease or reduced hepatic blood flow. The most common adverse effects are gastrointestinal disturbances (nausea, vomiting, diarrhea, constipation) and neurologic disorders (tremor, dizziness, sleep disturbances, psychosis, convulsions). About 40% of patients find these intolerable. The initial dosage is 100 to 200 mg every 8 hours. The maintenance dosage is 100 to 300 mg every 6 to 12 hours. All doses should be taken with food.

Tocainide

Like mexiletine, tocainide [Tonocard] is an oral analogue of lidocaine used to treat ventricular dysrhythmias. Effects on the EKG are minimal. Elimination is by hepatic metabolism and renal excretion. As with mexiletine, the most common side effects are gastrointestinal disturbances (especially nausea) and neurologic disorders (especially tremor). In addition, tocainide can cause serious blood dyscrasias, including a 2% incidence of agranulocytosis; hence, blood counts should be monitored. The drug can also cause pulmonary fibrosis and pneumonitis. Because of its serious adverse effects, tocainide should be reserved for patients with severe ventricular dysrhythmias that have not responded to safer drugs. The initial dosage is 200 to 400 mg every 8 hours. The maintenance dosage is 200 to 600 mg every 8 hours.

CLASS IC AGENTS

Class IC antidysrhythmics block cardiac sodium channels and thereby reduce conduction velocity in the atria, ventricles, and His-Purkinje system. In addition, these drugs delay ventricular repolarization, causing a small increase in the effective refractory period. All Class IC agents can exacerbate existing dysrhythmias and create new ones. Currently, only two Class IC agents are available: flecainide and propafenone. A third agent—encainide [Enkaid]—was voluntarily withdrawn from the market.

Flecainide

Flecainide [Tambocor] is employed for oral therapy of severe ventricular dysrhythmias. Like other Class IC agents, the drug decreases cardiac conduction and increases the effective refractory period. Prominent effects on the EKG are prolongation of the PR interval and widening of the QRS complex. Excessive QRS widening indicates a need for dosage reduction. Flecainide has prodysrhythmic effects. As a result, the drug can intensify existing dysrhythmias and can provoke new ones. In patients with asymptomatic ventricular tachycardia associated with acute myocardial infarction, flecainide caused a twofold *increase* in mortality. Flecainide decreases myocardial contractility and can thereby exacerbate or precipitate heart failure. Accordingly, the drug should not be combined with others that can decrease contractile force (e.g., beta blockers, verapamil). Elimination is by hepatic metabolism and renal excretion. Dosage is low initially (100 mg every 12 hours) and then gradually increased to a maximum of 400 mg/day. Because of its potential for serious side effects, flecainide should be reserved for severe ventricular dysrhythmias that have not responded to safer drugs. Patients should be monitored closely.

Propafenone

Propafenone [Rhythmol] is similar to flecainide in actions and uses. By blocking cardiac sodium channels, the drug decreases conduction velocity in the atria, ventricles, and His-Purkinje system. In addition, it causes a small increase in the ventricular effective refractory period. Prominent effects on the EKG are QRS widening and PR prolongation. Like flecainide, propafenone has prodysrhythmic actions that can exacerbate existing dysrhythmias and create new ones. It is not known if propafenone, like flecainide, increases mortality in patients with asymptomatic ventricular dysrhythmias following myocardial infarction. Propafenone has beta-adrenergic blocking properties and can thereby decrease myocardial contractility and promote bronchospasm. Accordingly, the drug should be used with caution in patients with congestive heart failure, A-V block, or asthma. Noncardiac adverse effects are generally mild and include dizziness, altered taste, blurred vision, and gastrointestinal symptoms (abdominal discomfort, anorexia, nausea, vomiting). Because of its prodysrhythmic actions, propafenone should be reserved for patients with life-threatening ventricular dysrhythmias that have not responded to safer drugs. Propafenone is dispensed in tablets (150 and 300 mg) for oral use. The dosage is 150 mg every 8 hours initially, and can be gradually increased to 300 mg every 8 hours.

OTHER CLASS I: MORICIZINE

Moricizine [Ethmozine] is a Class I antidysrhythmic drug approved for oral therapy of life-threatening ventricular dysrhythmias. This agent shares properties with other Class I drugs but doesn't quite fit any of the existing subclasses (IA, IB, and IC). Like other Class I agents, moricizine blocks cardiac sodium channels and thereby decreases conduction velocity in the atria, ventricles, and His-Purkinje system. Prominent effects on the EKG are QRS widening and PR prolongation. The most common adverse effects are dizziness, nausea, and headache. Like other antidysrhythmic drugs, moricizine is prodysrhythmic. In addition, moricizine can cause bradycardia, heart block, and congestive failure. Interactions with digoxin, diuretics, beta blockers, calcium channel blockers, angiotensin-converting enzyme inhibitors, and warfarin have not been reported. Because of its potential for adverse cardiac effects, moricizine should be reserved for life-threatening ventricular dysrhythmias that have not responded to safer drugs. The dosage is 200 mg every 8 hours initially, and may be gradually increased to a maximum of 300 mg every 8 hours.

CLASS II: BETA BLOCKERS

Class II consists of beta-adrenergic blocking agents. At this time only three beta blockers—propranolol, acebutolol, and esmolol—are approved for treating dysrhythmias. The basic pharmacology of these drugs is discussed in Chapter 18. Discussion here is limited to treatment of dysrhythmias.

Propranolol

Propranolol [Inderal] is considered a nonselective beta-adrenergic antagonist, since it blocks both beta$_1$- and beta$_2$-adrenergic receptors. As discussed in Chapter 18, beta$_1$ blockade affects the heart, and beta$_2$ blockade affects the bronchi.

Effects on the Heart and EKG. Blockade of cardiac beta$_1$ receptors attenuates sympathetic stimulation of the heart. The result is (1) decreased automaticity of the S-A node, (2) decreased conduction velocity through the A-V node, and (3) decreased myocardial contractility. The reduction in A-V conduction velocity translates to a prolonged P-R interval on the EKG.

It is worth noting that cardiac beta$_1$ receptors are functionally coupled to calcium channels, and that beta$_1$ blockade causes these channels to close. Hence, the effects of beta blockers on heart rate, A-V conduction, and contractility all result from decreased calcium influx. Because beta blockers and verapamil (a calcium channel blocker) both decrease calcium entry, the effects of these drugs on the heart are very similar.

Therapeutic Use. Propranolol is especially useful for treating dysrhythmias caused by excessive sympathetic stimulation of the heart. Among these dysrhythmias are sinus tachycardia, severe recurrent ventricular tachycardia, exercise-induced tachydysrhythmias, and paroxysmal atrial tachycardia provoked by emotion or exercise. In patients with supraventricular tachydysrhythmias, propranolol has two beneficial effects: (1) suppression of excessive discharge of the S-A node, and (2) slowing of ventricular rate by decreasing transmission of atrial impulses through the A-V node.

Adverse Effects. Beta blockers are generally well tolerated. Principal adverse effects concern the heart and bronchi. By blocking cardiac beta$_1$ receptors, propranolol can cause *congestive heart failure, A-V block*, and *sinus arrest. Hypotension* can occur secondary to reduced cardiac output. In patients with asthma, blockade of beta$_2$ receptors in the lung can cause *bronchospasm*. Because of its cardiac and pulmonary effects, propranolol is contraindicated for patients with asthma, sinus bradycardia, high-degree heart block, or congestive heart failure.

Dosage and Administration. Propranolol can be administered orally and, in life-threatening emergencies, by IV injection. Dosages with either route show wide individual variation. Oral dosages range from 10 to 80 mg every 6 to 8 hours. The usual intravenous dose is 1 to 3 mg injected at a rate of 1 mg/min.

Acebutolol

Acebutolol [Sectral] is a cardioselective beta blocker approved for oral therapy of ventricular premature beats (VPBs). Adverse effects are like those of propranolol: bradycardia, congestive heart failure, heart block, and—despite cardioselectivity—bronchospasm. Accordingly, acebutolol is contraindicated for patients with congestive heart failure, severe bradycardia, A-V heart block, and asthma. Acebutolol can also cause adverse immunologic reactions; titers of antinuclear antibodies may rise, resulting in myalgia, arthralgia, and arthritis. For suppression of VPBs, the initial dosage is 200 mg twice daily. Usual maintenance dosages range from 600 to 1200 mg/day.

Esmolol

Esmolol [Brevibloc] is a cardioselective beta blocker with a very short half-life (9 minutes). Administration is by IV infusion. The drug is employed for immediate control of ventricular rate in patients with atrial flutter and atrial fibrillation. Use is short-term only (e.g., in patients with dysrhythmias associated with surgery). The most common adverse reaction is hypotension. However, like other beta blockers, esmolol can also cause bradycardia, heart block, congestive heart failure, and bronchospasm. In addition, pain can occur at the infusion site. Treatment is begun with a loading dose of 500 μg/kg infused over 1 minute. The usual maintenance infusion rate is 100 μg/kg/min.

CLASS III: DRUGS THAT DELAY REPOLARIZATION

Three Class III antidysrhythmics are available: bretylium, amiodarone, and sotalol. All three drugs delay repolarization of fast potentials. Hence, all three prolong the action potential duration and the effective refractory period and, by doing so, prolong the QT interval. In addition, each drug can affect the heart in other ways. Hence, these agents are not interchangeable.

Bretylium

Bretylium [Bretylol] is used only for short-term therapy of severe ventricular dysrhythmias. The drug's principal adverse effect is profound hypotension.

Effects on the Heart and EKG. Therapeutic effects result from blockade of potassium channels in Purkinje fibers and ventricular muscle (see Fig.

44–2A). By doing so, bretylium delays repolarization and thereby prolongs both the action potential duration and the effective refractory period. Because ventricular repolarization is delayed, the QT interval on the EKG is prolonged.

When first administered, bretylium is taken up by sympathetic neurons, where it causes a transient increase in catecholamine release followed by blockade of further release. In the heart, the initial increase in release can briefly exacerbate dysrhythmias. In blood vessels, the extended blockade of release produces hypotension.

Adverse Effects. Profound and persistent *hypotension* is the most troubling side effect of therapy. This reaction is common, occurring in up to 66% of those treated. Blood pressure may fall in subjects who are supine as well as standing. Hypotension results from blockade of norepinephrine release in sympathetic neurons that promote contraction of vascular smooth muscle. Patients should undergo continuous monitoring of blood pressure. If hypotension develops, blood pressure may be raised with dopamine or norepinephrine.

Therapeutic Use. Bretylium is indicated for short-term therapy of ventricular fibrillation and recurrent ventricular tachycardia in patients who have been refractory to more conventional therapy (cardioversion, lidocaine). For these patients, bretylium may be life-saving.

Preparations, Dosage, and Administration. Bretylium tosylate [Bretylol] is dispensed in solution (50 mg/ml). The drug must be diluted for certain applications. In all cases, the EKG and blood pressure should be monitored continuously.

Intravenous. For nonemergency treatment, bretylium is administered by slow IV infusion. Rapid injection is reserved for emergencies. To manage ventricular fibrillation, the following protocol may be employed: (1) rapid IV injection of a 5 mg/kg dose, (2) rapid IV injection of additional doses (10 mg/kg) until the dysrhythmia has been controlled, and (3) slow IV infusion of maintenance doses (5 to 10 mg/kg) every 6 hours. (Maintenance doses are infused slowly because rapid administration results in nausea and vomiting. Initial doses are injected rapidly, despite the risk of nausea and vomiting, because of the need for rapid rhythm control.)

Intramuscular. Bretylium is used undiluted for IM injection. The initial dose is 5 to 10 mg/kg. Dosing may be repeated every 6 to 8 hours. Injection sites should be rotated.

Amiodarone

Amiodarone [Cordarone] is a Class III antidysrhythmic drug that has complex effects on the heart. Serious side effects are common, and may persist for months after therapy has stopped. In the United States, the drug is approved only for oral therapy of life-threatening ventricular dysrhythmias. Because of its severe toxicity, amiodarone is considered a drug of last resort. Patients must be followed closely.

Effects on the Heart and EKG. Amiodarone has complex effects on the heart. Like bretylium, amiodarone delays repolarization, and thereby prolongs the action potential duration and the ERP. The underlying cause of these effects may be blockade of potassium channels. Additional cardiac effects include reduced automaticity in the S-A node, reduced contractility, and reduced conduction velocity in the A-V node, ventricles, and His-Purkinje system. These effects occur secondary to blockade of sodium channels, calcium channels, and beta receptors. Prominent effects on the EKG are QRS widening and prolongation of the PR and QT intervals. Amiodarone also acts on coronary and peripheral blood vessels to promote dilation.

Pharmacokinetics. Amiodarone is highly lipid soluble and accumulates in many tissues, especially the liver and lungs. Elimination is by hepatic metabolism and excretion in the bile. Amiodarone has an extremely long half-life, ranging from 25 to 110 days. Because of its slow elimination, amiodarone continues to act long after administration has ceased.

Adverse Effects. Amiodarone produces many serious adverse effects. Since the drug's half-life is protracted, toxicity can continue for weeks or months after drug withdrawal.

Pulmonary Toxicity. Pulmonary toxicity (pneumonitis, alveolitis, pulmonary fibrosis) is the most serious adverse effect. Symptoms (dyspnea, cough, chest pain) resemble those of congestive heart failure and pneumonia. Pulmonary toxicity develops in 2% to 17% of those treated and carries a 10% risk of mortality. Patients at highest risk are those receiving long-term, high-dose therapy. A baseline chest x-ray and pulmonary function test are required. Pulmonary function should be monitored throughout treatment.

Cardiotoxicity. Amiodarone may cause a paradoxical *increase* in dysrhythmic activity. In addition, by suppressing the S-A and A-V nodes, the drug can cause sinus bradycardia and A-V heart block. By reducing contractility, amiodarone can precipitate congestive heart failure.

Other Adverse Effects. Virtually all patients develop *corneal microdeposits*, which may cause photophobia or blurred vision. Between 2% and 5% of patients experience *blue-gray discoloration of the skin*. *Gastrointestinal reactions* (anorexia, nausea, vomiting) are common. Possible *CNS reactions* include ataxia, dizziness, tremor, mood alteration, and hallucinations. *Hepatitis* and *thyroid dysfunction* (hypothyroidism, hyperthyroidism) have occurred; hence, all patients should undergo periodic liver and thyroid tests.

Therapeutic Use. Although amiodarone is very effective, toxicity limits its use. In the United States the drug is approved only for long-term therapy of two life-threatening ventricular dysrhythmias: recurrent ventricular fibrillation and recurrent hemodynamically unstable ventricular tachycardia. Treatment should be reserved for patients who have not responded to safer drugs. Outside the United States amiodarone is also used to treat atrial dysrhythmias.

Drug Interactions. Amiodarone can increase plasma levels of several drugs, including quinidine, procainamide, phenytoin, digoxin, diltiazem, and warfarin. Dosages of these agents may require reduction.

Preparations, Dosage, and Administration. Amiodarone [Cordarone] is available in 200-mg tablets for oral use. Treatment should be initiated in a hospital setting. The following schedule is used for loading: 800 to 1600 mg daily for 1 to 3 weeks followed by 600 to 800 mg daily for 4 weeks. The daily maintenance dosage is 100 to 400 mg.

Sotalol

Actions and Uses. Sotalol [Betapace] is a beta blocker that also delays repolarization. Hence, the drug has combined Class II and Class III properties. Prodysrhythmic properties are pronounced. Sotalol is approved only for ventricular dysrhythmias, such as sustained ventricular tachycardia, that are considered life-threatening. The drug is *not* approved for hypertension or angina pectoris (the primary indications for other beta-adrenergic blockers).

Pharmacokinetics. Sotalol is administered orally and undergoes nearly complete absorption. The drug is excreted unchanged in the urine. Its half-life is 12 hours.

Adverse Effects. The major adverse effect is *torsades de pointes*, a serious dysrhythmia that develops in about 5% of patients. The risk of this dysrhythmia is increased by hypokalemia and by other drugs that prolong the QT interval.

At therapeutic doses, sotalol produces substantial beta blockade. Hence, the drug can cause *bradycardia*, *A-V block*, *congestive heart failure*, and *bronchospasm*. Accordingly, the usual contraindications to beta blockers apply.

Preparations, Dosage, and Administration. Sotalol is dispensed in tablets (80, 160, and 240 mg) for oral use. Treatment should start in a hospital. The initial dosage is 80 mg twice daily. The usual maintenance dosage is 160 to 320 mg/day in two or three divided doses. The dosing interval should be increased in patients with renal impairment.

CLASS IV: CALCIUM CHANNEL BLOCKERS

Verapamil

Verapamil [Calan, Isoptin, Verelan] is a calcium channel blocking agent used to treat supraventricular dysrhythmias. This drug is the only calcium channel blocker currently approved for antidysrhythmic use. The basic pharmacology of verapamil is discussed in Chapter 38. Consideration here is limited to treatment of dysrhythmias.

Effects on the Heart and EKG. Blockade of cardiac calcium channels has three effects: (1) reduction of S-A nodal automaticity, (2) delay of A-V nodal conduction, and (3) reduction of myocardial contractility. Note that these effects are identical to those of the beta blockers (which makes sense in that beta blockers promote cardiac calcium channel closure). The principal effect of verapamil on the EKG is prolongation of the PR interval, reflecting suppression of A-V conduction.

Therapeutic Uses. Verapamil has two antidysrhythmic uses. First, the drug can slow ventricular rate in patients with atrial fibrillation or atrial flutter. Second, verapamil can terminate supraventricular tachycardia caused by an A-V nodal reentrant circuit. In both cases, benefits derive from suppressing A-V nodal conduction. With intravenous administration, effects can be seen in 2 to 3 minutes. Verapamil is not active against ventricular dysrhythmias.

Adverse Effects. Although generally safe, verapamil *can* cause undesired effects. Blockade of cardiac calcium channels can cause *bradycardia*, *A-V block*, and *congestive heart failure*. Blockade of calcium channels in vascular smooth muscle can cause vasodilation, resulting in *hypotension* and *edema*. Blockade of calcium channels in intestinal smooth muscle can produce *constipation*.

Drug Interactions. Like verapamil, *digoxin* decreases A-V conduction, thereby increasing the risk of A-V block. Also, verapamil delays elimination of digoxin, and can thereby cause digoxin accumulation.

Since verapamil and the *beta blockers* have nearly identical suppressant effects on the heart, the combination of these agents presents a risk of bradycardia, heart block, and congestive heart failure.

Preparations, Dosage, and Administration. Administration may be intravenous or oral. Intravenous therapy is preferred for initial treatment. Oral therapy is used for maintenance.

Intravenous. Verapamil is dispensed in solution (5 mg/2 ml) for IV use. The initial dose is 5 to 10 mg injected slowly (over 2 to 3 minutes). If the dysrhythmia persists, an additional 10 mg may be administered in 30 minutes. An IV infusion (0.375 mg/min) can be used for maintenance. Intravenous verapamil can cause serious adverse cardiovascular effects. Accordingly, blood pressure and the EKG should be monitored, and equipment for resuscitation should be immediately available.

Oral. Verapamil is available in standard and sustained-release tablets for oral use. The maintenance dosage is 40 to 120 mg three or four times a day.

OTHER ANTIDYSRHYTHMIC DRUGS

Digoxin

Although its primary indication is heart failure, digoxin [Lanoxin] is also used to treat supraventricular dysrhythmias. The basic pharmacology of digoxin is discussed in Chapter 42. Consideration here is limited to treatment of dysrhythmias.

Effects on the Heart. Digoxin suppresses dysrhythmias by decreasing conduction through the A-V node and by decreasing automaticity in the S-A node. The drug decreases A-V conduction by (1) a direct depressant effect on the A-V node, and (2) acting in the CNS to increase vagal (parasympathetic) impulses to the A-V node. Digoxin decreases automaticity of the S-A node by increasing vagal traffic to the node and by decreasing sympathetic traffic. It should be noted that although digoxin decreases automaticity in the S-A node, this drug can *increase* automaticity in *Purkinje fibers*. The latter effect contributes to the dysrhythmias that are *caused* by digoxin.

Effects on the EKG. By slowing A-V conduction, digoxin prolongs the PR interval. The QT interval may be shortened, reflecting accelerated repolarization of the ventricles. Depression of the S-T segment is common. The T wave may be depressed or even inverted. There is little or no change in the QRS complex.

Adverse Effects and Interactions. The major adverse effect is *cardiotoxicity (dysrhythmias)*. The risk of dysrhythmias is increased by hypokalemia, which can result from concurrent therapy with diuretics (thiazides and high-ceiling agents). Accord-

ingly, it is essential that potassium levels be kept within the normal range (3.5 to 5 mEq/L). The most common adverse effects are gastrointestinal disturbances (anorexia, nausea, vomiting, abdominal discomfort). CNS responses (fatigue, visual disturbances) are also relatively common.

Antidysrhythmic Uses. Digoxin is used only for supraventricular dysrhythmias. The drug is inactive against ventricular dysrhythmias.

Atrial Fibrillation and Atrial Flutter. Digoxin is used to slow ventricular rate in patients with atrial fibrillation and atrial flutter. Ventricular rate is decreased by reducing the number of atrial impulses that pass through the A-V node. It should be noted that although atrial fibrillation and flutter respond to digoxin and other drugs, cardioversion is the treatment of choice.

Supraventricular Tachycardia. Digoxin may be employed acutely and chronically to treat supraventricular tachycardia (SVT). Acute therapy is used to abolish the dysrhythmia. Chronic therapy is used to prevent its return. Digoxin suppresses SVT by increasing cardiac vagal tone and by decreasing sympathetic tone.

Dosage and Administration. Oral therapy is generally preferred. The initial dosage is 1 to 1.5 mg administered in three or four doses over 24 hours. The maintenance dosage is 0.125 to 0.5 mg/day.

Adenosine

Adenosine [Adenocard] is an expensive, intravenous drug used to terminate paroxysmal supraventricular tachycardia. Adverse effects are minimal because the drug is rapidly cleared from the blood.

Effects on the Heart and EKG. Adenosine decreases automaticity in the S-A node and greatly slows conduction through the A-V node. The most prominent EKG change is prolongation of the PR interval, which occurs because of delayed A-V conduction.

Therapeutic Use. Adenosine is approved only for termination of *paroxysmal supraventricular tachycardia*, including Wolff-Parkinson-White syndrome. The drug is not active against atrial fibrillation, atrial flutter, or ventricular dysrhythmias.

Pharmacokinetics. Adenosine has an extremely short plasma half-life (several seconds) owing to rapid uptake by cells and deactivation by circulating adenosine deaminase. Because of its rapid clearance from the blood, adenosine must be administered by IV bolus, as close to the heart as possible.

Adverse Effects. Adverse effects are short-lived, lasting for less than 1 minute. The most common effects are *sinus bradycardia*, *dyspnea* (from bronchoconstriction), *hypotension* and *facial flushing* (from vasodilation), and *chest discomfort* (perhaps from stimulation of pain receptors in the heart).

Drug Interactions. *Methylxanthines* (aminophylline, caffeine) block receptors for adenosine. Hence, asthma patients taking aminophylline or theophylline need larger doses of adenosine, and even then adenosine may not work.

Preparations, Dosage, and Administration. Adenosine [Adenocard] is dispensed in solution (6 mg/2 ml vial) for bolus IV administration. The injection should be made as close to the heart as possible, and should be followed by a saline flush. The initial dose is 6 mg. If there is no response in 1 or 2 minutes, 12 mg may be tried and repeated once. If a response is going to occur, it should happen as soon as the drug reaches the A-V node.

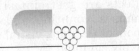

Summary of Major Nursing Implications

Summaries are limited to the major antidysrhythmic drugs. Summaries for beta blockers, calcium channel blockers, phenytoin, and digoxin appear in other chapters.

QUINIDINE

 Preadministration Assessment

Therapeutic Goal

The usual goal is long-term suppression of atrial and ventricular dysrhythmias.

Baseline Data

Obtain a baseline EKG and laboratory evaluation of liver function. Determine blood pressure.

Identifying High-Risk Patients

Quinidine is *contraindicated* for patients with a *history of hypersensitivity to quinidine or other cinchona alkaloids* and for patients with *complete heart block, digoxin intoxication,* or *conduction disturbances associated with marked QRS widening and QT prolongation.* Exercise *caution* in patients with *partial A-V block, congestive heart failure, hypotensive states,* and *hepatic dysfunction.*

 Implementation: Administration

Routes

Usual route: oral.
Rare routes: IM and IV.

Administration

Before giving full therapeutic doses, assess for hypersensitivity by giving a small test dose (200 mg PO or IM).

Advise patients to take quinidine with meals. Warn patients not to crush or chew sustained-release formulations.

Dosing must account for the particular quinidine salt being used: 200 mg of quinidine *sulfate* is equivalent to 275 mg of quinidine *gluconate* or quinidine *polygalacturonate.*

 Ongoing Evaluation and Interventions

Evaluating Therapeutic Effects

Monitor for beneficial changes in the EKG. Plasma drug levels should be kept between 2 and 5 µg/ml.

Minimizing Adverse Effects

Diarrhea. Diarrhea and other gastrointestinal disturbances occur in one third of patients and frequently force drug withdrawal. These effects can be reduced by administering quinidine with meals.

Cinchonism. Inform patients about symptoms of cinchonism (tinnitus, headache, nausea, vertigo, disturbed vision) and instruct them to notify the physician if these develop.

Cardiotoxicity. Monitor the EKG for signs of cardiotoxicity, especially widening of QRS complex (by 50% or more) and excessive prolongation of the QT interval. Monitor pulses for significant changes in rate or regularity. If cardiotoxicity develops, withhold quinidine and notify the physician.

Arterial Embolism. Embolism may occur during therapy of atrial fibrillation. The risk can be reduced by pretreatment with anticoagulants. Observe for signs of thromboembolism (e.g., sudden chest pain, dyspnea) and report these immediately.

Minimizing Adverse Interactions

Digoxin. Quinidine can double digoxin levels. When these drugs are combined, digoxin dosage should be reduced. Monitor patients for digoxin toxicity (dysrhythmias).

PROCAINAMIDE

Preadministration Assessment

Therapeutic Goal

Procainamide is indicated for acute and long-term management of ventricular and supraventricular dysrhythmias. Because of toxicity with long-term use, quinidine is preferred to procainamide for chronic suppression.

Baseline Data

Obtain a baseline EKG, complete blood counts, and laboratory evaluations of liver and kidney function. Determine blood pressure.

Identifying High-Risk Patients

Procainamide is *contraindicated* for patients with *systemic lupus erythematosus, complete A-V heart block,* and *second- or third-degree A-V block in the absence of an electronic pacemaker.* Exercise *caution* in patients with *hepatic or renal dysfunction* or a *history of procaine allergy.*

Implementation: Administration

Routes

Oral, IM, IV.

Administration

Instruct patients to administer procainamide at evenly spaced intervals around the clock. Warn patients not to crush or chew sustained-release preparations.

When switching from IV to oral therapy, allow 3 hours to elapse between stopping the infusion and giving the first oral dose.

Give IM injections deep into the gluteal muscle.

Ongoing Evaluation and Interventions

Evaluating Therapeutic Effects

Monitor the EKG for beneficial changes. Plasma drug levels should be kept between 3 and 10 μg/ml.

Minimizing Adverse Effects

Systemic Lupus Erythematosus–like Syndrome. Prolonged therapy can produce a syndrome resembling SLE. Inform patients about manifestations of SLE (joint pain and inflammation; hepatomegaly; unexplained fever; soreness of the mouth, throat, or gums) and instruct them to notify the physician if these develop. If SLE is diagnosed, procainamide should be discontinued. If discontinuation is impossible, signs and symptoms can be controlled with a nonsteroidal anti-inflammatory drug (e.g., aspirin) or with a glucocorticoid. The ANA titer should be measured periodically; if it rises, withdrawal of procainamide should be considered.

Blood Dyscrasias. Procainamide can cause *agranulocytosis, thrombocytopenia,* and *neutropenia.* Death has occurred. Obtain complete blood counts weekly during the first 3 months of treatment and periodically thereafter. Instruct patients to inform the physician at the first sign of infection (fever, chills, sore throat), bruising, or bleeding. If subsequent blood counts indicate hematologic disturbance, discontinue procainamide immediately.

Cardiotoxicity. Procainamide can cause dysrhythmias. Monitor pulses for changes in rate or regularity. Monitor the EKG for excessive QRS widening (greater than 50%) and for PR prolongation. If these occur, withhold procainamide and notify the physician.

Arterial Embolism. Embolism may occur during therapy of atrial fibrillation. The risk can be reduced by pretreatment with anticoagulants. Observe for signs of thromboembolism (e.g., sudden chest pain, dyspnea) and report these immediately.

LIDOCAINE

Preadministration Assessment

Therapeutic Goal

Management of ventricular dysrhythmias.

Baseline Data

Obtain a baseline EKG and determine blood pressure.

Identifying High-Risk Patients

Lidocaine is *contraindicated* for patients with *Stokes-Adams syndrome, Wolff-Parkinson-White syndrome,* and *severe degrees of S-A, A-V, or intraventricular block in the absence of electronic pacing.* Exercise *caution* in patients with *hepatic dysfunction or impaired hepatic blood flow.*

Implementation: Administration

Routes

Usual: IV.
Emergencies: IM.

Administration

Intravenous. Make certain the lidocaine preparation is labeled for IV use (i.e., is devoid of preservatives and catecholamines). Dilute concentrated preparations with 5% dextrose in water.

The initial dose is 50 to 100 mg (1 mg/kg) infused at a rate of 25 to 50 mg/

min. For maintenance, monitor the EKG and adjust the infusion rate on the basis of cardiac response. The usual rate is 1 to 4 mg/min.

Intramuscular. Reserve for emergencies. The usual dose is 300 mg injected into the deltoid muscle. Switch to IV lidocaine as soon as possible.

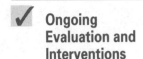

Ongoing Evaluation and Interventions

Evaluating Therapeutic Effects

Continuous EKG monitoring is required for evaluation. Plasma drug levels should be kept between 1.5 and 5 µg/ml.

Minimizing Adverse Effects

Excessive doses can cause convulsions and respiratory arrest. Equipment for resuscitation should be available. Convulsions can be managed with diazepam or phenytoin.

DRUGS SUMMARIZED IN OTHER CHAPTERS

PHENYTOIN. See Chapter 22.

PROPRANOLOL, ACEBUTOLOL, ESMOLOL. See Chapter 18.

VERAPAMIL. See Chapter 38.

DIGOXIN. See Chapter 42.

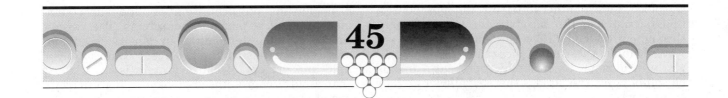

45

Prophylaxis of Coronary Artery Disease: Drugs Used to Lower Plasma Lipoproteins

Coronary artery disease (CAD) is characterized by deposition of fatty plaque on the arterial wall. By restricting coronary blood flow, CAD can produce anginal pain. If complete vessel blockage occurs, myocardial infarction (heart attack) will result.

The risk of developing CAD is increased by elevated levels of certain plasma lipoproteins, structures that transport cholesterol and triglycerides in the blood. The lipoprotein most clearly related to CAD is known as low-density lipoprotein (LDL). Clinical studies have shown conclusively that measures that reduce elevated levels of LDL can significantly reduce the risk of CAD. The primary method for lowering LDL levels is modification of diet. Drugs are indicated only when dietary measures prove insufficient.

PLASMA LIPOPROTEINS: PHYSIOLOGY AND PATHOPHYSIOLOGY

FUNCTION AND STRUCTURE OF THE LIPOPROTEINS

Function. Lipoproteins serve as carriers for transporting lipids (cholesterol, triglycerides) in

559

the blood. Like all other nutrients and metabolites, lipids must use the bloodstream for movement throughout the body. However, since lipids are not water soluble, these substances cannot dissolve directly in plasma. Lipoproteins represent a means of solubilizing the lipids, thereby allowing their transport.

Structure. The basic structure of lipoproteins is depicted in Figure 45–1. As indicated, lipoproteins are tiny, spherical structures that consist of a *lipid core* surrounded by a *protein shell*. The primary lipids within the core are *cholesterol* and *triglycerides*. Since protein molecules are hydrophilic (water soluble), and since the protein shell completely covers the lipid core, the entire structure is soluble in plasma.

CLASSES OF LIPOPROTEINS AND THEIR INFLUENCE ON CORONARY ARTERY DISEASE

There are six major classes of plasma lipoproteins. Distinctions among these classes are based on size, density, protein content, transport function, and predominant core lipids (cholesterol or triglycerides). From a pharmacologic perspective, the features of most concern are *lipid content* and *transport function*.

The topic of lipoprotein *density* deserves comment. This topic is of interest for two reasons. First, naming of lipoproteins is based on their density. Second, differences in density provide the basis for the physical isolation and subsequent measurement of plasma lipoproteins. The various classes of lipoproteins differ in density as a result of dissimilarities in their percent composition of lipid and protein. Because protein is more dense than lipid, lipoproteins that have a high percentage of protein (and a low percentage of lipid) have a relatively high density. Conversely, lipoproteins with a lower percentage of protein have a lower density.

Of the six major classes of lipoproteins, only three are of particular relevance to coronary atherosclerosis. These classes are named (1) very-low-density lipoproteins, (2) low-density lipoproteins, and (3) high-density lipoproteins. Properties of these three classes are summarized in Table 45–1.

Very-Low-Density Lipoproteins (VLDL)

VLDL are produced in the liver and have a lipid core composed primarily of *triglycerides*. The physiologic role of VLDL is *delivery of triglycerides* to adipose tissue and muscle. Of the total triglyceride content of plasma, most can be accounted for by VLDL.

The role of VLDL in atherosclerosis remains unclear. Although several studies suggest a link between elevated levels of VLDL and the development of atherosclerosis, this link has not been firmly established. Regardless of their contribution to atherosclerosis, high levels of triglycerides (>500 mg/dl) *are* associated with an increased risk of *pancreatitis*. Patients at risk of pancreatitis

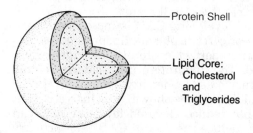

GENERAL LIPOPROTEIN STRUCTURE

Figure 45–1. Composition of plasma lipoproteins. In the general formula for triglycerides, RCOO—, R'COO—, and R"COO— represent fatty acids (saturated or unsaturated) that are usually 16 or 18 carbons in length.

RCOO—CH₂
R'COO—CH
R"COO—CH₂

TRIGLYCERIDE
(general formula)

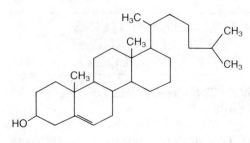

CHOLESTEROL

Table 45–1. Properties of Those Plasma Lipoproteins That Affect Atherosclerosis			
Lipoprotein Class*	Major Core Lipids	Transport Function	Influence on Atherosclerosis
VLDL	Triglycerides	*Delivery* of triglycerides to tissues	Elevated levels *probably contribute* to atherosclerosis.
LDL	Cholesterol†	*Delivery* of cholesterol to tissues	Elevated levels *definitely contribute* to atherosclerosis.
HDL	Cholesterol‡	Facilitates *removal* of cholesterol from tissues	Elevated levels *protect against* atherosclerosis.

*VLDL = very-low-density lipoproteins; LDL = low-density lipoproteins; HDL = high-density lipoproteins.
†LDL carry 60% to 75% of plasma cholesterol.
‡HDL carry 20% to 30% of plasma cholesterol.

should receive a VLDL-lowering drug (e.g., nicotinic acid).

Low-Density Lipoproteins (LDL)

LDL can be looked upon as by-products of VLDL metabolism, since many of the lipid and protein molecules used in the formation of LDL are remnants of VLDL degradation. In contrast to VLDL, whose primary core lipids are triglycerides, the predominant core lipid of LDL is *cholesterol*. As a rule, LDL account for the majority (between 60% and 75%) of all cholesterol present in plasma. The function of LDL is *delivery of cholesterol to the liver and other tissues*.

Cells that require cholesterol meet their needs through LDL absorption. This absorption is accomplished through endocytosis (engulfment), and requires the presence of *LDL receptors* on the cell surface. When cellular demand for cholesterol increases, cells meet this demand by synthesizing more LDL receptors, thereby increasing their capacity for LDL uptake. If a cell is unable to increase its production of LDL receptors, it will be unable to increase LDL absorption.

Long-term studies have established a solid link between elevated levels of LDL and development of CAD. Furthermore, it is clear that reducing LDL levels can decrease development of CAD, and may also cause regression of coronary atherosclerosis. For men who are over 45 years old, the risk of CAD becomes substantially increased when total plasma cholesterol rises above 200 mg/dl. For individuals with elevated levels of LDL, it is estimated that a 25% reduction in plasma LDL content would reduce the risk of serious CAD by 50%. Drugs employed to lower LDL levels include cholestyramine, colestipol, and nicotinic acid.

High-Density Lipoproteins (HDL)

As with LDL, *cholesterol* is the primary lipid present in the core of HDL. Under normal circumstances, the cholesterol present in HDL accounts for 20% to 30% of the total cholesterol in plasma. In contrast to LDL, whose function is the delivery of cholesterol to tissues, the role of the HDL is *promotion of cholesterol removal*.

The influence of HDL on CAD is dramatically different from that of LDL (and also VLDL). Whereas elevations in levels of LDL (and perhaps VLDL) *increase* the risk of CAD, elevation of HDL levels is associated with a *reduced* incidence of CAD. That is, it appears that elevation of HDL levels may actively *protect* against CAD. At this time, we have no drugs that act specifically to raise HDL levels.

LDL-CHOLESTEROL VERSUS HDL-CHOLESTEROL

From the foregoing, it is clear that not all cholesterol in plasma has the same impact on CAD. As discussed above, a rise in cholesterol associated with *LDL increases* the risk of CAD. In contrast, a rise in cholesterol associated with *HDL* appears to *lower* the risk of CAD. Hence, the impact of cholesterol on atherosclerosis depends upon the lipoprotein with which cholesterol is associated. Consequently, when speaking of plasma cholesterol levels, it is desirable to distinguish between cholesterol that is associated with HDL and cholesterol that is associated with LDL. We will use the terms *HDL-cholesterol* and *LDL-cholesterol* to make this distinction.

CHOLESTEROL TESTING AND FOLLOW-UP

Given the clear relationship between high cholesterol and CAD, it is recommended that all adults undergo periodic cholesterol evaluation. For individuals with existing CAD, the guidelines for cholesterol testing and follow-up are different from the guidelines for individuals without CAD. The guidelines presented here reflect recommendations in the Second Report of the National Cholesterol Education Program Expert Panel on Detection, Evaluation, and Treatment of High Blood Cholesterol in Adults.

Individuals Without CAD

Total Cholesterol and HDL-Cholesterol. All adults over the age of 20 should be tested for *total blood cholesterol* at least every 5 years; when possible, *HDL-cholesterol* should be determined at the same time. Measurements can be made without prior fasting. Classification of *total blood cholesterol* in individuals without CAD is as follows: <200 mg/dl = *desirable blood cholesterol,* 200 to 239 mg/dl = *borderline high-risk blood cholesterol,* and >240 mg/dl = *high-risk blood cholesterol.* An *HDL-cholesterol* level of less than 35 mg/dl is classified as *low HDL-cholesterol* (which is undesirable). As indicated in the top half of Table 45–2, follow-up to this initial screen is based on (1) the total cholesterol level, (2) the presence of low HDL-cholesterol (<35 mg/dl is a risk factor for CAD), and (3) the presence of additional risk factors for CAD. If these considerations suggest a risk of CAD, the individual should then be evaluated for *LDL-cholesterol.*

LDL-Cholesterol. Management decisions for lowering blood cholesterol are based on LDL-cholesterol levels, *not* on levels of total cholesterol or HDL-cholesterol. Hence, if screening for total cholesterol and HDL-cholesterol suggests that the patient may be at risk, an LDL-cholesterol determination is required. Blood for the determination should be drawn after fasting for 9 to 12 hours. An LDL-cholesterol level below 130 mg/dl is classified as desirable, and no treatment is needed. Conversely, levels above 130 mg/dl require intervention. Management guidelines are summarized in the bottom half of Table 45–2. Note that the recommended follow-up depends on (1) the LDL-cholesterol level, and (2) the presence or absence of other CAD risk factors (e.g., hypertension, smoking, diabetes mellitus, suboptimal levels of HDL-cholesterol).

Individuals with Existing CAD

Individuals with evidence of CAD are at highest risk. Accordingly, guidelines for cholesterol testing and follow-up are more stringent than for individuals without CAD. Patients with existing CAD should be evaluated *annually.* An *LDL-cholesterol* determination is required. As indicated in Table 45–3, an LDL-cholesterol level below 100 mg/dl is considered *optimal,* and no treatment is needed. Conversely, levels above 100 mg/dl are classified as *higher than optimal* and require intervention; the goal is to reduce LDL-cholesterol to less than 100 mg/dl. Note that in patients with existing CAD, the acceptable level of LDL-cholesterol (100 mg/dl) is not as high as the acceptable level in individuals without CAD (130 mg/dl).

MANAGEMENT OF HIGH LDL-CHOLESTEROL

NONDRUG THERAPY

Dietary Therapy. Diet modification is the cornerstone of treatment for reducing LDL-cholesterol levels. Depending on the severity of LDL-cholesterol elevation, diet modification may be the only treatment needed.

Dietary therapy has two objectives: (1) reduction of plasma LDL-cholesterol, and (2) reduction of body weight for individuals who are obese. To achieve these objectives, the patient should (1) limit *total fat* to 30% or less of caloric intake, (2) limit *saturated fats* (animal fats and some vegetable oils) to 10% or less of caloric intake, and (3) limit *cholesterol* to 300 mg/day or less. If these measures fail to reduce LDL-cholesterol to an acceptable level, consumption of saturated fat and cholesterol should be restricted further: saturated fat should be limited to 7% of caloric intake, and cholesterol should not exceed 200 mg/day. Patients should be given instruction and encouragement on diet modification. Consultation with a dietician may be appropriate. A list of specific foods to choose or avoid is presented in Table 45–4.

Reducing Risk Factors. Major risk factors for CAD are summarized in Table 45–5. These should be identified, and corrected when possible. *Cigarette smoking* raises LDL-cholesterol and lowers HDL-cholesterol, thereby increasing the risk of CAD; patients should be forcefully encouraged to quit smoking. *Diabetes mellitus, hypertension,* and *obesity* all carry an increased risk of CAD; these conditions should be treated.

A *sedentary lifestyle* carries an increased risk of CAD. Conversely, regular exercise lowers the risk of CAD. Running and swimming, for example, can decrease LDL-cholesterol and elevate HDL-cholesterol, thereby reducing CAD risk. When appropriate, an exercise program should be instituted.

Risk factors that cannot be corrected, but none-

Table 45–2. Cholesterol Testing and Follow–up for Individuals Without CAD

Total Cholesterol

mg/dl	Classification	Recommended Follow-up
<200	Desirable blood cholesterol	For patients with HDL-cholesterol ≥35 mg/dl: Repeat tests of total and HDL-cholesterol within 5 years For patients with HDL-cholesterol <35 mg/dl: Obtain lipoprotein analysis; further management based on LDL-cholesterol level
200–239	Borderline high-risk blood cholesterol	For patients with HDL-cholesterol ≥35 mg/dl and less than two CAD risk factors*: provide dietary information and recheck total and HDL-cholesterol within 1 to 2 years For patients with HDL-cholesterol <35 mg/dl or two or more risk factors: obtain lipoprotein analysis; further management based on LDL-cholesterol level
>240	High-risk blood cholesterol	Obtain lipoprotein analysis; further management based on LDL-cholesterol level

LDL-Cholesterol

mg/dl	Classification	Recommended Follow-up
<130	Desirable LDL-cholesterol	Retest total and HDL-cholesterol within 5 years
130–159	Borderline high-risk LDL-cholesterol	For patients with less than two CAD risk factors*: recheck LDL-cholesterol annually For patients with two or more CAD risk factors: institute dietary therapy to bring LDL-cholesterol below 130 mg/dl
160–189	High-risk LDL-cholesterol	For patients with less than two CAD risk factors: institute dietary therapy to bring LDL-cholesterol below 160 mg/dl For patients with two or more risk factors: institute dietary therapy, followed by drug therapy if needed, to bring LDL-cholesterol below 130 mg/dl
>190	High-risk LDL-cholesterol	For patients with less than two CAD risk factors: institute dietary therapy, followed by drug therapy if needed, to bring LDL-cholesterol below 160 mg/dl For patients with two or more risk factors: institute dietary therapy followed by drug therapy to bring LDL-cholesterol below 130 mg/dl

CAD = coronary artery disease.
*CAD risk factors: see Table 45–5.
Based on recommendations in the Summary of the Second Report of the National Cholesterol Education Program Adult Treatment Panel, published in JAMA 269(23):3015–3023, 1993.

Table 45–3. LDL-Cholesterol Testing and Follow-up for Patients with Evidence of CAD*

LDL-Cholesterol† (mg/dl)	Classification	Recommended Follow-up
<100	Optimal	Provide instruction on diet and exercise; repeat LDL-cholesterol measurement annually
100–129	Higher than optimal	Institute dietary therapy, followed by drug therapy if needed, to bring LDL-cholesterol to 100 mg/dl or less
≥130	Higher than optimal	Institute drug therapy to bring LDL-cholesterol to 100 mg/dl or less

*Based on recommendations in the Summary of the Second Report of the National Cholesterol Education Program Adult Treatment Panel, published in JAMA 269(23):3015–3023, 1993.
†Average of two measurements made 1 to 8 weeks apart; measurements are made following an 8- to 12-hour fast.

Table 45–4. Recommended Dietary Modifications to Lower Serum Cholesterol

Food Type	Recommendation	
	Choose	*Decrease*
Fish, chicken, turkey, and lean meats	Fish; poultry without skin; lean cuts of beef, lamb, pork, or veal; shellfish	Fatty cuts of beef, lamb, or pork; spare-ribs; organ meats; regular cold cuts; sausage; hot dogs
Skim and low-fat milk, cheese, yogurt, and dairy products	Skim and 1% fat milk (liquid, powdered, evaporated), buttermilk	4% fat milk (regular, evaporated, condensed), 2% fat milk, cream, half and half, imitation milk products, most nondairy creamers, whipped toppings
	Nonfat (0%) or low-fat yogurt	Whole-milk yogurt
	Low-fat cottage cheese (1% or 2% fat)	Whole-milk cottage cheese (4% fat)
	Low-fat cheeses, farmer or pot cheeses (all of these cheeses should be no more than 2 to 6 gm of fat per ounce)	All natural cheeses (e.g., blue, Roquefort, Camembert, cheddar, Swiss)
		Cream cheese (including low-fat and "light" types), sour cream (including low-fat and "light" types)
	Sherbet, sorbet	Ice cream
Eggs	Egg whites (2 whites = 1 whole egg in recipes), cholesterol-free egg substitutes	Egg yolks
Fruits and vegetables	Fresh, frozen, canned, and dried fruits and vegetables	Vegetables prepared in butter, cream, and other sauces
Breads and cereals	Homemade baked goods using unsaturated oils sparingly, angel food cake, low-fat crackers, low-fat cookies	Commercial baked goods: pies, cakes, muffins, doughnuts, croissants, biscuits, high-fat crackers, high-fat cookies
	Rice, pasta	Egg noodles
	Whole-grain breads and cereals (oatmeal, whole wheat, rye, bran, multigrain, etc)	Breads in which eggs are a major ingredient
Fats and oils	Unsaturated vegetable oils: corn, olive, rapeseed (canola oil), safflower, sesame, soybean, sunflower	Butter, coconut oil, palm oil, palm kernel oil, lard, bacon fat
	Margarine (regular or diet), shortening made from one of the unsaturated oils listed above	
	Mayonnaise, salad dressings made with one of the unsaturated oils listed above, low-fat dressings	Dressings made with egg yolk
	Seeds and nuts	Coconut
	Baking cocoa	Chocolate

From the National Cholesterol Education Program Adult Treatment Panel report, published in Arch. Intern. Med. 148:36–69, 1988.

theless should be identified, include a *family history of premature CAD*, a *history of cerebrovascular or peripheral vascular disease*, and *advancing age* (≥45 for men, ≥55 for women).

Low HDL-cholesterol (<35 mg/dl) is an independent risk factor for CAD. Unfortunately, we have no specific method for raising HDL-cholesterol at this time. As indicated in Table 45–5, *high* HDL-cholesterol (≥60 mg/dl) is a *negative* risk factor; that is, high HDL-cholesterol protects against CAD.

DRUG THERAPY

*Drugs are not the first-line therapy for lowering LDL-cholesterol. Rather, drugs should be employed only if dietary therapy and an exercise program have failed to reduce LDL-cholesterol to an acceptable level—and then only if the combination of ele-*vated LDL-cholesterol and other risk factors justifies drug use. Specific guidelines for implementing drug therapy are presented in Tables 45–2 and 45–3. When drugs are employed, it is essential that dietary therapy continue; beneficial effects of diet and drugs are additive, and drugs alone may be unable to produce adequate cholesterol reductions.

The objective of drug therapy is to lower LDL-cholesterol without also lowering HDL-cholesterol. At this time, the preferred drugs for reducing LDL-cholesterol are *cholestyramine* and *colestipol*. Alternatives include *nicotinic acid* (niacin), *lovastatin*, and *gemfibrozil*. For some patients, single-drug therapy is effective. Others may require a combination of drugs. Since LDL-cholesterol levels will return to pretreatment values if drugs are withdrawn, *treatment must continue lifelong*; patients must be made aware of this requirement. It is important to note that the principal benefit of drug therapy is *prophylaxis*: drugs are much more effec-

Table 45–5. Risk Factors for CAD (Other Than High LDL-Cholesterol)*

Positive Risk Factors†
Age (years)
    Male ≥45
    Female ≥55
Family history of premature CAD
Cigarette smoking
Hypertension
Diabetes mellitus
Low HDL-cholesterol (<35 mg/dl)
 	
Negative Risk Factor
High HDL-cholesterol (≥60 mg/dl)

*Net risk status is determined by adding the number of positive risk factors and then subtracting one risk factor if HDL-cholesterol is ≥60 mg/dl (since high HDL-cholesterol protects against CAD). †*Obesity* and *physical inactivity* are not listed as separate risk factors. *Obesity* is not listed because it operates through other risk factors that are included (hypertension, hyperlipidemia, low HDL-cholesterol, and diabetes mellitus); however, obesity is nonetheless a target for intervention. Although *physical inactivity* is not listed, it too is a target for intervention. Adapted from the Summary of the Second Report of the National Cholesterol Education Program Adult Treatment Panel, published in JAMA 269(23):3015–3023, 1993.

tive at preventing or retarding development of CAD than they are at promoting regression of coronary atherosclerosis that has already occurred.

Periodic monitoring of cholesterol is required. Levels should be measured monthly early in treatment and at longer intervals thereafter.

PHARMACOLOGY OF THE LIPID-LOWERING DRUGS

The principal lipid-lowering drugs are *cholestyramine, colestipol, nicotinic acid, gemfibrozil,* and *lovastatin*. All of these drugs can reduce LDL-cholesterol levels. In addition to the major lipid-lowering drugs, four other drugs are available: *clofibrate, probucol, pravastatin,* and *simvastatin*.

BILE ACID–BINDING RESINS: CHOLESTYRAMINE AND COLESTIPOL

The bile acid–binding resins are employed to lower LDL-cholesterol levels. Two bile acid–binding resins are available: *cholestyramine* [Questran, Cholybar] and *colestipol* [Colestid]. Since these drugs are alike in practically all respects, we will discuss them jointly. Both agents are unusually safe.

Effect on Plasma Lipoproteins

The principal response to bile acid–binding resins is a reduction in LDL-cholesterol levels. LDL levels begin to fall during the first week of therapy, and maximum reductions (about a 20% drop) develop within 1 month. If these drugs are discontinued, LDL-cholesterol will return to pretreatment levels in 3 to 4 weeks.

In some patients, bile acid–binding resins may increase levels of VLDL. In most cases, this elevation is brief and mild. However, if VLDL levels are already elevated prior to treatment, the increment induced by bile acid–binding resins may be sustained and substantial. Accordingly, bile acid–binding resins are not drugs of choice for lowering LDL-cholesterol in patients whose VLDL levels are also elevated.

Pharmacokinetics

Bile acid–binding resins are biologically inert. These drugs are insoluble in water, cannot be absorbed from the gastrointestinal tract, and are impervious to digestive enzymes. The drugs are administered orally and simply pass through the intestine to be excreted intact.

Mechanism of Action

The bile acid–binding resins lower LDL-cholesterol through an indirect mechanism. Following ingestion, these drugs form an insoluble complex with bile acids present in the intestine; this complex prevents the reabsorption of bile acids, and thereby accelerates their excretion. Since bile acids are normally reabsorbed, the increased excretion of bile acids creates a demand for increased bile acid synthesis. This synthesis takes place in the liver. Since bile acids are made from cholesterol, liver cells must have an increased cholesterol supply if they are to increase bile acid production. The required cholesterol is provided by LDL. To avail themselves of more LDL-cholesterol, liver cells increase their number of LDL receptors, thereby increasing their capacity for LDL uptake. The resultant increase in LDL absorption from plasma is the action that is ultimately responsible for the LDL-lowering effects of the bile acid–binding resins. It should be noted that the ability of liver cells to make LDL receptors is critical to the therapeutic effects of the resins; individuals who are genetically incapable of increasing LDL receptor synthesis are unable to benefit from bile acid–binding resin therapy.

Therapeutic Use

The bile acid–binding resins are drugs of first choice for lowering elevated levels of LDL-cholesterol. When used in conjunction with a low-cholesterol diet, these agents can produce a 15% to 20% reduction in LDL-cholesterol levels. LDL levels can be reduced even further (up to a total of 50%) by adding nicotinic acid to the regimen. By lowering plasma levels of LDL-cholesterol, the bile acid–binding resins can significantly decrease morbidity and mortality from CAD.

Adverse Effects

The bile acid–binding resins cannot be absorbed from the gastrointestinal tract and, therefore, have no systemic side effects. As a result, these resins are the safest of the lipoprotein-lowering drugs.

Adverse effects are limited to the gastrointestinal tract. *Constipation* is the principal undesired response. This can be minimized with a diet high in fiber and fluids. If necessary, a mild laxative may be used. Other effects on the gastrointestinal tract include *bloating, indigestion,* and *nausea.* Rarely, these resins decrease fat absorption, an action that may result in *decreased uptake of fat-soluble vitamins* (vitamins A, D, E, and K). Vitamin supplements may be required.

Drug Interactions

In addition to binding bile acids, the bile acid–binding resins can form complexes with drugs. Medications that become bound to these resins cannot be absorbed, making them unavailable for systemic effects. Drugs known to form complexes with these resins include thiazide diuretics, digoxin, warfarin, and some antibiotics. To reduce formation of complexes, oral medications should be administered either 1 hour before or 4 hours after the bile acid–binding resin.

Preparations, Dosage, and Administration

Cholestyramine. Cholestyramine is dispensed in powdered form [Questran, Questran Light] and in a bar [Cholybar]. With either form, the usual adult dosage is 4 to 12 gm twice a day. Patients should be instructed to mix powdered cholestyramine with fluid, since swallowing it dry can cause esophageal irritation and impaction. Appropriate liquids for mixing include water, fruit juices, and soups; pulpy fruits with a high fluid content (e.g., apple sauce, crushed pineapple) may also be used. The bars should be chewed thoroughly.

Colestipol. Colestipol hydrochloride [Colestid] is dispensed in granular form in packets (5 gm) and in bottles (300 and 500 gm). The usual adult dosage is 10 to 20 gm/day administered in one or two doses. Patients should be instructed to mix the granules with fluids or pulpy fruits before ingestion.

NICOTINIC ACID (NIACIN)

Nicotinic acid has the ability to reduce levels of LDL and VLDL. Unfortunately, this drug also causes a variety of side effects. Hence, despite its ability to lower lipoprotein levels, nicotinic acid is of limited clinical utility.

Effect on Plasma Lipoproteins

Nicotinic acid lowers levels of LDL and VLDL, while causing a modest increase in levels of HDL. VLDL levels begin to fall within the first 4 days of therapy. Maximum VLDL reductions range from 20% to 80%. Reductions in LDL levels develop more slowly, taking 3 to 5 weeks to reach maximum. When used alone, nicotinic acid lowers LDL-cholesterol by 10% to 15%. If a bile acid–binding resin is added to the regimen, a 40% to 60% decrease in LDL may be achieved.

Mechanism of Action

The primary effect of nicotinic acid is to decrease the production of VLDL. Reductions in LDL levels occur secondary to

VLDL decline. (Since LDL are by-products of VLDL metabolism, and since nicotinic acid decreases the amount of VLDL available to be metabolized, a fall in VLDL will cause LDL to fall as well.) There appear to be several mechanisms by which nicotinic acid decreases VLDL production. Notable among these is inhibition of lipolysis in adipose tissue.

Therapeutic Use

Because it lowers both LDL and VLDL, nicotinic acid is effective in practically all forms of hyperlipoproteinemia. However, because nicotinic acid causes a high incidence of side effects, some of which are hazardous, this drug has limited applications. Nicotinic acid is the current drug of choice for lowering VLDL levels in patients at risk of pancreatitis. This agent is also the drug of first choice for patients with concurrent elevations in VLDL and LDL.

Nicotinic acid (niacin) also has a role as a vitamin. The doses employed to correct niacin deficiency are much smaller than those employed to lower lipoprotein levels. The role of nicotinic acid as a vitamin is discussed in Chapter 71.

Adverse Effects

The most frequent adverse reactions involve the skin (flushing, itching) and gastrointestinal tract (gastric upset, nausea, vomiting, diarrhea). *Intense flushing* of the face, neck, and ears occurs in practically all patients receiving nicotinic acid in pharmacologic doses. This reaction diminishes in several weeks, and can be attenuated by taking aspirin (75 to 300 mg) 30 minutes before each dose. (Aspirin reduces flushing by preventing the synthesis of prostaglandins, the apparent mediators of this flushing response.)

In addition to its common side effects, nicotinic acid may induce more serious reactions. Nicotinic acid can *injure the liver*, causing jaundice and other symptoms; liver function should be assessed before treatment and periodically thereafter. Disruption of carbohydrate metabolism can result in *hyperglycemia* and *reduced glucose tolerance*; frequent determinations of blood glucose are needed. Disruption of uric acid metabolism can cause *gouty arthritis*. Because of these effects, nicotinic acid must be used with caution in patients with hepatic disease, diabetes, and gout.

Preparations, Dosage, and Administration

Nicotinic acid (niacin) is marketed generically and under multiple trade names. Three formulations are available: tablets, timed-release capsules, and an elixir. The usual maintenance dosage is 1 to 2 gm three times a day, administered with or after meals. (Note: When nicotinic acid is taken as a vitamin, the dosage is only about 25 mg/day—much lower than the dosage employed to lower plasma lipoproteins.)

GEMFIBROZIL

Gemfibrozil [Lopid] decreases levels of VLDL and raises levels of HDL. The drug does not reduce

LDL-cholesterol. Gemfibrozil is a relatively new drug and knowledge of its long-term safety is lacking.

Effects on Plasma Lipoproteins

Gemfibrozil decreases plasma triglyceride content by lowering levels of VLDL. Maximum reductions in VLDL range from 40% to 55%, and are achieved within 3 to 4 weeks of treatment. Gemfibrozil can raise HDL-cholesterol by about 25%. The drug has little effect on LDL-cholesterol levels.

Mechanism of Action

The mechanism by which gemfibrozil lowers VLDL levels is not known. Gemfibrozil can decrease lipolysis in adipose tissue and can reduce uptake of fatty acids by the liver. Both actions can decrease hepatic synthesis of triglycerides. Since triglycerides are the primary core lipids within VLDL, there is speculation that the ability of gemfibrozil to decrease triglyceride production may be the mechanism by which this agent lowers LDL levels. There is no explanation as to how gemfibrozil increases levels of HDL.

Therapeutic Uses

The principal indication for gemfibrozil is elevation of plasma VLDL and triglyceride content. Treatment is limited to patients who have not responded adequately to weight loss and dietary measures. Gemfibrozil can be used to lower LDL-cholesterol, but other drugs (e.g., cholestyramine, colestipol, lovastatin) are more effective.

Adverse Effects

Gemfibrozil is well tolerated. The most common reactions are rashes and gastrointestinal disturbances (nausea, abdominal pain, diarrhea).

Gallstones. Gemfibrozil increases biliary cholesterol saturation, thereby increasing the risk of gallstones. Patients should be informed about manifestations of gallbladder disease (e.g., upper abdominal discomfort, intolerance of fried foods, bloating) and instructed to notify the physician if these develop. Patients with pre-existing gallbladder disease should not receive this drug.

Liver Disease. Gemfibrozil may disrupt liver function. Cancer of the liver may also be a risk. Periodic tests of liver function are required.

Drug Interactions

Warfarin. *Gemfibrozil displaces warfarin from plasma albumin,* thereby increasing anticoagulant effects. Prothrombin time should be measured frequently to assess coagulation status. Warfarin dosage may need to be reduced.

Lovastatin. Gemfibrozil increases the risk of lovastatin-induced myopathy. Patients should not receive this drug combination.

Preparations, Dosage, and Administration

Gemfibrozil [Lopid] is dispensed in 300-mg capsules and 600-mg tablets. The usual adult dosage is 600 mg twice daily, administered 30 minutes before the morning and evening meals.

LOVASTATIN

Lovastatin [Mevacor] is the first member of a new class of lipid-lowering drugs—the HMG-CoA reductase inhibitors. These are the most effective drugs we have for lowering LDL-cholesterol levels. Since its introduction in 1989, lovastatin has become our most widely used lipid-lowering drug.

Effect on Plasma Lipoproteins

Lovastatin is an inhibitor of HMG-CoA reductase, the rate-limiting enzyme in cholesterol biosynthesis. The drug decreases total plasma cholesterol, LDL-cholesterol, VLDL-cholesterol, and total triglycerides. Levels of HDL-cholesterol remain unchanged or increase. Reductions in LDL-cholesterol are significant within 2 weeks and maximal within 4 to 6 weeks. Responses can be enhanced by concurrent therapy with cholestyramine or colestipol. Upon cessation of treatment, serum cholesterol returns to pretreatment levels.

Pharmacokinetics

Lovastatin is administered orally, and about 30% of each dose is absorbed. Most of an absorbed dose is extracted from the blood on its first pass through the liver, the principal site at which lovastatin acts. The drug undergoes rapid hepatic metabolism followed by excretion in the bile. Only a small fraction of each dose reaches the general circulation. Lovastatin crosses the blood-brain barrier and the placenta.

Therapeutic Use

Lovastatin is used to lower LDL-cholesterol in patients who have not responded adequately to a program of dietary therapy and exercise. Although the ability of lovastatin to reduce LDL-cholesterol is well documented, the drug's impact on morbidity and mortality from CAD has not been established. Furthermore, safety with long-term use is unknown.

Adverse Effects

Lovastatin is generally well tolerated. The most common effects, which are usually mild and transient, include gastrointestinal disturbances (nausea, cramps, constipation, diarrhea, abdominal pain), headache, and rash. More serious reactions (see below) are relatively rare.

Hepatotoxicity. Liver injury, as evidenced by elevations in serum transaminase levels, has developed in about 2% of patients treated for 1 year or longer. Jaundice and other clinical signs were absent. Because of the risk of liver injury, hepatic function should be assessed before treatment, every 4 to 6 weeks during the first 3 months of treatment, every 6 to 8 weeks for the next 12 months, and periodically thereafter. If serum transaminase levels rise to three times normal and remain at this height, lovastatin should be discontinued. Transaminase levels will decline to pretreatment levels following drug withdrawal. Caution should be exercised in patients with liver disease and in those who consume alcohol to excess.

Myopathy. Muscle injury coupled with elevation of creatine phosphokinase (CPK) has developed in about 0.5% of patients. If lovastatin is not withdrawn, the condition may progress to severe *myositis* (muscle inflammation) and *rhabdomyolysis* (muscle disintegration or dissolution), possibly associated with acute renal failure. The risk of these reactions is increased by concurrent use of gemfibrozil, nicotinic acid, cyclosporine (an immunosuppressant), and possibly erythromycin. Patients should be instructed to notify the physician if unexplained muscle pain or tenderness is noted. Lovastatin should be withdrawn if myositis is diagnosed or if CPK levels become excessive.

Long-Term Toxicity. Lovastatin suppresses biosynthesis of cholesterol, a compound required for synthesis of all cell membranes and several hormones. We do not yet know if prolonged suppression of cholesterol synthesis can adversely affect these critical processes.

Use in Pregnancy and Lactation

Lovastatin is classified in FDA Pregnancy Category X: the risks to the fetus outweigh any potential benefits of treatment. When administered to pregnant rats in doses 500 times greater than the maximal recommended dosage for humans, lovastatin produced fetal skeletal malformations. Teratogenic effects in humans have not been reported. However, because lovastatin inhibits synthesis of cholesterol, and since cholesterol is required for synthesis of cell membranes and several hormones, there is concern for human fetal injury nonetheless. Moreover, there is no compelling reason not to discontinue lipid-lowering drugs during pregnancy. Women of childbearing age should be informed about the potential for fetal harm and warned against becoming pregnant.

Lovastatin is contraindicated for use during breast-feeding. Although it is not known whether lovastatin can enter human milk, the drug has been shown to enter the milk of rats. Prudence dictates avoidance of the drug by nursing mothers.

Drug Interactions

Studies indicate that beneficial responses to lovastatin can be enhanced by concurrent therapy with a *bile acid–binding resin* (cholestyramine or colestipol). The risk of muscle injury is increased by concurrent use of *cyclosporine, gemfibrozil, nicotinic acid,* or *erythromycin.*

Preparations, Dosage, and Administration

Lovastatin [Mevacor] is dispensed in 10-, 20-, and 40-mg tablets. The usual initial dosage is 20 mg/day taken with the evening meal. Maintenance dosages range from 20 to 80 mg/day administered in single or divided doses.

PRAVASTATIN AND SIMVASTATIN

Actions and Uses. Pravastatin [Pravachol] and simvastatin [Zocor] are the newest members of the HMG-CoA reductase inhibitor family. Like lovastatin, these drugs decrease total plasma cholesterol, LDL-cholesterol, VLDL-cholesterol, and total triglycerides. Levels of HDL-cholesterol remain unchanged or increase. Pravastatin and simvastatin are approved for reducing total cholesterol and LDL-cholesterol when dietary measures alone have been insufficient. However, since these drugs have no apparent advantages over lovastatin, and since clinical experience with lovastatin is greater, there is no strong reason for using these newer drugs instead of lovastatin when an HMG-CoA reductase inhibitor is indicated.

Adverse Effects. Both drugs are well tolerated. The most common adverse effects are headache and gastrointestinal complaints (nausea, vomiting, diarrhea, abdominal pain). These effects occur more frequently with pravastatin than with simvastatin. With both drugs, as with lovastatin, there is a low (2%) incidence of *liver injury*, as evidenced by greater than threefold elevations in serum transaminases. Liver function should be assessed before treatment and at regular intervals thereafter. Like lovastatin, both drugs can cause *myalgia*; however, reports of severe myopathy have been rare (less than 0.1% incidence). Possible adverse consequences of long-term suppression of cholesterol synthesis are not known.

Preparations, Dosage, and Administration. *Pravastatin* [Pravachol] is dispensed in tablets (10 and 20 mg) for oral administration. The usual initial dosage is 10 to 20 mg once daily at bedtime. Maintenance dosages range from 10 to 40 mg once daily at bedtime.

Simvastatin [Zocor] is dispensed in tablets (5, 10, 20, and 40 mg] for oral administration. The initial dosage is 5 to 10 mg once daily in the evening. Maintenance dosages range from 5 to 40 mg once daily in the evening.

CLOFIBRATE

After years of use, this drug has failed to display a convincing ability to reduce mortality from myocardial infarction. Moreover, long-term therapy is associated with serious side effects, some of which may increase mortality. Consequently, clofibrate should be employed only when clearly indicated, and then only if the perceived benefits outweigh the risks.

Effect on Plasma Lipoproteins. The most frequent response to clofibrate is a reduction in VLDL levels, which decline by 20% within 2 to 5 days of the onset of treatment. A modest decrease in LDL-cholesterol also occurs. However, if the decline in VLDL levels is especially large, a compensatory *increase* in LDL-cholesterol may take place.

Under special circumstances, the effects of clofibrate may be more dramatic than just described. In patients with *familial dysbetalipoproteinemia* (an uncommon, genetically based disorder of lipoprotein metabolism), clofibrate can produce as much as an 80% reduction in triglyceride levels, together with a 50% reduction in total plasma cholesterol. These reductions are *not* associated with significant reductions in VLDL, LDL, or HDL levels.

Mechanism of Action. The mechanism by which clofibrate lowers lipoprotein levels is not clear. The drug has the ability to increase intravascular breakdown of VLDL, and this may contribute to therapeutic effects. In addition, clofibrate may accelerate the removal of VLDL breakdown products from plasma. The drug has no consistent effect on lipoprotein synthesis.

Therapeutic Uses. Clofibrate is indicated for patients with *familial dysbetalipoproteinemia* or *severe hypertriglyceridemia*. However, because of the risk of serious adverse effects, use should be restricted to patients who have failed to respond to dietary measures and safer drugs.

Adverse Effects. *Acute Effects.* Short-term effects are usually minor. The most common responses are *gastrointestinal disturbances*. Clofibrate may also produce a severe *flu-like syndrome*, characterized by cramping and muscle weakness.

Chronic Effects. Long-term use of clofibrate has been associated with a 36% increase in deaths from noncardiovascular causes.

Prolonged treatment increases the incidence of *cholelithiasis* (gallstones). These stones may require surgical removal, and not all patients survive surgery.

Clofibrate is associated with a variety of *cardiovascular disorders*. These include dysrhythmias, cardiomegaly, angina pectoris, intermittent claudication, pulmonary embolism, and peripheral vascular disease.

Large doses of clofibrate cause liver cancer in rodents. The carcinogenic potential in humans is not known. As a precaution, periodic tests of liver function should be performed.

Drug Interactions. Clofibrate can displace other drugs from albumin, thereby increasing their effects. This interaction is especially significant with *phenytoin* (an anticonvulsant) and *warfarin* (an anticoagulant). Dosage reductions for these drugs may be required.

Use in Pregnancy and Lactation. Although clofibrate has not been shown to affect the developing fetus, the drug can cross the placenta and is *contraindicated during pregnancy*. Women who intend to become pregnant should discontinue clofibrate several months before attempting conception. Clofibrate enters breast milk and is *contraindicated for nursing mothers*.

Preparations, Dosage, and Administration. Clofibrate [Atromid-S] is available in 500-mg capsules for oral use. The usual adult dosage is 1 gm twice a day.

PROBUCOL

Probucol [Lorelco] is a relatively new lipoprotein-lowering drug. This agent elicits moderate reductions in LDL-cholesterol and, unfortunately, lowers HDL-cholesterol as well. Probucol is highly lipid soluble and remains in the body for months after discontinuation. Probucol is a third-line antihyperlipidemic drug.

Effect on Plasma Lipoproteins. Probucol produces a 10% to 15% reduction in LDL-cholesterol; HDL-cholesterol is reduced to the same extent or more. Maximum reductions in both lipoproteins take 1 to 3 months to develop. Probucol has little or no effect on VLDL.

Pharmacokinetics. Administration is oral. About 10% of each dose is absorbed. Probucol is highly lipid soluble and, hence, extremely difficult to excrete. Following discontinuation, probucol may remain in the body for 6 months or more.

Therapeutic Use. Probucol is a third-line drug for lowering LDL-cholesterol. Use is limited to patients who have not responded to dietary measures and more desirable medications (bile acid–binding resins, nicotinic acid, lovastatin). Probucol is not a preferred agent for two reasons: (1) no proof exists that the drug protects against CAD, and (2) by lowering HDL-cholesterol, probucol may promote development of CAD rather than reduce it.

Adverse Effects. Acute reactions are generally mild. *Gastrointestinal disturbances* (diarrhea, flatulence, abdominal pain, nausea, vomiting) are most common, occurring in about 10% of those treated.

Probucol can cause *cardiac dysrhythmias*. The drug prolongs the QT interval. Serious dysrhythmias have occurred when the QT interval was especially prolonged. An electrocardiogram (EKG) should be taken prior to treatment, 6 months later, and annually thereafter. Probucol should not be given to individuals with myocardial injury or ventricular dysrhythmias.

Preparations, Dosage, and Administration. Probucol [Lorelco] is dispensed in 250- and 500-mg tablets for oral use. The usual adult dosage is 500 mg twice daily taken with the morning and evening meals.

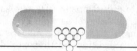

Summary of Major Nursing Implications

IMPLICATIONS THAT APPLY TO ALL DRUGS THAT LOWER LDL-CHOLESTEROL

 Preadministration Assessment

Baseline Data

Obtain laboratory values for total cholesterol, LDL-cholesterol, HDL-cholesterol, and triglycerides (VLDL).

Identifying CAD Risk Factors

The patient history and physical examination should identify CAD risk factors. These include *smoking, obesity, age* (men ≥45 yr, women ≥55 yr), *a family history of premature CAD*, a *personal history of cerebrovascular or peripheral vascular disease, reduced levels of HDL-cholesterol* (below 35 mg/dl), *diabetes mellitus*, and *hypertension*.

 Measures to Enhance Therapeutic Effects

Dietary Therapy

Diet modification should precede and accompany drug therapy for elevated LDL-cholesterol. Inform patients about the importance of diet in controlling cholesterol levels and arrange for dietary counseling. Provide patients with the following dietary guidelines: (1) restrict total dietary fat to 30% (or less) of caloric intake, (2) restrict saturated fats to 10% (or less) of caloric intake, and (3) restrict cholesterol to 300 mg/day. If these restrictions fail to reduce cholesterol to a desirable level, saturated fats should be reduced further (to 7% of caloric intake) and cholesterol should be restricted to 200 mg/day.

Exercise

Regular exercise can reduce LDL-cholesterol and elevate HDL-cholesterol, thereby reducing the risk of CAD. Help the patient establish an appropriate exercise program.

Reduction of CAD Risk Factors

Correctable CAD risk factors should be addressed. Encourage *cigarette smokers* to quit. Encourage *obese* patients to lose weight. Disease states that promote CAD—*diabetes mellitus* and *hypertension*—must be treated.

Promoting Compliance

Drug therapy for elevated LDL-cholesterol must continue lifelong; if drugs are withdrawn, cholesterol levels will return to pretreatment values. Inform patients about the need for continuous therapy and encourage them to adhere to the prescribed regimen.

BILE ACID–BINDING RESINS: CHOLESTYRAMINE AND COLESTIPOL

In addition to the implications discussed below, *see above* for implications that apply to all drugs that lower LDL-cholesterol.

 Preadministration Assessment

Therapeutic Goal

Bile acid–binding resins, in conjunction with dietary therapy and an exercise program, are used to reduce elevated levels of LDL-cholesterol.

Baseline Data

Obtain laboratory values for total cholesterol, LDL-cholesterol, HDL-cholesterol, and triglycerides (VLDL).

 Implementation: Administration

Route

Oral.

Administration

Instruct patients to mix *cholestyramine powder* and *colestipol granules* with water, fruit juice, soup, or pulpy fruit (e.g., apple sauce, pineapple) to reduce the risk of esophageal irritation and impaction. Inform patients that these resins are not water soluble and, hence, mixtures will be cloudy suspensions, not clear solutions.

Instruct patients to chew *cholestyramine bars* thoroughly.

 Ongoing Evaluation and Interventions

Evaluating Therapeutic Effects

Cholesterol levels should be monitored monthly early in treatment and at longer intervals thereafter.

Minimizing Adverse Effects

Constipation. Inform patients that constipation can be minimized by increasing dietary fiber and fluids. A mild laxative may be used if needed. Instruct patients to notify the physician if constipation becomes bothersome.

Vitamin Deficiency. Absorption of fat-soluble vitamins (A, D, E, and K) may be impaired. Vitamin supplements may be required.

Minimizing Adverse Interactions

Bile acid–binding resins can bind to other drugs and prevent their absorption. Administer other medications 1 hour before or 4 hours after the resin.

NICOTINIC ACID (NIACIN)

In addition to the implications discussed below, *see above* for implications that apply to all drugs that lower LDL-cholesterol.

 Preadministration Assessment

Therapeutic Goal

Nicotinic acid, in conjunction with dietary therapy and an exercise program, is used to reduce elevated levels of LDL-cholesterol, VLDL, and triglycerides.

Baseline Data

Obtain laboratory values for total cholesterol, LDL-cholesterol, HDL-cholesterol, and triglycerides (VLDL). Obtain a baseline test of liver function.

Identifying High-Risk Patients

Nicotinic acid is *contraindicated* for patients with *active liver disease.* Exercise *caution* in patients with *diabetes mellitus* and *gout.*

Implementation: Administration

Route

Oral.

Administration

Instruct patients to take nicotinic acid with meals to reduce GI upset.

Implementation: Measures to Enhance Therapeutic Effects

Dietary Therapy

Diet modification should precede and accompany drug therapy for elevated triglycerides and VLDL. Inform patients about the importance of diet in controlling lipid levels and arrange for dietary counseling. In addition to the guidelines presented above for all drugs that reduce LDL-cholesterol, patients with *hypertriglyceridemia* should restrict consumption of alcohol and other sources of triglycerides.

Ongoing Evaluation and Interventions

Evaluating Therapeutic Effects

Blood lipid levels should be monitored monthly early in treatment and at longer intervals thereafter.

Minimizing Adverse Effects

Flushing. Nicotinic acid causes flushing of the face, neck, and ears in most patients. Advise patients that flushing can be reduced by taking aspirin (75 to 300 mg) 30 minutes before each dose.

Liver Dysfunction. Nicotinic acid may injure the liver, causing jaundice or other symptoms. Liver function should be assessed before treatment and periodically thereafter.

Hyperglycemia. Nicotinic acid may cause hyperglycemia and reduced glucose tolerance. Blood glucose should be monitored frequently. Exercise caution in patients with diabetes.

Hyperuricemia. Nicotinic acid can elevate blood levels of uric acid. Exercise caution in patients with gout.

GEMFIBROZIL

Preadministration Assessment

Therapeutic Goal

Gemfibrozil, in conjunction with dietary therapy, is used to reduce elevated levels of VLDL. The drug is not very effective at lowering LDL-cholesterol.

Baseline Data

Obtain laboratory values for total cholesterol, LDL-cholesterol, HDL-cholesterol, and triglycerides (VLDL).

Identifying High-Risk Patients

Gemfibrozil is *contraindicated* for patients with *liver disease*, *severe renal dysfunction*, and *gallbladder disease*.

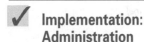

Route

Oral.

Administration

Instruct patients to administer gemfibrozil 30 minutes before the morning and evening meals.

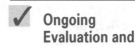

Evaluating Therapeutic Effects

Obtain periodic tests of blood lipids.

Minimizing Adverse Effects

Gallstones. Gemfibrozil increases gallstone development. Inform patients about manifestations of gallbladder disease (e.g., upper abdominal discomfort, intolerance of fried foods, bloating) and instruct them to notify the physician if these develop.

Liver Disease. Gemfibrozil may disrupt liver function. Cancer of the liver may also be a risk. Obtain periodic tests of liver function.

Minimizing Adverse Interactions

Warfarin. Gemfibrozil enhances the effects of warfarin, thereby increasing the risk of bleeding. Obtain frequent measurements of prothrombin time, and observe the patient for signs of bleeding. Reduction of warfarin dosage may be required.

Lovastatin. Gemfibrozil increases the risk of lovastatin-induced myopathy. This combination should be avoided.

LOVASTATIN

In addition to the implications discussed below, *see above* for implications that apply to all drugs that lower LDL-cholesterol.

Therapeutic Goal

Lovastatin, in combination with dietary therapy and an exercise program, is used to lower elevated levels of LDL-cholesterol.

Baseline Data

Obtain baseline values for total cholesterol, LDL-cholesterol, HDL-cholesterol, and triglycerides (VLDL).

Identifying High-Risk Patients

Lovastatin is *contraindicated* for patients with *active liver disease* and for *women who are pregnant or breast-feeding.*

Implementation: Administration

Route

Oral.

Administration

Instruct the patient to administer lovastatin with food.

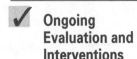

Ongoing Evaluation and Interventions

Evaluating Therapeutic Effects

Cholesterol levels should be monitored monthly early in treatment and at longer intervals thereafter.

Minimizing Adverse Effects

Hepatotoxicity. Lovastatin can injure the liver, but jaundice and other clinical signs do not occur. Liver function should be assessed every 4 to 6 weeks during the first 3 months of treatment and periodically thereafter. If serum transaminase becomes persistently excessive (more than 3 times normal) lovastatin should be discontinued.

Myopathy. Lovastatin can cause muscle injury associated with elevation of CPK. If the drug is not withdrawn, the condition may progress to severe myositis or rhabdomyolysis. Inform patients about the risk of myopathy and instruct them to notify the physician if unexplained muscle pain or tenderness develops. If myopathy is diagnosed or if CPK levels are excessive, lovastatin should be withdrawn. Concurrent use of gemfibrozil, nicotinic acid, cyclosporine, and erythromycin increases the risk of myopathy.

Long-Term Toxicity. The potential adverse effects of long-term suppression of cholesterol biosynthesis are not known.

Use in Pregnancy and Lactation

Lovastatin is contraindicated for use during pregnancy and lactation. Women of childbearing age should be informed about the potential for fetal harm and warned against becoming pregnant.

Minimizing Adverse Interactions

The risk of muscle injury is increased by concurrent use of *cyclosporine, gemfibrozil, nicotinic acid,* and *erythromycin.* Combined use of these drugs with lovastatin should be avoided.

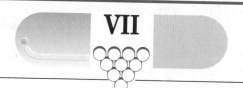

Drugs That Affect the Blood

46

Anticoagulant, Antiplatelet, and Thrombolytic Drugs

The drugs discussed in this chapter are used to prevent formation of thrombi (intravascular blood clots) and to remove thrombi that have already formed. These drugs act in several ways: some suppress coagulation, some inhibit platelet aggregation, and some promote clot dissolution. All of these drugs interfere with normal hemostasis. As a result, all carry a significant risk of hemorrhage.

PHYSIOLOGY AND PATHOPHYSIOLOGY OF COAGULATION

HEMOSTASIS

Hemostasis is the physiologic process by which bleeding is stopped. Hemostasis occurs in two stages: (1) formation of a platelet plug, followed by (2) reinforcement of the platelet plug with fibrin. Both processes are set in motion by injury to a blood vessel.

Stage One: Formation of a Platelet Plug. Platelet aggregation is initiated when platelets come in contact with collagen on the exposed surface of a damaged blood vessel. In response to contact with collagen, platelets adhere to the site of vessel injury. Following adhesion to the vessel wall, platelets release *adenosine diphosphate* (ADP), a substance that causes more platelets to stick to the developing mass. In addition to ADP, platelets release *thromboxane A₂* (TXA₂), an inducer of platelet aggregation that is more powerful than ADP. Under the influence of TXA₂ and ADP, a platelet plug quickly forms and bleeding is stopped. This plug is unstable, however, and must be reinforced with fibrin if protection is to last.

Stage Two: Fibrin Production. Fibrin is produced by way of two convergent pathways (Fig. 46–1), each consisting of a series of cascading reactions. These pathways are referred to as the *intrinsic system* and the *extrinsic system*. The intrinsic system is so named because all necessary clotting factors are present within the vascular system. The extrinsic system is so named because tissue thromboplastin, a factor from outside the vascular system, is required for the extrinsic system to work. As Figure 46–1 indicates, the two systems converge at factor Xa, after which they employ the same final series of reactions. Both systems are required for optimal production of fibrin.

Characteristic of both the intrinsic and extrinsic systems is the fact that each reaction in these sequences serves to enhance the reaction that follows (see Fig. 46–1). Looking at the intrinsic system, we can see that the reaction cascade begins with the conversion of clotting factor XII into its active form, XIIa. The active form of factor XII then stimulates the conversion of factor XI into its active form (XIa), and so on. Hence, once the sequence is initiated, it becomes self-sustaining and self-reinforcing.

Important to our understanding of anticoagulant drugs is the fact that *four coagulation factors—factors VII, IX, X, and prothrombin—require vitamin K for their synthesis.* These factors are highlighted in colored boxes in Figure 46–1. The significance of the vitamin K–dependent factors will become apparent when we discuss warfarin (an oral anticoagulant).

Keeping Hemostasis Under Control. To protect against widespread coagulation, the body must inactivate any clotting factors that stray from the site of blood vessel injury. This inactivation is accomplished with *antithrombin III*, a protein that forms a complex with clotting factors, thereby inhibiting their activity. The clotting factors that can be neutralized by antithrombin III appear in uncolored boxes in Figure 46–1. As we shall see, antithrombin III is intimately involved in the action of *heparin*, an injectable anticoagulant drug.

Physiologic Removal of Clots. As healing of an injured vessel proceeds, removal of the clot is eventually necessary. The body accomplishes this with *plasmin*, an enzyme that digests the fibrin meshwork of the clot. Plasmin is produced through the activation of its precursor, *plasminogen*. The *thrombolytic* drugs—streptokinase, urokinase, alteplase, and anistreplase—act by promoting conversion of plasminogen into plasmin.

THROMBOSIS

A thrombus is a blood clot formed within a blood vessel or within the chambers of the heart. Thrombosis (thrombus formation) reflects pathologic functioning of hemostatic mechanisms.

Arterial Thrombosis. Formation of an arterial thrombus begins with adhesion of platelets to the arterial wall. Following adhesion, these platelets release ADP and TXA₂, thereby attracting additional platelets to the developing thrombus. With continued platelet aggregation, occlusion of the artery takes place. As blood flow comes to a stop, the coagulation cascade is initiated, causing the original plug to become reinforced with fibrin. The pathologic consequence of an arterial thrombus is localized tissue injury owing to lack of perfusion.

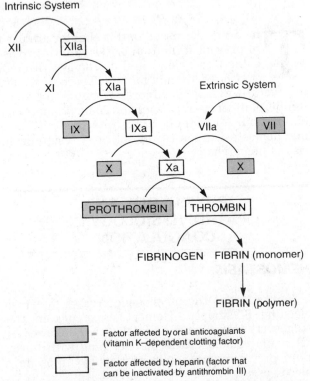

Figure 46–1. Outline of the coagulation cascade showing factors affected by anticoagulant drugs. Common names for factors shown: VII = proconvertin, IX = Christmas factor, X = Stuart factor, XI = plasma thromboplastin antecedent, and XII = Hageman factor.

Venous Thrombosis. Venous thrombi develop at sites where blood flow is slow. Stagnation of blood initiates the coagulation cascade, resulting in the production of fibrin. This fibrin enmeshes red blood cells and platelets to form the thrombus. The typical venous thrombus has a long tail that can break off to produce an *embolus*. Such emboli travel within the vascular system and become lodged at far-away sites, frequently in the pulmonary arteries. Hence, unlike an arterial thrombus, whose harmful effects are localized, injury from a venous thrombus occurs secondary to embolization at a site distant from the original thrombus.

OVERVIEW OF DRUGS USED TO TREAT THROMBOEMBOLIC DISORDERS

The drugs considered in this chapter fall into three major categories: (1) anticoagulants, (2) antiplatelet drugs, and (3) thrombolytic drugs. *Anticoagulants* (heparin, warfarin) are drugs that disrupt the coagulation cascade, and thereby suppress production of fibrin. *Antiplatelet* drugs (e.g., aspirin) inhibit platelet aggregation. *Thrombolytic* drugs (e.g., streptokinase) promote lysis of fibrin, and thereby cause dissolution of thrombi. Characteristic features of these drug classes are summarized in Table 46–1.

Although the anticoagulants and the antiplatelet drugs both suppress thrombosis, they do so by different mechanisms. As a result, these drugs differ in their effects and applications. The *antiplatelet drugs* are most effective at preventing *arterial* thrombosis. In contrast, *anticoagulants* (heparin and warfarin) act to prevent *venous* thrombosis.

PARENTERAL ANTICOAGULANTS

HEPARIN

Heparin is a rapid-acting anticoagulant administered only by injection. Heparin differs from the oral anticoagulants in several respects, including mechanism of action, time course of effects, indications, and management of overdosage.

Source

Heparin is present in a variety of mammalian tissues. The heparin employed clinically is prepared from two sources: lungs of cattle and intestines of pigs. The anticoagulant activity of heparin from either source is equivalent. Although heparin occurs naturally, its physiologic role is unknown.

Chemistry

Heparin is a large polymer composed of repeating units of two disaccharides (Fig. 46–2). Each heparin molecule contains 8 to 15 disaccharide units. An important feature of heparin's structure is the presence of many negatively charged groups (see Fig. 46–2). Because of these negative charges, heparin is highly polar and, therefore, cannot readily cross membranes.

Mechanism of Anticoagulant Action

Heparin suppresses coagulation by helping antithrombin III inactivate thrombin and other clotting factors. As depicted in Figure 46–3, heparin accomplishes this in two ways. First, heparin causes a configurational change in antithrombin III that greatly increases the ability of antithrombin III to interact with and inactivate thrombin. Second, heparin serves as a template to which both antithrombin III and thrombin can bind, thereby facilitating interaction between these two compounds. In addition to helping antithrombin III inactivate thrombin, heparin helps antithrombin III inactivate most other active clotting factors (see Fig. 46–1). By promoting the inactivation of clotting factors, heparin ultimately suppresses formation of fibrin. Since fibrin forms the framework of thrombi in *veins*, heparin is especially useful for prophylaxis of *venous thrombosis*. Because heparin, in combination with antithrombin III, acts directly to inhibit clotting factor activity, the anticoagulant effects of heparin develop *quickly* (within minutes of IV administration). This contrasts with the oral anticoagulants, whose full effects take *days* to develop.

Pharmacokinetics

Absorption and Distribution. Because of its polarity and large size, heparin is unable to cross membranes, including those of the gastrointestinal (GI) tract. Consequently, heparin cannot be absorbed if given orally, and, therefore, must be given by injection (IV or SC). Since it cannot cross membranes, heparin does not traverse the placenta and does not enter breast milk.

Metabolism and Excretion. Heparin undergoes hepatic metabolism followed by renal excretion. Under normal conditions, the half-life of heparin is short (about 1.5 hours). However, in patients with hepatic or renal disease, the half-life is prolonged.

Time Course of Effects. Therapy is initiated with a bolus IV injection and effects begin immediately. Duration of action is brief (hours) and varies with dosage. Effects are prolonged in patients with hepatic or renal impairment.

Table 46–1. Overview of Drugs Used to Treat Thromboembolic Disorders			
Drug Class	**Prototype**	**Drug Action**	**Therapeutic Effect**
Anticoagulants: parenteral	Heparin	↓ Fibrin formation (by promoting inactivation of clotting factors)	Prevention of venous thrombosis
Anticoagulants: oral	Warfarin	↓ Fibrin formation (by decreasing synthesis of clotting factors)	Prevention of venous thrombosis
Antiplatelet drugs	Aspirin	↓ Platelet aggregation	Prevention of arterial thrombosis
Thrombolytic drugs	Streptokinase	Promotion of fibrin digestion	Removal of newly formed thrombi

Therapeutic Uses

Heparin is the preferred anticoagulant for use during *pregnancy* and in situations that require rapid onset of anticoagulant effects, including *pulmonary embolism, evolving stroke,* and *massive deep vein thrombosis.* In addition, heparin is required for patients undergoing *open heart surgery* and *renal dialysis*; during these procedures, heparin serves to prevent coagulation in devices of extracorporeal circulation (heart-lung machines, dialyzers). Low-dose therapy is used to *prevent postoperative venous thrombosis.* Heparin may also be useful for treating *disseminated intravascular coagulation* (DIC), a complex disorder in which fibrin clots form throughout the vascular system and in which bleeding tendencies may be present; bleeding can occur because massive fibrin production consumes available supplies of clotting factors. Heparin is also used as an adjunct to thrombolytic therapy of *acute myocardial infarction.*

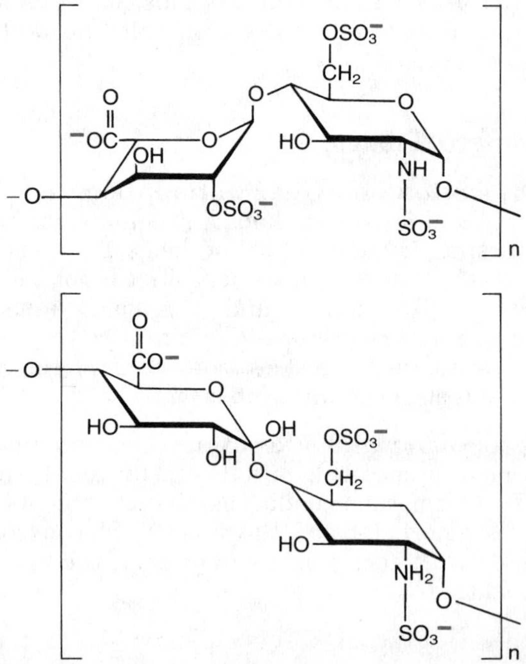

Adverse Effects

Hemorrhage. Bleeding develops in about 10% of patients and is the principal complication of treatment. Hemorrhage can occur at any site and may be fatal. Patients should be monitored closely for signs of blood loss. These include reduced blood pressure, increased heart rate, bruises, petechiae, hematomas, red or black stools, cloudy or discolored urine, pelvic pain (suggestive of ovarian hemorrhage), headache or faintness (suggestive of cerebral hemorrhage), and lumbar pain (suggestive of adrenal hemorrhage). If bleeding develops, heparin should be withdrawn. Severe overdosage can be treated with *protamine sulfate* (see below).

The risk of hemorrhage can be decreased in several ways. First, dosage should be carefully controlled so that the activated partial thromboplastin time (see below) does not exceed two times the control value. In addition, candidates for heparin therapy should be screened for risk factors (see *Warnings and Contraindications*). Lastly, antiplatelet drugs (e.g., aspirin) should be avoided.

Thrombocytopenia. Heparin may decrease platelet counts. Moderate reductions in platelet counts are common and result from heparin-induced platelet aggregation. Severe reductions are rare and result from development of antiplatelet antibodies. If severe thrombocytopenia develops (platelet count $<100,000/mm^3$) heparin should be discontinued. If anticoagulant therapy must be maintained, an oral anticoagulant (warfarin) may be substituted for heparin. Platelet counts should be obtained before treatment and frequently thereafter.

Figure 46–2. Structure of heparin. Each heparin molecule contains 8 to 10 sequences of each of the disaccharide units shown. The negatively charged groups are a major cause of heparin's inability to cross membranes.

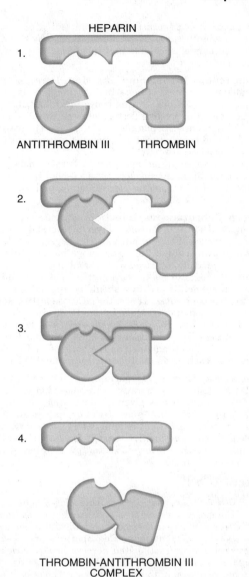

Figure 46–3. Mechanism of heparin action. *(1)* Heparin, thrombin, and antithrombin III are free in the blood. *(2)* Binding of heparin to antithrombin III causes a configurational change in antithrombin III that increases its ability to interact with thrombin. *(3)* Thrombin forms a complex with heparin and antithrombin III, after which thrombin and antithrombin III react, causing permanent inactivation of thrombin. *(4)* The thrombin–antithrombin III complex dissociates from heparin, freeing heparin to act again.

Hypersensitivity Reactions. Since commercial heparin is extracted from animal tissue, these preparations may be contaminated with antigens that can promote allergy. Possible allergic responses include chills, fever, and urticaria. Anaphylactic reactions are rare. To minimize the risk of severe reactions, patients should receive a small test dose of heparin prior to the full therapeutic dose.

Other Adverse Effects. Subcutaneous administration may produce *local irritation* and *hematoma. Vasospastic reactions* that persist for several hours may develop after 1 or more weeks of treatment. Long-term therapy may cause *osteoporosis.*

Warnings and Contraindications

Warnings. Heparin must be used with extreme caution in all patients for whom there is a high likelihood of bleeding. Included in this group are individuals with *hemophilia, increased capillary permeability, dissecting aneurysm, peptic ulcer disease, severe hypertension,* or *threatened abortion.* Heparin must also be used cautiously in patients with *severe disease of the liver or kidneys.*

Contraindications. Heparin is contraindicated for patients with *thrombocytopenia* and *uncontrollable bleeding.* In addition, heparin should be avoided both *during and immediately after surgery of the eye, brain, or spinal cord. Lumbar puncture* and *regional anesthesia* are additional contraindications.

Drug Interactions

In heparin-treated patients, platelet aggregation is the major remaining defense against hemorrhage. Drugs that depress platelet function (e.g., aspirin, ibuprofen, indomethacin) will weaken this defense and must be employed with caution.

Protamine Sulfate for Heparin Overdosage

Protamine sulfate is an antidote to severe heparin overdosage. Protamine is a small protein that has multiple positively charged groups. These charged groups bond ionically with the negatively charged groups on heparin, thereby forming a heparin-protamine complex that is devoid of anticoagulant activity. Neutralization of heparin occurs immediately and lasts for 2 hours, after which additional protamine may be needed. Protamine is administered by slow intravenous injection (no faster than 20 mg/min or 50 mg in 10 min). Dosage can be estimated by employing the knowledge that 1 mg of protamine will inactivate 100 units of heparin. Hence, for each 100 units of heparin in the body, 1 mg of protamine should be injected.

Laboratory Monitoring

The objective of anticoagulant therapy is to reduce blood coagulability to a level that is low enough to prevent thrombosis, but not so low as to promote spontaneous bleeding. Achieving this objective requires careful control of dosage based on frequent tests of coagulation. The laboratory test employed most commonly to monitor heparin therapy is the *activated partial thromboplastin time* (APTT). The normal value for APTT is 40 seconds. At therapeutic levels, heparin will increase the APTT by a factor of 1.5 to 2, making the APTT 60 to 80 seconds. Since heparin has a rapid onset and brief duration of action, if an APTT value should fall outside the therapeutic range, coagulability can be quickly corrected through an adjustment in dosage: if the APTT is too long (>80 seconds), the dosage should be lowered; conversely, if the APTT is too short (<60 seconds), the dosage should be increased. Measurements of APTT should be made frequently (every 4 to 6 hours) during the initial phase of therapy. Once an effective dosage has been established, one APTT measurement a day will suffice.

Unitage and Preparations

Unitage. Heparin is prescribed in units, not in milligrams. The heparin unit is an index of anticoagulant activity, and is defined as the amount of heparin that will prevent 1.0 ml of sheep plasma from coagulating for 1 hour. Heparin is prescribed in units because heparin preparations tend to differ from one another in anticoagulant activity when compared on a milligram basis.

Preparations. Two salts of heparin are available: (1) *heparin sodium* [Liquaemin Sodium] and (2) *heparin calcium* [Calciparine]. *Heparin sodium* is available in concentrations that range from 1000 to 40,000 units/ml. *Heparin calcium* is dispensed in single-dose (5000 units) prefilled syringes. Heparin calcium is a relatively new form of heparin and is reported to carry a lower risk of local hematoma than heparin sodium. Heparin sodium, however, is still the more frequently used salt. The heparin salts are dispensed in single-dose vials; multiple-dose vials; and unit-dose, preloaded syringes that have their own needles.

Heparin sodium [Hep-Lock] is dispensed in dilute form (10 and 100 units/ml) for use in heparin locks. These preparations are too weak to produce systemic anticoagulant effects.

Dosage and Administration

General Considerations. Heparin is administered by injection only. Two routes are employed: (1) intravenous (either intermittent or continuous) and (2) subcutaneous. Intramuscular injection will cause hematoma and must not be used. Heparin is not administered orally because heparin is too large and too polar to undergo intestinal absorption.

Dosage varies with the specific application. Postoperative prophylaxis of thrombosis, for example, requires relatively small doses. In other situations, such as open heart surgery, much larger doses are required. The dosages given below are for "general anticoagulant therapy." As a rule, the APTT should be employed as a guideline for dosage determination; increases in APTT of 1.5- to 2-fold are therapeutic. Since heparin is dispensed in widely varying concentrations, the label must be read carefully to insure that dosing is correct.

Intermittent Intravenous Therapy. Intermittent intravenous heparin is administered via an indwelling rubber-capped needle (heparin lock). Therapy is initiated with a dose of 10,000 units. Subsequent doses of 5000 to 10,000 units are given every 4 to 6 hours. The APTT should be taken 1 hour before each injection until dosage is stabilized. To avoid venous injury, the site of the heparin lock should be moved every 2 or 3 days.

When heparin is administered intermittently, plasma levels of the drug will fluctuate. These fluctuations may result in alternating periods of excessive and insufficient anticoagulant effects.

Continuous Intravenous Infusion. Intravenous infusion provides steady levels of heparin and, therefore, is preferred to intermittent injections. Dosing is begun with a bolus of 5000 to 10,000 units; this loading dose is followed by infusion at a rate of 1000 units/hr. During the initial phase of treatment, the APTT should be measured once every 4 hours and the infusion rate adjusted accordingly. To decrease the risk of overdosage, when heparin solutions are prepared, the amount made up should be sufficient for no more than a 6-hour infusion. Heparin should be infused using an electric pump, and the rate should be checked every 30 to 60 minutes.

Deep Subcutaneous Injection. Subcutaneous injections are made deep into the fatty layer of the abdomen (but not within 2 inches of the umbilicus). The heparin solution should be withdrawn using a 20- to 22-gauge needle. This needle is then discarded and replaced with a small needle (1/2 to 5/8 inch, 25- or 26-gauge) to make the injection. Following administration, firm but gentle pressure should be applied to the injection site for 1 to 2 minutes. The initial SC dose is 10,000 to 20,000 units (preceded immediately by an IV loading dose of 5000 units). The initial SC dose is followed by either (1) 8000 to 10,000 units every 8 hours, or (2) 15,000 to 20,000 units every 12 hours. Dosage is adjusted on the basis of APTT taken 4 to 6 hours after each injection. Injection sites should be rotated.

Low-Dose Therapy. Heparin in low doses is given for prophylaxis against postoperative thromboembolism. The initial dose (5000 units SC) is given 2 hours prior to surgery. Additional doses of 5000 units are given every 8 to 12 hours for 7 days (or until the patient is ambulatory). Low-dose heparin is also employed as adjunctive therapy for patients with myocardial infarction. During low-dose therapy, monitoring of APTT is not usually required.

ENOXAPARIN

Enoxaparin [Lovenox] is a low-molecular-weight form of heparin. (The molecular weight of enoxaparin ranges from 2000 to 8000 daltons, whereas the molecular weight of heparin ranges from 2000 to 40,000 daltons.) Enoxaparin is prepared by depolymerization of unfractionated porcine heparin. However, although enoxaparin is made from heparin, these drugs are not interchangeable on a unit-for-unit basis. The only approved indication for enoxaparin is prevention of deep vein thrombosis following hip replacement surgery. For this indication, the recommended dosage is 30 mg twice daily administered by deep SC injection. Dosing should begin as soon after surgery as possible, and no longer than 24 hours after. The average duration of treatment is 7 to 10 days. At the low doses employed to prevent postoperative thrombosis, enoxaparin does not significantly alter bleeding time, platelet function, prothrombin time, or activated partial thromboplastin time. Accordingly, there is usually no need for daily laboratory monitoring. In the event of overdosage, hemorrhage can be controlled with protamine sulfate, using 1 mg of protamine for each milligram of enoxaparin administered.

ORAL ANTICOAGULANTS

The oral anticoagulants, like heparin, are used to prevent thrombosis. In contrast to heparin, the oral agents have a delayed onset of action, which makes them inappropriate for emergency use. However, because they don't require injection, these drugs are well suited for long-term prophylaxis. As with heparin, oral anticoagulants carry a significant risk of hemorrhage. This risk is amplified by the many drug interactions to which the oral agents are subject. In the United States, only two oral anticoagulants are available: *warfarin* and *anisindione*. Of these, warfarin is by far the most frequently prescribed.

WARFARIN

Warfarin [Coumadin, others] is the oldest member of the oral anticoagulant family and will serve as our prototype for the group.

History

The history of warfarin underscores the potential hazards of the oral anticoagulants. The story of warfarin began with the observation that ingestion of spoiled clover silage could induce bleeding in cattle; the causative agent was identified as bishydroxycoumarin (dicumarol). Research into derivatives of dicumarol resulted in the synthesis of warfarin. When warfarin was first developed, clinical use was ruled out because of concerns about hemorrhage. Instead of becoming a medicine, warfarin was used to kill rats. The drug proved especially effective in this application and remains one of our most widely used rodenticides. Clinical interest in warfarin was renewed following the report of a failed suicide attempt using huge doses of a warfarin-based rat poison. The clinical trials triggered by that event soon demonstrated that warfarin could be employed safely in humans.

Mechanism of Action

Warfarin suppresses coagulation by acting as an *antagonist of vitamin K*. Four clotting factors (factors VII, IX, X, and prothrombin) require vitamin K for their synthesis. By antagonizing vitamin K, warfarin blocks the biosynthesis of these vitamin K-dependent factors.

Pharmacokinetics

Absorption, Distribution, and Elimination. Warfarin is readily absorbed following oral administration. Once in the bloodstream, about 99% of warfarin becomes bound to albumin. This binding provides the basis of several drug interactions. Those warfarin molecules that remain free (unbound) can readily cross membranes, including those of the placenta and milk-producing glands. Warfarin undergoes hepatic metabolism followed by excretion in the urine and feces.

Time Course of Effects. Although warfarin acts quickly to inhibit clotting factor synthesis, noticeable anticoagulant effects are delayed. This delay occurs because warfarin has no effect on clotting factors that are already present at the time of drug administration. Until these clotting factors decay, coagulation remains unaffected. Since decay of clotting factors occurs with a half-life of 6 hours to 2.5 days (depending on the clotting factor under consideration), initial responses to warfarin may not be evident until 8 to 12 hours after administration. Peak effects do not develop for several days.

After warfarin is discontinued, coagulation remains inhibited for 2 to 5 days. This residual effect is due to the long half-life of warfarin (1.5 to 2 days). Because warfarin leaves the body slowly, synthesis of new clotting factors remains suppressed, despite cessation of drug administration.

Therapeutic Uses

Warfarin is employed most frequently for long-term prophylaxis of thrombosis. Specific indications are (1) prevention of venous thrombosis and associated pulmonary embolism, (2) prevention of thromboembolism in patients with prosthetic heart valves, and (3) prevention of thrombosis during atrial fibrillation. For all of these indications, warfarin is the oral anticoagulant of choice. Because onset of effects is delayed, warfarin is not useful in emergencies. When rapid action is needed, therapy can be initiated with heparin.

Monitoring Treatment

The anticoagulant effects of warfarin are evaluated by monitoring *prothrombin time* (PT)—a coagulation test that is especially sensitive to alterations in vitamin K–dependent factors. The average pretreatment value for PT is 12 seconds. Treatment with warfarin prolongs PT.

Traditionally, PT test results have been reported as a *PT ratio*, which is simply the ratio of the patient's PT to a control PT. However, there is a serious problem with this form of reporting: test results can vary widely among laboratories. The underlying cause of variability is thromboplastin, a critical reagent employed in the PT test. To insure that test results among different laboratories are comparable, results are now reported in terms of an *international normalized ratio* (INR). The INR is determined by multiplying the observed PT ratio by a correction factor specific to the particular thromboplastin preparation employed in the test.

The objective of treatment is to raise the INR to an appropriate value. Recommended INR ranges are summarized in Table 46–2. As indicated, an INR of 2 to 3 is appropriate for most patients—although for some patients the target INR is 3 to 4.5. If the INR is below the recommended range, warfarin dosage should be increased. Conversely, if the INR is above the recommended range, the dosage should be reduced. Unfortunately, since

Table 46–2. Monitoring Oral Anticoagulant Therapy: Recommended Ranges of Prothrombin Time-Derived Values

Condition Being Treated	Recommended Ranges	
	Observed PT Ratio*	INR†
Acute myocardial infarction‡	1.3–1.5	2.0–3.0
Atrial fibrillation‡	1.3–1.5	2.0–3.0
Valvular heart disease‡	1.3–1.5	2.0–3.0
Pulmonary embolism, treatment	1.3–1.5	2.0–3.0
Venous thrombosis§	1.3–1.5	2.0–3.0
Tissue heart valves‡	1.3–1.5	2.0–3.0
Mechanical heart valves‡	1.5–2.0	3.0–4.5
Systemic embolism		
Prevention	1.3–1.5	2.0–3.0
Recurrent	1.5–2.0	3.0–4.5

*Observed PT Ratio = ratio of patient's prothrombin time (PT) to a control PT value. In this particular case, the reagent used to determine the control PT value is one of the preparations of rabbit brain thromboplastin employed in the United States. Had a different preparation of thromboplastin been used, the observed PT ratio could be very different.
†INR = international normalized ratio. This value is calculated from the observed PT ratio. The INR is equivalent to the PT ratio that would have been obtained if the patient's PT had been compared to a PT value obtained using the International Reference Preparation, a standardized human brain thromboplastin prepared by the World Health Organization. In contrast to PT ratios, INR values are comparable from one laboratory to the next throughout the United States and the rest of the world.
‡For prevention of systemic embolism.
§Prophylaxis in high-risk surgery; treatment.

warfarin has a delayed onset and prolonged duration of action, the INR cannot be altered quickly: once the dosage has been changed, the desired INR may take a week or more to be reached.

PT must be determined frequently during warfarin therapy. PT should be measured daily during the first 5 days of treatment, twice a week for the next 1 to 2 weeks, once a week for the next 1 to 2 months, and every 2 to 4 weeks thereafter. In addition, PT should be determined whenever a drug that interacts with warfarin is added to or deleted from the regimen.

Concurrent therapy with heparin can influence PT values. To minimize this influence, blood for PT determinations should be drawn no sooner than 5 hours after an *intravenous* injection of heparin, and no sooner than 24 hours after a *subcutaneous* injection.

Adverse Effects

Hemorrhage. Bleeding is the major complication of warfarin therapy. Hemorrhage can occur at any site. Patients should be monitored closely for signs of bleeding. For specific signs, refer to the discussion of heparin-induced hemorrhage. If bleeding develops, warfarin should be discontinued. Severe overdosage can be treated with *vitamin K* (see below). Patients should be encouraged

to carry identification (e.g., MedicAlert bracelet) to inform emergency health care personnel of warfarin use.

Several measures can reduce the risk of bleeding. Candidates for treatment must be carefully screened for risk factors (see *Warnings and Contraindications*). Prothrombin time must be measured frequently. A variety of drugs can potentiate warfarin's effects (see below); these must be used with extreme care. Patients should be given detailed verbal and written instructions regarding signs of bleeding, dosage size and timing, and scheduling of PT tests. When a patient is incapable of accurate self-medication, a responsible individual must supervise therapy. Patients should be advised to keep a written record of each drug administration, rather than relying on memory. A soft toothbrush can reduce gingival bleeding. An electric razor can reduce cuts from shaving.

Warfarin will intensify bleeding during surgery and dental procedures. Dentists and surgeons must be informed of warfarin use. Patients anticipating elective procedures should discontinue warfarin several days prior to the appointment. If an emergency procedure must be performed, injection of vitamin K will help suppress bleeding.

Fetal Hemorrhage and Teratogenesis from Use During Pregnancy. Warfarin can cross the placenta and affect the developing fetus. Fetal hemorrhage and death have occurred. In addition, the drug can cause fetal malformation, central nervous system (CNS) defects, and optic atrophy. Accordingly, *warfarin is classified in FDA Pregnancy Category X: the risks to the developing fetus outweigh any possible benefits of treatment.* Women of child-bearing age should be informed about the potential for teratogenesis and advised to postpone pregnancy. If pregnancy occurs, the possibility of termination should be discussed. If an anticoagulant is needed during pregnancy, heparin, which does not cross the placenta, should be employed.

Use During Lactation. Warfarin enters breast milk. Women should be advised against breast-feeding.

Other Adverse Effects. Adverse effects other than hemorrhage are uncommon. Possible undesired responses include *skin necrosis, alopecia, urticaria, dermatitis, fever, GI disturbances,* and *red-orange discoloration of urine,* which must not be confused with hematuria.

Drug Interactions

General Considerations. Warfarin is subject to a large number of clinically significant drug interactions—perhaps more than any other drug. As a result of these interactions, anticoagulant effects may be reduced to the point of permitting thrombosis, or they may be increased to the point of causing hemorrhage. Patients must be informed about the potential for hazardous interactions, and instructed to avoid all drugs not specifically approved by the physician. This prohibition includes prescription drugs and over-the-counter preparations.

Interactions between warfarin and other drugs are summarized in Table 46–3. As indicated, the interactants fall into three major categories: (1) *drugs that increase anticoagulant effects*, (2) *drugs that promote bleeding*, and (3) *drugs that decrease anticoagulant effects*. The major mechanisms by which anticoagulant effects can be *increased* are (1) displacement of warfarin from plasma albumin, and (2) inhibition of the hepatic enzymes that degrade warfarin. The major mechanisms for *decreasing* anticoagulant effects are (1) acceleration of warfarin degradation through induction of hepatic drug-metabolizing enzymes, (2) increased synthesis of clotting factors, and (3) inhibition of warfarin absorption. Mechanisms by which drugs can *promote bleeding*, and thereby complicate anticoagulant therapy, include (1) inhibition of platelet aggregation, (2) inhibition of the coagulation cascade, and (3) generation of gastrointestinal ulcers.

The existence of an interaction between warfarin and another drug does not absolutely preclude using the combination. This interaction does mean, however, that such combinations must be used with due caution. The potential for harm is greatest when an interacting drug is being added to or deleted from the regimen. At these times, prothrombin time must be monitored, and the dosage of warfarin must be adjusted to compensate for the impact of removing or adding an interacting drug.

Specific Interacting Drugs. Of the many drugs listed in Table 46–3, a few are especially likely to produce interactions of clinical significance. Four of these agents are discussed below.

Heparin. The interaction of heparin with warfarin is obvious: being an anticoagulant itself, heparin will directly increase the bleeding tendencies brought on by warfarin. Combined therapy with heparin plus warfarin must be performed with care.

Aspirin. Aspirin inhibits platelet aggregation. By blocking aggregation, aspirin can suppress formation of the platelet plug that initiates hemostasis. To make matters worse, aspirin can act directly on the GI tract to cause ulcers, thereby initiating bleeding. Hence, when the antifibrin effects of warfarin are coupled with the antiplatelet and ulcerogenic effects of aspirin, the potential for hemorrhagic disaster is substantial. Accordingly, patients should be warned specifically against using any product that contains aspirin. Drugs similar to aspirin (e.g., indomethacin, ibuprofen) should be avoided as well.

Phenylbutazone. Phenylbutazone, an antiarthritic drug, can interact with warfarin in several ways. Phenylbutazone can displace warfarin from albumin, and it can inhibit warfarin degradation. In addition, phenylbutazone can suppress platelet aggregation and induce gastric ulcers. All of these interactions increase the chances of a hemorrhagic event.

Barbiturates. Barbiturates (e.g., phenobarbital) are powerful inducers of hepatic drug-metabolizing enzymes. Hence, barbiturates can accelerate warfarin degradation, thereby decreasing anticoagulant effects. Accordingly, if a barbiturate is added to the regimen, warfarin dosage must be increased. Of equal importance, when barbiturates are withdrawn, causing rates of drug metabolism to decline, a compensatory decrease in warfarin dosage must be made.

Other Notable Interactions. Vitamin K increases clotting factor synthesis, and can thereby decrease anticoagulant effects. *Rifampin* (a drug for tuberculosis) and glutethimide (a CNS depressant) can stimulate drug metabolism, and can thereby reduce anticoagulant effects. Conversely, *cimetidine* (a drug for ulcers) and *disulfiram* (a drug for treating alcoholism) can inhibit warfarin metabolism, and can thereby increase anti-

Table 46–3. Interactions Between Warfarin and Other Drugs		
Drug Category	**Mechanism of Interaction**	**Representative Interacting Drugs**
Drugs that *increase* the effects of warfarin	Displacement of warfarin from albumin	Aspirin and other salicylates Phenylbutazone Sulfonamides Chloral hydrate
	Inhibition of warfarin degradation	Cimetidine Disulfiram Phenylbutazone Sulfonamides
	Decreased synthesis of clotting factors	Oral antibiotics
Drugs that *promote bleeding*	Inhibition of platelet aggregation	Aspirin and other salicylates Dipyridamole Phenylbutazone Indomethacin
	Inhibition of clotting factors	Heparin Antimetabolites
	Promotion of ulcer formation	Aspirin Indomethacin Phenylbutazone Glucocorticoids
Drugs that *decrease* the effects of warfarin	Induction of drug-metabolizing enzymes	Barbiturates Carbamazepine Glutethimide Phenytoin
	Promotion of clotting factor synthesis	Vitamin K_1 Oral contraceptives
	Reduction of warfarin absorption	Cholestyramine Colestipol

coagulant effects. *Sulfonamides* (antibacterial drugs) and *chloral hydrate* (a CNS depressant) can increase the effects of warfarin by displacing it from albumin.

Warnings and Contraindications

Like heparin, warfarin is *contraindicated* for patients with *severe thrombocytopenia* or *uncontrollable bleeding* and for patients undergoing *lumbar puncture, regional anesthesia,* or *surgery of the eye, brain,* or *spinal cord.* Also like heparin, warfarin must be used with extreme *caution* in patients at high risk of bleeding, including those with *hemophilia, increased capillary permeability, dissecting aneurysm, GI ulcers,* and *severe hypertension,* and in women anticipating *abortion.* In addition, warfarin is contraindicated in the presence of *vitamin K deficiency, liver disease,* and *alcoholism*—conditions that can disrupt hepatic synthesis of clotting factors. Also, warfarin is contraindicated during *pregnancy* and *lactation.*

Vitamin K₁ for Warfarin Overdosage

The effects of warfarin overdosage can be overcome with vitamin K_1 (phytonadione). Vitamin K_1 is an antagonist of warfarin action and will reverse warfarin-induced inhibition of clotting factor synthesis. (Vitamin K_3—menadione—has no effect on warfarin action.) For mild bleeding, vitamin K_1 should be administered orally; a dose of 10 to 20 mg will cause prothrombin levels to normalize within 24 hours. If bleeding is severe, parenteral vitamin K_1 (5 to 50 mg) is indicated. If vitamin K fails to control bleeding, levels of clotting factors can be raised quickly by infusing fresh whole blood, fresh frozen plasma, or plasma concentrates of the vitamin K–dependent factors.

Therapy with vitamin K is not without problems. The residual effects of vitamin K will hamper restoration of anticoagulant therapy once bleeding has been arrested. This problem can be minimized by keeping vitamin K dosage low. Also, intravenous vitamin K has been associated with severe anaphylactoid reactions. Accordingly, IV administration should be employed only if other routes are not feasible and only if the potential benefits outweigh the risks. The pharmacology of vitamin K is discussed at length in Chapter 71.

Contrasts Between Warfarin and Heparin

Although heparin and warfarin are both anticoagulants, these drugs have several important differences. Whereas administration of warfarin is oral, heparin must be given by injection. Although both drugs decrease fibrin formation, they do so by different mechanisms: heparin works through antithrombin III, whereas warfarin inhibits synthesis of vitamin K–dependent clotting factors.

Heparin and warfarin differ markedly with respect to time course of action: effects of heparin begin and fade rapidly, whereas effects of warfarin begin slowly but then persist for several days. Different tests are used to monitor therapy: changes in APTT are used to monitor heparin treatment, whereas changes in PT are used to monitor warfarin. Lastly, these drugs differ with respect to management of overdosage: protamine is given to counteract heparin; vitamin K_1 is given to counteract warfarin. These differences are summarized in Table 46–4.

Preparations, Dosage, and Administration

Warfarin sodium [Coumadin, Panwarfin, Sofarin] is dispensed in tablets (1, 2, 2.5, 5, 7.5, and 10 mg) for oral use. The initial dosage is 10 to 15 mg/day. Maintenance doses range from 2 to 15 mg daily and are determined by the target INR value: for most patients, dosage should be adjusted to produce an INR of 2 to 3.

ANISINDIONE

Anisindione [Miradon] has actions and uses like those of warfarin. However, since the incidence of severe side effects with this drug is much greater than with warfarin, use of anisindione is rare. The drug is dispensed in 50-mg tablets for oral administration. The initial dose is 300 mg. Maintenance dosages range from 25 to 250 mg/day.

ANTIPLATELET DRUGS

Antiplatelet drugs are agents that suppress platelet aggregation. Since a platelet core constitutes the bulk of an *arterial* thrombus, the principal indication for the antiplatelet drugs is prevention of thrombosis in *arteries.* In contrast, the

---

Table 46–4. Summary of Contrasts Between Heparin and Warfarin

	Heparin	Warfarin
Mechanism of action	Promotes action of antithrombin III	Inhibits synthesis of vitamin K–dependent clotting factors
Route	Intravenous or subcutaneous	Oral
Onset	Rapid (minutes)	Slow (hours)
Duration	Brief (hours)	Prolonged (days)
Monitoring	APTT*	PT†
Antidote for overdosage	Protamine	Vitamin K₁

*Activated partial thromboplastin time.
†Prothrombin time. Test results are reported in terms of a PT ratio or in terms of an INR (international normalized ratio).

principal indication for heparin and warfarin is prevention of thrombosis in *veins*. The antiplatelet drug employed most frequently is aspirin.

ASPIRIN

The basic pharmacology of aspirin is discussed in Chapter 61. Consideration here is limited to the use of aspirin to prevent arterial thrombosis.

Mechanism of Antiplatelet Action. Aspirin suppresses platelet aggregation by causing *irreversible inhibition of cyclooxygenase,* an enzyme required by platelets to synthesize thromboxane A$_2$ (TXA$_2$). As noted earlier in the chapter, TXA$_2$ acts on platelets to promote aggregation. In addition, TXA$_2$ acts on vascular smooth muscle to promote vasoconstriction. Both actions promote hemostasis. By inhibiting cyclooxygenase, aspirin suppresses TXA$_2$-mediated vasoconstriction and platelet aggregation, thereby reducing the risk of arterial thrombosis. Since platelets lack the machinery to synthesize new cyclooxygenase, the effects of a single dose of aspirin persist for the life of the platelet (5 to 7 days).

In addition to inhibiting the synthesis of TXA$_2$, aspirin can inhibit the synthesis of *prostacyclin* by the blood vessel wall. Since prostacyclin has effects that are exactly opposite to those of TXA$_2$—namely, suppression of platelet aggregation and promotion of vasodilation—suppression of prostacyclin synthesis can partially counteract the beneficial effects of aspirin therapy. Fortunately, aspirin is able to inhibit synthesis of TXA$_2$ at doses that are lower than those needed to inhibit synthesis of prostacyclin. Accordingly, if we keep the dosage of aspirin *low* (325 mg/day or less), we can minimize inhibition of prostacyclin production, while maintaining inhibition of TXA$_2$ production.

Indications for Antiplatelet Therapy. Antiplatelet therapy with aspirin has three applications of proven efficacy: (1) prevention of acute myocardial infarction (MI) in patients with unstable angina, (2) prevention of reinfarction in patients who have experienced an acute MI, and (3) prevention of stroke in patients with a history of transient ischemic attacks (TIAs). In all three situations, prophylactic therapy with aspirin can reduce the incidence of morbidity and mortality.

Dosing. Dosages for antiplatelet therapy should be low—325 mg/day or less. Doses of 160 to 325 mg/day are effective for reducing the risk of reinfarction following an acute MI. To reduce the incidence of TIAs, doses of 30 to 325 mg/day have been employed.

TICLOPIDINE

Actions and Uses. Ticlopidine [Ticlid] is an oral antiplatelet drug approved only for prevention of thrombotic stroke. The drug is at least as effective as aspirin, but is much more expen-

sive and carries a risk of neutropenia and agranulocytosis. In contrast to aspirin, ticlopidine acts by inhibiting ADP-mediated platelet aggregation, and not by inhibiting synthesis of thromboxane A$_2$. Suppression of aggregation persists for the life of the platelet.

Pharmacokinetics. Ticlopidine is well absorbed following oral administration. Antiplatelet effects begin within 48 hours and become maximal in about a week. The drug undergoes extensive hepatic metabolism followed by renal excretion. Ticlopidine has a long half-life (4 to 5 days) and effects persist for a week or more after drug withdrawal.

Adverse Effects. The most common effects are gastrointestinal disturbances (diarrhea, abdominal pain, flatulence, nausea, dyspepsia) and dermatologic reactions (rash, purpura, pruritus).

The most serious effects are hematologic. *Neutropenia* develops in 2.4% of those treated, and is sometimes severe. *Agranulocytosis* has occurred rarely. Both effects reverse within 1 to 3 weeks after drug withdrawal. Complete blood counts and a white cell differential should be obtained every 2 weeks through the first 3 months of treatment and at any sign of infection after this time. Ticlopidine should be withdrawn if neutropenia or agranulocytosis develop.

Preparations and Dosage. Ticlopidine [Ticlid] is dispensed in 250-mg tablets for oral administration. The recommended dosage is 250 mg twice a day, administered with food.

DIPYRIDAMOLE

Dipyridamole [Persantine] suppresses platelet aggregation, perhaps by increasing plasma levels of adenosine. The drug is approved only for prevention of thromboembolism following heart valve replacement surgery. For this application, the drug is always employed in combination with warfarin. The recommended dosage is 75 to 100 mg 4 times a day.

THROMBOLYTIC DRUGS

As their name implies, the thrombolytic drugs act to remove thrombi that have already formed. This contrasts with the anticoagulants, which act to prevent thrombus formation. Four thrombolytic drugs are available: streptokinase, urokinase, alteplase, and anistreplase. All four carry a risk of serious bleeding and, therefore, should be administered only by a clinician skilled in their use. Thrombolytic agents are employed acutely and only for severe thrombotic disease. Because of their mechanism of action (see below), these agents are also known as *fibrinolytics*.

STREPTOKINASE

Streptokinase [Kabikinase, Streptase] was the first thrombolytic drug available and will serve as our prototype for the group.

Mechanism of Action

Streptokinase acts by an indirect mechanism. The drug first binds to *plasminogen* to form a complex. This complex then acts on other molecules of plasminogen (a proenzyme present in blood) to cause their conversion into *plasmin*, an enzyme that digests the fibrin meshwork of clots. In addition to digesting clots, plasmin degrades fibrinogen and other clotting factors; these actions do not contribute to lysis of thrombi, but they do increase the risk of hemorrhage.

Therapeutic Uses

Streptokinase has three major indications: (1) acute coronary thrombosis (acute myocardial infarction), (2) deep vein thrombosis, and (3) massive pulmonary emboli. In all three situations, timely intervention is essential. For example, for treatment of coronary thrombosis, results are best when thrombolytic therapy is started within 4 to 6 hours of the onset of symptoms. Thrombolytic therapy of coronary thrombosis is discussed further in Chapter 43 (Management of Myocardial Infarction).

Pharmacokinetics

Streptokinase may be administered by IV infusion or by infusion directly into an occluded coronary artery. Because of rapid inactivation, the drug has a plasma half-life of only 12 to 18 minutes.

Adverse Effects

Bleeding. Bleeding is the major complication of treatment. Bleeding occurs for two reasons: (1) plasmin can destroy pre-existing clots, and can thereby promote recurrence of bleeding at sites of recently healed injury, and (2) by degrading clotting factors, plasmin can disrupt the coagulation cascade, and thereby interfere with new clot formation in response to vascular injury. Likely sites of bleeding include recent wounds, sites of needle puncture, and sites at which invasive procedures have been performed. Anticoagulants and antiplatelet drugs increase the risk of hemorrhage. High-dose therapy with these drugs must be avoided until thrombolytic effects have abated.

Management of bleeding depends on the severity. Oozing at sites of cutaneous puncture can be controlled with a pressure dressing. If severe bleeding occurs, streptokinase should be discontinued. Patients that require blood replacement can be given whole blood or blood products (packed red blood cells, fresh-frozen plasma). As a rule, blood replacement will restore hemostasis. If not, excessive fibrinolysis can be reversed with IV *aminocaproic acid* [Amicar], a compound that prevents activation of plasminogen and directly inhibits plasmin.

Several measures can reduce the risk of bleeding. These include (1) minimizing physical manipulation of the patient, (2) avoiding subcutaneous and intramuscular injections, (3) minimizing inva-

sive procedures, (4) avoiding concurrent use of anticoagulants (heparin, warfarin), and (5) avoiding concurrent use of antiplatelet drugs (e.g., aspirin).

Because of the risk of bleeding, streptokinase is absolutely contraindicated for patients with active internal bleeding, intracranial neoplasm, a history of a cerebrovascular accident, known bleeding diathesis, severe uncontrolled hypertension, or recent surgery of the CNS. Relative contraindications include recent thoracic or abdominal surgery, recent serious trauma, recent history of GI bleeding, organ biopsy, lumbar puncture, puncture of an uncompressible blood vessel, and advanced age. In addition, streptokinase should be avoided during the postpartum period.

Allergic Reactions. Streptokinase is a foreign protein extracted from cultures of streptococci. Since most individuals have antibodies to streptococci, allergic reactions can occur. The most common reactions are urticaria, itching, flushing, and headache. These can be treated with antihistamines. Severe anaphylaxis is rare.

Fever. Temperature elevation of 1.5°F or more occurs in one third of those treated. Only 3.5% of patients develop temperatures above 104°F. Acetaminophen—not aspirin—should be given to lower temperature.

Preparations, Dosage, and Administration

Streptokinase [Kabikinase, Streptase] is dispensed as a powder and must be reconstituted for use. Solutions are prepared with either 0.9% saline or 5% dextrose.

Dosage is prescribed in units. Therapy is usually initiated with an IV loading dose of 1.5 million units infused over 60 minutes. After the loading dose, infusion is continued for 1 to 3 days at a rate of 100,000 U/hr.

For treatment of an evolving myocardial infarction, streptokinase may be infused through a catheter placed in the occluded coronary artery. This technique offers two benefits: (1) high levels of streptokinase are achieved at the site where the drug is needed, and (2) high drug levels are avoided at other sites, thereby minimizing generalized bleeding. Timing of therapy is critical: streptokinase is most effective when therapy is initiated within 6 hours of the onset of symptoms.

OTHER THROMBOLYTIC DRUGS

Alteplase, urokinase, and anistreplase are similar to streptokinase with regard to mechanism of action, indications, and ability to promote bleeding. Principal differences among these drugs relate to half-life, source, antigenicity, and cost. Properties of these drugs are summarized in Table 46–5.

Alteplase

Alteplase [Activase], also known as tissue-type plasminogen activator (tPA), is produced commercially by recombinant DNA technology. The commercial preparation is identical to naturally occur-

	Drug			
Property	**Streptokinase**	**Anistreplase (APSAC)**	**Alteplase (tPA)**	**Urokinase**
Trade name(s)	Kabikinase, Streptase	Eminase	Activase	Abbokinase
Description	Streptokinase is a compound that forms an active complex with plasminogen	Anistreplase is an equimolar complex of acetylated streptokinase and human plasminogen	Alteplase is identical to human tissue plasminogen activator, an enzyme that converts plasminogen into plasmin	Urokinase is an enzyme that converts plasminogen to plasmin
Source	Streptococcal culture	Streptococcal culture (for streptokinase); human plasma (for plasminogen)	Recombinant DNA technology	Cultured human fetal kidney cells
Mechanism of action	All four drugs act directly or indirectly to cause the conversion of plasminogen to plasmin, an enzyme that digests the fibrin meshwork of thrombi			
Fibrin specificity	Minimal	Minimal	Moderate	Moderate
Adverse effects				
Bleeding	Yes	Yes	Yes	Yes
Allergic reactions	Yes	Yes	No	No
Half-life (minutes)	12–18	40–60	2–6	15–20
Typical dose	1.5 million units	30 units	100 mg	2 million units
Administration	IV infusion: 60 min	Slow IV injection: 2–5 min	10-mg IV bolus, with the remainder over 90 min	1 million units by IV bolus, then 1 million units IV over 1 hr
Cost (to pharmacy) for one course of treatment	$300	$2000	$2300	$3800

Table 46–5. Properties of Thrombolytic Drugs

ring human tPA, an enzyme that promotes conversion of plasminogen to plasmin, which then acts to digest clots. Low therapeutic doses produce selective activation of plasminogen that is bound to fibrin in thrombi. As a result, activation of plasminogen in the general circulation is minimal. However, despite selective activation of fibrin-bound plasminogen, bleeding tendencies with alteplase are equivalent to those seen with the other thrombolytic drugs. Since alteplase is devoid of foreign proteins, the drug does not cause allergic reactions. Alteplase has a short half-life (about 5 minutes) owing to rapid hepatic inactivation. The recommended dosage is 100 mg infused over 3 hours (60 mg the first hour, 20 mg the second hour, and 20 mg the third hour). Alternatively, an "accelerated" schedule may be used, in which two thirds of the dose is given in the first 30 minutes, and the remainder given over the next hour. Doses in excess of 100 mg are associated with an increased risk of intracranial bleeding and should be avoided. Alteplase is an expensive drug: a 100-mg dose costs about $2300. This compares with about $300 for an equivalent dose of streptokinase.

Urokinase

Urokinase [Abbokinase] is an enzyme found in human urine. Commercial urokinase is prepared by extraction from cultures of human fetal kidney cells. Like streptokinase, urokinase promotes the conversion of plasminogen into its active form (plasmin). As with streptokinase, bleeding is the principal adverse effect. Since urokinase is human derived, it is not antigenic. Accordingly, allergic reactions do not occur. Urokinase has a short half-life (15 to 20 minutes) owing to rapid inactivation by the liver. For treatment of myocardial infarction, the drug is given in an initial IV bolus (1 million units) followed by infusion of another 1 million units over the next hour. Because of its high cost (see Table 46–5), urokinase is used much less frequently than streptokinase.

Anistreplase (APSAC)

Anistreplase [Eminase] is an acylated complex of streptokinase plus human plasminogen. The streptokinase is obtained from streptococcal culture; the human plasminogen is obtained by extraction from human plasma. Because it is acylated, the plasminogen in anistreplase is inactive. Once in the body, the drug undergoes gradual deacylation followed by conversion to plasmin, which then acts to digest fibrin in clots. In addition to degrading fibrin in thrombi, anistreplase can degrade circulating fibrinogen. Both actions (digestion of fibrin and degradation of fibrinogen) promote bleeding. Clinical experience indicates that the risk of bleeding complications with anistreplase is the same as with the other thrombolytic drugs. Since anistreplase contains streptokinase (a foreign protein), the drug can cause allergic reactions. Anistreplase differs from the other thrombolytics in that it can be administered by slow IV *injection* instead of by *infusion*. This makes anistreplase more convenient to use. The recommended dosage is 30 units injected over 2 to 5 minutes. Like urokinase and alteplase, anistreplase is expensive, costing over $2000 for one course of treatment. An alternative name for anistreplase is *anisoylated plasminogen-stretokinase activator complex* or *APSAC*.

STREPTOKINASE VERSUS ALTEPLASE: THE GUSTO TRIAL

The GUSTO trial (Global Utilization of Streptokinase and tPA for Occluded Coronary Arteries) is the largest study ever conducted on the treatment of acute myocardial infarction. Over 41,000 patients from 15 countries participated. Although complete results of GUSTO have not been published as of this writing, preliminary results, which were presented in the spring of 1993, suggest that *mortality* from MI in patients receiving alteplase (tPA) is lower than in patients receiving streptokinase (SK)—although the risk of *hemorrhagic stroke* is higher with tPA. However, as discussed below, the apparent superiority of tPA as seen in GUSTO may not be relevant to everyday clinical practice.

In GUSTO, each participant received one of the following treatments (30-day mortality rates are in parentheses):

1. tPA + IV heparin (6.3%)
2. SK + IV heparin (7.4%)
3. SK + SC heparin (7.2%)
4. SK + tPA + IV heparin (7.0%)

As the mortality figures indicate, 7.4 of each 100 patients who received SK (plus IV heparin) died within 30 days. In contrast, only 6.3 of each 100 patients who received tPA (plus IV heparin) died within 30 days. Hence, by using tPA instead of SK, we might expect to save 1 additional life for each 100 patients.

What the above figures don't indicate is timing of tPA administration with respect to onset of MI symptoms. In GUSTO, nearly 90% of patients received treatment within 2 to 4 hours of symptom onset. Among patients who received tPA within 2 hours of symptom onset, the death rate was only 5.4%; among those treated 2 to 4 hours after symptom onset, the rate increased to 6.6%; and among those treated 4 to 6 hours after symptom onset, the rate jumped to 9.4%. Not only do these figures underscore the importance of early treatment of MI, they also bring into question the relevance to GUSTO to ordinary clinical practice—since, in usual practice, very few patients present as early as those in GUSTO. Furthermore, among patients who present *after* 4 hours, GUSTO showed no significant difference in mortality between treatment with tPA and treatment with SK. Hence, although tPA may be superior to SK when these drugs are employed under *ideal* conditions, tPA may not be superior in everyday practice. When this observation is coupled with two others—the much higher cost of tPA and the greater incidence of hemorrhagic stroke with tPA—the desirability of tPA over SK is not entirely obvious.

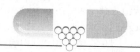

Summary of Major Nursing Implications

HEPARIN

 Preadministration Assessment

Therapeutic Goal

The objective of therapy is to prevent thrombosis without inducing spontaneous bleeding.

Heparin is the preferred anticoagulant for use during *pregnancy* and in situations that require rapid onset of effects, including *pulmonary embolism, evolving stroke,* and *massive deep vein thrombosis.* Other indications include *open heart surgery, renal dialysis,* and *disseminated intravascular coagulation.* Low doses are used to *prevent postoperative venous thrombosis* and to *enhance thrombolytic therapy of myocardial infarction.*

Baseline Data

Obtain baseline values for blood pressure, heart rate, complete blood cell counts, platelet counts, hematocrit, and activated partial thromboplastin time (APTT).

Identifying High-Risk Patients

Heparin is *contraindicated* for patients with *severe thrombocytopenia* or *uncontrollable bleeding* and for patients undergoing *lumbar puncture, regional anesthesia,* or *surgery of the eye, brain, or spinal cord.*

Use with extreme *caution* in patients at high risk of bleeding, including those with *hemophilia, increased capillary permeability, dissecting aneurysm, gastrointestinal ulcers,* or *severe hypertension.* Caution is also needed in patients with severe hepatic or renal dysfunction.

 Implementation: Administration

Routes

Intravenous (continuous infusion or intermittent) and subcutaneous. Avoid IM injections!

Administration

General Considerations. Dosage is prescribed in units, not milligrams. Heparin preparations vary widely in concentration; read the label carefully to insure correct dosing.

Intermittent IV Administration. Administer through a heparin lock every 4 to 6 hours. APTT should be determined before each dose during the early phase of treatment, and daily thereafter. Rotate the injection site every 2 to 3 days.

Continuous IV Infusion. Administer with a constant infusion pump or some other approved volume control unit. Policy may require that dosage be double-checked by a second person. Check the infusion rate every 30 to 60 minutes. During the early phase of treatment, APTT should be determined every 4 hours. Check the site of needle insertion periodically for extravasation.

Deep SC Injection. Perform SC injections into the fatty layer of the abdomen (but not within 2 inches of the umbilicus). Withdraw heparin solution using a 20- to 22-gauge needle and then discard that needle and replace it with a small needle (1/2 to 5/8 inch, 25- or 26-gauge) to make the injection. Apply firm but gentle pressure to the injection site for 1 to 2 minutes following administration. Rotate and record injection sites.

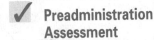

Ongoing Evaluation and Interventions

Evaluating Treatment

Periodic determinations of APTT are used to evaluate treatment. Heparin should increase the APTT by 1.5 to 2 fold.

Minimizing Adverse Effects

Hemorrhage. Heparin overdosage may cause hemorrhage. Monitor the patient closely for signs of bleeding. These signs include lowering of blood pressure, elevation of heart rate, discoloration of urine or stools, bruises, petechiae, hematomas, persistent headache or faintness (suggestive of cerebral hemorrhage), pelvic pain (suggestive of ovarian hemorrhage), and lumbar pain (suggestive of adrenal hemorrhage). Laboratory data suggesting hemorrhage include reductions in the hematocrit and blood cell counts. If bleeding occurs, heparin should be discontinued. Severe overdosage can be treated with *protamine sulfate* administered by slow IV injection. The risk of bleeding can be reduced by insuring that the APTT does not exceed two times the control value.

Thrombocytopenia. Heparin can decrease platelet counts, thereby increasing the risk of bleeding. Platelet counts should be monitored. If they drop below 100,000/mm^3, heparin should be discontinued.

Hypersensitivity Reactions. Allergy may develop to antigens in heparin preparations. To minimize the risk of severe reactions, administer a small test dose prior to the full therapeutic dose.

Minimizing Adverse Interactions

Antiplatelet Drugs. Concurrent use of *antiplatelet drugs* (e.g., aspirin) increases the risk of bleeding. Use these agents with caution.

WARFARIN

Preadministration Assessment

Therapeutic Goal

The goal of therapy is to prevent thrombosis without inducing spontaneous bleeding. Specific indications include (1) prevention of venous thrombosis and associated pulmonary embolism, (2) prevention of thromboembolism in patients with prosthetic heart valves, and (3) prevention of thrombosis during atrial fibrillation.

Baseline Data

Obtain a thorough medical history, making sure to identify use of any medications that might interact adversely with warfarin. Obtain baseline values of vital signs and prothrombin time.

Identifying High-Risk Patients

Warfarin is *contraindicated* in the presence of *vitamin K deficiency*, *liver disease, alcoholism, thrombocytopenia, uncontrollable bleeding, pregnancy*, and *lactation* and for patients undergoing *lumbar puncture, regional anesthesia*, or *surgery of the eye, brain, or spinal cord*.

Use with extreme *caution* in patients at high risk of bleeding, including those with *hemophilia, increased capillary permeability, dissecting aneurysm, gastrointestinal ulcers*, and *severe hypertension*.

Implementation: Administration

Route

Oral.

Administration

For most patients, dosage is adjusted to maintain an international normalized ratio (INR) value of 2 to 3. Maintain a flow chart for hospitalized patients indicating INR values and dosage size and timing.

Implementation: Measures to Enhance Therapeutic Effects

Promoting Compliance

Safe and effective therapy requires rigid adherence to the dosing schedule. Achieving this adherence requires active and informed participation by the patient. Provide the patient with detailed written and verbal instructions regarding the purpose of treatment, dosage size and timing, and the importance of strict adherence to the dosing schedule. Also, provide the patient with a chart on which to keep an ongoing record of warfarin use. If the patient is incompetent (e.g., mentally ill, alcoholic, senile), insure that a responsible individual supervises treatment.

Nondrug Measures

Advise the patient to (1) avoid prolonged immobility, (2) elevate the legs when sitting, (3) avoid garments that can restrict blood flow in the legs, (4) participate in exercise activities, and (5) wear support hose. These measures will reduce venous stasis, and will thereby reduce the risk of thrombosis.

Ongoing Evaluation and Interventions

Evaluating Therapeutic Effects

Evaluate therapy by monitoring *prothrombin time* (PT). Test results are reported in terms of an INR. For most patients, the target INR is 2 to 3. If the INR is below this range, dosage should be increased. Conversely, if the INR is above this range, dosage should be reduced.

Prothrombin time should be measured frequently: daily during the first 5 days, twice a week for the next 1 to 2 weeks, once a week for the next 1 to 2 months, and every 2 to 4 weeks thereafter. In addition, PT should be determined whenever a drug that interacts with warfarin is added to or deleted from the regimen.

If heparin is being employed concurrently, blood for PT determinations should be drawn no sooner than 5 hours after IV administration of heparin, and no sooner than 24 hours after SC administration.

Minimizing Adverse Effects

Hemorrhage. Hemorrhage is the major complication of warfarin therapy. Warn patients about the danger of hemorrhage and inform them about signs of bleeding. These signs include lowering of blood pressure, elevation of heart rate, discoloration of urine or stools, bruises, petechiae, hematomas, persistent headache or faintness (suggestive of cerebral hemorrhage), pelvic pain (suggestive of ovarian hemorrhage), and lumbar pain (suggestive of adrenal hemorrhage). Laboratory data suggesting hemorrhage include reductions in the hematocrit and blood cell counts.

Instruct the patient to withhold warfarin and notify the physician if signs of bleeding are noted. Advise the patient to wear some form of identification (e.g., Medic Alert bracelet) indicating warfarin use.

To reduce the incidence of bleeding, advise the patient to avoid excessive consumption of alcohol. Suggest use of a soft toothbrush to prevent bleeding from the gums. Advise patients to shave with an electric razor.

Warfarin will intensify bleeding during surgical or dental procedures. Instruct the patient to make certain that the dentist or surgeon is aware that warfarin is being taken. Warfarin should be discontinued several days prior to elective procedures. If emergency surgery must be performed, vitamin K_1 can help reduce bleeding.

Warfarin-induced bleeding can be controlled with vitamin K_1. If bleeding is minor, oral vitamin K will suffice. For severe bleeding, vitamin K is given by injection. The physician may advise the patient to keep a supply of vitamin K on hand for use in emergencies, but only after consultation with a physician.

Use in Pregnancy and Lactation. Warfarin can cross the placenta, causing fetal hemorrhage and malformation. Inform women of child-bearing age about potential risks to the fetus, and warn them against becoming pregnant. If pregnancy develops, termination should be considered.

Warfarin enters breast milk and may harm the nursing infant. Warn women against breast-feeding.

Minimizing Adverse Interactions

Inform patients that warfarin is subject to a large number of potentially dangerous drug interactions. Instruct patients to avoid all drugs—prescription and nonprescription—that have not been specifically approved by the physician. Prior to treatment, take a complete medication history to identify any drugs that might interact adversely with warfarin.

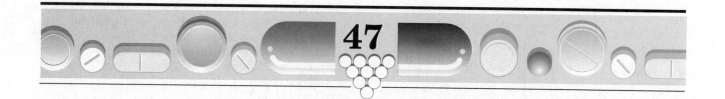

47

Drugs for Deficiency Anemias

Anemia is defined as a decrease in erythrocyte number, size, or hemoglobin content. Causes include blood loss, hemolysis, bone marrow dysfunction, and deficiencies of substances essential for hematopoiesis (red blood cell formation and maturation). Most deficiency anemias result from a deficiency in iron, vitamin B$_{12}$, or folic acid. Iron deficiency anemia is much more common than anemia due to a deficiency of vitamin B$_{12}$ or folic acid.

In discussing the deficiency anemias, we will limit our scope to deficiencies of iron, vitamin B$_{12}$, and folic acid. Iron is considered first, followed by vitamin B$_{12}$, and then folic acid. To facilitate discussion, we will start the chapter with a review of red blood cell development.

RED BLOOD CELL DEVELOPMENT

Red blood cells begin development in the bone marrow, and reach maturity in the blood. As developing red cells grow and divide, they evolve through four principal stages (Fig. 47–1). In their earliest stage, red cells lack hemoglobin and are known as *proerythroblasts*. In the next stage, red cells gain hemoglobin and are called *erythroblasts*. Both the erythroblasts and the proerythroblasts reside in the bone marrow. After the erythroblast stage, red cells evolve into *reticulocytes* (immature erythrocytes) and enter the systemic circulation. Following the reticulocyte stage, circulating red

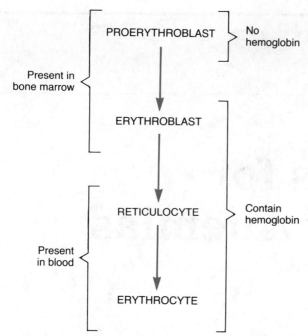

Figure 47–1. Stages of red blood cell development.

cells reach full maturity and are referred to as *erythrocytes*.

Red blood cell development requires the cooperative interaction of several factors: the bone marrow must be healthy; erythropoietin (a stimulant of red cell maturation) must be present; iron must be available for hemoglobin synthesis; and other factors, including vitamin B_{12} and folic acid, must be available to support synthesis of deoxyribonucleic acid (DNA). If any of these factors is absent or amiss, anemia will result.

IRON DEFICIENCY

Iron deficiency is the most common cause of nutrition-related anemia. Worldwide, people with iron deficiency number in the hundreds of millions. In the United States, between 5% and 10% of the population is estimated to be iron deficient.

BIOCHEMISTRY AND PHYSIOLOGY OF IRON

In order to understand the consequences of iron deficiency as well as the rationale behind iron therapy, we must first understand the biochemistry and physiology of iron. This information is reviewed below.

Metabolic Functions

Iron is essential to the function of hemoglobin, myoglobin (the oxygen-storing molecule of muscle), and a variety of iron-containing enzymes. From a quantitative perspective, the most significant use of iron is in hemoglobin: between 70% and 80% of all iron in the body is dedicated to hemoglobin production. Although the iron in myoglobin and certain enzymes is clearly important, the amount involved is small.

Fate in the Body

The major pathways for iron movement and utilization are shown in Figure 47–2. In the discussion below, the circled numbers refer to the circled numbers in the figure.

Uptake and Distribution. The life cycle of iron begins with ① the uptake of iron into mucosal cells of the small intestine. These cells absorb between 5% and 20% of dietary iron; the maximum absorptive capacity is 3 to 4 mg of iron per day. Iron in the ferrous form (Fe^{++}) is absorbed more readily than iron in the ferric form (Fe^{+++}). Food greatly reduces absorption.

Following uptake, iron can either ②ₐ undergo storage within mucosal cells in the form of *ferritin* (a complex consisting of iron plus a protein used for iron storage) or ②ᵦ undergo binding to *transferrin* (the iron transport protein) for distribution throughout the body.

Utilization and Storage. Iron that is bound to transferrin can undergo one of three fates. The majority of transferrin-bound iron is ③ₐ taken up by cells of the bone marrow for incorporation into hemoglobin. Small amounts are ③ᵦ taken up by the liver and other tissues for storage as ferritin; these stores make up about 18% of the iron in the body. Lastly ③𝒸, some of the iron in plasma is taken up by muscle (for production of myoglobin) and some is taken up by all tissues (for production of iron-containing enzymes). These last two uses account for about 10% of the iron in the body.

Recycling. As Figure 47–2 depicts, iron associated with hemoglobin undergoes continuous recycling. Following hemoglobin production in bone marrow, iron re-enters the circulation ④ as a component of hemoglobin in erythrocytes. (The iron in circulating erythrocytes accounts for about 70% of total body iron.) After approximately 120 days of useful life, red cells are catabolized ⑤. Iron released by this process re-enters the plasma bound to transferrin ⑥—and then the cycle begins anew.

Elimination. Excretion of iron is minimal. Under normal circumstances, only 1 mg of iron is excreted per day. At this rate, if none of the lost iron were replaced, body stores would decline by only 10% per year.

Iron leaves the body by several routes. Most excretion occurs via the bowel: iron in ferritin is lost as mucosal cells slough; iron also enters the bowel

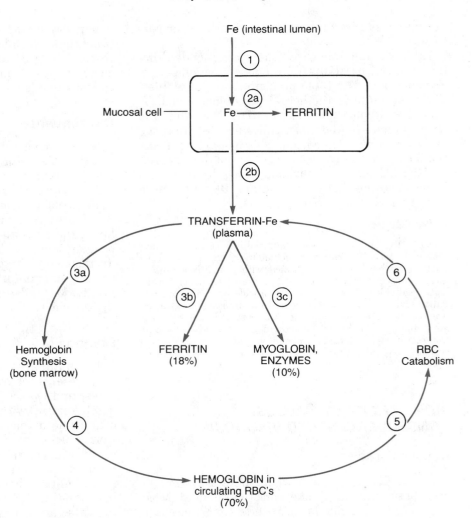

Figure 47–2. Fate of iron in the body. Pathways labeled with circled numbers are explained in the text. Values in parentheses indicate percentage of total body stores. Elimination of iron is not shown since most iron is rigidly conserved. (Fe = iron, RBC = red blood cell)

in the bile. Small amounts of iron are excreted in the urine and sweat.

It should be noted that although very little iron leaves the body as a result of excretion (i.e., normal physiologic loss), substantial amounts can leave the body because of blood loss. Hence, menorrhagia (excessive menstrual flow), hemorrhage, and blood donations can all cause significant reductions in iron levels.

Regulation of Body Iron Content. The amount of iron in the body is regulated through control of intestinal iron absorption. As noted, most of the iron that enters the body stays in the body. Hence, if all dietary iron were readily absorbed, body iron content could rapidly build to toxic levels. Such *excessive buildup is prevented through control of iron uptake: as body stores rise, uptake of iron declines; conversely, as body stores become depleted, uptake is allowed to increase.* For example, when body stores of iron are high, only 2% to 3% of dietary iron is absorbed. In contrast, when body stores are depleted, iron absorption may rise to as high as 20%. Although it is well established that iron absorption fluctuates as a function of need, we do not understand the mech-

anisms by which the rate of absorption is regulated.

Daily Requirements

Requirements for iron are determined largely by the rate at which the body is making erythrocytes. When red cell production is low, iron needs are small; conversely, when red cell production is high, requirements for iron are high as well. Accordingly, infants and children—individuals whose rapid growth rate requires massive red cell synthesis—have iron requirements that are quite high (relative to body weight). In contrast, the daily iron needs of adults are relatively low. Adult males need only 10 mg of dietary iron per day. Adult females need somewhat more, to compensate for iron loss during menstruation.

During pregnancy, requirements for iron increase dramatically. This increase results from (1) expansion of maternal blood volume, and (2) production of red blood cells by the fetus. In most cases, the iron needs of pregnant women are too great to be met by diet alone. Consequently, iron supplements (about 30 mg/day) are recommended during pregnancy and for 2 to 3 months after parturition.

Table 47–1 summarizes the recommended dietary allowances (RDAs) of iron as a function of age. For each age, the table presents two iron values. The first value is the actual physiologic need for iron. The second value is the RDA. Note that the RDA values are about ten times greater than the values for physiologic need. This disparity reflects the fact that, on average, only 10% of dietary iron is absorbed. Hence, if physiologic requirements are to be met, the diet must contain 10 times more iron than the body actually needs.

Dietary Sources

Iron is available in foods of plant and animal origin. Foods that are especially rich in iron include liver, egg yolk, brewer's yeast, and wheat germ. Other foods with a high iron content include muscle meats, fish, fowl, cereal grains, beans, and green leafy vegetables. Foods that do not provide much iron include milk and most nongreen vegetables. Since iron can be extracted from cooking utensils, the use of iron pots and pans can augment dietary iron. Except for individuals who have very high iron requirements (infants, pregnant women, those undergoing chronic blood loss), the average diet is sufficient to meet iron needs.

IRON DEFICIENCY: CAUSES, CONSEQUENCES, AND DIAGNOSIS

Causes

Iron deficiency results when there is an imbalance between iron uptake and iron demand. Most commonly, this imbalance results from increased demand, and not from reduced uptake. The most common causes of increased iron demand (and resulting iron deficiency) are (1) blood volume expansion during pregnancy coupled with red blood cell synthesis by the developing fetus, (2) blood volume expansion during infancy and early childhood, and (3) chronic blood loss, which is usually of gastrointestinal (GI) or uterine origin. Rarely, iron deficiency results from reduced iron uptake; potential causes include gastrectomy and sprue.

Consequences

Iron deficiency has multiple effects, the most conspicuous being *iron deficiency anemia*. In the absence of iron for hemoglobin synthesis, red blood cells become *microcytic* (small) and *hypochromic* (pale in color). The reduced oxygen-carrying capacity of blood results in listlessness, fatigue, and pallor of the skin and mucous membranes. If tissue oxygenation is severely compromised, tachycardia, dyspnea, and angina may result. In addition to causing anemia, iron deficiency impairs myoglobin production and reduces synthesis of iron-containing enzymes.

Diagnosis

The hallmarks of iron deficiency anemia are (1) the presence of microcytic, hypochromic erythrocytes, and (2) the absence of hemosiderin (aggregated ferritin) within bone marrow. Additional laboratory data that can help confirm a diagnosis of iron deficiency anemia include reduced red cell count, reduced hemoglobin and hematocrit values, reduced serum iron content, and increased serum iron-binding capacity (IBC). (Serum IBC measures iron binding by transferrin. An increase in IBC indicates an increase in the amount of transferrin that is not carrying any iron and, hence, signals reduced iron availability.)

When a diagnosis of iron deficiency anemia is made, it is imperative that the underlying cause be determined. This is especially true when the

Table 47–1. Recommended Dietary Allowances for Iron			
	Age (years)	Physiologic Requirement for Iron (mg/day)	RDA* for Iron (mg/day)
Infants	0–0.5	0.6	6
	0.5–1	1.0	10
Children	1–10	1.0	10
Males	11–18	1.2	12
	18+	1.0	10
Females	11–50	1.5	15
	50+	1.0	10
Pregnant and 2–3 months postpartum	—	5	30†

*Since only a small fraction of dietary iron is absorbed, the RDA is higher than the actual physiologic need.
†Iron requirements during pregnancy cannot be met through dietary sources alone; supplements are recommended.

suspected cause of deficiency is blood loss of GI origin. Such blood loss may be indicative of peptic ulcer disease or GI cancer, conditions that demand immediate treatment.

ORAL IRON PREPARATIONS I: FERROUS SULFATE

Ferrous sulfate is the least expensive of the oral iron preparations and is the standard against which other oral preparations are measured. Ferrous sulfate will serve as our prototype for the group.

Indications

Ferrous sulfate is the drug of choice for treating iron deficiency anemia. This compound is also employed for prophylaxis of iron deficiency in people whose need for iron cannot be met by diet alone (e.g., pregnant women, individuals experiencing chronic blood loss).

Adverse Effects

Gastrointestinal Disturbances. The most significant adverse effects of oral iron preparations involve the GI tract. These effects, which are dose dependent, include nausea, pyrosis (heartburn), bloating, constipation, and diarrhea. Gastrointestinal reactions are most intense during the initial phase of therapy, and become less disturbing with continued drug use. Because of their effects on the GI tract, oral iron preparations can aggravate peptic ulcers, regional enteritis, and ulcerative colitis. Accordingly, patients with these disorders should not take iron orally. In addition to its other GI effects, oral iron may impart a dark green or black coloration to stools. This effect is harmless and should not be interpreted as a sign of bleeding.

Staining of Teeth. Liquid iron preparations can stain the teeth. This effect can be prevented by (1) diluting liquid preparations with juice or water, (2) administering the iron through a straw or with a dropper, and (3) rinsing the mouth after administration.

Toxicity

Iron in large amounts is toxic. Poisoning is almost always the result of accidental or intentional overdose; poisoning from proper therapeutic use of iron is rare. Death from iron poisoning is most likely to occur in the very young. Death in adults is uncommon. For children, the lethal dose of elemental iron is between 2 and 10 gm. To reduce the chances of pediatric poisoning, iron should be stored in child-proof containers and kept out of reach.

Symptoms. The effects of iron poisoning are complex. Early reactions include nausea, vomiting, diarrhea, and shock. These responses are followed by acidosis, gastric necrosis, hepatic failure, pulmonary edema, and vasomotor collapse.

Diagnosis and Treatment. With rapid diagnosis and treatment, mortality from iron poisoning is low (about 1%). Serum iron should be measured and the intestine x-rayed to determine the presence of unabsorbed tablets. Induction of vomiting will remove iron from the stomach. Acidosis and shock should be treated as required.

If the plasma level of iron is high (above 500 μg/dl) it should be lowered using *deferoxamine*. Deferoxamine absorbs iron and thereby prevents toxic effects. The pharmacology of deferoxamine is discussed in Chapter 93 (Management of Poisoning).

Drug Interactions

Interaction of iron with other drugs can alter the absorption of iron, the other agent, or both. *Antacids* reduce the absorption of iron. Coadministration of iron with *tetracyclines* decreases the absorption of both agents. *Ascorbic acid* (vitamin C) promotes iron absorption but also increases its adverse effects. Accordingly, attempts to promote iron uptake by combining iron with ascorbic acid offer no advantage over a simple increase in iron dosage.

Formulations

Oral iron is available in several dosage forms (Table 47–2). Some of these formulations (timed- or sustained-release capsules and tablets) are intended to reduce gastric disturbances. Unfortunately, although side effects may be lowered, these dosage forms have disadvantages: iron may be released at inconstant rates, causing variable, unpredictable absorption; in addition, these preparations are expensive. Ordinary tablets do not have these drawbacks.

Dosage and Administration

General Considerations. Dosing with oral iron is complicated by the fact that the oral iron salts differ from one another with regard to percentage of elemental iron (see Table 47–2). Ferrous *sulfate*, for example, contains 20% iron by weight. In contrast, ferrous *gluconate* contains only 11.6% iron. Consequently, in order to provide equivalent amounts of elemental iron, we must use different doses of these iron preparations. For example, if we wished to provide 100 mg of elemental iron, we would need to administer a 500-mg dose of ferrous *sulfate*. To provide this same amount of elemental iron using ferrous *fumarate*, only a 300-mg dose would be required. In the discussion below, dosage values refer to milligrams of *elemental* iron, and not to milligrams of any particular iron salt needed to provide that amount of elemental iron.

Food affects therapy with oral iron in two ways. First, food helps protect against iron-induced GI distress. Second, food decreases absorption of iron by 50% to 70%. Hence, we have a dilemma: *absorption is best* when iron is taken *between* meals, but *side effects are lowest* when iron is taken *with* meals. As a rule, it is recommended that iron be

Table 47–2. Oral Iron Preparations

Iron Salt	Dosage Forms	% Iron (by weight)	Dose Providing 100 mg Iron
Ferrous sulfate	C, E, L, Sy, T, T-TR	20	500 mg
Ferrous sulfate (dried)	C, C-TR, T, T-SR	~30	330 mg
Ferrous fumarate	Su, T, T-Ch, T-TR, L	33	300 mg
Ferrous gluconate	C, E, T, T-SR	11.6	860 mg

C = capsule; C-TR = capsule, timed-release; E = elixir; L = liquid; Sy = syrup; Su = suspension; T = tablet; T-Ch = tablet, chewable; T-SR = tablet, sustained-release; and T-TR = tablet, timed-release

administered *between* meals, thereby maximizing absorption; if necessary, the dosage can be lowered to render GI effects more acceptable.

For two reasons, it may be desirable to take iron *with* food during *initial* therapy. First, since the GI effects of iron are most intense as treatment commences, the salving effects of food can be especially beneficial at this time. Second, by reducing GI discomfort during the early phase of therapy, administering iron with food can help promote compliance.

Use in Iron Deficiency Anemia. Dosing with oral iron represents a compromise between a desire to replenish lost iron rapidly and a desire to keep adverse GI effects to a minimum. For most adults, this compromise can best be achieved with doses of 65 mg administered three times a day, yielding a total daily dose of approximately 200 mg. Since there is a ceiling to intestinal absorption of iron, doses above this level provide only modest increase in therapeutic effect. On the other hand, at dosages greater than 200 mg/day, GI disturbances become disproportionately high. Hence, elevation of the daily dosage above 200 mg would augment adverse effects without offering a significant increase in benefits. When treating iron deficiency in infants and children, a typical dosage is 5 mg/kg/day administered in three or four divided doses.

Timing of iron administration is important: doses should be spaced evenly throughout the day. This schedule provides the bone marrow with a continuous iron supply, thereby maximizing red cell production.

Duration of therapy is determined by the therapeutic objective. If correction of anemia is the sole objective of treatment, a few months of therapy will be sufficient. However, if the objective also includes replenishment of ferritin, treatment must continue for an additional 4 to 6 months. It should be noted, however, that drugs are usually unnecessary for ferritin replenishment; in most cases, diet alone is sufficient. Accordingly, once anemia has been corrected, pharmaceutical iron can usually be discontinued.

Prophylactic Use of Iron. Pregnancy is the principal indication for prophylactic iron therapy. A daily dose of 30 mg taken between meals is recommended. Other candidates for iron prophylaxis include infants, children, and women experiencing menorrhagia.

ORAL IRON PREPARATIONS II: FERROUS GLUCONATE AND FERROUS FUMARATE

In addition to ferrous sulfate, two other iron salts—ferrous gluconate and ferrous fumarate—are available for oral use. Except for differences in percentage of iron content (see Table 47–2), all of these preparations are equivalent. Hence, when dosage is adjusted to provide equal amounts of elemental iron, ferrous gluconate and ferrous fumarate produce pharmacologic effects identical to those of ferrous sulfate: all three agents produce equivalent therapeutic responses, and all three cause the same degree of GI distress. Patients who fail to respond to one of these agents will not respond to the others. Patients who cannot tolerate the GI effects of one agent will find the others intolerable too.

PARENTERAL IRON: IRON DEXTRAN

Iron dextran is the only parenteral iron preparation available in the United States. This preparation is a complex consisting of ferric hydroxide and dextrans (polymers of glucose). The rate of response to parenteral iron is equal to that seen with oral iron. Iron dextran is dangerous—fatal anaphylactic reactions have occurred—and should be used only when circumstances demand.

Indications

Iron dextran is reserved for patients with a clear diagnosis of iron deficiency and for whom oral iron is either ineffective or intolerable. Primary candidates for parenteral iron are patients who, because of intestinal disease, are unable to absorb iron administered orally. Iron dextran is also indicated when blood loss is so great (500 to 1000 ml/week) that oral iron cannot be absorbed rapidly enough to meet hematopoietic needs. Parenteral iron may also be employed when there is concern that oral iron might exacerbate pre-existing disease of the stomach or bowel. Lastly, parenteral iron can be employed for the rare patient for whom the GI effects of oral iron are intolerable.

Adverse Effects

Anaphylactic Reactions. Potentially fatal anaphylaxis is the most serious adverse effect of iron dextran. Although these reactions are rare, the possibility of their occurrence demands that iron dextran be used only when clearly required. Whenever iron dextran is administered, injectable epinephrine and facilities for resuscitation should be at hand.

Other Adverse Effects. Iron dextran can cause headache, fever, urticaria, and arthralgia. More serious reactions—circulatory failure and cardiac arrest—have also occurred. When administered IM, iron dextran can cause persistent pain and prolonged, localized discoloration. Very rarely, tumors have developed at sites of IM injection. Intravenous administration may result in lymphadenopathy and phlebitis.

Preparations, Dosage, and Administration

Preparations. Iron dextran [InFeD] is dispensed in 10-ml vials and 2-ml ampuls, all containing 50 mg/ml of elemental iron.

Dosage. Dosage determination is complex. Dosage will vary depending on the degree of anemia, the weight of the patient, and the presence of persistent bleeding. For the patient with iron deficiency anemia who is not losing blood, the following equation provides a guideline for estimating total iron dosage:

$$\text{mg iron} = 0.66 \times \text{kg body weight} \times \left(100 - \frac{\text{hemoglobin value in g/dl}}{14.8}\right)$$

Administration. Iron dextran may be administered IM or IV. Intravenous administration is preferred. This route is just as effective as IM administration but causes fewer anaphylactic reactions and other adverse effects.

Intravenous. To minimize anaphylactic reactions, intravenous iron dextran should be administered by the following protocol: (1) administer a tiny test dose (25 mg over 5 minutes) and observe the patient for at least 15 minutes; (2) if the test dose appears safe, slowly administer a larger dose (500 mg over a 10- to 15-minute interval); and (3) if the 500-mg dose is uneventful, additional doses may be given as needed.

Intramuscular. Intramuscular iron dextran has significant drawbacks and should be avoided. Disadvantages include persistent pain and discoloration at the injection site, possible development of tumors, and greater risk of anaphylaxis than that associated with IV administration. When IM administration must be performed, iron dextran should be injected deep into each buttock using the Z-track technique. (Z-track injection keeps the iron dextran deep in the muscle, thereby minimizing leakage and surface discoloration.) As with IV iron dextran, a small test dose should precede the full therapeutic dose.

GUIDELINES FOR TREATING IRON DEFICIENCY

Assessment. Prior to initiation of therapy, the cause of iron deficiency must be determined. This information is required if treatment is to be appropriate. Potential causes of iron deficiency include pregnancy, bleeding, inadequate diet, and, rarely, reduced intestinal absorption.

The objective of therapy is to increase the production of hemoglobin and erythrocytes. When therapy is successful, reticulocytes will increase within 4 to 7 days; within 1 week, increases in hemoglobin and the hematocrit will be apparent; and within 1 month, hemoglobin levels will rise by at least 2 gm/dl. If these responses fail to occur, the patient should be evaluated for (1) compliance, (2) continued bleeding, (3) inflammatory disease (which can interfere with hemoglobin production), and (4) malabsorption of oral iron.

Routes of Administration. Iron preparations are available for oral, intravenous, and intramuscular administration. Oral iron (e.g., ferrous sulfate) is preferred to parenteral iron (iron dextran). Oral administration is safer than parenteral administration while being just as effective. Parenteral iron should be used only when oral iron is ineffective or intolerable. Of the two parenteral routes, IV is safer and preferred.

Duration of Therapy. Therapy with oral iron should be continued until hemoglobin levels become normal (about 15 gm/dl). This phase of treatment may require 1 to 2 months. After this time, continued treatment can help to replenish stores of ferritin. However, for most patients, diet alone is sufficient to replenish these stores.

Therapeutic Combinations. As a rule, combinations of antianemic agents should be avoided. Combining oral iron with parenteral iron can lead to iron toxicity. Accordingly, use of oral iron should cease prior to giving iron injections. Combinations of iron with vitamin B_{12} or folic acid should be avoided; these combinations can confuse interpretation of hematologic responses.

VITAMIN B_{12} DEFICIENCY

The term *vitamin B_{12}* refers not to a single agent but rather to a group of compounds that have very similar structures. These compounds are large molecules that contain an atom of cobalt. Because of this cobalt atom, members of the vitamin B_{12} family are known as *cobalamins*.

The most prominent consequences of vitamin B_{12} deficiency are *anemia* and *injury to the nervous system*. Anemia reverses rapidly following vitamin B_{12} administration. Neurologic damage takes longer for repair and, in some cases, may never fully reverse. Additional effects of B_{12} deficiency include GI disturbances and impaired production of white blood cells and platelets.

BIOCHEMISTRY AND PHYSIOLOGY OF VITAMIN B_{12}

In order to understand the consequences of vitamin B_{12} deficiency and the rationale behind therapy, we must first understand the normal biochemistry and physiology of this vitamin. This background information is reviewed below.

Metabolic Function

Vitamin B_{12} is essential for synthesis of DNA. Accordingly, vitamin B_{12} is required for the growth and division of virtually all cells in the body. The mechanism by which this vitamin influences DNA synthesis is depicted in Figure 47–3. As indicated, vitamin B_{12} helps catalyze the conversion of folic acid to its active form. Active folic acid then participates in several reactions essential for DNA synthesis. Hence, *it is by permitting utilization of folic acid that vitamin B_{12} influences cell growth and division*—and it is the absence of usable folic acid that underlies the blood cell abnormalities seen during vitamin B_{12} deficiency.

Fate in the Body

Absorption. Absorption of vitamin B_{12} requires the presence of *intrinsic factor*, a compound secreted by parietal cells of the stomach. Following ingestion, vitamin B_{12} forms a complex with intrinsic factor. Upon reaching the ileum, the B_{12}–intrinsic factor complex interacts with specific receptors on the intestinal wall, causing the complex to be absorbed. In the absence of intrinsic factor, absorption of vitamin B_{12} is nearly impossible.

Distribution and Storage. Following absorption, the complex of vitamin B_{12} with intrinsic factor dissociates. Free B_{12} then binds to *transcobalamin II* for transport via the blood to tissues. Most vitamin B_{12} goes to the liver and is stored. Total body stores of B_{12} are minute, ranging from 1 to 10 mg.

Elimination. Excretion of vitamin B_{12} takes place at an extremely slow rate; daily losses are on the order of only 0.05% of total body stores. Because B_{12} is excreted so slowly, *years* are required for B_{12} deficiency to develop—even when virtually no replenishment of lost B_{12} has been taking place.

Daily Requirements

Because very little vitamin B_{12} is excreted, and because body stores are small to begin with, daily requirements for this vitamin are miniscule. The average adult needs only 3 μg of B_{12} per day. Children need even less.

Dietary Sources

The ability to biosynthesize vitamin B_{12} is limited to microorganisms; higher plants and animals are unable to synthesize this compound. The organisms that make B_{12} reside in the soil, sewage, and the intestines of humans and other animals. Unfortunately, vitamin B_{12} produced in the human GI tract is unavailable for absorption. Consequently, humans must obtain the majority of their B_{12} by consuming animal products. Liver and dairy products are especially good sources.

VITAMIN B_{12} DEFICIENCY: CAUSES, CONSEQUENCES, AND DIAGNOSIS

Causes

In the majority of cases, vitamin B_{12} deficiency is the result of impaired absorption. Insufficient B_{12} in the diet is rarely a cause of deficiency. Potential causes of poor absorption include (1) regional enteritis, (2) celiac disease (a malabsorption syndrome involving abnormalities in the intestinal villi), and (3) development of antibodies directed against the vitamin B_{12}–intrinsic factor complex.

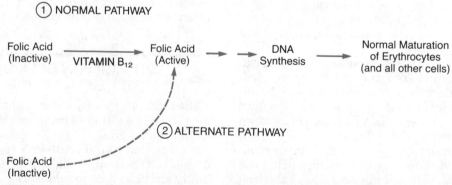

Figure 47–3. Relationship of folic acid and vitamin B_{12} to DNA synthesis and cell maturation. Folic acid, an essential factor for DNA synthesis, requires activation to be usable. ① Under normal circumstances, activation of folic acid occurs via a vitamin B_{12}–dependent pathway. Hence, vitamin B_{12} deficiency prevents folic acid utilization, resulting in defective DNA synthesis and disruption of cell growth and division. ② When folic acid is present in large amounts, activation can occur via an alternative pathway, thereby bypassing the requirement for vitamin B_{12}.

Most frequently, impaired absorption of vitamin B_{12} occurs secondary to a lack of intrinsic factor. The principal causes of intrinsic factor deficiency are atrophy of gastric parietal cells and surgery of the stomach (total gastric resection).

When vitamin B_{12} deficiency is caused by an absence of intrinsic factor, the resulting syndrome is called *pernicious anemia*—a term suggesting a highly destructive or fatal condition. Pernicious anemia is an old term that refers back to the days when, for most patients, vitamin B_{12} deficiency had no effective therapy. Hence, the condition was uniformly fatal. Today, vitamin B_{12} deficiency secondary to lack of intrinsic factor can be managed successfully. Hence, the label *pernicious* no longer bears its original ominous connotation.

Consequences

Many of the consequences of vitamin B_{12} deficiency result from disruption of DNA synthesis. Tissues that are affected most are those that have a high proportion of cells undergoing growth and division. Accordingly, vitamin B_{12} deficiency has profound effects on the bone marrow (the site where blood cells are produced) and on the epithelial cells lining the mouth and GI tract.

Megaloblastic Anemia. The most conspicuous consequence of vitamin B_{12} deficiency is an anemia in which large numbers of *megaloblasts* (oversized erythroblasts) appear in the bone marrow, and in which *macrocytes* (oversized erythrocytes) appear in the blood. These strange cells are produced because of impaired DNA synthesis: lacking sufficient DNA, growing cells are unable to divide; hence, as erythroblasts mature and their division is prevented, oversized cells result. Most megaloblasts die within the bone marrow; only a few evolve into the macrocytes that can be seen in the systemic circulation. Because of these unusual cells, the anemia associated with vitamin B_{12} deficiency is often referred to as either *megaloblastic* or *macrocytic* anemia.

Severe anemia is the manifestation of B_{12} deficiency that is most likely to prove fatal. Anemia causes peripheral and cerebral hypoxia. Heart failure and dysrhythmias are the most frequent causes of death.

It is important to note that the hematologic effects of vitamin B_{12} deficiency can be reversed with large doses of folic acid. As indicated in Figure 47–3, when folic acid is present in large amounts, some of it can be activated by a pathway that is independent of vitamin B_{12} (pathway ② in the figure). This route of activation bypasses the metabolic block caused by vitamin B_{12} deficiency, thereby permitting DNA synthesis to proceed.

Neurologic Damage. Deficiency of vitamin B_{12} causes demyelination of neurons, primarily in the spinal cord and brain. This neuronal injury can produce a variety of signs and symptoms. Early manifestations include paresthesias (tingling, numbness) of the hands and feet and a reduction in deep tendon reflexes. Late-developing responses include loss of memory, mood changes, hallucinations, and psychosis. If vitamin B_{12} deficiency is prolonged, neurologic damage can become permanent.

The precise mechanism by which vitamin B_{12} deficiency results in neuronal damage is unknown. We do know, however, that *neurologic damage is not related to effects on folic acid or DNA*. That is to say, the mechanism that underlies neuronal damage is different from the mechanism by which vitamin B_{12} deficiency disrupts hematopoiesis. Consequently, although administration of large doses of folic acid can correct the hematologic consequences of vitamin B_{12} deficiency, folic acid will not affect the neurologic picture.

Other Effects. As noted above, vitamin B_{12} deficiency can adversely affect virtually all tissues in which a high proportion of cells are undergoing growth and division. Hence, in addition to disrupting the production of erythrocytes, lack of vitamin B_{12} also prevents the bone marrow from making leukocytes (white blood cells) and thrombocytes (platelets). Loss of these blood cells can lead to infection and spontaneous bleeding. Disruption of DNA synthesis can also suppress division of the cells that form the epithelial lining of the mouth, stomach, and intestine, thereby causing oral ulceration and a variety of gastrointestinal disturbances.

Diagnosis

When megaloblastic anemia occurs, it may be due to vitamin B_{12} deficiency or to other causes, especially a lack of folic acid. Hence, if therapy is to be appropriate, a definitive diagnosis must be made.

Two tests are particularly helpful for establishing a diagnosis of vitamin B_{12} deficiency. The first test is obvious: measurement of plasma B_{12} content. The second procedure, known as the Schilling test, measures vitamin B_{12} absorption. (The Schilling test is performed by administering a small dose of radiolabeled vitamin B_{12}, after which the urine is monitored for the appearance of radioactivity. If the urine remains free of radioactivity, we can conclude that vitamin B_{12} absorption is impaired.) The combination of megaloblastic anemia plus low plasma vitamin B_{12} plus evidence of B_{12} malabsorption permits a clear diagnosis of vitamin B_{12} deficiency.

VITAMIN B_{12} PREPARATIONS I: CYANOCOBALAMIN

Cyanocobalamin is a purified, crystalline form of vitamin B_{12}. This compound is the drug of choice for treating all forms of vitamin B_{12} deficiency.

Adverse Effects

Cyanocobalamin is generally devoid of serious adverse effects. One potential response, *hypokalemia*, may occur as a natural consequence of increased erythrocyte production. Erythrocytes incorporate significant amounts of potassium. Hence, as large numbers of new red cells are produced, levels of free potassium may fall.

Dosage and Administration

Parenteral. Parenteral forms of cyanocobalamin can be administered by *intramuscular* or *deep subcutaneous* injection. *Cyanocobalamin must not be given intravenously.* Intramuscular and SC injections rarely cause pain or other local reactions.

Parenteral administration is required for all patients who are unable to absorb oral vitamin B_{12}. If the cause of malabsorption is irreversible (e.g., parietal cell atrophy, total gastrectomy), parenteral therapy must be continued for life. A typical dosing schedule for megaloblastic anemia is 30 μg/day for 5 to 10 days followed by 100 to 200 μg monthly until remission is complete. After anemia has been corrected, the patient will require monthly maintenance doses of 100 μg lifelong.

Oral. Oral cyanocobalamin is employed almost exclusively as a dietary supplement. The usual supplemental dose is 6 μg/day. Oral preparations are not useful for treating B_{12} deficiency caused by malabsorption.

VITAMIN B_{12} PREPARATIONS II: MISCELLANEOUS PREPARATIONS

Hydroxocobalamin. Hydroxocobalamin is very similar to cyanocobalamin. Both drugs are alike in structure and therapeutic effects. Hydroxocobalamin differs from cyanocobalamin in that hydroxocobalamin can be administered only by IM injection. Of greater importance, hydroxocobalamin can stimulate the production of antibodies directed against the vitamin B_{12}–transcobalamin II complex. Accordingly, hydroxocobalamin is not recommended.

Liver Extracts. Liver extracts have large amounts of vitamin B_{12}. Although these extracts can be used to treat vitamin B_{12} deficiency, purified cyanocobalamin is by far the treatment of choice. Administration of liver extracts is by IM injection.

GUIDELINES FOR TREATING VITAMIN B_{12} DEFICIENCY

Route of B_{12} Administration. Parenteral administration is required for all patients who are unable to absorb vitamin B_{12} given orally. In this group are patients with pernicious anemia (i.e., lack of intrinsic factor) and those with ileal disease. The *oral* route is used only when intestinal absorption is unimpaired.

Treatment of Moderate B_{12} Deficiency. The primary manifestations of moderate B_{12} deficiency are megaloblasts in the bone marrow and macrocytes in peripheral blood. Moderate deficiency does not cause leukopenia, thrombocytopenia, or neurologic complications. Moderate deficiency can be managed with vitamin B_{12} alone; no other measures are required.

Treatment of Severe B_{12} Deficiency. Severe deficiency produces multiple effects, all of which must be attended to. Unlike mild B_{12} deficiency, in which erythrocytes are the only blood cells affected, severe deficiency disrupts production of all blood cells. Loss of erythrocytes leads to hypoxia, cerebrovascular insufficiency, and congestive heart failure; loss of leukocytes encourages infection; and loss of thrombocytes promotes bleeding. In addition to causing serious hematologic deficits, severe B_{12} deficiency has adverse effects on the nervous system and GI tract.

Treatment of severe deficiency involves the following: (1) IM injection of vitamin B_{12} and folic acid (the folic acid accelerates recovery of hematologic deficits); (2) administration of 2 to 3 units of packed red blood cells (to correct anemia quickly); (3) transfusion of platelets (to suppress bleeding); and (4) therapy with antibiotics if infection has developed.

Following treatment with vitamin B_{12} plus folic acid, recovery from anemia occurs quickly. Within 1 to 2 days, megaloblasts disappear from the bone marrow; within 3 to 5 days, reticulocyte counts become elevated; by the 10th day, the hematocrit begins to rise; and within 2 to 3 weeks, the hematocrit becomes normal.

Recovery from neurologic damage is slow and depends on how long the damage had been present. Patients with deficits that have been present for only 2 to 3 months tend to recover with relative haste. Patients with deficits that have been present for many months or for years recover more slowly: months may pass before *any* improvement is apparent, and complete recovery may never occur.

Long-Term Treatment. For patients who lack intrinsic factor, or who suffer from some other permanent cause of vitamin B_{12} malabsorption, *lifelong treatment with vitamin B_{12} is required.* These people must be made aware of their condition, and arrangements should be made to insure monthly receipt of an injection. During prolonged therapy, the effectiveness of treatment should be periodically assessed: plasma levels of vitamin B_{12} should be measured every 3 to 6 months, blood samples should be examined for the return of macrocytes, and blood counts should be performed.

Potential Hazard of Folic Acid. If care is not exercised, use of folic acid in patients with vitamin B_{12} deficiency can result in exacerbation of the neurologic consequences of vitamin B_{12} deficiency. Recall that folic acid, by itself, can reverse the hematologic effects of B_{12} deficiency—but will not alleviate neurologic deficits. By correcting the most obvious manifestation of B_{12} deficiency (anemia), folic acid can obscure the fact that a deficiency of B_{12} still exists. *By masking B_{12} deficiency, use of folic acid can lead to undertreatment with B_{12} itself, and can thereby permit neurologic damage to progress.* Clearly, folic acid is not a substitute for vitamin B_{12}, and vitamin B_{12} deficiency should never be treated with folic acid alone. Whenever folic acid is employed during treatment of vitamin B_{12} deficiency, extra care must be taken to insure that vitamin B_{12} dosage is adequate.

FOLIC ACID DEFICIENCY

In one respect, folic acid deficiency is identical to a vitamin B_{12} deficiency: in both states, *megaloblastic anemia* is the most conspicuous pathology. However, in other important ways, folic acid deficiency and vitamin B_{12} deficiency are dissimilar (Table 47–3 provides a summary). Consequently, when a patient presents with megaloblastic anemia, it is essential to determine whether the cause is a deficiency of folic acid, vitamin B_{12}, or both.

PHYSIOLOGY AND BIOCHEMISTRY OF FOLIC ACID

Metabolic Function

As we noted when discussing vitamin B_{12}, folic acid (also known as *folate*) is an essential factor for DNA synthesis; without folic acid, DNA replication and cell division become disrupted.

In order to be usable, dietary folic acid must first be converted into an active form. Under normal conditions, activation occurs via a pathway employing vitamin B_{12} (see Fig. 47–3). However, when large amounts of folate are ingested, some of this folic acid can be activated via an alternative pathway—one that does not employ vitamin B_{12}. Hence, even in the absence of vitamin B_{12}, if sufficient amounts of folic acid are consumed, active folate will be available for DNA synthesis.

Fate in the Body

Folic acid is absorbed in the early segment of the small intestine. Following absorption, folic acid is transported to the liver and other tissues, where it is either used or stored.

Folic acid in the liver undergoes extensive enterohepatic recirculation. That is, folate from the liver is excreted into the intestine, after which it is reabsorbed and then returned to the liver through the hepatic-portal circulation. This enterohepatic recirculation helps salvage up to 200 μg of folate/day. Accordingly, this process is an important means of maintaining folic acid stores.

In contrast to vitamin B_{12}, folic acid is not conserved rigidly; every day, significant amounts are excreted. As a result, if intake of folic acid were to cease, signs of deficiency would develop rapidly (within weeks if body stores were already low when intake stopped).

Daily Requirements

The RDA of folic acid is 200 μg/day for adult males, 180 μg/day for adult females who do *not* plan on becoming pregnant soon, and 400 μ/day if they *do* plan on becoming pregnant soon. The RDA increases to 400 μg/day during pregnancy and is 280

Table 47–3. Vitamin B_{12} Deficiency versus Folic Acid Deficiency		
	Vitamin B_{12} Deficiency	**Folic Acid Deficiency**
Usual cause	Vitamin B_{12} malabsorption from lack of intrinsic factor	Low dietary folic acid
Primary hematologic effect	Megaloblastic anemia	Megaloblastic anemia
Neurologic effect	Damage to brain and spinal cord	None
Diagnosis	Low plasma vitamin B_{12}; low vitamin B_{12} absorption (Schilling test)	Low plasma folic acid
Treatment (usual route)	Cyanocobalamin (IM)	Folic acid (PO)
Usual duration of therapy	Lifelong	Short-term

μg/day for nursing mothers. Individuals with malabsorption syndromes (e.g., tropical sprue) may require as much as 2000 μg (2 mg) per day; at these high doses, folate will be taken up in sufficient quantity despite impairment of absorption.

Dietary Sources

Folic acid is present in all foods. Green vegetables, liver, and yeast are especially rich sources. It should be noted, however, that with prolonged cooking, folic acid is destroyed.

FOLIC ACID DEFICIENCY: CAUSES, CONSEQUENCES, AND DIAGNOSIS

Causes

Folic acid deficiency has two principal causes: (1) poor diet (especially as seen in alcoholics), and (2) malabsorption secondary to intestinal disease. Rarely, certain drugs may cause folate deficiency.

Alcoholism. Alcoholism, either acute or chronic, may be the most common cause of folate deficiency. Deficiency results for two reasons: (1) insufficient folic acid in the diet, and (2) derangement of enterohepatic recirculation because of alcohol-induced injury to the liver. Fortunately, with improved diet and reduced alcohol consumption, alcohol-related folate deficiency can often be reversed.

Sprue. Sprue is an intestinal malabsorption syndrome that decreases folic acid uptake. Since sprue does not block folate absorption entirely, deficiency can be corrected by giving large doses of folic acid orally.

Drugs. Plasma levels of folic acid may be lowered by *oral contraceptives* and by two anticonvulsants: *phenytoin* and *primidone*. Activation of folic acid may be reduced by *trimethoprim* (an antibiotic) and by *pyrimethamine* (an antimalarial agent). However, none of these interactions is likely to be of clinical significance.

Consequences

With the important exception that folic acid deficiency does not injure the nervous system, the effects of folate deficiency are identical to those caused by deficiency of vitamin B_{12}. Hence, as with vitamin B_{12} deficiency, the most prominent consequence of folate deficiency is *megaloblastic anemia*. In addition, like vitamin B_{12} deficiency, lack of folic acid may result in leukopenia, thrombocytopenia, and damage to the oral and gastrointestinal mucosa. Since we have already observed that many of the consequences of vitamin B_{12} deficiency result from depriving cells of active folic acid, the similarities between folate deficiency and vitamin B_{12} deficiency should come as no surprise.

Diagnosis

When patients present with megaloblastic anemia, it is essential to distinguish between folic acid deficiency and vitamin B_{12} deficiency as causative factors. This distinction can be made by comparing plasma levels of folate and vitamin B_{12}. If folic acid levels are low and vitamin B_{12} levels are normal, a diagnosis of folic acid deficiency is suggested. Conversely, if folate levels are normal and B_{12} is low, B_{12} deficiency would be the likely diagnosis. A decision *against* folic acid deficiency would be strengthened if neurologic deficits were observed.

FOLIC ACID PREPARATIONS

Nomenclature

Nomenclature regarding folic acid preparations can be confusing and deserves comment. Two forms of folic acid are available. One form is *inactive* as administered (but undergoes activation once it has been absorbed). The second form is *active* to start with. Both forms of folic acid have several generic names: the *inactive form* is referred to as *folacin, folate, pteroylglutamic acid,* and *folic acid*; the *active* form is referred to as *leucovorin calcium, folinic acid,* and *citrovorum factor*. The inactive form is by far the most commonly used preparation.

Folic Acid (Pteroylglutamic Acid)

Chemistry. Folic acid is inactive as administered and cannot support DNA synthesis. Activation takes place rapidly following absorption.

Indications. Folic acid has three applications: (1) treatment of megaloblastic anemia resulting from folic acid deficiency, (2) prophylaxis of folate deficiency, especially during pregnancy and lactation, and (3) initial treatment of severe megaloblastic anemia resulting from vitamin B_{12} deficiency.

Adverse Effects. Oral folic acid is nontoxic. Massive dosages (e.g., as much as 15 mg/day) have been taken with no ill effects.

Warning. If taken in sufficiently large doses, folic acid can correct the hematologic consequences of vitamin B_{12} deficiency, thereby masking the fact that a deficiency in vitamin B_{12} still exists. Since folic acid will not prevent the neurologic consequences of vitamin B_{12} deficiency (despite correcting the hematologic picture), this masking effect may allow irreversible damage to the nervous system. To reduce the chances of this problem, folate should not be used indiscriminately; unless specifically indicated, consumption of folic acid should not exceed 0.1 mg/day. Furthermore, whenever folic acid is given to patients known to have a deficiency in vitamin B_{12}, special care must be taken to insure that the vitamin B_{12} dosage is adequate.

Drug Interactions. Folic acid is generally devoid of significant drug interactions. If taken in greatly excessive dosage, folic acid may decrease the effects of phenytoin (an anticonvulsant), thereby allowing seizures. A variety of drugs (oral contraceptives, phenytoin, primidone, trimethoprim, and pyrimethamine) may reduce the effectiveness of folic acid. However, these interactions are rarely of clinical significance.

Formulations and Routes of Administration. Folic acid [Folvite] is available in tablets (0.1 to 1.0 mg) and as an injection (5 and 10 mg/ml). The injection may be administered IM, IV, or SC. As a rule, oral therapy is preferred to parenteral. Injections are reserved for patients with severely impaired absorption.

Dosage. For treatment of folate-deficient megaloblastic anemia in adults, the usual oral dosage is 1 to 2 mg a day. Once clinical symptoms have resolved, a maintenance dosage of 0.4 mg/day is given. For prophylaxis during pregnancy and lactation, doses of 1.0 mg/day may be used.

Leucovorin Calcium (Folinic Acid)

Leucovorin calcium is an active form of folic acid used primarily as an adjunct to cancer chemotherapy. Leucovorin is *not* used routinely to correct folic acid deficiency. Although leucovorin *could* be used to treat folate deficiency, folic acid is just as effective and less expensive. The role of leucovorin in the treatment of cancer is discussed in Chapter 91.

GUIDELINES FOR TREATING FOLIC ACID DEFICIENCY

Choice of Treatment Modality. The modality for treating folic acid deficiency should be matched with the cause. If folic acid deficiency is due to poor diet, the deficiency should be corrected by dietary measures—not with drugs. Ingestion of one fresh vegetable or one glass of fruit juice a day will usually correct the deficiency. In contrast, when folate deficiency is the result of malabsorption, diet alone

cannot correct the deficiency, and a pharmaceutical preparation of folate will be needed.

Route of Administration. Oral administration is preferred for most patients. Unlike vitamin B_{12}, folic acid is rarely administered by injection. Even in the presence of intestinal disease, oral folic acid can be effective, providing that the dosage is sufficiently high.

Prophylactic Use of Folic Acid. Folic acid should be taken prophylactically only when clearly appropriate. The principal indications are pregnancy and lactation. Since folic acid may mask vitamin B_{12} deficiency, indiscriminate use of folate should be avoided.

Treatment of Severe Deficiency. Folic acid deficiency can produce severe megaloblastic anemia. To insure a rapid response, therapy should be initiated with an IM injection of folic acid and vitamin B_{12}. (Because of the metabolic interrelationship between folic acid and vitamin B_{12}, the combination of these agents helps accelerate recovery.) After the initial injection, treatment should be continued with folic acid alone. Folic acid should be given orally in a dosage of 1 to 2 mg/day for 1 to 2 weeks. After this, maintenance doses of 0.4 mg/day may be required.

Therapy is evaluated by monitoring the hematologic picture. When treatment has been effective, megaloblasts will disappear from the bone marrow within 48 hours; the reticulocyte count will increase measurably within 2 to 3 days; and the hematocrit will begin to rise in the second week.

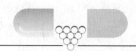

Summary of Major Nursing Implications

IRON PREPARATIONS

Ferrous Sulfate	Ferrous Gluconate
Ferrous Fumarate	Iron Dextran

Except where indicated, the implications summarized below apply to all of the iron preparations.

 Preadministration Assessment

Therapeutic Goal

Prevention or treatment of iron deficiency anemias.

Baseline Data

Prior to treatment, assess the degree of anemia. Fatigue, listlessness, and pallor indicate mild anemia; dyspnea, tachycardia, and angina suggest severe anemia. Laboratory findings indicative of anemia are subnormal hemoglobin levels, subnormal hematocrit, subnormal hemosiderin in bone marrow, and the presence of microcytic, hypochromic erythrocytes.

The cause of iron deficiency (e.g., pregnancy, occult bleeding, menorrhagia, inadequate diet, malabsorption) must be determined.

Identifying High-Risk Patients

All iron preparations are *contraindicated* for *patients with anemias other than iron-deficiency anemia.*

Iron dextran is *contraindicated* for *patients who have had a severe allergic reaction to this preparation in the past.*

Use *oral* preparations with *caution* in patients with *peptic ulcer disease, regional enteritis,* and *ulcerative colitis.*

 Implementation: Administration

Routes

Oral (ferrous sulfate, ferrous fumarate, ferrous gluconate).
Parenteral (iron dextran).

Oral Administration

Food reduces GI distress from oral iron but also greatly reduces absorption. Instruct the patient to administer oral iron between meals to maximize uptake. If GI distress is intolerable, the dosage may be reduced. If absolutely necessary, oral iron may be administered with meals.

Liquid preparations can stain the teeth. Instruct the patient to dilute liquid preparations with juice or water, administer them through a straw, and rinse the mouth afterward.

Warn the patient not to crush or chew sustained-release preparations.

Warn the patient against ingesting iron salts together with antacids or tetracyclines.

Inform the patient that oral iron salts are not identical. Warn the patient against changing from one salt to another.

Parenteral Administration

Iron dextran may be given IV and IM. Intravenous administration is safer and preferred.

Intravenous. To minimize anaphylactic reactions, follow this protocol: (1) inject 1 or 2 drops as a test dose and observe the patient for at least 15 minutes, (2) if the test dose appears safe, infuse 500 mg over 10 to 15 minutes, (3) if the 500-mg dose proves uneventful, give additional doses as needed.

Intramuscular. Intramuscular injection can cause significant adverse reactions (anaphylaxis, persistent pain, localized discoloration, promotion of tumors) and is generally avoided. Make injections deep into each buttock using the Z-track technique. Give a small test dose before giving the full therapeutic dose.

Advise the patient whose diet is poor in iron to increase consumption of iron-rich foods (e.g., liver, egg yolks, brewer's yeast, wheat germ, muscle meats, fish, fowl).

Implementation: Measures to Enhance Therapeutic Effects

Ongoing Evaluation and Interventions

Evaluating Therapeutic Responses

Evaluate treatment by monitoring the blood. Reticulocyte number should increase within 4 to 7 days, hemoglobin content and the hematocrit should begin to rise within 1 week, and hemoglobin levels should rise by at least 2 gm/dl within 1 month. If these responses do not occur, evaluate the patient for compliance, persistent bleeding, inflammatory disease, and malabsorption.

Minimizing Adverse Effects

Gastrointestinal Disturbances. Forewarn patients about possible GI reactions (nausea, vomiting, constipation, diarrhea) and inform them that these will diminish over time. If GI distress is severe, the dosage may be reduced, or, if absolutely necessary, iron may be administered with food.

Forewarn patients that iron will impart a harmless dark green or black coloration to stools.

Anaphylactic Reactions. Parenteral *iron dextran* can cause potentially fatal anaphylaxis. Before giving the drug, insure that injectable epinephrine and facilities for resuscitation are immediately available. After administration, observe the patient for 60 minutes. Follow the administration protocol described above.

Management of Acute Toxicity

Iron poisoning can be fatal to young children. Instruct parents to store iron out of reach and in child-proof containers. If poisoning occurs, rapid treatment is imperative. Induce vomiting to remove iron from the stomach. Administer deferoxamine if plasma levels of iron exceed 500 µg/ml. Manage acidosis and shock as required.

CYANOCOBALAMIN (VITAMIN B₁₂)

Preadministration Assessment

Therapeutic Goal

Correction of megaloblastic anemia and other sequelae of vitamin B₁₂ deficiency.

Baseline Data

Assess the extent of vitamin B_{12} deficiency. Record signs and symptoms of anemia (e.g., pallor, dyspnea, palpitations, fatigue). Determine the extent of neurologic damage. Assess GI involvement.

Baseline laboratory data include plasma vitamin B_{12} levels, erythrocyte and reticulocyte counts, and hemoglobin and hematocrit values. Bone marrow may be examined for megaloblasts. The physician may order a Schilling test to assess vitamin B_{12} absorption.

Identifying High-Risk Patients

Use with *caution* in patients receiving *folic acid.*

✓ Implementation: Administration

Routes

Oral, IM, SC.

Parenteral administration is required for most patients. Oral administration is effective only for patients with modest dietary deficiency.

Administration

Most patients require monthly injections for life.

✓ Implementation: Measures to Enhance Therapeutic Effects

Promoting Compliance

Patients with permanent impairment of vitamin B_{12} absorption (e.g., those with pernicious anemia) require lifelong vitamin B_{12} therapy. As a result, compliance is a major concern. To promote compliance, educate patients about the nature of their condition and impress upon them the need for regular monthly injections. Schedule appointments conveniently.

Improving Diet

When vitamin B_{12} deficiency is not due to impaired absorption, a change in diet may accelerate recovery. Advise the patient to increase consumption of vitamin B_{12}–rich foods (e.g., muscle meats, dairy products).

✓ Ongoing Evaluation and Interventions

Evaluating Therapeutic Effects

Success is gaged by improvements in hematologic and neurologic status. Over a period of 2 to 3 weeks, megaloblasts should disappear, reticulocyte counts should rise, and the hematocrit should normalize. Neurologic damage may take months to improve; in some cases, full recovery may never occur.

For patients receiving long-term therapy, vitamin B_{12} levels should be measured every 3 to 6 months, and blood counts should be performed.

Minimizing Adverse Effects

Hypokalemia may develop during the first days of therapy. Monitor serum potassium levels and observe the patient for signs of potassium insufficiency (e.g., muscle weakness, dysrhythmias).

Minimizing Adverse Interactions

Folic acid can mask hematologic symptoms of vitamin B_{12} deficiency, resulting in undertreatment and progression of neurologic injury from B_{12} insufficiency. When folic acid and cyanocobalamin are used concurrently, special care must be taken to insure that the cyanocobalamin dosage is adequate.

FOLIC ACID (FOLACIN, FOLATE, PTEROYLGLUTAMIC ACID)

 Preadministration Assessment

Therapeutic Goal

Folic acid is used for (1) treatment of megaloblastic anemia resulting from folic acid deficiency, (2) initial treatment of severe megaloblastic anemia resulting from vitamin B_{12} deficiency, and (3) prevention of folic acid deficiency (especially during pregnancy).

Baseline Data

Assess the extent of folate deficiency prior to treatment. Record signs and symptoms of anemia (e.g., pallor, dyspnea, palpitations, fatigue). Determine the extent of gastrointestinal damage.

Baseline laboratory data include serum folate levels, erythrocyte and reticulocyte counts, and hemoglobin and hematocrit values. In addition, bone marrow may be evaluated for megaloblasts. To rule out vitamin B_{12} deficiency, vitamin B_{12} determinations and a Schilling test may be ordered.

Identifying High-Risk Patients

Folic acid is *contraindicated* for patients with *pernicious anemia* (except during the acute phase of treatment). Inappropriate use of folic acid by these patients can mask signs of vitamin B_{12} deficiency, thereby allowing further neurologic deterioration.

 Implementation: Administration

Routes

Oral, SC, IV, and IM. Oral administration is most common and preferred. Injections are employed only when intestinal absorption is severely impaired.

 Implementation: Measures to Enhance Therapeutic Effects

Improving Diet

Advise the patient whose diet is deficient in folic acid to increase consumption of folate-rich foods (e.g., green vegetables, liver, yeast). Warn the patient that prolonged cooking destroys folic acid. If alcoholism underlies dietary deficiency, counseling should be offered.

 Ongoing Evaluation and Interventions

Evaluating Therapeutic Effects

Evaluate therapy by monitoring hematologic status. Within 2 weeks, megaloblasts should disappear, reticulocyte counts should increase, and the hematocrit should begin to rise.

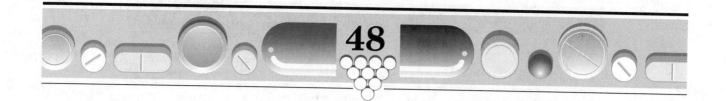

48

Hematopoietic Growth Factors

EPOETIN ALFA (ERYTHROPOIETIN)

FILGRASTIM (GRANULOCYTE COLONY-STIMULATING FACTOR)

SARGRAMOSTIM (GRANULOCYTE-MACROPHAGE COLONY-STIMULATING FACTOR)

Hematopoiesis is the process by which new blood cells are produced. This process is regulated in part by hematopoietic growth factors—naturally occurring hormones that (1) stimulate the proliferation and differentiation of hematopoietic stem cells, and (2) enhance function in the mature forms of those cells (neutrophils, monocytes, macrophages, and erythrocytes). In a laboratory setting, hematopoietic growth factors can cause stem cells to form colonies of mature blood cells. Because of this action, hematopoietic growth factors are also known as *colony-stimulating factors.* Therapeutic applications of hematopoietic growth factors include: (1) acceleration of neutrophil repopulation after cancer chemotherapy, (2) acceleration of bone marrow recovery after autologous bone marrow transplantation, and (3) stimulation of erythrocyte production in patients with chronic renal failure.

The names used for the hematopoietic growth factors are a potential source of confusion. At this time, three hematopoietic growth factors are available for clinical use. The *biologic* names of these three hormones are *erythropoietin, granulocyte colony-stimulating factor* (G-CSF), and *granulocyte-macrophage colony-stimulating factor* (GM-CSF). In addition to their biologic name, each compound has two types of *pharmacologic* names: a *generic* name and one or more *proprietary* (trade) names. The generic and trade names for the three growth factors are listed in Table 48–1. Keep in mind that the biologic, generic, and trade names for each compound all refer to the identical item.

613

Table 48–1. Nomenclature for Hematopoietic Growth Factors		
	Pharmacologic Names	
Biologic Name	**Generic Name**	**Trade Name**
Granulocyte colony-stimulating factor (G-CSF)	Filgrastim	Neupogen
Granulocyte-macrophage colony-stimulating factor (GM-CSF)	Sargramostim	Leukine, Prokine
Erythropoietin (EPO)	Epoetin alfa	Epogen, Procrit

EPOETIN ALFA (ERYTHROPOIETIN)

Epoetin alfa [Epogen, Procrit] is a drug produced by recombinant DNA technology. Chemically, the compound is a glycoprotein containing 165 amino acids. The protein portion of epoetin alfa is identical to that of human erythropoietin, a naturally occurring hormone. Epoetin alfa is used to maintain erythrocyte counts in (1) patients with chronic renal failure, (2) HIV-infected patients taking zidovudine, and (3) patients with nonmyeloid malignancies who have anemia secondary to chemotherapy.

Physiology

Erythropoietin is a glycoprotein hormone that stimulates production of red blood cells (erythrocytes). The hormone is produced by peritubular cells in the proximal tubules of the kidney. In response to anemia or hypoxia, circulating levels of erythropoietin rise dramatically, triggering an increase in erythrocyte synthesis. However, since production of erythrocytes requires iron, folic acid, and vitamin B_{12}, the response to erythropoietin will be minimal if any of these factors is deficient.

Therapeutic Uses

Anemia of Chronic Renal Failure. Epoetin alfa can reverse anemia associated with chronic renal failure (CRF). The drug is effective in patients on dialysis and in patients who do not yet require dialysis. Treatment virtually eliminates the need for transfusions. Initial effects can be seen within 1 to 2 weeks. The hematocrit reaches normal levels (30% to 33%) in 2 to 3 months. Patients experience an improved quality of life and increased energy levels. Unfortunately, treatment does not delay the progression of renal deterioration.

For therapy to be effective, iron stores must be adequate. Transferrin saturation should be at least 20%, and ferritin concentration should be at least 100 ng/ml. If pretreatment assessment shows these values to be low, they must be restored with iron supplements.

HIV-Infected Patients Taking Zidovudine. Epoetin alfa is approved for treating anemia caused by therapy with zidovudine (AZT) in patients with HIV infection (AIDS). For these patients, treatment can maintain or elevate erythrocyte counts, and reduce the need for transfusions. However, if endogenous levels of erythropoietin are at or above 500 mU/ml, raising them further with epoetin is not likely to be of benefit.

Chemotherapy-Induced Anemia. One formulation of epoetin [Procrit] is used to treat chemotherapy-induced anemia in patients with *nonmyeloid malignancies*, thereby reducing or eliminating the need for periodic transfusions. Since transfusions require hospitalization, whereas epoetin can be self-administered at home, epoetin therapy can spare patients considerable inconvenience. Because epoetin works slowly (the hematocrit may take 2 to 4 weeks to recover), transfusions are still indicated when rapid replenishment of red blood cells is required. Please note that epoetin is *not* approved for patients with *leukemias and other myeloid malignancies* because it may stimulate proliferation of these cancers.

Investigational Use. Epoetin has been used with success on an investigational basis to increase the harvest of red blood cells for autologous transfusion in patients anticipating elective surgery.

Pharmacokinetics

Epoetin alfa is administered parenterally (IV or SC). The drug cannot be given orally because, being a glycoprotein, it would be degraded in the gastrointestinal tract. The plasma half-life of the drug is highly variable and is not changed by dialysis.

Adverse Effects and Interactions

Epoetin alfa is generally well tolerated. Although the drug is a protein, no serious allergic reactions have been reported. The most significant adverse effect is hypertension. There are no significant drug interactions.

Hypertension. In patients with CRF, epoetin is frequently associated with an increase in blood pressure. The extent of hypertension is directly related to the rate of rise in the hematocrit. To minimize the risk of hypertension, blood pressure should be monitored and, if necessary, controlled with antihypertensive drugs. If hypertension cannot be controlled, the dosage of epoetin should be reduced. In patients with pre-existing hypertension (a common complication of CRF), it is imperative that blood pressure be under control prior to epoetin use. About 30% of dialysis patients receiving epoetin require an adjustment in their antihypertensive therapy once the hematocrit has been normalized.

Monitoring

The hematocrit should be determined prior to treatment and twice weekly thereafter until the target level has been reached and a maintenance dose established. Complete blood counts with a differential should be done routinely. Blood chemistry—BUN, uric acid, creatinine, phosphorous, and potassium—should be monitored. Iron should be measured periodically and maintained at an adequate level.

Preparations, Dosage, and Administration

Epoetin alfa [Epogen, Procrit] is dispensed in 1-ml vials (2000, 3000, 4000, and 10,000 units) for SC and IV injection. Vials should not be shaken; epoetin is a protein that can be denatured by agitation. Use only one dose per vial and discard the unused portion. Don't mix epoetin with other drugs. Store at 2°C to 8°C; don't freeze.

Patients With Chronic Renal Failure. Initial dosage is 50 to 100 U/kg 3 times a week. Administration is by IV bolus (for dialysis patients) and by IV bolus or SC injection (for nondialysis patients). Dosage should be reduced when the therapeutic endpoint is reached (hematocrit of 30% to 33%) or if the rate of rise in the hematocrit exceeds 4 units in 2 weeks. Once the target hematocrit has been achieved, an individualized maintenance dosage should be established: for dialysis patients, the median maintenance dosage is 75 U/kg 3 times a week; for nondialysis patients, the median maintenance dosage is 75 to 100 U/kg once a week. If the hematocrit rises above 36%, epoetin should be temporarily withheld.

HIV-Infected Patients Taking Zidovudine. Prior to treatment, measure the endogenous erythropoietin level. If this level is already at or above 500 mU/ml, epoetin alfa is unlikely to be of benefit.

Therapy is begun at 100 U/kg (IV or SC) three times a week. If the response is insufficient, the dosage may be increased by increments of 50 to 100 U/kg until a maximum of 300 U/kg 3 times a week has been reached. When the hematocrit has been restored to the desired level, an individualized maintenance dosage should be established.

Patients Receiving Cancer Chemotherapy. The initial dosage is 150 U/kg SC three times a week. If the response is inadequate by 8 weeks, the dosage may be increased to 300 U/kg three times a week.

FILGRASTIM (GRANULOCYTE COLONY-STIMULATING FACTOR)

Filgrastim [Neupogen] is a drug produced by recombinant DNA technology. This agent is essentially identical in structure and actions to human granulocyte colony- stimulating factor (G-CSF), a naturally occurring hormone. Filgrastim is used to reduce infection in patients undergoing cancer chemotherapy.

Physiology

G-CSF acts on cells in the bone marrow to increase production of neutrophils (granulocytes). In addition, it enhances phagocytic and cytotoxic actions of mature neutrophils. The hormone is produced by monocytes, fibroblasts, and endothelial cells in response to inflammation and allergic challenge. This suggests that the hormone's natural role is to help fight infections and cancer.

Therapeutic Uses

Patients Undergoing Cancer Chemotherapy. Filgrastim has been approved by the Food and Drug Administration (FDA) to reduce the risk of infection in patients undergoing cancer chemotherapy. Many anticancer drugs act on the bone marrow to suppress production of neutrophils, thereby greatly increasing the risk of infection. By stimulating production of neutrophils, filgrastim can decrease the risk of infection. Clinical trials have shown that the drug (1) reduces the incidence of severe neutropenia (absolute neutrophil counts below 500/mm^3), (2) produces a dose-dependent increase in circulating neutrophils, (3) reduces the incidence of infection, (4) reduces the need for hospitalization, and (5) reduces the need for intravenous antibiotics. Unfortunately, this useful drug is very expensive: the cost to the pharmacist for a single course of treatment is $1800 to $2800. Because the drug stimulates proliferation of bone marrow cells, it should not be used in patients with cancers that originated in the marrow.

Investigational Uses. Filgrastim can reverse *zidovudine-induced neutropenia* in HIV-infected patients. However, the drug does not reduce the incidence of opportunistic infections in these people.

Filgrastim provides effective treatment for *congenital neutropenia* (Kostmann's syndrome), a condition characterized by pronounced neutropenia and frequent, severe infections. Therapy causes resolution of existing infections and decreases the incidence of subsequent infections. Because treatment is chronic, the cost is extremely high.

Pharmacokinetics

Administration is parenteral (IV or SC). Filgrastim cannot be used orally because, being a protein, it would be destroyed in the gastrointestinal tract. Other aspects of the drug's kinetics are unremarkable.

Adverse Effects and Interactions

When used on a short-term basis, filgrastim is generally devoid of serious adverse effects. There are no drug interactions of note.

Bone Pain. Filgrastim causes bone pain in about 25% of those treated. Pain is dose-related and usually of mild-to-moderate intensity. In most cases, relief can be achieved with a nonopioid analgesic (e.g., acetaminophen). If not, an opioid may be tried.

Leukocytosis. When administered in doses greater than 5 μg/kg/day, filgrastim has caused white cell counts to rise above 100,000/mm³ in 2% of patients. Although no adverse effects were associated with this degree of leukocytosis, avoidance of leukocytosis would be prudent nonetheless. Excessive white cell counts can be avoided by obtaining complete blood counts twice weekly during treatment, and reducing filgrastim dosage if leukocytosis develops.

Other Adverse Effects. Treatment frequently causes elevation of plasma uric acid, lactate dehydrogenase, and alkaline phosphatase. These increases are usually moderate and reverse spontaneously. Long-term therapy has caused splenomegaly in some patients.

Preparations, Dosage, and Administration

Filgrastim [Neupogen] is dispensed in solution (300 μg/ml) in 1- and 1.6-ml vials. Administration is IV and SC. The usual dosage is 5 μg/kg once daily. Therapy should start no sooner than 24 hours after termination of chemotherapy, and should continue for up to 2 weeks after the expected chemotherapy-induced nadir, or until the absolute neutrophil count has reached 10,000/mm³. The drug is stored at 2° to 8°C—not frozen. Prior to administration, filgrastim can be kept at room temperature for up to 6 hours. It should not be agitated. Only 1 dose per vial should be used, and the vial should not be re-entered. A complete blood count and platelet count should be obtained prior to treatment and twice weekly during treatment.

SARGRAMOSTIM (GRANULOCYTE-MACROPHAGE COLONY-STIMULATING FACTOR)

Sargramostim [Leukine, Prokine], like filgrastim and epoetin, is produced by recombinant DNA technology. This drug is nearly identical in structure and actions to human granulocyte-macrophage colony-stimulating factor (GM-CSF), a naturally occurring hormone. Sargramostim is given to accelerate bone marrow recovery in patients undergoing bone marrow transplants.

Physiology

GM-CSF acts on cells in the bone marrow to increase production of neutrophils, monocytes, macrophages, and eosinophils. In addition, the hormone acts on the mature forms of these cells to enhance their function. For example, GM-CSF acts on neutrophils and macrophages to increase their chemotactic, antifungal, and antiparasitic actions. Also, the hormone acts on monocytes and polymorphonuclear leukocytes to enhance their actions against cancer cells. GM-CSF is synthesized by T lymphocytes, monocytes, fibroblasts, and endothelial cells. Like G-CSF, GM-CSF is produced in response to inflammation and allergic challenge, suggesting that its natural role is to help fight infections and cancers.

Therapeutic Uses

Adjunct to Autologous Bone Marrow Transplantation. Sargramostim can accelerate myeloid recovery in cancer patients who have undergone an autologous bone marrow transplant (BMT) following high-dose chemotherapy (with or without concurrent irradiation). The drug is approved for promoting myeloid recovery following BMT in patients with acute lymphoblastic leukemia, non-Hodgkin's lymphoma, and Hodgkin's disease. In these patients, sargramostim can (1) accelerate neutrophil engraftment, (2) reduce the duration of antibiotic use, (3) reduce the duration of infectious episodes, and (4) reduce the duration of hospitalization. Therapy is expensive: the cost to the pharmacist for a 21-day course of sargramostim is more than $4000.

Treatment of Failed Bone Marrow Transplants. Sargramostim is approved for patients in whom an autologous or allogenic BMT has failed to take. For these patients, the drug can produce a significant increase in survival time.

Investigational Uses. In *HIV-infected patients*, sargramostim can reverse neutropenia caused by zidovudine (a drug that inhibits HIV replication) and by ganciclovir (a drug for cytomegalovirus retinitis).

In patients with *aplastic anemia* (a syndrome characterized by pancytopenia and high mortality from infection and bleeding), sargramostim can increase neutrophil counts and reduce the incidence and severity of infections.

Sargramostim is beneficial for patients with *myelodysplastic syndrome* (MDS), a chronic disorder characterized by greatly reduced hematopoiesis. Patients with MDS are neutropenic, thrombocytopenic, and anemic, putting them at high risk for serious infections and bleeding. The syndrome has a mortality rate of 66%—and those who survive often develop leukemia. Treatment with sargramostim can increase counts of neutrophils, eosinophils, and monocytes. However, the premalignant clone still exists, and may eventually cause leukemia.

Pharmacokinetics

Sargramostim is administered by IV infusion. Since the drug is a protein and would be degraded in the digestive tract, it cannot be administered by mouth. Other aspects of the drug's kinetics are unremarkable.

Adverse Effects and Interactions

Sargramostim is generally well tolerated. A variety of acute reactions have been observed, including *diarrhea, weakness, rash, malaise,* and *bone pain* that can be managed with nonopioid analgesics (e.g., acetaminophen). *Pleural and pericardial effusions* have occurred, but only when sargramostim dosage was massive (16 times the recommended dosage). There are no drug interactions of note.

Leukocytosis and Thrombocytosis. Stimulation of the bone marrow can produce excessive elevations in white blood cells and platelets. Complete blood counts should be done twice weekly during therapy. If the white cell count rises above 50,000/mm^3, if the absolute neutrophil count rises above 20,000/mm^3, or if the platelet count rises above 500,000/mm^3, sargramostim should be interrupted or the dosage reduced.

Preparations, Dosage, and Administration

Preparations. Sargramostim [Leukine, Prokine] is dispensed as a powder (250 and 500 μg) in single-use vials to be reconstituted for IV infusion.

Reconstitution and Storage. To reconstitute the powder, add 1 ml of sterile water and swirl gently; don't shake. To prepare the final solution for infusion, dilute the reconstituted concentrate in either (1) 0.9% sodium chloride (if the final concentration of sargramostim is to be 10 μg/ml or more) or in (2) 0.9% sodium chloride plus 0.1% albumin (if the final concentration is to be less than 10 μg/ml). Since the solution contains no antibacterial preservatives, it should be used as soon as possible—and no later than 6 hours after preparation. Sargramostim (powder, reconstituted concentrate, final IV solution) should be kept at 2° to 8° C (never frozen) until used.

Dosage and Administration. For acceleration of myeloid recovery after an autologous bone marrow transplant, the recommended dosage is 250 μg/m^2 (as a 2-hour IV infusion) administered once daily for 21 days beginning 2 to 4 hours after the bone marrow infusion.

For patients in whom an autologous or allogenic bone marrow transplant has failed or in whom engraftment has been delayed, the recommended dosage is 250 μg/m^2 (as a 2-hour IV infusion) administered once daily for 14 days. After a 7-day drug-free interval, the 14-day series of infusions can be repeated if needed. After another 7-day interval, the 14-day series can be repeated once more if needed. If the graft still has not taken, further treatment is unlikely to be of benefit.

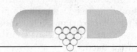

Summary of Major Nursing Implications

EPOETIN ALFA (ERYTHROPOIETIN)

 Preadministration Assessment

Therapeutic Goal

Restoration and maintenance of erythrocyte counts in (1) patients with chronic renal failure, (2) HIV-infected patients receiving zidovudine, and (3) cancer chemotherapy patients.

Baseline Data

All Patients. Obtain blood pressure, blood chemistry (BUN, uric acid, creatinine, phosphorus, potassium), complete blood counts with differential and platelet count, hematocrit, degree of transferrin saturation (should be at least 20%), and ferritin concentration (should be at least 100 ng/ml).

HIV-Infected Patients. Obtain an erythropoietin level. (If the level is already above 500 mU/ml, epoetin is unlikely to be of help.)

Identifying High-Risk Patients

Epoetin alfa is *contraindicated* for patients with *uncontrolled hypertension, hypersensitivity to mammalian cell-derived products or albumin*, and *cancers of myeloid origin*.

 Implementation: Administration

Routes

Subcutaneous, intravenous.

Handling and Storage

Epoetin alfa is dispensed in single-use vials; don't re-enter the vial; discard the unused portion. Don't agitate. Don't mix with other drugs. Store at 2° to 8° C; don't freeze.

Administration and Dosage

Patients with Chronic Renal Failure. Initial dosage is 50 to 100 U/kg three times a week. For dialysis patients, administer by IV bolus. For nondialysis patients, administer by IV bolus or SC injection.

If the rate of rise in the hematocrit exceeds 4 units in 2 weeks, reduce the dosage. When the therapeutic endpoint is reached (hematocrit of 30% to 33%), reduce the dosage to maintenance amount: for dialysis patients, the median maintenance dosage is 75 U/kg three times a week; for nondialysis patients, the median maintenance dosage is 75 to 100 U/kg once a week. If the hematocrit rises above 36%, temporarily withhold epoetin.

HIV-Infected Patients Taking Zidovudine. Initial dosage is 100 U/kg (IV or SC) three times a week. If the rise in the hematocrit is insufficient, increase the dosage by increments of 50 to 100 U/kg until a maximum of 300

U/kg three times a week has been reached. Establish an individualized maintenance dosage once the therapeutic endpoint is achieved.

Cancer Chemotherapy Patients. Initial dosage is 150 U/kg three times a week.

Ongoing Evaluation and Interventions

Monitoring Summary

Determine the hematocrit twice weekly until the target level has been reached and a maintenance dosage established. Obtain complete blood counts with a differential and platelet counts routinely. Monitor blood chemistry, including BUN, uric acid, creatinine, phosphorus, potassium. Monitor iron stores and maintain at an adequate level. Monitor blood pressure.

Minimizing Adverse Effects

Hypertension. Monitor blood pressure and, if necessary, control with antihypertensive drugs. If hypertension cannot be controlled, reduce epoetin dosage. In patients with pre-existing hypertension (a common complication of chronic renal failure), make certain that blood pressure is controlled prior to epoetin use.

FILGRASTIM
(GRANULOCYTE COLONY-STIMULATING FACTOR)

Preadministration Assessment

Therapeutic Goal

Filgrastim is given to reduce the risk of infection in cancer patients by accelerating neutrophil recovery following high-dose chemotherapy.

Baseline Data

Obtain complete blood counts and platelet counts.

Identifying High-Risk Patients

Filgrastim is *contraindicated* for patients with *hypersensitivity to E. Coli–derived proteins.*

Implementation: Administration

Routes

Subcutaneous, intravenous.

Handling and Storage

Filgrastim is dispensed in single-use vials; don't re-enter the vial; discard the unused portion. Don't agitate. Store at 2° to 8°C; don't freeze. Prior to administration, filgrastim may be kept at room temperature for up to 6 hours.

Administration

Begin treatment no sooner than 24 hours after termination of chemotherapy and continue for up to 2 weeks after the expected chemotherapy-induced nadir, or until the absolute neutrophil count has reached 10,000/mm³.

Ongoing Evaluation and Interventions

Evaluating Therapeutic Effects

Obtain complete blood counts twice weekly. Discontinue treatment when the absolute neutrophil count reaches 10,000/mm³.

Minimizing Adverse Effects

Bone Pain. Evaluate for bone pain and treat with a nonopioid analgesic (e.g., acetaminophen). Consider a more powerful (opioid) analgesic if pain is not relieved.

Leukocytosis. Massive doses of filgrastim can cause leukocytosis (white blood cell counts above 100,000/mm³). If leukocytosis develops, reduce filgrastim dosage.

SARGRAMOSTIM (GRANULOCYTE-MACROPHAGE COLONY-STIMULATING FACTOR)

Preadministration Assessment

Therapeutic Goal

Acceleration of myeloid recovery in cancer patients who have undergone an autologous bone marrow transplant following high-dose chemotherapy (with or without concurrent irradiation).

Treatment of patients for whom an autologous or allogenic bone marrow transplant has failed to take.

Baseline Data

Obtain complete blood counts with differential and platelet count.

Identifying High-Risk Patients

Sargramostim is *contraindicated* in the presence of *hypersensitivity to yeast-derived products* and *excessive leukemic myeloid blasts in bone marrow or peripheral blood*. Exercise *caution* in patients with *cardiac disease*, *hypoxia*, *peripheral edema*, or *pleural or pericardial effusion*.

Implementation: Administration

Route

Intravenous (by infusion).

Handling, Reconstitution, and Storage

Sargramostim is dispensed in single-use vials; don't re-enter the vial; discard the unused portion. Don't agitate. Don't mix with other drugs.

To reconstitute, add 1 ml of sterile water and swirl gently; don't shake. To prepare the final solution for infusion, dilute the reconstituted concentrate in either 0.9% sodium chloride (if the final concentration of sargramostim is to be 10 μg/ml or more) *or* in 0.9% sodium chloride plus 0.1% albumin (if the final concentration is to be less than 10 μg/ml). Administer as soon as possible—and no later than 6 hours after preparation.

Store sargramostim (powder, reconstituted concentrate, final IV solution) at 2° to 8° C until used.

Administration and Dosage

For acceleration of myeloid recovery after an autologous bone marrow transplant, give 250 μg/m² (as a 2-hour IV infusion) once daily for 21 days beginning 2 to 4 hours after the bone marrow infusion.

For patients in whom an autologous or allogenic bone marrow transplant has failed, give 250 μg/m² (as a 2-hour IV infusion) once daily for 14 days.

After a 7-day drug-free interval, the 14-day series of infusions can be repeated if needed. After another 7-day interval, the 14-day series can be repeated once more if needed.

Minimizing Adverse Effects

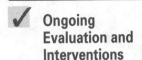
Ongoing Evaluation and Interventions

Leukocytosis and Thrombocytosis. Obtain complete blood counts with a differential and platelet counts twice weekly. If the white blood cell count rises above 50,000/mm^3, if the absolute neutrophil count rises above 20,000/mm^3, or if the platelet count rises above 500,000/mm^3, temporarily interrupt sargramostim or reduce its dosage.

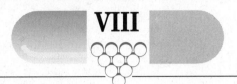

VIII

Endocrine Drugs

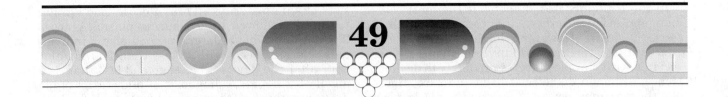

Drug Therapy of Diabetes

Our topic in this chapter is drug therapy of diabetes mellitus. We will begin by discussing diabetes itself, after which we will focus on insulin, the principal drug used for treatment. We will also discuss the oral hypoglycemic agents, a group of second-line antidiabetic drugs.

DIABETES MELLITUS: OVERVIEW OF THE DISEASE AND ITS TREATMENT

The term *diabetes mellitus* is derived from the Greek word for *fountain* and the Latin word for *honey*. Hence, the name *diabetes mellitus* describes one of the prominent symptoms of untreated diabetes: production of large volumes of glucose-rich urine. In this chapter we will use the term *diabetes mellitus* interchangeably with the term *diabetes*.

Diabetes is primarily a disorder of carbohydrate metabolism. Symptoms result from a deficiency of insulin or from resistance to insulin's actions. The principal characteristics of diabetes are (1) elevation of fasting blood glucose, (2) glycosuria, and (3) reduced glucose tolerance (i.e., reduced ability to respond appropriately to massive glucose intake). In addition to its effects on carbohydrate metabolism, diabetes is associated with derangements of protein and fat metabolism. Chronic diabetes can result in blindness, kidney disease, neuropathy, and accelerated atherosclerosis.

625

In the United States, diabetes is the most common endocrine disorder, and the third leading cause of death. However, thanks to recent advances in treatment, morbidity and mortality associated with chronic diabetes are likely to decline. Hence, although diabetes still has no cure, rigorous therapy may permit a productive life of near normal duration and quality.

DIAGNOSIS

Elevation of plasma glucose levels is the principal diagnostic sign of diabetes. In nondiabetics, *fasting* glucose levels are less than 115 mg/dl. If fasting glucose levels routinely exceed 140 mg/dl, diabetes is indicated.

When measurement of fasting blood glucose is insufficient to make a definitive diagnosis, a *glucose tolerance test* can be performed. This test consists of administering an oral glucose load (75 gm to adults) followed by measuring plasma glucose levels 1 and 2 hours later. In nondiabetic individuals, glucose levels will be less than 200 mg/dl 1 hour after the glucose challenge and less than 140 mg/dl at 2 hours. A diagnosis of diabetes is made if plasma glucose levels exceed 200 mg/dl for *both* the 1-hour and 2-hour determinations.

TYPES OF DIABETES MELLITUS

There are two principal forms of diabetes: (1) insulin-dependent diabetes mellitus (IDDM), and (2) noninsulin-dependent diabetes mellitus (NIDDM). Several less common forms (e.g., gestational diabetes) have also been identified. The distinguishing characteristics of IDDM and NIDDM are summarized in Table 49–1 and discussed below.

Table 49–1. Characteristics of the Major Forms of Diabetes Mellitus

Characteristics	Type of Diabetes Mellitus	
	Insulin-Dependent (IDDM)	*Noninsulin-Dependent (NIDDM)*
Alternative names	Type I diabetes mellitus, juvenile-onset diabetes mellitus, ketosis-prone diabetes mellitus	Type II diabetes mellitus, adult-onset diabetes mellitus
Age of onset	Usually childhood or adolescence	Usually over age 35
Speed of onset	Abrupt	Gradual
Family history	Usually negative	Frequently positive
Prevalence	5% to 10% of diabetics have IDDM	90% of diabetics have NIDDM
Etiology	Unknown. Possible causes include heredity, viral infection, and autoimmune disease	Unknown—but there is a strong familial association, suggesting heredity as the underlying cause
Primary defect	Loss of pancreatic beta cells	Insulin resistance and/or inappropriate insulin secretion
Insulin levels	Reduced early in the disease, and completely absent later	Levels may be low (indicating deficiency), normal, or high (indicating resistance)
Treatment	Insulin replacement is mandatory, along with strict dietary control; oral hypoglycemic drugs are not effective	Exercise and a reduced calorie diet may be sufficient; if not, an oral hypoglycemic agent or insulin is required
Blood glucose	Levels fluctuate widely in response to infection, exercise, and changes in caloric intake and insulin dose	Levels are more stable than in IDDM
Symptoms	Polyuria, polydipsia, polyphagia, weight loss	May be asymptomatic
Body composition	Usually thin and undernourished	Frequently obese
Ketosis	Common, especially if insulin dosage is insufficient	Uncommon

Insulin-Dependent Diabetes Mellitus

IDDM accounts for 5% to 10% of all cases of diabetes. Approximately 1 million Americans have this disorder. IDDM is known by three alternative names: *type I diabetes mellitus, juvenile-onset diabetes mellitus,* and *ketosis-prone diabetes mellitus.* As a rule, IDDM develops during childhood or adolescence. Onset of symptoms is usually abrupt.

The primary defect in IDDM is *destruction of pancreatic beta cells*—the cells responsible for insulin synthesis. Insulin levels are *reduced* early in the disease and *completely absent* later. The underlying cause of beta cell destruction is not known. Suggested causes include viral infection and autoimmunity (development of antibodies directed against the patient's own beta cells). In addition, genetic factors appear to predispose certain individuals to IDDM.

Noninsulin-Dependent Diabetes Mellitus

NIDDM is the most prevalent form of diabetes. Approximately 10 million Americans (about 5% of the population) are known to have this disease. NIDDM has two alternative names: *type II diabetes mellitus* and *adult-onset diabetes mellitus.* The disease usually begins in middle age and progresses gradually. Obesity is almost always present. In contrast to IDDM, NIDDM carries little risk of ketoacidosis. However, NIDDM does carry the same long-term risks as IDDM (see below).

Symptoms result from a combination of insulin resistance and failure of appropriate insulin secretion. In contrast to patients with IDDM, patients with NIDDM are capable of insulin synthesis. In fact, insulin levels tend to be normal or even slightly elevated. However, although insulin is still produced, its secretion is no longer tightly coupled to plasma glucose content: release of insulin is delayed and peak output is subnormal. Furthermore, the target tissues of insulin (liver, muscle, adipose tissue) exhibit insulin resistance. Resistance appears to result from two causes: (1) reduced binding of insulin to its receptors, and (2) reduced receptor responsiveness. Although the underlying cause of NIDDM is not known, there is a strong familial association, suggesting that heredity may be a major factor.

OVERVIEW OF TREATMENT

Insulin-Dependent Diabetes Mellitus

The goal of therapy is to maintain glucose levels within an acceptable range. This will prevent acute complications and will reduce or prevent long-term complications. Glycemic control is accomplished with an integrated program of *diet, exercise,* and *insulin replacement.*

Proper diet, balanced by insulin replacement, is the cornerstone of treatment. Since patients with IDDM are usually thin, the goal of diet is to maintain weight—not lose weight. The recommended diet consists of 55% to 60% carbohydrates (unrefined or fiber-containing refined), 15% protein, and no more than 30% fat (primarily unsaturated and monosaturated). Cholesterol should be limited to 300 mg/day. Total caloric intake should be spread evenly throughout the day, with meals spaced 4 to 5 hours apart.

Unless specifically contraindicated, regular exercise should be part of the treatment program. Exercise can increase cellular responsiveness to insulin, and may also increase glucose tolerance. Since strenuous exercise can produce hypoglycemia, close oversight is needed to establish a safe balance between exercise, glucose intake, and insulin dosage. Exercise should be avoided if glycemic control is unstable.

Survival requires daily administration of insulin. Before insulin replacement therapy became available, people with IDDM invariably died within a few years of the onset of disease; the cause of death was ketoacidosis. It is essential to coordinate insulin dosage with caloric intake. If caloric intake is too great or too small with respect to insulin dosage, hyperglycemia or hypoglycemia will result.

It should be noted that *oral hypoglycemic* agents (e.g., tolbutamide), which can be helpful for patients with NIDDM, are *not* effective for patients with IDDM.

Noninsulin-Dependent Diabetes Mellitus

As with IDDM, the goal of therapy with NIDDM is to maintain blood glucose levels within an acceptable range. However, for patients with NIDDM, the core of treatment is *diet and exercise alone*; insulin or oral hypoglycemics are employed only as adjuncts. Since patients are often obese, the usual dietary goal is to promote weight loss and establish a more lean body composition. Clinical experience has shown that dietary measures, by themselves, often normalize insulin release and decrease insulin resistance. Frequently, these beneficial responses precede loss of weight. Exercise provides the additional benefit of promoting glucose uptake by muscle, even when insulin is low or absent.

If diet and exercise fail to produce adequate glycemic control, pharmacotherapy will be needed. Either an *oral hypoglycemic agent* (e.g., tolbutamide) or *insulin* may be employed. It must be stressed, however, that drugs should be used only as a *supplement* to caloric restriction and exercise; drugs are not a substitute for the nondrug measures.

SHORT-TERM COMPLICATIONS OF DIABETES

Acute complications are seen primarily in patients with IDDM. Principal concerns are *hyperglycemia* and *hypoglycemia*. Hyperglycemia results when insulin dosage is insufficient. Conversely, hypoglycemia results when insulin dosage is excessive. *Ketoacidosis*, a potentially fatal acute complication, develops when hyperglycemia is allowed to persist. All three of these complications are discussed further later in the chapter.

LONG-TERM COMPLICATIONS OF DIABETES

The long-term sequelae of diabetes take years or even decades to develop. More than 90% of diabetic deaths result from long-term complications—not from hypoglycemia or ketoacidosis. Ironically, insulin can be viewed as having made long-term complications possible: prior to the discovery of insulin, diabetics died long before chronic disorders could arise. There is strong evidence linking most of the long-term complications to *chronic hyperglycemia*. Hence, with rigorous control of blood glucose, development of these disorders should be minimized.

Macrovascular Disease. Cardiovascular complications are the leading cause of death among diabetics. Diabetes carries an increased risk of *hypertension, myocardial infarction,* and *stroke.* Much of this pathology is due to atherosclerosis, which develops earlier in diabetics than in nondiabetics and progresses at an accelerated rate. Macrovascular complications appear to result primarily from alterations in lipid metabolism, rather than from hyperglycemia.

Microvascular Disease. *Microangiopathy* is common; the basement membrane of capillaries thickens, causing blood flow in the microvasculature to decline. Poor circulation can be prominent in the lower limbs, resulting in chronic skin ulcers and even gangrene. In addition, diabetic microangiopathy is a contributor to blindness and kidney disease (see below). Microvascular complications are directly related to the degree and duration of hyperglycemia.

Retinopathy. Diabetes is the major cause of blindness among American adults. Visual losses result most commonly from damage to retinal capillaries. Microaneurysms may occur, followed by scarring and proliferation of new vessels; the overgrowth of new retinal capillaries reduces visual acuity. Capillary damage may also impair vision by causing local ischemia, with resultant death of retinal cells. Retinopathy appears to be accelerated by hyperglycemia, hypertension, and smoking. Accordingly, these risk factors should be controlled or eliminated.

Nephropathy. Diabetic nephropathy is characterized by proteinuria, reduced glomerular filtration, and increased arterial blood pressure. This syndrome is the primary cause of morbidity and mortality in patients with IDDM. There is strong evidence that tight glycemic control can delay—or even reverse—renal dysfunction. Diabetic nephropathy can be managed by renal dialysis. If the injured kidney is replaced with a transplant, the new kidney is likely to fail within a few years unless tight control of diabetes is established.

Neuropathy. Nerve degeneration often begins early in the course of diabetes, but symptoms are usually absent for years. Both sensory and motor nerves may be affected. Symptoms of diabetic neuropathy include tingling sensations in the fingers and toes, pain, suppression of reflexes, and loss of sensation (especially vibratory sensation). Impotence in males is common. Although the cause of nerve damage is unknown, hyperglycemia and lack of insulin are likely candidates. Good glycemic control may partially restore nerve function.

Gastroparesis. Diabetic gastroparesis affects 20% to 30% of patients with long-standing diabetes. Manifestations include nausea, vomiting, delayed gastric emptying, and abdominal distention secondary to atony of the gastrointestinal (GI) tract. Injury to the autonomic nerves that control GI motility may be the underlying cause. Symptoms can be reduced with *metoclopramide* [Reglan], a drug that promotes gastric emptying.

DIABETES AND PREGNANCY

Before the discovery of insulin, virtually all babies born to diabetic mothers died during infancy. Although insulin therapy has greatly improved this picture, successful management of the diabetic pregnancy remains a challenge. Three factors contribute to the problem. First, the placenta produces hormones that can antagonize insulin's actions. Second, production of cortisol, a hormone that promotes hyperglycemia, increases threefold during pregnancy. Both of these factors increase the need for insulin. Third, since glucose can pass freely from the maternal circulation to the fetal circulation, hyperglycemia in the mother will stimulate secretion of fetal insulin; the resultant hyperinsulinemia can have multiple adverse effects on the developing fetus.

Successful management of the diabetic pregnancy demands that proper glucose levels be maintained in *both* the fetus and the mother; failure to do so may be teratogenic or otherwise detrimental to the fetus. Achieving glucose control requires diligence on the part of the mother and her physician.

Blood glucose levels must be monitored six to seven times a day. Insulin dosage and food intake must be adjusted accordingly.

Since fetal death occurs frequently near term, it is desirable that delivery take place as soon as development of the fetus will permit. Hence, when tests indicate sufficient fetal maturation, it is common practice to deliver the infant early—either by cesarean section or by induction of labor with drugs.

Gestational diabetes is defined as diabetes that appears during pregnancy and then subsides rapidly after delivery. Gestational diabetes is managed in much the same manner as any other diabetic pregnancy: blood glucose should be monitored and then controlled with insulin and diet. In most cases, the diabetic state disappears almost immediately after delivery. In these cases, insulin should be discontinued. If the diabetic condition persists beyond parturition, it is no longer considered gestational and should be rediagnosed and treated accordingly.

INSULIN

PHYSIOLOGY

Structure. The structure of insulin is depicted in Figure 49–1. As indicated, insulin consists of two amino acid chains: the "A" (acidic) chain and the "B" (basic) chain. The A and B chains are linked to each other by two disulfide bridges.

Biosynthesis. Insulin is synthesized in the pancreas by beta cells in the islets of Langerhans. The immediate precursor of insulin is called *proinsulin* (see Fig. 49–1). Proinsulin consists of insulin itself plus a peptide loop that runs from the A chain to the B chain. This loop is referred to as *connecting peptide* or *C-peptide*. In the final step of insulin synthesis, C-peptide is clipped from the proinsulin molecule.

Measurement of plasma C-peptide levels offers a way to assess residual capacity for insulin synthesis. Since commercial insulin preparations are devoid of C-peptide, and since endogenous C-peptide is only present as a by-product of insulin biosynthesis, the presence of C-peptide in the blood of a diabetic indicates that the pancreas is still producing some insulin of its own.

Secretion. The principal stimulus for insulin release is glucose. Under normal conditions, there is tight coupling between elevations in plasma glucose content and increased secretion of insulin. Insulin release may also be triggered by amino acids, fatty acids, and ketone bodies.

The sympathetic nervous system provides additional control of insulin release. Activation of beta$_2$-adrenergic receptors in the pancreas *promotes* secretion of insulin. Conversely, activation of pancreatic alpha-adrenergic receptors *inhibits* insulin release.

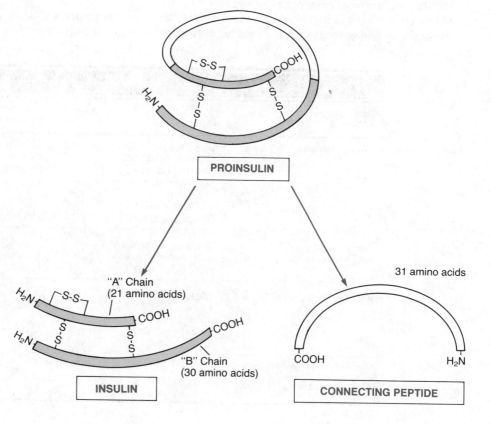

Figure 49–1. Conversion of proinsulin to insulin and connecting peptide.

Metabolic Actions. The metabolic actions of insulin are primarily *anabolic* (i.e., conservative or constructive). Insulin promotes energy conservation and buildup of energy stores. The hormone also promotes cell growth and division.

Insulin acts in two ways to promote anabolic effects. First, insulin stimulates cellular transport (uptake) of glucose, amino acids, nucleotides, and potassium. Second, insulin promotes synthesis of complex organic molecules. Under the influence of insulin (and other factors), glucose is converted into glycogen, amino acids are assembled into proteins, nucleotides are compiled into nucleic acids (DNA and RNA), and fatty acids are incorporated into triglycerides. The principal metabolic actions of insulin are summarized in Table 49–2.

METABOLIC CONSEQUENCES OF INSULIN DEFICIENCY

Insulin deficiency puts the body into a *catabolic* mode (i.e., a metabolic state that favors the breakdown of complex molecules into their simple constituents). Hence, in the absence of insulin, glycogen is converted into glucose, proteins are degraded into amino acids, and fats (triglycerides) are converted to glycerol (glycerin) and free fatty acids. These catabolic effects contribute to the signs and symptoms of diabetes. Note that the catabolic effects produced by insulin deficiency are opposite to the anabolic effects seen when insulin levels are normal.

Insulin deficiency promotes *hyperglycemia* by three mechanisms: (1) increased glycogenolysis, (2) increased gluconeogenesis, and (3) reduced glucose utilization. *Glycogenolysis*, by definition, generates free glucose by breaking down glycogen. The raw materials that allow increased *gluconeogenesis* are the amino acids and fatty acids produced by degradation of proteins and fats. *Reduced glucose utilization* occurs because insulin deficiency decreases cellular uptake of glucose, and decreases conversion of glucose to glycogen.

Diabetic ketoacidosis occurs secondary to disruption of glucose and fat metabolism. This potentially fatal syndrome is discussed separately later in the chapter.

THERAPEUTIC USES

The principal indication for insulin is *diabetes mellitus*; the drug is required by all patients with IDDM and by some who have NIDDM. Intravenous insulin is used to treat *diabetic ketoacidosis*. Because of its ability to promote cellular uptake of potassium (and thereby lower plasma potassium levels), insulin infusion is employed to treat *hyperkalemia*. The use of insulin in diabetes is discussed further later in the chapter.

PREPARATIONS

Insulin is available in several forms. These preparations differ from one another with respect to time course of action, route of administration, concentration, insulin source, and degree of purity.

The Six Basic Insulin Preparations

There are six basic preparations of insulin: "natural" insulin and five modified insulins. Effects of

Table 49–2. Metabolic Actions of Insulin		
Substances Affected	**Insulin Action**	**Site of Action**
Carbohydrates	↑ Glucose uptake	Muscle, adipose tissue
	↑ Glucose oxidation	Muscle
	↑ Glucose storage	Muscle, liver
	↑ Glycogen synthesis	
	↓ Glycogenolysis	
	↓ Gluconeogenesis*	Liver
Amino acids and proteins	↑ Amino acid uptake	Muscle
	↓ Amino acid release	Muscle
	↑ Protein synthesis	Muscle
Lipids	↑ Triglyceride synthesis	Adipose tissue
	↓ Release of FFA† and glycerol	Adipose tissue
	↑ Oxidation of FFA to ketoacids‡	Liver

*Because of decreased delivery of substrate (fatty acids and amino acids) to the liver.
†Free fatty acids.
‡Because of decreased delivery of FFA to the liver.

the modified insulins begin more slowly than those of natural insulin but last longer. The effects of the modified insulins have been prolonged by two processes: (1) complexing insulin with a protein, and (2) altering the physical state of insulin itself. When classified according to time course of action, the insulin preparations fall into three groups: rapid acting, intermediate acting, and long acting (Table 49–3). Characteristics of the six basic preparations are discussed below.

(1) Regular Insulin (Insulin Injection). Regular insulin, also known as insulin injection, is unmodified, crystalline insulin. As shown in Table 49–3, regular insulin is the *fastest acting* of the insulin preparations and has the *shortest duration* of action. Regular insulin is dispensed as a clear solution, and is the only form of insulin that can be administered *intravenously*.

In the past, preparations of regular insulin were unstable at room temperature and, therefore, required constant refrigeration. The stability of formulations available today has been greatly improved. As a result, insulin bottles in *current use* (usually a 2- to 4-week supply) do not need to be kept cold, although exposure to sunlight and extreme heat must be avoided.

(2) and (3) Isophane Insulin Suspension (NPH Insulin) and Protamine Zinc Insulin Suspension (PZI). Isophane insulin and PZI are preparations in which insulin has been conjugated with *protamine* (a large protein). The presence of protamine decreases the solubility of these prepa-

rations and, therefore, retards their absorption. As a result, onset of action is delayed, and duration of action is prolonged. Isophane insulin is classified as an intermediate-acting preparation, and PZI is classified as long acting (see Table 49–3). Since protamine is a foreign protein, it may cause allergic reactions in some patients.

(4), (5), and (6) Semilente Insulin, Lente Insulin, and Ultralente Insulin. In the "Lente" series of insulins, solubility has been altered by modifying the physical state of insulin itself; no foreign proteins are employed. *Semilente insulin* (prompt insulin zinc suspension) is the fastest-acting member of the series (see Table 49–3). The insulin in this preparation is amorphous (noncrystalline) and present as particles of small size. In *Ultralente insulin* (extended insulin zinc suspension), insulin is present as large crystals; these crystals dissolve slowly, giving Ultralente insulin a long duration of action. *Lente insulin* (insulin zinc suspension) is a stable mixture composed of 70% Ultralente insulin and 30% Semilente insulin. This preparation has an intermediate duration of action. Because no modifying proteins are present, the Lente insulins are less allergenic than NPH insulin and PZI.

Sources of Insulin

Much of commercial insulin is prepared by extraction from beef pancreas or pork pancreas. Insulin from both sources is similar in structure to human insulin: pork insulin is identical to human

Table 49–3. The Six Basic Types of Insulin: Time Course and Mixing Compatibility

Class	Generic Name (Alternative Generic Name)	Onset (hr)	Peak (hr)	Duration (hr)	May Be Mixed With:
Short-acting	Regular insulin (insulin injection)	0.5–1	2–4	6–8	All insulins
	Semilente insulin (insulin zinc suspension, prompt)	1–1.5	4–8	12–16	Regular insulin, Lente insulin, Ultralente insulin
Intermediate-acting	NPH insulin (isophane insulin suspension)	1–1.5	6–12	18–24	Regular insulin
	Lente insulin (insulin zinc suspension)	1–2	6–12	18–24	Regular insulin, Semilente insulin, Ultralente insulin
Long-acting	PZ1 insulin (protamine zinc insulin suspension)	4–8	14–24	28–36	Regular insulin
	Ultralente insulin (insulin zinc suspension extended)	4–8	10–30	36 +	Regular insulin, Lente insulin, Semilente insulin

Time Course of Action

insulin with the exception of one amino acid; beef insulin contains three amino acids that differ from those of human insulin. Because beef and pork insulins are not identical to human insulin, antibodies against these foreign insulins may develop.

Two processes have been developed to synthesize insulin that is indistinguishable from that made by the human pancreas. One of these procedures is *semisynthetic*. In this process, enzymes are employed to convert pork insulin into human insulin. This is accomplished by clipping off the terminal amino acid (alanine) from the B chain of pork insulin and replacing it with threonine.

The second method employs *recombinant DNA technology*. In this process, genes that code for the A and B chains of human insulin are introduced into *Escherichia coli*. The separate chains are then synthesized by the bacteria, after which the chains are linked chemically to form insulin.

There is very little clinical difference between *human insulin* (semisynthetic or recombinant) and *pork insulin that has been highly purified*. Hence, for most patients, it would appear that the advantages of using human insulin may be relatively minor. Table 49–4 indicates the source—beef, pork, beef plus pork, or "human"—of commercial insulin preparations.

Purity of Insulin Preparations

At one time, insulin prepared from animal sources (beef or pork pancreas) contained substantial amounts of *proinsulin* and other contaminants—impurities that tended to promote adverse reactions (e.g., allergic responses, lipoatrophy). Thanks to technologic advances, the insulins produced today are of much greater purity than those of the past. In the United States, *standard* insulin preparations now contain no more than 25 parts per million (ppm) of proinsulin, the major contaminant of commercial preparations. Preparations that bear the label *purified* contain less than 10 ppm of proinsulin. None of the purified preparations is considered antigenic. The degree of purity of commercial insulin preparations is indicated in Table 49–4. It should be noted that categories of purity do not apply to the human insulins (since these preparations have no proinsulin at all).

Concentration

Insulin is available in three concentrations: 40 U/ml (U-40), 100 U/ml (U-100), and 500 U/ml (U-500). As indicated in Table 49–4, each of the six basic types of insulin is available in U-40 and U-100 formulations. Only regular insulin is also marketed in a U-500 preparation.

For routine therapy, U-100 insulins are preferred. Although U-40 insulins are still produced, their use has declined. In the interests of reducing dosing errors, the American Diabetes Association has recommended that the U-40 preparations be abandoned in favor of universal use of U-100 insulin.

U-500 insulin is reserved for patients with insulin resistance (patients who need doses in excess of 200 units a day). The high concentration of the U-500 preparation permits the administration of a large insulin dose in a volume that is manageable.

Choice of an Insulin Preparation

When selecting an insulin preparation, four factors require consideration: (1) concentration, (2) time course of action, (3) purity, and (4) source. With respect to concentration, all patients (except those with insulin resistance) can be treated satisfactorily with U-100 insulins. Factors that underlie decisions about insulin time course are complex and beyond the scope of this text.

The therapeutic significance of insulin purity and species of origin is yet to be established. Most patients can be managed well with beef or pork insulin of standard purity (i.e., less than 25 ppm proinsulin). Clinical differences between human insulin and purified pork insulin are minimal; hence, there is usually no strong basis for selecting between them.

There are some patients for whom human insulin or purified pork insulin may be of special benefit. These are (1) patients experiencing local allergic reactions, (2) patients with insulin-induced lipoatrophy, (3) pregnant patients, and (4) newly diagnosed patients, since, if there indeed are long-term benefits to using less antigenic insulins, new patients are likely to benefit most.

Once an insulin preparation has been selected, *the patient must not arbitrarily change to an insulin of different species of origin or degree of purity*. Such changes can result in altered glycemic control and should be made only in collaboration with the physician.

ADMINISTRATION AND STORAGE

Routes of Administration

Insulin must be given by injection. (Because of its peptide structure, insulin would be inactivated by the digestive system if it were given by mouth.) *All* insulins may be injected *subcutaneously*. Only *regular insulin* (U-40 and U-100) may also be administered *intravenously* and *intramuscularly*. The *U-500* preparation of *regular insulin* may be injected SC or IM; however, because of the risk of severe allergic reactions, this preparation should *not* be administered IV.

In emergencies, *regular* insulin (and *only* regular insulin) may be administered *intravenously*. Since regular insulin forms a true *solution*, it is safe for intravenous use. In contrast, all other in-

Table 49–4. Insulin Preparation

Insulin Type and Trade Name	Source	Purified*	Concentration (U/ml)
Regular Insulin			
Regular Iletin I	Beef-pork	No	40, 100
Regular Insulin	Pork	No	100
Beef Regular Iletin II	Beef	Yes	100
Pork Regular Iletin II	Pork	Yes	100
Regular Purified Pork Insulin	Pork	Yes	100
Velosulin (pork)	Pork	Yes	100
Humulin R	Human†	NA	100
Humulin BR (buffered)‡	Human†	NA	100
Novolin R	Human§	NA	100
Novolin R Penfill‖	Human§	NA	100
Velosulin (human)	Human§	NA	100
Regular (concentrated) Iletin II, U-500	Pork	Yes	500
Semilente Insulin			
Semilente Iletin I	Beef-pork	No	40, 100
Semilente Insulin	Beef	No	100
Isophane (NPH) Insulin			
NPH Iletin I	Beef-pork	No	40, 100
NPH Insulin	Beef	No	100
Beef NPH Iletin II	Beef	Yes	100
NPH Purified (pork)	Pork	Yes	100
Pork NPH Iletin II	Pork	Yes	100
Insulatard NPH (pork)	Pork	Yes	100
Insulatard NPH (human)	Human§	NA	100
Humulin N	Human†	NA	100
Novolin N	Human§	NA	100
Novolin N Penfill‖	Human§	NA	100
Lente Insulin			
Lente Iletin I	Beef-pork	No	40, 100
Lente Insulin	Beef	No	100
Lente Iletin II (beef)	Beef	Yes	100
Lente Iletin II (pork)	Pork	Yes	100
Lente Purified Pork Insulin	Pork	Yes	100
Humulin L	Human†	NA	100
Novolin L	Human§	NA	100
Protamine Zinc Insulin			
Protamine, Zinc, & Iletin I	Beef-pork	No	40, 100
Protamine, Zinc, & Iletin II (beef)	Beef	Yes	100
Protamine, Zinc, & Iletin II (pork)	Pork	Yes	100
Ultralente Insulin			
Ultralente Iletin I	Beef-pork	No	40, 100
Ultralente Insulin	Beef	No	100
Humulin U Ultralente	Human†	NA	100
70% NPH/30% Regular Insulin			
Mixtard	Pork	Yes	100
Mixtard Human 70/30	Human§	NA	100
Humulin 70/30	Human†	NA	100
Novolin 70/30	Human§	NA	100
Novolin 70/30 PenFill‖	Human§	NA	100

*Yes (purified) = less than 10 ppm proinsulin; No ("unpurified") = 10 to 25 ppm proinsulin; NA = not applicable to human insulin
†Produced by recombinant DNA technology.
‡For use only in external insulin infusion pumps.
§Semisynthetic (produced by enzymatic modification of pork insulin).
‖For use with *NovoPen*.

sulin preparations consist of particles in *suspension*—not solution; introduction of these particles into the bloodstream could produce serious adverse effects. When administered by IV infusion, insulin can adsorb to the infusion set, thereby reducing the dosage that the patient receives. Since the extent of adsorption is not predictable, monitoring the therapeutic response is essential. If emergency treatment by the intravenous route is impossible, regular insulin may be administered IM instead.

Syringe and Needle Selection

The insulin syringe should correspond to the concentration of the preparation to be injected. To facilitate matching, a simple color code is employed. Bottles of U-40 insulins are identified with *red caps*, and syringes for injecting U-40 insulins bear *red markings*. The color *orange* is used to identify bottles and syringes for U-100 insulins. For SC injections, the needle should be 25- or 26-gauge and 1/2 to 3/4 inch long.

Preparation for Injection

With the exception of regular insulin, all insulin preparations consist of particles in suspension. Hence, to insure correct dosing, these particles must be evenly dispersed prior to loading the syringe. Dispersion is accomplished by rolling the insulin vial between the palms of the hands. Mixing must be *gentle*, since vigorous agitation will cause frothing and render accurate dosing impossible. If granules or clumps remain after gentle agitation, the vial should be discarded.

Unlike insulin suspensions, which are cloudy, regular insulin is a clear and colorless solution. Because it is a solution, regular insulin can be administered without prior mixing. If a preparation of regular insulin becomes cloudy or discolored, or if a precipitate develops, that preparation should be discarded.

Before loading the syringe, the bottle cap should be swabbed with alcohol. Air bubbles should be eliminated from the syringe and needle after loading. The skin should be cleaned with alcohol prior to injection.

Sites of Injection

The most common sites of SC injection are the upper arms, thighs, and abdomen. Since rates of absorption vary among these sites, it is recommended that injections be made using only one general locale (e.g., thigh or abdomen). Regardless of whether one general locale or several are used, specific sites of injection within the locale should be rotated. This practice will reduce the incidence of lipohypertrophy (see below). About 1 inch should be allowed between sites of injection. Ideally, each site should be used only once every month.

Mixing Insulins

When the treatment plan calls for the use of two different insulin preparations (e.g., regular insulin plus NPH insulin), it is usually desirable to mix the preparations together (rather than injecting them separately), since this will eliminate the need for an additional injection. However, although mixing insulins offers convenience, it can alter the time course of the response. Accordingly,

to insure a consistent response, insulins should be mixed according to established guidelines (see below). Also, only those insulins that are compatible with each other should be mixed. Mixing compatibility is summarized in Table 49–3.

All Types of Insulin. Mixtures should be made only among insulins of like concentration. That is, U-100 insulins should be mixed only with other U-100 insulins, and U-40 insulins should be mixed only with other U-40 insulins.

Regular Insulin. Regular insulin is compatible with all other insulin preparations. When preparing a mixture of regular insulin with another insulin preparation, the regular insulin should be drawn into the syringe first. This sequence will avoid contaminating the stock vial of regular insulin with insulin of another type.

NPH Insulin. This preparation is compatible only with regular insulin. Mixtures of NPH and regular insulin may be prepared by the patient, or may be purchased premixed (70% NPH/30% regular). Mixtures of regular and NPH insulin are stable and do not alter the kinetics of either component. In the past, NPH insulins contained an excess of protamine, which could react with regular insulin to alter its time course of action. This reaction does not occur with the NPH preparations in use today.

Lente Insulins. The Lente insulins (Semilente, Lente, and Ultralente) may be mixed with one another or with regular insulin. When the Lente insulins are mixed with one another, no change in time course occurs. In contrast, when Lente insulins are mixed with regular insulin, zinc present in the Lente-type insulin can complex with the regular insulin, thereby delaying and prolonging its actions. Since this reaction begins soon after mixing, these mixtures should be injected immediately to avoid altering the regular insulin.

Storage

Insulin in *unopened vials* should be stored *under refrigeration* until needed. Vials should not be frozen. When stored unopened under refrigeration, insulin can be used up to the expiration date on the vial.

The vial in current use can be kept at room temperature for up to 1 month without significant loss of activity. Direct sunlight and extreme heat must be avoided. Partially filled vials should be discarded after several weeks if left unused. Injection of insulin stored at room temperature causes less pain than cold insulin.

Mixtures of insulin prepared in *vials* are stable for 1 month at room temperature and for 3 months under refrigeration.

Mixtures of insulin in *prefilled syringes* (plastic or glass) should be stored in a refrigerator, where they will be stable for at least 1 week, and perhaps 2. The syringe should be stored vertically with the needle pointing up to avoid clogging the needle. Prior to administration, the syringe should be agitated gently to resuspend the insulin.

INSULIN THERAPY OF DIABETES MELLITUS

Insulin is given to all patients who have IDDM and to some who have NIDDM. In addition, insulin is employed to manage gestational diabetes. In treating these disorders, the objective is to maintain blood glucose levels within an acceptable range (premeal and bedtime values between 80 and 140 mg/dl in older children and adults, and between 100 and 200 mg/dl in children under 5 years). When therapy is successful, both hyperglycemia and hypoglycemia will be avoided—and the long-term complications of diabetes will be minimized.

Tight Glucose Control: Benefits and Drawbacks

The process of maintaining glucose levels within a normal range is referred to as *tight glucose control*. Until recently, it was assumed—but not proved—that tight glucose control would reduce the long-term complications of diabetes. Now, there is no longer any doubt: the *Diabetes Control and Complications Trial*, a 9-year study whose results were announced in the summer of 1993, has shown conclusively that tight glucose control can greatly reduce the long-term complications of diabetes. In this study, patients with Type I diabetes (IDDM) received either (1) *conventional* insulin therapy (i.e., one or two injections/day) or (2) *intensive* insulin therapy (four injections/day). The patients who received intensive therapy experienced a 50% decrease in clinically significant kidney disease, a 60% decrease in neuropathy, and a 76% decrease in serious ophthalmic complications. Moreover, onset of ophthalmic problems was delayed, and progression of existing problems was slowed. All of these benefits were correlated with improved glycemic control. Hence, with rigorous control of blood glucose, the high degree of morbidity traditionally associated with diabetes can be markedly reduced. Although the participants in this study were Type I diabetics, we can assume that tight glucose control would be of similar benefit to Type II diabetics, who are at risk for the same long-term complications experienced by Type I diabetics.

Unfortunately, intensive insulin therapy has its drawbacks. The greatest concern is *hypoglycemia*: since glucose levels are kept relatively low, the possibility of hypoglycemia secondary to a modest insulin overdosage is significantly increased. Other disadvantages are greater inconvenience, increased complexity, and a need for greater patient motivation. Lastly, intensive therapy is more expensive: whereas traditional therapy costs about $2000 a year, intensive therapy costs about $4000.

Intensive therapy is discussed further under *Dosing Schedules*.

Dosage

To achieve tight glucose control, insulin dosage must be closely matched with insulin needs. If caloric intake is increased, insulin dosage must be increased as well. When a meal is missed or is low in calories, the dosage of insulin must be decreased. Dosage must undergo additional adjustments to meet specialized needs. For example, insulin needs are *increased* by infection, stress, obesity, the adolescent growth spurt, and pregnancy (after the first trimester). Conversely, insulin needs are *decreased* by exercise and pregnancy (during the first trimester). To insure that insulin dosage is coordinated with insulin requirements, the patient and physician must work together to establish an integrated program of nutrition, exercise, and insulin replacement therapy.

Total daily dosages may range from 0.1 U/kg body weight to more than 2.5 U/kg. For patients with IDDM, initial dosages typically range from 0.5 to 0.6 U/kg/day. For patients with NIDDM, initial dosages typically range from 0.2 to 0.6 U/kg/day.

Dosing Schedules

The schedule of insulin administration helps determine the extent to which tight glucose control is achieved. Three dosing schedules are compared below. These modes are referred to as (1) conventional therapy, (2) intensified conventional therapy, and (3) continuous subcutaneous insulin infusion.

Conventional Therapy. Several dosing schedules fall under the heading of conventional therapy. A representative schedule is summarized in Table 49–5. In this schedule, a combination of regular insulin (a fast-acting preparation) plus Lente insulin (an intermediate-acting preparation) is administered 15 to 30 minutes before breakfast and again before the evening meal. No insulin is administered with the noon meal. Typically, two thirds of the total daily dose is given in the morning, and the remainder is given late in the day. Dosage remains rigidly fixed from one day to the next.

Conventional therapy does not provide tight glucose control. The weak point of this schedule is that there is no provision for adjusting insulin dosage in response to ongoing alterations in insulin needs. Hence, if a particular meal is abnormally large, insulin levels will be insufficient and hyperglycemia will result. Conversely, if a meal is delayed, reduced in size, or missed entirely, hypoglycemia will follow.

Intensified Conventional Therapy (ICT). This form of therapy is designed to provide tight glucose control. A representative regimen is presented in Table 49–5. In this regimen, the patient injects Ultralente insulin (a long-acting preparation) in the evening and also injects regular insulin (a rapid-acting preparation) prior to each meal. The *Ultralente* preparation provides a *basal* level

Table 49–5. Insulin Therapy of Diabetes Mellitus: Conventional versus Intensified Conventional Therapy

	Insulin Type and Dosing Schedule			
Regimen	**Breakfast**	**Lunch**	**Supper**	**Bedtime**
Conventional Therapy*	Regular + lente	None	Regular + lente	None
Intensified Conventional Therapy†	Regular	Regular	Regular	Ultralente

*Dosage is *fixed* (2/3 daily total in AM, 1/3 daily total in PM). As a result, flexibility of timing and composition of meals is not possible.
†Dosage of regular insulin is *adjusted for each meal;* hence, timing and composition of meals can be varied.

of insulin throughout the night and the following day. The mealtime doses of *regular* insulin accommodate the *acute* needs that occur at times of caloric loading. Note that insulin is injected *four times each day,* rather than just twice as in conventional therapy.

The most significant feature of ICT is *adaptability.* Unlike conventional therapy, in which doses never change, the preprandial doses given in ICT are adjusted to match the caloric content of each meal: if no meal is eaten, no insulin is administered; if a meal is delayed, so is the dose of regular insulin; if a meal is larger than usual, the insulin dose is increased proportionately. Since insulin dosage is determined by the timing and size of each meal, ICT offers patients a degree of glycemic control and dietary flexibility that is not possible with conventional therapy.

Home blood glucose monitoring (HBGM) is an essential component of ICT. This procedure is discussed below under *Monitoring Therapy.*

Continuous Subcutaneous Insulin Infusion (CSII). CSII is accomplished using a portable infusion pump connected to an indwelling subcutaneous catheter. The only form of insulin employed for CSII is regular insulin. To provide a basal level of insulin, the pump is set to infuse the hormone continuously at a slow but steady rate. To accommodate insulin needs created by eating, the pump is triggered manually to provide a bolus dose of insulin matched in size to the caloric content of each meal. Hence, like ICT, CSII can adapt to changes in insulin needs. As with ICT, home monitoring of blood glucose is an essential component of treatment. Studies to date indicate that CSII and ICT are about equal in their abilities to provide tight glucose control.

CSII is not free of undesired effects. The most troubling concern is severe hypoglycemia, which has occurred when pump malfunction caused the infusion of excessive doses of insulin. CSII has also produced local allergic reactions and infections at the site of needle insertion. Furthermore, CSII is expensive.

Achieving Tight Glucose Control

Intensified conventional therapy is the method of choice for achieving tight glucose control. Although CSII is promising, this technique is difficult to use. Also, CSII poses greater risks than ICT. Tight control of blood glucose cannot be achieved with conventional insulin therapy.

As we have seen, the primary requirement for achieving tight glucose control is a method of insulin delivery that permits adjustments in dosage to accommodate ongoing variations in insulin needs. ICT and CSII meet this criterion. In addition to an adaptable method of insulin delivery, achieving tight glucose control requires the following:

1. Careful attention to all elements of the treatment program (diet, exercise, insulin replacement therapy)
2. A defined glycemia target (ideally, 80 to 140 mg/dl)
3. Home monitoring of blood glucose
4. A high degree of patient motivation
5. Extensive patient education

Tight glucose control cannot be achieved without the informed participation of the patient. Accordingly, patients must receive thorough instruction on the following:

1. The nature of diabetes
2. The importance of tight glucose control
3. The major components of the treatment routine (insulin, diet, exercise)
4. Procedures for purchasing of insulin, syringes, and needles
5. The importance of avoiding arbitrary changes in insulin source or purity
6. Methods of insulin storage
7. Procedures for mixing insulins
8. Calculation of dosage adjustments
9. Techniques of insulin injection
10. Measurement of blood glucose content.

In the final analysis, responsibility for managing

diabetes rests with the patient. The health care team can design a treatment program and can provide education and guidance. However, tight glucose control will be achieved only if the patient is actively involved in his or her own therapy.

MONITORING TREATMENT

Several tests may be used to evaluate glycemic control. These include measurement of glucose in urine, measurement of glucose in blood, and measurement of glycosylated hemoglobin. As discussed below, daily monitoring of blood glucose content is the preferred procedure. However, with current technology, this test may not be practical for all patients.

Urine Glucose Monitoring. Until recent years, this procedure had been the mainstay for assessing glycemic control. Urine testing is inexpensive and easy for patients to perform. Unfortunately, urine testing is also of limited utility. There is a poor correlation between urine glucose concentration and blood glucose levels. Furthermore, a negative urine glucose test tells us only that blood glucose is below 180 mg/dl, the typical threshold for spilling glucose from blood to urine. What a negative test does *not* tell us is *how much* below the threshold the glucose level is. Hence, a patient with a negative urine glucose test could be hypoglycemic, normoglycemic, or even slightly hyperglycemic; without some other means of evaluation, we cannot distinguish among these possibilities. Accordingly, although urine testing is superior to no testing at all, it is clearly inferior to blood glucose monitoring.

Home Blood Glucose Monitoring (HBGM). HBGM is the current standard for self-monitoring. The test is performed by placing a drop of blood on a chemically treated strip, which is then read by a small machine. The test is rapid, relatively inexpensive, and can be performed in almost any setting. Information on blood glucose content provides a basis for "fine tuning" insulin dosage. HBGM is far superior to measuring glucose in urine: with HBGM, hyperglycemia can be detected long before blood glucose levels are high enough to cause spilling of glucose into urine. Furthermore, HBGM can detect *hypo*glycemia, something that urinary measurements simply can't do.

HBGM does have certain drawbacks. These tests are more expensive than urine tests, and are more difficult to perform. Also, the machines employed require periodic calibration, and patients require education on how to apply test results. Because of these disadvantages, HBGM may not be practical for patients with limited economic resources, or for patients who are unable or unwilling to learn how to use the device and apply the results.

Glycosylated Hemoglobin. Glucose interacts with hemoglobin to form glycosylated derivatives, the most prevalent of which is named *hemoglobin A_{1c}*. With *prolonged* hyperglycemia, levels of hemoglobin A_{1c} gradually increase. Since red blood cells have a long life span (120 days), levels of *hemoglobin A_{1c}* reflect *average* glucose levels over an extended time. Hence, by measuring *hemoglobin A_{1c}* every 3 to 4 months, we can get a picture of *long-term* glycemic control. These measurements can be a useful adjunct to daily blood glucose monitoring.

COMPLICATIONS OF INSULIN THERAPY

Hypoglycemia

Hypoglycemia will occur whenever insulin levels exceed insulin needs. A major cause of insulin excess is overdosage. Imbalance between insulin levels and insulin needs can also result from reduced intake of food, vomiting and diarrhea (which reduce absorption of nutrients), excessive consumption of alcohol (which promotes hypoglycemia), unaccustomed exercise (which promotes glucose uptake and utilization), and parturition (which reduces insulin requirements).

Diabetic patients and their families should be familiar with the signs and symptoms of hypoglycemia. Some symptoms result from activation of the sympathetic nervous system, whereas others arise from the central nervous system (CNS). When glucose levels fall *rapidly*, activation of the sympathetic nervous system occurs, resulting in tachycardia, palpitations, sweating, and nervousness. However, if the decline in glucose is *gradual*, symptoms may be limited to those of CNS origin. Mild CNS symptoms include headache, confusion, drowsiness, and fatigue. If hypoglycemia is severe, convulsions, coma, and death may follow.

Rapid treatment of hypoglycemia is mandatory; if hypoglycemia is allowed to persist, irreversible brain damage or death may result. In conscious patients, glucose levels can be restored with oral sugar supplements (e.g., orange juice, sugar cubes, honey, candy). However, if the swallowing reflex or the gag reflex is suppressed, nothing should be administered by mouth. In cases of severe hypoglycemia, intravenous glucose is the preferred therapy. If glucose is unavailable, parenteral *glucagon* is an alternative method of treatment.

In anticipation of hypoglycemic episodes, diabetics should always have an oral carbohydrate available (e.g., Life Savers, candy, sugar cubes). Many physicians recommend that patients keep glucagon on hand as well. Patients should carry some sort of identification (e.g., MedicAlert bracelet) to inform emergency personnel of their condition.

Both severe hypoglycemia and diabetic ketoacidosis (see below) can produce coma. Of these two causes of diabetic coma, hypoglycemia is the more common. Since treatment of these two conditions is very different (hypoglycemia involves withholding insulin, whereas ketoacidosis requires insulin administration), it is essential that coma from these causes be differentiated. The most definitive diagnosis is made by measuring plasma or urinary levels of glucose: in hypoglycemic coma, glucose levels are very low; in ketoacidosis, glucose levels are very high.

Other Complications

Lipodystrophies. Altered deposition of subcutaneous fat (lipodystrophy) can occur at sites of insulin injection. Two types of change may be seen: (1) *lipoatrophy* (loss of subcutaneous fat), and (2) *lipohypertrophy* (accumulation of subcutaneous fat).

Lipoatrophy produces a depression in the skin at the site of insulin injection. The cause of atrophy appears to be immunologic. Accordingly, fat atrophy is most likely with use of insulin preparations that have a high concentration of antigenic contaminants. Because the insulin preparations in use today are much purer than those used in the past, the incidence of lipoatrophy is now low. When lipoatrophy occurs, subcutaneous fat can often be restored by injecting a highly purified insulin preparation (e.g., purified pork insulin or human insulin) directly into the site of fat loss.

Lipohypertrophy occurs at sites of frequent insulin injection. Fat accumulates because insulin stimulates fat synthesis. When use of the site is discontinued, excess fat will eventually be lost. Lipohypertrophy can be minimized through systematic rotation of injection sites.

Allergic Reactions. Insulin injection can produce local and systemic allergic responses. Fortunately, serious reactions are rare.

With local reactions, the injection site becomes red and hardened. These reactions are usually *delayed*, taking several hours to develop. Local reactions occur in response to a *contaminant* in the insulin preparation, and not to the insulin itself. Accordingly, local allergy is more likely with use of less purified insulin products.

Systemic reactions take place *rapidly*, and are characterized by the widespread appearance of red and intensely itchy welts. Breathing difficulty may develop. Systemic reactions occur in response to insulin itself, and *not* to a contaminant. Beef insulin, which differs from human insulin by three amino acids, is the most frequent cause of systemic allergy. Generalized reactions are least likely with pork and human insulins. If severe allergy develops in a patient who nonetheless must continue insulin use, a desensitization procedure can be performed. This process entails giving small initial doses of purified pork or human insulin, followed by a series of progressively larger doses.

DRUG INTERACTIONS

Hypoglycemic Agents. Drugs with the ability to lower blood glucose levels can intensify hypoglycemia induced by insulin. Drugs that promote hypoglycemia include *sulfonylureas*, *alcohol* (used acutely), and *beta-adrenergic blocking agents*. When these drugs are combined with insulin, special care must be taken to insure that blood glucose content does not fall too low.

Hyperglycemic Agents. Drugs with the ability to increase blood glucose, such as *thiazide diuretics*, *glucocorticoids*, and *sympathomimetics*, can counteract the therapeutic effects of insulin. When these agents are combined with insulin, an increase in insulin dosage may be required.

Beta-Adrenergic Blocking Agents. Beta blockers can delay awareness of insulin-induced hypoglycemia by masking those signs that are associated with stimulation of the sympathetic nervous system (e.g., tachycardia, palpitations). Furthermore, since beta blockade impairs glycogenolysis, and since glycogenolysis is one means by which the diabetic can counteract a fall in blood glucose, beta blockers can make insulin-induced hypoglycemia even worse.

Digoxin. The risk of severe dysrhythmias during treatment with digoxin is greatly increased by hypokalemia. Since insulin can lower plasma levels of potassium (by promoting potassium uptake into cells), insulin can increase the risk of digoxin-induced dysrhythmias. Accordingly, when insulin and digoxin are combined, special care must be taken to keep potassium levels within a normal range.

ORAL HYPOGLYCEMICS (SULFONYLUREAS)

As their name suggests, the oral hypoglycemics are drugs that can be administered by mouth to lower plasma glucose content. These agents can be used to treat patients with NIDDM but are *not* effective for patients with IDDM.

All of the available oral hypoglycemics belong to a chemical family known as *sulfonylureas*. The sulfonylureas are derivatives of the sulfonamide antibiotics, but lack antimicrobial activity.

Individual sulfonylureas can be classified as *first-generation agents* or *second-generation agents*. Both generations can reduce glucose levels to the same extent. The principal difference between the two groups lies with their potencies: maximally effective doses of the second-generation sulfonylureas are much lower than those of the first-generation drugs. However, although differences in potency are large, these differences are of minimal clinical significance. The first- and second-generation sulfonylureas are listed in Table 49–6.

TOLBUTAMIDE

Tolbutamide [Orinase], a first-generation agent, will serve as our prototype for the sulfonylurea family. As with the other sulfonylureas, use of tolbutamide is restricted to patients with NIDDM.

Mechanism of Action

Tolbutamide produces its *initial* effects by stimulating the release of insulin from pancreatic islets. Accordingly, tolbutamide will be ineffective if the pancreas is incapable of insulin synthesis. It is for this reason that tolbutamide is of no value to insulin-dependent diabetics.

With *prolonged* use, tolbutamide provides the additional benefit of enhancing cellular sensitivity to insulin. Although the mechanism of this effect is not known, one hypothesis is that chronic exposure to tolbutamide increases the number of insulin receptors.

Pharmacokinetics

Tolbutamide is readily absorbed following oral administration. Plasma levels peak within 3 to 5 hours. The drug undergoes extensive hepatic metabolism followed by urinary excretion. Because of its mode of elimination, tolbutamide must be used with caution in patients with hepatic or renal impairment. Tolbutamide has a relatively short half-life (about 6 hours) and, therefore, must be administered two to three times a day.

Therapeutic Use

Oral hypoglycemics are employed only in the treatment of NIDDM. These drugs are of no help to patients with IDDM. Sulfonylureas should be employed only if blood glucose cannot be lowered by a program of caloric restriction and exercise. In addition, when these agents are to be used, they should be employed as an *adjunct* to nondrug therapy—not as a substitute. It should be noted that although sulfonylureas are capable of lowering plasma glucose levels, there is no evidence that these agents prevent or decrease the long-term complications of diabetes.

There is disagreement among practitioners regarding the precise role of sulfonylureas in NIDDM therapy. Some physicians consider these agents to be drugs of first choice. For these clinicians, a sulfonylurea is the first drug to try when NIDDM cannot be controlled by diet and exercise alone. In contrast, other practitioners consider sulfonylureas to be the least desirable treatment for NIDDM. These physicians prescribe oral agents only when diet and exercise have proved ineffective, and the patient is unwilling or unable to use insulin.

With prolonged use, tolbutamide and other oral hypoglycemics may lose their ability to lower blood

Generic Name [Trade Name]	Onset (hr)	Duration (hr)	Dosage*
First-Generation Agents			
Tolbutamide [Orinase]	1	6–12	Initial: 1–2 gm/day in 1 to 3 doses Maximum: 2–3 gm/day in 1 to 3 doses
Acetohexamide [Dymelor]	1	12–24	Initial: 0.25–1.5 gm/day in 1 or 2 doses Maximum: 1.5 gm/day in 1 or 2 doses
Tolazamide [Tolinase]	4–6	12–24	Initial: 100–200 mg/day with breakfast Maximum: 0.75–1 gm in 2 divided doses
Chlorpropamide [Diabinese]	1	24–72	Initial: 250 mg once a day Maximum: 750 mg once a day
Second-Generation Agents			
Glipizide [Glucotrol]	1	12–24	Initial: 5 mg once a day with breakfast Maximum: 40 mg/day in 2 divided doses
Glyburide Nonmicronized [DiaBeta, Micronase]	2–4	12–24	Initial: 2.5–5 mg/day with breakfast Maximum: 20 mg/day in 1 or 2 doses
Micronized [Glynase PresTab]	1	24	Initial: 1.5–3 mg/day with breakfast Maximum: 12 mg/day in 1 or 2 doses

Table 49–6. Oral Hypoglycemic Agents

*The dosages listed are for nonelderly patients. Elderly patients should use smaller doses.

glucose. This loss may result from progression of the underlying disease or from development of drug resistance. If loss of glycemic control occurs, insulin therapy will be required. Insulin is also likely to be needed at times of stress (e.g., trauma, surgery, fever, infection).

Adverse Effects

Hypoglycemia. Tolbutamide and all other sulfonylureas can cause excessive lowering of blood glucose. Although hypoglycemia is usually mild, some fatalities have occurred. Hypoglycemia is sometimes persistent, requiring infusion of dextrose for several days. Hypoglycemic reactions are most likely in patients with kidney or liver dysfunction, since accumulation of tolbutamide may occur. If signs of hypoglycemia develop (fatigue, excessive hunger, profuse sweating, palpitations) the physician should be notified.

Cardiovascular Toxicity. There has been controversy regarding the possibility of adverse cardiovascular reactions to oral hypoglycemics. In 1970, the University Group Diabetes Program (UGDP) published results indicating that sulfonylureas carried an increased risk of mortality from cardiovascular causes. In the UGDP study, cardiovascular mortality was 2.5 times greater among subjects treated with a combination of diet plus tolbutamide than among control subjects who received dietary therapy alone. The UGDP study has been criticized on several grounds, including design, patient selection, dosing, and compliance. Subsequent clinical trials by other groups have failed to confirm the conclusions of the UGDP report. The American Diabetes Association, which initially endorsed the UGDP study, has since withdrawn its support.

Other Adverse Effects. Tolbutamide may induce *allergic skin reactions* (e.g., itching, rash). If these persist, the drug should be discontinued. *Hematologic reactions* (thrombocytopenia, leukopenia, anemia) occur rarely and are usually benign. *Gastrointestinal disturbances* (nausea, vomiting, anorexia), which are relatively uncommon, can be decreased by administering tolbutamide with food. Additional adverse effects include headache, fatigue, weakness, and paresthesias.

Drug Interactions

Drugs That Can Intensify Hypoglycemia. A variety of drugs, acting by diverse mechanisms, can intensify hypoglycemic responses to sulfonylureas. Included are *nonsteroidal anti-inflammatory drugs, sulfonamide antibiotics, ethanol* (used acutely), *ranitidine,* and *cimetidine.* Caution must be exercised when a sulfonylurea is used in combination with these drugs.

Drugs that Can Counteract Hypoglycemia. A number of drugs can decrease the hypoglycemic response to sulfonylureas. Among these drugs are *calcium channel blockers, combination oral contra-*ceptives, glucocorticoids, phenothiazines,* and *thiazide diuretics.* When tolbutamide and these drugs are used concurrently, special care must be taken to avoid hyperglycemia.

Beta-Adrenergic Blocking Agents. Beta blockers can interfere with tolbutamide's action by suppressing insulin release. (Recall that activation of beta receptors is one way to promote insulin release.) Since beta blockers can also mask sympathetic responses (e.g., tachycardia, tremors) to declining blood glucose, use of beta blockers can delay awareness of tolbutamide-induced hypoglycemia.

Alcohol. When alcohol is combined with tolbutamide, a disulfiram-like reaction may occur. This syndrome includes flushing, palpitations, and nausea. Disulfiram reactions are discussed fully in Chapter 33. As noted above, alcohol can also potentiate the hypoglycemic effects of tolbutamide. Patients taking tolbutamide must be warned against alcohol consumption.

Use in Pregnancy and Lactation

Oral hypoglycemics should be avoided during pregnancy. Although adequate studies in humans are lacking, sulfonylureas are known to be teratogenic in animals. Furthermore, since sulfonylurea therapy during pregnancy often fails to provide good glycemic control, and since even mild hyperglycemia may be hazardous to the fetus, insulin is generally preferred to sulfonylureas for managing the diabetic pregnancy.

It is especially important to avoid tolbutamide near term. Newborns exposed to sulfonylureas at the time of delivery have experienced severe hypoglycemia lasting as long as 4 to 10 days. Hence, if an oral hypoglycemic has been taken during pregnancy, it should be discontinued at least 48 hours prior to the anticipated time of delivery.

Tolbutamide should not be taken by women who are nursing. The drug is excreted into breast milk, posing a risk of hypoglycemia to the infant. If a woman wishes to breast-feed, she should substitute insulin for the sulfonylurea.

Preparations, Dosage, and Administration

Tolbutamide [Orinase] is dispensed in 250- and 500-mg tablets. Because of its short half-life, the drug is usually administered in divided daily doses. The usual starting dosage is 1 to 2 gm/day administered in one to three doses. The maximum dosage is 2 to 3 gm/day.

OTHER SULFONYLUREAS

In addition to tolbutamide, five other sulfonylureas are available (see Table 49–6). All of these drugs have similar actions and side effects, and they all share the same application: treatment of noninsulin-dependent diabetes. All sulfonylureas can cause hypoglycemia.

The oral hypoglycemics differ significantly from one another with respect to duration of action. For example, the shortest-acting sulfonylurea (tolbutamide) has effects that last only 6 to

12 hours. In contrast, chlorpropamide, the longest-acting oral hypoglycemic, has effects that may last as long as 3 days. Time courses and dosages are summarized in Table 49–6.

DIABETIC KETOACIDOSIS: PATHOGENESIS AND TREATMENT

Ketoacidosis is the most severe manifestation of insulin deficiency. This syndrome is characterized by hyperglycemia, production of ketoacids, hemoconcentration, acidosis, and coma. Before insulin became available, practically all insulin-dependent diabetics died from ketoacidosis.

Pathogenesis

Diabetic ketoacidosis is brought on by derangements of glucose and fat metabolism. Altered glucose metabolism causes hyperglycemia, water loss, and hemoconcentration. Altered fat metabolism causes production of ketoacids. Figure 49–2 outlines the sequence of metabolic events by which ketoacidosis develops. Note that in its final stages, the syndrome consists of hemoconcentration and shock, in addition to ketoacidosis itself. The alterations in fat and glucose metabolism that lead to ketoacidosis are described in detail below.

Altered Fat Metabolism. Alterations in fat metabolism lead to production of ketoacids. As indicated in Figure 49–2, insulin deficiency promotes lipolysis (breakdown of fats) in adipose tissue. The products of lipolysis are glycerol and free fatty acids (FFA). Both of these metabolites are transported to the liver. In the liver, oxidation of FFA results in the production of two ketoacids (beta-hydroxybutyric acid and acetoacetic acid), which are also referred to as *ketone bodies*. Accumulation of ketoacids puts the body in a state of ketosis. Ketosis can be detected by an odor of decaying apples that ketones impart to the urine. As buildup of ketoacids increases, frank acidosis develops. At this point, the patient's condition changes from ketosis to ketoacidosis. (Ketoacidosis can be distinguished from ketosis by the presence of hyperventilation.) Acidosis contributes to the development of shock.

Alterations in Glucose Metabolism. Deranged glucose metabolism leads to hyperglycemia, water loss, and hemoconcentration. As shown in Figure 49–2, insulin deficiency has two direct effects on the metabolism of glucose: (1) an increase in glucose production, and (2) a decrease in glucose utilization. (The glycerol released by lipolysis is a substrate for glucose synthesis and, therefore, helps to increase glucose production.) Since more glucose is being made, and less is being used, plasma levels of glucose rise, causing hyperglycemia. Glycosuria develops when plasma glucose content becomes so high that the amount of glucose filtered by the glomeruli of the kidney exceeds the capacity of the renal tubules for glucose reuptake. As the concentration of glucose in the urine increases, osmotic diuresis develops, resulting in the loss of large volumes of water. Dehydration is worsened because of vomiting brought on by ketosis. Vomiting is a direct source of fluid loss and, more importantly, is an impediment to rehydration with oral fluids. (It should be noted that along with loss of water, sodium and potassium are also lost. These positive ions are excreted in conjunction with ketone bodies, compounds that carry a negative charge.) As dehydration becomes more severe, hemoconcentration develops. Hemoconcentration causes cerebral dehydration, which, together with acidosis, leads to shock.

Treatment

Diabetic ketoacidosis is a life-threatening emergency. Treatment is directed at the following: restoration of insulin levels, correction of acidosis, replacement of lost water and sodium, and normalization of potassium and glucose levels. Details of therapy are presented below.

Insulin Infusion. Insulin levels are restored by infusing regular insulin at a rate of 0.1 U/kg/hr. Use of an infusion pump is recommended. The total dose should range from 35 to 40 units. (This dose is much lower than the 500 to 1000 units employed in the past.) The dosing objective is to achieve an optimum blood level of insulin (about 100 to 150 μU/ml). Dosage is not determined by the degree of glycemia or ketonemia.

Intravenous infusion of insulin is preferred to subcutaneous injection. When insulin is administered SC, insulin levels cannot be lowered quickly in response to excessive dosing; hence, avoiding hypoglycemia may be difficult. In contrast, since insulin levels will drop quickly when an infusion is terminated, infusion permits better regulation of blood glucose content.

Bicarbonate for Acidosis. Acidosis is a serious problem with a straightforward solution. Severe acidosis (pH less than 7.1 and plasma bicarbonate less than 10 mEq/L) is corrected by administering sodium bicarbonate IV. pH will equilibrate about 30 minutes after bicarbonate administration. When acidosis is moderate, no specific treatment is needed.

Water and Sodium Replacement. Dehydration and sodium loss are both corrected with intravenous saline. Depending on the specific needs of the patient, either 0.9% or 0.45% saline may be employed. Adults usually require between 8 and 10 L of fluid during the first 12 hours of treatment. In elderly patients and patients with heart disease, central venous pressure should be monitored.

Potassium Replacement. Loss of potassium is a serious problem and must be corrected. Potassium can be replenished through oral or IV administration. Since hypokalemia predisposes the patient to dysrhythmias, EKG monitoring is essential.

Treatment of potassium loss is tricky. This is because *plasma* potassium levels may be normal even though *intracellular* potassium is very low. When insulin is administered, causing cellular uptake of potassium to increase, severe hypokalemia can develop as plasma potassium rushes into potassium-depleted cells. Because of this relationship between insulin administration and plasma potassium levels, the following guidelines apply: (1) if plasma potassium is normal, no potassium should be administered until plasma levels decline in response to insulin; (2) if plasma potassium is low, potassium should be given immediately (and then readministered if potassium levels fall following insulin administration).

Normalization of Glucose Levels. Treatment of ketoacidosis with insulin may convert *hyper*glycemia into *hypo*glycemia. Because cellular uptake of glucose is impaired by insulin deficiency, ketoacidosis is likely to be associated with a *reduction* in *intracellular* glucose—despite *elevations* in *plasma* glucose content. Under these conditions, insulin administration will cause plasma glucose to rush into the glucose-depleted cells, thereby causing plasma levels of glucose to drop precipitously. If insulin therapy induces hypoglycemia, plasma glucose can be restored by administering either glucagon or glucose itself.

GLUCAGON (FOR INSULIN OVERDOSAGE)

Glucagon is a polypeptide hormone produced by alpha cells of the pancreatic islets. The hormone increases plasma levels of glucose and relaxes smooth muscle of the GI tract. The drug can be used to elevate blood glucose levels following insulin overdosage.

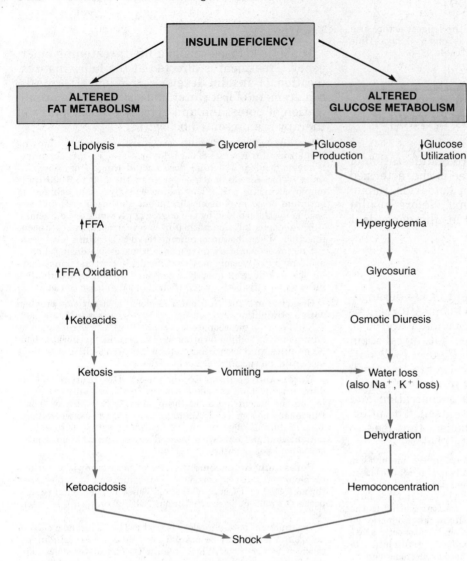

Figure 49–2. Pathogenesis of diabetic ketoacidosis. The syndrome of ketoacidosis is caused by derangements of fat and glucose metabolism that occur in response to lack of insulin. (FFA = free fatty acids)

Actions. Glucagon has effects on carbohydrate metabolism that are exactly opposite to those of insulin. Specifically, glucagon promotes the breakdown of glycogen, reduces glycogen synthesis, and stimulates biosynthesis of glucose. Hence, whereas insulin acts to lower plasma glucose content, glucagon causes glucose levels to rise. In addition, glucagon acts on gastrointestinal smooth muscle to promote relaxation.

Therapeutic Uses. Glucagon is used to treat hypoglycemia resulting from insulin overdosage. In unconscious patients, arousal usually occurs within 20 minutes of glucagon injection. If no response occurs by this time, intravenous dextrose (glucose) must be administered. Once consciousness has been produced, oral carbohydrates should be given; these will help prevent recurrence of hypoglycemia and will help restore hepatic glycogen content.

Glucagon cannot correct hypoglycemia resulting from starvation. Since glucagon acts, in large part, by promoting glycogen breakdown, and since starvation depletes glycogen stores, glucagon cannot elevate glucose levels in individuals who are starved.

Adverse Effects. Serious untoward effects are rare. Nausea and vomiting occur infrequently. Animal studies indicate no adverse effects on the fetus. However, adequate data in pregnant women are lacking.

Preparations, Dosage, and Administration. Glucagon is administered parenterally (IM, SC, and IV). The drug is dispensed in powder form and must be reconstituted to a concentration of 1 mg/ml using the diluent supplied by the manufacturer. A dose of 0.5 to 1 mg is usually effective.

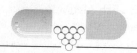

Summary of Major Nursing Implications

INSULIN

Preadministration Assessment

Therapeutic Goal

Insulin is required by all patients with IDDM and by some with NIDDM. The goal of therapy is to maintain plasma glucose levels within an acceptable range (premeal and bedtime values between 80 and 140 mg/dl in older children and adults, and between 100 and 200 mg/dl in children under 5 years).

Baseline Data

Assess for clinical manifestations of diabetes (e.g., polyuria, polydipsia, polyphagia, weight loss) and for indications of hyperglycemia. Baseline laboratory tests include fasting blood glucose, a glucose tolerance test, urinary glucose and ketones, and serum electrolytes.

Identifying High-Risk Patients

Special care is needed in patients taking drugs that can raise or lower blood glucose levels, such as *sympathomimetics, beta blockers, glucocorticoids,* and *sulfonylureas.*

Patients with a history of severe *allergic reactions to insulin derived from beef or pork pancreas* should be treated with one of the human insulins.

Maintaining glycemic control during *pregnancy* is both very important and very difficult.

Implementation: Administration

Routes

All insulins may be administered SC. None are given PO. *Regular* insulin (U-40 and U-100) may be administered IM and IV, in addition to SC. U-500 regular insulin may be administered SC and IM, but not IV.

Syringe and Needle Selection

Teach the patient to use a syringe that corresponds with the concentration of insulin to be administered: a U-40 syringe (identified by red markings) is used for U-40 insulins (identified by red bottle caps); a U-100 syringe (orange markings) is used for U-100 insulins (orange bottle caps).

Inform the patient that needles for SC injection should be 25- or 26-gauge and 1/2- to 3/4-inch long.

Preparation for Subcutaneous Injection

Teach the patient to prepare for SC injections as follows:

1. Before loading the syringe, disperse insulin *suspensions* (i.e., all forms of insulin except regular insulin) by rolling the vial gently between the palms. Vigorous agitation will cause frothing and must be avoided. If granules or clumps remain after mixing, discard the vial.

2. *Regular insulin* is a clear solution and, therefore, can be administered

without mixing. If a preparation becomes cloudy or discolored, or if a precipitate develops, discard the vial.

    3. Before loading the syringe, swab the bottle cap with alcohol.

    4. Eliminate air bubbles from the syringe and needle after loading.

    5. Cleanse the skin with alcohol prior to injection.

Sites of Injection

Provide the patient with the following instruction regarding sites of SC injection:

    1. Usual sites of injection are the upper arms, thighs, and abdomen. To minimize variability in responses, it is preferable to make all injections in just one of these areas.

    2. Rotate the injection site within the general area employed (i.e., abdomen, thigh, or upper arm). Allow about 1 inch between sites. If possible, use each site just once every month.

Mixing Insulins

Teach the patient the following guidelines for mixing insulins:

    1. *All Types of Insulin.* Mix U-40 insulins only with other U-40 insulins, and U-100 insulins only with other U-100 insulins.

    2. *Regular insulin* may be mixed with all other types of insulin. When preparing a mixture, draw the regular insulin into the syringe first to avoid contaminating the vial of regular insulin with insulin of a different type.

    3. *NPH insulin* is compatible only with regular insulin. Mixtures may be prepared by the patient or purchased premixed (70% NPH/30% regular).

    4. *Lente insulins* (Semilente, Lente, Ultralente) may be combined with one another or with regular insulin. Mixtures of Lente insulins with regular insulin should be injected immediately after being prepared.

Insulin Storage

Teach the patient the following about insulin storage:

    1. Store *unopened vials* of insulin in the refrigerator, but do not freeze. When stored under these conditions, insulin can be used up to the expiration date on the vial.

    2. The *vial in current use* can be stored at *room temperature* for up to 1 month, but must be kept out of direct sunlight and extreme heat. Discard partially filled vials after several weeks if left unused.

    3. *Mixtures* of insulin prepared in *vials* may be stored for 1 month at room temperature, and for 3 months under refrigeration.

    4. *Mixtures* of insulin in *prefilled syringes* (plastic or glass) should be stored in a refrigerator, where they will be stable for at least one week, and perhaps two. Store the syringe vertically (needle pointing up) to avoid clogging the needle. Gently agitate the syringe prior to administration to resuspend the insulin.

Dosage Adjustment

The dosing goal is to maintain blood glucose levels within an acceptable range. Dosage must be adjusted to balance changes in caloric intake and other factors that can either decrease insulin needs (strenuous exercise, pregnancy during the first trimester) or increase insulin needs (illness, trauma, stress, the adolescent growth spurt, pregnancy after the first trimester).

Regular insulin can adsorb in varying amounts onto IV infusion sets.

Dosage adjustments made to compensate for losses are based on the therapeutic response.

Implementation: Measures to Enhance Therapeutic Effects

Patient and Family Education

Patient and family education is an absolute requirement for safe and successful glycemic control. Provide patients and their families with thorough instruction on (1) the nature of diabetes, (2) the importance of tight glucose control, (3) the major components of the treatment routine (insulin, diet, exercise), (4) procedures for purchasing insulin, syringes, and needles, (5) methods of insulin storage, (6) procedures for mixing insulins, (7) calculation of dosage adjustments, (8) techniques of insulin injection, (9) rotation of injection sites, (10) measurement of blood and/or urinary glucose content, (11) the signs and management of hypoglycemia, (12) the signs and management of hyperglycemia, (13) the special problems of diabetic pregnancy, and (14) the procedure for obtaining Medic-Alert registration. Warn patients against making arbitrary changes to an insulin of different purity or species of origin.

Ongoing Evaluation and Interventions

Evaluating Therapeutic Effects

Whenever practical, home blood glucose monitoring (HBGM) should be employed to evaluate treatment. Teach the patient how to use the HBGM measuring device and encourage him or her to monitor blood glucose daily. Urinary glucose may be monitored as an alternative, but these measurements are much less useful than HBGM. The physician may request periodic measurements of hemoglobin A_{1c} as a means of assessing long-term glycemic control.

Minimizing Adverse Effects

Hypoglycemia. Hypoglycemia will occur whenever insulin levels exceed insulin needs. Inform the patient about potential causes of hypoglycemia (e.g., reduced food intake, vomiting, diarrhea, excessive consumption of alcohol, unaccustomed exercise, termination of pregnancy) and teach the patient and family members to recognize the early signs and symptoms of hypoglycemia (tachycardia, palpitations, sweating, nervousness, headache, confusion, drowsiness, fatigue).

Rapid treatment is mandatory. If the patient is conscious, oral carbohydrates are indicated (e.g., orange juice, sugar cubes, honey, candy). However, if the swallowing reflex or gag reflex is suppressed, nothing should be administered PO. For unconscious patients, IV glucose is the treatment of choice. If glucose is unavailable, parenteral glucagon may be used.

Hypoglycemic coma must be differentiated from coma of diabetic ketoacidosis (DKA). The differential diagnosis is made by measuring plasma or urinary glucose content: hypoglycemic coma is associated with very low levels of glucose, whereas high levels signify DKA.

Lipoatrophy. Loss of subcutaneous fat can occur at sites of insulin injection. Inform the patient that lipoatrophy can be reversed by injecting a highly purified insulin preparation (e.g., purified pork or human insulin) directly into the site of fat loss.

Lipohypertrophy. Accumulation of subcutaneous fat can occur at sites of frequent insulin injection. Inform the patient that lipohypertrophy can be minimized by systematic rotation of the injection site.

Local Allergic Reactions. Reddening or hardening may occur at sites of insulin injection. These reactions can be minimized by using highly purified insulin preparations.

Systemic Allergic Reactions. Systemic reactions (widespread urticaria, impairment of breathing) are rare. Systemic allergy is most common with beef insulin and is less likely with pork or human insulin. If systemic allergy develops, it can be reduced through desensitization (i.e., administration of small initial doses of purified pork or human insulin followed by a series of progressively larger doses).

Minimizing Adverse Interactions

Hypoglycemic Agents. Several drugs, including *sulfonylureas, alcohol* (used acutely), and *beta-adrenergic blocking* agents can intensify hypoglycemia induced by insulin. When any of these drugs is combined with insulin, special care must be taken to insure that blood glucose content does not fall too low.

Hyperglycemic Agents. Several drugs, including *thiazide diuretics, glucocorticoids,* and *sympathomimetics* can elevate blood glucose, and can thereby counteract the therapeutic effects of insulin. When these agents are combined with insulin, increased insulin dosage may be required.

Beta-Adrenergic Blocking Agents. Beta blockade can mask sympathetic responses (e.g., tachycardia, palpitations, tremors) to declining blood glucose, and can thereby delay awareness of insulin-induced hypoglycemia. Also, since beta blockade impairs glycogenolysis, beta blockers can make insulin-induced hypoglycemia even worse.

Digoxin. By lowering plasma levels of potassium (secondary to increased cellular uptake of potassium), insulin can increase the risk of digoxin-induced dysrhythmias. Accordingly, when insulin and digoxin are used concurrently, special care must be taken to keep plasma potassium levels within a physiologic range.

Management of Diabetic Ketoacidosis

Treatment is directed at the following: restoration of insulin levels, correction of acidosis, replacement of lost water and sodium, restoration of potassium levels, and normalization of glucose metabolism.

Intravenous Insulin. Restore insulin levels with intravenous insulin (0.1 U/kg/hr). The total dose usually ranges from 35 to 40 units. Use of an infusion pump is recommended.

Intravenous Sodium Bicarbonate. Correct severe acidosis (pH less than 7.1, plasma bicarbonate less than 10 mEq/L) with IV sodium bicarbonate. When acidosis is less severe, no specific treatment is needed.

Intravenous Saline. Replenish lost salt and water with IV saline (0.9% or 0.45%). The usual adult requirement is between 8 and 10 L of fluid during the first 12 hours of treatment.

Potassium Replacement. Replenish potassium with oral or IV supplements. If plasma potassium is normal, withhold potassium until levels decline under the influence of insulin. If plasma potassium is low, administer potassium immediately (and then readminister if levels fall in response to insulin).

Normalization of Glucose Levels. Treatment of DKA with insulin may convert *hyper*glycemia into *hypo*glycemia. If hypoglycemia develops, restore plasma glucose content by administering glucagon or glucose.

ORAL HYPOGLYCEMICS (SULFONYLUREAS)

Tolbutamide	Chlorpropamide
Acetohexamide	Glipizide
Tolazamide	Glyburide

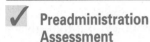

Preadministration Assessment

Therapeutic Goal

Sulfonylureas are used as an adjunct to caloric restriction and exercise to maintain glycemic control in patients with NIDDM. These drugs are *not* useful for patients with IDDM.

Identifying High-Risk Patients

These drugs are *contraindicated* for women who are *pregnant* or *breast-feeding*. Use with *caution* in patients with *kidney or liver dysfunction*. Sulfonylureas should not be used in conjunction with *alcohol*.

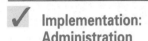

Implementation: Administration

Route

Oral.

Administration

Advise patients to administer with food if GI upset occurs.

Note that dosages for the second-generation agents are much lower than dosages for first-generation agents (see Table 49–6).

Implementation: Measures to Enhance Therapeutic Effects

Sulfonylureas are intended only as supplemental therapy of NIDDM. Encourage patients to maintain their established program of exercise and caloric restriction.

Ongoing Evaluation and Interventions

Minimizing Adverse Effects

Hypoglycemia. Inform patients about signs of hypoglycemia (palpitations, tachycardia, sweating, fatigue, excessive hunger) and instruct them to notify the physician if these occur. Treat severe hypoglycemia with IV glucose.

Minimizing Adverse Interactions

Drugs That Can Intensify Hypoglycemia. Several drugs, including *nonsteroidal anti-inflammatory drugs, sulfonamide antibiotics, ethanol* (used acutely), *ranitidine*, and *cimetidine*, can intensify hypoglycemia caused by sulfonylureas. Exercise caution when using a sulfonylurea in combination with these drugs.

Drugs That Can Counteract Hypoglycemia. Several drugs, including *calcium channel blockers, combination oral contraceptives, glucocorticoids, phenothiazines*, and *thiazide diuretics*, can decrease hypoglycemic responses to sulfonylureas. When a sulfonylurea is combined with these drugs, exercise caution to avoid hyperglycemia.

Beta-Adrenergic Blocking Agents. Beta blockade can mask sympathetic responses (e.g., tachycardia, tremors) to declining blood glucose, and can thereby can delay awareness of tolbutamide-induced hypoglycemia. Also, since beta blockade impairs glycogenolysis, beta blockers can make hypoglycemia even worse.

Alcohol. Concomitant use of alcohol and a sulfonylurea can cause a disulfiram-like reaction (flushing, palpitations, nausea). Warn the patient against alcohol ingestion.

Use in Pregnancy and Lactation

Pregnancy. Discontinue sulfonylureas during pregnancy. If a hypoglycemic agent is needed, insulin is the drug to use.

Lactation. Sulfonylureas are excreted into breast milk, posing a risk of hypoglycemia to the nursing infant. Women who choose to breast-feed should substitute insulin for the sulfonylurea.

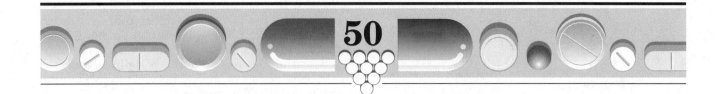

Drugs for Thyroid Disorders

Thyroid hormones have profound effects on metabolism, cardiac function, growth, and development. These hormones stimulate the metabolic rate of most cells, and increase the force and rate of cardiac contractions. During infancy and childhood, thyroid hormones promote maturation; an absence of these hormones can produce dwarfism and permanent mental impairment. Fortunately, most abnormalities of thyroid function can be effectively treated.

We will begin our study of thyroid drugs by reviewing thyroid physiology. Next we will review the pathophysiology of hypothyroid and hyperthyroid states. With this background, we will then discuss the agents used to treat thyroid disorders.

THYROID PHYSIOLOGY

Chemistry and Nomenclature

The thyroid gland produces two active hormones: *triiodothyronine* (T$_3$) and *thyroxine* (T$_4$, tetraiodothyronine). As Figure 50–1 shows, the structures of these hormones are nearly identical, the only difference being that T$_4$ contains four atoms of iodine, whereas T$_3$ contains only three. The biologic effects of T$_3$ and T$_4$ are qualitatively similar. However, when compared on a molar basis, T$_3$ is more potent than T$_4$.

The preparations of T$_3$ and T$_4$ employed clinically are manmade. These synthetic compounds have structures identical to those of the naturally

649

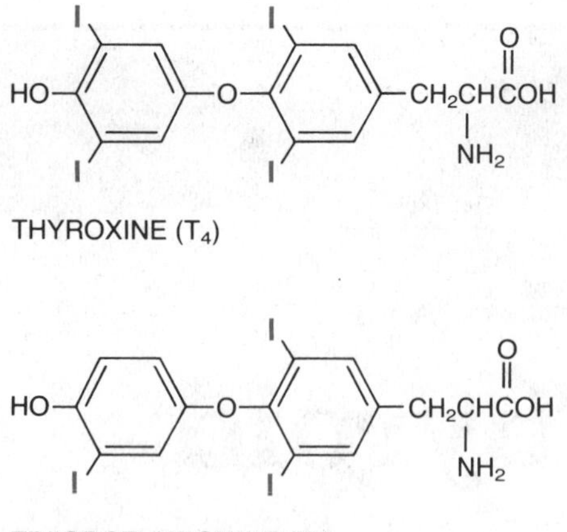

Figure 50–1. Structural formulas of the thyroid hormones.

occurring hormones. Synthetic T_3 has the generic name *liothyronine*; the generic name of synthetic T_4 is *levothyroxine*. A fixed ratio mixture of T_3 plus T_4, known as *liotrix*, is also available.

Thyroid Hormone Actions

Thyroid hormones have three principal actions: (1) stimulation of energy use, (2) stimulation of the heart, and (3) promotion of growth and development. Stimulation of energy use elevates the basal metabolic rate, resulting in increased oxygen consumption and increased heat production. Stimulation of the heart increases both the rate and force of contraction, resulting in increased cardiac output. Thyroid effects on growth and development are profound: thyroid hormones are essential for normal development of the brain and other components of the nervous system; these hormones also have a significant impact on maturation of skeletal muscle.

Synthesis and Fate of Thyroid Hormones

Synthesis. Synthesis of thyroid hormones takes place in four basic steps (Fig. 50–2). The circled numbers in the figure correspond with the step numbers below.

Step 1. Formation of thyroid hormone begins with the active transport of *iodide* into the thyroid. Under normal circumstances, this uptake process produces concentrations of iodide within the thyroid that are 20 to 50 times greater than the concentration of iodide in plasma. When plasma iodide levels are extremely low, intrathyroid iodide content may reach levels that are more than 100 times greater than those of plasma.

Step 2. Following uptake, iodide undergoes oxidation to *iodine*, the active form of iodide. Oxidation of iodide is catalyzed by an enzyme called *peroxidase*.

Step 3. In step three, activated iodine becomes incorporated into tyrosine residues that are bound to *thyroglobulin*, a large glycoprotein molecule. As indicated in the figure, one tyrosine molecule may receive either one or two atoms of iodine, resulting in the production of monoiodotyrosine (MIT) and diiodotyrosine (DIT), respectively.

Step 4. The final step of thyroid hormone synthesis consists of the coupling of iodinated tyrosines. Coupling of one DIT with one MIT forms T_3 (step 4A); coupling of one DIT with another DIT forms T_4 (step 4B).

Fate. Thyroid hormones are released from the thyroid gland by a proteolytic process. The amount of T_4 released is substantially greater than the amount of T_3. However, much of the T_4 that is released undergoes conversion into T_3 by enzymes in peripheral tissues. In fact, conversion of T_4 into T_3 accounts for the majority (about 80%) of the T_3 found in the bloodstream.

Greater than 99% of the T_3 and T_4 in plasma is bound to plasma proteins. Consequently, only a tiny fraction of circulating thyroid hormone is free to produce biologic effects.

Thyroid hormones are eliminated primarily by hepatic metabolism. Because T_3 and T_4 are extensively bound to plasma proteins, metabolism takes place slowly. As a result, the half-lives of these hormones are prolonged: T_3 has a half-life of 1 to 2 days, and T_4 has a half-life of approximately 1 week.

Regulation of Thyroid Function by the Hypothalamus and the Anterior Pituitary

The functional relationship between the hypothalamus, anterior pituitary, and thyroid is shown schematically in Figure 50–3. As the figure indicates, thyrotropin-releasing hormone (TRH), secreted by the hypothalamus, acts on the pituitary to cause secretion of thyrotropin (thyroid-stimulating hormone, TSH). TSH then acts on the thyroid to stimulate all aspects of thyroid function: thyroid size is enlarged, iodine uptake is augmented, and synthesis and release of thyroid hormones are increased. In response to rising plasma levels of T_3 and T_4, further release of TSH by the pituitary is suppressed. The stimulatory effect of TSH on the thyroid followed by the inhibitory effect of thyroid hormones on the pituitary represents a typical negative feedback loop.

Influence of Iodine Levels on Thyroid Function

Low Iodine. When iodine availability is diminished, production of thyroid hormones decreases. The ensuing drop in thyroid hormone levels promotes release of TSH. In response to increased

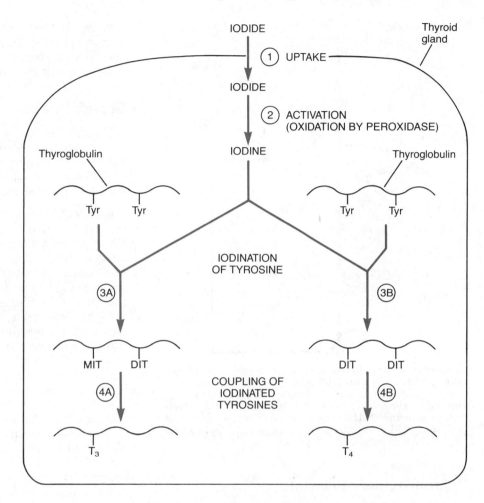

Figure 50–2. Steps in thyroid hormone synthesis. The reactions at each step (circled numbers) are explained in the text. (Tyr = tyrosine, MIT = monoiodotyrosine, DIT = diiodotyrosine, T_3 = triiodothyronine, T_4 = thyroxine)

levels of TSH, thyroid size increases (causing goiter), and the ability of the thyroid to concentrate iodine increases as well. If the iodine deficiency is not too severe, the increased capacity for iodine uptake will permit production of thyroid hormones in amounts sufficient to return plasma levels of T_3 and T_4 to normal values.

High Iodine. The effect of extremely high iodine levels on thyroid function is opposite to the effect of low iodine: uptake of iodide is suppressed, and synthesis and release of thyroid hormone decline. The mechanisms underlying these effects are not understood.

THYROID PATHOPHYSIOLOGY

HYPOTHYROIDISM

Hypothyroidism can occur at any age. In the adult, mild deficiency of thyroid hormone is referred to simply as hypothyroidism; severe deficiency in adults is called *myxedema*. When hypothyroidism occurs in infancy, the resulting condition is known as *cretinism*.

Hypothyroidism in Adults

Clinical Presentation. Hypothyroidism in adults produces a characteristic set of signs and symptoms. The face is pale, puffy, and expressionless. The skin is cold and dry. The hair is brittle. Heart rate and temperature are lowered. The patient may complain of lethargy, fatigue, and intolerance to cold. Mentality may be impaired. Thyroid enlargement (goiter) may occur if reduced levels of T_3 and T_4 promote excessive release of TSH.

Causes. Hypothyroidism in the adult is usually due to malfunction of the thyroid itself. Causes of gland malfunction include autoimmune disease, insufficient iodine in the diet, surgical removal of the thyroid, and destruction of the thyroid by radioactive iodine. Adult hypothyroidism may also result from deficient secretion of TSH and TRH.

Therapeutic Strategy. Hypothyroidism in adults requires replacement therapy with thyroid hormones. In almost all cases, treatment must continue for life. For mild deficiency, oral hormones are employed. For severe deficiency, IV therapy may be required. When replacement doses are adequate, therapy will eliminate all signs and symptoms of thyroid deficiency.

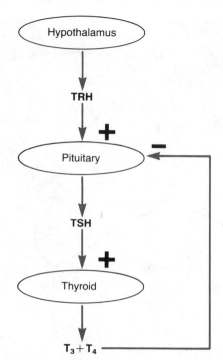

Figure 50–3. Regulation of thyroid function. TRH from the hypothalamus stimulates release of TSH from the pituitary. TSH stimulates all aspects of thyroid function, including release of T_3 and T_4. T_3 and T_4 act on the pituitary to suppress further TSH release. (TRH = thyrotopin-releasing hormone, TSH = thyrotropin [thyroxid-stimulating hormone], T_3 = triiodothyronine, T_4 = thyroxine)

Hypothyroidism in Infants

Clinical Presentation. Thyroid deficiency in infants (cretinism) causes mental retardation and derangement of growth. In the absence of thyroid hormones, the child develops a large and protruding tongue, potbelly, and dwarfish stature. Development of the nervous system, bones, teeth, and muscles is impaired.

Causes. Cretinism usually results from a failure in thyroid development. Other causes include autoimmune disease, severe iodine deficiency, TSH deficiency, and exposure to radioactive iodine *in utero*.

Therapeutic Strategy. Hypothyroidism in newborns requires replacement therapy with thyroid hormones. If treatment is initiated within a few days of birth, physical and mental development will be normal. However, if therapy is delayed for several months, some permanent retardation will be evident, although the physical effects of thyroid deficiency will reverse. Replacement therapy must continue for life.

HYPERTHYROIDISM

There are two major forms of hyperthyroidism: *Graves' disease* and *Plummer's disease*. Of the two,

Graves' disease is the more common. Signs and symptoms of both are similar; the principal difference is that Graves' disease may cause exophthalmos, whereas Plummer's disease does not.

Graves' Disease

Graves' disease is the most common cause of excessive thyroid hormone secretion. This disorder occurs most frequently in women 20 to 40 years of age. The incidence of Graves' disease in females is six times greater than in males.

Clinical Presentation. Most clinical manifestations of Graves' disease result from elevated levels of thyroid hormone. Heart beat is rapid and strong; dysrhythmias and angina may develop. The central nervous system is stimulated, resulting in rapid thought flow and speech, nervousness, and insomnia. Skeletal muscles may weaken and atrophy. Metabolic rate is raised, resulting in increased heat production, increased body temperature, intolerance to heat, and skin that is warm and moist. Appetite is increased. However, despite increased food consumption, weight loss will occur if caloric intake fails to match the increase in metabolic rate. Collectively, the above signs and symptoms are referred to as *thyrotoxicosis*.

In addition to thyrotoxicosis, victims of Graves' disease often present with *exophthalmos* (protrusion of the eyeballs). The cause of exophthalmos is obscure. However, we do know that this condition is not caused by increased levels of thyroid hormones.

If levels of thyroid hormones are extremely high, *thyroid storm* may result. This syndrome is characterized by hyperthermia, severe tachycardia, and profound weakness. Unconsciousness, coma, and heart failure may occur.

Cause. Thyroid stimulation in Graves' disease is caused by thyroid-stimulating immunoglobulins (TSIs). These immunoglobulins are antibodies produced by an autoimmune process. TSIs increase thyroid activity by stimulating receptors for TSH. That is, TSIs mimic the effects of TSH on thyroid function. TSIs are not responsible for exophthalmos.

Therapeutic Modalities. Treatment for Graves' disease is directed at decreasing the production of thyroid hormones. Three modalities are employed: (1) surgery (subtotal thyroidectomy), (2) radiation therapy, and (3) antithyroid drugs. Of the three approaches, surgical removal of thyroid tissue and radiation are the most definitive. Since exophthalmos is not the result of hyperthyroidism per se, this condition will not be improved by lowering thyroid hormone production. If exophthalmos is severe, it can be treated with high doses of oral glucocorticoids.

Thyroid storm can be life-threatening and requires immediate treatment. High doses of iodine will suppress thyroid hormone release; propranolol will control heart rate; and digitalis can improve cardiac function in the event of heart failure. Additional measures include sedation, cooling, and administration of fluids.

Plummer's Disease

Plummer's disease (toxic nodular goiter) is the result of thyroid adenoma. Clinical manifestations are much like those of Graves' disease, except that Plummer's disease does not produce exophthalmos. Plummer's disease is a persistent condition that rarely undergoes spontaneous remission. Accordingly, surgery and radiation, which provide long-term control, are often preferred over drugs for treatment.

THYROID FUNCTION TESTS

Several laboratory tests can be used to evaluate thyroid function. Three of these are described below.

Serum T$_4$ Test. The serum T$_4$ test measures total (bound plus free) *thyroxine*. Since serum T$_4$ levels reflect overall thyroid activity, this test is useful for initial screening of thyroid function: levels of T$_4$ will be low in *hypo*thyroid patients and high in *hyper*thyroid patients. The test can also be used to monitor thyroid-hormone replacement therapy; all thyroid preparations, except liothyronine, should cause T$_4$ levels to rise.

Serum T$_3$ Test. The T$_3$ test measures total (bound plus free) *triiodothyronine*. This test is useful for diagnosing the various forms of hyperthyroidism, since, in these disorders, levels of T$_3$ often rise sooner and to a greater extent than do levels of T$_4$. T$_3$ determinations can also be employed to monitor thyroid-hormone replacement therapy; all thyroid preparations should cause an increase in levels of T$_3$.

Serum Thyrotropin. Serum TSH levels can be used to evaluate replacement therapy in hypothyroidism. In hypothyroid patients, levels of thyroid hormone are insufficient to suppress TSH secretion; hence, in the absence of treatment, TSH levels will be high. If replacement therapy is adequate, a decline in TSH levels will be measured.

Measurement of serum TSH can be used to distinguish between primary hypothyroidism and secondary hypothyroidism: in primary (thyroidal) hypothyroidism, TSH levels will be high, whereas in secondary hypothyroidism (hypothyroidism resulting from anterior pituitary dysfunction) TSH levels will be low.

THYROID HORMONE PREPARATIONS

Thyroid hormones are available as pure, synthetic compounds, and as extracts of animal thyroid glands. All of these preparations have qualitatively similar effects. The synthetic preparations are more stable and better standardized than are the animal-gland extracts. As a result, the synthetics are generally preferred to the natural products. Properties of the thyroid hormone preparations are summarized in Table 50–1.

LEVOTHYROXINE (T$_4$)

Levothyroxine [Levothroid, Synthroid, Levoxine] is a synthetic preparation of thyroxine (T$_4$), a naturally occurring thyroid hormone. The structure of levothyroxine is identical to that of the natural hormone. Levothyroxine is the drug of choice for most patients who require thyroid hormone replacement. Consequently, levothyroxine will serve as our prototype for the thyroid hormone preparations.

Pharmacokinetics

Absorption. Absorption of oral levothyroxine is variable. Depending upon the preparation, absorption may range from 42% to 74%.

Conversion to T$_3$. Much of an administered dose of levothyroxine is converted to T$_3$ in the body. As a result, levothyroxine can produce nearly normal levels of both T$_3$ and T$_4$. Hence, for most patients, there is no need to give T$_3$ along with levothyroxine.

Half-life and Plasma Levels. The half-life of levothyroxine is prolonged (about 7 days). From a clinical perspective, this long half-life has advantages as well as disadvantages. On the negative side, about 1 month (four half-lives) is required for plasma levels of levothyroxine to reach plateau. As a result, onset of full effects is delayed. On the positive side, a long half-life causes hormone levels to remain steady between doses. This property makes levothyroxine especially desirable for lifelong therapy.

Therapeutic Uses

Levothyroxine is indicated for all forms of hypothyroidism, regardless of their cause. The drug is used for cretinism, myxedema coma, ordinary hypothyroidism in adults and children, and simple goiter. Levothyroxine is also used to treat hypothyroidism resulting from insufficient TSH (secondary to pituitary malfunction) and from insufficient TRH (secondary to hypothalamic malfunction). In addition, levothyroxine is used to insure proper levels of thyroid hormones following thyroid surgery, irradiation, and treatment with antithyroid drugs.

Thyroid hormones should not be taken to treat

Generic Name	**Trade Names**	**Dosage Forms**	**Equivalent Dosage**	**Description**	
Levothyroxine	Levothroid, Synthroid, Levoxine	Tablets, injection	50–60 μg	Synthetic preparation of T_4 identical to the naturally occurring hormone	
Liothyronine	Cytomel, Triostat	Tablets, injection	15–37 μg	Synthetic preparation of T_3 identical to the naturally occurring hormone	
Liotrix	Euthroid, Thyrolar	Tablets	60 μg	Synthetic T_4 plus synthetic T_3 in a 4:1 fixed ratio	
Thyroglobulin	Proloid	Tablets	60 mg	Purified extract of hog thyroid	
Thyroid	Armour Thyroid, S-P-T, Thyrar	Tablets, capsules	60 mg	Desiccated animal thyroid glands	

Table 50–1. Thyroid Hormone Preparations

obesity. These hormones will accelerate metabolism and promote weight reduction only if the dosage is high enough to establish a pathologic (hyperthyroid) state.

Adverse Effects

When administered in appropriate dosage, levothyroxine rarely causes adverse effects. If the dosage is excessive, *thyrotoxicosis* may be produced. Signs and symptoms include tachycardia, angina, tremor, nervousness, insomnia, hyperthermia, heat intolerance, and sweating. The patient should be informed about these signs and instructed to notify the physician if they develop. If the dosage is especially large, *thyroid storm* may occur.

Drug Interactions

Oral Anticoagulants. Levothyroxine accelerates the degradation of vitamin K–dependent clotting factors. As a result, effects of oral anticoagulants will be enhanced. If thyroid hormone replacement therapy is instituted in a patient who has been taking oral anticoagulants, dosage of the anticoagulant should be reduced.

Catecholamines. Thyroid hormones increase cardiac responsiveness to catecholamines (e.g., epinephrine, dopamine, dobutamine). This increases the risk of catecholamine-induced dysrhythmias. Caution must be exercised when administering catecholamines to patients receiving levothyroxine and other thyroid preparations.

Other Interactions. Levothyroxine can increase requirements for *insulin* and *digitalis.* Hence, when converting patients from a hypothyroid to a euthyroid state, doses of insulin and digitalis may need to be increased. *Cholestyramine* binds to levothyroxine, thereby reducing levothyroxine absorption; to

prevent this interaction, levothyroxine should be administered no sooner than 4 hours after cholestyramine.

Dosage and Administration I: General Considerations

Routes of Administration. Levothyroxine is almost always administered by mouth. Oral doses should be taken on an empty stomach to enhance absorption. Doses are usually taken in the morning before breakfast.

Intravenous administration is used for myxedema coma and for patients who cannot take levothyroxine orally. Intravenous doses are about one half the size of oral doses.

Evaluation. The goal of thyroid hormone replacement therapy is to provide a dosage that will compensate precisely for the existing thyroid deficit. Determining this dosage is accomplished using a combination of clinical judgment and laboratory tests. When therapy is successful in adults, clinical evaluation should reveal a reversal of the signs and symptoms of thyroid deficiency—and an absence of signs of thyroid excess. Successful therapy of infants is reflected in normalization of intellectual function and normalization of growth and development. Monthly determinations of height (length) provide a good index of success.

Laboratory determinations of serum TSH are an important means of evaluation. Successful therapy will cause elevated TSH levels to fall. These levels will begin their decline within hours of the onset of therapy and will continue to drop as plasma levels of thyroid hormone build up. If an adequate dosage is established, TSH levels will remain suppressed for the duration of treatment.

For some patients, serum T_4 must be used to evaluate levothyroxine therapy. In young children,

TSH secretion may remain high even though levels of thyroid hormone have been restored. In such patients, TSH determinations are not helpful. For these patients, serum T_4 levels can be employed to evaluate dosage; when the dosage is appropriate, T_4 levels will be in the normal to high-normal range.

Duration of Therapy. For most hypothyroid patients, replacement therapy must be continued for life. Treatment provides symptomatic relief but does not produce cure. The patient must be made fully aware of the chronic nature of the condition. In addition, the patient should be forewarned that although therapy will cause symptoms to improve, these improvements do not constitute a reason to interrupt or discontinue drug use.

Dosage and Administration II: Specific Applications

Hypothyroidism in Adults. The dosage should be low initially and then increased gradually until full replacement doses have been achieved. A typical dosing schedule consists of 50 μg daily (PO) for 2 weeks followed by 100 μg daily for 2 additional weeks; thereafter, daily doses of 150 μg are taken for life.

Myxedema Coma. Myxedema coma is a rare but serious condition and requires rapid treatment. Levothyroxine is administered intravenously in a dose of 200 to 500 μg. If required, an additional dose of 100 to 300 μg can be given 1 day later. Adrenal corticosteroids (e.g., hydrocortisone) are also required.

Cretinism. In cretinism, thyroid hormone dosage *decreases* with age. For infants less than 6 months old, the dosage is 10 μg/kg/day; for children aged 6 to 8 months, 8 μg/kg/day; for children aged 1 to 5 years, 6 μg/kg/day; and for children aged 5 to 10 years, 4 μg/kg/day.

Simple Goiter. In simple goiter, the thyroid is enlarged and levels of thyroid hormones are reduced. Thyroid enlargement is caused by TSH that has been released in response to low levels of thyroid hormone in the blood. When treating simple goiter, the goal is to provide full replacement doses of thyroid hormone so as to suppress further TSH release. This goal can usually be achieved with 100 to 200 μg of levothyroxine/day.

LIOTHYRONINE (T_3)

Liothyronine [Cytomel, Triostat] is a synthetic preparation of triiodothyronine (T_3), a naturally occurring thyroid hormone. The structure of liothyronine is identical to that of thyroid-derived T_3. The effects of liothyronine are qualitatively similar to those of levothyroxine.

Contrasts with Levothyroxine. Liothyronine differs from levothyroxine in three important ways: (1) liothyronine has a shorter half-life and shorter duration of action, (2) liothyronine has a more rapid onset of action, and (3) liothyronine is more expensive. Because of its high price and relatively brief duration of action, liothyronine is less desirable than levothyroxine for long-term use. However, because its effects develop quickly, liothyronine may be superior to levothyroxine in situations that require speedy results (e.g., myxedema coma).

Evaluation. As with levothyroxine, the dosage of liothyronine is adjusted on the basis of clinical evaluation and laboratory data. Two laboratory tests are useful: serum T_3 and serum TSH. Since liothyronine is not converted into T_4, plasma levels of T_4 remain low. Hence, T_4 levels cannot be used to assess treatment.

Dosage and Administration. Liothyronine is usually administered by mouth, although IV administration may also be employed. Dosage of liothyronine is about one-half the dosage of levothyroxine.

OTHER THYROID PREPARATIONS

Liotrix

Liotrix is a mixture of synthetic T_4 plus synthetic T_3 in a 4:1 fixed ratio. (This ratio is similar to the ratio of these hormones in plasma.) The rationale for use of liotrix is that this mixture can produce plasma levels of T_4 and T_3 similar to those that occur naturally. However, since levothyroxine alone produces the same ratio of T_4 to T_3, liotrix offers no advantage over levothyroxine for most indications.

Dosing with liotrix can be confusing. Two brands of liotrix are available—Euthroid and Thyrolar—and both use the same designations for tablet strength ($\frac{1}{2}$, 1, 2, 3). However, although the designations are the same, tablets with a particular designation (e.g., $\frac{1}{2}$) produced by one manufacturer do not contain the same amount of hormone as tablets with that same designation produced by the other manufacturer. Because of these differences, care should be taken if patients are switched from one brand of liotrix to the other, or from liotrix to a different thyroid preparation.

Natural Thyroid Products

Thyroid. Thyroid consists of desiccated animal thyroid glands. Standardization of this preparation is based on content of iodine, levothyroxine, and liothyronine; the ratio of levothyroxine to liothyronine is not less than 5:1. Thyroid is dispensed in tablets ranging from 16 to 325 mg. Capsules are also available. For practical purposes, thyroid is obsolete: use is limited to those patients who have been taking the preparation for years. Thyroid is rarely prescribed for patients starting therapy today.

Thyroglobulin. Thyroglobulin [Proloid] is a purified extract of hog thyroid glands. Like thyroid, thyroglobulin is standardized on the basis of its content of iodine, levothyroxine, and liothyronine; the ratio of levothyroxine to liothyronine is at least 2.8:1. Thyroglobulin is available in tablets ranging from 32 to 200 mg.

DRUGS USED TO TREAT HYPERTHYROIDISM

There are three major categories of thyroid inhibitors: (1) thioamide derivatives (propylthiouracil, methimazole), (2) iodides, and (3) radioactive iodine. In addition to these agents, propranolol can be used to treat hyperthyroid patients.

PROPYLTHIOURACIL

Propylthiouracil (PTU) inhibits thyroid hormone synthesis. This drug is a member of the thioamide category of antithyroid drugs and will serve as prototype for the group. Only one other thioamide (methimazole) is currently employed.

Mechanism of Action

The therapeutic effects of PTU result from blockade of thyroid hormone synthesis. Blockade of synthesis occurs in two ways: (1) PTU prevents the oxidation of iodide, thereby inhibiting incorporation of iodine into tyrosine, and (2) PTU prevents the coupling of iodinated tyrosines. Propylthiouracil causes these effects by inhibiting peroxidase, the enzyme that catalyzes both reactions.

It should be noted that although PTU prevents thyroid hormone synthesis, PTU does not destroy existing stores of the hormone. Once therapy has begun, 1 to 2 weeks may be required for existing stores to become depleted. Until depletion occurs, therapeutic effects will not be evident.

Pharmacokinetics

Propylthiouracil is rapidly absorbed following oral administration, and therapeutic effects begin within 30 minutes. The plasma half-life of PTU is short (about 2 hours). As a result, PTU must be administered several times each day. The drug can cross the placenta and can enter breast milk.

Therapeutic Uses

Propylthiouracil has three applications in the management of hyperthyroidism. First, PTU can be used alone as the sole form of therapy for Graves' disease. Second, PTU can be employed as an adjunct to radiation therapy; PTU is administered to control hyperthyroidism until the effects of radiation become manifest. Third, PTU can be given to suppress thyroid hormone synthesis in preparation for thyroid gland surgery (subtotal thyroidectomy).

Adverse Effects

Adverse responses to PTU are relatively rare. However, severe adverse effects can occur.

Agranulocytosis. Agranulocytosis is the most serious toxicity of PTU. This reaction is rare and usually occurs during the first 2 months of therapy. Sore throat and fever may be the earliest indications of the reaction. Patients should be instructed to report these signs immediately. Since agranulocytosis often develops rapidly, periodic blood counts are of minimal value for early detection. If agranulocytosis occurs, PTU should be discontinued. When discovered early, agranulocytosis is usually reversible.

Hypothyroidism. Excessive dosing with PTU may convert the patient from a hyperthyroid state to a hypothyroid state. If this occurs, the dosage

should be reduced. Temporary administration of thyroid hormone may be required.

Pregnancy and Lactation. Propylthiouracil crosses the placenta and has caused neonatal hypothyroidism and goiter. Accordingly, the drug must be used judiciously during pregnancy. To minimize effects on the fetus, the dosage should be kept as low as possible. As an alternative, some physicians recommend treatment with full doses of PTU combined with thyroid hormone replacement therapy. However, this practice is controversial. Propylthiouracil enters breast milk and is contraindicated for nursing mothers.

Other Adverse Effects. The most common undesired effect of PTU is rash. The drug may also cause nausea, arthralgia, headache, dizziness, and paresthesias.

Preparations, Dosage, and Administration

Propylthiouracil is available in 50-mg tablets for oral administration. Because of its short half-life, PTU is usually administered in multiple daily doses. A typical adult *maintenance* dosage is 50 mg every 8 hours. *Initial* doses may total up to 900 mg daily.

METHIMAZOLE

Methimazole, like propylthiouracil, is a member of the thioamide family of antithyroid drugs. This agent has the same mechanism of action, uses, and adverse effects as PTU. Methimazole crosses the placenta more readily than PTU. Hence, if a thioamide must be used in pregnancy, PTU is preferred. Like PTU, methimazole is contraindicated for nursing mothers. Methimazole is dispensed in tablets (5 and 10 mg) under the trade name Tapazole. The usual adult maintenance dosage is 5 to 15 mg/day administered in 3 divided doses.

IODIDE PRODUCTS (NONRADIOACTIVE)

Three iodide preparations are available for thyroid therapy. All three have the same mechanism of action and similar pharmacologic effects. However, because these preparations differ from one another in their traditional applications, each will be discussed separately.

Strong Iodine Solution (Lugol's Solution)

Description. Lugol's solution is a mixture containing 5% elemental iodine and 10% potassium iodide. The iodine undergoes reduction to iodide within the gastrointestinal tract prior to absorption.

Mechanism of Action. When present in high concentrations, iodide has a paradoxical suppressant effect on the thyroid. This suppression is brought about in three ways. First, high concentrations of iodide decrease iodine uptake by the thyroid. Second, high concentrations of iodide inhibit thyroid hormone synthesis by suppressing both the iodination of tyrosine and the coupling of iodinated tyrosine residues. Third, high concentrations of iodine inhibit release of thyroid hormone into the bloodstream. All three actions combine to decrease circulating levels of T_3 and T_4.

Unfortunately, the effects of iodide on thyroid function cannot be sustained indefinitely: with long-term iodide administration, suppressant effects become weaker. Accordingly, iodide is rarely used alone to produce thyroid suppression.

Therapeutic Use. Strong iodine solution is given to hyperthyroid individuals to suppress thyroid function in preparation for thyroid surgery. Initial effects can usually be observed within 24 hours; peak effects develop within 10 to 15 days. In most cases, plasma levels of thyroid hormone are reduced with PTU prior to therapy with iodine. Iodine solution (together with more PTU) is then administered for the last 10 days prior to subtotal thyroid removal.

In addition to its use for thyroid suppression, strong iodine solution is employed as an antiseptic (see Chapter 85).

Adverse Effects. Chronic ingestion of iodine can produce *iodism*. Signs and symptoms include a brassy taste, a burning sensation in the mouth and throat, soreness of the teeth and gums, frontal headache, coryza (nasal inflammation and sneezing), salivation, and various skin eruptions. All of these manifestations fade rapidly upon discontinuation of iodine use.

Overdosage. Iodine is corrosive and overdosage will injure the gastrointestinal tract. Symptoms include abdominal pain, vomiting, and diarrhea. Swelling of the glottis may result in asphyxiation. Treatment consists of gastric lavage (to remove iodine from the stomach) and administration of sodium thiosulfate (to reduce iodine to iodide).

Dosage and Administration. When used to prepare hyperthyroid patients for thyroidectomy, strong iodine solution is administered in a dosage of 2 to 6 drops three times daily for 10 days immediately preceding surgery. Iodine solution should be mixed with juice or some other beverage to disguise its unpleasant taste.

Sodium Iodide (IV)

Intravenous sodium iodide is employed for the acute management of *thyrotoxic crisis*. Benefits derive from the ability of high concentrations of iodide to rapidly suppress thyroid hormone release. In the treatment of thyrotoxicosis, sodium iodide is used in combination with propylthiouracil and propranolol. Sodium iodide for IV use is dispensed as a 10% solution in 10-ml ampuls. The daily dosage ranges from 250 to 500 mg.

Although intravenous sodium iodide rarely causes adverse effects, *severe hypersensitivity reactions* have occurred. These reactions may develop immediately or they may be delayed by several hours. The most characteristic feature of these reactions is angioedema. Skin eruptions, serum sickness, and edema of the larynx may also develop. Death has occurred. There is no specific antidote to these hypersensitivity reactions; hence, treatment is purely supportive.

Potassium Iodide

Potassium iodide [Thyro-Block] taken orally can be used to protect the thyroid gland in the event of a radiation emergency. If a nuclear accident should release radioactive iodine into the environment, thyroidal uptake of this radioactive iodide would damage the gland. By administering large doses of nonradioactive iodide, uptake of radioactive material can be blocked. The dosage for potassium iodide is 130 mg/day for all people over the age of 1 year; children less than 1 year old should receive 65 mg daily. Duration of use is likely to last from 3 to 10 days. Potassium iodide tablets for blocking radioactive iodine uptake are available only through state and federal agencies.

RADIOACTIVE IODINE (^{131}I)

Physical Properties

^{131}I, a radioactive isotope of stable iodine, emits a combination of beta particles and gamma rays. Radioactive decay of ^{131}I takes place with a half-life of 8 days. Hence, after 56 days (7 half-lives), less than 1% of the radioactivity in a dose of ^{131}I remains.

Use in Graves' Disease

^{131}I can be used to destroy thyroid tissue in patients with hyperthyroidism. The objective is to produce clinical remission without causing complete destruction of the gland. Unfortunately, delayed hypothyroidism, due to excessive thyroid damage, is a frequent complication of therapy.

Effect on the Thyroid. Like stable iodine, ^{131}I is concentrated in the thyroid gland. Destruction of thyroid tissue is produced primarily by emission of beta particles. (The gamma rays from ^{131}I are relatively harmless.) Since beta particles have a very limited ability to penetrate any type of physical barrier, these particles do not travel outside the thyroid; hence, damage to surrounding tissue is minimal.

Reduction of thyroid function is gradual. Initial effects of ^{131}I take several days or weeks to become apparent. Full effects take 2 to 3 months to develop.

Not all patients respond satisfactorily to a single ^{131}I treatment. About 66% of patients with Graves' disease are cured with a single exposure to ^{131}I; others require 2 or more treatments.

Advantages and Disadvantages of ^{131}I Therapy. The advantages of ^{131}I treatment are considerable: (1) cost is low; (2) patients are spared the risks, discomfort, and expense of thyroid surgery; (3) death from ^{131}I treatment has never occurred, nor is it ever likely to; and (4) no tissue other than the thyroid is injured (patients should be re-assured of this fact).

Treatment with ^{131}I is not without drawbacks. First, the effect of treatment is delayed, taking several months to achieve a maximum. Second, and more important, treatment is associated with a significant incidence of delayed *hypothyroidism*. Hypothyroidism results from excessive dosage and occurs in 10% of patients within the first year following ^{131}I exposure. An additional 2% to 3% develop hypothyroidism each year thereafter.

Who Should Be Treated and Who Should Not. Patients over the age of 30 may be candidates for ^{131}I therapy. ^{131}I is also indicated for patients who have not responded adequately to antithyroid drugs or to subtotal thyroidectomy.

Children are considered inappropriate candidates. The likelihood of delayed hypothyroidism is higher in children than in adults. Also, there is concern that administration of ^{131}I to young patients may carry a slight risk of causing cancer. It should be noted, however, that there is no evidence that the use of ^{131}I in the treatment of Graves' disease has ever caused cancer of the thyroid or any other tissue.

Iodine 131 is contraindicated in pregnancy and lactation. Exposure of the fetus to ^{131}I after the first trimester may damage the immature thyroid, and exposure to radiation at any point in fetal life carries a risk of generalized developmental harm. Since ^{131}I enters breast milk, women receiving this agent should not breast-feed.

Dosage. Dosage of ^{131}I is determined by thyroid gland size and by the rate of thyroidal iodine uptake. In the treatment of Graves' disease, the dosage usually ranges between 4 and 10 mCi.

Use in Thyroid Cancer

^{131}I can be used to destroy malignant thyroid cells. However, since most forms of thyroid cancer do not accumulate iodine,

only a small percentage of patients are candidates for ^{131}I therapy.

The doses of ^{131}I used to treat cancer are large, ranging from 50 to 150 mCi. These doses are much higher than those used to treat Graves' disease. Because high amounts of radioactivity are involved, body wastes must be disposed of properly. In addition, adverse effects from large doses of ^{131}I can be severe: radiation sickness may occur; leukemia may be produced; and bone marrow function may be depressed, resulting in leukopenia, thrombocytopenia, and anemia.

Diagnostic Use

^{131}I can be employed to diagnose a variety of thyroid disorders, including hyperthyroidism, hypothyroidism, and goiter. Following ^{131}I administration, the thyroid is scanned for uptake of radioactivity; the amount and location of ^{131}I uptake reveals the extent of thyroid activity. Doses used for diagnosis are miniscule (less than 1 mCi for children, and less than 10 mCi for adults). These tracer doses pose virtually no threat to health.

Preparations

^{131}I is dispensed in capsules and solution for oral administration. Both preparations are odorless and tasteless. Capsules contain between 0.8 and 100 mCi of ^{131}I. Vials of oral solution contain between 3.5 and 150 mCi of ^{131}I. Capsules and oral solutions are available generically (as sodium iodide ^{131}I) and under the trade name Iodotope.

PROPRANOLOL

Propranolol can suppress tachycardia and other symptoms of hyperthyroidism. Relief of these symptoms results from beta-adrenergic blockade; propranolol does not reduce levels of T_3 or T_4. One advantage of propranolol is that its effects occur rapidly, unlike those of propylthiouracil and ^{131}I. In the absence of contraindications (e.g., asthma, congestive heart failure), patients experiencing thyrotoxicosis should receive propranolol immediately; administration may be oral or intravenous. The dosage is highly individualized, ranging from 40 to 240 mg/day in divided doses. The basic pharmacology of propranolol is discussed Chapter 18.

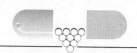

Summary of Major Nursing Implications

LEVOTHYROXINE

 Preadministration Assessment

Therapeutic Goal
Resolution of signs and symptoms of hypothyroidism.

Baseline Data
Obtain plasma levels of TSH and T_4.

 Implementation: Administration

Routes
Oral, IV.

Administration
Oral. Instruct the patient to take levothyroxine on an empty stomach, preferably in the morning before breakfast. Not all products have equal bioavailability; warn the patient against switching from one brand to another.

Make certain that the patient understands that replacement therapy must continue for life. Caution the patient against discontinuing treatment without consulting the physician.

Intravenous. Intravenous administration is reserved for treatment of myxedema coma and for patients who cannot take levothyroxine orally.

 Ongoing Evaluation and Interventions

Evaluating Therapeutic Effects
Adults. Clinical evaluation should reveal reversal of signs of thyroid deficiency and an absence of signs of thyroid excess (e.g., tachycardia). Laboratory tests should indicate normal plasma levels of TSH and T_4.

Infants. Clinical evaluation should reveal normalization of intellectual function, growth, and development. Monthly measurements of height provide a good index of thyroid sufficiency. Laboratory tests should show normal plasma levels of TSH and T_4. (Note: TSH levels may remain abnormal in some children, despite adequate dosing.)

Minimizing Adverse Effects
Thyrotoxicosis. Overdosage may cause thyrotoxicosis. Inform patients about symptoms of thyrotoxicosis (tachycardia, angina, tremor, nervousness, insomnia, hyperthermia, heat intolerance, sweating) and instruct them to notify the physician if these develop.

Minimizing Adverse Interactions
Oral Anticoagulants. Levothyroxine can intensify the effects of the oral anticoagulants. Dosages of oral anticoagulants should be reduced.

Catecholamines. Thyroid hormones sensitize the heart to catecholamines (e.g., epinephrine, dopamine, dobutamine) and may thereby promote dysrhythmias. Exercise caution when catecholamines and levothyroxine are used concomitantly.

LIOTHYRONINE (T₃)

With the exceptions noted below, the nursing implications for liothyronine are the same as those for levothyroxine.

Evaluation of Therapeutic Effects

Success is indicated by resolution of the signs and symptoms of hypothyroidism and by normalization of plasma T_3 and TSH levels. T_4 levels cannot be used to evaluate therapy.

PROPYLTHIOURACIL

Preadministration Assessment

Therapeutic Goals

PTU therapy has three indications: (1) reduction of thyroid hormone production in Graves' disease, (2) control of hyperthyroidism until the effects of radiation on the thyroid become manifest, and (3) suppression of thyroid hormone production prior to subtotal thyroidectomy.

Baseline Data

Obtain plasma levels of T_3 and T_4.

Identifying High-Risk Patients

PTU is contraindicated for nursing mothers. Use with caution during pregnancy.

Implementation: Administration

Route

Oral.

Administration

Instruct the patient to take PTU at regular intervals around the clock (usually every 8 hours).

Ongoing Evaluation and Interventions

Summary of Monitoring

Evaluate treatment by monitoring for weight gain, decreased heart rate, and other indications that levels of thyroid hormone have declined. Laboratory tests should indicate a decrease in plasma content of T_3 and T_4.

Minimizing Adverse Effects

Agranulocytosis. Inform patients about early signs of agranulocytosis (fever, sore throat) and instruct them to notify the physician if these develop. If follow-up blood tests reveal leukopenia, PTU should be withdrawn.

Hypothyroidism. PTU may cause excessive reductions in thyroid hormone synthesis. If signs of hypothyroidism develop or if plasma levels of T_3

and T_4 become subnormal, PTU dosage should be reduced. Supplemental thyroid hormone may be needed.

Use in Pregnancy and Lactation. PTU can cause fetal hypothyroidism and goiter; use with caution during pregnancy. PTU is contraindicated for nursing mothers.

STRONG IODINE SOLUTION (LUGOL'S SOLUTION)

Preadministration Assessment

Therapeutic Goal

Suppression of thyroid hormone production in preparation for subtotal thyroidectomy.

Baseline Data

Obtain tests of thyroid function.

Route

Oral.

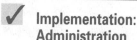

Implementation: Administration

Administration

Advise the patient to dilute strong iodine solution with fruit juice or some other beverage to increase palatability.

Minimizing Adverse Effects

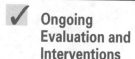

Ongoing Evaluation and Interventions

Mild Toxicity. Inform patients about symptoms of iodism (brassy taste, burning sensations in the mouth, soreness of gums and teeth) and instruct them to discontinue treatment and notify the physician if these occur. Symptoms fade upon drug withdrawal.

Severe Toxicity. Iodine solution can cause corrosive injury to the gastrointestinal tract. Instruct the patient to discontinue drug use and notify the physician immediately if severe abdominal distress develops. Treatment includes gastric lavage and administration of sodium thiosulfate.

RADIOACTIVE IODINE (^{131}I)

Use in Graves' Disease

Therapeutic Goal. Suppression of thyroid hormone production.

Identifying High-Risk Patients. ^{131}I is contraindicated during pregnancy and lactation.

Dosage and Administration. ^{131}I is administered in capsules or an oral liquid. The dosing objective is to reduce thyroid hormone production without causing complete thyroid destruction. The dosage for Graves' disease is 4 to 10 mCi.

Promoting Therapeutic Effects. Responses take 2 to 3 months to develop fully. Propylthiouracil may be required during this interval.

Minimizing Adverse Effects. Excessive thyroid destruction can cause *hypothyroidism.* Patients who develop thyroid insufficiency need thyroid hormone supplements.

Use in Thyroid Cancer

High doses (50 to 150 mCi) are required. These doses can cause radiation sickness, leukemia, and bone marrow depression. Monitor for these effects. Body wastes will be contaminated with radioactivity and must be disposed of appropriately.

Diagnostic Use

^{131}I is used to diagnose hyperthyroidism, hypothyroidism, and goiter. Diagnostic doses are so small (less than 10 mCi) as to be virtually harmless.

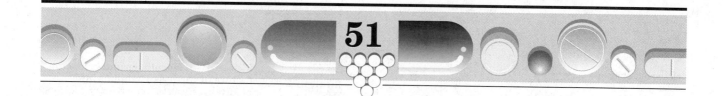

51

Drugs Related to Hypothalamic and Pituitary Function

The hypothalamus and pituitary are intimately related both anatomically and functionally. Working together, these structures help regulate practically all bodily processes. To achieve their widespread effects, the hypothalamus and pituitary employ at least 15 hormones and regulatory factors (Fig. 51–1). The endocrinology of these two structures is exceedingly complex. Fortunately, from the perspective of therapeutics, the picture is much less imposing. This is because the clinical applications of the hypothalamic and pituitary hormones are limited. In this chapter, our emphasis will be on three agents: growth hormone, antidiuretic hormone, and prolactin. Additional hypothalamic and pituitary hormones of therapeutic interest are considered briefly here and discussed at greater length in other chapters.

OVERVIEW OF HYPOTHALAMIC AND PITUITARY ENDOCRINOLOGY

Anatomic Considerations

The pituitary sits in a depression in the skull located just below the third ventricle of the brain; the hypothalamus is located immediately above (see Fig. 51–1). The pituitary has two divisions:

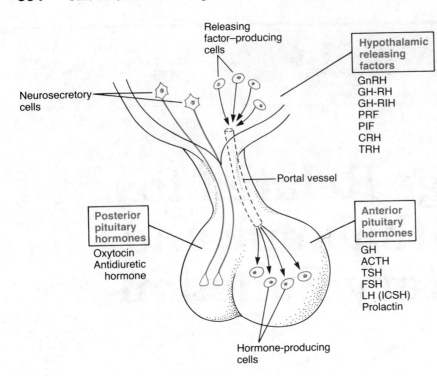

Figure 51–1. Hormones and releasing factors of the hypothalamus and pituitary. *Hypothalamic-releasing factors.* GnRH = gonadotropin-releasing hormone, GH-RH = growth hormone–releasing hormone, GH-RIH = growth hormone–release inhibiting hormone (somatostatin), PRF = prolactin-releasing factor, PIF = prolactin-inhibiting factor, CRH = corticotropin-releasing hormone, TRH = thyrotropin-releasing hormone.

Anterior pituitary hormones. GH = growth hormone, ACTH = adrenocorticotropic hormone, TSH = thyroid-stimulating hormone, FSH = follicle-stimulating hormone, LH (ICSH) = luteinizing hormone (interstitial cell–stimulating hormone).

the *anterior pituitary* (or *adenohypophysis*) and the *posterior pituitary* (or *neurohypophysis*). Both divisions are under hypothalamic control. As indicated in Figure 51–1, the hypothalamus communicates with the *anterior* pituitary by way of release-regulating factors delivered through a system of portal blood vessels; communication with the *posterior* pituitary is neuronal.

Hormones of the Anterior Pituitary

The anterior pituitary produces six major hormones. Production and release of these hormones is controlled largely by the hypothalamus. Functions of the anterior pituitary hormones are summarized briefly as follows:

Growth hormone (GH) stimulates growth in practically all tissues and organs.

Adrenocorticotropic hormone (ACTH) acts on the adrenal cortex to promote synthesis and release of adrenocortical hormones.

Thyrotropin (TSH, thyroid-stimulating hormone) acts on the thyroid gland to promote synthesis and release of thyroid hormones.

Follicle-stimulating hormone (FSH) acts on the ovary to promote follicular growth and development. In the testes, FSH promotes spermatogenesis.

Luteinizing hormone (LH) acts in women to promote ovulation and development of the corpus luteum. In men, LH, which is also known as *interstitial cell-stimulating hormone*, acts on the testes to promote androgen production.

Prolactin stimulates milk production after parturition.

Hormones of the Posterior Pituitary

The posterior pituitary has only two hormones: *oxytocin* and *antidiuretic hormone* (ADH). The principal function of oxytocin is to facilitate uterine contractions at term. Antidiuretic hormone promotes renal conservation of water.

Although oxytocin and ADH are considered hormones of the posterior pituitary, these agents are actually synthesized in the hypothalamus. The cells that make oxytocin and ADH are called neurosecretory cells. As indicated in Figure 51–1, these cells originate in the hypothalamus and project their axons to the posterior pituitary. Oxytocin and ADH are produced within the bodies of these cells, and then transported down the axons to the cell terminals for storage. When appropriate stimuli impinge upon the bodies of the neurosecretory cells, impulses are sent down the axon, causing the hormones to be released.

Hypothalamic Release-Regulating Factors

The hypothalamus bears the primary responsibility for regulating the release of hormones from the *anterior* pituitary. To accomplish this, the hypothalamus employs eight different release-regulating factors (see Fig. 51–1). Most of these factors *stimulate* the release of anterior pituitary hormones. However, two of these factors regulate release by exerting an *inhibitory* influence. As indicated in Figure 51–1, the hypothalamic release-regulating factors are delivered to the anterior pituitary via portal blood vessels. Although the hypothalamic releasing factors are of extreme physiologic importance, only two of these factors (thyrotropin-releasing hormone and gonadotropin-releasing hormone) have clinical applications. These are the only hypothalamic release-regulating factors that we will discuss in this chapter.

Feedback Regulation of the Hypothalamus and Anterior Pituitary

With few exceptions, the release of hypothalamic and anterior pituitary hormones is regulated by a *negative feedback loop*. Such a loop is illustrated in Figure 51–2. In this example, the loop begins with the secretion of releasing-factor X from the hypothalamus. Factor X then acts on the anterior pituitary to stimulate the release of hormone A. Hormone A then acts on its target gland to promote the release of hormone B. Hormone B has two actions: (1) it produces its designated biologic effects, and (2) it acts on the hypothalamus and pituitary to inhibit further release of factor X and hormone A. This feedback inhibition of the hypothalamus and pituitary suppresses further release of hormone B itself, thereby keeping levels of hormone B within an appropriate range.

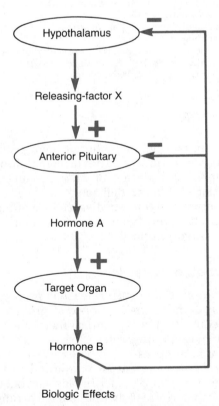

Figure 51–2. Negative feedback regulation of the hypothalamus and anterior pituitary. The feedback loop works as follows: Factor X stimulates the pituitary to release hormone A, which stimulates its target organ, causing release of hormone B. Hormone B then acts on the hypothalamus and pituitary to suppress further release of factor X and hormone A, thereby suppressing further release of hormone B itself.

DRUGS RELATED TO ANTERIOR PITUITARY FUNCTION

GROWTH HORMONE

Growth hormone is a large polypeptide hormone (191 amino acids) produced by the anterior pituitary. As its name suggests, this hormone helps regulate growth. An absence of growth hormone during childhood results in *dwarfism*. Excessive growth hormone results in *giantism*.

Physiologic Effects

Promotion of Growth. Growth hormone stimulates the growth of practically all organs and tissues. If administered prior to epiphyseal closure, growth hormone increases bone length, producing a corresponding increase in height. The size and number of muscle cells are increased, resulting in enlargement of muscle mass. The internal organs are stimulated to grow in proportion to overall body growth. The only organs that do not respond noticeably to growth hormone are the brain and eyes.

Promotion of Protein Synthesis. For growth to occur, cells must increase their production of protein. Growth hormone facilitates this process by increasing amino acid uptake and utilization. Since amino acids have substantial nitrogen content, increased protein synthesis results in net nitrogen retention. This retention is reflected in reduced urinary nitrogen excretion. Increased amino acid utilization also causes blood urea nitrogen (BUN) to fall.

Effect on Carbohydrate Metabolism. Administration of growth hormone reduces glucose utilization. Hence, plasma levels of glucose tend to rise. When growth hormone is administered to nondiabetics, elevation of blood glucose stimulates release of insulin, thereby maintaining plasma levels of glucose within a normal range. In contrast, when growth hormone is administered to diabetics, insulin cannot be released; hence, the hyperglycemic action of growth hormone is unopposed, and plasma glucose levels may climb dramatically.

Growth Hormone Deficiency

Growth hormone is essential for normal growth of children; hormone deficiency results in *dwarfism*. In children who are growth hormone deficient, growth is retarded to an equal extent in all parts of the body. Hence, the dwarf, although tiny, is of normal proportions. Dwarfism is not associated with mental impairment. In contrast to normal individuals, whose growth ceases at puberty, the dwarf continues to grow throughout life. The only treatment for growth hormone deficiency is replacement therapy with *human* growth hormone. Growth hormone from animal sources is not effective.

Therapeutic Use

The only approved indication for growth hormone is treatment of children whose growth has been retarded because of proven growth hormone deficiency. Except in experimental protocols, growth hormone should not be given to promote growth in children who are short for reasons unrelated to lack of growth hormone. Also, this agent should not be given during or after epiphyseal closure. To avoid this misuse, epiphyseal status should be assessed annually.

Treatment is prolonged, and responses are usually satisfactory. Height and weight should be measured monthly to assess treatment; an annual height increase of 7 cm is average. Therapy should continue until a satisfactory adult height has been achieved, until epiphyseal closure occurs, or until a response can no longer be elicited. Efficacy of therapy declines as the patient grows older, and is usually lost entirely by ages 20 to 24 years. If treatment fails to promote growth, growth hormone should be discontinued and the diagnosis of growth hormone deficiency should be re-evaluated.

Adverse Effects and Interactions

Hyperglycemia. Growth hormone is diabetogenic. When used in patients with pre-existing diabetes, significant hyperglycemia may result. Glucose levels should be monitored and insulin dosage should be adjusted accordingly.

Hypothyroidism. Growth hormone therapy is associated with a decline in thyroid function. Function of the thyroid should be assessed periodically. If thyroid hormone levels are subnormal, replacement therapy should be instituted.

Antibodies to Growth Hormone. Somatrem, one of the two growth hormone preparations available, is antigenic. Quite often, somatrem stimulates formation of antibodies directed against itself and against pituitary-derived growth hormone. Fortunately, these antibodies rarely decrease the effectiveness of treatment.

Poverty. Growth hormone is expensive. One year of treatment with somatrem can cost $10,000 to $20,000.

Interaction with Glucocorticoids. Glucocorticoids can oppose the growth-stimulating effects of growth hormone. Patients receiving growth hormone should not be given glucocorticoids in doses that exceed the equivalent of 10 to 15 mg/M² of hydrocortisone.

Preparations

Somatrem. Somatrem [Protropin] is a form of growth hormone produced by recombinant DNA technology. With the exception of one amino acid, the structure of somatrem is identical to that of growth hormone produced by the human pituitary. The biologic activity of somatrem is indistinguishable from that of the naturally occurring hormone.

Somatropin. Like somatrem, somatropin [Humatrope], is produced by recombinant DNA technology. The structure of somatropin is identical to that of growth hormone produced by the human pituitary.

Dosage and Administration

Growth hormone is administered parenterally (IM and SC). It cannot be used orally because of rapid inactivation by the digestive system. Intramuscular administration has been traditional. However, studies indicate that SC administration is less painful than IM while being just as safe and effective.

Growth hormone is dispensed as a lyophilized powder for reconstitution with 1 to 5 ml of diluent. Mix gently; *do not shake*. Do not inject the drug if the preparation is cloudy or contains particulate matter.

Dosage is individualized. For *somatrem* [Protropin], the maximum recommended dosage is 0.26 IU/kg (0.1 mg/kg) three times a week. For *somatropen* [Humatrope], the maximum recommended dosage is 0.16 IU/kg (0.06 mg/kg) three times a week.

PROLACTIN

Prolactin is a polypeptide hormone produced by the anterior pituitary. The principal function of prolactin is stimulation of milk production after parturition. Prolactin deficiency is generally without symptoms (except for disturbance of lactation). In contrast, overproduction of prolactin causes multiple adverse effects.

Regulation of Release

Regulation of prolactin release is predominantly *inhibitory*. Under the influence of prolactin-inhibiting factor (PIF), a regulatory molecule produced by the hypothalamus, release of prolactin from the pituitary is suppressed. When release of PIF declines, release of prolactin is allowed to increase. Although the identity of PIF has not been established with certainty, available data strongly suggest that PIF is *dopamine*. Another hypothalamic factor, known as prolactin-releasing factor (PRF), acts to promote prolactin release. However, the stimulatory influence of PRF is usually dominated by PIF-mediated inhibition. The most powerful stimulus to prolactin release is suckling, an action that presumably suppresses hypothalamic release of PIF.

Prolactin Hypersecretion

Excessive secretion of prolactin produces adverse effects in males and females. Women may experience amenorrhea, galactorrhea (excessive milk flow), and infertility. In men, libido and potency are reduced, and occasionally galactorrhea occurs. Puberty may be delayed in boys and girls. Causes of prolactin hypersecretion include pituitary adenoma, injury to the hypothalamus, and certain drugs (e.g., antipsychotics, estrogens).

Bromocriptine for Suppression of Prolactin Release

Excessive secretion of prolactin can be reduced with bromocriptine, a dopaminergic agonist. By binding to dopaminergic receptors in the pituitary, bromocriptine exerts the same inhibitory influence on prolactin release as does PIF. Bromocriptine is used to inhibit prolactin release in postpartum women, and to decrease the release of prolactin by pituitary adenomas. The usual dosage is 2.5 mg administered two to three times daily. Adverse effects are common early in therapy and include nausea, vomiting, dizziness, and hypotension. Other uses of bromocriptine include management of infertility (see Chapter 57) and treatment of Parkinson's disease (see Chapter 21).

THYROTROPIN

Thyrotropin (thyroid-stimulating hormone, TSH) is a hormone produced by the anterior pituitary. The physiologic role of thyrotropin is stimulation of thyroid gland function. In promoting thyroid function, thyrotropin causes (1) increased thyroidal uptake of iodine, (2) increased synthesis of thyroid hormones, (3) increased release of thyroid hormones, and (4) thyroid growth.

Thyrotropin is employed clinically to diagnose thyroid failure. Specifically, thyrotropin is used to differentiate primary hypothyroidism (failure of the thyroid gland itself) from secondary hypothyroidism (hypothyroidism resulting from insufficient production of thyrotropin by the pituitary). Testing is performed as follows: thyrotropin is administered (IM or SC) in a dose of 10 IU for 1 to 3 days; 24 hours after the last dose, radioactive iodine is administered, and thyroidal uptake of the radioactive iodine is then measured. In patients with primary hypothyroidism, the thyroid is unable to respond to thyrotropin; hence, uptake of radioactive iodine is low. In contrast, if lack of endogenous thyrotropin is the cause of hypothyroidism, administration of the test doses of thyrotropin will promote substantial iodine uptake. Thyrotropin used for diagnosis of thyroid failure is marketed under the trade name Thytropar. (Thyroid disease and its treatment are discussed in Chapter 50.)

CORTICOTROPIN

Corticotropin (adrenocorticotropic hormone, ACTH) is a polypeptide hormone produced by the anterior pituitary. This hormone acts on the adrenal cortex to stimulate the production and release of adrenocortical hormones (e.g., cortisol, aldosterone). The principal use of corticotropin is diagnosis of adrenocortical dysfunction. A synthetic analogue of corticotropin, called cosyntropin, is available. Corticotropin and cosyntropin,

along with the hormones of the adrenal cortex, are discussed in Chapter 53.

GONADOTROPINS

The anterior pituitary produces two gonadotropic hormones: *follicle-stimulating hormone* (FSH) and *luteinizing hormone* (LH). (It should be noted that LH is also known as *interstitial cell–stimulating hormone* or ICSH.) LH and FSH are produced by the pituitaries of males and females and serve to regulate gonadal function in both sexes. In women, FSH acts on the ovary to promote follicular growth and development. In men, FSH supports sperm production. The role of LH in women is to promote ovulation and formation of the corpus luteum. In men, LH stimulates testosterone synthesis by Leydig cells of the testicular interstitium. Plasma levels of LH and FSH are relatively stable in males. In females, levels of both hormones vary with the phase of the menstrual cycle. The physiology of LH and FSH in females is discussed further in Chapter 55.

LH and FSH are employed clinically to treat infertility in men and women. In women, fertility is increased by promoting follicular development and ovulation. In men, increased fertility results from enhancement of spermatogenesis. The preparation of gonadotropins employed therapeutically is called menotropins. Menotropins is an extract of the urine of postmenopausal women and contains equal amounts of LH and FSH activity. The use of menotropins in the management of infertility is discussed further in Chapter 57.

DRUGS RELATED TO POSTERIOR PITUITARY FUNCTION

ANTIDIURETIC HORMONE

Antidiuretic hormone (ADH) is a tripeptide hormone that acts on the kidney to cause reabsorption (conservation) of water. Deficiency of ADH produces *diabetes insipidus*, a condition in which large volumes of dilute urine are produced.

Physiology

Actions. Antidiuretic hormone promotes renal conservation of water. The hormone accomplishes this by acting on the collecting ducts of the kidney to increase their permeability to water, which results in increased water reabsorption. Because water is withdrawn from the tubular urine (back into the extracellular space), urine that entered the collecting ducts in a relatively dilute state becomes highly concentrated by the time it leaves.

In addition to its renal actions, ADH can stimulate contraction of vascular smooth muscle and the smooth muscle of the gastrointestinal (GI) tract. Because of its ability to cause vasoconstriction, ADH is known alternatively as *vasopressin*. It should be noted that the plasma levels of ADH required to cause smooth muscle contraction are higher than those that occur physiologically.

Production and Storage. Antidiuretic hormone is produced within the cell bodies of neurosecretory cells of the hypothalamus, and is then transported down the axons of those cells to their terminals in the posterior pituitary. ADH is stored in these terminals until released.

Regulation of Release. Release of ADH is regulated by the hypothalamus, the brain center responsible for maintaining body fluids at their proper osmolality. When the hypothalamus senses that osmolality has risen too high, it instructs the posterior pituitary to release ADH. The resultant increase in water reabsorption dilutes body fluids, causing osmolality to decline. Release of ADH can also be stimulated by hypotension and by a reduction in plasma volume.

Diabetes Insipidus

Causes, Signs, and Symptoms. Diabetes insipidus is a syndrome caused by partial or complete deficiency of ADH. The syndrome is characterized by polydipsia (excessive thirst) and excretion of large volumes of dilute urine. The deficiency of ADH may be inherited or it may result from head trauma, neurosurgery, cancer, and other causes.

Treatment. Therapy of diabetes insipidus is dependent on the extent of ADH deficiency. When the deficiency is total, ADH replacement therapy is required; treatment is usually lifelong. When the deficiency is only partial, medications other than ADH may be employed. The primary agents used are (1) *chlorpropamide*, which promotes ADH release and increases renal responsiveness to ADH, and (2) *clofibrate*, which simply promotes ADH release.

Of the ADH preparations available, *desmopressin* is the agent of choice for treating diabetes insipidus. Desmopressin is preferred over other ADH preparations because of its prolonged duration of action, ease of administration, and lack of significant side effects. Response to treatment is rapid, and urine volume quickly drops to normal amounts. Desmopressin is administered by nasal spray, usually twice daily. Because desmopressin is expensive, and because excessive dosing can result in water intoxication (see below), the smallest effective dosage should be employed.

Antidiuretic Hormone Preparations

Three preparations with ADH activity are available: *vasopressin*, *desmopressin*, and *lypressin*. Vasopressin is identical in structure to naturally occurring ADH; desmopressin and lypressin are structural analogues of natural ADH. These three preparations differ from one another with respect to duration of action, routes of administration, and therapeutic applications (Table 51–1). These agents also differ in their ability to cause vasoconstriction (see *Cardiovascular Effects*). All three agents may be employed to treat diabetes insipi-

dus. However, because of its prolonged effects, convenient route (intranasal), and freedom from significant side effects, desmopressin is the drug of choice.

Adverse Effects

Water Intoxication. Excessive water retention can cause water intoxication. Early signs include drowsiness, listlessness, and headache. Severe intoxication progresses to convulsions and terminal coma. Patients experiencing early symptoms of intoxication should notify the physician. Treatment of water intoxication includes restriction of fluid intake and diuretic therapy.

A major cause of water intoxication is failure to reduce water intake once ADH therapy has begun. Since treatment prevents continued fluid loss, failure to decrease fluid intake will result in water buildup and intoxication. Hence, at the onset of treatment, patients should be instructed to reduce their accustomed fluid intake.

Cardiovascular Effects. Because of its powerful vasoconstrictor actions, *vasopressin* can cause severe adverse cardiovascular effects. Desmopressin and lypressin, which possess only weak pressor activity, do not adversely affect hemodynamics. By constricting arteries of the heart, vasopressin can cause angina pectoris and even myocardial infarction—especially if given to patients with coronary insufficiency. In addition, vasopressin may cause gangrene by decreasing blood flow in the periphery. Because it can reduce cardiac perfusion, vasopressin must be used with extreme caution in patients with coronary artery disease. This warning does not apply to desmopressin and lypressin.

OXYTOCIN

Oxytocin is produced by neurosecretory cells of the hypothalamus, and is then transported down the axons of these cells for storage in the posterior pituitary. Oxytocin has two physiologic roles: (1) promotion of uterine contraction during labor, and (2) stimulation of milk ejection during breast-feeding. The principal therapeutic application of oxytocin is induction of labor near term. In addition, the hormone can be used by nursing mothers to promote milk ejection. The physiology, pharmacology, and applications of oxytocin are discussed in Chapter 58.

DRUGS RELATED TO HYPOTHALAMIC FUNCTION

Of the seven regulatory factors found in the hypothalamus, only two—gonadotropin-releasing hormone (Gn-RH) and thyrotropin-releasing hormone (TRH)—have clinical applications. Gn-RH and its synthetic analogues are used to treat prostatic cancer and endometriosis, and to induce ovulation. TRH is used to diagnosis thyroid disorders.

GONADOTROPIN-RELEASING HORMONE

Gonadotropin-releasing hormone is produced by the hypothalamus and promotes release of gonadotropins (LH and FSH) from the pituitary. Four preparations of Gn-RH are available: *leuprolide*, *goserelin*, *nafarelin*, and *gonadorelin*. The actions and uses of gonadorelin and nafarelin are discussed in Chapter

Generic Name [Trade Name]	Routes	Duration of Antidiuretic Action (hours)	Therapeutic Uses	Usual Adult Dosage
Desmopressin [DDAVP, Concentraid]	Intranasal, SC, IV	8–20	Diabetes insipidus	0.1 ml (10 μg intranasally 2 times/day **or** 0.25–0.5 ml SC or IV twice daily
			Hemophilia*	0.3 μg/kg IV over 15–30 min
Lypressin [Diapid]	Intranasal	3–8	Diabetes insipidus	1–2 sprays (about 2–4 pressor units) into each nostril 4 times/day
Vasopressin [Pitressin Synthetic]	IM, SC†	2–8	Diabetes insipidus	5–10 units IM or SC 3–4 times/day
			Postoperative abdominal distention	5 units IM initially; then 10 units IM every 3–4 hours
			Abdominal radiography (to dispel gas shadows)	10 units 2 hr before and again 30 min before the procedure
			Bleeding esophageal varices‡	20 units by intra-arterial or IV infusion
Vasopressin tannate [Pitresin Tannate]	IM	24–96	Diabetes insipidus	1.5–5 units every 1–3 days

*Desmopressin controls bleeding by increasing levels of clotting factor VIII.
†Sometimes administered intranasally or IV.
‡Investigational use.

57 (Drug Therapy of Infertility). Leuprolide and goserelin are discussed in Chapter 91 (Representative Anticancer Drugs).

THYROTROPIN-RELEASING HORMONE

Thyrotropin-releasing hormone is produced by the hypothalamus and acts on the pituitary to stimulate release of thyrotropin (thyroid-stimulating hormone, TSH). A synthetic preparation of TRH, called *protirelin*, is used clinically. Protirelin is thought to be identical to TRH made by the hypothalamus. Protirelin is employed in the diagnosis of thyroid, pituitary, and hypothalamic disorders. Testing is performed by injecting protirelin (IV) and then sampling the blood for increases in TSH content. Interpretation of test findings can be difficult and will not be discussed here. Protirelin is marketed under the trade names Thypinone and Relefact-TRH. For a general discussion of thyroid physiology and pharmacology, refer to Chapter 50.

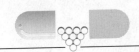

Summary of Major Nursing Implications

GROWTH HORMONE: SOMATREM AND SOMATROPIN

 Preadministration Assessment

Therapeutic Goal

Normalization of growth and development in children with proven growth hormone deficiency.

Baseline Data

Assess developmental status (height, weight, etc.). Obtain thyroid function tests.

Identifying High-Risk Patients

Growth hormone is contraindicated during and after *epiphyseal closure*. Use with caution in patients with *diabetes mellitus* and *hypothyroidism*.

 Implementation: Administration

Routes

IM, SC.

Administration

Reconstitute the lyophilized powder with 1 to 5 ml of diluent. *Mix gently; do not shake.* Do not inject if the preparation is cloudy or contains particulate matter.

 Ongoing Evaluation and Interventions

Evaluating Treatment

Monitor height and weight monthly; an annual height increase of 7 cm is average. Continue therapy until a satisfactory adult height has been achieved, until epiphyseal closure occurs, or until a response can no longer be elicited (usually by age 20 to 24).

If no stimulation of growth occurs, discontinue treatment and re-evaluate the diagnosis of growth hormone deficiency.

Minimizing Adverse Effects and Interactions

Hyperglycemia. Growth hormone can elevate plasma glucose content in diabetics. Increase insulin dosage as needed.

Hypothyroidism. Growth hormone may suppress thyroid function. Assess thyroid function before treatment and periodically thereafter. If levels of thyroid hormone fall, institute replacement therapy.

Interaction with Glucocorticoids. Glucocorticoids can oppose the growth-stimulating effects of growth hormone.

Dosage of glucocorticoids should not exceed the equivalent of 10 to 15 mg/M^2 of hydrocortisone.

ANTIDIURETIC HORMONE

Desmopressin

Lypressin

Vasopressin

The nursing implications summarized here apply only to the use of ADH preparations for *diabetes insipidus*.

 Preadministration Assessment

Therapeutic Goal

Normalization of urinary water excretion in patients with diabetes insipidus.

Baseline Data

Determine fluid and electrolyte status.

Identifying High-Risk Patients

Use *vasopressin* with caution in patients with coronary artery disease and other vascular diseases.

 Implementation: Administration

Routes

IM, IV, SC, intranasal. The route depends upon the preparation being used (see Table 51–1).

Administration

Teach the patient the technique for intranasal administration. To promote compliance, make certain that the patient understands that treatment of diabetes mellitus is lifelong.

 Ongoing Evaluation and Interventions

Evaluating Therapeutic Effects

Teach the patient to monitor and record daily intake and output of fluid. If ADH dosage is correct, urine volume should rapidly drop to normal.

Minimizing Adverse Effects

Water Intoxication. Excessive retention of water can produce water intoxication; this is most likely at the beginning of therapy. Instruct patients to decrease their accustomed fluid intake at the start of treatment. Inform patients about early signs of water intoxication (drowsiness, listlessness, and headache) and instruct them to notify the physician if these occur. Treatment includes fluid restriction and diuretic therapy.

Cardiovascular Effects. *Vasopressin*, but not desmopressin or lypressin, is a powerful vasoconstrictor. Excessive vasoconstriction can produce angina pectoris, myocardial infarction, and gangrene (from extravasation of IV vasopressin). Vasopressin must be used with caution, especially in patients with coronary insufficiency.

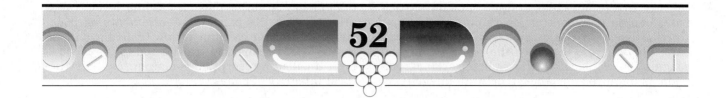

52

Drugs Affecting Calcium Levels and Utilization

CALCIUM PHYSIOLOGY

CALCIUM PATHOPHYSIOLOGY
    Hypercalcemia
    Hypocalcemia
    Rickets
    Osteomalacia
    Osteoporosis
    Paget's Disease of Bone
    Hypoparathyroidism
    Hyperparathyroidism

DRUGS USED TO TREAT DISORDERS INVOLVING CALCIUM
    Vitamin D
    Calcium Salts
    Calcitonin
    Other Drugs that Affect Calcium

It is difficult to overemphasize the biologic importance of calcium, an element critical to the functional integrity of nerve, muscle, bone, the heart, and the coagulation of blood. Since these calcium-dependent processes can be seriously disrupted by alterations in calcium availability, the body must maintain calcium levels within narrow limits. To regulate calcium, three factors are employed: parathyroid hormone, vitamin D, and calcitonin. When these regulatory mechanisms fail, hypercalcemia or hypocalcemia results.

In approaching our study of drugs that influence the availability and utilization of calcium, we will begin by reviewing calcium physiology. Next we will discuss the syndromes produced by disruption of calcium metabolism. Having established this background, we will then discuss the pharmacologic agents used to treat calcium-related disorders.

CALCIUM PHYSIOLOGY

Actions

Calcium is critical to the function of the nervous system, muscular system, cardiovascular system, and skeletal system. In the nervous system, calcium helps regulate excitability and transmitter

673

release. In the muscular system, calcium participates in excitation-contraction coupling and in contraction itself. In the cardiovascular system, calcium plays a role in myocardial contraction and coagulation of blood. In the skeletal system, calcium is required for the structural integrity of bone.

Body Stores

Calcium in Bone. The vast majority of calcium in the body (>98%) is present in bone. Calcium is deposited in bone in the form of *hydroxyapatite* crystals. The calcium component of bone undergoes constant turnover: under the influence of several hormones, calcium may be resorbed from bone back into the blood, and calcium from the blood may be deposited in bone.

Calcium in Blood. The normal value for total serum calcium is 10 mg/dl (2.5 mM, 5 mEq/L). Of this total, about 50% is bound to proteins and other substances and, therefore, is unavailable for use. The remaining 50% is present as free, ionized calcium. It is the free calcium that participates in physiologic processes.

Absorption and Excretion

Absorption. Absorption of calcium takes place in the small intestine. Under normal conditions, about one third of ingested calcium is absorbed. Absorption can be increased by parathyroid hormone and vitamin D (see below). In contrast, glucocorticoids can decrease calcium absorption. Also, a variety of foods (e.g., spinach, whole grain cereals, bran) contain compounds that can interfere with calcium absorption.

Excretion. Excretion of calcium is primarily renal. The amount lost is determined by glomerular filtration and by the extent of tubular reabsorption. Excretion of calcium can be reduced by parathyroid hormone and vitamin D (see below). Excretion of calcium can be increased with a loop diuretic (e.g., furosemide) and by loading with sodium. Calcitonin also augments calcium elimination (see below). In addition to renal excretion, substantial amounts of calcium can be lost through lactation.

Regulation of Serum Calcium Levels

Blood levels of calcium are tightly controlled. The body maintains calcium levels by adjusting the rates of three processes: (1) absorption of calcium from the intestine, (2) excretion of calcium by the kidney, and (3) resorption or deposition of calcium in bone. Regulation of these processes is under the control of three factors: parathyroid hormone, vitamin D, and calcitonin. It should be noted

that preservation of plasma calcium levels takes priority over the calcium requirements of bone. Hence, if serum calcium is low, calcium will be resorbed from bone and transferred to the blood—even if calcium resorption compromises the structural integrity of bone.

Parathyroid Hormone. Parathyroid hormone (PTH) is released from the parathyroid glands in response to low levels of plasma calcium. The effect of PTH is to restore these reduced levels to normal. Parathyroid hormone elevates serum calcium by three mechanisms: (1) PTH acts on bone to promote calcium resorption, (2) PTH acts on the kidney to promote reabsorption of calcium that had been filtered by the glomerulus, and (3) by causing the activation of vitamin D, PTH promotes calcium absorption from the intestine. In addition to its effects on calcium, PTH acts to *reduce* plasma levels of phosphate.

Vitamin D. Vitamin D is similar to PTH both in its effects on calcium levels and in the mechanisms by which these effects are produced. Like PTH, vitamin D increases plasma calcium content. Also like PTH, vitamin D elevates plasma calcium levels by (1) increasing calcium absorption from the intestine, (2) increasing calcium resorption from bone, and (3) decreasing calcium excretion by the kidney. In contrast to PTH, vitamin D acts to *elevate* plasma levels of phosphate. The actions of vitamin D are discussed further later in the chapter.

Calcitonin. Calcitonin, a hormone produced by the thyroid gland, decreases plasma levels of calcium. Hence, calcitonin acts in opposition to PTH and vitamin D. Calcitonin is released from the thyroid gland when serum calcium levels rise too high. Calcitonin lowers serum calcium by inhibiting the resorption of calcium from bone and by increasing calcium excretion by the kidney. Unlike PTH and vitamin D, calcitonin does not influence calcium absorption.

CALCIUM PATHOPHYSIOLOGY

HYPERCALCEMIA

Clinical Presentation. Hypercalcemia is usually asymptomatic. When symptoms are present, they often involve the kidney (damage to tubules and collecting ducts), gastrointestinal tract (nausea, vomiting, constipation), and central nervous system (lethargy and depression). Hypercalcemia may also result in dysrhythmias and calcium deposition in soft tissues.

Causes. Hypercalcemia may arise from a variety of causes. Life-threatening elevations in plasma calcium are most frequently associated with cancer. Hyperparathyroidism is another common cause of severe hypercalcemia (see below). Additional causes include vitamin D intoxication, sarcoidosis, and use of thiazide diuretics.

Treatment. Hypercalcemia can be managed with a variety of drugs. When serum calcium must be lowered rapidly, a combination of intravenous saline plus a loop diuretic (e.g., furosemide) is the treatment of choice. Other agents for lowering calcium include phosphates (which promote calcium deposition in bone and reduce calcium absorption); EDTA (which binds calcium and promotes its excretion); corticosteroids (which reduce intestinal calcium absorption); and a group of drugs—calcitonin, plicamycin, phosphates, corticosteroids, and etidronate—that inhibit resorption of calcium from bone.

HYPOCALCEMIA

Clinical Presentation and Cause. Hypocalcemia enhances neuromuscular excitability. As a result, tetany, convulsions, laryngospasm, and spasm of other muscles may occur. Hypocalcemia is caused most frequently by a deficiency of either parathyroid hormone, vitamin D, or dietary calcium.

Treatment. Severe hypocalcemia is corrected by infusing an intravenous calcium preparation (e.g., calcium gluconate). Once calcium levels have been restored, an oral calcium salt (e.g., calcium carbonate) can be given for maintenance. Vitamin D should be included in the regimen if there is a coexisting deficiency of this vitamin.

RICKETS

Rickets is a disease of childhood brought on by insufficient dietary vitamin D or limited exposure to sunlight. This disease is extremely rare in the United States. Rickets is characterized by defective bone growth and skeletal deformities. Bone abnormalities are caused as follows: (1) vitamin D deficiency results in reduced calcium absorption; (2) in response to hypocalcemia, parathyroid hormone (PTH) is released; (3) PTH restores serum calcium by promoting calcium resorption from bone, thereby causing bones to soften; and (4) stress on the softened bones caused by weight bearing results in deformity. Treatment consists of vitamin D replacement therapy.

OSTEOMALACIA

Osteomalacia is the adult equivalent of rickets. Like rickets, this condition results from insuffi-cient vitamin D. In the absence of vitamin D, mineralization of bone is impaired, resulting in back pain, bowing of the legs, fractures of the long bones, and kyphosis ("hunchback" curvature of the spine). Treatment consists of vitamin D replacement therapy.

OSTEOPOROSIS

Clinical Presentation. Osteoporosis is characterized by a progressive loss of bone mass. The marrow becomes enlarged, the bone cortex is reduced in thickness, and structural weakness develops. Kyphosis and reductions in height occur owing to compression and collapse of the vertebrae. Patients are predisposed to vertebral crush fractures and fractures of the hip. Osteoporosis is very common in postmenopausal women; estrogen deficiency appears to be the primary cause.

Treatment. Therapy of osteoporosis is largely prophylactic; no available treatment will reverse bone loss that has already occurred. Oral calcium supplements may be used to insure adequate calcium intake. In postmenopausal women, estrogens can help retard loss of bone. Calcitonin may also be employed. However, this agent is expensive and the need for parenteral administration makes it inconvenient for long-term use.

PAGET'S DISEASE OF BONE

Clinical Presentation. Paget's disease of bone is a chronic condition seen most frequently in people over 40 years old. The disease is characterized by (1) increased bone resorption, (2) replacement of the resorbed bone with abnormal bone, and (3) increased blood flow to the areas of bone affected. Although many patients are asymptomatic, about 25% experience bone pain and osteoarthritis; skeletal deformity may also occur. Weakening of bone may lead to fractures. Neurologic complications may occur secondary to compression of the spinal cord, spinal nerves, and cranial nerves. Rarely, increased blood flow to bone may be so great as to cause high-output heart failure. Increased bone turnover causes elevation in serum alkaline phosphatase (reflecting increased bone deposition) and increased urinary hydroxyproline (reflecting increased bone resorption).

Treatment. Asymptomatic patients are usually not treated. Mild pain can be managed with analgesics and anti-inflammatory agents. When the disease is more severe, calcitonin or etidronate is employed; both agents suppress the accelerated turnover of bone. Calcitonin (IM or SC) is the drug of choice for rapid relief of pain. Etidronate, which is cheaper than calcitonin and administered orally, may be the preferred drug for prolonged therapy.

HYPOPARATHYROIDISM

Reductions in parathyroid hormone (PTH) usually result from inadvertent removal of the parathyroids during surgery on the thyroid gland. Lack of PTH causes hypocalcemia, which in turn may produce paresthesias, tetany, muscle spasm, laryngospasm, and convulsions. Symptoms can be relieved with vitamin D and, if necessary, calcium supplements.

HYPERPARATHYROIDISM

Clinical Presentation and Cause. Primary hyperparathyroidism usually results from parathyroid adenoma. The resulting increase in PTH secretion causes hypercalcemia and lowers serum phosphate. Hypercalcemia can cause skeletal muscle weakness, constipation (from decreased smooth muscle tone), and CNS symptoms (lethargy, depression). Hypercalciuria and hyperphosphaturia are also present and may cause renal calculi. Loss of calcium and phosphate from bone may be sufficient to produce bone abnormalities.

Treatment. Primary hyperparathyroidism is usually treated by surgical resection of the parathyroid glands. If surgery is contraindicated, hypercalcemia can be managed with a combination of oral neutral phosphate, a low-calcium diet, and high fluid intake.

DRUGS USED TO TREAT DISORDERS INVOLVING CALCIUM

VITAMIN D

The term *vitamin D* refers to two compounds: (1) *ergocalciferol* (vitamin D_2), and (2) *cholecalciferol* (vitamin D_3). Vitamin D_3 is the form of vitamin D produced naturally in humans when the skin is exposed to sunlight. Vitamin D_2 is a form of vitamin D that occurs in the plant kingdom. Vitamin D_2 is used as a drug and to fortify foods. Both forms of vitamin D produce nearly identical effects. Therefore, rather than distinguishing between these compounds, we will use the term *vitamin D* to refer to vitamins D_2 and D_3 collectively.

Physiologic Actions

Vitamin D is an important regulator of calcium and phosphorous homeostasis. Vitamin D increases blood levels of both elements, primarily by increasing their intestinal absorption and by promoting their mobilization from bone. In addition, vitamin D reduces renal excretion of calcium and phosphate; however, the quantitative significance of this effect is not clear. With usual doses of vitamin D, there is no net loss of calcium from bone; decalcification of bone occurs only when serum calcium concentrations cannot be maintained by increasing intestinal calcium absorption.

Vitamin D Deficiency

Insufficient dietary vitamin D produces *rickets* in children and *osteomalacia* in adults. Signs and symptoms of these conditions are described above. Administration of vitamin D can completely reverse the symptoms of both conditions, unless permanent deformity has already developed.

Sources and Daily Requirements

Vitamin D is obtained by exposure to sunlight and through the diet. In the United States, vitamin D is present as an additive in a variety of foods, including milk, other dairy products, cereals, and candy. Because of these supplements, Americans rarely experience nutritional vitamin D deficiency.

The recommended dietary allowance (RDA) for vitamin D decreases with age: for people 24 years old and younger, the RDA is 400 international units (IU); for people over 24, the RDA decreases to 200 IU. Since substantial amounts of vitamin D may be present in the diet, and since vitamin D in excess can be harmful, supplements should not be taken unless the diet has first been evaluated and judged to be vitamin D deficient.

Activation of Vitamin D

In order to affect calcium and phosphate metabolism, vitamin D must first undergo activation. The extent of this activation is carefully regulated, and is determined by calcium availability: when plasma calcium levels fall, activation of vitamin D is increased. The pathways for activating vitamins D_2 and D_3 are shown in Figure 52–1.

Let's begin consideration of vitamin D activation by focusing on the natural human vitamin (vitamin D_3). As shown in Figure 52–1, vitamin D_3 (cholecalciferol) is produced in the skin through the action of sunlight on provitamin D_3 (7-dehydrocholesterol). Neither provitamin D_3 nor vitamin D_3 itself possesses significant biologic activity. In the next reaction, enzymes in the liver convert cholecalciferol into calcifediol; calcifediol serves as a transport form of vitamin D_3 and possesses only slight biologic activity. In the final step of vitamin D activation, calcifediol is converted into the highly active calcitriol. This reaction occurs in the kidney and can be stimulated by (1) parathyroid hormone, (2) reductions in dietary vitamin D, and (3) decline in plasma levels of calcium.

Vitamin D_2 is activated by the same enzymes that activate vitamin D_3. As we saw with vitamin

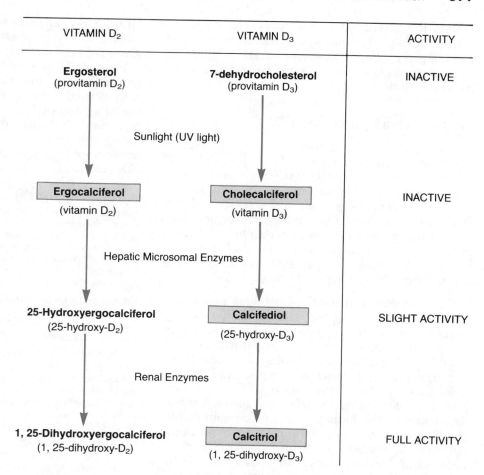

	VITAMIN D₂	VITAMIN D₃	ACTIVITY

Figure 52–1. Vitamin D activation. *Ergosterol* is found in yeasts and fungi. *7-Dehydrocholesterol* is present in the skin. (Colored boxes indicate forms of vitamin D used therapeutically.)

D₃, only the last compound in the series (in this case 1,25-dihydroxyergocalciferol) displays significant biologic activity.

Pharmacokinetics

Vitamin D is administered orally and absorbed from the small intestine. Bile is essential for absorption. Hence, in the absence of sufficient bile, IM administration may be required. Vitamin D is transported in the blood complexed with vitamin D-binding protein. Storage of vitamin D occurs primarily in the liver. As discussed above, vitamin D undergoes metabolic activation. Reactions that occur in the liver produce the major transport form of vitamin D. A later reaction in the kidney produces the fully active vitamin. Excretion of vitamin D is via the bile. Very little vitamin D leaves in urine.

Viewing Vitamin D as a Hormone

Although referred to as a vitamin, vitamin D has all the characteristics of a hormone. With sufficient exposure to sunlight, the body can manufacture all the vitamin D it needs. Hence, under ideal conditions, external sources of vitamin D are probably unnecessary. Following its production in the skin, vitamin D travels to other locations (liver and kidney) for activation. Like other hormones, activated vitamin D then travels to various sites in the body (bone, intestine, kidney) to exert its regulatory actions. Also like other hormones, vitamin D undergoes feedback regulation: as plasma levels of calcium fall, activation of vitamin D increases; when plasma levels of calcium return to normal, the rate of vitamin D activation declines.

Drug Interactions

Antiseizure Drugs. Two antiseizure drugs—*phenobarbital* and *phenytoin*—can promote osteomalacia and rickets. Previously, it was thought that these responses were the result of increased vitamin D breakdown occurring secondary to induction of hepatic drug-metabolizing enzymes. However, since levels of calcitriol (the active form of vitamin D) remain normal during anticonvulsant therapy, this explanation is inadequate. Current evidence suggests that the derangements of bone mineralization that can occur during phenobarbital and phenytoin therapy are the result of increased resistance to vitamin D in target organs—and not the result of accelerated vitamin D destruction.

Cardiac Glycosides. Excessive elevations in calcium levels can cause dysrhythmias in patients receiving digitalis. When vitamin D is given to these patients, special care must be taken to avoid hypercalcemia.

Toxicity (Hypervitaminosis D)

Vitamin D toxicity (hypervitaminosis D) can be produced by doses of vitamin D in excess of 1000 IU/day in infants and 60,000 IU/day in adults. Poisoning occurs most commonly in children; causes include accidental ingestion and excessive administration of vitamin D by parents. Doses of potentially toxic magnitude are also encountered clinically. When these huge doses are used, the margin of safety is small, and patients should be monitored closely for signs of poisoning.

Clinical Presentation. Most signs and symptoms of vitamin D toxicity occur secondary to hypercalcemia. Early responses include weakness, fatigue, nausea, vomiting, and constipation. With persistent hypercalcemia, kidney function is affected, resulting in polyuria, nocturia, and proteinuria. Calcium deposition in soft tissues can damage the heart, blood vessels, and lungs; calcium deposition in the kidneys can cause nephrolithiasis. Very large doses of vitamin D can cause decalcification of bone, resulting in osteoporosis; mobilization of bone calcium can occur despite the presence of high calcium concentrations in blood. In children, vitamin D poisoning can suppress growth for 6 or more months.

Treatment. Treatment consists of immediate discontinuation of vitamin D, high fluid intake, and institution of a low-calcium diet. Glucocorticoids may be given to suppress calcium absorption. If hypercalcemia is severe, renal excretion of calcium can be accelerated using a combination of intravenous saline and furosemide.

Therapeutic Uses

The primary indications for vitamin D are nutritional rickets, osteomalacia, and hypoparathyroidism. Other applications include vitamin D-resistant rickets, vitamin D-dependent rickets, and renal osteodystrophy.

Preparations, Dosage, and Administration

There are five preparations of vitamin D. Four of these (ergocalciferol, cholecalciferol, calcifediol, calcitriol) are identical to forms of vitamin D that occur naturally. The fifth preparation (dihydrotachysterol) is a synthetic derivative of vitamin D_2. (The naturally occurring preparations are highlighted in colored boxes in Fig. 52–1.) Individual vitamin D preparations differ in their clinical applications. Indications for specific preparations are given below.

Vitamin D is usually administered by mouth. Intramuscular injections (of ergocalciferol) may also be used. Dosage is usually prescribed in international units (IU). (One IU is equivalent to the biologic activity in 0.025 μg of vitamin D_3.) Daily dosages of vitamin D range from 400 IU (for dietary supplementation) to as high as 500,000 IU (for vitamin D–resistant rickets).

Ergocalciferol (Vitamin D_2). Ergocalciferol [Calciferol, Drisdol] is used for hypoparathyroidism, vitamin D-resistant rickets, and familial hypophosphatemia. Ergocalciferol is dispensed in capsules (50,000 IU), tablets (50,000 IU), solution (8000 IU/ml), and as an injection (500,000 IU/ml). The dosage for vitamin D-resistant rickets ranges from 12,000 to 500,000 IU daily. The dosage for hypoparathyroidism ranges from 50,000 to 200,000 IU daily (together with 4 gm of calcium lactate given 6 times/day).

Cholecalciferol (Vitamin D_3). Vitamin D_3 [Delta-D] is given as a dietary supplement and for the prophylaxis and treatment of vitamin D deficiency. Cholecalciferol is available in tablets containing 400 IU and 1000 IU.

Calcifediol (25-hydroxy-D_3). Calcifediol [Calderol] is indicated for the management of metabolic bone disease and hypocalcemia in patients undergoing chronic renal dialysis. Calcifediol is available in capsules (20 and 50 μg) for oral use. Initial dosage is 300 to 350 μg/week (administered in divided doses on a daily or every-other-day schedule). For maintenance, daily doses of 50 to 100 μg are adequate for most patients.

Calcitriol (1, 25-dihydroxy-D_3). Calcitriol [Rocaltrol, Calcijex] is indicated for treatment of hypoparathyroidism and for management of hypocalcemia in patients undergoing chronic renal dialysis. The drug is dispensed in capsules (0.25 and 0.5 μg) and as an injection (1 and 2 μg/ml). For dialysis patients, daily doses of 0.5 to 1.0 μg are usually adequate. The initial dosage for hypoparathyroidism is 0.25 μg/day.

Dihydrotachysterol (DHT). DHT is a synthetic derivative of vitamin D_2. DHT is interesting in that, unlike vitamin D_2 and D_3, it doesn't require renal enzymes for activation; metabolic conversation by the liver is all that is needed to render DHT fully active. DHT is indicated for hypoparathyroidism, postoperative tetany, and tetany of unknown cause. DHT is available in tablets (0.125, 0.2, and 0.4 mg), capsules (0.125 mg), and oral solutions (0.2 and 0.25 mg/ml). Preparations are marketed under the trade names DHT and Hytakerol.

CALCIUM SALTS

Calcium salts are available in oral and parenteral formulations for treatment of hypocalcemic states. The various calcium salts differ in their percentage of elemental calcium. These differences must be accounted for when determining dosage.

Oral Calcium Salts

Therapeutic Uses. Oral calcium preparations are used to treat mild hypocalcemia. In addition, calcium salts are taken as dietary supplements. People who may need supplementary calcium include children, adolescents, the elderly, and women who are pregnant or breast-feeding.

Although there is controversy over the ability of lifelong calcium supplements to prevent osteoporosis in women, many women take calcium supplements in hopes that they may work. For prophylaxis of osteoporosis, some physicians recommend that mature women take 1000 mg of calcium daily before menopause, and 1500 mg daily afterward. Estrogen replacement therapy is a proven method of reducing postmenopausal osteoporosis.

Adverse Effects. When calcium is taken chronically in high doses (3 to 4 gm/day), *hypercalcemia* can result. Hypercalcemia is most likely in patients who are also receiving large doses of vitamin D. Signs and symptoms include gastrointestinal disturbances (nausea, vomiting, constipation), renal dysfunction (polyuria, nephrolithiasis), and CNS effects (lethargy, depression). In addition, hypercalcemia may cause cardiac dysrhythmias and deposition of calcium in soft tissue. Hypercalcemia can be minimized with frequent monitoring of plasma calcium content.

Drug Interactions. *Corticosteroids* reduce absorption of oral calcium. Calcium binds to *tetracyclines*, thereby decreasing tetracycline absorption. To minimize this interaction, calcium and tetracyclines should be administered at least 1 hour apart. *Thiazide diuretics* decrease renal calcium excretion and may thereby cause hypercalcemia.

Food Interactions. Certain foods contain substances that can suppress calcium absorption. One such substance—oxalic acid—is found in spinach, rhubarb, Swiss chard, and beets. Phytic acid, another depressant of calcium absorption, is present in bran and whole grain cereals. Oral calcium should not be administered with these foods.

Preparations and Dosage. The calcium salts available for oral administration are listed in Table 52–1. Note that the dosage required to provide a particular amount of elemental calcium differs among preparations. Recommended dosages for prophylaxis against bone loss due to aging are 1.0 to 1.5 gm/day. Chewable tablets are preferred to standard tablets because of more consistent bioavailability.

Parenteral Calcium Salts

Therapeutic Use. Parenteral calcium salts are given to raise calcium levels rapidly in patients with symptoms of severe hypocalcemia (i.e., hypocalcemic tetany). Three parenteral preparations are available: *calcium chloride, calcium gluconate,* and *calcium gluceptate.* Calcium gluconate (IV) is the agent of choice.

Adverse Effects. *Calcium chloride* is highly irritating. Intramuscular injection may cause necrosis and sloughing; hence, this route must never be used. When the drug is administered IV, care must be taken to avoid extravasation, since local infiltration can produce severe injury. Although less of an irritant than calcium chloride, *calcium gluconate* can produce pain, sloughing, and abscess formation if administered IM. Overdosage with any of the calcium salts can produce signs and symptoms of hypercalcemia (weakness, lethargy, nausea, vomiting, coma, death).

Drug Interactions. Parenteral calcium may cause severe bradycardia in patients taking *digoxin.* Accordingly, calcium infusions should be done slowly and cautiously in these patients. Several classes of compounds—*phosphates, carbonates, sulfates, tartrates*—may cause calcium to precipitate and, therefore, should not be added to parenteral calcium solutions.

Dosage and Administration. All three parenteral calcium salts may be given IV; only calcium gluceptate should be given IM. Solutions of calcium salts should be warmed to body temperature prior to administration. Intravenous injections should be done slowly (0.5 to 2 ml/min). Dosage forms and dosages are summarized in Table 52–2.

CALCITONIN

Calcitonin is indicated for hypercalcemia and Paget's disease of bone. In humans, calcitonin is

Table 52–1. Oral Calcium Salts			
Generic Name	**Trade Names**	**Calcium Content**	**Dose Providing 500 mg Calcium**
Calcium acetate	Phos-Ex, PhosLo	25%	2.0 gm
Calcium carbonate	Various names	40%	1.3 gm
Calcium citrate	Citracal	21%	2.4 gm
Calcium glubionate	Neo-Calglucon	6.6%	7.6 gm
Calcium gluconate*	—	9%	5.5 gm
Calcium lactate	—	13%	3.8 gm
Dibasic calcium phosphate	—	23%	2.2 gm
Tricalcium phosphate	Posture	39%	1.3 gm

*Also available in parenteral form (see Table 52–2).

		Table 52–2. Calcium Salts for Parenteral Administration		
Generic Name	Dosage Form	Calcium per ml of Solution	Route	Usual Adult Dosage Range
Calcium chloride	10% solution	27 mg	IV	5–10 ml (135–270 mg Ca)
Calcium gluconate*	10% solution	9 mg	IV	5–20 ml (45–180 mg Ca)
Calcium gluceptate	22% solution	18 mg	IV	5–20 ml (90–360 mg Ca)
			IM	2–5 ml (36–90 mg Ca)

*Also available in an oral formulation (see Table 52–1).

produced by parafollicular cells of the thyroid. Two forms of calcitonin are employed clinically: (1) *salmon calcitonin* (synthetic calcitonin derived from salmon), and (2) *human calcitonin* (synthetic calcitonin identical to thyroid-derived calcitonin). The salmon hormone produces the same metabolic effects as human calcitonin but has a longer half-life and greater milligram potency.

Use in Paget's Disease of Bone

Mechanism and Actions. Calcitonin is helpful in moderate-to-severe Paget's disease and is the drug of choice for rapid relief of pain associated with this disorder. Calcitonin produces its therapeutic effects by acting directly on osteoclasts to inhibit resorption of bone. Beneficial effects on bone turnover are reflected in (1) decreased plasma levels of alkaline phosphatase, (2) increased urinary excretion of hydroxyproline, and (3) reduced blood flow to bone. In addition, serum levels of calcium and phosphorus are reduced. Neurologic symptoms resulting from spinal cord compression may be relieved.

Development of Resistance. When taken for a year or longer, *salmon* calcitonin often loses effectiveness. In many such cases, patients have high levels of antibodies directed against the hormone. These antibodies may be responsible for the loss of therapeutic effect. In patients who have antibodies to salmon calcitonin, human calcitonin remains effective.

Use in Hypercalcemia

Calcitonin can lower plasma calcium content in patients with hypercalcemia secondary to hyperparathyroidism, vitamin D toxicity, and cancer. Levels of calcium (and phosphorus) are lowered due to inhibition of bone resorption. Although calcitonin is effective against hypercalcemia, this hormone is not a preferred treatment.

Adverse Effects

Serious reactions are uncommon. About 10% of patients experience nausea; this response diminishes with time. An additional 10% have inflammatory reactions at the site of injection. Flushing of the face and hands may occur.

Preparations, Dosage, and Administration

Preparations and Routes. *Salmon calcitonin* [Calcimar, Miacalcin] is dispensed in 2-ml vials (200 IU/ml) and 1-ml ampuls (100 IU/ml) for IM and SC administration. *Human calcitonin* [Cibacalcin] is dispensed in 0.5 mg vials for SC administration.

Dosage. Paget's disease may be treated with salmon calcitonin or human calcitonin. With salmon calcitonin, the initial dosage is 100 IU/day (IM or SC); the maintenance dosage is 50 IU 3 times/week. With human calcitonin, the dosage is 0.5 to 1.0 mg (SC) administered either daily or 2 to 3 times/week; therapy is discontinued when symptoms are relieved (in 6 months to 1 year).

Only salmon calcitonin is approved for hypercalcemia. Doses range from 4 to 8 IU/kg (IM or SC) administered every 6 to 12 hours.

OTHER DRUGS THAT AFFECT CALCIUM

Drugs Used to Treat Hypercalcemia

Furosemide. Furosemide, a loop diuretic, promotes renal excretion of calcium. This action is useful for treating *hypercalcemic emergencies*. In managing such emergencies, isotonic saline (IV) must be given prior to furosemide. Furosemide dosage for adults is 80 to 100 mg every 1 to 2 hours as needed; the infusion rate must not exceed 4 mg/min. To avoid fluid and electrolyte imbalance, urinary losses must be measured and replaced. The basic pharmacology of furosemide is discussed in Chapter 35 (Diuretics).

Glucocorticoids. Glucocorticoids reduce intestinal absorption of calcium. This action can be useful in the treatment of hypercalcemia. For severe hypercalcemia, parenteral therapy is indicated (e.g., 100 to 500 mg hydrocortisone sodium succinate IV daily). Since glucocorticoids can produce serious adverse effects when used on a chronic basis, the risks of long-term treatment must be carefully weighed against the benefits. The basic pharmacology of the glucocorticoids is discussed in Chapter 62 (Glucocorticoids in Nonendocrine Diseases).

Inorganic Phosphates. Phosphates lower plasma levels of calcium, and can be employed to treat hypercalcemia. Suggested mechanisms for reducing plasma calcium include (1) decreased bone resorption, (2) increased bone formation, and (3) decreased intestinal absorption of calcium (secondary to decreased renal activation of vitamin D). Intravenous use of phosphates is hazardous and limited to treatment of life-threatening hypercalcemia. Oral administration is considerably safer.

Oral phosphates are given to treat mild-to-moderate hypercalcemia. These agents should not be given to patients whose kidney function is impaired or whose serum phosphate level is elevated. Oral phosphates should not be combined with antacids that contain aluminum, magnesium, or calcium; all of these elements bind phosphate and will prevent its absorption. Initial treatment should provide 1 to 2 gm of phosphorus/day. Doses are reduced when serum calcium levels normalize.

Edetate Disodium (EDTA). Edetate disodium is a chelating agent that binds calcium in the blood; this interaction rapidly reduces the plasma concentration of free calcium. The EDTA-calcium complex is filtered by the glomerulus but not reabsorbed by the kidney tubules; hence, renal excretion of calcium is increased. Although EDTA is highly effective at reducing hypercalcemia, this agent is also very toxic: EDTA can cause profound hypocalcemia, resulting in tetany, convulsions, dysrhythmias, and death. Severe nephrotoxicity can also occur. Because of its toxicity, EDTA is used only for life-threatening hypercalcemic crisis. The usual adult dose is 40 mg/kg infused over 4 to 6 hours. The total daily dose must not exceed 3 gm.

Plicamycin. Plicamycin [Mithracin] is a cytotoxic antibiotic produced by several species of *Streptomyces*. Although used primarily for testicular cancer, plicamycin is also indicated for hypercalcemia. Plicamycin lowers plasma calcium levels by acting directly on bone to prevent calcium resorption. For management of hypercalcemia, relatively low doses are employed (e.g., 25 µg/kg/day for 3 to 4 days). Calcium-lowering effects may be visible within 1 to 2 days, and may persist for several days to 3 or more weeks. Plicamycin lowers platelet counts and reduces levels of several clotting factors; both actions result in bleeding tendencies.

Gallium Nitrate. Gallium nitrate [Ganite] is used to treat hypercalcemia of malignancy. In addition, the drug is under investigation for use in Paget's disease of bone and postmenopausal osteoporosis. Gallium reduces calcium levels by preventing bone resorption; it may also increase bone formation. Gallium is highly nephrotoxic and must not be used with other nephrotoxic drugs, such as amphotericin B and the aminoglycosides. To minimize kidney damage, the patient must be hydrated with intravenous fluids before treatment. Renal function must be monitored. The usual single dose is 100 to 200 mg/M². This dose is diluted in 1 L of 5% dextrose or 0.9% sodium chloride and infused over 24 hours. The dose is repeated daily for 5 days.

Miscellaneous Agents That Affect Calcium

Etidronate. Etidronate [Didronel], a biphosphonate, is used to treat *Paget's disease of bone*. This agent binds to hydroxyapatite, the basic inorganic component of bone, and decreases both the accretion and dissolution of bone mineral content; turnover of bone is reduced by about 50%. Bone pain is usually lessened, although some patients experience increased discomfort. The incidence of Paget's fractures may decline. Evidence of improvement may be delayed for 1 to 3 months; maximal effects develop in about 6 months. Benefits often persist for a year or more following a single course of therapy. When compared with calcitonin, etidronate has the advantages of being orally administered and relatively inexpensive.

Etidronate is administered by mouth, usually as a single daily dose. Less than 6% is absorbed. About half the absorbed dose is rapidly excreted by the kidneys; the remaining 50% becomes incorporated into bone. For treatment of Paget's disease, the usual adult dosage is 5 mg/kg/day for no more than 6 months. Repeated treatments can be given, but not until 90 days have elapsed since the end of the prior course.

Etidronate has been used investigationally for *postmenopausal osteoporosis*. In postmenopausal women with osteoporosis and vertebral compression fractures, treatment has increased bone mass and reduced the incidence of new fractures. The dosing schedule employed was 400 mg/day for 2 weeks repeated every 3 to 3.5 months.

Pamidronate. Pamidronate [Aredia], like etidronate, is a biphosphonate compound. The drug is approved for treating *hypercalcemia of malignancy*. In addition, the drug is under study for use in *Paget's disease of bone, hyperparathyroidism,* and *postmenopausal osteoporosis*. Pamidronate has the same mechanism of action as etidronate: the drug avidly binds hydroxyapatite crystals in bone, thereby blocking calcium resorption. Pamidronate remains bound until the bone is remodeled. For hypercalcemia of malignancy, the initial dose is 60 to 90 mg (IV) infused over 24 hours. This dose is repeated in 7 days if needed. The most common adverse effects are transient leukopenia and fever. Other adverse effects include nausea and mild thrombophlebitis at the infusion site.

Estrogens. Estrogen replacement therapy provides effective *prophylaxis of postmenopausal osteoporosis*. However, estrogens will not reverse bone loss that has occurred prior to treatment. Estrogen therapy is indicated following natural menopause and menopause resulting from surgical removal of the ovaries. The use of estrogens for prophylaxis of osteoporosis is discussed further in Chapter 55 (Estrogens and Progestins).

Thiazide Diuretics. Unlike most diuretics, thiazides *reduce* renal excretion of calcium. Because of their ability to cause calcium retention, thiazides may be useful as adjuncts to vitamin D and calcium in the treatment of *hypoparathyroidism*. The basic pharmacology of the thiazides is discussed in Chapter 35 (Diuretics).

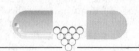

Summary of Major Nursing Implications

VITAMIN D

✓ **Preadministration Assessment**

Therapeutic Goal

Treatment of rickets, osteomalacia, and hypoparathyroidism.

Baseline Data

The physician may order serum levels of vitamin D, calcium, phosphorus, and alkaline phosphatase as well as a 24-hour urinary calcium determination. Assess dietary vitamin D and calcium content.

Identifying High-Risk Patients

Vitamin D is *contraindicated* in the presence of *hypercalcemia, hypervitaminosis D*, and *malabsorption syndrome*. Exercise *caution* in patients taking *digoxin*.

✓ **Implementation: Administration**

Routes

Oral, IM.

Administration

Instruct the patient to swallow oral preparations intact, without crushing or chewing.

✓ **Implementation: Measures to Enhance Therapeutic Effects**

Therapeutic responses to vitamin D require adequate calcium intake. Assess dietary calcium content and adjust to insure calcium sufficiency.

Encourage the patient to comply with the entire treatment regimen: vitamin D dosing; consumption of adequate dietary vitamin D and calcium.

✓ **Ongoing Evaluation and Interventions**

Monitoring Summary

Monitor serum calcium, serum phosphorous, and urinary calcium.

Minimizing Adverse Interactions

Antiseizure Drugs. *Phenobarbital* and *phenytoin* can reduce the effects of vitamin D; patients may require increased vitamin D doses.

Digoxin. Vitamin D-induced hypercalcemia can cause dysrhythmias in patients taking digoxin. Monitor serum calcium and make certain it remains normal.

Management of Toxicity

Large therapeutic doses may cause hypervitaminosis D, a syndrome characterized by hypercalcemia, hypercalciuria, decalcification of bone, and deposition of calcium in soft tissues. Monitor serum calcium content; levels should stay below 10 mg/dl. Monitor serum phosphorus and urinary calcium as well. If vitamin D toxicity develops, have the patient discontinue vitamin D immediately, increase fluid intake, and institute a low-calcium diet. In severe cases, calcium excretion can be accelerated with IV saline plus furosemide.

ORAL CALCIUM SALTS

Calcium Acetate   Calcium Gluconate

Calcium Carbonate   Calcium Lactate

Calcium Citrate   Dibasic Calcium Phosphate

Calcium Glubionate

 Preadministration Assessment

Therapeutic Goal

Treatment of mild hypocalcemia; supplementation of dietary calcium; possible prophylaxis of postmenopausal osteoporosis.

Baseline Data

Obtain a serum calcium level.

Identifying High-Risk Patients

Calcium salts are *contraindicated* for patients with *hypercalcemia, renal calculi,* and *hypophosphatemia.*

 Implementation: Administration

Route

Oral.

Dosage

Individual calcium salts differ from one another as to their percentage of elemental calcium. As a result, the dose required to provide a specific amount of calcium differs between the salts. Make certain that the patient does not switch arbitrarily to a different preparation.

Administration

Advise the patient to take oral calcium salts with a large glass of water; administration with or after meals promotes absorption. Advise the patient to avoid foods that can suppress calcium absorption (e.g., spinach, Swiss chard, beets, bran, whole grain cereals).

 Ongoing Evaluation and Interventions

Minimizing Adverse Effects

Prolonged therapy can cause *hypercalcemia.* Inform patients about signs of hypercalcemia (nausea, vomiting, constipation, frequent urination, lethargy, depression) and instruct them to notify the physician if these occur. Hypercalcemia can be minimized with frequent monitoring of serum calcium.

Minimizing Adverse Interactions

Glucocorticoids. These drugs reduce calcium absorption; increased calcium dosage may be required.

Tetracyclines. Calcium binds to tetracyclines, thereby reducing tetracycline absorption. Instruct the patient to separate administration of tetracyclines and calcium by at least 1 hour.

Thiazide Diuretics. Thiazides decrease renal excretion of calcium. A reduction in calcium dosage may be needed to avoid hypercalcemia.

PARENTERAL CALCIUM SALTS

Calcium Chloride
Calcium Gluconate
Calcium Gluceptate

 Preadministration Assessment

Therapeutic Goal

Reversal of clinical manifestations of hypocalcemia.

Baseline Data

Assess for signs and symptoms of hypocalcemia (tetany, convulsions, laryngospasm, and spasm of other muscles). Obtain measurement of serum calcium.

Identifying High-Risk Patients

Parenteral calcium is *contraindicated* for patients with *hypercalcemia* and *ventricular fibrillation*. Use with extreme *caution* in patients taking *digoxin*.

 Implementation: Administration

Routes

IM, IV. All parenteral calcium salts may be given IV; only *calcium glubionate* and *calcium gluceptate* should be given IM.

Administration

Warm solutions to body temperature prior to infusion or IM injection. Perform IV injections slowly (0.5 to 2 ml/minute).

Drugs that contain phosphate, carbonate, sulfate, and tartrate groups can cause calcium to precipitate; do not mix these drugs with parenteral calcium solutions.

Calcium chloride may cause necrosis and sloughing if solutions become extravasated. Monitor the infusion closely.

Ongoing Evaluation and Interventions

Evaluating Therapeutic Effects

Evaluate the patient for reductions in tetany, muscle spasm, laryngospasm, paresthesias, and other symptoms of severe hypocalcemia.

Minimizing Adverse Effects

Overdosage can produce acute *hypercalcemia*, resulting in nausea, vomiting, weakness, lethargy, coma, and possibly death. Avoid hypercalcemia through careful control of dosage.

Minimizing Adverse Interactions

Parenteral calcium may cause severe bradycardia in patients taking *digoxin*. Infuse calcium slowly and cautiously in these patients.

CALCITONIN

Preadministration Assessment

Therapeutic Goal

Treatment of Paget's disease of bone and hypercalcemia.

Baseline Data

The physician may order measurements of serum alkaline phosphatase, calcium, and phosphorus, as well as a 24-hour urinary hydroxyproline.

Identifying High-Risk Patients

Salmon calcitonin is *contraindicated* for patients allergic to this preparation.

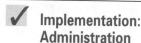
Implementation: Administration

Routes

Human calcitonin: SC.
Salmon calcitonin: IM, SC. Administration by outpatients is SC, not IM.

Administration

Teach patients how to inject calcitonin SC, and instruct them to rotate the sites of injection.

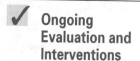
Ongoing Evaluation and Interventions

Evaluating Therapeutic Effects

Paget's Disease of Bone. Monitor for reductions in bone pain, serum alkaline phosphatase levels, and 24-hour urinary hydroxyproline value.

Hypercalcemia. Monitor for reductions in serum calcium and phosphorus levels.

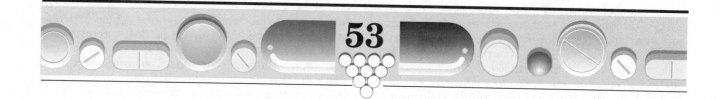

Drugs for Disorders of the Adrenal Cortex

The hormones of the adrenal cortex affect multiple physiologic processes, including maintenance of glucose availability, regulation of water and electrolyte balance, development of sexual characteristics, and life-preserving responses to stress. As one might guess, when production of adrenal hormones goes awry, the consequences can be profound. The two most familiar forms of adrenocortical dysfunction are *Cushing's syndrome*, caused by adrenal hormone excess, and *Addison's disease*, caused by adrenal hormone deficiency.

In approaching the drugs used for disorders of the adrenal cortex, we will begin by reviewing adrenocortical endocrinology. After that, we will discuss the disease states associated with adrenal hormone excess and insufficiency. Having established this background, we will discuss the agents used for diagnosis and treatment of adrenocortical disorders.

PHYSIOLOGY OF THE ADRENOCORTICAL HORMONES

The adrenal cortex produces three classes of steroid hormones: *glucocorticoids, mineralocorticoids,* and *androgens*. Glucocorticoids influence carbohy-

687

drate metabolism and other processes; mineralocorticoids modulate salt and water balance; adrenal androgens contribute to expression of sexual characteristics. When referring to either the glucocorticoids or the mineralocorticoids, the terms *corticosteroids*, *adrenocorticoids*, or *corticoids* may be used. These terms are *not* used in reference to adrenal androgens.

GLUCOCORTICOIDS

Glucocorticoids are so named because of their ability to increase the availability of glucose. Of the several glucocorticoids produced by the adrenal cortex, *cortisol* is the most important. The structural formula of cortisol is shown in Figure 53–1.

When considering the glucocorticoids, it is important to distinguish between *physiologic effects* and *pharmacologic effects*. Physiologic effects occur at *low* levels of glucocorticoids (i.e., the levels produced by release of glucocorticoids from healthy adrenals or by administration of exogenous glucocorticoids in low doses). *Pharmacologic* effects occur at *high* levels of glucocorticoids. These are the levels achieved when exogenous glucocorticoids are administered in the large doses required to treat disorders unrelated to adrenocortical function (e.g., allergic reactions, asthma, inflammation). In this chapter, we will limit discussion to the *physiologic* role of glucocorticoids. The use of glucocorticoids for *nonendocrine* purposes (which is the major application of these agents) is discussed in Chapter 62.

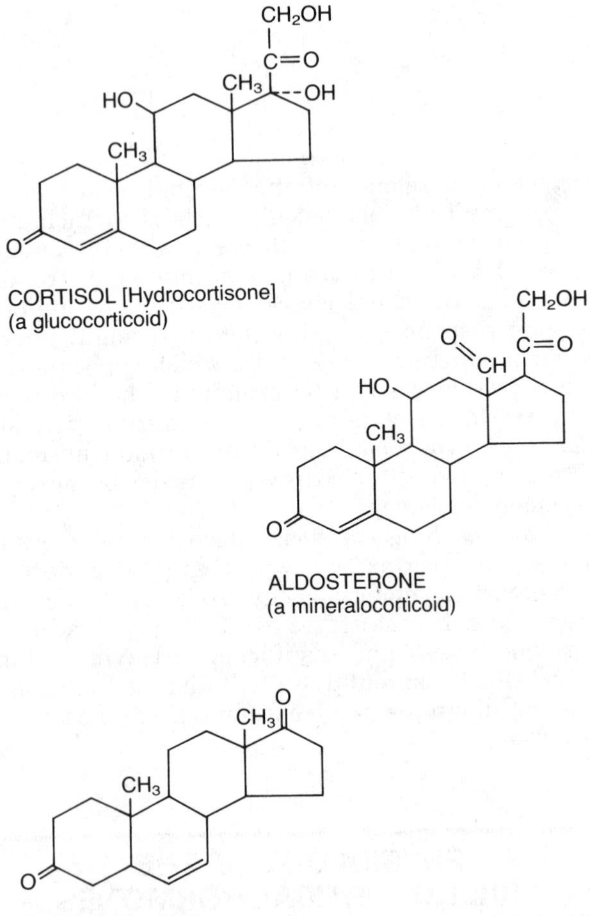

Physiologic Effects

Carbohydrate Metabolism. Supplying the brain with glucose is essential for survival. Glucocorticoids help meet this need. Glucocorticoids promote glucose availability in three ways: (1) stimulation of gluconeogenesis, (2) reduction of peripheral glucose utilization, and (3) promotion of glucose storage (in the form of glycogen). All three actions increase glucose availability during fasting, and thereby help insure that the brain will not be deprived of its primary source of energy.

The effects of glucocorticoids on carbohydrate metabolism are opposite to those of insulin: whereas insulin lowers plasma levels of glucose, glucocorticoids cause glucose levels to rise. When present chronically in high concentrations, glucocorticoids produce symptoms much like those of diabetes.

Protein Metabolism. Glucocorticoids promote protein catabolism (breakdown). This action, which is opposite to that of insulin, provides amino acids for glucose synthesis. If present at high levels for a prolonged time, glucocorticoids will cause thinning of the skin, muscle wasting, and negative nitrogen balance.

Fat Metabolism. Glucocorticoids promote lipolysis (fat breakdown). When present at high levels for an extended period (as occurs in Cushing's syndrome), glucocorticoids cause fat redistribution, giving the patient a potbelly, "moon face," and a "buffalo hump" on his or her back.

Cardiovascular System. Glucocorticoids are required to maintain the functional integrity of the vascular system. When levels of glucocorticoids are depressed, capillary permeability is increased, the ability of vessels to constrict is reduced, and blood pressure falls.

Glucocorticoids have multiple effects on blood cells. These hormones increase red blood cell counts and levels of hemoglobin. Of the white blood cells, only the polymorphonuclear leukocytes increase; circulating numbers of lymphocytes, eosinophils, basophils, and monocytes are lowered.

Skeletal Muscle. Glucocorticoids support function of striated muscle, primarily by maintaining circulatory competence. In the absence of sufficient

CORTISOL [Hydrocortisone]
(a glucocorticoid)

ALDOSTERONE
(a mineralocorticoid)

ANDROSTENEDIONE
(an androgen)

Figure 53–1. Structural formulas of representative adenocortical hormones.

levels of glucocorticoids, muscle perfusion decreases, causing work capacity to decrease as well.

Central Nervous System (CNS). Glucocorticoids affect mood, CNS excitability, and the electroencephalogram. Glucocorticoid insufficiency is associated with depression, lethargy, and irritability. Rarely, outright psychosis occurs. In contrast, when present in excess, glucocorticoids can produce generalized excitation and euphoria.

Stress. In response to stress (e.g., anxiety, exercise, trauma, infection, surgery), the adrenal cortex secretes increased amounts of glucocorticoids, and the adrenal medulla secretes increased amounts of epinephrine. Working together, glucocorticoids and epinephrine serve to maintain blood pressure and plasma glucose content. If glucocorticoid levels are insufficient, hypotension and hypoglycemia can occur. If the stress is extreme (e.g., trauma, surgery, severe infection), glucocorticoid deficiency can result in circulatory collapse and death. Accordingly, it is essential that patients with adrenal insufficiency be given glucocorticoid supplements when severe stress occurs.

Regulation of Synthesis and Secretion

Adrenal storage of glucocorticoids is minimal; hence, glucocorticoids must be synthesized as they are needed. Accordingly, the amount of glucocorticoid released from the adrenals per unit time closely approximates the amount being made.

Synthesis and release of glucocorticoids are regulated by a negative feedback loop (Fig. 53–2). The loop begins with the release of corticotropin-releasing factor (CRF) from the hypothalamus. CRF acts on the anterior pituitary to cause release of adrenocorticotropic hormone (ACTH), which stimulates the adrenal cortex, causing synthesis and release of cortisol and other glucocorticoids. Following release, cortisol acts in two ways: (1) it promotes its designated biologic effects, and (2) it acts on the hypothalamus and pituitary to suppress further release of CRF and ACTH. Hence, as cortisol levels rise, they act to suppress further stimulation of glucocorticoid production, thereby keeping plasma levels of glucocorticoids within an acceptable range.

The hypothalamic-pituitary-adrenal system is activated by signals from the CNS. These signals turn the system on by causing the hypothalamus to release CRF. As indicated in Figure 53–2, two modes of activation are involved. One mode provides a basal level of stimulation. Basal stimulation follows a circadian rhythm, peaking in the early morning and reaching a nadir late in the evening. The second mode of activation is stress. Stressful events that can activate the loop include injury, infection, and surgery. The signals generated by stress produce intense stimulation of the hypothalamus. The resultant release of CRF and

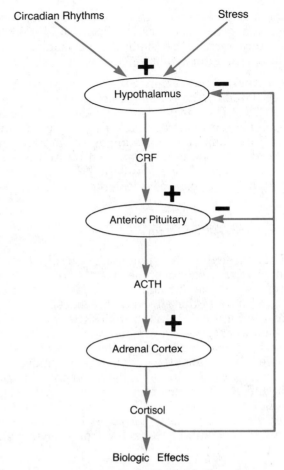

Figure 53–2. Negative feedback regulation of glucocorticoid synthesis and secretion. (CRF = corticotropin-releasing factor, ACTH = adrenocorticotropic hormone)

ACTH can cause plasma levels of cortisol to increase by a factor of 10. Because stress is such a powerful stimulus, it overrides feedback inhibition by cortisol.

MINERALOCORTICOIDS

The mineralocorticoids influence renal processing of sodium, potassium, and hydrogen. Of the mineralocorticoids made by the adrenal cortex, *aldosterone* is the most important.

Physiologic Effects. Aldosterone acts on the collecting ducts of the nephron to promote sodium reabsorption in exchange for secretion of potassium and hydrogen. The total amount of hydrogen and potassium lost equals the amount of sodium reabsorbed. It should be noted that as sodium is reabsorbed, water is reabsorbed along with it. In the absence of aldosterone, renal excretion of sodium and water is greatly increased, whereas excretion of potassium and hydrogen is reduced. As a result, aldosterone insufficiency causes hyponatremia, hyperkalemia, acidosis, cellular dehydration, and reduction of extracellular fluid volume. Left uncorrected, the condition can lead to renal failure, circulatory collapse, and death.

Control of Secretion. Secretion of aldosterone is regulated by the renin-angiotensin system—not by ACTH. The mechanisms by which the renin-angiotensin system regulates aldosterone are discussed in Chapter 37. It is important to note that since aldosterone is not regulated by ACTH, conditions in which secretion of ACTH is altered do not affect the release of aldosterone.

ADRENAL ANDROGENS

The adrenal cortex produces several steroids that have androgenic properties. *Androstenedione* is representative of these compounds. Under normal conditions, the effects of the adrenal androgens are minimal. In adult males the influence of adrenal androgens is overshadowed by the effects of testosterone produced by the testes. In adult females, a metabolite of the adrenal androgens (testosterone) contributes to development of sexual hair and maintenance of normal libido. Although adrenal androgens normally have very little effect, when secretion of these hormones is excessive, as occurs in congenital adrenal hyperplasia, virilizing actions can be pronounced.

PATHOPHYSIOLOGY OF THE ADRENOCORTICAL HORMONES

ADRENAL HORMONE EXCESS

Cushing's Syndrome

Causes. Signs and symptoms of Cushing's syndrome result from excess levels of circulating glucocorticoids. Principal causes of the excess are (1) hypersecretion of ACTH by pituitary adenomas (Cushing's disease), (2) hypersecretion of glucocorticoids by adrenal adenomas and carcinomas, and (3) administration of exogenous glucocorticoids in the large doses used to treat arthritis and other nonendocrine disorders.

Clinical Presentation. Cushing's syndrome is characterized by obesity, hyperglycemia, glycosuria, hypertension, fluid and electrolyte disturbances, osteoporosis, muscle weakness, myopathy, hirsutism, menstrual irregularities, and decreased resistance to infection. The skin is weakened, resulting in striae (stretch marks) and increased susceptibility to injury. Fat undergoes redistribution to the abdomen, face, and upper back, giving the patient a characteristic potbelly, "moon face," and "buffalo hump." Psychiatric changes are common.

Treatment. Treatment of Cushing's syndrome is directed at the cause. The treatment of choice for adrenal adenoma and carcinoma is surgical removal of the diseased gland. If bilateral adrenalectomy is performed, replacement therapy with glucocorticoids and mineralocorticoids will be needed. For patients with inoperable adrenal carcinoma, treatment with *mitotane* is indicated. Mitotane is an anticancer drug that produces selective destruction of adrenocortical cells. The pharmacology of mitotane is discussed in Chapter 91.

When Cushing's syndrome is caused by pituitary adenoma, surgery is the preferred form of treatment. Partial removal of the pituitary often lowers ACTH secretion to safe levels, while leaving other pituitary functions intact. If partial adenectomy is unsuccessful, the remainder of the pituitary may be removed. Alternatively, pituitary irradiation may be employed.

The role of drugs in treating Cushing's syndrome is limited. Most commonly, drugs are employed as adjuncts to radiation and surgery; drugs are rarely the primary therapeutic modality. Drugs can relieve symptoms by inhibiting corticosteroid synthesis. Two drugs that act by this mechanism—*aminoglutethimide* and *trilostane*—are discussed below.

Primary Hyperaldosteronism

Clinical Presentation and Causes. Hyperaldosteronism (excessive secretion of aldosterone) causes hypokalemia, metabolic alkalosis, and hypertension. Muscle weakness and changes in the electrocardiogram develop secondary to hypokalemia. Hyperaldosteronism is frequently caused by an aldosterone-producing adrenal adenoma. The condition may also result from bilateral adrenal hyperplasia.

Treatment. Management of hyperaldosteronism is dependent on the cause. When an adrenal adenoma is responsible, surgical resection of the adrenal is usually curative. When bilateral adrenal hyperplasia underlies hyperaldosteronism, an aldosterone antagonist is the preferred treatment. The antagonist employed most frequently is *spironolactone*, a drug we normally think of as a potassium-sparing diuretic. Under the influence of spironolactone, potassium levels may normalize in 2 weeks. To achieve full control of hypertension, an additional diuretic may be required. The basic pharmacology of spironolactone is discussed in Chapter 35 (Diuretics).

ADRENAL HORMONE INSUFFICIENCY

General Therapeutic Considerations

Adrenal hormone insufficiency can result from multiple causes, including destruction of the adrenals, inborn deficiencies of the enzymes required for corticosteroid synthesis, and reduced secretion of ACTH and CRF. Regardless of the cause, adrenal insufficiency requires lifelong replacement therapy with appropriate corticosteroids. All patients require a *glucocorticoid*. Some may require a *mineralocorticoid* as well. Of the glucocorticoids available, *cortisone* and *hydrocortisone* are drugs of first choice. When a mineralocorticoid is indicated, *fludrocortisone* is the drug of choice.

Replacement therapy should mimic normal patterns of corticosteroid secretion. For glucocorticoids, this can be accomplished by dividing the daily dosage, giving two thirds in the morning and one third in the evening. Mineralocorticoids can be administered once a day. Doses of glucocorticoids and mineralocorticoids should approximate the amounts normally secreted by the adrenals. It is important to note that when glucocorticoids are employed for replacement therapy, doses are much smaller than the doses employed to treat nonendocrine disorders.

At times of stress, patients must increase their glucocorticoid dosage. The importance of doing so cannot be overemphasized: *failure to increase the dosage can be fatal.* Recall that healthy adrenals increase their output of glucocorticoids in response to stress. For patients with adrenal insufficiency, the extra glucocorticoids that would normally be supplied by the adrenals must instead be supplied through supplemental dosing. For mild stress (e.g., upper respiratory infection), doubling the normal dosage should suffice. For severe stress (e.g., surgery), the dosage should be increased fivefold. To insure availability of glucocorticoids in emergencies, the patient should carry an adequate supply at all times. This supply should include an injectable preparation plus an oral preparation. Furthermore, the patient should wear some form of identification (e.g., MedicAlert bracelet) to inform emergency health personnel about glucocorticoid requirements.

Addison's Disease (Primary Adrenocortical Insufficiency)

Clinical Presentation and Causes. Addison's disease is characterized by weakness, emaciation, hypoglycemia, and increased pigmentation of the skin and mucous membranes. Hyperkalemia, hyponatremia, and hypotension are present as well. These symptoms result from a deficiency of glucocorticoids and mineralocorticoids occurring secondary to adrenal atrophy. Potential causes of adrenal atrophy include carcinoma, infection, and autoimmune disease.

Treatment. Replacement therapy with adrenocorticoids is required. *Hydrocortisone* and *cortisone* are the drugs of choice. Both agents exert a combination of mineralocorticoid and glucocorticoid ac-

tivity. Hence, therapy with either agent alone may be sufficient. If additional mineralocorticoid activity is needed, *fludrocortisone*, the only mineralocorticoid available, can be added to the regimen.

Secondary and Tertiary Adrenocortical Insufficiency

Secondary adrenocortical insufficiency results from decreased secretion of ACTH, and tertiary insufficiency results from decreased secretion of CRF. In both cases, adrenal secretion of glucocorticoids is diminished, whereas secretion of mineralocorticoids is usually not affected. Glucocorticoid insufficiency produces a characteristic set of symptoms: hypoglycemia, malaise, loss of appetite, and reduced capacity to respond to stress. For secondary and tertiary insufficiency, treatment consists of replacement therapy with a glucocorticoid (e.g., hydrocortisone, cortisone). A mineralocorticoid is needed rarely.

Acute Adrenal Insufficiency (Adrenal Crisis)

Clinical Presentation. Acute adrenal insufficiency is characterized by hypotension, dehydration, weakness, lethargy, and gastrointestinal symptoms (e.g., vomiting, diarrhea). Left untreated, the syndrome progresses to shock and then death.

Causes. Adrenal crisis may be brought on by adrenal failure, pituitary failure, and by failure to provide patients receiving replacement therapy with adequate doses of corticosteroids. Adrenal crisis may also be triggered by abrupt withdrawal from chronic, high-dose glucocorticoid therapy.

Treatment. Patients require rapid replacement of fluid, salt, and glucocorticoids. They also need glucose for energy. These needs are met by injecting 100 mg of hydrocortisone (as an IV bolus) followed by IV infusion of normal saline with dextrose. Additional hydrocortisone is given by infusion at a rate of 100 mg every 8 hours.

Congenital Adrenal Hyperplasia

Clinical Presentation and Causes. Congenital adrenal hyperplasia results from an inborn deficiency of enzymes needed for glucocorticoid synthesis. The capacity to make glucocorticoids is decreased, but not eliminated. In an attempt to enhance glucocorticoid synthesis, the pituitary releases amounts of ACTH that are much greater than normal. The resultant high levels of ACTH produce powerful stimulation of the adrenals, causing growth of the adrenals (hyperplasia) and increased synthesis of glucocorticoids and androgens. (Synthesis of mineralocorticoids is relatively unaffected.) Frequently, stimulation of glucocorticoid synthesis may be sufficient to bring levels of cortisol up to normal. Unfortunately, the amounts of ACTH required to normalize glucocorticoid production are so large that synthesis of adrenal androgens becomes excessive. In girls, increased androgen levels cause masculinization of the external genitalia. The ovaries, uterus, and fallopian tubes are not affected. Increased androgen levels in boys may cause precocious phallic enlargement. In children of both sexes, linear growth is accelerated. However, because androgens cause premature closure of the epiphyses, adult height is usually diminished.

Treatment. The therapeutic objective is to insure adequate levels of glucocorticoids while preventing excessive production of adrenal androgens. This goal is achieved through lifelong administration of glucocorticoids. *Hydrocortisone* and *cortisone* are the drugs of choice. By supplying glucocorticoids exogenously, we can suppress secretion of ACTH; since ACTH release is diminished, the adrenals are no longer stimulated to produce excessive quantities of androgens. As a rule, suppression of ACTH secretion can be achieved with daily doses of hydrocortisone equivalent to twice the amount secreted each day by normal adrenals. To assess the efficacy of therapy, children should be monitored every 3 months for growth rate and signs of virilization.

AGENTS FOR REPLACEMENT THERAPY IN ADRENOCORTICAL INSUFFICIENCY

Patients with adrenocortical insufficiency require replacement therapy with corticosteroids. A glucocorticoid is always required, and some patients require a mineralocorticoid as well. The principal glucocorticoids employed are *hydrocortisone* and *cortisone*. *Fludrocortisone* is the only mineralocorticoid available.

It should be noted that classification of a drug as a "glucocorticoid" or "mineralocorticoid" may be an oversimplification. That is, a drug that we classify as a glucocorticoid may also exhibit salt-retaining (mineralocorticoid) activity. Conversely, a drug that we classify as a mineralocorticoid may also display typical glucocorticoid activity.

HYDROCORTISONE

Hydrocortisone is a synthetic steroid whose structure is identical to that of cortisol, the principal glucocorticoid produced by the adrenal cortex (see Fig. 53–1). Hydrocortisone is a drug of choice for adrenocortical insufficiency and will serve as

our prototype of the glucocorticoids employed clinically. It should be noted that despite its classification as a glucocorticoid, hydrocortisone also has mineralocorticoid properties.

Therapeutic Uses

Replacement Therapy. Hydrocortisone is a preferred drug for all forms of adrenocortical insufficiency. *Oral* hydrocortisone is ideal for chronic replacement therapy. *Parenteral* administration is used to manage acute adrenal insufficiency, and to supplement oral doses at times of stress. Because of its mineralocorticoid actions, hydrocortisone can sometimes be used as sole therapy for adrenal insufficiency, even when salt loss is a symptom.

Nonendocrine Applications. Hydrocortisone and other glucocorticoids are used to treat a broad spectrum of nonendocrine disorders, ranging from allergic reactions to inflammation to cancer. The doses required in these disorders are considerably higher than the doses employed in replacement therapy. The use of glucocorticoids for nonendocrine diseases is discussed in Chapter 62.

Adverse Effects

When given in the low doses required for replacement therapy, hydrocortisone and other glucocorticoids are devoid of adverse effects. In contrast, when taken chronically in the large doses employed to treat nonendocrine disorders, glucocorticoids are highly toxic. The adverse effects of chronic, high-dose therapy include adrenal suppression and production of Cushing's syndrome. These and other adverse effects are discussed in Chapter 62.

Preparations, Dosage, and Administration

Preparations. For replacement therapy, four hydrocortisone preparations are used: hydrocortisone base, hydrocortisone cypionate, hydrocortisone sodium phosphate, and hydrocortisone sodium succinate. The base and the cypionate salt can be administered orally. Because they are insoluble, these preparations must not be administered IV. The sodium phosphate and sodium succinate salts are water soluble and can be used IV and IM.

Dosage and Administration. The oral route is employed for chronic treatment. Intravenous and IM administration are reserved for emergencies. For oral therapy of chronic adrenal insufficiency, the total daily dose ranges from 12 to 15 mg/m². This dose may be divided, giving two thirds in the morning and one third in the afternoon. For emergency treatment, IV doses of 50 to 100 mg are employed. When IV injections can't be used, IM doses of 100 to 250 mg may be given instead. Doses for nonendocrine disorders are given in Chapter 62.

CORTISONE

Cortisone is a prodrug that undergoes conversion to its active form—hydrocortisone (cortisol)—within the body. Like hydrocortisone itself, cortisone has both glucocorticoid and mineralocorticoid actions, and is a drug of choice for chronic adrenal insufficiency. In contrast to hydrocortisone, which can be administered orally, IV, and IM, cortisone can only be used orally and IM. Cortisone is insoluble in water and must never be administered IV. Absorption of intramuscular cortisone is unpredictable; hence, cortisone injections are not recommended for acute adrenal insufficiency. For management of chronic adrenal insufficiency, the usual oral dosage is 12 to 15 mg/m²/day.

FLUDROCORTISONE

Fludrocortisone is a potent mineralocorticoid that also possesses significant glucocorticoid activity. Fludrocortisone is the only mineralocorticoid available and is the drug of choice for chronic mineralocorticoid replacement.

Therapeutic Uses. Fludrocortisone is a preferred drug for treating Addison's disease, primary hypoaldosteronism, and congenital adrenal hyperplasia (when salt wasting is a feature of the syndrome). In most cases, fludrocortisone must be used in combination with a glucocorticoid (e.g., hydrocortisone, cortisone).

Adverse Effects. Adverse effects are a direct consequence of fludrocortisone's mineralocorticoid actions. When the dosage is too high, salt and water are retained in excess, while excessive amounts of potassium are lost. These effects on water and salt can result in expansion of blood volume, hypertension, edema, cardiac enlargement, and hypokalemia. Patients should be monitored for weight gain and elevation of blood pressure. If these changes occur, fludrocortisone should be temporarily withdrawn. Fluid and electrolyte imbalance should resolve spontaneously within days.

Preparations, Dosage, and Administration. Fludrocortisone acetate [Florinef Acetate] is available in 0.1-mg tablets for oral administration. The usual daily dose is 0.1 mg. If excessive salt retention occurs, the dose should be decreased to 0.05 mg.

AGENTS FOR DIAGNOSTIC TESTING OF ADRENOCORTICAL FUNCTION

CORTICOTROPIN AND COSYNTROPIN

Corticotropin and cosyntropin are compounds whose effects mimic those of human ACTH: both compounds act on the adrenal cortex to stimulate synthesis and secretion of cortisol and other adrenal corticosteroids. Corticotropin is prepared from animal pituitary glands and is nearly identical in structure to human ACTH. Cosyntropin is a synthetic polypeptide whose structure corresponds to the first 24 amino acids of ACTH. Since corticotropin, cosyntropin, and ACTH all produce equivalent stimulation of the adrenal cortex, we will use the term ACTH in reference to all three compounds.

Clinical Applications

ACTH is used primarily for diagnostic tests. For reasons discussed below, ACTH has only limited utility as a medication.

Diagnosis of Adrenal Insufficiency. Suspected adrenal insufficiency can be assessed by administering ACTH and then measuring plasma cortisol content. In patients with primary adrenocortical insufficiency, ACTH is unable to promote cortisol synthesis. Hence, plasma levels of the hormone will not be raised. If ACTH succeeds in elevating cortisol levels, primary adrenal insufficiency can be ruled out.

Therapeutic Uses. Because of its ability to stimulate glucocorticoid production, ACTH can, in theory, be used to treat a variety of conditions responsive to glucocorticoids. In practice, however, ACTH is rarely used for therapeutics. There are several reasons for this: (1) responses to ACTH are highly variable; (2) ACTH cannot be given orally, whereas glucocorticoids can; (3) ACTH can produce undesired side effects by stimulating production of adrenal androgens, and possibly aldosterone as well; (4) since the therapeutic effects of ACTH derive from enhanced glucocorticoid production, ACTH is only useful in patients with functioning adrenal glands; and (5) there is no evidence that treatment with ACTH offers any benefits over treatment with glucocorticoids themselves. Consequently, in most cases where ACTH might be employed, it is preferable to treat with glucocorticoids directly.

Preparations

There are three preparations of corticotropin and one of cosyntropin. *Corticotropin injection* [Acthar] is dispensed in 25- and 40-unit vials; routes are IM, SC, and IV. *Repository corticotropin* injection [H.P. Acthar Gel, ACTH-40, ACTH-80] is dispensed in 40- and 80-unit vials; routes are IM and SC. *Corticotropin zinc hydroxide* [Cortrophin-Zinc] is dispensed in 40-unit vials; administration is IM. *Cosyntropin* [Cortrosyn] is dispensed in 0.25-mg vials; routes are IM and IV.

DEXAMETHASONE

Dexamethasone is a synthetic steroid that has pronounced glucocorticoid properties and very little mineralocorticoid activity. The drug is used primarily to treat nonendocrine disorders. Dexamethasone is also employed in the diagnostic tests described below.

Overnight Dexamethasone Suppression Test

The overnight dexamethasone suppression test is used to diagnose Cushing's syndrome. This test is performed by administering 1 mg of dexamethasone at 11 PM followed by measurement of plasma cortisol levels at 8 o'clock the following morning. In normal individuals, dexamethasone acts on the pituitary to suppress release of ACTH, thereby suppressing synthesis and release of cortisol. If the patient has Cushing's syndrome, little or no suppression of cortisol production will occur.

Prolonged Dexamethasone Suppression Test

Once Cushing's syndrome has been diagnosed, the prolonged dexamethasone suppression test can be used to distinguish between excessive ACTH release as the cause versus dysfunction of the adrenal cortex itself. This test is performed as follows: first, baseline measurement of *urinary* 17-hydroxycorticosteroids is made (these compounds provide an index of adrenal corticosteroid production); second, dexamethasone is administered in 2-mg doses every 6 hours for 48 hours; and third, 24-hour urine is collected for determination of 17- hydroxycorticosteroids. If primary adrenal dysfunction is responsible for the symptoms of Cushing's syndrome, no suppression of 17-hydroxycorticosteroid production will occur. In contrast, if excessive ACTH release underlies Cushing's syndrome, prolonged administration of dexamethasone should produce some suppression of ACTH secretion and, therefore, should cause a small but measurable reduction in urinary 17-hydroxycorticosteroids.

It should be noted that the dexamethasone suppression test is not the best method for determining the underlying cause of Cushing's syndrome. The preferred procedure is to measure plasma ACTH and cortisol content directly. If plasma cortisol levels are high and ACTH levels are normal, adrenal dysfunction is responsible for the observed signs. If levels of both ACTH and cortisol are high, excessive ACTH secretion is likely to be the underlying problem.

INHIBITORS OF CORTICOSTEROID SYNTHESIS

Several drugs have been employed to inhibit excessive corticosteroid synthesis. Two of these drugs—aminoglutethimide and trilostane—are discussed below. Although these agents can relieve hypercortisolism in some patients, drugs are seldom the preferred form of therapy. Accordingly, the corticosteroid synthesis inhibitors are used rarely.

AMINOGLUTETHIMIDE

Actions. Aminoglutethimide blocks the conversion of cholesterol to pregnenolone, the first step in the synthesis of all adrenal steroids. As a result, production of glucocorticoids, mineralocorticoids, and androgens declines.

Therapeutic Use. Aminoglutethimide has been employed as a temporary means of decreasing excessive corticosteroid production in patients awaiting more definitive therapy (e.g., surgery). Duration of treatment is seldom greater than 3 months. In patients with adrenal adenoma, adrenal carcinoma, and ectopic ACTH-secreting tumors, morning plasma levels of cortisol are reduced by about 50%. Aminoglutethimide does not affect the underlying disease process. Hence, if therapy is stopped, excessive production of adrenal corticoids will resume.

Adverse Effects. Untoward effects are common. The most frequent are drowsiness, nausea, anorexia, and morbilliform rash. Additional effects include headache, dizziness, hematologic abnormalities, hypothyroidism, muscle pain, and fever. Masculinization may occur in females. Precocious sexual development may occur in males.

Preparations, Dosage, and Administration. Aminoglutethimide [Cytadren] is available in 250-mg tablets for oral use. The initial dosage is 250 mg every 6 hours. If steroid synthesis remains excessive, the dosage may be gradually increased, but should not exceed 2 gm/day.

TRILOSTANE

Actions and Use. Trilostane inhibits enzymes required for corticosteroid synthesis. As a result, secretion of cortisol and aldosterone is reduced. Like aminoglutethimide, trilostane is indicated for interim relief of hypercortisolism in patients awaiting more definitive treatment (e.g., surgery). Trilostane does not produce cure, and relapse will occur upon discontinuation of treatment.

Adverse Effects. About 25% of patients experience adverse effects. Gastrointestinal disturbances (abdominal pain, nausea, diarrhea) are most common. Other side effects include flushing, headache, and a burning sensation in membranes of the nose and mouth.

Use in Pregnancy. Trilostane can cause fetal harm. When taken by pregnant women, the drug can reduce progesterone levels, induce cervical dilatation, and cause termination of pregnancy. Pregnancy should be ruled out prior to trilostane use. Patients who become pregnant during treatment should be advised of the potential hazards to the fetus. Trilostane is classified under FDA Pregnancy Category X: the risks from use in pregnancy clearly outweigh any potential benefits.

Preparations, Dosage, and Administration. Trilostane [Modrastane] is available in 30- and 60-mg capsules for oral administration. The initial dosage is 30 mg four times a day. Daily dosage may be gradually increased to a maximum of 480 mg.

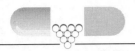 # Summary of Major Nursing Implications

---

GLUCOCORTICOIDS: HYDROCORTISONE AND CORTISONE

The nursing implications summarized here apply only to the use of glucocorticoids for *replacement therapy*. Nursing implications that pertain to use of glucocorticoids for *nonendocrine disorders* are summarized in Chapter 62.

Use in Addison's Disease

Administration. Instruct the patient to take two thirds of the daily dose in the morning and one third in the afternoon. Make certain that the patient understands that replacement therapy must continue lifelong.

Emergency Preparedness. Warn the patient that dosage must be increased at times of stress (e.g., infection, surgery, trauma). Advise the patient to carry an emergency supply of glucocorticoids at all times. This supply should include an injectable glucocorticoid plus an oral preparation. Advise the patient to wear identification (e.g., MedicAlert bracelet) to inform emergency medical personnel of glucocorticoid requirements.

Use in Congenital Adrenal Hyperplasia

To assess therapy, monitor the child at 3-month intervals for signs of excess androgen production (e.g., excessive growth rate, virilization in girls, precocious phallic enlargement in boys). Suppression of these effects indicates success.

Minimizing Adverse Effects

Excessive doses can produce symptoms of Cushing's syndrome. Observe the patient for signs of Cushing's syndrome and notify the physician if these develop.

FLUDROCORTISONE (A MINERALOCORTICOID)

Route

Oral.

Minimizing Adverse Effects

Excessive doses cause retention of sodium and water and excessive excretion of potassium, resulting in expansion of blood volume, hypertension, cardiac enlargement, edema, and hypokalemia. Inform patients about signs of salt and water retention (e.g., unusual weight gain, swelling of feet or lower legs), and instruct them to notify the physician if these occur. Treatment consists of temporary withdrawal of fludrocortisone; fluid and electrolyte balance should normalize within days.

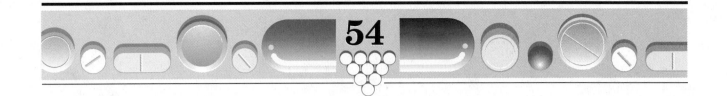

Androgens

A ndrogens are hormones produced by the testes, ovaries, and adrenal cortex. The major endogenous androgen is testosterone. The androgens are noted most for their ability to promote expression of male sex characteristics. However, androgens can also influence sexuality in females. In addition, the androgens have significant physiologic and pharmacologic effects unrelated to sex. The primary clinical application of the androgens is management of androgen deficiency in males. Principal adverse effects are virilization and hepatotoxicity.

TESTOSTERONE

Testosterone is the prototype of the androgen hormones. This compound is the principal endogenous androgen in males and females. In addition to its physiologic role, testosterone is representative of the androgens employed clinically. The structural formula of testosterone is shown in Figure 54–1.

BIOSYNTHESIS AND SECRETION

Males. Testosterone is made by Leydig cells of the testes. Daily production in men ranges from 2.5 to 10 mg. Synthesis of testosterone is promoted by two hormones of the anterior pituitary: follicle-stimulating hormone (FSH) and luteinizing hormone (LH). (Another name for LH is interstitial cell-stimulating hormone.) Production of testosterone is under negative-feedback control: rising

697

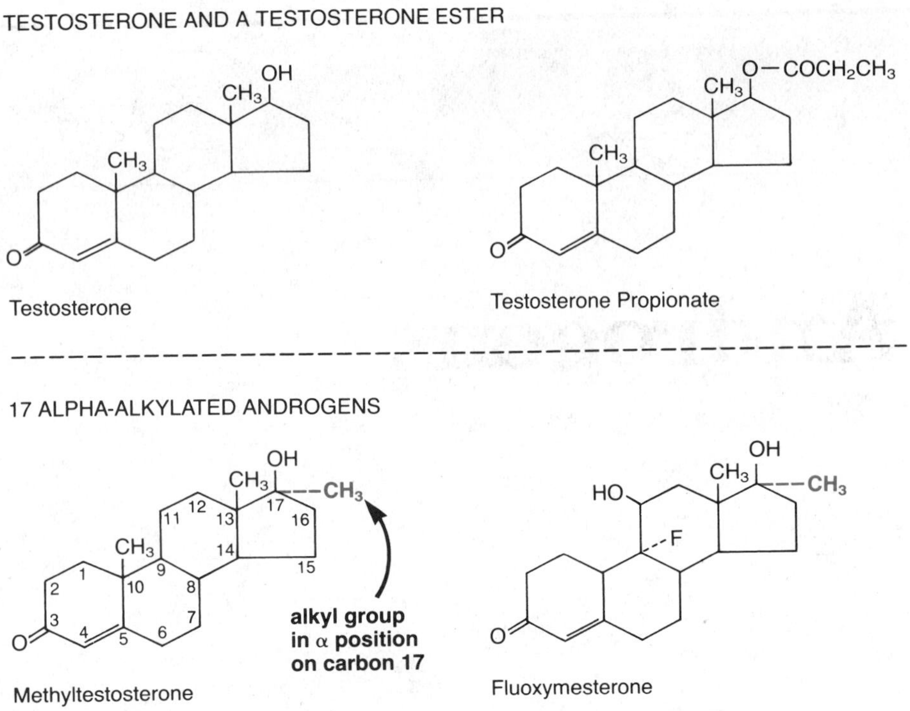

TESTOSTERONE AND A TESTOSTERONE ESTER

Testosterone

Testosterone Propionate

Figure 54–1. Structural formulas of representative androgens.

─ ─

17 ALPHA-ALKYLATED ANDROGENS

alkyl group in α position on carbon 17

Methyltestosterone

Fluoxymesterone

plasma levels of testosterone act on the pituitary to suppress further release of FSH and LH, thereby reducing the stimulus for further testosterone formation.

Some of the testosterone present in plasma is produced by the adrenals. However, androgenic activity attributable to the adrenals is much less than that of testicular origin. Hence, in men, adrenal androgens have minimal functional significance.

Females. In women, preandrogens (precursors of testosterone) are secreted by the adrenal cortex and by the ovaries. Conversion of these precursors into testosterone takes place in peripheral tissues. Synthesis of preandrogens by the adrenals is regulated by adrenocorticotropic hormone (ACTH). Ovarian production of preandrogens is under the control of LH. Total daily secretion of testosterone is about 0.25 mg—about 10 to 40 times less than the amount produced in men. In the event of ovarian or adrenocortical pathology (e.g., adenoma, carcinoma, hyperplasia), secretion of androgens can be greatly increased. Such increases may be sufficient to produce virilization.

MECHANISM OF ACTION

The effects of testosterone on its target tissues are mediated by specific receptors located in the cell cytoplasm. Following binding of testosterone to its receptor, the hormone-receptor complex migrates to the cell nucleus, and then acts on DNA to promote synthesis of specific messenger RNA

molecules. These, in turn, serve as templates for production of specific proteins. It is through these proteins that the effects of testosterone become manifest. It should be noted that in some tissues (e.g., prostate, seminal vesicles) androgen receptors do not interact with testosterone itself; in these tissues, testosterone must first be converted into a metabolite (dihydrotestosterone) in order to permit receptor binding.

PHYSIOLOGIC AND PHARMACOLOGIC EFFECTS

Effects on Sex Characteristics in Males

Pubertal Transformation. Increased production of testosterone brings on the transformations that signal puberty in males. Under the influence of testosterone, the testes enlarge, after which growth of the penis and scrotum occurs. Pubic and axillary hair appear, and hair on the trunk, arms, and legs assumes adult male patterns. Testosterone stimulates bone growth and growth of skeletal muscle, causing height and weight to increase rapidly. Testosterone also accelerates epiphyseal closure, causing bone growth to cease within a few years. The larynx enlarges, thereby deepening the voice. Sebaceous glands increase in number, causing the skin to become oily; acne results if the glands become clogged and infected. The final pubertal change is beard development. A period of several years is required for all of these transformations to take place.

Spermatogenesis. Androgens are required for the production of sperm by the seminiferous tubules, and for the maturation of sperm as they pass through the epididymis and vas deferens. Androgen deficiency causes sterility.

Effects on Sex Characteristics in Females

Under physiologic conditions, endogenous androgens have only moderate effects in females. Principal effects are promotion of clitoral growth and, perhaps, maintenance of normal libido. However, when production of androgens becomes excessive (e.g., in girls with congenital adrenal hyperplasia), virilization can take place. Masculinization can also occur in response to the therapeutic use of androgens (see below).

Anabolic Effects

Testosterone promotes growth of skeletal muscles. This anabolic effect results from the binding of androgens to the same type of receptor that mediates androgen actions in other tissues. In normal males, testosterone produced by the testes is sufficient to cause near maximal stimulation of the musculature. Hence, for healthy males, the increment in muscle mass that can be achieved through use of exogenous androgens is minimal. In contrast, when administered to males who are testosterone deficient, exogenous androgens can promote significant muscle development.

The effects of androgens on muscle growth in human females have not been documented; because of virilizing side effects, studies involving high-dose androgen treatment cannot be performed. However, experiments with laboratory animals do indicate that androgens can stimulate muscle growth in the female mammal. Hence, although clear proof is lacking, it seems likely that exogenous androgens can increase muscle mass in girls and women.

Erythropoietic Effects

Testosterone promotes the synthesis of erythropoietin, a hormone that acts on bone marrow to increase production of erythrocytes. This action of testosterone, together with the high levels of testosterone present in males, explains why men have a greater hematocrit than women. When women are given testosterone, the hematocrit rises and hemoglobin levels increase by an average of 4.3 gm/dl. In contrast, since men have high testosterone levels to begin with, the increase in plasma hemoglobin content that can be elicited with exogenous androgens is only 1 gm/dl.

CLINICAL PHARMACOLOGY OF THE ANDROGENS

In addition to testosterone, a number of other androgens are employed clinically. All of these agents can bind to androgen receptors, and, therefore, all can elicit similar responses. Major differences among individual androgens pertain to route of administration, pharmacokinetics, adverse effects, and specific applications.

CLASSIFICATION

The androgens fall into three basic categories: (1) testosterone and testosterone esters, (2) 17-alpha-alkylated compounds (noted for their hepatotoxicity), and (3) miscellaneous androgens. The androgens that belong to each of these classes are listed in Table 54–1.

When speaking of testosterone-like compounds, it is traditional to distinguish between "androgens" and "anabolic steroids." However, we will not make this distinction. It is now clear that the receptor type that mediates the anabolic actions of the androgens is the same receptor type that mediates the androgenic actions of these hormones. Consequently, it has not been possible to separate anabolic activity from androgenic activity: virtually all anabolic hormones are also androgenic. Accordingly, rather than creating two categories—androgens versus anabolic steroids—and assigning some agents to one category and some to the other, we will simply refer to all of the testosterone-like drugs as androgens.

THERAPEUTIC USES

Male Hypogonadism. Hypogonadism in males is the principal indication for androgens. In this condition, the testes fail to produce adequate amounts of testosterone. Hence, replacement therapy is required. Male hypogonadism may be hereditary or may result from other causes, including pituitary failure, hypothalamic failure, and primary dysfunction of the testes.

When complete hypogonadism occurs in boys, puberty will not take place unless exogenous androgens are supplied. To induce puberty, a long-acting parenteral preparation (e.g., testosterone enanthate, testosterone cypionate) is often chosen; injections are given IM every 2 to 4 weeks for 3 to 4 years. Under the influence of this therapy, the normal sequence of pubertal changes occurs: growth is accelerated, the penis enlarges, the voice deepens, and other secondary sex characteristics are expressed. As in normal males, these changes take place over several years.

Table 54–1. Androgens in Clinical Use

	Generic Name	Trade Name	Route	Usual Dosage
Testosterone and Testosterone Esters	Testosterone	Andro 100, Histerone, Tesamone	IM	10 to 25 mg 2 to 3 times weekly (for androgen deficiency)
	Testosterone cypionate	Depo-Testosterone, Andro-Cyp, others	IM	50 to 400 mg every 2 to 4 weeks (for androgen deficiency)
	Testosterone enanthate	Delatestryl, others	IM	50 to 400 mg every 2 to 4 weeks (for androgen deficiency)
	Testosterone propionate	Testex	IM	10 to 25 mg 2 to 4 times weekly (for androgen deficiency)
17-Alpha-Alkylated Androgens	Fluoxymesterone	Halotestin	PO	2 to 10 mg daily (for androgen deficiency)
	Methyltestosterone	Oreton Methyl, others	PO	Oral: 10 to 50 mg daily Buccal: 5 to 25 mg daily (for androgen deficiency)
	Oxandrolone	Oxandrin	PO	5 to 10 mg daily (for anabolic effects)
	Oxymetholone	Anadrol-50	PO	1 to 5 mg/kg daily (for anemia)
	Stanozolol	Winstrol	PO	6 mg daily (for hereditary angioedema)
Other Androgens	Danazol	Danocrine	PO	400 to 600 mg daily (for hereditary angioedema)
	Nandrolone decanoate	Deca-Durabolin, Androlone-D, others	IM	50 to 200 mg weekly (for anemia of renal disease)
	Nandrolone phenpropionate	Durabolin, Hybolin, Nandrobolic	IM	50 to 100 mg weekly (for breast carcinoma)
	Testolactone	Teslac	PO	250 mg 4 times daily (for breast carcinoma)

Androgen replacement therapy is also beneficial when testicular failure occurs in adult males. Treatment restores libido, increases ejaculate volume, and supports expression of secondary sex characteristics.

Delayed Puberty. In some boys, puberty fails to occur at the usual age. Most often, this failure reflects a familial pattern of delayed puberty, and is not indicative of pathology. Puberty can be expected to occur spontaneously, but at an age somewhat older than normal. Hence, although androgen therapy can be employed, treatment is not an absolute necessity. However, although therapy is not required, the psychologic pressures of delayed sexual maturation are sometimes greater than a boy (or his parents) can tolerate. In these cases, a limited course of androgen therapy is indicated.

Breast Cancer. Testosterone and other androgens have been used to provide palliation in women with advanced and metastatic breast carcinoma. The mechanism of palliation is not known. For treatment of breast cancer, high doses of androgens are required. As a result, some virilization is inevitable; the patient should be forewarned of this likelihood. (In contrast to their beneficial effects in women, androgens exacerbate breast cancer in males. Accordingly, androgens are contraindicated for use in men.)

Hereditary Angioedema. Hereditary angioedema is a disorder in which an inhibitor of the complement system is deficient. Lack of the inhibitor allows uncontrolled activation of the complement cascade, resulting in increased vascular permeability and angioedema (localized swelling of the subcutaneous tissue of the face, hands, feet, and genitalia). Androgens provide prophylaxis against this response by elevating plasma levels of the deficient inhibitor. For treatment of hereditary angioedema, *stanozolol* and *danazol* are the androgens of choice.

Anemias. Androgens may be used in men and women to treat anemias that have been refractory to other therapy. Anemias that may respond include aplastic anemia, anemia associated with renal failure, Fanconi's anemia, and anemia caused by cancer chemotherapy. Androgens help relieve anemia by promoting synthesis of erythropoietin, the renal hormone that stimulates production of red blood cells. In addition to increasing erythrocyte count, androgens may stimulate production of white blood cells and platelets.

Other Uses. Androgens can be administered postpartum to suppress lactation, thereby preventing breast engorgement in non-nursing mothers. However, it should be noted that bromocriptine is the preferred drug for this indication. Because of their anabolic actions, androgens may be able to counteract the catabolic actions of glucocorticoids (e.g., muscle wasting, thinning of the skin, demineralization of bone), which can occur during chronic, high-dose glucocorticoid therapy. Rarely, androgens are given to treat osteoporosis in postmenopausal women; however, evidence of efficacy is lacking.

ADVERSE EFFECTS

Virilization. This is the most common complication of androgen therapy. When taken in high doses by women, androgens can cause acne, deepening of the voice, proliferation of facial and body hair, male-pattern baldness, increased libido, clitoral enlargement, and menstrual irregularities. Clitoral growth, hair loss, and lowering of the voice may be irreversible. Masculinization can also occur in children: boys may experience growth of pubic hair, phallic enlargement, increased frequency of erections, and even priapism (persistent erection).

In girls, growth of pubic hair and clitoral enlarge-ment may occur. To prevent irreversible masculin-ization, androgens must be discontinued when vi-rilizing effects first appear. In the treatment of breast carcinoma, some virilization should be tol-erated.

Premature Epiphyseal Closure. When given to children, androgens can accelerate epiphyseal closure, thereby decreasing attainable adult height. To evaluate androgen effects on the epiph-yses, x-ray examination of the hand and wrist should be performed every 6 months.

Hepatotoxicity. Androgens can cause *chole-static hepatitis* and other disorders of the liver. Clinical *jaundice* may occur, but this is rare. Pa-tients receiving androgens should undergo periodic tests of liver function. If jaundice develops, it will reverse following discontinuation of androgen use. Androgens may also be carcinogenic: *hepatocellu-lar carcinoma* has developed in some patients fol-lowing prolonged use of these drugs.

It must be emphasized that not all androgens are hepatotoxic: liver damage is associated primar-ily with the *17-alpha-alkylated androgens*. As in-dicated in Figure 54–1 (see methyltestosterone), these androgens all share a structural feature in common—an alkyl group substituted on carbon 17 of the steroid nucleus. Because of their capacity to cause liver damage, *the 17-alpha-alkylated com-pounds should not be used chronically*. In contrast to the 17-alpha-alkylated androgens, the testoster-one esters (testosterone propionate, testosterone cypionate, testosterone enanthate) have never been associated with liver disease.

Effects on Cholesterol Levels. Androgens can lower plasma levels of HDL-cholesterol ("good cho-lesterol") and elevate plasma levels of LDL-choles-terol ("bad cholesterol"). These actions may in-crease the risk of atherosclerosis.

Use in Pregnancy. *Because of their ability to induce masculinization of the female fetus, andro-gens are contraindicated during pregnancy.* Poten-tial fetal changes include vaginal malformation, clitoral enlargement, and formation of a structure resembling the male scrotum. Virilization is most likely when androgens are taken during the first trimester. Women who become pregnant while using androgens should be apprised of the possible consequences to the fetus.

Edema. Edema can result from androgen-in-duced retention of salt and water. This complica-tion is of concern for patients with congestive heart failure and for those with a predisposition to de-velop edema from other causes. Treatment consists of discontinuing the androgen; a diuretic may also be needed.

Gynecomastia. Breast enlargement may occur in males receiving androgen replacement therapy. This paradoxical effect appears to result from con-version of certain androgens into estrogen.

Abuse Potential. As discussed below, andro-gens are frequently misused (abused) to enhance athletic performance. Because of their abuse po-tential, most androgens are now regulated under the Controlled Substances Act. Of the androgens listed in Tables 54–1, all but danazol and testolac-tone are classified as Schedule III drugs; danazol and testolactone are not regulated.

PREPARATIONS, DOSAGE, AND ADMINISTRATION

Individual androgens differ from one another in their applications. No single androgen is employed for all of the uses discussed above. Specific appli-cations of individual androgens are summarized in Table 54–2.

With respect to route of administration, individ-ual androgens fall into one of two categories: (1) orally usable drugs, and (2) drugs that must be given IM. Routes of administration for individual androgens are summarized in Table 54–1.

ANDROGEN (ANABOLIC STEROID) ABUSE BY ATHLETES

Many athletes take androgens (anabolic ste-roids) in an effort to enhance athletic performance. The potential benefits of this practice appear to be small. In contrast, the risks are substantial.

What can anabolic steroids do for the athlete? Unfortunately, the scientific answer to this ques-tion is equivocal. Studies *have* shown that steroids can increase lean muscle mass. However, the in-crease is small. (Weight gain occurs, but largely due to retention of water.) Furthermore, benefits occur only in athletes who (1) have undergone weight training prior to steroid use, (2) continue weight training during steroid use, and (3) con-sume a high-protein, high-calorie diet. Steroids have a clear effect on muscle growth in *young males and females of all ages*. In contrast, the ef-fects of exogenous androgens in *sexually mature males* are less certain, since levels of endogenous testosterone are already sufficient to produce func-tional saturation of androgen receptors. It *is* clear that for steroids to have *any* effect in adult males, *massive* doses are required.

Regardless of whether steroids actually enhance athletic performance, many athletes believe they do. *Perceived* benefits are (1) increased muscle mass and strength, (2) accelerated recovery time, permitting more frequent workouts, (3) accelerated healing after muscle injury, (4) heightened aggres-siveness, and (5) increased energy.

Who takes steroids? Steroid use is especially prevalent among football players, weight lifters,

Table 54–2. Applications of Individual Androgens

Androgens	Hypogonadism (male)	Delayed puberty (male)	Breast cancer (female)	Anemias	Hereditary angioedema	Catabolic states	Breast engorgement	Osteoporosis
Testosterone and Testosterone Esters								
Testosterone	✓	✓	✓					
Testosterone cypionate	✓	✓	✓					
Testosterone enanthate	✓	✓	✓					
Testosterone propionate	✓	✓	✓				✓	
17-Alpha-Alkylated Androgens								
Fluoxymesterone	✓		✓				✓	
Methyltestosterone	✓		✓				✓	
Oxandrolone						✓		✓
Oxymetholone				✓				
Stanozolol					✓			
Other Androgens								
Danazol					✓			
Nandrolone decanoate				✓				
Nandrolone phenpropionate			✓					
Testolactone			✓					

discus throwers, shot putters, and body builders. The drugs are also used by sprinters and athletes in endurance sports (e.g., cycling, Nordic skiing). Steroids are used by athletes of all ages (professionals, and athletes in college, high school, and junior high). Use is not limited to males: some females also take these drugs, despite masculinizing effects.

The potential for adverse effects is significant. Salt and water retention can lead to hypertension. Reduction of HDL-cholersterol and elevation of LDL-cholesterol may accelerate development of atherosclerosis. When administered in the high doses used by athletes, androgens suppress release of LH and FSH, resulting in testicular shrinkage, decreased spermatogenesis, and reduced testosterone production. In females, androgens can cause menstrual irregularities and virilization (growth of facial hair, deepening of the voice, decreased breast size, uterine atrophy, clitoral enlargement, male-pattern baldness); hair loss, growth of facial hair, and voice change may be irreversible. In boys and girls, androgens promote premature epiphyseal closure, thereby reducing attainable adult height. In boys, androgens can induce premature puberty. Because most of the androgens that athletes take are 17-alpha-alkylated compounds, hepatotoxicity (cholestatic hepatitis, jaundice, hepatocellular carcinoma) is an ever present danger. Adverse psychologic effects include hallucinations, delusions, manic episodes, depression, and excessive aggressiveness ("roid rage").

Long-term androgen use can lead to an "abuse" or "addiction" syndrome. Characteristics of the syndrome include preoccupation with androgen use and difficulty in stopping use. When androgens finally are discontinued, an abstinence syndrome can develop similar to that produced by withdrawal of alcohol, opioids, and cocaine. Because of their abuse potential, most androgens are now classified under Schedule III of the Controlled Substances Act. Of the androgens produced in the United States (Table 54–1), all are regulated except for danazol and testolactone.

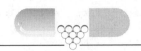

Summary of Major Nursing Implications

ANDROGENS

 Preadministration Assessment

Therapeutic Goals

Males: treatment of hypogonadism and delayed puberty.
Females: treatment of breast cancer and breast engorgement.
Males and females: treatment of anemias, hereditary angioedema, catabolic states, and osteoporosis.

Identifying High-Risk Patients

Androgens are *contraindicated* during *pregnancy* and for *males who have breast cancer*. Also, androgens are *contraindicated* for *enhancing athletic performance*.

 Implementation: Administration

Routes

PO, IM.

Administration

Advise patients to take oral androgens with food if gastrointestinal upset occurs.

 Ongoing Evaluation and Interventions

Minimizing Adverse Effects

Virilization. Virilization may occur in women, girls, and boys. Inform female patients about signs of virilization (deepening of the voice, acne, changes in body or facial hair, menstrual irregularities), and instruct them to notify the physician if these occur. Irreversible changes may be avoided if androgens are withdrawn early. In the treatment of breast carcinoma, some virilization should be tolerated.

Premature Epiphyseal Closure. Accelerated bone maturation can decrease attainable adult height. Monitor effects on epiphyses with x-rays of the hand and wrist twice yearly.

Hepatotoxicity. The *17-alpha-alkylated androgens* can cause cholestatic hepatitis, jaundice, and other liver disorders. Rarely, liver cancer develops. Obtain periodic tests of liver function. Inform patients about signs of liver dysfunction (jaundice, malaise, anorexia, fatigue, nausea), and instruct them to notify the physician if these occur. Liver function normalizes following cessation of drug use. Avoid long-term use of 17-alpha-alkylated preparations.

Edema. Salt and water retention may result in edema. Inform patients about signs of salt and water retention (swelling of the extremities, unusual weight gain), and instruct them to notify the physician if these occur. Treatment consists of androgen withdrawal and, if necessary, use of a diuretic.

Teratogenesis. Androgens can cause masculinization of the female fetus. Rule out pregnancy prior to androgen use. Warn women against becoming pregnant while taking androgens.

55

Estrogens and Progestins

E strogens and progestins are hormones that promote the maturation and ongoing activity of female reproductive organs. In addition, these hormones promote development of secondary sex characteristics in females. The principal endogenous estrogen is *estradiol*. *Progesterone* is the major progestational hormone. Both hormones are produced by the ovaries. During pregnancy, large amounts are also produced by the placenta.

Clinical applications of the female sex hormones fall into two major categories: (1) contraception, and (2) noncontraceptive uses. In this chapter, we will focus on noncontraceptive applications. For the estrogens, these applications include treatment of menopausal symptoms, osteoporosis, prostatic carcinoma, and carcinoma of the breast. For the progestins, the principal noncontraceptive indications are amenorrhea, dysfunctional uterine bleeding, endometrial carcinoma, and endometriosis. The use of estrogens and progestins for contraception is the subject of Chapter 56.

THE MENSTRUAL CYCLE

Since much of the clinical pharmacology of the estrogens and progestins is related to their actions during the menstrual cycle, an understanding of the menstrual cycle is essential to an understanding of the hormones. Accordingly, we will begin our discussion of female sex hormones with a review of

705

the menstrual cycle. The anatomic and hormonal changes that take place during the cycle are summarized in Figure 55–1.

Ovarian and Uterine Events. The menstrual cycle consists of a coordinated series of ovarian and uterine events. In the ovary, the following sequence occurs: (1) several ovarian follicles ripen; (2) one of the ripe follicles ruptures, causing ovulation; (3) the ruptured follicle evolves into a corpus luteum; and (4) if fertilization of the ovum does not occur, the corpus luteum dissolves. As these ovarian events are taking place, parallel events take place in the uterus: (1) while ovarian follicles ripen, the endometrium prepares for nidation (implantation of a fertilized ovum) by increasing in thickness and vascularity; (2) following ovulation, the uterus continues its preparation by increasing secretory activity; and (3) if nidation fails to occur, the thickened endometrium breaks down, causing menstruation, and the cycle begins anew.

The Roles of Estrogens and Progesterone. The uterine changes that take place during the menstrual cycle are brought about under the influence of estrogens and progesterone produced by the ovaries. During the first half of the cycle, estrogens are secreted by the maturing ovarian follicles. As suggested by Figure 55–1, these estrogens act on the uterus to cause proliferation of the endometrium. At midcycle, one of the ovarian follicles ruptures and then evolves into a corpus luteum. For most of the second half of the cycle, estrogens and progesterone are produced by the newly formed corpus luteum. These hormones maintain the endometrium in its hypertrophied state. At the end of the cycle, the corpus luteum atrophies, causing production of estrogens and progesterone to decline. In response to the diminished supply of ovarian hormones, the endometrium breaks down.

The Role of Pituitary Hormones. Two anterior pituitary hormones—follicle-stimulating hormone (FSH) and luteinizing hormone (LH)—play central roles as regulators of the menstrual cycle. During the first half of the cycle, FSH acts on the developing ovarian follicles, causing the follicles to grow and secrete estrogens. The resultant rise in estrogen levels exerts a negative feedback influence on the pituitary, thereby suppressing further FSH release. At midcycle, LH levels rise abruptly (see Fig. 55–1). This LH surge, which is triggered by rising estrogen levels, causes one of the mature follicles to swell rapidly, burst, and release its ovum. (Why only one follicle undergoes ovulation remains a mystery.) Following ovulation, LH acts on the newly formed corpus luteum to promote secretion of estrogens and progesterone.

From the foregoing, it is clear that precisely timed alterations in the secretion of FSH and LH are responsible for coordinating the structural and secretory changes that occur throughout the men-

strual cycle. However, despite considerable research, we still do not know how FSH secretion and LH secretion are regulated.

ESTROGENS

BIOSYNTHESIS

Females. In premenopausal women, the ovary is the principle organ of estrogen production. During the follicular phase of the menstrual cycle, estrogens are synthesized by ovarian follicles under the direction of FSH; during the luteal phase of the cycle, estrogens are synthesized by the corpus luteum under the direction of LH. The major estrogen produced by the ovaries is *estradiol*. In the periphery, some of the estradiol secreted by the ovaries is converted into *estrone* and *estriol*; these estrogens are less potent than estradiol itself. Estrogens are eliminated by a combination of hepatic metabolism and urinary excretion.

During pregnancy, large quantities of estrogens are produced by the placenta. Excretion of these hormones results in high levels of estrogens in the urine. (The urine of pregnant mares is extremely rich in estrogens and serves as a commercial source of these hormones.)

Males. Estrogen production is not limited to females. In the human male, small amounts of testosterone are converted into estradiol and estrone by the testes. Enzymatic conversion of testosterone in peripheral tissues (e.g., liver, fat, skeletal muscle) results in additional estrogen production. Underscoring the capacity of males to produce estrogen is the curious fact that stallions, despite their reputation for virility, excrete even greater quantities of urinary estrogens than do pregnant mares.

PHYSIOLOGIC AND PHARMACOLOGIC EFFECTS

Effects on Primary and Secondary Sex Characteristics of Females

Estrogens support the development and maintenance of the female reproductive tract and secondary sex characteristics. These hormones are required for the growth and maturation of the uterus, vagina, fallopian tubes, and breasts. In addition, estrogens direct development of pubic and axillary hair as well as pigmentation of the nipples and genitalia.

Estrogens have a profound influence on physiologic processes related to reproduction. During the follicular phase of the menstrual cycle, estrogens cause proliferation of the vaginal and uterine epithelium; secretions by the cervical glands are in-

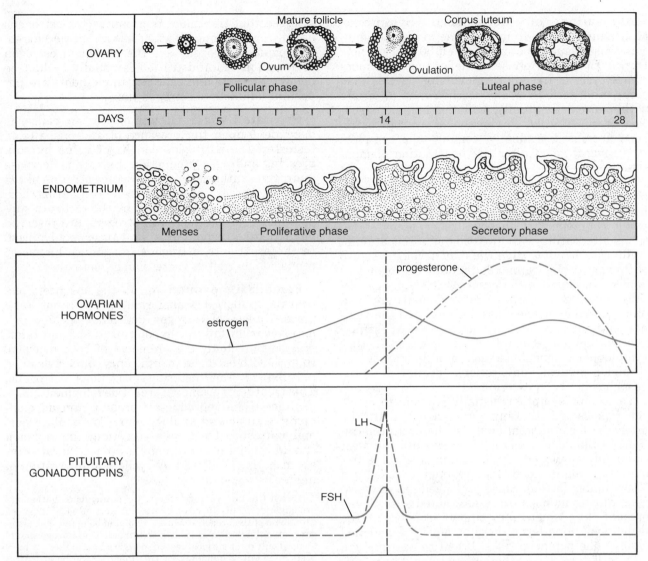

Figure 55–1. The menstrual cycle: anatomic and hormonal changes. (LH = luteinizing hormone, FSH = follicle-stimulating hormone)

creased; and breast enlargement is induced. Estrogens increase vaginal acidity by promoting deposition of glycogen in the vaginal epithelium. At the end of the menstrual cycle, a decline in estrogen levels can bring on menstruation. However, it is the fall in progesterone levels at the end of the cycle that normally causes breakdown of the endometrium and resultant menstrual bleeding. Following menstruation, estrogens promote endometrial restoration. Although the effects of estrogens on the release of pituitary gonadotropins are not completely understood, it is clear that high levels of estrogen can suppress release of FSH. During pregnancy, estrogens stimulate uterine growth and blood flow. In addition, estrogens (along with progestins) act on the breasts to promote development of the acini.

Metabolic Actions

Estrogens are responsible for the *rapid growth of the long bones* that occurs during puberty. Estro-

gens also direct epiphyseal closure, thereby bringing linear growth to a halt.

Estrogens have favorable effects on cholesterol levels: levels of low-density lipoprotein (LDL) cholesterol are reduced, while levels of high-density lipoprotein (HDL) cholesterol are elevated. There is speculation, but no proof, that these effects on cholesterol metabolism may explain the reduced incidence of myocardial infarction observed in premenopausal women. Additional metabolic effects of the estrogens include *fluid retention* and *protein anabolism* (buildup).

CLINICAL PHARMACOLOGY

Therapeutic Uses

In this chapter, discussion is limited to the noncontraceptive uses of estrogens. Use of estrogens for contraception is discussed in Chapter 56.

Alleviation of Menopausal Symptoms. Menopause results from a decline in ovarian follicles. Onset usually occurs at about 50 years of age. During the initial phase of menopause, the menstrual cycle is irregular; anovulatory cycles may occur, and periods of amenorrhea may alternate with menses. Eventually, ovulation and menstruation cease entirely. Production of ovarian estrogens decreases gradually, coming to a complete stop several years after the termination of menstruation.

Loss of estrogen is responsible for several of the physiologic changes that characterize menopause. In most women, estrogen decline brings on *vasomotor symptoms*; hot flushes (flashes) occur, sometimes alternating with sweating or a sensation of chilliness. *Atrophic vaginitis* may develop because of changes in the vaginal epithelium. Estrogen loss is also associated with *degenerative changes in estrogen-dependent tissues*: the endometrium atrophies, uterine muscle mass declines, and the vaginal epithelium becomes reduced in thickness and glycogen content. The role of estrogen loss in other symptoms of menopause (e.g., muscle cramps, arthralgia, anxiety, palpitations, dizziness, faintness) has not been determined.

Vasomotor symptoms usually respond to estrogen replacement therapy. Oral estrogens are the preferred form of treatment. Of the oral preparations available, *conjugated estrogens* are the most commonly employed. Cyclic administration is frequently recommended. This regimen is discussed below under *Dosing*. Since prolonged use of estrogens during menopause is associated with development of endometrial carcinoma (see below), the benefits of long-term therapy must be weighed against the potential risks. If estrogens are given on a long-term basis, the patient should be evaluated every 6 to 12 months to determine the need for continued treatment. Since vasomotor symptoms decline spontaneously over time, estrogen therapy can often be gradually reduced, and then discontinued entirely.

Like vasomotor symptoms, atrophic vaginitis is responsive to estrogen therapy. For this condition, estrogens may be administered orally or in a vaginal cream.

Prophylaxis of Osteoporosis. Osteoporosis is characterized by demineralization and weakening of the bones. Compression fractures of the vertebrae are common. Fractures of the hip and wrist can be caused by minimal trauma. Osteoporosis occurs in a majority (about 70%) of elderly white females; males and black females rarely experience this disorder. The condition develops following surgical removal of the ovaries and after menopause. Estrogen deficiency appears to be the principal cause.

In postmenopausal women, estrogen replacement therapy decreases bone loss and reduces the incidence of fractures. However, it must be stressed that treatment is prophylactic: estrogens do not reverse bone loss that has already occurred. Conjugated estrogens are the preferred estrogen preparation. Administration is usually cyclic (see below). Exercise and calcium supplements are important adjuncts to estrogen therapy.

Prostate Cancer. Growth of prostate cancer is dependent upon the presence of androgens (e.g., testosterone). Estrogens can be of value by suppressing androgen production. Estrogens decrease androgen synthesis by suppressing secretion of LH (also known as interstitial cell-stimulating hormone), the hormone required by the testes to support androgen production. Estrogens are reserved for patients in whom prostate cancer is advanced. In these patients, estrogens can induce histologic remission as well as regression of metastases.

Female Hypogonadism. In the absence of estrogens, pubertal transformation will not take place. Causes of estrogen deficiency include primary ovarian failure, hypopituitarism, and bilateral oophorectomy (i.e., removal of both ovaries). In girls with estrogen insufficiency, puberty can be induced by administering exogenous estrogens. This treatment promotes breast development, maturation of the reproductive organs, and development of pubic and axillary hair. To simulate normal patterns of estrogen secretion, the regimen should consist of continuous low-dose therapy (for about a year) followed by cyclic administration of higher estrogen doses.

Breast Cancer. Estrogen therapy can provide palliation and prolongation of life in postmenopausal women with advanced carcinoma of the breast. However, it should be noted that estrogens are not a preferred form of treatment. These drugs should be used only after surgical resection and radiation therapy have been ruled out. Candidates for treatment should be at least 5 years postmenopausal; use of estrogens prior to this time may *promote* tumor growth rather than impede it. Biopsy of the neoplasm should show the presence of estrogen receptors; cancers that lack receptors for estrogens are unlikely to respond to estrogen treatment. The estrogen employed most frequently is *diethylstilbestrol* (DES). Doses are large—usually 30 to 75 times greater than those used for estrogen replacement therapy.

Other Uses. Estrogens may be given to treat *dysfunctional uterine bleeding*, but progestins are preferred for this indication. Estrogens may be used to *suppress postpartum lactation*. However, painful engorgement of the breasts is uncommon, and rarely requires drug therapy. Furthermore, when drugs are indicated, bromocriptine is the agent of choice (see Chapter 51). Estrogens have been used in the past *to prevent habitual or threatened abortion*. This practice has been abandoned because it is both ineffective and potentially harmful to the fetus (see below).

Adverse Effects

Gastrointestinal Disturbances. *Nausea* is the most frequent undesired response to the estrogens. Fortunately, this reaction diminishes with continued drug use, and is rarely so severe as to necessitate cessation of therapy. Nausea can be minimized by administering estrogens with food and by initiating therapy with low doses. If taken in large doses, estrogens may cause anorexia, vomiting, and diarrhea.

Endometrial Carcinoma. Prolonged use of estrogens by postmenopausal women is associated with an increased risk of endometrial carcinoma. Estrogen users develop this cancer at a rate 4 to 14 times greater than that seen in nonusers. As dosage size and duration of treatment increase, the risk of endometrial carcinoma increases as well. Consequently, when estrogens are given to relieve menopausal symptoms, the lowest effective dosage should be established, and this dosage should be administered for the shortest time necessary. If a woman receiving estrogens should develop persistent or recurrent vaginal bleeding, she should be evaluated to determine if endometrial carcinoma is the cause. All patients should undergo an endometrial biopsy every 2 to 3 years.

Concurrent use of a progestin decreases the risk of estrogen-associated endometrial cancer. Progestins decrease the risk of cancer by promoting more complete shedding of the endometrium when estrogens are withdrawn each month.

Breast Cancer. Estrogens are not carcinogenic and they do not *cause* breast cancer. However, estrogens can *promote* the growth of certain tumors that have estrogen receptors. Accordingly, estrogen-dependent breast cancer must be ruled out before initiating treatment.

Other Adverse Effects. Use of estrogens during menopause produces a small increase in the risk of *gallbladder disease*. Treatment of breast cancer and bone metastases can result in severe *hypercalcemia*. Estrogens may cause *jaundice* in patients with pre-existing liver dysfunction. Central nervous system reactions include *headache, dizziness*, and *depression*.

Adverse Effects Associated with Use During Pregnancy

Use of estrogens during pregnancy can cause cancer and developmental abnormalities. Women who become pregnant while taking estrogens should be apprised of the risks to the fetus. *Estrogens are classified in FDA Pregnancy Category X: the risks of use during pregnancy clearly outweigh any potential benefit.*

Cancer. Diethylstilbestrol (DES), a nonsteroidal estrogen, has caused vaginal and cervical cancer in women who were exposed to this drug during fetal life (i.e., in women whose mothers took DES during pregnancy). Estimates of the incidence of vaginal and cervical cancer resulting from *in utero* exposure to DES range from 0.01% to 0.1%. These cancers appear most commonly when women who were exposed to DES reach 19 years of age; after the age of 30, the chance of developing these malignancies is very low. Although DES is the only estrogen clearly linked to induction of va-

ginal and cervical cancers, there is no reason to believe that other estrogens do not present a similar risk.

Birth Defects. Use of DES during pregnancy has produced genital abnormalities (e.g., testicular hypoplasia) in the male fetus. Abnormal semen production has also occurred. There have been no reports of cancer in males following *in utero* exposure to DES.

Drug Interactions

The interactions of estrogens with other drugs are probably similar to those seen with the oral contraceptives. These interactions are discussed in Chapter 56.

Classification of the Estrogens Used Clinically

The estrogens can be divided into two principal categories: (1) *steroidal estrogens* (natural and semisynthetic estrogens), and (2) *nonsteroidal estrogens* (synthetic estrogens). The steroidal estrogens can be subdivided into two classes: (1) preparations that contain estrone, and (2) preparations that contain estradiol and its derivatives. The estrogen preparations that belong to these groups are listed in Table 55–1. This table also presents routes of administration, therapeutic uses, and usual dosages. Structural formulas of representative estrogens are shown in Figure 55–2.

Routes of Administration

Traditional Routes. The principal routes of administration are *oral* and *intramuscular*. With only one exception (conjugated estrogens), preparations that are used orally are not administered IM, and vice versa. As a rule, the oral preparations, because of their convenience, are preferred to parenteral estrogens. In addition to oral and IM use, some estrogens may be applied *intravaginally*. One preparation—conjugated estrogens—may be administered *intravenously*.

Transdermal Administration. *Estradiol* is available in a transdermal patch formulation, marketed under the trade name *Estraderm*. The estradiol-containing patch is applied to the skin of the trunk (but not the breasts), allowing estrogen to be absorbed through the skin and then directly into the bloodstream. When compared with oral administration, the patches have two significant advantages: (1) the total dosage of estrogen is greatly reduced, and (2) the serum levels of estrogen produced by the patches more closely resemble premenopausal estrogen levels than do the serum levels produced by oral estrogens.

Table 55-1: Estrogens: Dosage Forms, Routes, Indications, and Dosages

Class		Generic Name	Trade Name	Dosage Form	Route	Indications	Dosages
Steroidal Estrogens	*Estrone-Containing Preparations*	Estrone	Theelin, Kestrone 5	Aqueous suspension	IM	Female hypogonadism	0.1–2 mg/wk
						Prostate cancer	2–4 mg 2–3 times/wk
		Estropipate[a]	Ogen, Ortho-Est	Tablets	PO	Menopausal symptoms	0.625–5 mg qd, in cycle[e]
						Female hypogonadism	1.25–7.5 mg qd, in cycle[e]
		Estrogenic substance[b]	Ogen Gynogen, others	Cream Injection	Vaginal IM	Atrophic vaginitis Female hypogonadism	2–4 gm qd 0.1–2 mg/wk
						Prostate cancer	2–4 mg 2–3 times/wk
		Conjugated estrogens[c]	Premarin	Tablets	PO	Menopausal symptoms	1.25 mg qd, in cycle[e]
						Female hypogonadism	2.5–7.5 mg qd, in cycle[e]
						Atrophic vaginitis	0.3–1.25 mg qd, in cycle[e]
						Osteoporosis	0.625 mg qd, in cycle[e]
						Breast cancer	10 mg tid, in cycle[e]
						Prostate cancer	1.25–2.5 mg tid
				Injection	IV, IM	Uterine bleeding	25 mg
				Cream	Vaginal	Atrophic vaginitis	2–4 gm qd
		Esterified estrogens[d]	Estratab, Menest	Tablets	PO	Menopausal symptoms	0.3–1.25 mg qd, in cycle[e]
						Female hypogonadism	2.5–7.5 mg qd, in cycle[e]
						Prostate cancer	1.25–2.5 mg tid
						Breast cancer	10 mg tid
	Estradiol and Derivatives	Estradiol	Estrace	Tablets	PO	Menopausal symptoms	1–2 mg qd, in cycle[e]
						Female hypogonadism	1–2 mg qd, in cycle[e]
						Prostate cancer	1–2 mg tid
						Breast cancer	10 mg tid
			Estraderm	Transdermal system	Trans-dermal	Menopausal symptoms	Apply 10- or 20-cm² system twice weekly, in cycle[e]
						Female hypogonadism	Same dose as in menopause
						Atrophic vaginitis	Same dose as in menopause
			Estrace	Cream	Vaginal	Atrophic vaginitis	2–4 gm qd for 1–2 wk, then 1 gm 1–3 times/wk for maintenance
		Estradiol cypionate	Depo-Estradiol, others	Injection	IM	Menopausal symptoms	1–5 mg every 3–4 wk
						Female hypogonadism	1.5–2 mg once a month
		Estradiol valerate	Delestrogen, others	Injection	IM	Menopausal symptoms	10–20 mg every 4 wk
						Female hypogonadism	10–20 mg every 4 wk
						Prostate cancer	30 mg every 1–2 wk
		Ethinyl estradiol[f]	Estinyl	Tablets	PO	Menopausal symptoms	0.02–0.05 mg qd in cycle[e]
						Breast cancer	1 mg tid
						Prostate cancer	0.15–2 mg qd

Table 55–1. Estrogens: Dosage Forms, Routes, Indications, and Dosages *Continued*							
Class	**Generic Name**	**Trade Name**	**Dosage Form**	**Route**	**Indications**	**Dosages**
Nonsteroidal Estrogens	Chlorotrianisene	Tace	Capsules	PO	Menopausal symptoms	12–25 mg qd, in cycle[e]
					Female hypogonadism	12–25 mg qd, in cycle[e]
					Prostate cancer	12–25 mg qd
	Dienestrol	DV	Cream	Vaginal	Atrophic vaginitis	Apply 1 or 2 times/day for 1–2 wk, then 1–3 times weekly for maintenance
	Diethylstilbestrol[f]	Generic only	Tablets	PO	Breast cancer	15 mg qd
					Prostate cancer	1–3 mg qd (initially)
	Diethylstilbestrol diphosphate	Stilphostrol	Tablets	PO	Prostate cancer	50 mg PO tid (initially);
			Injection	IV		250–500 mg IV once or twice/week (for maintenance)
	Quinestrol	Estrovis	Tablets	PO	Menopausal symptoms	100 μg qd for 7 days, then 7 days off, then 100 μg/wk for maintenance
					Female hypogonadism	Same dose as in menopause

[a]Estropipate is crystalline estrone sulfate stabilized with piperazine.
[b]This preparation consists primarily of estrone.
[c]This preparation consists of 50% to 65% sodium estrone sulfate plus 20% to 35% sodium equilin sulfate.
[d]This preparation consists of 75% to 85% sodium estrone sulfate plus 6% to 15% sodium equilin sulfate.
[e]In cycle = 3 weeks of drug, then 7–10 days off, then repeat the sequence. Studies indicate that addition of a progestin during the last 10 to 13 days of estrogen use will decrease endometrial hyperplasia and possibly the risk of endometrial cancer.
[f]For use in contraception, see Chapter 56.

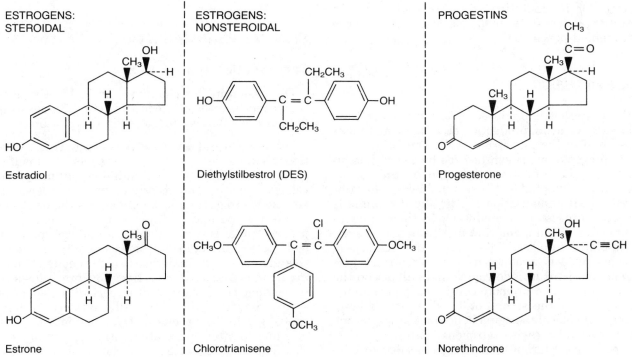

Figure 55–2. Structural formulas of representative estrogens and progestins.

Dosing

Cyclic Administration. When estrogens are taken for replacement therapy (e.g., treatment of menopausal symptoms or female hypogonadism), cyclic administration is often employed. The purpose of this dosing schedule is to simulate estrogen secretion during the normal menstrual cycle. In the cyclic regimen, estrogen is administered daily for 3 weeks and then discontinued for 1 week. This sequence is then repeated for as long as therapy is indicated. Addition of a progestin during the last 10 days of estrogen use promotes monthly uterine breakdown. By doing so, the progestin decreases the risk of endometrial carcinoma. When used to reduce symptoms of menopause, estrogens should be administered in the lowest effective dosage and for the shortest time required.

Dosing in Cancer Patients. Use of estrogens to treat cancer differs from other applications. As indicated in Table 55–1, the dosages employed are substantially higher than those used for other indications. In addition, administration is not cyclic. Since cyclic therapy is not required, a long-acting intramuscular preparation (e.g., estradiol valerate) may be preferred to oral estrogens.

PROGESTINS

Progestins are compounds that have actions like those of progesterone, the principal endogenous progestational hormone. As their name implies, the progestins act prior to gestation to prepare the uterus for implantation of a fertilized ovum. In addition, progestins help maintain the uterus throughout pregnancy.

BIOSYNTHESIS

Progesterone is produced by the ovaries and the placenta. Ovarian production occurs during the second half of the menstrual cycle. During this period, progesterone is synthesized by the corpus luteum. Production of progesterone by the corpus luteum is regulated by LH secreted by the anterior pituitary. If implantation of a fertilized ovum fails to occur, progesterone production by the corpus luteum ceases, and menstrual flow begins. However, if implantation does take place, the developing trophoblast will produce its own luteotropic hormone (chorionic gonadotropin) that will act on the corpus luteum to promote continued progesterone secretion. By the second or third month of pregnancy, the placenta begins to produce progesterone of its own (along with estrogens). After this time, ovarian progesterone is no longer needed to support gestation. Placental synthesis of progesterone and estrogens continues throughout the remainder of pregnancy.

PHYSIOLOGIC AND PHARMACOLOGIC EFFECTS

Effects on the Endometrium and Endocervical Glands. Progesterone secreted during the second half of the menstrual cycle converts the endometrium from a proliferative state into a secretory state. At the end of the menstrual cycle, progesterone production ceases. The resultant abrupt fall in progesterone levels is the principal stimulus for the onset of menstruation. In addition to affecting the endometrium, progesterone acts on the endocervical glands, causing their secretions to become scant and viscous. This action is opposite to that of estrogen, which promotes the flow of profuse, watery secretions.

Effects During Pregnancy. As noted above, progesterone levels increase during pregnancy. These high levels of progesterone are thought to have two actions that help to sustain pregnancy. First, progesterone inhibits uterine contraction. Second, progesterone may suppress the maternal immune response, thereby preventing immune rejection of the fetus.

Other Effects. Pharmacologic doses of progesterone can suppress release of pituitary gonadotropins (LH and FSH). This prevents maturation of follicles and ovulation. Also, individual progestin preparations display varying degrees of estrogenic, androgenic, and anabolic activity.

CLINICAL PHARMACOLOGY

Therapeutic Uses

Discussion in this chapter is limited to the noncontraceptive uses of progestins. Use of progestins for contraception is considered in Chapter 56.

Dysfunctional Uterine Bleeding. This condition occurs when progesterone levels are insufficient to balance the stimulatory influence of estrogen on the endometrium. In the absence of sufficient progesterone, estrogen puts the endometrium in a state of continuous proliferation. Since progesterone is unavailable to induce monthly endometrial breakdown, the excessively proliferative endometrium undergoes spontaneous sloughing at irregular intervals. Irregular breakdown of the endometrium can result in periodic episodes of severe menstrual bleeding. Alternatively, chronic spotting may be produced. Dysfunctional uterine bleeding is often associated with anovulatory cycles. The disorder occurs most commonly in adolescents and in women approaching menopause.

Table 55–2. Progestins: Trade Names, Dosage Forms, Routes, Uses, and Dosage

Generic Name	Trade Name	Dosage Form	Route	Therapeutic Uses and Usual Dosage	
Progesterone*	Various names	Oily or aqueous solution	IM	Amenorrhea	5–10 mg/day for 6–8 days
				Dysfunctional uterine bleeding	5–10 mg/day for 6 days
Hydroxyprogesterone caproate	Duralutin, others	Oily solution	IM	Amenorrhea	375 mg initially (may require estrogen priming)
				Dysfunctional uterine bleeding	Same dosage as amenorrhea
				Endometrial cancer	1-gm doses given 1–7 days/week
Medroxyprogesterone acetate*	Amen, Curretab, Provera, Cycrin	Tablets	PO	Amenorrhea	5–10 mg/day for 5–10 days
				Dysfunctional uterine bleeding	5–10 mg/day for 5–10 days
	Depo-Provera	Aqueous suspension	IM	Endometriosis	150 mg every 3 months
				Endometrial cancer	0.4–1.0 gm/week
Megestrol acetate	Megace	Tablets	PO	Breast cancer	40 mg 4 times daily
				Endometrial cancer	40–320 mg/day in divided doses
Norethindrone*	Norlutin	Tablets	PO	Amenorrhea	5–20 mg/day on days 5–25 of the menstrual cycle
				Dysfunctional uterine bleeding	Same dosage as for amenorrhea
				Endometriosis	10 mg/day (initially); 30 mg/day for maintenance
Norethindrone acetate*	Aygestin, Norlutate	Tablets	PO	Amenorrhea	2.5–10 mg/day on days 5–25 of the menstrual cycle
				Dysfunctional uterine bleeding	Same dosage as for amenorrhea
				Endometriosis	5 mg/day (initially); 15 mg/day for maintenance

*For use in contraception, see Chapter 56.

Treatment has two objectives: the initial goal is cessation of hemorrhage; the long-term goal is to establish a regular monthly cycle. Excessive bleeding can be stopped by administering a progestin for several days. Dosing may be continued for 2 weeks for sustained suppression. When progestin administration is stopped, withdrawal bleeding will take place. This bleeding is likely to be profuse and associated with cramping.

Cyclic therapy is employed to establish a regular monthly cycle. In this regimen, administration of an oral progestin is initiated 5 days after the onset of each menstrual period and continued for the next 20 days. This form of therapy promotes a repeating pattern of endometrial proliferation followed by endometrial breakdown and menstruation.

Amenorrhea. Progestins can induce menstrual flow in selected women who are experiencing amenorrhea. If endogenous estrogen levels are adequate, treatment with a progestin for 5 to 10 days will be followed by withdrawal bleeding when the progestin is discontinued. If estrogen levels are low, it may be necessary to induce endometrial proliferation with an estrogen prior to giving the progestin. Cyclic therapy can be used to promote regular monthly flow. This form of treatment consists of estrogen administration for 25 days coupled with progestin administration on days 15 through 25. The regimen is repeated beginning on the first day of each month.

Endometriosis. Endometriosis is a disorder in which endometrial tissue has become implanted in an abnormal location (e.g., uterine wall, ovary, extragenital sites). This condition is painful and a frequent cause of infertility and spontaneous abortion. Endometriosis can be treated surgically, or growth of the implants can be suppressed with drugs. When drug therapy is indicated, the medication most commonly employed is *danazol*. This agent inhibits synthesis of estrogens and progesterone, thereby depriving the implant of the hormones required to support its growth.

Before danazol became available, progestins (alone or in combination with an estrogen) were the preferred pharmacologic therapy of endometriosis. Continuous (noncyclic) treatment for 6 to 9 months can often produce symptomatic relief as well as regression of ectopic endometrial growths. Progestins that have been used against endometriosis include medroxyprogesterone acetate (MPA) and norethindrone.

Hypoventilation. Progestins can stimulate respiration in males and females. This ability has been put to use in treating patients with hypoventilation secondary to extreme obesity and chronic obstructive pulmonary disease.

Threatened or Habitual Miscarriage. High doses of progestins had once been used in efforts to prevent threatened or habitual miscarriage. There is no evidence that this treatment is effective. Furthermore, high doses of progestins pose a risk to the fetus (see below). Consequently, progestin use during pregnancy should usually be avoided. Progestins may be administered during pregnancy when production of progestins by the ovary is inadequate. These replacement doses should be kept low, and then discontinued when production of progestins by the placenta becomes sufficient to support the pregnancy.

Premenstrual Syndrome. Premenstrual syndrome (PMS) is characterized by enlargement and tenderness of the breasts, fluid retention, abdominal bloating, muscle pain, headache, insomnia, and emotional symptoms (irritability, anxiety, depression). These symptoms appear prior to menstruation but not at other times during the menstrual cycle. The cause of PMS is unknown, although hormonal changes (progesterone insufficiency and relative estrogen excess) are suspected.

Various nondrug and drug therapies have been tried. For many women, nondrug approaches are sufficient. These include education and supportive counseling, altered diet (high content of protein and complex carbohydrates and low content of caffeine, sodium, and refined sugar), and improved sleep hygiene (supplemented with diphenhydramine, if needed).

A number of drugs have been employed in attempts to relieve symptoms of PMS. *Progesterone* has been used for years on the theory that it may produce a favorable hormonal balance. *Pyridoxine* (vitamin B₆) has been employed to alleviate depression associated with PMS. *Diuretics* (e.g., spironolactone) have been used to decrease fluid retention and abdominal bloating. *Bromocriptine* has been used to reduce breast tenderness, bloating, and depression. *Aspirin, acetaminophen,* and *ibuprofen* have been used to reduce headache, dysmenorrhea, cramps, muscle pain, and joint pain. It should be noted, however, that there have been few controlled studies to demonstrate the efficacy of these treatments. Furthermore, even in uncontrolled studies, none of these drugs has been universally effective.

Endometrial Carcinoma. Progestins can induce beneficial responses (palliation, regression of tumor size, remission) in women with metastatic endometrial carcinoma. Several months of treatment may be required before a response is observed. The progestins employed for this indication are *medroxyprogesterone acetate* (MPA) and *megestrol acetate.* MPA is given once weekly by IM injection; megestrol acetate is administered daily by mouth. In addition to its use against endometrial carcinoma, megestrol acetate may provide palliation for women with cancer of the breast.

Adverse Effects

Teratogenic Effects. Administration of progestins in high doses during the first 4 months of pregnancy has been associated with an increased incidence of birth defects (limb reductions, heart defects, masculinization of the female fetus). Accordingly, use of progestins during early pregnancy is not recommended. Women who become pregnant while taking progestins should be apprised of the potential risk to the fetus.

Gynecologic Effects. Because of their actions on the endometrium, progestins can cause breakthrough bleeding, spotting, and amenorrhea. Other effects include breast tenderness and alteration of cervical secretions. To facilitate evaluation of potential adverse drug responses, the patient should undergo examination of the breasts and pelvic organs prior to therapy. In addition, Papanicolaou smears should be obtained and evaluated. Patients should be instructed to report any episodes of abnormal vaginal bleeding.

Other Adverse Effects. Progestins have been associated with depression, jaundice, edema, lethargy, photosensitivity, nausea, and exacerbation of acute intermittent porphyria.

Preparations, Dosage, and Administration

The progestins employed for noncontraceptive purposes are listed in Table 55–2. Included in this table are dosage forms, routes of administration, usual dosages, and therapeutic applications. Several of the progestins presented in Table 55–2 are also employed for contraception. The contraceptive uses of these and other progestins are discussed in Chapter 56.

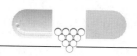

Summary of Major Nursing Implications

ESTROGENS

 Preadministration Assessment

Therapeutic Goal

Estrogens are used to alleviate *menopausal symptoms* and to treat *female hypogonadism, breast cancer, prostatic cancer,* and *dysfunctional uterine bleeding.*

Baseline Data

Assessment should include a breast examination, pelvic examination, Papanicolaou smear, lipid profile, mammography, and blood pressure measurement. If the goal of therapy is treatment of menopausal symptoms, menopause should be verified.

Identifying High-Risk Patients

Estrogens are *contraindicated* during *pregnancy* and for patients with *estrogen-dependent cancer; undiagnosed abnormal vaginal bleeding; active thrombophlebitis* or *thromboembolic disorders;* or a history of *estrogen-associated thrombophlebitis, thrombosis,* or *thromboembolic disorders.*

 Implementation: Administration

Routes

Oral, IM, IV, transdermal, and intravaginal. Routes for specific estrogens are given in Table 55–1.

Administration

Transdermal. Give the patient the following instructions for using the estradiol transdermal system: (1) apply the transdermal patch to an area of clean, dry, intact skin on the abdomen or some other region of the trunk (but not the breasts or waistline); press the patch firmly in place and hold for 10 seconds; (2) if the patch falls off, re-apply the same patch or, if necessary, apply a new patch; (3) remove the old patch and apply a new one twice weekly; and (4) rotate the application site such that the same site is not used more than once each week. Inform the patient that transdermal administration is usually employed in a cyclic dosing schedule (see below).

Intravaginal. Instruct the patient to apply the estrogen preparation high into the vagina using the applicator provided.

Dosing Schedules

Cyclic. Long-term cyclic administration is employed for prophylaxis of osteoporosis and for treatment of female hypogonadism, female castration, and primary ovarian failure. *Short-term* cyclic administration is used to relieve symptoms of menopause.

Instruct the patient to administer the estrogen in a repeating sequence consisting of 3 weeks of drug use followed by 1 week in which no drug is taken.

Frequently, a progestin is added to each cycle during the last 10 days of estrogen administration.

Continuous. Chronic, noncyclic administration is used in the treatment of neoplastic disease (prostate cancer, breast cancer).

 Ongoing Evaluation and Interventions

Monitoring Summary

The patient should receive a yearly follow-up breast and pelvic exam. An endometrial biopsy should be performed every 2 to 3 years.

Minimizing Adverse Effects

From Use During Pregnancy. *In utero* exposure to estrogens can cause genital abnormalities in males and vaginal cancer in females. Accordingly, *estrogens are contraindicated during pregnancy.* Inform women of child-bearing age about the potential risks to the fetus. Instruct the patient to discontinue estrogens immediately if pregnancy is suspected.

Endometrial Carcinoma. Estrogen therapy during menopause increases the risk of endometrial carcinoma. To reduce this risk, estrogens should be used on a cyclic schedule in the lowest effective dosage for the shortest time necessary. Evaluate the need for continuing treatment every 6 months. The risk of endometrial carcinoma can be further reduced by adding a progestin to each cycle during the last 10 days of estrogen administration. Instruct the patient to notify the physician if persistent or recurrent vaginal bleeding develops so that the possibility of endometrial carcinoma can be evaluated. The patient should receive an endometrial biopsy every 2 to 3 years.

Nausea. Nausea is common but diminishes with time. Inform the patient that nausea can be reduced by taking estrogens with food.

Effects Resembling Those Caused by Oral Contraceptives. Use of estrogens for noncontraceptive purposes can produce adverse effects similar to those caused by oral contraceptives (e.g., abnormal vaginal bleeding, hypertension, benign hepatic adenoma, reduced glucose tolerance). Nursing implications regarding these responses are summarized in Chapter 56.

Minimizing Adverse Interactions

The interactions of estrogens are probably similar to those seen with the oral contraceptives. Implications regarding these interactions are summarized in Chapter 56.

PROGESTINS

 Preadministration Assessment

Therapeutic Goal

Progestins are used to treat *dysfunctional uterine bleeding, amenorrhea,* and *endometriosis.*

Baseline Data

The physical examination should include breast and pelvic examinations. A Papanicolaou smear should be obtained.

Identifying High-Risk Patients

Progestins are *contraindicated* in the presence of *undiagnosed abnormal vaginal bleeding, thrombophlebitis, thromboembolic disorders, severe liver disease,* and *carcinoma of the breast and reproductive organs.* Progestins should be avoided during *pregnancy.*

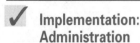

Implementation: Administration

Routes

Oral, IM.

Administration

Advise the patient to take oral progestins with food if gastrointestinal upset occurs.

Ongoing Evaluation and Interventions

Minimizing Adverse Effects

Teratogenic Effects. Progestins can cause birth defects (limb reductions, heart defects, masculinization of the female fetus) if taken during the first 4 months of pregnancy. Inform women of child-bearing age about the potential risks to the fetus. Instruct the patient to discontinue progestins immediately if pregnancy is suspected.

Gynecologic Effects. Inform the patient about potential side effects (breakthrough bleeding, spotting, amenorrhea, alteration of cervical secretions, breast tenderness). Instruct the patient to notify the physician if abnormal vaginal bleeding occurs.

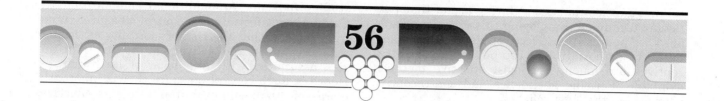

56

Contraceptive Agents

B irth control can be accomplished by interfering with the reproductive process at any step from gametogenesis to nidation (implantation of a fertilized ovum). Pharmacologic modes of contraception include oral contraceptives (OCs), levonorgestrel implants, long-acting intramuscular contraceptives, spermicides, a progesterone-containing intrauterine device, and gossypol (an investigational agent that suppresses sperm production). In addition to drugs, conception can be prevented by surgery (tubal ligation, vasectomy, hysterectomy), mechanical devices (condom, diaphragm, cervical cap, intrauterine device), and avoiding intercourse during periods of fertility (calendar method, temperature method, cervical mucus method).

Our principal focus in this chapter is on oral contraceptives. These agents are among the most effective forms of birth control and are one of our most widely used families of drugs. In preparing to study these agents and other forms of contraception, you should review Chapter 55, paying special attention to information on the menstrual cycle and the physiologic and pharmacologic effects of the estrogens and progestins.

EFFECTIVENESS AND SAFETY OF BIRTH CONTROL METHODS

EFFECTIVENESS

The effectiveness of a birth control method can be expressed in terms of the percentage of accidental pregnancies that occur during use of that particular technique. Employing this criterion, Table 56–1 compares the effectiveness of the major modes of birth control. As can be seen, oral contraceptives are among the most effective methods available. Periodic abstinence and contraceptive sponges are the least reliable.

Note that Table 56–1 contains two columns of figures, one labeled *optimal* and the other *typical*. The *optimal* figures are the pregnancy rates that are likely when a method of birth control is employed exactly as it should be (i.e., consistently and with proper technique). The *typical* figures represent pregnancy rates observed in actual practice. The higher pregnancy rates reported in the typical column are largely an indication that methods of birth control are not always used when and as they should be.

SAFETY

The issue of the relative safety of birth control measures is complex. Contributing to this complexity is the fact that much of our information on the adverse effects of oral contraceptives (OCs) was gathered at a time when these agents were employed in doses higher than those employed today. Hence, it is very likely that OCs, as currently prescribed, are considerably safer than published studies indicate. An additional complication regarding the safety of birth control measures stems from the fact that the risk of mortality associated with pregnancy and delivery is greater than the risk associated with any form of birth control. Hence, a birth control measure that is inherently more safe than others, but is also less effective, may become relatively less safe when the dangers associated with a greater pregnancy rate are factored into the equation.

Keeping the above provisos in mind, we can make the following observations on birth control safety. Of the contraceptive methods available, OCs produce the broadest spectrum of adverse effects, ranging from nausea to menstrual irregularity to rare thromboembolic disorders. Despite their wide variety of undesired actions, when used by nonsmoking women with normal cardiovascular function, OCs produce no greater mortality than other active forms of birth control. The lowest mortality rate is seen when barrier methods (diaphragm, condom, cervical cap) are used together with abortion (if contraceptive failure should occur). In women who have pelvic inflammatory disease, symptoms will be exacerbated by use of an intrauterine device (IUD).

SELECTING A BIRTH CONTROL METHOD

Several factors should be considered when choosing a method of birth control. Chief among these are *effectiveness*, *safety*, and *personal preference*. As indicated in Table 56–1, OCs are highly effective. However, although other methods may be less effective than OCs, when used correctly and consistently, these methods can still provide from 95% to 99% protection against pregnancy. Hence, if OCs are unacceptable, alternatives of reasonable effectiveness are available.

When factoring safety into the choice of a birth control method, several guidelines apply. Oral contraceptives should be avoided by women with certain cardiovascular disorders (see below) and should be used with caution by women who smoke heavily. For women in these categories, a barrier method or an IUD would be preferable to OCs. Although OCs are both effective and convenient, they can also produce many side effects; women who consider the benefit-to-risk ratio unfavorable should be advised about alternative contraceptive techniques. Women who have pelvic inflammatory disease (PID) should not use an IUD.

Personal preference is a major factor in providing the motivation needed for consistent implementation of a birth control method. Since even the best form of contraception will be ineffective if improperly practiced, the importance of personal preference cannot be stressed too strongly. Practi-

Table 56–1. Effectiveness of Birth Control Methods

Birth Control Method	Failure Rate (%)*	
	Optimal†	Typical‡
Oral contraceptives		
Combination pills	0.1	3
Progestin-only pills	0.5	2
Intrauterine device		3
Progesterone T	2.0	
Copper T 380A	0.8	
Depot intramuscular progestin:		
Medroxyprogesterone acetate	0.3	0.3
Levonorgestrel subdermal implant [Norplant]	0.04	0.04
Condom (without spermicide)	2	12
Spermicide alone	3	21
Diaphragm with spermicide	6	18
Cervical cap with spermicide	5	18
Sponge with spermicide	6–9	18–28
Female sterilization	0.2	0.4
Male sterilization	0.1	0.15
Periodic abstinence	2–10	20
No birth control	Pregnancy rate would be 80% to 85%	

*Failure rate = percent of women who have an accidental pregnancy during first year of use.
†Optimal = failure rate that would be expected if the birth control method were practiced exactly as it should be.
‡Typical = failure rate usually observed in actual practice.

tioners should take pains to educate clients about the various contraceptive methods available so that expressions of preference can be based on understanding.

Additional factors that bear on selection of a birth control method include family planning goals, age, frequency of sexual intercourse, and the individual's capacity for compliance. If family planning goals have already been met, sterilization of either the male or female partner may be desirable. For women who engage in coitus frequently, OCs or progestin implants can be a reasonable choice. Conversely, when sexual activity is limited, use of a spermicide, condom, or diaphragm may be most appropriate. Since barrier methods combined with spermicides can offer some protection against venereal disease (as well as providing contraception), these combinations may be of special benefit to individuals who have multiple partners. If compliance is a problem (as it can be with OCs, condoms, and diaphragms), an IUD or progestin implant can offer reliable protection.

ORAL CONTRACEPTIVES

CLASSIFICATION

There are two principal categories of OCs: (1) those that contain both an estrogen and a progestin, known as *combination OCs,* and (2) those that contain only a progestin, known as "minipills" or *progestin-only OCs.* Of the two groups, combination OCs are by far the most widely used.

The combination OCs have three subgroups: *monophasic, biphasic,* and *triphasic.* In a monophasic regimen, the daily estrogen and progestin dosage remains constant throughout the monthly cycle of use. In a biphasic regimen, the estrogen dosage remains constant, but the progestin dosage is increased during the second half of the cycle. In triphasic regimens, the monthly cycle is divided into three segments. In all triphasic regimens, the progestin dosage changes for each segment of the cycle; in one regimen, the estrogen dosage varies also.

COMBINATION ORAL CONTRACEPTIVES

Since their introduction in the late 1950's, combination OCs have become one of our most widely prescribed families of drugs. As indicated in Table 56–1, these agents are nearly 100% effective, making them one of the most efficacious forms of birth control available. Not only are these drugs highly effective, they are very safe, although minor side effects are relatively common.

Chemistry

Combination OCs consist of an *estrogen* plus a *progestin.* Only two estrogens are employed: *ethinyl estradiol* and *mestranol* (see Table 56–3). In contrast, several progestins are used, *norethindrone* being employed most often.

Mechanism of Action

Combination OCs decrease fertility in several ways. The principal effect of these agents is *inhibition of ovulation.* The precise mechanism by which inhibition occurs is not known. In addition, OCs can promote thickening of the cervical mucus, thereby creating a barrier to the passage of sperm. Also, OCs can modify the endometrium, making it less favorable for nidation.

Adverse Effects

Combination OCs can cause a wide variety of adverse effects. However, although many types of effects may be produced, severe effects are rare. Hence, when compared with the serious risks associated with pregnancy and childbirth, the risks of OCs are low.

Preadministration Assessment. Since OCs are taken by women who are healthy, and since OCs represent a potential health hazard, it is important that steps be taken to minimize any risks associated with OC use. Accordingly, a thorough physical examination should be performed prior to OC prescription. This examination should include blood pressure determination, examination of the breasts and pelvic organs, and a Papanicolaou smear. These tests should be repeated at least once a year.

Thrombotic Disorders. Combination OCs have been associated with venous and arterial thromboembolism, pulmonary embolism, myocardial infarction, and thrombotic stroke. These thrombotic disorders are caused by the *estrogen* component of combination OCs—not by the progestin. Thrombosis results at least in part from an increase in circulating levels of clotting factors. Thrombosis is not due to atherosclerosis.

In contrast to older OCs, the OCs available today carry a low risk of thrombosis. When combination OCs first became available, they contained *high* doses of estrogens (e.g., 100 μg ethinyl estradiol). As a result, these preparations carried a significant risk of thrombotic disorders. Because today's OCs contain *low* doses of estrogens—no more than 50 μg ethinyl estradiol, and usually less—the risk of thrombosis among users is only slightly greater than among nonusers.

The risk of thromboembolic phenomena from OCs is increased in the presence of other risk factors, especially *heavy smoking* and a *history of thromboembolism.* Additional risk factors include cerebrovascular disease, coronary artery disease, myocardial infarction, and surgery in which postoperative thrombosis might be expected.

Until recently, OCs were not recommended for women over the age of 35. This was because older clinical studies indicated a dramatic increase in the risk of thrombosis for this group. However, newer data show that today's low estrogen OCs may be used up to age 45 with no greater risk of thrombosis than among younger women.

Several measures can help minimize thromboembolic phenomena. First, the estrogen dose in OCs should be no greater than required for contraceptive efficacy. Second, OCs should not be prescribed for women who are heavy smokers, for women with a history of thromboembolism, or for women with other risk factors for thrombosis. Third, OCs should be discontinued at least 4 weeks prior to surgery in which postoperative thrombosis might be expected. Lastly, women should be informed about the symptoms of thrombosis and thromboembolism (e.g., leg tenderness or pain, sudden chest pain, shortness of breath, severe headache, sudden visual disturbance) and instructed to cease OC use and notify the physician if these occur.

Hypertension. The incidence of hypertension among OC users is three to six times greater than among nonusers. Oral contraceptives elevate blood pressure by increasing blood levels of both angiotensin (a potent vasoconstrictor) and aldosterone (a hormone that promotes salt and water retention). The risk of hypertension increases with age and with duration of OC use. Women taking OCs should undergo periodic determination of blood pressure. If hypertension develops, OCs should be discontinued. Blood pressure usually declines to pretreatment levels within a few months after OCs have been withdrawn.

Cancer. The risk of cancer from OCs appears to be extremely low. As discussed in Chapter 55, women who had been exposed to diethylstilbestrol (DES), a nonsteroidal estrogen, during fetal life are at increased risk of developing cervical and vaginal cancer upon maturing. To minimize this risk, OCs should be discontinued if contraceptive failure occurs. Although estrogen use by postmenopausal women is associated with an increased incidence of endometrial carcinoma (see Chapter 55), use of OCs appears to *protect* against this form of cancer. Oral contraceptive use is also associated with a reduction in ovarian cancer. In the past it was thought that OCs might cause breast cancer; in extensive later studies, no link between breast carcinoma and OCs has been found. However, since estrogens can promote the growth of existing breast carcinoma, women with this disease should not use OCs.

Teratogenic Effects. Birth defects can be produced by estrogens and progestins. Exposure of the male fetus to DES can cause testicular hypoplasia and abnormal semen production. Progestin use during early pregnancy has been associated with a variety of teratogenic defects (e.g., limb reductions, heart abnormalities, masculinization of the female fetus). Accordingly, if pregnancy should occur, OCs should be discontinued immediately.

Abnormal Uterine Bleeding. By inducing endometrial regression, OCs may decrease or eliminate menstrual flow during the initial months of use. Breakthrough bleeding and spotting may occur, especially when OCs with low estrogen and progestin content are employed. If bleeding irregularities persist, the possibility of malignancy should be investigated. If two consecutive periods are missed, the client should be evaluated for pregnancy. Following discontinuation of OC use, a period of 1 to 3 months may be required before normal menstruation resumes; in extreme cases, cyclic menses may not return for up to 1 year.

Effects Related to Estrogen or Progestin Imbalance. Many of the mild side effects of OCs result from an excess or deficiency in estrogen or progestin. Effects that can result from an excess of estrogen include nausea, breast tenderness, and edema. Progestin excess can produce increased appetite, fatigue, and depression. A deficiency in either class of hormone can cause menstrual irregularities. Side effects related to hormonal imbalance are summarized in Table 56–2. By making appropriate adjustments in the estrogen and progestin content of an OC regimen, many of these effects can be minimized.

Use in Pregnancy and Lactation. Because of their carcinogenic and teratogenic actions (see above), *OCs are contraindicated for use during pregnancy* (FDA Pregnancy Category X). Pregnancy should be ruled out prior to initiation of OC therapy. If pregnancy occurs during OC use, drug administration should cease immediately. OCs enter breast milk and also act to reduce milk production. Accordingly, OCs should not be taken by women who are breast-feeding.

Benign Hepatic Adenoma. Hepatic adenoma is a rare complication of OC use. Although nonmalignant, these tumors are highly vascular and, hence, can be the source of severe hemorrhage if they rupture. Women using OCs should undergo periodic palpation of the liver. If a mass is detected, further tests should be performed to establish a definitive diagnosis. If hepatic adenoma is diagnosed, OCs must be discontinued; spontaneous regression of the tumor usually follows.

Multiple Births. The incidence of twin births is increased in women who become pregnant shortly after discontinuing OCs. Women who desire preg-

Table 56-2. Side Effects Caused by an Excess or Deficiency in the Estrogen or Progestin Content of an Oral Contraceptive Regimen

Estrogen		Progestin	
Excess	*Deficiency*	*Excess*	*Deficiency*
Nausea	Early or midcycle	Increased appetite	Late breakthrough
Breast tenderness	breakthrough	Weight gain	bleeding
Edema	bleeding	Depression	Amenorrhea
Bloating	Increased spotting	Tiredness	Hypermenorrhea
Hypertension	Hypomenorrhea	Fatigue	
Mirgraine headache		Hypomenorrhea	
Cervical mucorrhea		Breast regression	
Polyposis		Monilial vaginitis	
		Acne, oily scalp*	
		Hair loss*	
		Hirsutism*	

*Caused by progestins that have androgenic activity.

nancy, but wish to reduce the chances of multiple births, should employ an alternative form of birth control for approximately 3 months after OCs have been withdrawn.

Glucose Intolerance. Oral contraceptives can elevate plasma glucose levels. This diabetogenic effect is caused by the *progestin* in OCs. Glucose intolerance is most likely in patients who are already diabetic or have experienced gestational diabetes. Since hypoglycemic agents (e.g., insulin) can control glucose elevations induced by OCs, the presence of diabetes does not preclude OC use. Prediabetic women should be monitored for development of hyperglycemia. Glucose intolerance may occur less with OCs that contain *desogestrel* or *norgestimate* as their progestin component.

Other Adverse Effects. Rarely, OCs cause *gallbladder disease* accompanied by jaundice. This condition reverses following termination of treatment. OCs can cause a variety of *ocular lesions* (e.g., retinal vascular occlusion, retinal edema, optic neuropathy). Accordingly, OCs should be withdrawn in the event of unexplained visual disturbance. *Melanoderma* (darkening of the skin) may occur during OC use; a reduction in dosage may cause pigmentation to decrease.

Summary of Contraindications and Precautions

Combinations OCs are *contraindicated* during pregnancy and for women with the following disorders (or a history thereof): thrombophlebitis, thromboembolic disorders, cerebrovascular accident, coronary artery disease, known or suspected breast carcinoma, known or suspected estrogen-dependent neoplasm, benign or malignant liver tumors, and undiagnosed abnormal genital bleeding.

These drugs should be used with *caution* by women with diabetes, women who are heavy smokers (more than 15 cigarettes a day), women who have risk factors for cardiovascular disease (e.g., hypertension, obesity, hypercholesterolemia), and women anticipating elective surgery in which postoperative thrombosis might be expected.

Noncontraceptive Benefits of Oral Contraceptives

Oral contraceptives decrease the risk of several diseases, including ovarian cancer, endometrial cancer, ovarian cysts, pelvic inflammatory disease, premenstrual syndrome, fibrocystic breast disease, toxic shock syndrome, and anemia. In addition, OCs favorably affect menstrual symptoms: cramps are reduced, menstrual flow is smaller and of shorter duration, and menses are more predictable.

Drug Interactions

Drugs That Reduce the Effects of Oral Contraceptives. The effectiveness of OCs can be decreased by a variety of drugs. *Rifampin* (given to treat tuberculosis) and several *anticonvulsants* (phenobarbital, phenytoin, primidone) can stimulate hepatic drug-metabolizing enzymes, and can thereby accelerate OC degradation. A number of antibiotics, including *tetracycline* and *ampicillin*, can also lower OC efficacy: by killing gut flora, these agents reduce enterohepatic recirculation of OCs, and thereby accelerate OC elimination. Women taking OCs in combination with any of the above agents should be alert for indications of reduced OC blood levels (e.g., breakthrough bleeding, spotting). If these signs appear, it may be necessary to increase OC dosage or use an alternative form of birth control.

Drugs Whose Effects Are Reduced by Oral Contraceptives. Oral contraceptives can reduce the effects of several drugs. By increasing levels of clotting factors, OCs can decrease the effectiveness of *oral anticoagulants* (e.g., warfarin). OCs can also reduce the effects of *insulin and other hypoglycemic agents*. Hence, when combined with OCs, anticoagulants and hypoglycemic agents may require greater than normal dosage.

Drugs Whose Effects Are Increased by Oral Contraceptives. Oral contraceptives can impair the hepatic metabolism of several agents, including *theophylline* (used for asthma) and *imipramine* (an antidepressant). Because of reduced metabolic breakdown, these drugs may accumulate to toxic levels. Accordingly, women taking these drugs in combination with OCs should be alert for signs of toxicity; a reduction in the dosage of theophylline or imipramine may be required.

Preparations

The combination OCs currently available are listed in Table 56–3. As shown in the table, the principal estrogen present in OCs is *ethinyl estradiol*. The most frequently employed progestin is *norethindrone*. The preparations in Table 56–3 are listed in order of increasing estrogen content. OCs with lower amounts of estrogen are less likely to produce serious side effects. The table also indicates which preparations belong to each of the three subgroups of combination OCs (monophasic, biphasic, triphasic). The biphasic and triphasic preparations reflect efforts to more closely simulate ovarian production of estrogens and progestins. However, these preparations offer little if any advantage over monophasic OCs.

Dosage and Administration

Dosing Schedules. Most OCs are taken in a sequence that consists of 21 days of OC use followed by 7 days on which either (1) no pill is taken, (2) an inert pill is taken, or (3) an iron-containing pill is taken. The sequence is begun on the fifth day of the menstrual cycle (i.e., 5 days after the onset of menses) and is repeated for as long as indicated. Successive cycles should commence every 28 days, regardless of whether breakthrough bleeding or spotting have occurred. Pills should be taken at the same hour every day (e.g., with a meal, at bedtime). During the first week of OC use, an additional form of birth control (e.g., condom, diaphragm) is recommended. Postpartum use of OCs can be initiated immediately after delivery, as long as breast-feeding is not intended. Dosing schedules for individual preparations are summarized in Table 56–3.

Adjustments to Estrogen and Progestin Dosage. In most cases, therapy is initiated with an OC whose estrogen content is equivalent to 35 μg of estrogen or less. If this low-estrogen preparation results in signs of estrogen deficiency (e.g., spotting, breakthrough bleeding), an OC with higher estrogen content may be substituted. Conversely, if signs of estrogen excess become apparent (e.g., nausea, edema, breast discomfort), a preparation with lower estrogen content may be selected. In a similar fashion, the progestin content of the regi-

men can be adjusted so as to alleviate symptoms of progestin excess or deficiency. When substituting one combination OC for another, the change can be made at the beginning of any new cycle; the change will not affect contraceptive efficacy.

What to Do in the Event of Missed Dosage. The chances of ovulation (and hence pregnancy) from missing one OC dose are quite small. However, the risk of pregnancy becomes progressively larger with each consecutive omission. If only one dose is missed, that dose should be taken together with the next scheduled dose. If two doses are missed, two doses should be taken per day on the following 2 days. If three doses are missed, a new cycle should be initiated, starting 7 days after the last pill was taken. An additional form of birth control should be used during the first 2 weeks of the new cycle.

PROGESTIN-ONLY ORAL CONTRACEPTIVES

Progestin-only OCs, also known as "minipills," contain a progestin (norethindrone or norgestrel) but have no estrogen. Because they lack estrogen, minipills do not cause thromboembolic disorders and most of the other adverse effects associated with combination OCs. Unfortunately, although somewhat safer than combination OCs, the progestin-only preparations are less effective and cause more menstrual irregularity (breakthrough bleeding, spotting, amenorrhea, inconsistent cycle length, variations in the volume and duration of monthly flow). Because of these drawbacks, minipills are considerably less popular than combination OCs. The three progestin-only preparations currently available are listed in Table 56–3.

Contraceptive effects of the minipill result largely from alteration of cervical secretions: under the influence of progestin, cervical glands produce a thick, sticky mucus that acts as a barrier to penetration by sperm. Progestins also modify the endometrium, making it less favorable for nidation. In comparison to combination OCs, minipills are relatively ineffective as inhibitors of ovulation; hence, suppression of ovulation is not a major mechanism by which minipills prevent conception.

Unlike combination OCs, whose administration is cyclic, progestin-only OCs are taken continuously. Use is initiated on day 1 of the menstrual cycle and a pill is taken every day thereafter. Each pill should be taken at the same time of day.

The following guidelines apply in the event of missed dosage. If one pill is missed, it should be taken as soon as remembered; the next pill should be taken as scheduled. If two pills are missed, one should be taken as soon as remembered and the other should be discarded; the next pill should be taken as originally scheduled. If three pills are

Table 56–3. Oral Contraceptives: Composition and Dosing Schedule

Trade Name	μg	Estrogen	mg	Progestin	Dosing Schedule Options*
Combination OCs: Monophasic					
Loestrin 1/20	20	Ethinyl estradiol	1	Norethindrone	A,C
Levlen	30	Ethinyl estradiol	0.15	Levonorgestrel	A,B
Nordette	30	Ethinyl estradiol	0.15	Levonorgestrel	A,B
Lo/Ovral	30	Ethinyl estradiol	0.3	Norgestrel	A,B
Loestrin 1.5/30	30	Ethinyl estradiol	1.5	Norethindrone	A,C
Desogen	30	Ethinyl estradiol	0.15	Desogestrel	B
Ortho-Cept	30	Ethinyl estradiol	0.15	Desogestrel	A,B
Demulen 1/35	35	Ethinyl estradiol	1	Ethynodiol diacetate	A,B
Ovocon-35	35	Ethinyl estradiol	0.4	Norethindrone	A,B
Brevicon	35	Ethinyl estradiol	0.5	Norethindrone	A,B
Genora	35	Ethinyl estradiol	0.5	Norethindrone	A,B
Modicon	35	Ethinyl estradiol	0.5	Norethindrone	A,B
Nelova	35	Ethinyl estradiol	0.5	Norethindrone	A,B
Genora 1/35	35	Ethinyl estradiol	1	Norethindrone	A,B
N.E.E. 1/35	35	Ethinyl estradiol	1	Norethindrone	A,B
Nelova 1/35E	35	Ethinyl estradiol	1	Norethindrone	A,B
Norcept-E 1/35	35	Ethinyl estradiol	1	Norethindrone	A,B
Norethin 1/35E	35	Ethinyl estradiol	1	Norethindrone	A,B
Norinyl 1+35	35	Ethinyl estradiol	1	Norethindrone	A,B
Ortho-Novum 1/35	35	Ethinyl estradiol	1	Norethindrone	A,B
Ortho-Cyclen	35	Ethinyl estradiol	0.250	Norgestimate	A,B
Ovral	50	Ethinyl estradiol	0.5	Norgestrel	A,B
Norlestrin 2.5/50	50	Ethinyl estradiol	2.5	Norethindrone acetate	A,C
Demulin 1/50	50	Ethinyl estradiol	1	Ethynodiol diacetate	A,B
Norlestrin 1/50	50	Ethinyl estradiol	1	Norethindrone acetate	A,B,C
Genora 1/50	50	Ethinyl estradiol	1	Norethindrone	A,B
Nelova 1/50M	50	Ethinyl estradiol	1	Norethindrone	A,B
Norethin 1/50M	50	Ethinyl estradiol	1	Norethindrone	A,B
Ovocon-50	50	Ethinyl estradiol	1	Norethindrone	A,B
Ortho-Novum 1/50	50	Mestranol	1	Norethindrone	A,B
Norinyl 1+50	50	Mestranol	1	Norethindrone	A,B
Combination OC: Biphasic					
Ortho-Novum 10/11,	35	Ethinyl estradiol	0.5	Norethindrone (pill 1)	D,E
Nelova 10/11	35	Ethinyl estradiol	1.0	Norethindrone (pill 2)	
Combination OCs: Triphasic					
Tri-Norinyl	35	Ethinyl estradiol	0.5	Norethindrone (pill 1)	F,G
	35	Ethinyl estradiol	1.0	Norethindrone (pill 2)	
Ortho-Novum 7/7/7	35	Ethinyl estradiol	0.5	Norethindrone (pill 1)	H,I
	35	Ethinyl estradiol	0.75	Norethindrone (pill 2)	
	35	Ethinyl estradiol	1.0	Norethindrone (pill 3)	
Tri-Levlen, Triphasil	30	Ethinyl estradiol	0.05	Levonorgestrel (pill 1)	J,K
	40	Ethinyl estradiol	0.075	Levonorgestrel (pill 2)	
	30	Ethinyl estradiol	0.125	Levonorgestrel (pill 3)	
Ortho Tri-Cyclen	35	Ethinyl estradiol	0.18	Norgestimate (pill 1)	H,I
	35	Ethinyl estradiol	0.215	Norgestimate (pill 2)	
	35	Ethinyl estradiol	0.25	Norgestimate (pill 3)	
Progestin-Only OCs					
Micronor			0.35	Norethindrone	L
Nor-Q.D.			0.35	Norethindrone	L
Orvette			0.075	Norgestrel	L

*Key to Dosing Schedule Options:
A = One pill daily for 21 days; 7 days with no pills.
B = One pill daily for 21 days; inert pills for 7 days.
C = One pill daily for 21 days; iron pills for 7 days.
D = Type 1 pills for 10 days; type 2 pills for 11 days; no pills for 7 days.
E = Same as D but with inert pills for the last 7 days (rather than no pills).
F = Type 1 pills for 7 days; type 2 pills for 9 days; type 1 pills for 5 days; no pills for 7 days.
G = Same as F but with inert pills for the last 7 days (rather than no pills).
H = Type 1 pills for 7 days; type 2 pills for 7 days; type 3 pills for 7 days; no pills for 7 days.
I = Same as H but with inert pills for the last 7 days (rather than no pills).
J = Type 1 pills for 6 days; type 2 pills for 5 days; type 3 pills for 10 days; no pills for 7 days.
K = Same as J but with inert pills for the last 7 days (rather than no pills).
L = One pill daily without interruption.

missed, administration should be discontinued, and use should not be resumed until menstruation occurs or until pregnancy has been ruled out. (Progestins are teratogenic and, therefore, must not be taken if there is any suspicion of conception.)

LONG-ACTING CONTRACEPTIVES

SUBDERMAL PROGESTIN IMPLANTS

A subdermal system [Norplant System] for delivery of levonorgestrel is available for long-term, reversible contraception. As indicated in Table 56–1, subdermal implants are the most effective contraceptives available. Unfortunately, they also have a high incidence of side effects.

Description. The Norplant System consists of 6 tiny silastic rubber capsules (2.4 mm × 34 mm), each containing 36 mg of levonorgestrel, a synthetic progestin. The capsules are surgically implanted on the inside of the upper arm through a small incision using local anesthesia. Levonorgestrel then diffuses slowly and continuously from the capsules, providing blood levels sufficient for contraception for up to 5 years. The capsules are removed after 5 years, and then replaced if continued contraception is desired.

Mechanism of Action. Subdermal levonorgestrel acts in much the same way as progestin-only OCs: cervical mucous is made thick and sticky, creating a barrier to migration of sperm; endometrial growth is suppressed, thereby discouraging nidation; and, in some women, ovulation is suppressed.

Pharmacokinetics. The daily release of levonorgestrel is about 80 μg initially and declines over time. Plasma drug levels vary widely among users. The drug is slowly metabolized by the liver. Following removal of the capsules, blood levels become undetectable within 10 to 14 days.

Adverse Effects. Menstrual irregularities are most common. Their incidence is as follows: prolonged bleeding or many bleeding days (28%), spotting (17%), amenorrhea (9.4%), irregular onset of bleeding (7.6%), and frequent bleeding onsets (7%). Other common reactions include breast discharge, cervicitis, musculoskeletal pain, abdominal discomfort, leukorrhea, and vaginitis, all of which have an incidence of 5% or more. In about 6% of users, removal of the implants has been difficult.

INTRAUTERINE PROGESTERONE CONTRACEPTIVE SYSTEM

The intrauterine contraceptive system [Progestasert] is an IUD that contains a 38-mg reservoir of progesterone. The device releases progesterone at a rate of 65 μg/day, an amount too small to elevate systemic progesterone levels. To insure that progesterone release remains adequate, a new device must be inserted annually; insertion should be performed during or shortly after menstruation so as to preclude installation during pregnancy. Although the mechanism by which contraception occurs remains obscure, it is clear that the progesterone IUD does not inhibit ovulation. Furthermore, since models of this IUD that lack progesterone are ineffective, we can conclude that localized actions of progesterone are required for contraceptive effects. It has been hypothesized that the device works by (1) altering the endometrium to prevent nidation, or (2) reducing the viability of sperm. Adverse effects associated with this IUD and others include bleeding and cramps during the first weeks of use, uterine perforation, and increased risk of pelvic inflammatory disease.

DEPOT MEDROXYPROGESTERONE ACETATE

Following a single IM injection, medroxyprogesterone acetate (MPA) [Depo-Provera], provides highly effective contraception for 3 or more months. Injections of 150 mg are repeated every 3 months to provide continuous protection. MPA prevents pregnancy in three ways: (1) suppression of ovulation, (2) thickening of the cervical mucus, and (3) alteration of the endometrium such that nidation is discouraged. When injections are discontinued, an average of 12 months is required for fertility to return, and some women may remain infertile for up to 2.5 years.

Adverse effects of MPA are typical of those seen with other progestins. Menstrual disturbances are common; cycles become irregular at first and, after 6 to 12 months, menstruation may cease entirely. Because the drug is used on a long-term basis, osteoporosis may be a concern. Other adverse effects include weight gain, abdominal bloating, headache, and depression. Although MPA has produced uterine and mammary cancers in animals, a large-scale study has shown no increase in the risk of uterine, ovarian, or breast cancer in women.

Although used worldwide for contraception for many years, MPA did not receive approval for contraceptive use in the United States until 1992. Approval had been withheld in large part because (1) MPA has caused cancer in laboratory animals, and (2) when undesired effects occur with MPA, they will be prolonged. These drawbacks are not seen with other forms of contraception (e.g., oral contraceptives). Furthermore, it had been argued that with the advanced health care system that exists in the United States, the need for a long-acting, injectable contraceptive was much smaller than in many other parts of the world. Despite these arguments, it is clear that MPA does have attractive features, most notably its high contraceptive efficacy (see Table 56–1) and its capacity for infrequent administration. With these qualities, MPA would seem to be a desirable form of birth control for (1) women who are incapable of using other methods reliably, and (2) women for whom other forms of contraception are contraindicated.

EMERGENCY POSTCOITAL CONTRACEPTION

Postcoital contraceptives, also known as "morning-after" pills, can prevent pregnancy when taken following intercourse. To be effective, these drugs should be taken no later than 72 hours after coitus. Because their side effects can be intense, postcoital contraceptives are not considered substitutes for traditional methods of birth control. Rather, these drugs should be reserved for isolated instances of unprotected intercourse; they might be used to prevent an unplanned and unwanted pregnancy resulting from sexual assault, contraceptive failure (e.g., torn condom), or occasional lack of forethought. Table 56–4 summarizes the postcoital drugs that have been used with success.

ETHINYL ESTRADIOL/NORGESTREL [OVRAL]

Ovral is a commercially available oral contraceptive that contains 50 μg of ethinyl estradiol (an estrogen) and 0.5 mg levo-

Table 56–4. Drugs for Emergency Postcoital Contraception

Drug	Dosage
Ethinyl estradiol + norgestrel (the combination is available as Ovral, an oral contraceptive)	100 µg ethinyl estradiol + 1 mg norgestrel (2 Ovral tablets) taken twice, 12 hours apart
Mifepristone (RU 486)*	600 mg in one dose
Diethylstilbestrol	25 mg bid for 5 days
Ethinyl estradiol	2.5 mg bid for 5 days
Conjugated estrogens	10 mg tid for 5 days
Estrone	5 mg tid for 5 days

*Not available in the United States.

norgestrel (a progestin). For postcoital contraception, 2 Ovral tablets are taken within 72 hours of coitus, and 2 more tablets are taken 12 hours later. Pregnancy is prevented by the estrogen in Ovral, which (1) acts on the fallopian tubes to impede migration of the ovum, and (2) alters the endometrium to discourage nidation. The contribution of the progestin is unknown. The high estrogen content of the regimen produces a high incidence of side effects: nausea (60%), vomiting (17%), headache (70%), and breast tenderness (46%). Since estrogens and progestins can harm a developing fetus, pre-existing pregnancy should be ruled out before Ovral is given.

MIFEPRISTONE (RU 486)

Mifepristone (RU 486) is a synthetic steroid that blocks receptors for progesterone. The drug is used for "morning-after" contraception and for termination of early pregnancy (abortion).

In addition, mifepristone is under investigation for treatment of recurrent breast cancer, certain meningiomas, Cushing's syndrome, and glaucoma. At this time, the drug is available only in France, the United Kingdom, and Sweden—not in the United States.

Postcoital Contraception. For postcoital contraception, mifepristone is given in a single, 600-mg oral dose no later than 72 hours after unprotected intercourse. Like Ovral, mifepristone prevents pregnancy by blocking nidation. Mifepristone would seem preferable to Ovral for two reasons. First, only one dose is required. Second, side effects occur less frequently: headache occurs in 49% of patients, nausea in 40%, breast tenderness in 27%, and vomiting in 3%. The major disadvantage of mifepristone is that onset of menstruation may be delayed, which can be very stressful to a woman concerned about the possibility of being pregnant.

Termination of Early Pregnancy. For termination of early pregnancy, mifepristone is employed in combination with a prostaglandin. Mifepristone is given first, and the prostaglandin is given 48 hours later. The combination stimulates uterine contractions, causing the conceptus to undergo detachment and expulsion. In the past, an *intramuscular* prostaglandin was used with mifepristone. However, an effective *oral* prostaglandin—*misoprostol*—is now available, making the procedure more convenient and less expensive. (As discussed in Chapter 66, misoprostol [Cytotec] is also used to prevent peptic ulcers in patients taking aspirin-like drugs.)

In a recent clinical study conducted in France, the abortion success rate with mifepristone-misoprostol was nearly 99%. (Success was defined as termination of pregnancy with complete expulsion of the conceptus.) All women in the study had amenorrhea for less than 50 days. Dosing was done as follows: each patient received a 600-mg oral dose of mifepristone and, if abortion had not occurred within 48 hours, each was given a 400-µg dose of misoprostol; a second dose of misoprostol (200 µg) was offered if abortion had not occurred by 4 hours after the first dose. Only 5.5% of the pregnancies terminated prior to dosing with misoprostol; with the addition of misoprostol (1 or 2 doses), the cumulative success rate was 98.7%. In the major-

Table 56–5. Spermicides

Formulation	Active Ingredient	Trade Name
Foam	Nonoxynol 9 (12.5%)	Delfen Contraceptive, Koromex
	Nonoxynol 9 (8%)	Because, Emko, Emko Pre-Fil
Jelly	Nonoxynol 9 (5%)	Ramses
	Nonoxynol 9 (3%)	Koromex
	Nonoxynol 9 (2%)	Gynol II Contraceptive*, Shur-Seal Gel
	Octoxynol 9 (2%)	Koromex*
	Octoxynol 9 (1%)	Ortho-Gynol Contraceptive*
Gel	Nonoxynol 9 (2%)	Conceptrol Disposable Contraceptive, Koromex Crystal Clear*
Cream	Nonoxynol 9 (5%)	Conceptrol Birth Control
	Nonoxynol 9 (2%)	Ortho Creme Contraceptive*
	Octoxynol 9 (3%)	Koromex*
Suppository	Nonoxynol 9 (2.27%)	Encare
	Nonoxynol 9 (100 mg)	Intercept Contraceptive Inserts, Semicid
Sponge	Nonoxynol 9 (1 g)	Today
Condom	Nonoxynol 9 (5.6%) (latex condom with spermicide-containing lubricant)	Excita Extra, Koromex, Ramses Extra, Sheik Elite

*Intended for use only in combination with a diaphragm.

ity of patients (69%), abortion occurred within 4 hours of the first misoprostol dose.

The principal adverse effect of mifepristone-misoprostol is prolonged bleeding, which may persist for 1 to 2 weeks. Rarely, a transfusion is required. About 80% of patients experience transient cramping, beginning 1 hour after taking misoprostol; about 15% require a nonopioid analgesic for relief. Other common side effects are nausea (40%), vomiting (15%), and diarrhea (10%).

The Future of Mifepristone in the United States. Unlike many drugs, which are unavailable in the United states for medical and scientific reasons, mifepristone is unavailable for political and ideological reasons—specifically, strong opposition from antiabortion groups. In support of the drug are many women's organizations and some major physicians' groups, including the American Medical Organization. Although mifepristone is not yet available in the U.S., it may be within a few years. The drug's European manufacturer (Roussel-UCLAF) recently agreed to license mifepristone to the Population Council, a nonprofit U.S. organization; once the license is granted, the Council will select a U.S. manufacturer, sponsor an application to the FDA, and conduct a large-scale U.S. clinical trial. Because extensive clinical studies have already been conducted outside the United States, mifepristone may receive FDA approval more rapidly than most drugs, perhaps within 2 to 3 years from the start of the process.

OTHER POSTCOITAL CONTRACEPTIVES

In addition to Ovral and mifepristone (RU 486), Table 56–4 lists four other regimens for postcoital contraception. All four consist of an estrogen taken in high doses for 5 days. Because high doses are taken for an extended time, side effects (nausea, vomiting, breast tenderness) are more severe than with Ovral or mifepristone.

SPERMICIDES

Spermicides are dispensed in the form of foams, gels, creams, and suppositories; a spermicide-impregnated sponge is also available. All of these preparations can be purchased without a prescription. When used alone, and especially when used in combination with a diaphragm or condom, spermicides can provide very effective contraception (see Table 56–1). As indicated in Table 56–5, spermicidal preparations employ either *nonoxynol 9* or *octoxynol 9* as their active ingredient. Adverse effects are minimal. Most studies show no relationship between spermicide use and birth defects.

Correct use of spermicides is required for contraceptive efficacy. The spermicide must be applied prior to coitus, but no more than 1 hour in advance. Suppositories should be inserted a minimum of 10 to 15 minutes before intercourse to allow time for dispersion. The spermicide should be re-applied each time intercourse is anticipated. Douching should be postponed for at least 6 hours following coitus.

The contraceptive sponge differs somewhat from other spermicidal preparations. The sponge acts in three ways to prevent conception: it (1) releases spermicide (nonoxynol 9), (2) provides a barrier to sperm, and (3) absorbs seminal fluid. Unlike other spermicides, which must be re-applied every time intercourse is to take place, a single sponge provides contraception for repeated coitus over a 24-hour period. A sponge should remain in place no longer than 1 day. The most common adverse effects are vaginal irritation and dryness.

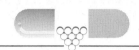

Summary of Major Nursing Implications

COMBINATION ORAL CONTRACEPTIVES

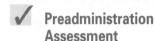

**Preadministration
Assessment**

Therapeutic Goal

Prevention of unwanted pregnancy.

Baseline Data

A thorough physical examination should be performed, including pelvic and breast examinations, palpation of the liver, and blood pressure measurement. Laboratory tests should include a Papanicolaou smear.

Assess for a history of hypertension, diabetes, thrombophlebitis, thromboembolic disorders, cerebrovascular disease, coronary artery disease, breast carcinoma, estrogen-dependent neoplasm, and benign or malignant liver tumors.

Identifying High-Risk Patients

Combinations OCs are *contraindicated* during *pregnancy* and for women with the following disorders (or a history thereof): *thrombophlebitis, thromboembolic disorders, cerebrovascular disease, coronary artery disease, myocardial infarction, known or suspected breast carcinoma, known or suspected estrogen-dependent neoplasm, benign or malignant liver tumors, and undiagnosed abnormal genital bleeding.*

Combination OCs should be used with *caution* in women with *diabetes,* women *who smoke heavily* (more than 15 cigarettes a day), women *who have risk factors for cardiovascular disease* (e.g., hypertension, obesity, hypercholesterolemia), and women anticipating *elective surgery in which postoperative thrombosis might be expected.*

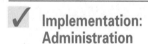

**Implementation:
Administration**

At the Start of OC Use

Caution the client that an additional form of birth control (e.g., condom, diaphragm) should be employed during the first week of OC use.

Dosing Schedule

Provide the client with the following instructions on administration: (1) initiate administration 5 days after the onset of menstruation, (2) the administration sequence consists of 21 days of drug use followed by 7 days off (for the 7 "off" days, the manufacturer may provide inert tablets, iron-containing tablets, or no tablets), and (3) take pills at the same time each day (e.g., with a meal, at bedtime).

Responding to Missed Doses

Provide the client with the following instructions regarding missed doses: (1) if only one dose is missed, take the omitted dose together with the next scheduled dose, (2) if two doses are missed, take two doses per day on the following 2 days, and (3) if three doses are missed, initiate a new cycle (starting 7 days after the last pill was taken) and use an additional form of contraception (e.g., condom, diaphragm) during the first 2 weeks of the new cycle.

Postpartum Use

Inform the client that OCs can be initiated immediately after delivery if breast-feeding is not intended.

Promoting Compliance

Counsel the client about the importance of taking OCs as prescribed. Encourage the client to read the package insert provided with combination OCs.

✔ **Ongoing Evaluation and Interventions**

Monitoring Summary

Periodic examinations should include breasts, pelvic organs, abdominal organs, blood pressure, and a Papanicolaou smear.

Minimizing Adverse Effects

Thrombotic Disorders. Because of their estrogen content, combination OCs increase the risk of thrombosis and thromboembolism. To minimize thrombosis and thromboembolism, (1) use OCs of low estrogen content, (2) avoid use of OCs by women with known risk factors for thrombotic disorders, and (3) discontinue OCs at least 4 weeks prior to elective surgeries in which postoperative thrombosis might be expected. Inform the client about symptoms of thrombosis and thromboembolism (e.g., leg tenderness or pain, sudden chest pain, shortness of breath, severe headache, sudden visual disturbance) and instruct her to notify the physician if these develop.

Hypertension. Perform periodic determinations of blood pressure. If hypertension is detected, discontinue OCs. Blood pressure will usually normalize within a few months.

Abnormal Uterine Bleeding. During initial use, combination OCs may reduce or eliminate menstrual flow; breakthrough bleeding or spotting may also occur. Menstrual irregularities may be greater with low-estrogen preparations.

Instruct the client to notify the physician if two consecutive periods are missed; the possibility of pregnancy must be evaluated.

Instruct the client to notify the physician if bleeding irregularities persist; the possibility of malignancy must be investigated.

Inform the client that menstruation may take several months to normalize following OC withdrawal.

Effects Related to Estrogen or Progestin Imbalance. An excess or deficiency in estrogen or progestin levels can cause specific side effects (see Table 56–2). By adjusting the estrogen or progestin content of the OC regimen, these effects can be reduced or eliminated. Substitution of one combination OC for another can be made at the beginning of any new cycle.

Use in Pregnancy and Lactation. OCs are contraindicated during pregnancy: these agents are carcinogenic and can cause fetal malformation. Pregnancy should be ruled out prior to OC use. Inform the client that in the event of contraceptive failure, OC use should cease immediately.

Inform the client that oral contraceptives enter breast milk and can reduce milk production. Instruct her not to breast-feed while taking OCs.

Benign Hepatic Adenoma. Women taking OCs should undergo periodic palpation of the liver; if a mass is detected, further tests are required for definitive diagnosis. If benign hepatoma is present, OC use must cease; regression of the tumor usually follows.

Glucose Intolerance. Oral contraceptives can elevate plasma glucose levels. Advise the diabetic client to monitor blood glucose content closely; an increase in dosage of insulin or oral hypoglycemic medication may be needed. Monitor the prediabetic client for hyperglycemia.

Multiple Births. The incidence of twin births is increased when conception takes place shortly after termination of OC use. Advise the client to employ another form of birth control for 3 months after termination of OC use if she wishes to reduce the chances of multiple births.

Minimizing Adverse Interactions

Drugs that Reduce Oral Contraceptive Levels. Several *anticonvulsants* (phenobarbital, phenytoin, primidone) and certain *antibiotics* (e.g., rifampin, tetracycline, ampicillin) can accelerate OC elimination. Advise the client who is taking OCs in combination with these agents to be alert for indications of reduced OC levels (e.g., breakthrough bleeding, spotting) and to notify the physician if these occur. An increase in OC dosage or use of an alternative method of birth control may be required.

Drugs Whose Effects Are Reduced by Oral Contraceptives. Oral contraceptives can reduce the effects of some drugs, including *oral anticoagulants* (e.g., warfarin) and *insulin and other hypoglycemic agents*. When combined with OCs, oral anticoagulants and hypoglycemic agents may require greater than normal dosages.

Drugs Whose Effects Are Increased by Oral Contraceptives. Oral contraceptives can increase blood levels of several drugs, including *theophylline* and *imipramine*. Women using these drugs in combination with OCs should be alert for signs of toxicity; dosage reduction for theophylline or imipramine may be required.

PROGESTIN-ONLY ORAL CONTRACEPTIVES

✓ **Preadministration Assessment**

Therapeutic Goal

Prevention of unwanted pregnancy.

Identifying High-Risk Patients

Progestin-only pills are *contraindicated* during *pregnancy*.

✓ **Implementation: Administration**

Dosing Schedule

Instruct the client to initiate OC use on day 1 of the menstrual cycle and to take one pill every day thereafter. Pills should be taken at the same time each day (e.g., with a meal or at bedtime).

Responding to Missed Doses

Provide the client with the following instruction regarding missed doses: (1) if one pill is missed, take it as soon as the omission is noticed, (2) if two pills are missed, take one pill as soon as the omission is noticed, discard the second pill, and take the next scheduled pill at its normal time, and (3) if three pills are missed, terminate OC use. Do not resume use until menstruation occurs or until pregnancy has been ruled out.

 Ongoing Evaluation and Interventions

Minimizing Adverse Effects

Menstrual Irregularities. Breakthrough bleeding, spotting, amenorrhea, inconsistent cycle length, and variations in the amount and duration of monthly flow are common and unavoidable. Forewarn the patient of these effects.

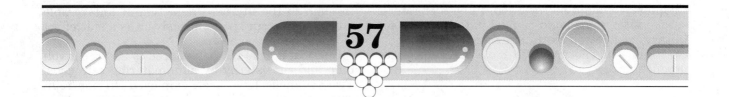

Drug Therapy of Infertility

*I*nfertility is defined as a decrease in the ability to reproduce. This contrasts with *sterility*, which is the complete absence of reproductive ability. About 15% of couples attempting to have children experience infertility. Failure to conceive may be due to reproductive dysfunction of the male partner, the female partner, or both. When medical treatment is implemented, approximately one half of infertile couples achieve pregnancy. To date, drug therapy of female infertility has been considerably more successful than drug therapy of male infertility.

In treating infertility, the chances of success are greatly enhanced by accurate diagnosis. A variety of diagnostic procedures may be employed, including semen analysis, determination of basal body temperature patterns, measurement of estrogen and progesterone levels, endometrial biopsy, and evaluation of fallopian tube patency. A complete medical history of both partners is essential. This history should include information on frequency and timing of coitus and use of drugs that might lower fertility.

In approaching the drugs employed to increase fertility, we will begin with a discussion of causes of reproductive dysfunction. Following this we will discuss the fertility-promoting drugs. In preparation for the study of these agents, the following from Chapter 55 should be reviewed: information on the menstrual cycle and information on the biosynthesis and physiologic and pharmacologic effects of the female hormones (estrogens and progestins). In addition, the section on testosterone in

733

Chapter 54 should be reviewed. In both chapters, special attention should be paid to the roles of pituitary gonadotropins (luteinizing hormone, follicle-stimulating hormone) in male and female reproduction.

INFERTILITY: CAUSES AND TREATMENT STRATEGIES

FEMALE INFERTILITY

Female infertility can result from disruption of any phase of the reproductive process. The most critical phases are follicular maturation, ovulation, transport of the ovum through the fallopian tubes, fertilization of the ovum, nidation, and growth and development of the conceptus. These events cannot take place unless the ovaries, uterus, hypothalamus, and pituitary are functioning properly and in concert. If the activity of any of these structures is disturbed, fertility can be impaired. The causes of female infertility that respond to drug therapy are discussed below.

Anovulation and Failure of Follicular Maturation

In the absence of adequate hormonal stimulation, ovarian follicles will not ripen and ovulation will not take place. Frequently, these causes of infertility can be corrected with drugs. The agents used to promote follicular maturation and/or ovulation are *clomiphene*, *gonadorelin*, *menotropins*, and *human chorionic gonadotropin* (HCG). Clomiphene and gonadorelin induce follicular maturation and ovulation by promoting release of FSH and LH from the pituitary; in some cases, induction of ovulation requires co-treatment with HCG. Menotropins is used in conjunction with HCG: menotropins acts directly on the ovary to promote follicular development; after the follicle has matured, HCG is given to induce ovulation. Since HCG acts on the mature follicle to cause ovulation, the drug is used only after follicular maturation has been induced with another agent (menotropins or clomiphene). The pharmacology of clomiphene, gonadorelin, menotropins, and HCG is discussed below.

Unfavorable Cervical Mucus

In the periovulatory period, the cervical glands normally secrete large volumes of thin, watery mucus. These secretions, which are produced under the influence of estrogen, facilitate passage of sperm through the cervical canal. If the cervical mucus is scant or of inappropriate consistency (thick, sticky), sperm will be unable to pass through to the uterus. Production of unfavorable mucus may occur spontaneously or as a side effect of clomiphene (see below).

Cervical mucus can be restored to its proper volume and consistency by administering estrogens. Two regimens have been employed. In one regimen, ethinyl estradiol is given beginning early in the menstrual cycle (on day 6, 7, or 8) and continued through day 12 or 13; dosages range from 20 to 80 µg/day. In the second regimen, conjugated estrogens are administered from day 5 through day 15 of the cycle; dosages range from 2.5 to 5 mg/day. When used to counteract the effects of clomiphene on the cervical mucus, estrogens are administered for 10 days beginning 1 day after the last clomiphene dose.

Hyperprolactinemia

Elevation of prolactin levels may be caused by a pituitary adenoma or by disturbed regulation of the healthy pituitary. Amenorrhea, galactorrhea, and infertility may all occur in association with excessive prolactin secretion. The mechanism by which hyperprolactinemia impairs fertility is not known. Hyperprolactinemia can be treated with *bromocriptine* (see below).

Luteal Phase Defect

The term *luteal phase defect* refers to a group of disorders in which secretion of progesterone by the corpus luteum is insufficient to maintain endometrial integrity. Dysfunction of the corpus luteum may be spontaneous or may occur secondary to hyperprolactinemia or to use of clomiphene. Luteal phase defect can be diagnosed by making serial determinations of plasma progesterone levels or by taking a biopsy of the endometrium.

Progesterone is the preferred therapy for luteal phase defect. This hormone will correct the defect regardless of its etiology. Only progesterone itself should be used; synthetic progestins are teratogenic and may also induce degeneration of the corpus luteum. Progesterone treatment should commence after ovulation has occurred, and should continue through the first 8 to 10 weeks of pregnancy (i.e., until the placenta has developed the capacity to make its own progestins).

Progesterone may be administered by IM injection (12.5 mg/day) or in a vaginal suppository (25 mg twice daily). Because progesterone injections are both painful and inconvenient, the suppositories are preferred.

Endometriosis

Endometriosis is a condition in which endometrial tissue has become implanted in an abnormal location (e.g., uterine wall, ovary, extragenital sites). These implants respond to hormonal stimulation in much the same fashion as the normally situated endometrium. Endometriosis is a common cause of infertility and, when pregnancies do occur, the rate of spontaneous abortion is high (about 50%).

The mechanism by which endometriosis reduces fertility is not always clear. In some cases, infertility results from ovarian or tubal adhesions that impede transport of the ovum. However, when endometriosis is mild, visible causes of infertility are frequently absent.

Endometriosis can be treated surgically, with drugs, or with a combination of both modalities. All three approaches can increase fertility. In recent years, the drug employed most frequently has been *danazol*. Before danazol became available, progestins (alone and in combination with an estrogen) were the preferred pharmacologic therapy. Most recently, *nafarelin* (a synthetic analogue of gonadotropin-releasing hormone) has been used with success. Danazol and nafarelin are discussed further below.

Androgen Excess

Overproduction of androgens can decrease fertility. Excess androgens may be of ovarian or adrenal origin. The most common condition associated with androgen excess is polycystic ovary (PCO). This condition is characterized by the presence of multiple polycystic follicles within a thickened capsule; ovulation is absent. *Clomiphene* is the treatment of choice for PCO. If clomiphene alone fails to induce ovulation, addition of HCG to the regimen may improve results. If the androgen excess is of adrenal origin, a combination of *clomiphene plus dexamethasone* (a glucocorticoid) may prove effective; dexamethasone decreases adrenal androgen synthesis by suppressing release of adrenocorticotropic hormone from the pituitary.

MALE INFERTILITY

For about 30% of couples that experience infertility, failure to conceive is due entirely to reproductive dysfunction in the male. Male infertility is due most often to (1) decreased density or motility of sperm, or to (2) semen of abnormal volume or quality. The most obvious manifestation of male infertility is impotence (inability to achieve erection). In most cases, infertility in males is not associated with an identifiable endocrine disorder. Unfortunately, male infertility is generally unresponsive to drugs.

Hypogonadotropic Hypogonadism

A few males may be incapable of spermatogenesis because of insufficient gonadotropin secretion. In these rare cases, drug therapy may be helpful.

If the gonadotropin deficiency is only partial, sperm counts can be increased using HCG (alone or in combination with menotropins). If the deficiency is severe, treatment with androgens is required (see Chapter 54). If therapy with HCG and menotropins is intended, the patient should be informed that treatment will be prolonged (3 to 4 years) and very expensive.

Impotence

Inability to achieve erection is the most conspicuous cause of male infertility. In recent years, vasoactive drugs (phentolamine, papaverine, alprostadil) have been given to produce erection. Use of these agents is discussed later in the chapter.

Idiopathic Male Infertility

Idiopathic infertility is defined as infertility for which no cause can be identified. It is estimated that 25% to 40% of male infertility is idiopathic. Since the cause is unknown, specific drug therapy is impossible. Accordingly, treatment is empiric (trial and error). Several drugs, including androgens, clomiphene, and HCG, have been administered in hopes of improving idiopathic infertility in males. Unfortunately, none of these agents has been especially successful.

DRUGS USED TO TREAT INFERTILITY

The majority of drugs used to increase fertility are directed at improving reproductive function in females. Drugs can increase female fertility by helping promote the following: (1) maturation of ovarian follicles, (2) ovulation, (3) production of favorable cervical mucus, (4) control of endometriosis, and (5) reduction of excessive prolactin levels. The ability of drugs to increase fertility in males is limited. In some cases, therapy may improve semen and sperm production. Recently, drugs have been given with success to facilitate erection.

CLOMIPHENE

Therapeutic Use. Clomiphene [Clomid, Serophene] is used to promote follicular maturation and ovulation in selected infertile women.

Mechanism of Fertility Promotion. Clomiphene blocks receptors for estrogen. By blocking these receptors in the hypothalamus and the pituitary, clomiphene makes it appear to these structures that estrogen levels are low. In response, the pituitary increases secretion of gonadotropins (LH and FSH) and these hormones then stimulate the ovary, promoting follicular maturation and ovulation. In properly selected patients, the ovulation rate is about 90%. Because of its mechanism of action, clomiphene can induce ovulation only if the pituitary is capable of producing LH and FSH, and only if the ovaries are capable of responding to these hormones. Success is impossible in women with primary failure of either the ovaries or the pituitary. Accordingly, ovarian and pituitary function should be verified prior to clomiphene therapy. If treatment produces follicular maturation but ovulation fails to occur, it may be possible to induce ovulation by adding HCG to the regimen (see below). The occurrence of ovulation can be determined by three methods: (1) monitoring for an increase in basal body temperature, (2) monitoring for an increase in progesterone levels, and (3) examining a biopsy of the endometrium for evidence of secretory transformation.

Adverse Effects. Common side effects include hot flushes (similar to the vasomotor responses of menopause), nausea, abdominal discomfort, bloating, and breast engorgement. Some patients experience visual disturbances (blurred vision, visual flashes), which reverse following clomiphene withdrawal. Multiple births (usually twins) occur in 8% to 10% of clomiphene-facilitated pregnancies. Patients should be informed of this possibility.

Excessive stimulation of the ovaries can produce ovarian enlargement. This reaction is most likely in women with polycystic ovaries. Hyperstimulation of the ovaries can be minimized by avoiding unnecessarily large clomiphene doses. If undue ovarian enlargement occurs, administration of clomiphene should cease. The ovaries will regress to normal size following drug withdrawal.

Some actions of clomiphene may *interfere* with conception. Luteal phase defect may be induced. This response can be corrected by administering progesterone. Because of its antiestrogenic actions, clomiphene may force the production of scant and viscous cervical mucus; estrogen therapy will render cervical secretions more hospitable to sperm.

It is recommended that clomiphene be avoided during pregnancy. Although no human fetal defects have been reported, clomiphene has produced developmental abnormalities in animals.

Preparations, Dosage, and Administration. Clomiphene [Clomid, Serophene] is dispensed in 50-mg tablets for oral use. The initial course of treatment consists of 50 mg once daily for 5 days. If cyclic menstrual bleeding has been occurring, therapy should begin on the fifth day after the onset of menses. If menstruation has been absent, therapy can commence at any time (assuming that pregnancy has been ruled out). If the first course of treatment fails to induce ovulation, a second 5-day course (using 100 mg/day) may be tried. The second course may begin as early as 30 days after the previous course. Doses may be increased in subsequent courses. However, doses above 100 mg/day are rarely needed. Once a dose that induces ovulation has been established, that dose should be used for a maximum of three cycles. If pregnancy has not occurred, further treatment is unlikely to increase the chances of success. When ovulation does occur, it is usually within 5 to 10 days after the last clomiphene dose; patients should be instructed to have coitus at least every other day during this time.

MENOTROPINS

Menotropins [Pergonal] (also known as human menopausal gonadotropin or HMG) is a hormonal preparation having equal amounts of LH and FSH activity. Commercial menotropins is prepared by extraction from the urine of postmenopausal women.

Therapeutic Actions and Use. Menotropins is employed in conjunction with HCG to promote follicular maturation and ovulation. Menotropins acts directly on the ovaries to cause maturation of follicles. Once follicles have ripened, HCG is administered to induce ovulation.

Menotropins is employed when gonadotropin secretion by the pituitary is insufficient to provide adequate ovarian stimulation. Candidates for menotropins therapy must have ovaries capable of responding to FSH and LH; menotropins will be of no help in the presence of primary ovarian failure. Among properly selected patients, the rate of ovulation approaches 100%. It should be noted that therapy with menotropins is not cheap: a single cycle of treatment can cost between $500 and $1500 (in addition to physicians' fees and laboratory costs). Menotropins has also been used to treat infertility in males (hypogonadotropic hypogonadism, idiopathic male infertility).

Adverse Effects. The most serious adverse response is *ovarian hyperstimulation syndrome*, a condition characterized by sudden enlargement of the ovaries. Mild-to-moderate ovarian enlargement is common, occurring in about 20% of patients. This condition is benign and resolves spontaneously upon discontinuation of drug use. Of greater concern is ovarian enlargement that occurs rapidly and that may be accompanied by ascites, pleural effusion, and considerable pain. If this manifestation of ovarian stimulation occurs, menotropins should be withdrawn and the patient hospitalized. Treatment is usually supportive (bed rest, analgesics, fluid and electrolyte replacement). If rupture of ovarian cysts occurs, surgery may be required to stop bleeding. Enlargement of the ovaries is most likely during the first 2 weeks of treatment. To insure early detection, the patient should be examined at least every other day during the interval of menotropins use, and for 2 weeks after termination of treatment. Ovarian stimulation can be minimized by keeping the dosage as low as possible. In addition to causing excessive ovarian stimulation, menotropins may produce *spontaneous abortion* (in about 25% of menotropins-facilitated pregnancies) and *multiple births* (15% of pregnancies result in twins; 5% of pregnancies have three or more conceptuses).

Monitoring Therapy. Ovarian responses to menotropins must be monitored in order to determine timing of HCG administration and to minimize the risk of ovarian enlargement. Responses can be followed by measuring serum estrogen levels and by ultrasonography of the developing follicles. When estrogen levels rise to twice the pretreatment baseline, or when ultrasonography indicates that follicles have enlarged to 16 to 20 mm, administration of menotropins should cease and HCG should be injected. However, if estrogen production is excessive (serum levels three to four times the pretreatment baseline), HCG should not be administered, since there is a risk of ovarian hyperstimulation under these conditions. In addition, HCG should be withheld if ultrasonography indicates the presence of four or more mature follicles.

Preparations, Dosage, and Administration. Menotropins [Pergonal] is dispensed as a powder to be reconstituted with sterile saline immediately prior to use. Each ampule contains 75 international units (IU) of FSH activity and 75 IU of LH activity. Administration is by IM injection.

Menotropins is used sequentially with HCG: after follicular maturation has been induced with menotropins, HCG is injected to promote ovulation. For the initial cycle, the contents of one menotropins ampule is injected daily for 9 to 12 days. When estrogen measurements indicate follicular maturation has occurred, menotropins is discontinued; HCG (5000 to 10,000 USP units) is injected 24 hours after the last menotropins dose. Ovulation occurs 2 to 3 days after injection of HCG. Accordingly, patients should be instructed to have intercourse on the eve of HCG injection and on the following 2 to 3 days. If there is evidence of ovulation but conception does not take place, treatment should be repeated for two more courses using the same menotropins dosage. If treatment remains ineffective, two additional courses may be tried, using twice as much menotropins as previously. If there is still no conception, further treatment is unlikely to help.

GONADORELIN

Therapeutic Use and Mechanism of Action. Gonadorelin [Lutrepulse] is a synthetic polypeptide identical in structure to human gonadotropin-releasing hormone (Gn-RH). The drug is given to treat infertility resulting from hypothalamic failure to secrete Gn-RH.

Under physiologic conditions, Gn-RH is secreted from the hypothalamus in a *pulsatile* pattern; following secretion, the hormone acts on the pituitary to promote release of LH and FSH, which, in turn, act on the ovary to promote follicular maturation and ovulation. To be effective, gonadorelin must be administered in "pulses" that mimic physiologic secretion of Gn-RH. When administered in this pattern, the drug is able to promote follicular maturation and ovulation.

Adverse Effects. Because administration is via an indwelling intravenous catheter, there is a risk of inflammation, infection, phlebitis, and hematoma at the site of infusion. Like menotropins, gonadorelin can cause hyperstimulation of the ovaries,

but the risk is much lower with gonadorelin. There is a 12% incidence of multiple births, twins being most common.

Preparations, Dosage, and Administration. Gonadorelin acetate [Lutrepulse] is dispensed as a lyophilized powder to be reconstituted for IV use. The drug is administered through an indwelling catheter, usually in a forearm vein, using a portable infusion pump (Lutrepulse pump) supplied by the manufacturer. The initial dosing schedule is 5 μg every 90 minutes for 21 days or until ovulation occurs. If pregnancy occurs, administration may be continued for an additional 2 weeks to support the corpus luteum. Throughout the procedure, the catheter should be moved every 24 hours. Treatment is expensive, costing $750 to $1000 per cycle.

HUMAN CHORIONIC GONADOTROPIN

Human chorionic gonadotropin (HCG) is a polypeptide hormone produced by the placenta. HCG is similar in structure and identical in action to luteinizing hormone (LH).

Therapeutic Use. HCG is used to induce ovulation in women who are infertile because of ovulatory failure. The drug causes ovulation by simulating the midcycle LH surge. When HCG is used to promote ovulation, follicular maturation must first be induced with another agent, usually menotropins. HCG can also be used in conjunction with clomiphene when treatment with clomiphene alone has failed to promote ovulation.

Adverse Effects. The most severe adverse response to HCG is *ovarian hyperstimulation syndrome*. If this reaction occurs, hospitalization and discontinuation of HCG are indicated. HCG may also provoke *rupture of ovarian cysts* with resultant bleeding into the peritoneal cavity. *Multiple births* may be induced; the patient should be informed of this possibility. Additional adverse effects include *edema, pain at the site of injection*, and *central nervous system disturbances* (headache, irritability, restlessness, fatigue).

Preparations, Dosage, and Administration. Commercial HCG is prepared by extraction from the urine of pregnant women. HCG is dispensed as a powder and must be reconstituted for use. Administration is by IM injection. The usual dose for induction of ovulation is 5000 to 10,000 USP units.

Prior to giving HCG, follicular maturation must be induced with another agent (menotropins or clomiphene). When used in conjunction with menotropins, HCG is injected 1 day after the last menotropins dose. When used as an adjunct to clomiphene, HCG is administered 7 to 9 days after the last clomiphene dose.

BROMOCRIPTINE

Therapeutic Uses. Bromocriptine [Parlodel] is used to correct amenorrhea and infertility associated with excessive prolactin secretion. If galactorrhea is present, this consequence of hyperprolactinemia may also be corrected. When the source of excessive prolactin is a pituitary adenoma, bromocriptine can induce regression of the tumor, in addition to reducing prolactin secretion. Continuous treatment can suppress tumor growth for years. Bromocriptine is also used in Parkinson's disease (see Chapter 21) and to suppress postpartum lactation in women who choose not to breast-feed.

Mechanism of Fertility Promotion. Bromocriptine stimulates receptors for dopamine. By stimulating dopamine receptors in the anterior pituitary, bromocriptine inhibits prolactin secretion. Reductions in prolactin levels are accompanied by normalization of the menstrual cycle and a return of fertility. The mechanism by which lowering of prolactin levels leads to a return of ovulation is not known.

Adverse Effects. When bromocriptine is given to treat infertility, adverse effects are frequent but usually mild. Nausea occurs in 50% of patients. Headache, dizziness, fatigue, and abdominal cramps are also common. Orthostatic hypotension may occur, but is rare at the doses employed to decrease prolactin secretion. Teratogenic effects have not been reported. Adverse effects can be minimized by taking bromocriptine with meals and by initiating treatment at low doses.

Preparations, Dosage, and Administration. Bromocriptine mesylate [Parlodel] is dispensed in 2.5-mg tablets and 5-mg capsules. Dosing is begun at 2.5 mg once a day and then gradually increased to 2.5 mg two or three times a day. All doses should be administered with food. Normalization of the menstrual cycle may occur rapidly (within a few days) or may require up to 2 months of treatment. As soon as pregnancy is achieved, use of bromocriptine should cease. As a rule, administration should not resume until after delivery. If treatment is not reinstated, hypersecretion of prolactin is almost certain to recur within a year.

DRUGS FOR ENDOMETRIOSIS: DANAZOL AND NAFARELIN

Danazol

Therapeutic Use. Danazol [Danocrine] is used to treat *endometriosis and associated infertility*. Treatment leads to complete resolution of endometrial implants in the majority of patients. In most cases, ovulation is restored within 1 to 3 months after danazol has been discontinued. Since danazol may temporarily impair the ability of the endometrium to support pregnancy, attempts at conception should be postponed for about 3 months following danazol withdrawal. It should be noted that when endometriosis is mild, danazol may *reduce* fertility rather than increase it. In addition to the therapy of endometriosis, danazol has been used to treat *angioneurotic edema* and *fibrocystic breast disease*.

Mechanism of Fertility Promotion. Danazol acts by multiple mechanisms to induce regression of endometrial implants. First, danazol inhibits several of the enzymes required for synthesis of ovarian hormones, thereby depriving the implant of the hormonal environment needed for its maintenance. Second, danazol suppresses secretion of pituitary gonadotropins (FSH and LH), thereby further decreasing the availability of ovarian hormones. Lastly, danazol may act directly on the implant to block ovarian hormone receptors. All of these actions result in atrophy of ectopic endometrial tissue. The normal endometrium atrophies as well.

Adverse Effects and Interactions. Danazol is weakly androgenic and may induce virilization. Potential manifestations include acne, deepening of the voice, and growth of facial hair. These effects are usually reversible upon cessation of treatment. If taken during pregnancy, danazol may cause masculinization of the female fetus. Danazol may also cause edema and, consequently, should be used cautiously in patients with cardiac and renal disorders. Liver dysfunction has been reported; liver function should be assessed before therapy and periodically thereafter. Danazol may intensify the effects of oral anticoagulants (e.g., warfarin).

Preparations, Dosage, and Administration. Danazol [Danocrine] is dispensed in capsules (50, 100, and 200 mg) for oral administration. A dosage of 200 to 300 mg twice daily is usually effective. To insure that danazol is not taken during pregnancy, therapy should be initiated at the time of menstruation. The usual course of treatment is 3 to 9 months.

Nafarelin

Nafarelin [Synarel], a synthetic analogue of gonadotropin-releasing hormone (Gn-RH), is used to treat endometriosis. The drug is available only in a nasal spray formulation.

Mechanism of Action. Ectopic endometrial implants, like the normal endometrium, are dependent on ovarian hormones. Nafarelin suppresses endometriosis by indirectly suppressing ovarian hormone production.

How does nafarelin suppress production of ovarian hormones? *Initial* doses of nafarelin actually *increase* hormone production. This increase occurs because nafarelin, like endogenous Gn-RH, acts on the pituitary to promote release of FSH and LH, which, in turn, act on the ovary to stimulate hormone production. However, in contrast to endogenous Gn-RH, which has a short half-life and is released in a pulsatile fashion, nafarelin has a long half-life and is administered on a continuing basis. As a result, nafarelin causes *continuous* stimulation of pituitary Gn-RH receptors. This continuous stimulation has the paradoxical effect of *suppressing* FSH and LH release, thereby depriving the ovary of the stimulation needed for hormone production.

Therapeutic Use. Nafarelin is approved for treatment of *endometriosis*. The drug is about as effective as danazol for this application. Nafarelin reduces the area of endometriosis, improves symptoms, and increases the rate of pregnancy. Because of concern about bone loss (see below), nafarelin should not be used for more than 6 months.

It must be stressed that nafarelin, like danazol, does not produce cure. Within 6 months after discontinuation of treatment, symptoms return in up to 50% of women who had previously been rendered symptom free.

Adverse Effects. Most undesired effects are secondary to estrogen deficiency. Common responses include hot flushes, vaginal dryness, decreased libido, mood changes, and headache. Nasal irritation also occurs. Nafarelin is teratogenic and must not be used during pregnancy.

The adverse effect of greatest concern is *bone loss.* After 3 to 6 months of treatment, bone mass and mineral content have decreased in some patients. To minimize the risk of osteoporosis, the manufacturer recommends that treatment last no longer than 6 months.

Preparations, Dosage, and Administration. Nafarelin [Synarel] is dispensed in a spray for intranasal administration. (The drug cannot be given orally because of rapid degradation by gastrointestinal enzymes.) For treatment of endometriosis, the initial dosage is 200 μg (one spray) in the morning and another 200 μg in the evening. Doses should alternate between nostrils. Treatment should begin between days 2 and 4 of the menstrual cycle.

INTRACAVERNOUS INJECTIONS FOR IMPOTENCE

Papaverine plus Phentolamine

Therapeutic Use. The combination of papaverine (a smooth muscle relaxant) plus phentolamine (an alpha-adrenergic blocking agent) can counteract impotence when injected directly into the corpus cavernosum of the penis. Erection develops within minutes and lasts for 2 to 4 hours. In clinical trials, erection suitable for coitus was produced in 65% to 100% of males whose impotence was of neurologic or vascular origin.

Mechanism of Action. Papaverine and phentolamine produce erection by (1) increasing arterial inflow to the penis, and (2) decreasing venous outflow. Arterial inflow is augmented by alpha-adrenergic blockade (causing arterial dilation) and by the direct relaxant action of papaverine on arterial smooth muscle. Venous outflow is reduced, probably because relaxation of corporal smooth muscle results in occlusion of the venules that drain the corporal spaces.

Adverse Effects. *Priapism* (persistent erection) occurs in about 10% of patients. Persistent erection can be relieved by aspiration of blood from the corpus followed by irrigation with a solution containing a vasoconstrictor (e.g., epinephrine, phenylephrine, metaraminol). Development of painless *fibrotic nodules* in the corpus is common. Other adverse effects include *orthostatic hypotension with dizziness, transient paresthesias, ecchymosis* (extravasation of blood into subcutaneous tissue), and *difficulty in achieving orgasm or ejaculation.*

Dosage and Administration. For males with psychogenic or neurogenic impotence, erection can be achieved by injecting as little as 0.1 ml of a solution containing 30 mg of papaverine/ml and 1.0 mg of phentolamine/ml. A 1-ml syringe with a 27-gauge or 28-gauge, ⅜-inch needle is used. Injections are made directly into the corpus cavernosum through the lateral aspect of the shaft of the penis. These injections are nearly painless and can be administered by the patient.

Alprostadil (Prostaglandin E₁)

Like the combination of phentolamine plus papaverine, alprostadil can produce erection in impotent males when injected directly into the corpus carvernosum. Alprostadil is as effective as phentolamine plus papaverine and causes a lower incidence of priapism and fibrotic nodules. Unfortunately, alprostadil is also more painful: transient testicular pain is common while the erection develops and may be severe. Doses range from 5 to 40 μg.

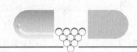

Summary of Major Nursing Implications

CLOMIPHENE

The implications summarized here apply only to the use of clomiphene for promoting maturation of ovarian follicles and ovulation. (Clomiphene has also been used investigationally to increase fertility in males.)

 Preadministration Assessmemt

Therapeutic Goal

Promotion of follicular maturation and ovulation in carefully selected patients.

Baseline Data

Take a complete health and gynecologic history; a pelvic examination and an endometrial biopsy are required. Ovarian and pituitary function must be confirmed. Pregnancy must be ruled out.

Identifying High-Risk Patients

Clomiphene is *contraindicated* during *pregnancy* and in women with *liver disease* and *abnormal uterine bleeding of undetermined origin*.

 Implementation: Administration

Route

Oral.

Administration Schedule

If cyclic menstrual bleeding has been occurring, therapy should begin 5 days after the onset of menses. If menstruation has been absent, treatment can begin at any time.

The initial course of treatment consists of 50 mg doses once daily for 5 days. If ovulation fails to occur, additional courses may be tried, each beginning no sooner than 30 days after the previous course.

Timing of Coitus

Advise the patient to have coitus at least every other day during the 5- to 10-day period that follows the last clomiphene dose.

Adjunctive Use of HCG

If ovulation fails to occur under the influence of clomiphene alone, injection of HCG 7 to 9 days after the last clomiphene dose may yield success.

 Ongoing Evaluation and Interventions

Evaluating Therapeutic Effects

Successful induction of ovulation is evaluated by monitoring for an increase in basal body temperature or plasma progesterone levels or by examining an endometrial biopsy for evidence of secretory transformation.

Minimizing Adverse Effects

Ovarian Enlargement. Instruct the patient to notify the physician if pelvic pain occurs (an indication of ovarian enlargement). If ovarian enlargement is diagnosed, clomiphene should be withdrawn, after which ovarian size usually regresses spontaneously.

Reduced Fertility. Clomiphene may cause luteal phase defect; this response can be corrected with progesterone. Alteration of cervical mucus may occur; estrogens can be used to restore the volume and fluidity of cervical secretions.

Multiple Births. Inform the patient that multiple births (usually twins) are not uncommon in clomiphene-facilitated pregnancies.

Visual Disturbances. Forewarn the patient about possible visual disturbances (blurred vision, visual flashes), and instruct her to notify the physician if these occur. Visual aberrations cease following drug withdrawal.

Other Adverse Effects. Common side effects include hot flushes (similar to the vasomotor responses of menopause), nausea, abdominal discomfort, bloating, and breast engorgement. Forewarn the patient about these effects, and instruct her to notify the physician if these reactions are especially disturbing.

MENOTROPINS

The implications summarized here refer only to the use of menotropins (together with HCG) for induction of follicular maturation and ovulation. (Menotropins is also used to treat certain forms of infertility in males.)

 Preadministration Assessment

Therapeutic Goal

Induction of follicular maturation and ovulation (in conjunction with HCG) in carefully selected patients.

Baseline Data

A thorough gynecologic and endocrinologic evaluation should precede treatment. Ovarian function must be verified. Obtain a baseline value for serum estrogen.

Identifying High-Risk Patients

Menotropins is *contraindicated* in the presence of *pregnancy*, *primary ovarian failure*, *thyroid dysfunction*, *adrenal dysfunction*, *ovarian cysts*, and *ovarian enlargement* (other than that due to polycystic ovary syndrome).

 Implementation: Administration

Route

Intramuscular.

Administration

Reconstitute powdered menotropins with sterile saline immediately prior to injection.

Menotropins is employed sequentially with HCG. Administer menotropins for 9 to 12 days (to promote follicular maturation). Twenty-four hours after the last dose, inject HCG. Ovulation follows in 2 to 3 days.

Serum estrogen content and ultrasonography are used to assess follicular maturation; upon follicular maturation, menotropins is discontinued and HCG is injected. If estrogen production is excessive (three to four times the pretreatment baseline) or if ultrasonography indicates the presence of four or more mature follicles, HCG should be withheld.

Timing of Coitus

Advise the patient to have intercourse on the eve of HCG injection and on the following 2 to 3 days (i.e., during the probable period of ovulation).

Minimizing Adverse Effects

Ongoing Evaluation and Interventions

Ovarian Hyperstimulation Syndrome. Rapid ovarian enlargement can occur, sometimes associated with ascites, pleural effusion, and pain. If ovarian enlargement is excessive, discontinue menotropins and hospitalize the patient. Treatment is supportive (bed rest, analgesics, fluid and electrolyte replacement). If ovarian cysts rupture, surgery may be required to stop bleeding. To insure early detection of ovarian enlargement, the patient should be examined at least every other day during menotropins use and for 2 weeks following drug withdrawal. Since HCG can intensify ovarian stimulation, if serum estrogen levels rise to three to four times the pretreatment baseline (suggesting existing hyperstimulation of the ovaries), HCG should not be given.

Other Adverse Effects. Forewarn the patient that treatment may result in *spontaneous abortion*. Inform the patient that *multiple births* are relatively common in menotropins-facilitated pregnancies.

HUMAN CHORIONIC GONADOTROPIN

The implications summarized here apply only to the use of HCG in the treatment of female infertility.

Therapeutic Goal

Preadministration Assessment

Induction of ovulation in women who are infertile because of anovulation. Pretreatment with menotropins or clomiphene is required.

Route

Implementation: Administration

Intramuscular.

Administration

HCG must be used in conjunction with menotropins or clomiphene. When used with menotropins, HCG is injected 1 day after the last menotropins dose. When used with clomiphene, HCG is administered 7 to 9 days after the last clomiphene dose.

Minimizing Adverse Effects

Ongoing Evaluation and Interventions

Ovarian Hyperstimulation Syndrome. See implications for menotropins.

Multiple Births. Inform the patient that multiple births are common in HCG-facilitated pregnancies.

BROMOCRIPTINE

The implications summarized here refer only to the use of bromocriptine for hyperprolactinemia. They do not apply to treatment of Parkinson's disease or to suppression of lactation.

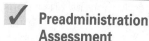

Preadministration Assessment

Therapeutic Goal

Treatment of female infertility occurring secondary to hyperprolactinemia.

Identifying High-Risk Patients

Bromocriptine is *contraindicated* during *pregnancy* and in patients with *severe ischemic heart disease* or *peripheral vascular disease.*

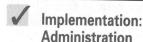

Implementation: Administration

Route

Oral.

Administration

Instruct the patient to take bromocriptine with food.

Normalization of the menstrual cycle may occur within a few days or may require up to 2 months of treatment.

Bromocriptine should be withdrawn when pregnancy is achieved, and administration should not resume until after delivery.

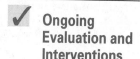

Ongoing Evaluation and Interventions

Minimizing Adverse Effects

Nausea. Inform the patient that nausea can be reduced by taking bromocriptine with meals.

Other Adverse Effects. Headache, dizziness, fatigue, and abdominal cramps can be reduced by initiating therapy at low doses.

DANAZOL

The implications summarized here refer only to the use of danazol in the treatment of endometriosis. (Danazol may also be used to treat angioneurotic edema and fibrocystic breast disease.)

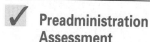

Preadministration Assessment

Therapeutic Goal

Regression of ectopic endometrial implants (endometriosis) and reversal of infertility occurring secondary to endometriosis.

Baseline Data

Obtain tests of liver function.

Identifying High-Risk Patients

Danazol is *contraindicated* during *pregnancy* and for women with *undiagnosed genital bleeding* or *severe impairment of cardiac, renal, or hepatic function.*

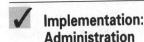

Implementation: Administration

Route

Oral.

Administration

Initiate therapy during menstruation. Treatment typically lasts 3 to 9 months. Ovulation and fertility are usually restored 1 to 3 months after danazol withdrawal.

Minimizing Adverse Effects

Ongoing Evaluation and Interventions

Impairment of Pregnancy. Danazol may temporarily impair the ability of the endometrium to support pregnancy. Caution the patient to avoid conception for about 3 months following danazol withdrawal.

Virilization. Danazol is weakly androgenic. Inform the patient about signs of masculinization (acne, deepening of the voice, growth of facial hair), and instruct her to notify the physician if these occur. Virilization usually reverses following danazol withdrawal.

Use in Pregnancy. If taken during pregnancy, danazol may cause masculinization of the female fetus. Warn the patient against becoming pregnant prior to danazol withdrawal.

Edema. Danazol may cause edema. Use with caution in the presence of cardiac and renal disease.

Liver Dysfunction. Liver dysfunction has been reported. Liver function should be assessed prior to danazol use and periodically throughout the course of treatment.

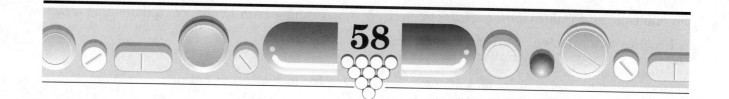

58

Uterine Stimulants and Relaxants

UTERINE STIMULANTS (OXYTOCICS)
    Oxytocin
    Ergot Alkaloids: Ergonovine and
        Methylergonovine
    Prostaglandins: Carboprost and
        Dinoprostone

UTERINE RELAXANTS (TOCOLYTICS)
    Beta$_2$-Adrenergic Agonists: Ritodrine and
        Terbutaline
    Other Uterine Relaxants

U terine contraction can be intensified or diminished with drugs. Drugs that stimulate contraction are known as *oxytocics*. Drugs that inhibit contraction are called *tocolytics*. Oxytocic agents have three applications: (1) induction or augmentation of labor, (2) control of postpartum bleeding or hemorrhage, and (3) induction of abortion. The tocolytic drugs have only one major use: suppression of preterm labor.

UTERINE STIMULANTS (OXYTOCICS)

There are three groups of uterine stimulants: (1) *oxytocin* (in a group by itself), (2) *prostaglandins*, and (3) *ergot alkaloids*. The principal indication for oxytocin is induction of labor; the principal use of prostaglandins is abortion; and the principal use of ergot alkaloids is control of postpartum bleeding.

OXYTOCIN

Oxytocin [Pitocin, Syntocinon] is a peptide hormone produced by the posterior pituitary. This hormone promotes uterine contraction during parturition and stimulates the milk-ejection reflex. The primary therapeutic use of oxytocin is induction of labor near term, a procedure for which oxytocin is the agent of choice.

Physiologic and Pharmacologic Effects

Uterine Stimulation. Oxytocin can increase the force, frequency, and duration of uterine contractions. The ability of the uterus to respond to oxytocin depends on the stage of gestation: early in pregnancy, uterine sensitivity to oxytocin is low; as pregnancy proceeds, the uterus becomes progressively more responsive; and just prior to term, a large and abrupt increase in responsiveness to oxytocin develops. These increases in sensitivity occur because the number of oxytocin receptors on uterine smooth muscle increases throughout pregnancy. Although uterine sensitivity to oxytocin is low early in pregnancy, oxytocin can still initiate and enhance contractions at this stage. However, the doses required are much larger than those needed to stimulate the uterus at term.

Despite the profound effects of oxytocin on uterine contractility, the precise role of oxytocin in natural labor and delivery has not been established. We do know that administration of exogenous oxytocin can elicit contractions identical to those seen during spontaneous labor. However, we also know that parturition can take place with virtually no oxytocin present, although labor will be prolonged. Furthermore, during normal labor or during labor induced artificially (through rupture of the membranes), only modest increases in plasma oxytocin levels are observed. From these observations we can conclude that although oxytocin is not absolutely required for parturition, it is likely that oxytocin serves to facilitate production of contractions. However, it is not certain that oxytocin is responsible for actually *initiating* the process of labor.

Milk Ejection. Milk is produced by glandular tissue of the breast and is later transferred, via small channels, into large sinuses within the breast. Once in these sinuses, milk is readily accessible to the suckling infant. Transfer of milk to the sinuses is brought about by the milk-ejection reflex: when the infant sucks on the breast, neuronal stimuli are sent to the posterior pituitary, causing release of oxytocin; oxytocin then causes contraction of the smooth muscle surrounding the small milk channels, thereby forcing milk into the large sinuses. In the absence of oxytocin, milk ejection does not occur.

Water Retention. Oxytocin is similar in structure to antidiuretic hormone (ADH), a compound that acts on the kidney to decrease excretion of water. Although less potent than ADH, oxytocin can promote renal retention of water.

Pharmacokinetics

Oxytocin is usually administered IV or IM; intranasal application is used for some indications. The plasma half-life of oxytocin is extremely short, ranging from 12 to 17 minutes. Elimination is by a combination of hepatic metabolism and renal excretion.

Use for Induction of Labor

Rationale. Induction of labor is reserved for those pregnancies in which early vaginal delivery is likely to decrease morbidity and mortality for either the mother or the infant. The most common reason for induction is premature rupture of the membranes. Other acceptable indications include severe maternal infection, diabetes mellitus, placental insufficiency, renal insufficiency, anemia, antepartum bleeding, and preeclampsia (at or near term). Labor should be induced only when the risk of continued pregnancy constitutes a greater risk to the mother and fetus than the risk of induction itself. Induction should not be performed for elective purposes (e.g., convenience of the obstetrician).

Precautions and Contraindications. Improper use of oxytocin can be hazardous. Uterine rupture may occur, which may result in death of the mother, infant, or both. The likelihood of trauma is especially high in the presence of cephalopelvic disproportion, fetal malpresentation, placental abnormalities, previous uterine surgery, and fetal distress. Oxytocin is contraindicated in pregnancies with any of these characteristics. Induction of labor in women of high parity (five or more pregnancies) carries a high risk of uterine rupture; oxytocin must be used with special caution in these patients.

Adverse Effect: Water Intoxication. When administered in large doses, oxytocin exerts an antidiuretic effect. If large volumes of fluid have been administered along with oxytocin, retention of water may produce intoxication. However, at the doses employed to induce labor, water intoxication is rare.

Dosage and Administration. For induction of labor, oxytocin is administered by intravenous infusion. The flow rate must be carefully controlled, preferably with an infusion pump. Solutions should be dilute (e.g., 10 mU/ml) and infused at an initial rate of no more than 1 to 2 mU/min. The infusion rate is then gradually increased (by increments of 1 to 2 mU/min every 30 to 60 minutes) until uterine contractions resembling those of spontaneous labor have been produced (i.e., contractions every 2 to 3 minutes and lasting 45 to 60 seconds). The infusion rate should rarely exceed 10 mU/min.

During oxytocin infusion, constant monitoring is required. The mother should be monitored for uterine contractility (frequency, duration, intensity), blood pressure, and pulse rate. The fetus should be monitored for heart rate and rhythm. In the event of significant maternal or fetal distress, the infusion should be stopped; this will cause contractions to diminish rapidly. Complications that usually require interruption of the infusion are (1) elevation of resting uterine pressure above 15 to 20 mm Hg, (2) contractions that persist for more than 1 minute, (3) contractions that occur more often than every 2 to 3 minutes, and (4) pronounced alteration in fetal heart rate or rhythm.

Additional Therapeutic Uses

Augmentation of Labor. Oxytocin may be employed if labor is *dysfunctional*. However, patients must be judiciously selected, and oxytocin dosage must be regulated with special care. As a rule, oxytocic agents should not be used to promote labor that is already in progress, even if that labor is proceeding slowly: by intensifying the force of contractions, oxytocin may cause uterine damage (laceration or rupture) or trauma to the infant.

Postpartum Use. Oxytocin can be administered after placental delivery to control bleeding or hemorrhage and to increase uterine tone. Administration may be IM or IV.

Milk Ejection. Oxytocin has been used to promote milk ejection in nursing mothers. When employed for this purpose, the drug is administered by nasal spray 2 to 3 minutes prior to breast-feeding. Unfortunately, this treatment frequently fails. In addition, since oxytocin acts only to cause milk ejection, this agent will be of no help in cases of insufficient milk production.

Abortion. Oxytocin has been employed during the second trimester for management of incomplete abortion. Intravenous infusion of 10 units at a rate of 10 to 20 mU/min is often effective in emptying the uterus. However, oxytocin is not the treatment of choice: during the first trimester, suction procedures are preferable to oxytocin; in the second trimester, prostaglandins are usually preferred.

Preparations

Oxytocin [Pitocin, Syntocinon] is available as an injection (10 U/ml) for IV and IM administration. The drug is also dispensed as a spray (40 U/ml) for intranasal application.

ERGOT ALKALOIDS: ERGONOVINE AND METHYLERGONOVINE

Ergot is a dried preparation of *Claviceps purpurea*, a fungus that grows on rye plants. The ergot alkaloids are compounds present in ergot. Ergot is capable of inducing powerful uterine contractions, a fact known to midwifes for centuries. Analysis of ergot has revealed the presence of several pharmacologically active constituents. Of these, *ergonovine* has proved the most effective uterine stimulant. A derivative of ergonovine—*methylergonovine*—has been synthesized and produces effects very much like those of the natural alkaloid. Because the actions of ergonovine and methylergonovine are so similar, we will consider these agents jointly.

Pharmacologic Effects

The ergot alkaloids produce their effects by acting at a variety of receptors (adrenergic, dopamin-

ergic, serotonergic). These drugs exert their most profound effects on uterine and vascular smooth muscle.

Effects on the Uterus. Ergot alkaloids stimulate uterine contraction. In small doses, these agents produce contractions of moderate strength that alternate with uterine relaxation of a normal degree and duration. With large doses, the force and frequency of contractions are greatly increased, and the extent of uterine relaxation is reduced; sustained contraction is not uncommon. Because contractions may be prolonged, *ergot alkaloids are not employed for induction of labor.*

Vascular Effects. Ergot alkaloids can cause constriction of arterioles and veins. This ability is the basis for using certain ergot alkaloids (ergotamine, dihydroergotamine) to treat migraine headache (see Chapter 29).

Pharmacokinetics

Regardless of route of administration, ergonovine and methylergonovine act rapidly. Uterine contractions begin within 60 seconds of IV injection, and within 10 minutes of oral and IM administration. Effects persist for several hours.

Therapeutic Uses

Postpartum Use. The ergot alkaloids are given postpartum and postabortion to increase uterine tone and decrease bleeding. The ability of these drugs to induce sustained uterine contraction makes them especially well suited for these purposes. Administration is usually delayed until after delivery of the placenta. The patient should be monitored for blood pressure, pulse rate, and uterine contractility. Cramping occurs as part of the therapeutic response, but may also indicate overdosage.

Augmentation of Labor. Because contractions may be both intense and prolonged, ergot alkaloids are not recommended for use during labor. If these drugs are given during labor, excessive uterine tone can cause trauma to the mother and fetus. Placental blood flow may be reduced, resulting in fetal hypoxia and uterine rupture. In addition, cervical laceration may occur.

Migraine. Ergot alkaloids relieve migraine in part by constricting dilated cerebral blood vessels. The two ergot preparations employed in migraine are ergotamine and dihydroergotamine. The pharmacology of these drugs and the treatment of migraine are discussed in Chapter 29 (Drugs for Headache).

Adverse Effects

When ergot alkaloids are given orally or IM, significant adverse effects are rare. In contrast, IV administration frequently results in *hypertension*. This reaction can be severe and may be associated with nausea, vomiting, and headache; convulsions and even death have occurred. Accordingly, IV injection should be reserved for emergencies. Furthermore, patients with pre-existing hypertension should not be given these drugs. Caution should be exercised in the presence of cardiovascular, renal, and hepatic disorders.

Contraindications

Ergot alkaloids are contraindicated for women who are pregnant, hypertensive, or hypersensitive to these drugs. These drugs are also contraindicated for induction of labor and for use in the presence of threatened or ongoing spontaneous abortion.

Preparations, Dosage, and Administration

Preparations. Ergonovine maleate [Ergotrate Maleate] and methylergonovine maleate [Methergine] are both dispensed in solution (0.2 mg/ml) for IV and IM administration, and in tablets (0.2 mg) for oral administration.

Dosage and Administration. Ergonovine and methylergonovine are usually administered IM or PO. Intravenous administration is hazardous and should be reserved for emergency control of postpartum hemorrhage. Administration is usually performed only after passage of the placenta. Dosage for both drugs is as follows: *intramuscular* (for control of postpartum bleeding), 0.2 mg initially, repeated in 2 to 4 hours if needed; *intravenous* (for control of uterine hemorrhage), 0.2 mg infused over 60 seconds or more; and *oral* (to minimize postpartum bleeding), 0.2 to 0.4 mg every 6 to 12 hours (usually for 2 days).

PROSTAGLANDINS: CARBOPROST AND DINOPROSTONE

Prostaglandins are synthesized in all tissues of the body, where they act as local hormones. Unlike true hormones, which travel to distant sites to produce their effects, prostaglandins act on the very tissues in which they are made; degradation of prostaglandins is so rapid that these agents rarely escape their tissue of origin intact. Although the prostaglandins produce a broad spectrum of physiologic effects (see Chapter 59), clinical use of these compounds is limited. At this time, the principal obstetric application of prostaglandins is induction of abortion.

Physiologic and Pharmacologic Effects

Uterine Stimulation. Prostaglandins, like oxytocin, can increase the force, frequency, and duration of uterine contractions. In the early months of pregnancy, the uterus is more responsive to prostaglandins than to oxytocin. During the second and third trimesters, prostaglandins can induce contractions of sufficient strength to cause complete evacuation of the uterus.

Like oxytocin, prostaglandins appear to have a physiologic role as promoters of uterine contraction, spontaneous labor, and delivery. Observations supporting this statement include: (1) exogenous prostaglandins can induce uterine contractions that are very similar in frequency and duration to those that occur spontaneously, (2) the ability of the uterus to synthesize prostaglandins increases at term, (3) the prostaglandin content of amniotic fluid, umbilical blood, and maternal blood increases at term and during labor, and (4) labor is delayed and prolonged by agents that inhibit prostaglandin synthesis.

Cervical Softening. Local application of prostaglandins produces cervical softening. This softening results from breakdown of collagen, and, hence, mimics the process by which natural cervical ripening occurs. Softening of the cervix is not dependent on uterine stimulation.

Therapeutic Uses

Termination of Pregnancy. Prostaglandins are used to induce second trimester abortion. Uterine contractions develop slowly. As a result, about 18 hours must pass before expulsion of the fetus takes place. Unlike other abortifacients, prostaglandins are not feticidal; hence, the aborted fetus may show transient signs of life. Prostaglandins have been proved teratogenic in animals. Therefore, if abortion fails, it is important that pregnancy be terminated by an alternative procedure (e.g., administration of oxytocin or hypertonic saline). Following passage of the fetus and placenta, the patient should be examined for possible cervical or uterine laceration.

Selection of an abortifacient depends on the duration of gestation. During the first trimester (weeks 1 to 12), suction is the procedure of choice; except for mifepristone (RU 486) (see Chapter 56) drugs are ineffective during this time. In the second trimester (weeks 13 to 20), dilation plus evacuation is the generally preferred procedure. However, several chemical agents may also be used, including prostaglandins, oxytocin, saline, and urea. (Oxytocin is not very effective but may be used as an adjunct to the prostaglandins.) Hypertonic solutions of saline and urea (administered by intra-amniotic instillation) produce abortion by acting as poisons to the placenta and fetus.

Other Applications. One prostaglandin (carboprost) is indicated for control of *postpartum hemorrhage*. This drug is reserved for bleeding that has been refractory to more conventional agents (oxytocin, ergot alkaloids). In these situations, carboprost may be lifesaving. Another prostaglandin (dinoprostone) is used to *initiate ripening of the cervix* (prior to induction of labor); also, the drug has been used investigationally for *induction of labor*.

Adverse Effects

Gastrointestinal Disturbances. Gastrointestinal reactions are extremely common and result from the ability of prostaglandins to stimulate the smooth muscle of the alimentary canal. Vomiting and diarrhea occur in up to 60% of those treated. Nausea also occurs frequently. These responses can be reduced by pretreatment with antiemetic and antidiarrheal medications.

Cervical or Uterine Laceration. Intense uterine contractions can result in cervical or uterine laceration. The patient should be examined thoroughly for trauma following expulsion of the fetus and placenta.

Other Adverse Effects. *Fever* is common. When hyperthermia develops, it is important to distinguish between drug-induced fever and pyrexia resulting from endometritis. With *dinoprostone*, there is a 10% incidence of headache, shivering, and chills.

Precautions and Contraindications

Prostaglandins are contraindicated for women with acute pelvic inflammatory disease and active disease of the heart, lungs, kidneys, or liver. These drugs should be used with caution in women with a history of asthma, hypotension, hypertension, diabetes, or uterine scarring.

Preparations, Dosage, and Administration

Carboprost Tromethamine. Carboprost tromethamine [Hemabate] is dispensed as an injection containing 250 µg of carboprost per ml. Administration is IM. For *induction of abortion* (weeks 13 to 20), the dosage is 250 µg initially followed by 250 µg every 1.5 to 3.5 hours as needed. For *control of postpartum bleeding*, a single 250 µg dose is injected.

Dinoprostone. Dinoprostone is available in two formulations: (1) 20-mg vaginal suppositories, and (2) a gel (0.5 mg dinoprostone/2.5 ml gel) in prefilled syringes with shielded endocervical catheters (10- and 20-mm tip). Dinoprostone suppositories [Prostin E2] are used for abortion. Dinoprostone gel [Prepidil] is used for cervical ripening.

For induction of *abortion* (weeks 12 to 20), one 20-mg vaginal suppository is inserted initially, followed by one suppository every 3 to 5 hours as needed.

For *cervical ripening*, 0.5 mg of dinoprostone gel is introduced into the cervical canal just below the level of the internal os. The drug is administered using the prefilled syringe supplied by the manufacturer and fitted with the appropriate endocervical catheter. If the desired response has not occurred within 6 hours, an additional 0.5-mg dose can be given. If necessary, a third 0.5-mg dose can be given 6 hours later.

UTERINE RELAXANTS (TOCOLYTICS)

Uterine relaxants (tocolytics) are given to prevent premature delivery (i.e., delivery prior to the 37th week of gestation). The drugs employed most frequently are beta$_2$-adrenergic agonists: ritodrine and terbutaline. These agents have largely replaced older tocolytics (magnesium sulfate, ethanol) for delaying preterm labor.

BETA$_2$-ADRENERGIC AGONISTS: RITODRINE AND TERBUTALINE

Two beta$_2$-adrenergic agonists—ritodrine and terbutaline—are used to delay preterm labor. Although both drugs are effective, only ritodrine has received FDA approval for this application.

Ritodrine

Ritodrine [Yutopar] is classified as a beta$_2$-selective adrenergic agonist. Despite this classification, ritodrine also stimulates beta$_1$-adrenergic receptors, although less readily than beta$_2$ receptors. By causing beta$_1$ and beta$_2$ stimulation, ritodrine can elicit all of the effects characteristic of other beta-adrenergic agonists. These effects are described fully in Chapter 17.

Effect on the Uterus. Stimulation of uterine beta$_2$ receptors relaxes uterine smooth muscle. Following oral or IV administration, ritodrine decreases both the intensity and frequency of uterine contractions. Ritodrine-induced relaxation can be prevented with a beta-adrenergic blocker (e.g., propranolol).

Therapeutic Use. The only indication for ritodrine is suppression of preterm labor. Delivery may be delayed for *weeks* (to permit full-term intrauterine development) or labor may be suppressed for just a few *days* (while glucocorticoids are given to promote maturation of the fetal lungs). Ritodrine is not given if gestation has been less than 20 weeks, and use of ritodrine beyond the 34th week of gestation is rare. Therapy is most effective early in pregnancy and early in labor. Efficacy in advanced labor is uncertain. Treatment is begun with an intravenous infusion (for about 12 hours). Thereafter, oral therapy is instituted to maintain suppression of labor.

Adverse Effects. Significant adverse effects with *oral* ritodrine are rare. The adverse effects described below are associated with *intravenous* administration.

Pulmonary Edema. Intravenous ritodrine has caused pulmonary edema. The risk appears higher when glucocorticoids are given concurrently, and when the infusion fluid is isotonic saline. Accordingly, 5% dextrose may be the preferred fluid. Some physicians recommend limiting total fluid intake to 2.5 L over 24 hours. The patient should be monitored for fluid overload. If pulmonary edema develops, the infusion should be discontinued and standard treatment implemented.

Tachycardia. Intravenous ritodrine almost always elevates maternal and fetal heart rate. Tachycardia results from stimulation of beta$_1$ receptors in the heart. Maternal and fetal heart rate should be monitored. Excessive tachycardia can usually be corrected by reducing the rate of infusion.

Hypotension. Blood pressure may be reduced because of vasodilation brought about by stimulation of beta$_2$ receptors on blood vessels. Hypotension can be minimized by keeping the patient in a left-lateral recumbent position.

Hyperglycemia. Intravenous ritodrine elevates blood glucose levels by stimulating beta$_2$ receptors in the liver. For most patients hyperglycemia is transient. However, hyperglycemia is likely to persist in insulin-dependent diabetics. Insulin infusion is usually required to prevent ketoacidosis in these patients.

Precautions and Contraindications. Ritodrine should be employed only if the benefits of continued pregnancy outweigh the risks associated with drug-induced delay of delivery. Conditions for which the risks are considered too high include eclampsia, severe preeclampsia, hemorrhage, chorioamnionitis, maternal heart disease, and gestation of less than 20-weeks' duration. In these cases ritodrine is contraindicated. In addition, ritodrine must be used with caution in the presence of hyperthyroidism (because of heightened cardiac sensitivity to beta$_1$ stimulants) and in women with insulin-dependent diabetes.

Preparations, Dosage, and Administration. Ritodrine hydrochloride [Yutopar] is dispensed as an injection (10 and 15 mg/ml) for intravenous administration and in tablets (10 mg) for oral administration.

Intravenous therapy is used initially to arrest labor rapidly; later, the patient is switched to oral ritodrine for long-term suppression. Infusion is begun at a rate of 0.1 mg/min. This rate may be increased gradually until contractions have ceased or until the maximum acceptable rate (0.35 mg/min) has been reached. Infusion is continued for 12 hours after labor has stopped. Oral therapy is begun 30 minutes prior to terminating the infusion. The initial oral dosage is 10 mg every 2 hours for 24 hours. After this, the dosage is 10 to 20 mg every 4 to 6 hours (to a maximum of 120 mg daily). Oral therapy is continued for as long as suppression of labor is considered desirable. If contractions recur, IV treatment can be reinstated.

Terbutaline

Terbutaline [Brethine, Bricanyl], is a beta$_2$-selective adrenergic agonist that is much like ritodrine in its actions, adverse effects, and potential uses. The principal indication for terbutaline is asthma (see Chapter 64). In addition, the drug is also widely used to delay preterm labor, although it is not FDA approved for this application. Therapy is initiated with an IV infusion at a rate of 10 μg/min; the rate is then gradually increased to a maximum of 80 μg/min. After contractions have been suppressed with IV therapy, oral therapy (2.5 mg every 4 to 6 hours) is used for maintenance. For delay of labor, terbutaline appears superior to ritodrine in two ways: (1) recurrence of labor during oral therapy with terbutaline is less common than during oral therapy with ritodrine, and (3) terbutaline is much less expensive than ritodrine.

OTHER UTERINE RELAXANTS

Magnesium Sulfate (Intravenous). The primary obstetric use of magnesium sulfate is control of seizures associated with eclampsia and severe preeclampsia. However, magnesium may also be given to suppress preterm labor. Magnesium sulfate causes uterine relaxation through a direct effect on uterine smooth muscle; both the force and frequency of contractions are reduced. Arrest of labor is achieved at plasma levels of magnesium ranging from 4 to 7 mEq/L. At levels greater than these, substantial inhibition of cardiac conduction and neuromuscular transmission may occur, resulting in cardiac arrest and respiratory depression. Because it does not sensitize the heart to catecholamines or promote hyperglycemia, magnesium sulfate may be preferred to beta$_2$ agonists for suppressing preterm labor in women with hyperthyroidism or diabetes.

Ethanol (Intravenous). Once used widely to inhibit preterm labor, intravenous ethanol is rarely given for this purpose today; availability of superior agents (e.g., ritodrine) has rendered ethanol obsolete. Ethanol is thought to decrease uterine contractions by inhibiting release of oxytocin from the pituitary. To suppress labor, ethanol must achieve plasma levels of 0.12% to 0.18%. At these levels, inebriation, nausea, and vomiting can be considerable. One of the limitations of ethanol is its short span of action: labor cannot be suppressed for more than a few hours, or at most a few days.

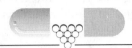 # Summary of Major Nursing Implications

---

OXYTOCIN

The implications summarized here apply only to the use of oxytocin for induction of labor, the principal use of this drug.

 Preadministration Assessment

Therapeutic Goal

Oxytocin is given to initiate or improve uterine contractions so as to achieve early vaginal delivery. Treatment is reserved for pregnancies in which induction is likely to decrease morbidity and mortality for the mother or the infant.

Baseline Data

The history should determine parity, previous obstetric problems, stillbirths, and abortions. Full maternal and fetal status should be assessed.

Identifying High-Risk Patients

Induction of labor is *contraindicated* in the presence of *cephalopelvic disproportion, fetal malpresentation, placental abnormality, previous major surgery to the uterus or cervix,* and *fetal distress.*

Use with *caution* in women of *high parity* (five or more pregnancies).

 Implementation: Administration

Route

Intravenous.

Administration

Administer by carefully controlled infusion, preferably with an infusion pump.

 Ongoing Evaluation and Interventions

Minimizing Adverse Effects

Uterine contractions of excessive intensity, frequency, and duration can cause maternal and fetal harm. Monitor uterine contractility (frequency, duration, intensity), maternal blood pressure, and fetal and maternal heart rate. Interrupt the infusion if any of the following occur: (1) resting intrauterine pressure rises above 15 to 20 mm Hg, (2) individual contractions persist longer than 1 minute, (3) contractions occur more often than every 2 to 3 minutes, and (4) fetal heart rate or rhythm changes significantly.

ERGOT ALKALOIDS: ERGONOVINE AND METHYLERGONOVINE

 Preadministration Assessment

Therapeutic Goal

Ergonovine and methylergonovine are used for prevention and treatment of postpartum and postabortion hemorrhage.

Identifying High-Risk Patients

Ergot alkaloids are contraindicated *during pregnancy, for induction of labor*, in women with *hypertension or allergy to ergot alkaloids*, and *in the presence of threatened or ongoing spontaneous abortion.*

**Implementation:
Administration**

Routes

Oral and IM administration are usual. Intravenous administration is hazardous and reserved for hemorrhagic emergencies.

Administration

As a rule, administration is postponed until after passage of the placenta. Perform IV injections slowly (over 60 seconds or more).

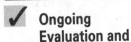

**Ongoing
Evaluation and
Interventions**

Evaluating Therapeutic Effects

Monitor blood pressure, pulse rate, and uterine activity. Report sudden increases in blood pressure, excessive uterine bleeding, and insufficient uterine tone. Cramping is normal but may also indicate overdosage.

Minimizing Adverse Effects

Significant adverse effects—*hypertension, nausea, vomiting, headache, convulsions, death*—usually occur only with IV administration. To minimize risk, infuse slowly (over 60 seconds or more) and reserve IV administration for emergencies.

PROSTAGLANDINS: CARBOPROST AND DINOPROSTONE

**Preadministration
Assessment**

Therapeutic Goal

Prostaglandins are used for *induction of abortion* (carboprost, dinoprostone), *control of postpartum hemorrhage* (carboprost), *induction of labor* (dinoprostone), and *initiation of cervical ripening* (dinoprostone).

Identifying High-Risk Patients

Prostaglandins are *contraindicated* for women with *acute pelvic inflammatory disease* and *active disease of the heart, lungs, kidneys, or liver*. These drugs should be used with *caution* in women with a *history of asthma, hypotension, hypertension, diabetes, or uterine scarring.*

**Implementation:
Administration**

Routes

Carboprost: intramuscular.
Dinoprostone: vaginal suppository, gel for intracervical instillation.

**Ongoing
Evaluation and
Interventions**

Evaluation of Therapeutic Effects

Termination of Pregnancy. Monitor and record intensity, frequency, and duration of contractions. If treatment fails to terminate pregnancy, an alternative procedure (e.g., use of oxytocin or hypertonic saline) should be employed.

Minimizing Adverse Effects

Gastrointestinal Disturbances. Nausea, vomiting, and diarrhea can be reduced by pretreatment with antiemetic and antidiarrheal drugs.

Fever. Fever may be prostaglandin-induced or it may indicate endometritis. If fever develops, a differential diagnosis must be made.

Cervical or Uterine Laceration. Use for abortion may result in cervical or uterine laceration. Examine the patient thoroughly for trauma following expulsion of the fetus and placenta.

RITODRINE AND TERBUTALINE: BETA₂-ADRENERGIC AGONISTS USED TO DELAY PRETERM LABOR

 Preadministration Assessment

Therapeutic Goal

Delay of preterm labor in pregnancies between 20 and 34 weeks' duration. An accurate determination of gestational age is required.

Baseline Data

Determine maternal heart rate, blood pressure, blood glucose, and fluid status. Determine fetal heart rate.

Identifying High-Risk Patients

Ritodrine is *contraindicated* in the presence of *eclampsia, severe preeclampsia, hemorrhage, chorioamnionitis, maternal heart disease,* and *gestation of less than 20 weeks' duration.* Exercise *caution* in women with *hyperthyroidism* and *insulin-dependent diabetes..*

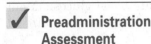 **Implementation: Administration**

Routes

Oral, IV.

Administration

Begin therapy with an IV infusion and continue the infusion for 12 hours after contractions cease. Begin oral maintenance therapy 30 minutes before terminating the infusion. Continue oral therapy for as long as suppression of labor is considered desirable. If contractions recur, reinstitute IV administration.

 Ongoing Evaluation and Interventions

Monitoring Summary

Monitor maternal blood pressure, heart rate, blood glucose, and fluid status. Monitor fetal heart rate.

Evaluating Therapeutic Effects

Warn the outpatient on oral therapy that contractions may resume. Instruct her to return to the hospital for intravenous therapy if oral therapy becomes ineffective.

Minimizing Adverse Effects

Significant adverse effects occur primarily with IV administration; side effects of oral therapy are usually minor.

Pulmonary Edema. Intravenous ritodrine may cause pulmonary edema. Monitor the patient for fluid overload. If pulmonary edema develops, discontinue the infusion.

Concurrent therapy with glucocorticoids increases the risk of edema, as does the use of isotonic saline for the infusion fluid. The risk may be reduced by using 5% dextrose for the infusion fluid and by limiting total fluid intake to 2.5 L over 24 hours.

Tachycardia. Intravenous treatment almost always causes maternal and fetal tachycardia. Monitor maternal and fetal heart rate and reduce the dosage if tachycardia is excessive.

Hypotension. Ritodrine- and terbutaline-induced vasodilation can cause hypotension. Monitor blood pressure. Hypotension can be minimized by having the patient assume a left-lateral recumbent position.

Hyperglycemia. Intravenous beta$_2$ agonists elevate blood glucose. Monitor blood glucose levels. Insulin-dependent diabetics are likely to require insulin infusion.

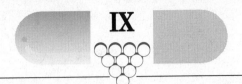

Prostaglandins and Related Drugs

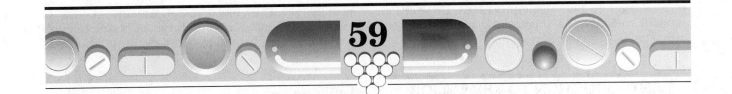

59

Eicosanoids: Prostaglandins and Related Agents

The eicosanoids—*prostaglandins, prostacyclin, thromboxane A₂*, and *leukotrienes*—constitute a diverse group of compounds with a broad spectrum of biologic actions. Eicosanoids of one type or another are found in virtually every tissue of the body. The eicosanoid family is so named because all of its members are derived from eicosanoic (20-carbon) fatty acids.

The eicosanoids are produced locally to elicit local effects. In contrast to some local hormones, which are synthesized and then stored for release at a later time, the eicosanoids are made "on demand." Degradation of the eicosanoids is usually rapid; these agents frequently have half-lives of less than 10 minutes.

Because of their many different effects, the eicosanoids are of great therapeutic interest. Drugs that can either mimic or prevent eicosanoid actions have the potential for producing multiple beneficial effects. Two important classes of medicines—the "aspirin-like" drugs and the glucocorticoids—act in large part by inhibiting eicosanoid synthesis. To date, only a few eicosanoids have been approved for therapeutic use, primarily as uterine stimulants. The clinical potential of many other eicosanoids is under investigation.

Our principal objective in this chapter is to establish an overview of the eicosanoid family. Emphasis is on the biosynthesis, pharmacologic effects, and possible roles of eicosanoids in physiologic and pathologic processes. In addition, we will consider the therapeutic potential of the eicosanoids.

INTRODUCTION TO THE MAJOR EICOSANOID CLASSES

There are four classes of eicosanoids: prostaglandins, thromboxanes, prostacyclins, and leukotrienes. The characteristic properties of these groups are discussed below.

Prostaglandins

The prostaglandins (PGs) were the first eicosanoids to be discovered. These compounds are present in most tissues of the body and can produce a wide variety of biologic effects. Prostaglandins were initially prepared by extraction from seminal fluid and from male accessory reproductive glands; hence, the family name.

The first two PGs to be isolated were named prostaglandin E (PGE) and prostaglandin F (PGF). The letters E and F refer to *ether* and *fosfate* (Swedish for phosphate), the solvents employed for extracting these PGs. As can be seen in Figure 59–1, PGE and PGF are structurally identical except in the configurations of their five-membered rings. In addition to prostaglandins E and F, six other types of prostaglandins have been identified. The eight PG groups currently known are named prostaglandins A through H. These prostaglandins are identified by the structures of their five-membered rings (Fig. 59–2).

The names of prostaglandins and other eicosanoids usually bear a numerical subscript (e.g., PGA_1, PGE_2). This subscript refers to the number of double bonds in the molecule. In humans, practically all endogenous eicosanoids contain two double bonds. Hence, their names bear the subscript 2. Figure 59–1 illustrates the use of numerical subscripts to indicate the number of double bonds in the eicosanoid molecule.

Thromboxanes

Thromboxane A_2 is the principal representative of the thromboxane family. This compound is found almost exclusively in platelets. The name *thromboxane* reflects the role of this agent as a promoter of thrombus formation (platelet aggregation). Thromboxane differs structurally from the prostaglandins in that it contains a six-membered ring (see Fig. 59–1).

Prostacyclin (Prostaglandin I₂)

Prostacyclin, also known as prostaglandin I_2, is in a class by itself. This compound is produced primarily within blood-vessel walls, and acts to cause vasodilation and inhibition of platelet aggregation. The structure of prostacyclin is shown in Figure 59–1.

Leukotrienes

The leukotrienes are so named because they were discovered in leukocytes, and because they can be classified chemically as trienes (molecules that contain three conjugated double bonds). Several subgroups of leukotrienes have been identified. These are named leukotrienes A, B, C, and D. The leukotrienes are mediators of inflammatory responses and severe allergic reactions (anaphylaxis). Production of leukotrienes is limited to the lungs, mast cells, leukocytes, and platelets. The structure of leukotriene C_4 is shown in Figure 59–1.

SYNTHESIS AND DEGRADATION OF EICOSANOIDS

Synthesis

The eicosanoids are produced in response to a variety of stimuli (e.g., chemicals, hormones, local trauma). Since these compounds are not stored in tissues, synthesis immediately precedes observed effects.

In humans, *arachidonic acid* (eicosatetraenoic acid) is the precursor of eicosanoid synthesis. Arachidonic acid employed for eicosanoid production is present in the body as an esterified component of cell-membrane phospholipids. Hence, before arachidonic acid can act as a substrate for eicosanoid synthesis, it must first be freed from the cell membrane. As indicated in Figure 59–3, liberation of arachidonic acid is accomplished by an enzyme named *phospholipase A_2*. This enzyme is activated by the various physical, chemical, and hormonal stimuli that induce eicosanoid synthesis.

Following liberation of arachidonic acid, the pathway of eicosanoid synthesis divides (see Fig. 59–3). One branch of the pathway is catalyzed by *lipoxygenase*; the other branch is catalyzed by *cyclooxygenase*. The lipoxygenase branch leads to the production of leukotrienes. The cyclooxygenase branch produces prostaglandins, prostacyclin, and thromboxane A_2. The cyclooxygenase branch contains two enzymes worth noting (in addition to cyclooxygenase itself). One of these enzymes— *thromboxane synthetase*—is required for production of thromboxane A_2. The other enzyme—*prostacyclin synthetase*—catalyzes the synthesis of prostacyclin (PGI_2). Production of prostaglandins E_2 and F_2 alpha, the principal PGs in the body, is catalyzed by isomerases that act on PGH.

The ability to synthesize specific eicosanoids

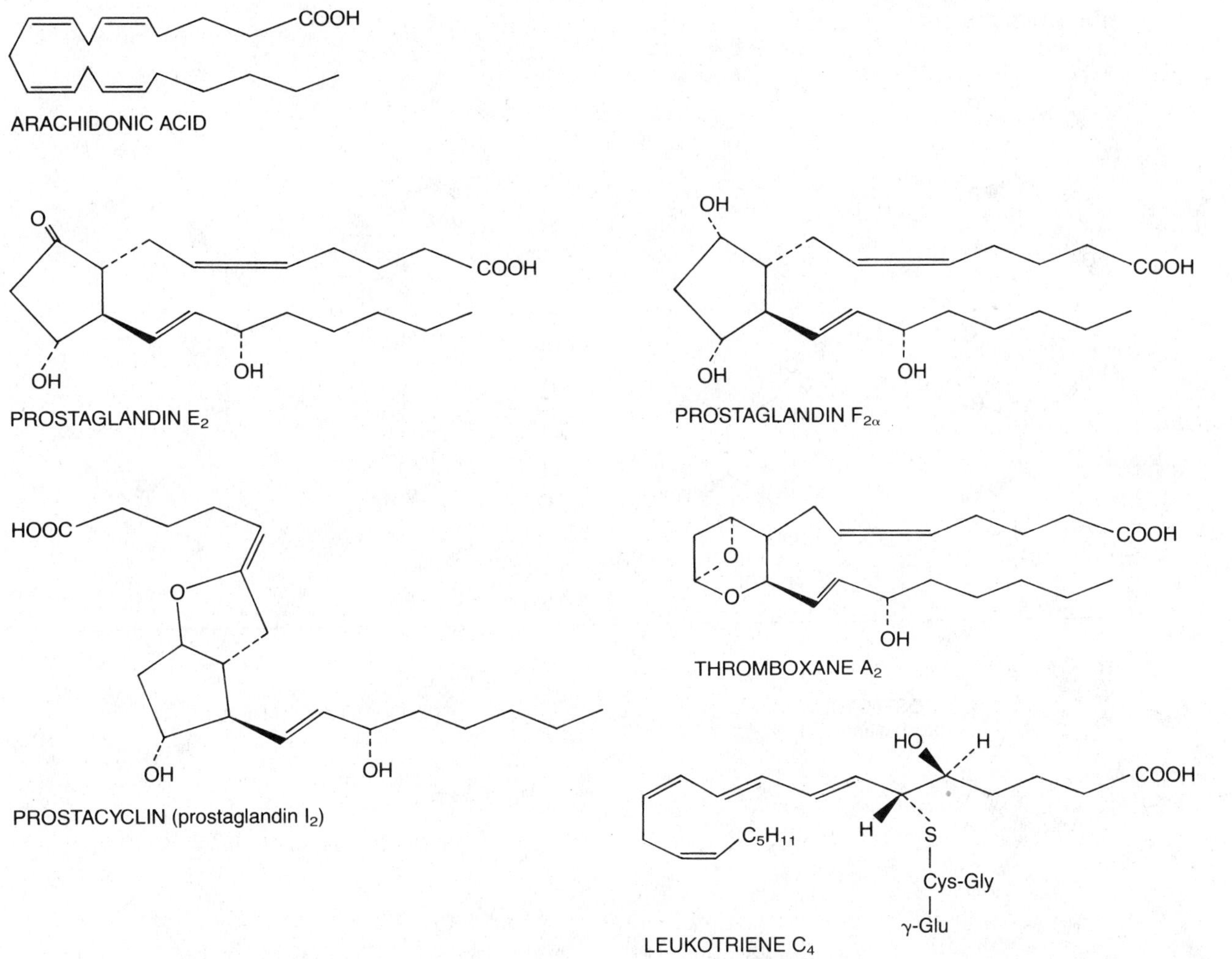

Figure 59–1. Structures of arachidonic acid and some representative eicosanoids.

varies among tissues. The lungs and spleen, for example, can manufacture all of the arachidonic acid products. This contrasts with platelets, which are equipped primarily for synthesis of thromboxane A_2, and with the blood vessel wall, where PGI_2 is the predominant eicosanoid produced.

Degradation

Enzymes for the inactivation of prostaglandins are widely distributed. Their presence has been demonstrated in the liver, lungs, spleen, kidneys, adipose tissue, and other sites. Degradative activity is especially high in the lungs; the lungs can, for example, produce 95% inactivation of PGE_2 in the blood during a single pass through the pulmonary circulation. Because enzymes for their degradation are so prevalent, PGs are rapidly cleared from the blood.

Thromboxane A_2 (TXA_2) and PGI_2 are chemically unstable. Both compounds undergo rapid, nonenzymatic conversion to inactive products. The half-life of TXA_2 is about 30 seconds; the half-life of PGI_2 is 3 minutes.

In contrast to PGs and TXA_2, leukotrienes are broken down slowly. This slow inactivation accounts for the persistent effects of these compounds.

PHARMACOLOGIC ACTIONS OF THE EICOSANOIDS

Eicosanoids can influence the function of virtually all tissues. In this section we will focus on the major responses that can be elicited by *pharmacologic* doses of eicosanoids. It should be kept in mind, however, that responses to exogenous eicosanoids do not necessarily reflect the roles played by eicosanoids produced in the body. For example, although we know that high doses of prostaglandins can produce luteolysis (regression of the corpus luteum), we cannot conclude from this observation that prostaglandins serve as physiologic regulators of the menstrual cycle. The possible physiologic roles of the eicosanoids are considered later in the chapter.

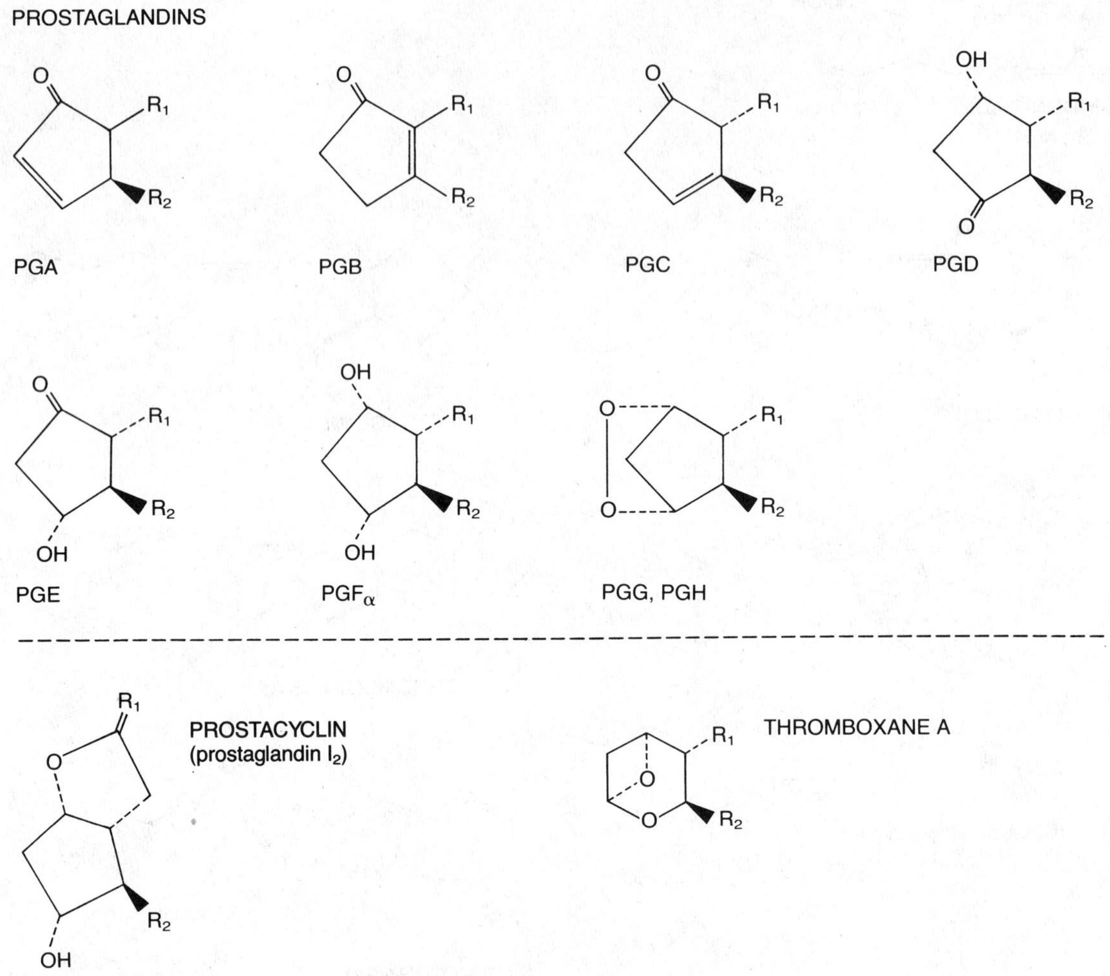

PROSTAGLANDINS

PGA   PGB   PGC   PGD

PGE   PGF$_\alpha$ PGG, PGH

PROSTACYCLIN
(prostaglandin I$_2$)

THROMBOXANE A

Figure 59–2. Ring structures of the eicosanoids.

MECHANISMS OF EICOSANOID ACTION

There is a growing body of evidence indicating that eicosanoids produce their effects by binding to membrane-bound receptors. Available data suggest that there are specific receptors for individual members of the eicosanoid family. In some cases, interaction of an eicosanoid with its receptor produces either an increase or a decrease in intracellular levels of cyclic adenosine 3',5'-monophosphate (cyclic AMP). These changes in cyclic AMP concentration then lead to alterations in cell function.

PHARMACOLOGIC ACTIONS OF INDIVIDUAL EICOSANOIDS

Prostaglandins

The prostaglandins can produce diverse pharmacologic effects. To minimize confusion, discussion is limited to PGE$_2$ and PGF$_2$ alpha, the predominant prostaglandins in humans.

Prostaglandin E$_2$. PGE$_2$ relaxes some smooth muscles and causes others to contract. Smooth muscle of the bronchi and trachea is relaxed; when administered by aerosol to patients with asthma, PGE$_2$ produces prominent bronchodilation. Prostaglandin E$_2$ also relaxes smooth muscle of blood vessels: administration of PGE$_2$ lowers total peripheral resistance and increases blood flow to most organs. Both effects occur secondary to vasodilation. In the uterus, PGE$_2$ acts as a smooth muscle stimulant; when administered to pregnant women, PGE$_2$ produces a dose-dependent increase in the intensity and frequency of uterine contractions.

PGE$_2$ has multiple effects on the gastrointestinal (GI) tract. This prostaglandin is a potent inhibitor of gastric secretion; following PGE$_2$ administration, gastric juice undergoes a reduction in acidity, volume, and pepsin content. In the stomach and small intestine, PGE$_2$ promotes secretion of mucus; this mucus helps protect the GI tract from self-

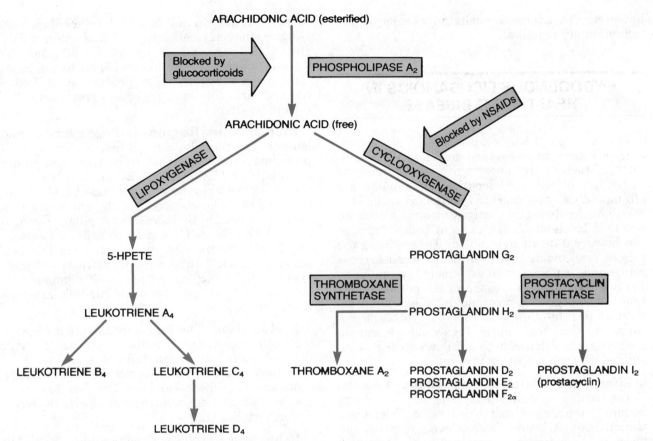

Figure 59–3. Biosynthesis of the eicosanoids. (NSAIDs = nonsteroidal anti-inflammatory drugs, 5-HPETE = 5-hydroperoxyeicosatetraenoic acid)

digestion. PGE_2 also stimulates secretion of water and electrolytes into the intestinal lumen. Lastly, PGE_2 acts in the intestine to promote contraction of longitudinal smooth muscle.

PGE_2 acts in the periphery to modulate pain. In the presence of PGE_2, the responsiveness of sensory nerves to painful stimuli (mechanical and chemical) is enhanced.

Prostaglandin F_2 Alpha. PGF_2 alpha causes contraction of bronchial, uterine, and intestinal smooth muscle. If administered to an individual with asthma, PGF_2 alpha will cause intense bronchoconstriction. This response is opposite to the effect of PGE_2. Like PGE_2, PGF_2 alpha can increase the intensity and frequency of uterine contractions. In the intestine, PGF_2 alpha causes circular smooth muscle to contract. In addition to stimulating smooth muscle, PGF_2 alpha acts in the ovary to promote luteolysis.

Thromboxane A_2

Thromboxane A_2 is produced almost exclusively by platelets. The compound is a powerful inducer of platelet aggregation. In addition, TXA_2 promotes contraction of all vascular smooth muscle.

Prostacyclin (PGI₂)

Prostacyclin has actions opposite to those of thromboxane: prostacyclin is an inhibitor of platelet aggregation and a potent vasodilator. Vasodilation is prominent in vessels of the heart, kidney, skeletal muscles, and lungs. Because of its vasodilator properties, prostacyclin produces hypotension when administered IV. Like PGE_2, prostacyclin inhibits gastric secretion and sensitizes afferent nerves to painful stimuli.

Leukotrienes

Leukotriene C_4 and *leukotriene D_4* have similar pharmacologic properties. Both of these eicosanoids are potent bronchoconstrictors. In addition, both compounds promote exudation of plasma by increasing capillary permeability. Together, these leukotrienes constitute what was once thought to be a single compound: slow-reacting substance of anaphylaxis (SRS-A). Unlike leukotrienes C_4 and D_4, *leukotriene B_4* does not affect the bronchi or the microvasculature. However, this compound does exert a powerful chemotactic effect (chemical attractant action) on polymorphonuclear leukocytes. As discussed below, the leukotrienes appear to have important roles as mediators of allergic and inflammatory reactions.

ENDOGENOUS EICOSANOIDS IN HEALTH AND DISEASE

The roles played by eicosanoids in physiologic and pathologic processes are not known with certainty. Much of the uncertainty stems from the instability of these compounds: eicosanoids are often produced and degraded with such speed that relationships between changes in endogenous eicosanoid levels and alterations in bodily function can be very difficult to establish. Determining the role of eicosanoids is also difficult because these compounds are present in extremely low amounts. Frequently, conjecture regarding the possible functions of endogenous eicosanoids is based on responses to inhibitors of eicosanoid synthesis. Because of the uncertainty regarding eicosanoid functions, the discussion that follows must be considered somewhat speculative.

Effects on Platelets and Blood Vessels. Thromboxane A_2 and prostacyclin have opposing actions on platelets and blood vessels: whereas thromboxane A_2 promotes platelet aggregation and vascular constriction, prostacyclin suppresses these responses. Hence, it has been suggested that the balance between thromboxane A_2 and prostacyclin may be an important factor in the regulation of hemostasis.

Thromboxane A_2 and prostacyclin may also be involved in certain pathologic conditions. Excessive production of thromboxane A_2 may contribute to thromboembolic disorders (by causing platelet aggregation) and to hypertension (by promoting vasoconstriction). Stimulation of prostacyclin synthesis may be a factor in hypotension seen during anaphylactic and septicemic shock.

Gastrointestinal Function. Administration of prostaglandins suppresses secretion of gastric acid and increases secretion of cytoprotective mucus. Both actions can help prevent erosion of the gastrointestinal wall. In light of these responses to exogenous prostaglandins, it has been suggested that endogenous prostaglandins may serve a physiologic role as regulators of acid and mucus secretion. This concept is supported by the observation that therapy with inhibitors of prostaglandin synthesis (e.g., aspirin, glucocorticoids) is associated with increased gastric acidity and ulcer formation.

Asthma. Several products of arachidonic acid (PGs, TXA_2, leukotrienes) have bronchoconstrictor properties, and are released by sensitized lung tissue in response to appropriate antigens. However, only the leukotrienes appear to be of pathologic significance. This statement is based on two observations: (1) aspirin and other inhibitors of *cyclooxygenase* (the enzyme leading to production of PGs and TXA_2) are *ineffective* as medications for asthma, whereas (2) inhibitors of *phospholipase A_2* (the enzyme required for production of leukotrienes) are *the most effective* treatments for asthma available.

Inflammatory Responses. Prostaglandins and leukotrienes contribute to all four classic signs of inflammation: calor (heat), rubor (redness), tumor (swelling), and dolor (pain). By inducing vasodilation, PGE_2 and prostacyclin increase blood flow to the area of inflammation, and thereby cause redness and warmth. By increasing capillary permeability, leukotrienes C_4 and D_4 contribute to swelling. Pain is heightened by the actions of PGE_2 on sensory nerves. Leukotriene B_4 attracts polymorphonuclear leukocytes to the site of inflammation; these white blood cells intensify the inflammatory response.

Fertilization. The high concentration of prostaglandins in human seminal fluid, coupled with the observation that some infertile males have semen that is low in PGs, suggests a role for these compounds in conception. However, despite considerable research, the contribution of PGs to fertilization remains unknown.

Labor and Delivery. Prostaglandins appear to have a role as promoters of uterine contraction during spontaneous labor. This statement is based on the following observations: (1) concentrations of PGs in blood and amniotic fluid increase at the time of labor, and (2) inhibitors of cyclooxygenase (i.e., inhibitors of PG synthesis) can prolong gestation and labor, and can interrupt labor when it occurs prematurely.

Neonatal Circulation. In premature infants, prostaglandins appear responsible for keeping the ductus arteriosus patent. This statement is based on the observation that inhibitors of PG synthesis cause the ductus arteriosus to close. The concept is further supported by the fact that exogenous prostaglandins can be used to *prevent* closure of the ductus arteriosus (see below).

EICOSANOIDS AND THERAPEUTICS

Because of their widespread and prominent effects, the eicosanoids are of great therapeutic interest. Drugs that can either *mimic* or *prevent* the actions of eicosanoids have the potential for producing a broad spectrum of beneficial effects.

Agents with the ability to *mimic* eicosanoid actions are the naturally occurring eicosanoids and their synthetic derivatives. Pharmaceutical chemists have created a large number of eicosanoid analogues in attempts to develop new therapeutic agents. Many of these compounds are undergoing clinical evaluation. At this point, however, only a few prostaglandins have received FDA approval for therapeutic use.

Two groups of drugs can *prevent* eicosanoid actions: (1) aspirin-like drugs (nonsteroidal anti-inflammatory drugs), and (2) glucocorticoids (steroidal anti-inflammatory drugs). Both groups prevent eicosanoid actions by inhibiting eicosanoid synthesis. Currently, there are no drugs available for clinical use that can prevent eicosanoid actions by acting as antagonists at eicosanoid receptors.

PROSTAGLANDINS IN CLINICAL USE

Prostaglandins have received much attention as potential therapeutic agents. As noted above, the only eicosanoids thus far approved for clinical use belong to the prostaglandin family. In the discussion below, we will consider the approved applications of the prostaglandins as well as their investigational uses.

Before proceeding, a note about prostaglandin nomenclature will be helpful. Throughout this chapter we have used *traditional* names (e.g., prostaglandin E_2, prostaglandin F_2 alpha) when referring to various PGs. Although these traditional names are widely employed, they are not the official generic names of the PGs. The official generic name (nonproprietary name) of PGE_2, for example, is *dinoprostone*. Trade names for this compound are *Prostin E_2* and *Prepidil*. Currently, there are five prostaglandins in clinical use. The traditional, generic, and trade names for these drugs are summarized in Table 59–1.

Uses Approved by the FDA

Applications Related to Stimulation of Uterine Contraction. Induction of *abortion* is the principal application of the prostaglandins. The agents approved for this use are *dinoprostone* and *carboprost tromethamine*. These drugs induce abortion by stimulating uterine contraction. When

employed for abortion, the prostaglandins produce a high incidence of nausea, vomiting, and diarrhea.

Carboprost tromethamine is indicated for control of *postpartum hemorrhage* (contraction of the uterus causes bleeding to cease).

Dinoprostone can be used for *induction of labor*. However, oxytocin is preferred for this use. Dinoprostone is also given to *initiate cervical ripening*.

The pharmacology of dinoprostone and carboprost tromethamine is discussed further in Chapter 58 (Uterine Stimulants and Relaxants).

Maintenance of a Patent Ductus Arteriosus. Neonates with certain heart defects depend upon a patent ductus arteriosus for survival; in the event of ductal closure, blood flow to the lungs and systemic circulation may become too low to support life. In the United States, alprostadil [Prostin VR Pediatric] is approved for keeping the ductus arteriosus patent. Alprostadil increases blood flow by relaxing the smooth muscle of the ductus wall, thereby causing the ductus arteriosus to dilate. Administration is by IV infusion. Apnea develops in 10% to 12% of infants treated. Accordingly, respiration must be monitored continuously, and ventilatory assistance must be immediately available. Alprostadil is indicated only as temporary therapy until corrective surgery can be performed. It is noteworthy that drugs that *inhibit* synthesis of endogenous prostaglandins will *promote* closure of the ductus arteriosus. One such inhibitor (indomethacin) is used clinically to accelerate closure in premature infants.

Prevention of NSAID-Induced Ulcers. Long-term therapy with aspirin and other nonsteroidal anti-inflammatory drugs (NSAIDs) can cause gastric ulcers. These ulcers result from reduced production of cytoprotective mucus and increased secretion of acid, both of which occur secondary to inhibition of prostaglandin synthesis by the NSAIDs. It should be no surprise, therefore, that administration of an exogenous prostaglandin can help prevent these ulcers. Currently, only one prostaglandin—*misoprostol* [Cytotec]—is approved by the FDA for prophylaxis of NSAID-induced gas-

Table 59–1. Names of Prostaglandins in Clinical Use		
Traditional Name*	**Generic Name†**	**Trade Name**
Prostaglandin E_1	Alprostadil	Prostin VR Pediatric
Prostaglandin E_2	Dinoprostone	Prostin E2, Prepidil
15 Methyl-prostaglandin F_2 alpha	Carboprost tromethamine	Hemabate
Prostacyclin (Prostaglandin I_2)	Epoprostenol	Cyclo-prostin, Flolan
—	Misoprostol	Cytotec

*This nomenclature was developed by the scientists who discovered and researched the prostaglandins.
†Official names assigned to the prostaglandins by the United States Adopted Names Council.

tric ulcers. The pharmacology of misoprostol is discussed in Chapter 66 (Drugs for Peptic Ulcer Disease).

Investigational Uses

Cardiovascular Applications. Epoprostenol [Flolan, Cyclo-prostin] is an inhibitor of platelet aggregation and a potent vasodilator. When given by intra-arterial infusion to patients with severe peripheral vascular disease, prostacyclin has produced dramatic and long-lasting improvement. The drug has also been used successfully for suppression of platelet aggregation during extracorporeal circulation (e.g., cardiopulmonary bypass, charcoal hemoperfusion, renal dialysis). The use of prostacyclin in the treatment of acute myocardial infarction, pulmonary hypertension, and variant angina pectoris is being investigated.

Prostaglandins A and A_2 have been given to lower blood pressure in patients with essential hypertension. Benefits derive from systemic vasodilation and from increased renal blood flow.

Treatment of Impotence. Alprostadil can induce erection in impotent males when injected directly into the corpus cavernosum of the penis. The use of alprostadil for impotence is discussed in Chapter 57 (Drug Therapy of Infertility).

INHIBITORS OF EICOSANOID SYNTHESIS

The inhibitors of eicosanoid synthesis fall into two major categories: (1) nonsteroidal anti-inflammatory drugs, and (2) steroidal anti-inflammatory drugs (glucocorticoids). These two groups differ with respect to mechanism of action, spectrum of effects, and clinical applications. The pharmacology of the nonsteroidal anti-inflammatory drugs is discussed in Chapter 61 (Aspirin-Like Drugs). The steroidal anti-inflammatory drugs are discussed in Chapter 62 (Glucocorticoids in Nonendocrine Diseases).

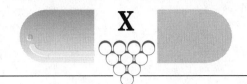

Drugs for Inflammation and Allergic Disorders

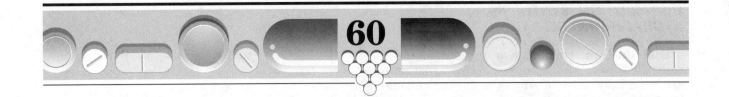

60

Histamine and Antihistamines

H istamine is an endogenous compound found in specialized cells throughout the body. This substance plays an important role in allergic reactions and regulation of gastric acid secretion. The antihistamines, one of our most widely used families of drugs, are agents that block histamine actions.

In order to understand the antihistamines, we must first understand histamine itself. Accordingly, we will begin the chapter with a discussion of histamine, emphasizing its contribution to allergic responses. Having established this background, we will then discuss the antihistamines.

HISTAMINE

Histamine is a locally acting substance with prominent and varied effects. In the vascular system, histamine dilates small blood vessels and increases capillary permeability. In the bronchi, histamine produces constriction. In the stomach, histamine stimulates secretion of acid. In the central nervous system (CNS), histamine acts as a neurotransmitter. Despite this impressive spectrum of effects, clinical applications for histamine itself are limited. Currently, use of histamine is restricted to diagnostic procedures. However, although its clinical utility is minimal, histamine is still of great medical interest because of its involvement in two common pathologic states: allergies and peptic ulcer disease.

DISTRIBUTION, SYNTHESIS, STORAGE, AND RELEASE

Distribution. Histamine is present in practically all tissues of the body. Levels of histamine are especially high in the skin, lungs, and gastrointestinal (GI) tract. The histamine content of plasma is relatively low.

Synthesis and Storage. Histamine is synthesized and stored in two types of cells: *mast cells* and *basophils*. Mast cells are present in the skin and other soft tissues; basophils are present in the blood. In both mast cells and basophils, histamine is stored in structures called secretory granules. (It should be noted that in addition to histamine, these secretory granules contain other substances that, like histamine, are mediators of allergic reactions.)

Release. Release of histamine from mast cells and basophils is produced by allergic and nonallergic mechanisms.

Allergic Release. The initial requirement for allergic release of histamine is the production of antibodies of the IgE class. These antibodies are generated in response to exposure to specific allergens (e.g., pollens, insect venoms, certain drugs). Following synthesis, the antibodies become attached to the outer surface of mast cells and basophils (Fig. 60–1). When the subject is re-exposed to the allergen, the allergen becomes bound by the antibodies. As indicated in Figure 60–1, binding of allergen to *adjacent* antibodies creates a bridge between those antibodies. By a mechanism that is not understood, this bridging process stimulates calcium mobilization. The calcium, in turn, causes the histamine-containing storage granules to fuse with the cell membrane and disgorge their contents into the extracellular space. Note that allergic release of histamine requires *prior exposure* to the allergen; an allergic reaction cannot occur during initial contact with an allergen.

Nonallergic Release. A number of agents (certain drugs, radiocontrast media, plasma expanders) can act directly on mast cells to cause histamine release. With these agents, no prior sensitization is needed. Cell injury can also cause direct release of histamine.

PHYSIOLOGIC AND PHARMACOLOGIC EFFECTS

Histamine acts through two types of receptors to produce its effects. These receptors are labeled H_1 and H_2. Responses to stimulation of these receptors are discussed below.

Effects of H_1 Stimulation

Vasodilation. Stimulation of H_1 receptors causes dilation of small blood vessels (arterioles

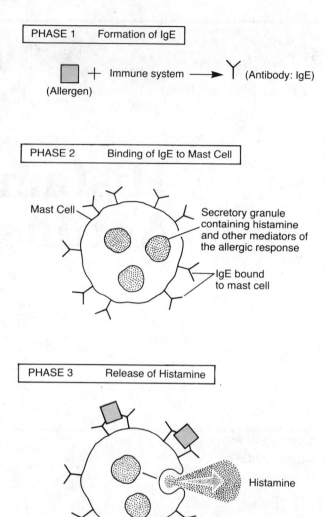

Figure 60–1. Release of histamine by allergen-antibody interaction.

and venules). Vasodilation is prominent in the skin of the face and upper body. In these areas, release of histamine causes the skin to become warm and flushed. If vasodilation is extensive, total peripheral resistance will be reduced and blood pressure will fall.

Increased Capillary Permeability. H_1 stimulation increases capillary permeability by causing contraction of capillary endothelial cells. This contraction produces openings between endothelial cells through which fluid, protein, and platelets can flow. Escape of fluid and protein into the interstitial space produces edema. If loss of intravascular fluid is substantial, a reduction in blood pressure may occur.

Bronchoconstriction. H_1 stimulation causes constriction of the bronchi. If histamine is administered to an individual with asthma, severe bronchoconstriction will follow. However, although *exogenous* histamine is clearly capable of inducing bronchial constriction, histamine is not the cause of the bronchoconstriction that occurs during a spontaneous asthma attack. Consequently, antihistamines are of no use in the treatment of asthma.

Other Effects. Stimulation of H_1 receptors located on sensory nerves can produce itching and pain. H_1 stimulation also promotes secretion of mucus. In the CNS, histamine appears to act as a neurotransmitter. The CNS receptors at which histamine acts may belong to the H_1 class.

Effects of H_2 Stimulation

The principal response to H_2-receptor stimulation is secretion of gastric acid. Histamine acts directly on parietal cells of the stomach to promote acid release. Histamine is the dominant regulator of gastric acidity. Acetylcholine and gastrin, two modulators of acid production, play a subordinate role; in the presence of H_2 blockade, acetylcholine and gastrin are unable to elicit acid secretion.

HISTAMINE IN ALLERGIC RESPONSES

Allergic reactions are mediated by histamine and other compounds (e.g., prostaglandins, leukotrienes). The intensity of an allergic reaction is determined by which of these substances is mediating the reaction.

Mild Allergy. The symptoms of mild allergy (e.g., rhinitis, itching, localized edema) are caused largely by histamine (acting at H_1 receptors). As a result, mild allergic conditions (e.g., hay fever, acute urticaria, mild transfusion reactions) are generally responsive to antihistamine therapy.

Severe Allergic Reactions (Anaphylaxis). Severe allergic reactions manifest as anaphylactic shock, a syndrome characterized by bronchoconstriction, hypotension, and edema of the glottis. Although histamine is involved in these responses, it is only a minor contributor; other substances (e.g., leukotrienes) are the principal causative agents. Since histamine has little to do with producing anaphylaxis, it follows that antihistamines will be of minimal value as treatment. The drug of choice for management of anaphylaxis is *epinephrine*. The rationale for using epinephrine is discussed in Chapter 17.

THE TWO TYPES OF ANTIHISTAMINES: H_1 ANTAGONISTS AND H_2 ANTAGONISTS

Antihistamines fall into two basic categories: H_1-receptor antagonists and H_2-receptor antagonists.

The H_1 antagonists block histamine actions only at H_1 receptors. The H_2 antagonists produce selective blockade at H_2 receptors. The principal application of the H_1 blockers is management of mild allergic disorders. The H_2 antagonists are used to treat gastric and duodenal ulcers. Since the H_2 antagonists do not block H_1 receptors, these drugs are of no use for allergies. In this chapter, our focus is on the H_1 antagonists. The H_2 blockers, which are important and widely used, are discussed in Chapter 66 (Drugs for Peptic Ulcer Disease).

H_1 ANTAGONISTS I: BASIC PHARMACOLOGY

The H_1 antagonists are the classic antihistamines. These agents were in use long before the H_2 blockers were developed. In fact, before H_2 blockers became available, the term H_1 antagonist did not exist; the drugs that we now call H_1 antagonists or H_1 blockers were simply referred to as antihistamines. Because of its historical use, the term *antihistamines* is still commonly employed as a synonym for the subgroup of histamine antagonists that produce selective H_1 blockade. In this chapter, we will respect tradition and continue to use the term *antihistamine* interchangeably with *H_1 blocker* and *H_1 antagonist*.

Although the many H_1 antagonists available have similar antihistaminic actions, these drugs differ significantly in their side effects. Because of these differences, selection of a prototype to represent the group is not feasible. Hence, rather than structuring discussion around one prototypic drug, we will discuss the H_1 antagonists collectively. Differences between individual antihistamines are addressed where appropriate.

Mechanism of Action

H_1 blockers bind selectively to H_1-histaminic receptors, thereby preventing the actions of histamine at these sites. The H_1 antagonists have no effect at H_2 receptors. Antihistamines do not act by preventing the release of histamine from mast cells or basophils.

It should be noted that although interaction of the classic antihistamines with *histaminic* receptors is limited to the H_1-receptor subtype, these drugs can also bind to *non*histaminic receptors. Of particular significance is the ability of certain antihistamines to bind to and block muscarinic receptors. Blockade of muscarinic receptors underlies several important side effects of these drugs.

Pharmacologic Effects

Peripheral Effects. The major effects of the H_1 antagonists can be attributed to preventing the actions of histamine at H_1 receptors. In arterioles and venules, H_1 blockers inhibit the dilator actions of histamine, and thereby reduce localized flushing. In capillary beds, the antihistamines prevent histamine-induced increases in permeability, thereby reducing edema. By blocking the actions of histamine at sensory nerves, H_1 antagonists reduce itching and pain. Blockade of H_1 receptors in mucous membranes suppresses secretion of mucus.

Effects on the Central Nervous System. Antihistamines can cause both excitation and depression of the CNS. At *therapeutic doses*, antihistamines usually produce CNS *depression*: reaction time is slowed, alertness is diminished, and drowsiness is likely. These effects are more pronounced with some antihistamines than with others; with the newest antihistamines—terfenadine, loratadine, and astemizole—CNS depression is negligible.

Stimulation of the CNS is most common following antihistamine overdosage. Convulsions frequently result. Very young children are especially sensitive to CNS stimulation by these drugs.

Other Pharmacologic Effects. Blockade of muscarinic cholinergic receptors by antihistamines can produce typical *anticholinergic* effects. These are discussed below under *Adverse Effects*. Several antihistamines can suppress nausea and vomiting (see below under *Motion Sickness*).

Therapeutic Uses

All of the H_1 antagonists are useful in treating allergic disorders. Some of these drugs are also indicated for other conditions (e.g., motion sickness, insomnia).

Mild Allergy. Antihistamines can reduce symptoms of mild allergies. In people with *seasonal allergic rhinitis* (hay fever), H_1 blockers can reduce sneezing, rhinorrhea, and itching of the eyes, nose, and throat. In patients with *acute urticaria*, these drugs can reduce redness, itching, and edema. The antihistamines can also reduce symptoms of *allergic conjunctivitis* and urticaria associated with mild *transfusion reactions*. In all of these conditions, benefits result from H_1-receptor blockade—and not from preventing allergen-induced release of histamine from mast cells and basophils. Since mild allergic reactions may be mediated by other substances in addition to histamine, relief of symptoms with antihistamines may not be complete.

Severe Allergy. As noted previously, the major symptoms of anaphylaxis (hypotension, laryngeal edema, bronchospasm) are caused by mediators other than histamine. Hence, although antihistamines may be employed as adjuncts to epinephrine in the treatment of anaphylaxis, the benefits of antihistamines are minimal.

Motion Sickness. Some antihistamines, such as promethazine [Phenergan] and dimenhydrinate [Dramamine], are labeled for use in motion sickness. The mechanism by which motion sickness is relieved is not known. Possible mechanisms include blockade of H_1 receptors in the CNS and blockade of CNS receptors for acetylcholine. Motion sickness and its treatment are discussed in Chapter 68. The antihistamines employed for motion sickness, along with their dosages, are listed in Table 68–1.

Insomnia. The ability of antihistamines to cause CNS depression has led to the use of these drugs for sedation. Practically every over-the-counter (OTC) sleep aid contains an H_1 antagonist (diphenhydramine or pyrilamine) as its active ingredient. However, although antihistamines can induce sleep when used in sufficient dosage, the doses recommended for OTC preparations are usually too small to be effective.

Common Cold. Despite their widespread presence in cold remedies, antihistamines are of practically no value as treatment for the common cold. These drugs neither prevent colds nor shorten their duration. Moreover, since histamine does not mediate symptoms of colds, H_1 blockade cannot even provide symptomatic relief. The only benefit that these drugs may offer is a moderate reduction in rhinorrhea, an effect that derives from the *anticholinergic* properties of the H_1 antagonists.

Adverse Effects

All of the H_1 blockers can produce undesired effects. As a rule, these responses are more a nuisance than a source of serious discomfort or danger. Frequently, side effects subside with continued drug use. Since individual antihistamines differ in their abilities to produce particular side effects (Table 60–1), adverse responses can be minimized by judicious drug selection.

Sedation. Sedation is the most common undesired effect of the antihistamines. Fortunately, tolerance to this effect often develops within a few days or weeks. If a preparation with a long half-life is being used, daytime sedation can be minimized by administering the entire daily dose at night. Patients should be advised to avoid driving and other hazardous activities if alertness is significantly impaired. Also, patients should be warned against use of alcohol and other CNS depressants since these agents will intensify the depressant effects of the H_1 antagonists.

Three antihistamines that have little or no sedative action are now available. These agents—astemizole, loratadine, and terfenadine—are unable to cross the blood-brain barrier and, therefore, do not alter CNS function. For patients experiencing disabling sedation with traditional H_1 antagonists,

Table 60–1. Pharmacologic Effects of H₁ Antagonists			
Drug	H₁–Blocking Activity	Sedative Effects	Anticholinergic Effects
Alkylamines			
Brompheniramine	+ + +	+	+ +
Chlorpheniramine	+ +	+	+ +
Dexchlorpheniramine	+ + +	+	+ +
Triprolidine	+ + to + + +	+	+ +
Ethanolamines			
Carbinoxamine	+ to + +	+ +	+ + +
Clemastine	+ to + +	+ +	+ + +
Diphenhydramine	+ to + +	+ + +	+ + +
Ethylenediamines			
Pyrilamine	+ to + +	+	±
Tripelennamine	+ to + +	+ +	±
Phenothiazines			
Methdilazine	+ + +	+	+ + +
Promethazine	+ + +	+ + +	+ + +
Trimeprazine	+ + +	+ +	+ + +
Piperidines			
Azatadine	+ +	+ +	+ +
Cyproheptadine	+ +	+	+ +
Diphenylpyraline	+ +	+	+ +
Phenindamine	+ +	*	+ +
Others: Nonsedating			
Astemizole	+ + to + + +	±	±
Loratadine	+ + to + + +	±	±
Terfenadine	+ + to + + +	±	±

± = low to none; + = low; + + = moderate; + + + = high
*May cause excitation.

therapy with a nonsedating antihistamine may be helpful. Unfortunately, the nonsedative agents are considerably more expensive than the traditional H₁ antagonists. The sedative properties of individual antihistamines are indicated in Table 60–1.

Nonsedative CNS Effects. In addition to sedation, antihistamines can cause dizziness, incoordination, confusional states, and fatigue. The elderly are especially sensitive to these reactions. In some patients, paradoxical excitation occurs, resulting in insomnia, nervousness, tremors, and even convulsions. CNS stimulation is most common in children and following overdosage.

Gastrointestinal Effects. Gastrointestinal disturbances are common. Responses include nausea, vomiting, loss of appetite, and diarrhea or constipation. These reactions can be minimized by administering antihistamines with meals.

Anticholinergic Effects. The H₁ antagonists possess weak atropine-like properties. These antimuscarinic actions can produce drying of mucous membranes in the mouth, nasal passages, and throat. Cholinergic blockade may also result in urinary hesitancy, constipation, and palpitations. If dry mouth becomes distressing, discomfort can be minimized by sucking on hard candy and by taking frequent sips of fluid. Antihistamines should be

used with caution in patients with asthma, since thickening of bronchial secretions may impair pulmonary function. Care should also be exercised in patients with other conditions that may be exacerbated by muscarinic blockade (e.g., urinary retention, prostatic hypertrophy, hypertension). The antimuscarinic efficacy of individual H₁ blockers is indicated in Table 60–1. As shown, the nonsedative antihistamines (astemizole, loratadine, and terfenadine) are also the least anticholinergic.

Cardiac Dysrhythmias. Potentially fatal cardiac dysrhythmias (ventricular fibrillation, torsades de pointes, others) have occurred rarely in patients taking *astemizole* and *terfenadine*, two of the nonsedative antihistamines. These serious reactions have usually occurred when dosage was excessive. Patients should be cautioned against exceeding the prescribed dosage, even if the prescribed dosage has failed to relieve allergic symptoms. In some cases, syncope (fainting) has preceded development of dysrhythmias. Patients who experience syncope should discontinue terfenadine and astemizole and undergo evaluation for potential dysrhythmias. With both drugs, the risk of dysrhythmias is increased by *severe hepatic dysfunction* and by concurrent use of *erythromycin, itraconazole,* or *ketoconazole.* Accordingly, terfenadine and astemizole are contraindicated for patients with liver disease and for patients receiving erythromycin, itraconazole, or ketoconazole.

Drug Interactions

Alcohol and other CNS depressants (e.g., barbiturates, benzodiazepines, opioids) can intensify the depressant effects of the H_1 antagonists. Patients should be advised against consumption of alcoholic beverages. If medications with CNS-depressant properties are combined with H_1 blockers, dosage of the depressant may need to be lowered.

Erythromycin, itraconazole, and *ketoconazole* increase the risk of serious dysrhythmias from terfenadine and astemizole. Accordingly, concurrent use of terfenadine or astemizole with these agents is contraindicated.

Use in Pregnancy and Lactation

Pregnancy. The margin of safety of antihistamines in pregnancy is not known. There have been reports of fetal malformation, but direct involvement of H_1 antagonists has not been proved. Given the uncertainty regarding the safety of these drugs, it is recommended that antihistamines be used only when clearly necessary, and only when the benefits of treatment outweigh the potential risks to the fetus. Antihistamines should be avoided late in the third trimester, since newborns are particularly sensitive to the adverse actions of these drugs.

Lactation. The H_1 antagonists can be excreted in breast milk, thereby posing a risk to the nursing infant. Since infants, and especially newborns, are unusually sensitive to antihistamines, these drugs should not be used by women who are breast-feeding.

Acute Toxicity

Although the antihistamines have a large margin of safety, acute poisoning is nonetheless common, owing to the widespread use of these drugs. CNS effects are prominent, especially anticholinergic reactions. Specific symptoms and treatment are described below.

Symptoms. The anticholinergic actions of H_1 blockers produce symptoms resembling those of atropine poisoning (dilated pupils, flushed face, hyperpyrexia, tachycardia, dry mouth, urinary retention). In children, CNS excitation is prominent, manifesting as hallucinations, incoordination, ataxia, and convulsions. In extreme cases, intoxication progresses to coma, cardiovascular collapse, and death.

Treatment. There is no specific antidote to antihistamine poisoning. Hence, treatment is directed at drug removal and management of symptoms. Emesis should be induced to expel the drug from the stomach. Following this, activated charcoal plus a cathartic are given to minimize absorption of any drug that remains in the GI tract. Convulsions should be treated with IV phenytoin. Anticonvulsants that have CNS-depressant

properties must be avoided. Hyperthermia can be reduced by application of ice packs or by sponge baths.

H_1 ANTAGONISTS II: PREPARATIONS

TRADITIONAL H_1 ANTAGONISTS

The traditional (sedative) H_1 antagonists can be classified in five major categories (alkylamines, ethanolamines, ethylenediamines, phenothiazines, and piperidines). As indicated in Table 60–1, these groups differ in antihistaminic efficacy and the ability to cause sedation and muscarinic blockade. Given these differences, it is often possible, through judicious drug selection, to produce effective H_1 blockade while minimizing undesired reactions.

Sedation can be a significant problem. CNS depression is most prominent with the ethanolamines (e.g., diphenhydramine) and phenothiazines (e.g., promethazine). Sedation is less prominent with the alkylamines (e.g., chlorpheniramine) and least likely with astemizole, loratadine, and terfenadine, the nonsedative antihistamines. For most patients, the alkylamines can provide effective H_1 blockade while causing only a modest reduction in alertness. For those who experience excessive sedation with an alkylamine, astemizole, loratadine, or terfenadine may be tried.

All of the H_1 blockers can be administered by mouth. In addition, some can be given parenterally or by rectal suppository. Routes and dosages for individual H_1 antagonists are summarized in Table 60–2.

NONSEDATIVE H_1 ANTAGONISTS

Three nonsedative antihistamines are available: terfenadine, astemizole, and loratadine. Sedation does not occur because these drugs are unable to cross the blood-brain barrier. Unfortunately, these agents are much more expensive than traditional antihistamines; they cost, for example, about 20 times more than chlorpheniramine, a representative traditional agent. Accordingly, it would seem prudent to reserve the nonsedative antihistamines for patients who experience too much sedation with the traditional drugs. Although the nonsedative antihistamines are generally well tolerated, two of them—terfenadine and astemizole—have been associated with fatal cardiac dysrhythmias, usually as a result of overdosage.

Terfenadine

Terfenadine [Seldane] was the first nonsedative antihistamine to become available and will serve

Generic Name	Trade Names	Routes	Usual Adult Oral Dosage
Alkylamines			
Brompheniramine	Dimetane, others	PO, IV, IM, SC	4 mg q4–6hr
Chlorpheniramine	Chlor-Trimeton, others	PO, IV, IM, SC	4 mg q4–6hr
Dexchlorpheniramine	Polaramine, others	PO	2 mg q4–6hr
Triprolidine	Actidil, Myidil	PO	2.5 mg q4–6hr
Ethanolamines			
Carbinoxamine	Clistin	PO	4–8 mg q6–8hr
Clemastine	Tavist	PO	1 mg q12 hr
Diphenhydramine	Benadryl, others	PO, IV, IM	25–50 mg q6–8hr
Ethylenediamines			
Pyrilamine	Nisaval	PO	25–50 mg q6–8hr
Tripelennamine	PBZ, Pelamine	PO	25–50 mg q4–6hr
Phenothiazines			
Methdilazine	Tacaryl	PO	8 mg q6–12hr
Promethazine	Phenergan, others	PO, IV, IM, R*	12.5–25 mg q6–24hr
Trimeprazine	Temaril	PO	2.5 mg q6hr
Piperidines			
Azatadine	Optimine	PO	1–2 mg q12hr
Cyproheptadine	Periactin	PO	4 mg q6–8hr
Diphenylpyraline	Hispril	PO	5 mg q12hr
Phenindamine	Nolahist	PO	25 mg q4–6hr
Others: Nonsedating			
Astemizole	Hismanal	PO	10 mg q24hr
Loratadine	Claritin	PO	10 mg q24hr
Terfenadine	Seldane	PO	60 mg q12hr

*R = Rectal suppository

as our prototype for the group. As noted above, sedation is minimal because the drug does not cross the blood-brain barrier. No synergism has been seen with alcohol and other CNS depressants. In addition to being nonsedative, terfenadine is essentially devoid of anticholinergic actions.

Although generally well tolerated, terfenadine can adversely affect the heart; *fatal dysrhythmias* have occurred, usually secondary to overdosage. Patients should be warned not to exceed the prescribed dosage. Furthermore, caution should be exercised in patients with pre-existing cardiac disease. The risk of dysrhythmias is increased by severe liver dysfunction and concurrent use of erythromycin, itraconazole, or ketoconazole.

Terfenadine is dispensed in 60-mg tablets for oral administration. The usual adult dosage is 60 mg twice daily.

Astemizole

Astemizole [Hismanal] is much like terfenadine. The drug does not cross the blood-brain barrier, does not produce signifi-

cant sedation, and does not intensify the effects of alcohol and other CNS depressants. Also, it has minimal anticholinergic actions.

Like terfenadine, astemizole has been associated with fatal cardiac dysrhythmias. Patients should be warned not to exceed the prescribed dosage. As with terfenadine, the risk of dysrhythmias is increased by severe liver disease and by concurrent use of erythromycin, itraconazole, or ketoconazole.

Astemizole is available in 60-mg tablets for oral administration. Absorption is reduced greatly (60%) in the presence of food; hence, the drug should be administered 1 hour before meals or 2 hours after. Astemizole has a long half-life (9 days)— much longer than that of terfenadine. As a result, astemizole is effective when given just once a day (whereas terfenadine must be given twice daily). Because of its long half-life, astemizole can take several days to reach effective plasma concentrations. To achieve therapeutic levels more quickly, a loading schedule is used. This schedule consists of 30 mg once on day 1, 20 mg once on day 2, and 10 mg once daily thereafter.

Loratadine

Loratadine [Claritin] is the newest of the nonsedative antihistamines. Like terfenadine and astemizole, loratadine does not cause significant sedation and does not intensify sedation from alcohol and other CNS depressants. Adverse cardiac effects have not been reported. Loratadine is available in 10-mg tablets for oral administration. The drug should be taken on an empty stomach. The usual adult dosage is 10 mg once daily.

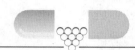

Summary of Major Nursing Implications

H₁ ANTAGONISTS

✓ Preadministration Assessment

Therapeutic Goal

Oral Therapy. Relief of symptoms of mild-to-moderate allergic disorders (e.g., seasonal rhinitis, allergic conjunctivitis, uncomplicated urticaria and angioedema).

Parenteral Therapy. Treatment of allergic reactions to blood or plasma; adjunctive therapy of anaphylaxis.

Identifying High-Risk Patients

Antihistamines are *contraindicated* during the *third trimester of pregnancy* and for *nursing mothers* and *newborns*. *Terfenadine* and *astemizole* are contraindicated for patients with *severe liver disease* and for patients taking *erythromycin*, *itraconazole*, or *ketoconazole*.

Exercise *caution* when treating *young children*, the *elderly*, and *patients with conditions that may be aggravated by muscarinic blockade, including asthma, urinary retention, open-angle glaucoma, hypertension*, and *prostatic hypertrophy*.

Use *astemizole* and *terfenadine* with *caution* in patients with *cardiac disease*.

✓ Implementation: Administration

Routes

All H₁ blockers can be administered orally. Some can also be administered parenterally or by rectal suppository (see Table 60–1).

Administration

Advise the patient to take all antihistamines (except astemizole) with food if GI upset occurs.

Instruct the patient to take *astemizole* at least 1 hour before eating or 2 hours after.

Warn the patient not to crush or chew enteric-coated preparations.

✓ Ongoing Evaluation and Interventions

Minimizing Adverse Effects

Sedation. For most patients, an antihistamine in the alkylamine group (see Table 60–1) can provide effective H₁ blockade with minimal sedation. If sedation is unacceptable with these agents, a nonsedative antihistamine (*astemizole, loratadine,* or *terfenadine*) can be used. With long-acting antihistamines, daytime sedation can be minimized by administering the entire daily dose in the evening. Caution the patient to avoid hazardous activities if sedation is substantial.

Anticholinergic Effects. Advise the patient that dryness of the mouth and throat can be reduced by sucking on hard candy and by taking frequent sips of liquids. Other atropine-like responses (urinary hesitancy, tachycardia, constipation) are not usually problems. *Astemizole, loratadine,* and *terfenadine* have minimal anticholinergic effects.

Gastrointestinal Distress. Advise the patient that GI disturbances (nausea, vomiting) can be minimized by taking antihistamines with meals.

Cardiac Dysrhythmias. *Astemizole* and *terfenadine* can cause potentially fatal cardiac dysrhythmias. Warn the patient not to exceed the prescribed dosage. Use with caution in patients with cardiac disease. Syncope has preceded dysrhythmias in some patients; if syncope occurs, discontinue astemizole and terfenadine and evaluate for potential dysrhythmias. The risk of dysrhythmias is increased by concurrent use of erythromycin, itraconazole, or ketoconazole; accordingly, concurrent use of these agents is contraindicated. The risk of dysrhythmias is also increased by severe liver disease, which is another contraindication for use of astemizole and terfenadine.

Minimizing Adverse Interactions

CNS Depressants. *Alcohol* and other *CNS depressants* can intensify the depressant actions of the H_1 antagonists. Warn the patient against consumption of alcohol. Dosages of CNS depressants (e.g., barbiturates, benzodiazepines, opioids) may need to be reduced. *Astemizole, loratadine,* and *terfenadine* have no CNS depressant effects and do not potentiate the actions of CNS depressants.

Antimicrobials. *Erythromycin, itraconazole,* and *ketoconazole* increase the risk of serious dysrhythmias from astemizole and terfenadine. Concurrent use of these agents is contraindicated.

Management of Toxicity

There is no specific antidote for antihistamine overdosage; treatment is directed at removal of the drug and management of symptoms. To remove the drug, give an emetic and, after vomiting has occurred, give activated charcoal and a cathartic. Treat hyperthermia with ice packs or with cooling sponge baths. Control convulsions with IV phenytoin.

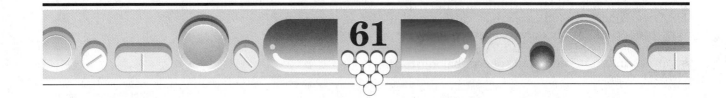

61

Aspirin-Like Drugs: Nonsteroidal Anti-inflammatory Drugs and Acetaminophen

NONSTEROIDAL ANTI-INFLAMMATORY DRUGS
    Aspirin
    Other Nonsteroidal Anti-inflammatory Drugs

ACETAMINOPHEN

The family of aspirin-like drugs consists of aspirin itself and a large number of related agents. Most of these drugs can produce three clinically useful effects: (1) suppression of inflammation, (2) relief of pain, and (3) reduction of fever. As discussed below, all three responses are produced through one central mechanism: inhibition of cyclooxygenase, the enzyme responsible for synthesis of prostaglandins. This same mechanism underlies the principal adverse effects of these drugs: (1) gastric ulceration, (2) suppression of platelet aggregation, and (3) induction of acute renal failure. Because of their pronounced anti-inflammatory actions, the aspirin-like drugs are commonly referred to as *nonsteroidal anti-inflammatory drugs* (to distinguish them from cortisone and other steroids used to treat inflammatory disorders). Because of their ability to relieve pain, these drugs are also known as *nonopioid analgesics* (to distinguish them from morphine and other opioid analgesics).

The aspirin-like drugs fall into two major categories: (1) agents that possess anti-inflammatory properties (nonsteroidal anti-inflammatory drugs, NSAIDs) and (2) agents that lack anti-inflammatory properties. With only one exception—acetaminophen—all of the aspirin-like drugs are able to suppress inflammation, and, hence, belong to the NSAID category.

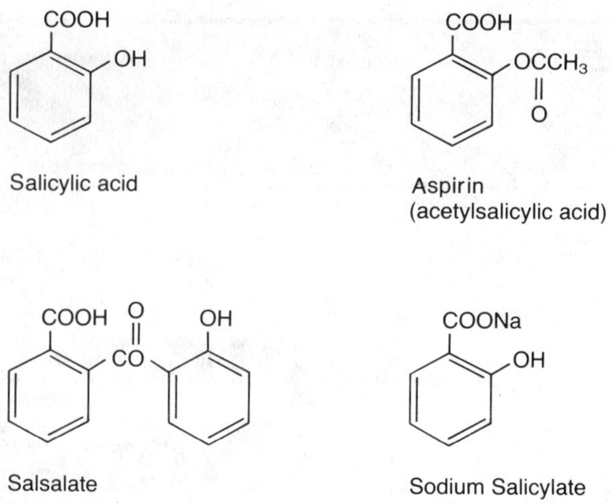

Figure 61–1. Structural formulas of aspirin and related salicylates.

NONSTEROIDAL ANTI-INFLAMMATORY DRUGS

The NSAIDs are a large and commonly prescribed family of drugs. These agents are a mainstay of treatment for inflammatory disorders (e.g., rheumatoid arthritis) and are used widely to relieve mild-to-moderate pain, suppress fever, and relieve symptoms of primary dysmenorrhea. All NSAIDs pose a risk of gastric ulceration, acute renal failure, and suppression of platelet aggregation. Aspirin, the oldest member of the family, will serve as our prototype for the group.

ASPIRIN

Aspirin is an important drug whose effectiveness is frequently unappreciated. Given that aspirin is available without prescription, widely advertised on television, and used somewhat casually by the general public, you may be surprised to hear that aspirin is considered a highly valuable and effective medication. The drug provides excellent relief of mild-to-moderate pain, reduces fever, and is the initial drug of choice for rheumatoid arthritis and other inflammatory disorders. You may also be surprised to discover that aspirin can cause serious toxicity (e.g., gastric ulceration).

Chemistry

Aspirin belongs to a chemical family known as *salicylates*. All members of this group are derivatives of salicylic acid (Fig. 61–1). Aspirin is produced by substituting an acetyl group onto salicylic acid. Because of this acetyl group, aspirin is commonly known as *acetylsalicylic acid*, or simply ASA.

Mechanism of Action

Although aspirin has been in use since 1899, it was not until 1970 that its mechanism of action began to be revealed. It is now clear that most of the therapeutic and adverse effects of aspirin result from *inhibition of cyclooxygenase*, an enzyme required for biosynthesis of *prostaglandins* and related metabolites of arachidonic acid (prostacyclin and thromboxane A_2).

As discussed in Chapter 59, prostaglandins and other metabolites of arachidonic acid produce a wide variety of biologic effects. These agents mediate inflammatory responses, increase the responsiveness of pain receptors, and promote fever. In the stomach, prostaglandins serve three functions: they suppress output of gastric acid, promote secretion of cytoprotective mucus and bicarbonate, and support normal submucosal blood flow. In platelets, thromboxane A_2 stimulates aggregation. In the kidney, prostaglandins promote vasodilation, thereby increasing renal blood flow.

By inhibiting synthesis of prostaglandins and thromboxane A_2, aspirin can produce beneficial effects and undesired effects. The principal benefits that derive from inhibiting cyclooxygenase are (1) suppression of inflammation, (2) relief of pain, and (3) reduction of fever. By decreasing prostaglandin synthesis in the stomach, aspirin increases gastric acidity, reduces secretion of cytoprotective mucus and bicarbonate, and reduces submucosal blood flow; this combination of effects can lead to gastric ulceration. Inhibition of thromboxane A_2 synthesis suppresses platelet aggregation, an effect that can be both beneficial and harmful: reduced platelet aggregation can help prevent myocardial reinfarction but can also promote bleeding. By decreasing prostaglandin synthesis in the kidney, aspirin can reduce renal blood flow, which in turn can lead to acute renal failure.

Pharmacokinetics

Absorption. Aspirin is absorbed rapidly and completely following oral administration. The principal site of absorption is the small intestine. When administered by rectal suppository, aspirin is absorbed slowly and blood levels are lower than with oral therapy.

Metabolism. Aspirin has a very short half-life (15 to 20 minutes) because of rapid conversion to salicylic acid, an active metabolite. The rate of salicylic acid inactivation depends on the amount present: at *low* therapeutic levels, salicylic acid has a half-life of approximately 2 hours; at *high* therapeutic levels, the half-life may exceed 20 hours.

Distribution. Salicylic acid is extensively bound to plasma albumin. At therapeutic levels, binding is between 80% and 90%. Aspirin undergoes distribution to all body tissues and fluids, including breast milk, fetal tissues, and the central nervous system (CNS).

Excretion. Salicylic acid and its metabolites are excreted by the kidneys. Excretion of salicylic acid is highly dependent on urinary pH. Accordingly, by raising the pH of urine from 6 to 8, we can increase the excretion of salicylic acid by a factor of 4.

Plasma Drug Levels. Low therapeutic doses of aspirin produce plasma salicylate levels in the range of 100 μg/ml. Anti-inflammatory doses produce salicylate levels of about 400 μg/ml. Signs of salicylism (toxicity) begin to appear when plasma salicylate levels exceed 200 μg/ml. Severe toxicity occurs at levels above 400 μg/ml.

Therapeutic Uses

Suppression of Inflammation. Aspirin is the initial drug of choice for treatment of rheumatoid arthritis, osteoarthritis, and juvenile arthritis. The drug is also indicated for other inflammatory disorders (e.g., rheumatic fever, tendinitis, bursitis). Dosages employed to suppress inflammation are considerably larger than the doses employed for analgesia or reduction of fever. The use of aspirin and other NSAIDs to treat arthritis is discussed in Chapter 63.

The precise mechanisms by which aspirin decreases inflammation have not been established. We do know that prostaglandins contribute to several (but not all) components of the inflammatory process. Hence, inhibition of prostaglandin synthesis provides a partial explanation of aspirin's anti-inflammatory effects. Other possible mechanisms include modulation of T-cell function, suppression of inflammatory cell infiltration, and stabilization of lysozymes.

Analgesia. Aspirin is our most widely used medication for relieving mild-to-moderate pain. Just how much analgesia is produced depends on the type of pain. Aspirin is most active against joint pain, muscle pain, and headache. For some forms of postoperative pain, aspirin can be more effective than opioids. However, aspirin is relatively inactive against severe pain of visceral origin. In contrast to the opioid analgesics, aspirin produces neither tolerance nor physical dependence. In addition, aspirin is less toxic than the opioids.

Aspirin relieves pain primarily by actions in the periphery. At sites of injury, prostaglandins act to sensitize pain receptors to mechanical and chemical stimulation. Aspirin reduces pain by suppressing biosynthesis of these prostaglandins. In addition to this peripheral mechanism, aspirin has actions in the CNS that contribute to pain relief.

Reduction of Fever. Aspirin is the drug of choice for reducing temperature in febrile individuals. However, because of the risk of Reye's syndrome (see below), *aspirin should not be used to treat fever in children suspected of having chickenpox or influenza.* Although aspirin readily reduces fever, the drug will not lower normal body temperature, nor will it lower temperature that has become elevated in response to physical activity or to a rise in external temperature.

Aspirin reduces fever (promotes heat loss) by causing dilation of cutaneous blood vessels, thereby increasing blood flow to the skin. Cutaneous vasodilation results from actions exerted in the hypothalamus, the brain region that regulates body temperature. Fever occurs when the "set point" of the hypothalamus becomes elevated. Set-point elevation is triggered by local synthesis of prostaglandins in response to an *endogenous pyrogen* (fever-promoting substance). Aspirin lowers the set point by inhibiting pyrogen-induced synthesis of prostaglandins. The reason that aspirin does not lower body temperature in afebrile individuals is that there is no pyrogen present to stimulate prostaglandin formation.

Dysmenorrhea. Aspirin can provide relief from primary dysmenorrhea. Benefits derive from inhibiting prostaglandin synthesis in uterine smooth muscle. (Prostaglandins promote uterine contraction. Hence, suppression of prostaglandin synthesis relieves cramping.) Some of the newer aspirin-like drugs (e.g., ibuprofen, naproxen) are superior to aspirin for relieving dysmenorrhea. The efficacy of the newer drugs is attributed to a greater ability to inhibit the particular form of cyclooxygenase present in uterine smooth muscle.

Suppression of Platelet Aggregation. As discussed above, synthesis of thromboxane A_2 by platelets promotes aggregation. Aspirin suppresses platelet aggregation by causing *irreversible* inhibition of platelet cyclooxygenase, the enzyme required for production of thromboxane A_2. Since platelets lack the machinery to synthesize new cyclooxygenase, the effects of a single dose of aspirin persist for the life of the platelet (about 8 days). When administered in low doses (160 mg/day) following myocardial infarction, aspirin can decrease the risk of reinfarction and death. In *men* who experience recurrent transient ischemic attacks (TIAs), aspirin can reduce both the frequency of attacks and the incidence of stroke. Unfortunately, the drug does not seem to suppress TIAs in women. The role of aspirin as *prophylaxis* against initial myocardial infarction is controversial: daily low-dose therapy appears to reduce the risk of myocardial infarction but may *increase* the risk of hemorrhagic stroke.

Adverse Effects

When administered in analgesic or antipyretic (fever-reducing) doses, aspirin rarely causes serious adverse effects. However, significant toxicity is common at the higher doses required to treat inflammatory disorders.

Gastrointestinal Effects. The most common side effects of aspirin are *gastric distress, heartburn*, and *nausea*. These reactions can be reduced by taking aspirin with food or with a full glass of water.

Occult gastrointestinal (GI) bleeding occurs frequently. In most cases, the amount of blood lost each day is insignificant. However, with chronic aspirin use, cumulative blood loss can result in anemia.

Long-term high-dose therapy can cause *gastric ulceration*. The FDA estimates that aspirin-induced ulcers and their complications are responsible for 10,000 to 20,000 deaths annually. Ulcers result from (1) increased secretion of acid and pepsin, (2) decreased production of cytoprotective mucus and bicarbonate, (3) decreased submucosal blood flow, and (4) the direct irritant action of aspirin on the gastric mucosa. The first three effects occur secondary to inhibition of prostaglandin synthesis. Injury to the stomach is most likely with aspirin preparations that dissolve slowly: because of slow dissolution, particulate aspirin becomes entrapped in folds of the stomach wall, causing prolonged exposure to high concentrations of the drug. Because aspirin-induced ulcers are often asymptomatic, perforation and upper GI hemorrhage can occur without premonitory signs. (Hemorrhage is due in part to erosion of the stomach wall and in part to suppression of platelet aggregation.) Factors that increase the risk of ulceration include (1) advanced age, (2) a history of peptic ulcer disease, (3) previous intolerance to aspirin or other NSAIDs, (4) cigarette smoking, and (5) a history of alcoholism. Because alcohol intensifies the irritant effects of aspirin, alcohol should not be consumed during aspirin therapy.

Aspirin-induced ulcers can be managed by discontinuing aspirin and giving an anti-ulcer medication—usually an *H₂-receptor antagonist* (e.g., cimetidine) or *sucralfate*. In some cases, it may be possible to continue aspirin therapy while treating the ulcer with *omeprazole*. The pharmacology of sucralfate, omeprazole and the H₂-receptor blockers is discussed in Chapter 66 (Drugs for Peptic Ulcer Disease).

The only drug approved for *prophylaxis* against aspirin-induced ulcers is *misoprostol*, a synthetic prostaglandin. Misoprostol helps prevent ulcers by (1) suppressing secretion of gastric acid, (2) promoting secretion of cytoprotective mucus and bicarbonate, and (3) maintaining normal submucosal blood flow. Because misoprostol can stimulate uterine contractions, the drug is absolutely contraindicated during pregnancy. The pharmacology of misoprostol is discussed in Chapter 66.

Bleeding. Aspirin can promote bleeding by suppressing platelet aggregation. After ingestion of just two aspirin tablets, bleeding time is doubled for approximately 1 week. (Recall that platelets are unable to replace aspirin-inactivated cyclooxygenase. Hence, prolongation of bleeding time persists for the life of the platelet.) Because of its effects on platelets, *aspirin is contraindicated for patients with bleeding disorders* (e.g., hemophilia, vitamin K deficiency, hypoprothrombinemia). In order to minimize blood loss during elective surgery and parturition, aspirin should be discontinued at least 1 week prior to these procedures. Care must be exercised when aspirin is used in conjunction with anticoagulants.

Renal Effects. For most patients, the risk of aspirin-induced renal dysfunction is very low. However, among patients with predisposing risk factors—advanced age, pre-existing renal dysfunction, hypovolemia, hepatic cirrhosis, or congestive heart failure—the incidence of aspirin-induced renal impairment may be as high as 20%.

Aspirin impairs kidney function by inhibiting the synthesis of prostaglandins that cause renal vasodilation. The resultant vasoconstriction decreases renal blood flow, decreases glomerular filtration rate, and promotes renal ischemia. These effects can combine to cause acute renal failure. Fortunately, aspirin does not affect renal function in most patients because, under normal conditions, prostaglandins do not participate in the regulation of renal blood flow. Rather, prostaglandins serve to maintain renal blood flow primarily in patients with the risk factors noted above.

Development of renal impairment is signaled by reduced urine output, weight gain despite use of diuretics, and a rapid rise in serum creatinine and blood urea nitrogen. If any of these signs is observed, aspirin should be withdrawn immediately. In most cases, kidney function then returns to its baseline level.

The risk of renal impairment can be reduced by identifying high-risk patients and treating them with the smallest aspirin dosages possible.

Salicylism. Salicylism is a syndrome that begins to develop when aspirin levels climb just slightly above the therapeutic level. Overt signs include *tinnitus* (ringing in the ears), *sweating, headache*, and *dizziness*. Acid-base disturbance may also occur (see below). If salicylism develops, aspirin should be withheld until symptoms subside; therapy should then resume but with a small reduction in dosage. In some cases, development of tinnitus can be used to adjust aspirin dosage: when tinnitus occurs, the maximum acceptable dose has been achieved. However, this guideline may be inappropriate for older patients, since they may fail to develop tinnitus even when aspirin levels become toxic.

Acid-base disturbance results from the effects of aspirin on respiration. When administered in high therapeutic doses, aspirin acts on the CNS to stimulate breathing. The resultant increased loss of CO_2 produces *respiratory alkalosis*. In response to alkalosis, the kidneys excrete increased amounts of bicarbonate. As a result, plasma pH returns to a normal value and a state of *compensated respiratory alkalosis* is produced.

Reye's Syndrome. This syndrome is a rare but serious illness of childhood that has a mortality rate of 20% to 30%. Epidemiologic data suggest a relationship between Reye's syndrome and use of aspirin by children who have influenza or chickenpox. However, a direct causal link has not been established. Because of the possible relationship between aspirin and development of Reye's syndrome, *it is recommended that aspirin (and other NSAIDs) be avoided by children and teenagers suspected of having influenza or chickenpox.*

Hypersensitivity Reactions. Hypersensitivity develops in about 0.3% of aspirin recipients. Reactions are most likely in adults who have certain predisposing conditions: asthma, hay fever, chronic urticaria, or nasal polyps. Hypersensitivity reactions are uncommon in children. The aspirin hypersensitivity reaction begins with profuse, watery rhinorrhea and may progress to generalized urticaria, bronchospasm, laryngeal edema, and shock. Despite its resemblance to severe anaphylaxis, this reaction is not allergic and is not mediated by the immune system. Since individuals who react to aspirin are also sensitive to most other NSAIDs, it is thought that hypersensitivity reactions are in some way related to inhibition of cyclooxygenase. However, it is not clear why the reaction is limited to those adults who have the predisposing conditions noted. As with severe anaphylactic reactions, *epinephrine* is the treatment of choice. Hypersensitivity to aspirin is a contraindication to using other drugs with aspirin-like properties.

Use in Pregnancy

Aspirin poses risks to the pregnant patient and the developing fetus. Accordingly, the drug is classified in FDA Pregnancy Category D: there is evidence of human fetal risk, but the potential benefits from use of the drug during pregnancy may outweigh the potential for harm. The principal risks to pregnant women are (1) anemia (from GI blood loss), and (2) postpartum hemorrhage. In addition, by inhibiting prostaglandin synthesis, aspirin may suppress spontaneous uterine contractions, and may thereby prolong gestation and labor.

Aspirin crosses the placenta and may adversely affect the fetus. Since prostaglandins help keep the ductus arteriosus patent, inhibition of prostaglandin synthesis by aspirin may induce premature closure of the ductus arteriosus. Aspirin therapy has also been associated with low birth weight, stillbirth, intracranial hemorrhage in premature infants, and neonatal death.

Summary of Precautions and Contraindications

Aspirin is contraindicated in patients with *peptic ulcer disease*, *bleeding disorders* (e.g., hemophilia, vitamin K deficiency, hypoprothrombinemia), and *hypersensitivity to aspirin itself or other NSAIDs*. In addition, the drug should be used with extreme caution by *pregnant women* and by *children who have chickenpox or influenza*. Caution should also be exercised when treating *elderly patients*, *patients who smoke cigarettes*, and patients with *congestive heart failure, hepatic cirrhosis, hypovolemia, renal dysfunction, asthma, hay fever, chronic urticaria, nasal polyps*, or a *history of alcoholism*. Aspirin should be withdrawn 1 week prior to elective surgery or the anticipated date of parturition.

Drug Interactions

Because of its widespread use, aspirin has been reported to interact with many other medications. However, most of these interactions have little clinical significance. Significant interactions are discussed below.

Oral Anticoagulants. The most important interactions of aspirin occur with oral anticoagulants (e.g., warfarin). Because aspirin suppresses platelet function and can decrease prothrombin production, aspirin will intensify the effects of anticoagulant drugs. Furthermore, since aspirin can initiate gastric bleeding, augmentation of anticoagulant effects can increase the risk of gastric hemorrhage. Accordingly, the combination of aspirin with an oral anticoagulant must be used with great care.

Glucocorticoids. Like aspirin, glucocorticoids promote gastric ulceration. Accordingly, the risk of ulcers is greatly increased when these drugs are combined—as may happen when treating arthritis. To reduce the risk of gastric ulceration, patients can be given *misoprostol* for prophylaxis.

Acute Poisoning

Aspirin overdosage is a common cause of poisoning. Although rarely fatal in *adults*, aspirin poisoning may prove lethal in *children*. The lethal dose for adults is 20 to 25 gm. In contrast, as little as 4 gm may be sufficient to kill a child.

Signs and Symptoms. Initially, aspirin overdosage produces a state of compensated respiratory alkalosis—the same state seen in mild salicylism. As poisoning progresses, respiratory excitation is replaced by respiratory depression. Acidosis, hyperthermia, sweating, and dehydration are prominent, and electrolyte imbalance is likely. Stupor and coma result from effects in the CNS. Death is usually from respiratory failure. The mechanisms that underlie these clinical manifestations are described below.

Many symptoms of aspirin overdosage occur secondary to *uncoupling of oxidative phosphorylation*, the process by which the energy released during oxidation of carbohydrates, fats, and proteins is used to form ATP from ADP. When oxidative phosphorylation becomes uncoupled, energy from metabolism of carbohydrates and other nutrients can no longer be transferred to ATP and stored. The consequences of this uncoupling are threefold: (1) Production of CO_2 is increased (secondary to the increased rates of metabolism that take place in futile attempts to form needed ATP). (2) There is increased production of lactic and pyruvic acids (as by-products of increased metabolism). (3) Production of heat is increased because the energy that would normally be used to make ATP is released in the form of heat. Increased heat production is responsible for hyperthermia and dehydration, two of the more serious consequences of aspirin overdosage.

The acidosis that characterizes aspirin poisoning results from multiple causes. Respiratory acidosis occurs because CO_2 production is increased and because toxic levels of salicylate act on the CNS to decrease respiration, thereby allowing even more CO_2 to accumulate. Respiratory acidosis remains uncompensated because bicarbonate stores become depleted during the initial phase of poisoning. Superimposed on respiratory acidosis is true metabolic acidosis. Metabolic acidosis results from (1) the acidity of aspirin and its metabolites, (2) increased production of lactic and pyruvic acids, and (3) accumulation of acidic products of metabolism (e.g., sulfuric and phosphoric acids) because of aspirin-induced impairment of renal excretion.

Acidosis is intensified by the following cycle: (1) Because of the pH partitioning effect, acidosis promotes penetration of salicylate into the CNS. (2) Increased entry of salicylate deepens respiratory depression. (3) Deepening of respiratory depression increases accumulation of CO_2, thereby increasing acidosis. (4) Increasing acidosis causes even more salicylate to enter the CNS, producing even further deepening of respiratory depression. This cycle continues until respiration ceases.

Treatment. Aspirin poisoning is an acute medical emergency that requires hospitalization. The immediate threats to life are respiratory depression, hyperthermia, dehydration, and acidosis. Treatment is largely symptomatic. If respiration is inadequate, mechanical ventilation should be instituted. External cooling (e.g., sponging with tepid water) can help reduce hyperthermia. Intravenous fluids are administered to correct dehydration; the composition of these fluids is determined by electrolyte and acid-base status. Slow infusion of bicarbonate is given to reverse acidosis. Several measures (induction of emesis, gastric lavage, administration of activated charcoal) can reduce further gastrointestinal absorption of aspirin. Alka-

linization of the urine with bicarbonate accelerates excretion of aspirin and salicylate. If necessary, hemodialysis or peritoneal dialysis can be used to remove salicylates from the body.

Formulations

Aspirin is available in several formulations, including plain and buffered tablets, enteric-coated preparations, and tablets used to produce a buffered solution. These different formulations reflect efforts to increase rates of absorption and decrease gastric irritation. For the most part, the clinical utility of the more complex formulations is no greater than that of plain aspirin tablets.

Aspirin Tablets (Plain). All brands are essentially the same with respect to analgesic efficacy, time of onset, and duration of action. Some of the less expensive tablets have greater particle size, which results in slower dissolution and prolonged contact with the gastric mucosa. These effects can augment gastric irritation. Over time, aspirin in tablets decomposes and emits an odor of vinegar (acetic acid); these tablets should be discarded.

Aspirin Tablets (Buffered). The amount of buffer in buffered aspirin tablets is too small to produce significant elevation of gastric pH. An equivalent effect on pH can be achieved by taking plain aspirin tablets with a glass of water or with food. Buffered aspirin tablets are no different from plain tablets with respect to analgesic effects and incidence of gastric distress. Buffered tablets may dissolve faster than plain tablets, resulting in a somewhat faster onset of action.

Buffered Aspirin Solution. A buffered aspirin solution is produced by dissolving effervescent aspirin tablets [Alka-Seltzer] in a glass of water. This solution has considerable buffering capacity due to its high content of sodium bicarbonate. Effects on gastric pH are sufficient to decrease the incidence of gastric irritation and bleeding. In addition, absorption is accelerated and peak blood levels are increased. Unfortunately, these benefits do not come without a price. The sodium content of buffered aspirin solution can be detrimental to individuals on a sodium-restricted diet. Also, absorption of bicarbonate can result in elevation of urinary pH, an effect that will accelerate aspirin excretion. Lastly, this highly buffered preparation is expensive. Because of this combination of benefits and drawbacks, the buffered aspirin solution is well suited for occasional use but is generally inappropriate for long-term therapy.

Enteric-Coated Preparations. These preparations dissolve in the intestine rather than the stomach, thereby reducing gastric irritation. Unfortunately, absorption from these formulations can be delayed and erratic. Patients should be advised not to crush or chew these preparations.

Timed-Release Tablets. These formulations offer no advantage over plain aspirin tablets. Since the half-life of salicylic acid is long to begin with, timed-release tablets cannot produce a significant increase in duration of action.

Rectal Suppositories. Suppositories have been employed for patients who cannot take aspirin orally. Absorption can be variable, resulting in plasma drug levels that are insufficient in some patients and excessive in others. Also, rectal irritation can occur. Because of these undesirable properties, aspirin suppositories are not generally recommended.

Dosage and Administration

Aspirin is almost always administered by mouth. Gastric irritation can be minimized by administering aspirin with a glass of water or with food. Dosage depends on the age of the patient and the condition being treated. Adult and pediatric dosages for major indications are summarized in Table 61–1.

OTHER NONSTEROIDAL ANTI-INFLAMMATORY DRUGS

In attempts to produce an aspirin-like drug with fewer gastrointestinal and hemorrhagic effects than aspirin, the pharmaceutical industry has produced a large number of drugs with actions very similar to those of aspirin. In the United States, over 20 NSAIDs are now available (Table 61–2). Like aspirin, all of the newer NSAIDs are inhibitors of prostaglandin synthesis. Consequently, all of these drugs display anti-inflammatory, analgesic, and antipyretic properties. In addition, they all

can promote gastric ulceration, bleeding, and renal failure—although the intensity of these effects may be less with some NSAIDs than with others. Patients who are hypersensitive to aspirin are likely to experience cross-hypersensitivity with the newer aspirin-like drugs. For most of the NSAIDs, safety during pregnancy has not been established. Hence, their use by pregnant women is not recommended.

The principal indications for the newer NSAIDs are rheumatoid arthritis and other inflammatory disorders. In addition, certain NSAIDs are used to treat fever, bursitis, tendinitis, mild-to-moderate pain, and primary dysmenorrhea (see Table 61–2).

Although individual NSAIDs differ from one another chemically, pharmacokinetically, and, to some extent, pharmacodynamically, all of these drugs are very similar clinically: they all produce essentially equivalent antirheumatic effects and they all present an essentially equal risk of serious adverse effects (gastric ulceration and renal failure). However, for reasons that are not understood, individual patients may respond better to one NSAID than to another. Furthermore, individual patients may tolerate one NSAID better than another. Accordingly, in order to optimize therapy for the individual patient, therapeutic trials with more than one NSAID may be needed.

Properties of individual NSAIDs are discussed below.

Nonacetylated Salicylates: Choline Salicylate, Magnesium Salicylate, Sodium Salicylate, and Salsalate

Similarities to Aspirin. The nonacetylated salicylates are similar to aspirin (an acetylated salicylate) in most respects. Like aspirin, these drugs inhibit prostaglandin synthesis and are employed to treat arthritis, moderate pain, and fever. Their most common adverse effects are gastrointestinal disturbances. As with aspirin, these drugs should not be given to children

Table 61–1. Aspirin Dosage		
Indication	**Adult Dosage**	**Pediatric Dosage**
Aches and pains; fever	325–650 mg every 4 hr	2 to 3 years old: 160 mg 4 to 5 years old: 240 mg 6 to 8 years old: 325 mg 9 to 10 years old: 405 mg 11 years old: 485 mg Over 11 years old: 650 mg *All of the above doses are administered every 4 hr*
Acute rheumatic fever	5–8 gm/day in divided doses	100 mg/kg/day (initially) then 75 mg/kg/day for 4 to 6 wk
Rheumatoid arthritis	3.6–5.4 gm/day in divided doses	90–130 mg/kg/day in divided doses at 4- to 6-hr intervals
Postmyocardial infarction	160 or 325 mg/day	
Prevention of transient ischemic attacks (in men)	650 mg 2 times/day or 325 mg 4 times a day	

Table 61–2. Clinical Pharmacology of the Nonsteroidal Anti-inflammatory Drugs

Generic Name [Trade Name]	Maximum Daily Dosage (mg)	Plasma Half-Life (hr)	Major Indications				
			Rheumatoid Arthritis	*Moderate Pain*	*Fever*	*Primary Dysmenorrhea*	*Bursitis/ Tendinitis*
Salicylates							
Aspirin (many trade names)	8000	0.2–0.3	A	A	A		
Choline salicylate [Arthropan]	5200	2–30*	A	A	A		
Magnesium salicylate [Magan]	4800	2–30*	A	A	A		
Sodium salicylate (generic)	3900	2–30*	A	A	A		
Salsalate [Disalcid, Mono-Gesic]	3000	2–30*	A	A	A		
Propionic Acid Derivatives							
Fenoprofen [Nalfon]	3200	2–3	A	A			
Flurbiprofen [Ansaid]	300	2.6–5	A	I	I	I	I
Ibuprofen [Motrin, Rufen, others]	3200	1.8–2.5	A	A	A	A	
Ketoprofen [Orudis]	300	1.4–2.2	A	A		A	
Naproxen [Naprosyn]	1500	12–16	A	A	I	A	A
Naproxen sodium [Anaprox]	1375	12–13	A	A	I	A	A
Oxaprozin [Daypro]	1800	50–60	A				
Other NSAIDs							
Diclofenac [Voltaren]	200	0.9–1.3	A	I			
Diflunisal [Dolobid]	1500	11–15	A	A			
Etodolac [Lodine]	1200	3–6	I	A			I
Indomethacin [Indocin]	200	3.9–5.3	A			I	A
Ketorolac [Toradol]	40	2.4–8.6		A			
Meclofenamate [Meclomen]	400	2–3	A	A			
Mefenamic acid [Ponstel]	1000	2–4		A		A	
Nabumetone [Relafen]	2000	21–31	A				
Piroxicam [Feldene]	20	35–79	A			I	
Phenylbutazone [Butazolidin, Azolid]	600	43–93	A				
Sulindac [Clinoril]	400	6–22	A				A
Tolmetin [Tolectin]	2000	0.7–1.3	A				

A = FDA approved indication; I = investigational use
*Half-life increases with increasing dosage.

with chickenpox or influenza, because of the possibility of precipitating Reye's syndrome.

Contrasts with Aspirin. In contrast to aspirin, *the nonacetylated salicylates cause little or no suppression of platelet aggregation.* Accordingly, these drugs are preferred to aspirin for use by surgical patients and by patients with bleeding disorders.

Because of its sodium content, *sodium salicylate* should be avoided by patients on a sodium-restricted diet (e.g., patients with hypertension or congestive heart failure).

Magnesium salicylate may accumulate to toxic levels in patients with chronic renal insufficiency. Accordingly, magnesium salicylate should be avoided by these people.

Salsalate is a prodrug that breaks down to release two molecules of salicylate in the alkaline environment of the small intestine. Because the stomach is not exposed to salicylate, salsalate produces less gastric irritation than aspirin.

Like salsalate, *choline salicylate* causes less gastric irritation than aspirin.

Preparations, Dosage, and Administration. *Choline salicylate* [Arthropan] is dispensed in solution (870 mg/5 ml) for oral use. The usual dosage is 870 mg every 3 to 4 hours.

Magnesium salicylate [Magan, others] is dispensed in caplets (325 and 500 mg) and tablets (545 and 600 mg) for oral administration. The usual dosage is 650 mg every 4 hours or 1090 mg every 8 hours. The maximum dosage is 4800 mg/day administered in three or four doses.

Sodium salicylate (generic) is dispensed in enteric coated tablets (325 and 650 mg) for oral use. The usual dosage is 325 to 650 mg every 4 hours.

Salsalate [Disalcid, Mono-Gesic, others] is dispensed in capsules (500 mg) and tablets (500 and 750 mg) for oral use. The usual dosage is 3000 mg/day in divided doses.

Ibuprofen

Ibuprofen [Advil, Motrin, Rufen, others] is the prototype of the *propionic acid derivatives.* (Other members of the family are listed in Table 61–2, and discussed individually below.) Like aspirin, ibuprofen inhibits prostaglandin synthesis and has anti-inflammatory, analgesic, and antipyretic actions. The drug is used to treat fever, mild-to-moderate pain, and arthritis. In addition, ibuprofen appears superior to most other NSAIDs for relief of primary dysmenorrhea. This property has been attributed to unusually effective inhibition of prostaglandin synthesis in uterine smooth muscle.

The incidence of adverse effects is low, and ibuprofen is generally well tolerated. The drug produces less gastric bleeding than aspirin and causes less inhibition of platelet aggregation. Consequently, ibuprofen is one of the safer NSAIDs for use with anticoagulants.

Ibuprofen is available in two formulations: (1) tablets (200 to 800 mg), and (2) a 20 mg/ml oral suspension [Children's Advil, Pedia-Profen] for pediatric patients. The dosage for arthritis ranges from 1.2 to 3.2 gm/day administered in three or four divided doses. The dosage for primary dysmenorrhea is 400 mg every 4 hours. Administration with meals or milk can reduce gastric distress.

Fenoprofen

Fenoprofen [Nalfon] belongs to the propionic acid family of NSAIDs. Like other NSAIDs, the drug inhibits synthesis of prostaglandins, thereby causing anti-inflammatory, analgesic, and antipyretic effects. Fenoprofen is indicated for arthritis and mild-to-moderate pain. The most common adverse effects are gastrointestinal disturbances. Fenoprofen is dispensed in capsules (200 and 300 mg) and tablets (600 mg) for oral use. The usual dosage for rheumatoid arthritis is 300 to 600 mg three or four times a day. The maximum daily dosage is 3.2 gm.

Flurbiprofen

Flurbiprofen [Ansaid] is chemically related to ibuprofen and the other derivatives of propionic acid. The drug is approved for treating arthritis and has been used on an investigational basis to treat bursitis, tendinitis, moderate pain, fever, and primary dysmenorrhea. The most common adverse effects are gastrointestinal disturbances (dyspepsia, nausea, diarrhea, abdominal pain). The risk of serious gastrointestinal effects (ulceration, perforation, hemorrhage) may be greater than with ibuprofen. Like other NSAIDs, flurbiprofen can exacerbate renal impairment. The drug is dispensed in tablets (50 and 100 mg) for oral administration. The usual dosage for rheumatoid arthritis is 200 to 300 mg/day administered in two to four divided doses.

Ketoprofen

Ketoprofen [Orudis] belongs to the propionic acid family of NSAIDs. The drug inhibits synthesis of prostaglandins and has anti-inflammatory, analgesic, and antipyretic effects. Indications are rheumatoid arthritis, mild-to-moderate pain, and primary dysmenorrhea. The most common adverse effects are dyspepsia (11.5%), nausea, vomiting, and abdominal pain. Ketoprofen is dispensed in capsules (25, 50, and 75 mg) for oral administration. The usual dosage for rheumatoid arthritis is 150 to 300 mg/day administered in three or four divided doses. The dosage for moderate pain or primary dysmenorrhea is 25 to 50 mg every 6 to 8 hours.

Naproxen and Naproxen Sodium

Actions and Uses. Naproxen [Anaprox] and naproxen sodium [Naprosyn] belong to the propionic acid family of NSAIDs. Because these drugs have prolonged half-lives (see Table 61–2), they needn't be administered as frequently as the other propionic acid derivatives (e.g., ibuprofen). Naproxen and naproxen sodium are approved for treating arthritis, bursitis, tendinitis, primary dysmenorrhea, and mild-to-moderate pain. In addition, they are used investigationally to reduce fever. Like other NSAIDs, they act primarily by inhibiting synthesis of prostaglandins.

Adverse Effects. Naproxen and naproxen sodium are among the better tolerated NSAIDs. The most common adverse effects are gastrointestinal disturbances. Like other NSAIDs, these drugs can compromise renal function by decreasing renal blood flow. Bleeding time can be prolonged secondary to reversible inhibition of platelet aggregation.

Preparations, Dosage, and Administration. *Naproxen* is dispensed in tablets (250, 375, and 500 mg) and as an oral suspension (25 mg/ml). The usual dosage for rheumatoid arthritis is 250 to 500 mg twice daily. The dosage for mild-to-moderate pain is 500 mg initially followed by 250 mg every 6 to 8 hours.

Naproxen sodium is dispensed in tablets (275 and 550 mg) for oral use. The usual dosage for rheumatoid arthritis is 275 to 550 mg twice daily. The dosage for mild-to-moderate pain is 550 mg initially followed by 275 mg every 6 to 8 hours.

Diclofenac

Diclofenac [Voltaren] is approved for treating rheumatoid arthritis, osteoarthritis, and ankylosing spondylitis. The drug has been used on an investigational basis to treat moderate pain. Like other NSAIDs, diclofenac produces its anti-inflammatory, analgesic, and antipyretic effects by inhibiting the synthesis of prostaglandins.

Diclofenac is well absorbed following oral administration, but undergoes extensive (40% to 50%) metabolism on its first pass through the liver. In blood, about 99.5% of the drug is protein bound, primarily to albumin. Diclofenac is metabolized by the liver and excreted in the urine.

The most common adverse effects are abdominal pain, dyspepsia, and nausea. Diclofenac can cause fluid retention, and this can exacerbate hypertension and congestive heart failure. The risk of liver dysfunction is greater than with other NSAIDs. Accordingly, patients should receive periodic tests of liver function, and should be instructed to report manifestations of liver injury (e.g., jaundice, fatigue, nausea).

Diclofenac is dispensed in enteric-coated tablets (25, 50, and

75 mg) for oral administration. The dosage for rheumatoid arthritis is 150 to 200 mg/day administered in two or three divided doses. The dosage for osteoarthritis is 100 to 150 mg/day administered in two or three divided doses.

Diflunisal

Diflunisal [Dolobid] is a derivative of salicylic acid. However, unlike the salicylates, diflunisal is not converted to salicylic acid in the body. The drug is indicated for mild-to-moderate pain and rheumatoid arthritis. Like other NSAIDs, the drug inhibits prostaglandin synthesis and can cause gastrointestinal disturbances, suppression of platelet aggregation, and impairment of kidney function. Diflunisal has a prolonged half-life (11 to 15 hours), which allows the drug to be administered only two or three times a day. Diflunisal is dispensed in tablets (250 and 500 mg) for oral use. For treatment of arthritis and mild-to-moderate pain, the *initial* dose is 500 to 1000 mg. *Maintenance* doses of 250 to 500 mg are administered every 8 to 12 hours.

Etodolac

Etodolac [Lodine] is indicated for osteoarthritis and moderate pain. The drug has been used on an investigational basis to treat rheumatoid arthritis, bursitis, and tendinitis. Like other NSAIDs, etodolac produces many of its effects by suppressing the synthesis of prostaglandins. The drug's most common adverse effects are dyspepsia (10%), nausea, vomiting, diarrhea, and abdominal pain. Clinical studies suggest that etodolac may cause less gastric ulceration and bleeding than other NSAIDs. Etodolac is dispensed in capsules (200 and 300 mg) for oral use. The recommended dosage for osteoarthritis is 800 to 1200 mg/day in divided doses. The dosage for moderate pain is 200 to 400 mg every 6 to 8 hours.

Indomethacin

Actions and Uses. Indomethacin [Indocin] is an effective anti-inflammatory agent approved for treating arthritis, bursitis, tendinitis, and, as discussed in Chapter 63, acute gouty arthritis. The drug can reduce pain and fever but is not routinely used for these effects because of its potential for toxicity.

Adverse Effects. Untoward effects are seen in 35% to 50% of those treated. About 20% of patients discontinue the drug. The most common adverse effect is *severe frontal headache*, which occurs in 25% to 50% of recipients. Other CNS effects (dizziness, vertigo, confusion) are also common. Seizures and psychiatric changes (e.g., depression, psychosis) have occurred. Mild gastrointestinal reactions (nausea, vomiting, indigestion) are experienced by 3% to 9% of users. More severe GI effects (ulceration with perforation, hemorrhage) may also develop. Hematologic reactions (neutropenia, thrombocytopenia, aplastic anemia) have occurred but are rare. Indomethacin suppresses platelet aggregation.

Precautions and Contraindications. Because of its adverse effects, indomethacin is contraindicated for infants and children under the age of 14, patients with peptic ulcer disease, and women who are pregnant or breast-feeding. Caution is required in patients with epilepsy and psychiatric disorders, in patients involved in hazardous activities, and in patients receiving anticoagulant therapy.

Pharmacokinetics. Indomethacin is well absorbed following oral administration and distributes to all body fluids and tissues. The drug is metabolized in the liver. Metabolites and parent drug are excreted in the urine and feces.

Preparations, Dosage, and Administration. Indomethacin [Indocin] is dispensed in standard capsules (25 and 50 mg), sustained-release capsules (75 mg), an oral suspension (5 mg/ml), and rectal suppositories (50 mg). For treatment of rheumatoid arthritis, the initial dosage is 25 mg two or three times a day. The maximum daily dosage is 200 mg. Gastrointestinal reactions can be reduced by administering indomethacin with meals. Dosages for treating gout are presented in Chapter 63.

Ketorolac

Actions and Uses. Ketorolac [Toradol] is the only *injectable* NSAID available in the United States for treatment of pain. In clinical trials, the drug has been as effective as morphine against postoperative pain while causing fewer adverse effects. Because of the risks associated with prolonged use, ketorolac is approved only for short-term therapy (5 days or less) of moderate-to-severe pain. Like other NSAIDs, ketorolac suppresses prostaglandin synthesis. This action is thought to underlie the drug's analgesic effects as well as its anti-inflammatory and antipyretic effects.

Pharmacokinetics. Ketorolac is administered orally and by IM injection. Analgesia begins within 10 minutes of IM injection and persists for up to 6 hours. The drug is eliminated by a combination of hepatic metabolism and urinary excretion. In young adults, ketorolac has a half-life of 4 to 6 hours. The half-life may be prolonged in the elderly and in patients with renal impairment.

Adverse Effects. The most common adverse effects are *gastrointestinal*: nausea (12%), dyspepsia (12%), diarrhea (3% to 9%), and abdominal distress, cramps, and pain (13%). With short-term intramuscular therapy, there have been no reports of peptic ulcers or gastrointestinal bleeding. However, these effects *have* occurred with long-term oral therapy.

Like other NSAIDs, ketorolac causes reversible suppression of platelet aggregation. Although IM ketorolac has not been associated with serious postoperative bleeding, the drug does prolong bleeding time and has caused hematomas.

In contrast to other NSAIDs, IM ketorolac has not been associated with anaphylactic reactions or acute renal failure.

Ketorolac lacks the serious adverse effects of the opioid (narcotic) analgesics. The drug does not cause respiratory depression, adverse cardiovascular effects, physical dependence, or tolerance. Ketorolac has no abuse potential and is not regulated under the Controlled Substances Act. Although ketorolac does cause constipation, the incidence is lower than with opioids.

Preparations, Dosage, and Administration. Ketorolac [Toradol] is available in 10-mg tablets for oral administration, and in preloaded syringes (15 and 30 mg/ml) for IM injection.

Intramuscular administration may be done on a PRN basis or on a fixed schedule. When a fixed schedule is employed, the initial (loading) dose is 30 or 60 mg. After this, maintenance doses of 15 or 30 mg (one-half the loading dose employed) are given every 6 hours. Treatment should be limited to 5 days or less. The maximum daily dosage is 150 mg on the first day and 120 mg on subsequent days. Ketorolac is eliminated slowly by the elderly and by patients with renal impairment; accordingly, dosages should be reduced in these people.

Oral therapy should be of limited duration. The usual dosage is 10 mg every 4 to 6 hours. The maximum daily dosage is 40 mg.

Mefenamic Acid

Mefenamic acid [Ponstel] is indicated for relief of primary dysmenorrhea and moderate pain. The principal adverse effect is diarrhea, which is sometimes severe. Mefenamic acid is dispensed in 250-mg capsules for oral administration. The dosage for primary dysmenorrhea is 500 mg initially followed by 250 mg every 6 hours. The drug should be administered with food or milk to reduce gastric distress. Duration of treatment is usually 2 to 3 days.

Nabumetone

Nabumetone [Relafen] is a prodrug that undergoes conversion to its active form (6-MNA) in the liver. Like other NSAIDs, 6-MNA inhibits biosynthesis of prostaglandins, and this action is thought to underlie many of the beneficial and adverse effects of the drug. Although nabumetone has antipyretic, analgesic, and anti-inflammatory properties, the drug is approved only for treatment of arthritis. Principal adverse effects are diarrhea (14%), abdominal cramps (13%), dyspepsia (12%), and nausea (3% to 9%). Because nabumetone is inactive as administered, the drug may cause less gastrointestinal ulceration and bleeding than other NSAIDs. Nabumetone is dispensed in 500- and 750-mg tablets for oral use. Treatment of rheumatoid arthritis is begun with a single dose of 1000 mg. After this, the daily dosage is 1500 to 2000 mg administered in one or two doses. Administration with food *increases* the rate of absorption.

Piroxicam

Piroxicam [Feldene] has anti-inflammatory, analgesic, and antipyretic properties. However, the drug is approved only for treatment of arthritis. The most outstanding feature of piroxicam is its long half-life (about 50 hours). Because the drug is eliminated so slowly, therapeutic effects can be maintained with once-a-day dosing. In general, piroxicam is better tolerated than aspirin. Undesired effects are seen in 11% to 46% of those treated, and between 4% and 12% discontinue therapy. Gastrointestinal reactions are most common, occurring in about 20% of recipients. The incidence of gastric ulceration is about 1%. Like aspirin, piroxicam inhibits platelet aggregation and prolongs bleeding time. The drug is dispensed in 10- and 20-mg capsules for oral administration. The usual dosage is 20 mg once a day.

Phenylbutazone

Actions and Uses. Phenylbutazone [Butazolidin, Azolid] is an effective anti-inflammatory agent, but toxicities (especially blood dyscrasias) limit its use. The drug should be employed only after trials with other NSAIDs have been unsuccessful, and only when the potential benefits outweigh the risks. The duration of treatment should be as brief as possible, preferably less than 1 week. Phenylbutazone can relieve fever and pain but should not be used for these conditions.

Adverse Effects. Untoward effects are common and lead to discontinuation of therapy by 10% to 15% of patients. The most frequent effects are nausea, vomiting, epigastric distress, and rashes. More serious effects include hypersensitivity reactions, gastric ulceration, ulcerative stomatitis, hepatitis, and nephritis. In addition, phenylbutazone can act on the kidney to cause retention of sodium, chloride, and water. These renal effects can result in peripheral edema, pulmonary edema, and congestive heart failure.

The most serious adverse effects are hematologic. Phenylbutazone can cause *leukopenia*, *agranulocytosis*, and *aplastic anemia*. Death from these reactions has an incidence of 2.2 per 100,000 patients. Toxicity may appear suddenly, or may develop days or even weeks after therapy has ceased. When treatment with phenylbutazone is prolonged, frequent blood tests are required. If a blood disorder develops, phenylbutazone should be discontinued immediately.

Contraindications. Because of its adverse effects, phenylbutazone is contraindicated for patients with hypertension, cardiac dysfunction, and renal disease. In addition, the drug is contraindicated for senile patients, patients under the age of 14, and patients with a history of peptic ulcer disease or hypersensitivity to other NSAIDs.

Drug Interactions. Phenylbutazone can intensify the effects of other drugs (e.g., oral anticoagulants, sulfonamides, sulfonylureas) by displacing them from binding sites on plasma proteins. The resultant increase in free drug can lead to toxicity. Care should be taken when these combinations are employed.

Pharmacokinetics. Phenylbutazone is administered orally and absorption is rapid. The drug undergoes extensive metabolism, and the metabolites are excreted in the urine. Elimination is slow, taking place with a half-time of 50 to 65 hours.

Preparations and Dosage. Phenylbutazone [Butazolidin, Azolid] is dispensed in 100-mg tablets and capsules for oral administration. For treatment of rheumatoid arthritis, the initial dosage is 300 to 600 mg/day administered in three or four divided doses. Once a response has developed, the dosage should be reduced. During long-term therapy, the maximum maintenance dosage is 400 mg/day.

Sulindac

Sulindac [Clinoril] is a prodrug that undergoes conversion to its active form within the body. The drug is approved for treating rheumatoid arthritis, tendinitis, bursitis, and acute gouty arthritis. Principal adverse effects are abdominal distress, dyspepsia, nausea, vomiting, and diarrhea. Gastric ulceration is less common than with some other NSAIDs, perhaps because sulindac is not active as administered. Like other NSAIDs, sulindac causes reversible inhibition of platelet aggregation, prolongs bleeding time, and causes acute renal failure. The drug is dispensed in 150- and 200-mg tablets for oral administration. The usual dosage is 150 mg administered twice daily with meals. The maximum daily dosage is 400 mg.

Tolmetin

Tolmetin [Tolectin] is used to treat arthritis and related inflammatory disorders. The drug has analgesic and antipyretic properties but is not employed for relief of fever or pain unrelated to inflammation. Adverse effects occur in 25% to 40% of those treated. Between 5% and 10% of patients discontinue the drug. Gastrointestinal effects (nausea, vomiting, indigestion) are most common. Gastric ulceration has occurred, but this reaction is less frequent than with aspirin. Nonetheless, caution should be exercised in patients with a history of peptic ulcer disease. Hypersensitivity reactions occur more frequently than with aspirin. Effects on the CNS (headache, dizziness, anxiety, drowsiness) are less severe and less frequent than with indomethacin. Unlike most other NSAIDs, tolmetin does not augment the effects of oral anticoagulants. The drug is dispensed in tablets (200 and 600 mg) and capsules (400 mg) for oral administration. For treatment of rheumatoid arthritis, the initial dosage is 400 mg three times a day. The maximum daily dosage is 2 gm. Gastrointestinal distress can be minimized by administering tolmetin with food.

ACETAMINOPHEN

Acetaminophen [Tylenol, others] is similar to aspirin in some respects but quite different in others. Acetaminophen has *analgesic* and *antipyretic* properties equivalent to those of aspirin. However, in contrast to aspirin and the other NSAIDs, *acetaminophen is devoid of clinically useful anti-inflammatory and antirheumatic actions*. In addition, acetaminophen does not suppress platelet aggregation, does not cause gastric bleeding, and does not decrease renal blood flow or cause renal failure. Furthermore, acetaminophen overdosage differs from overdosage with aspirin both in manifestations and treatment.

Mechanism of Action

Differences between the effects of acetaminophen and aspirin are thought to result from selective inhibition of prostaglandin synthesis: whereas aspirin can inhibit synthesis of prostaglandins in both the CNS and the periphery, inhibition by acetaminophen is limited to the CNS; acetaminophen has only minimal effects on prostaglandin synthesis at peripheral sites. By decreasing prostaglandin synthesis in the CNS, acetaminophen is able to reduce fever and pain. The inability of acetaminophen to inhibit prostaglandin synthesis outside the CNS may explain the absence of anti-inflammatory effects, gastric bleeding, and adverse effects on the kidneys and platelets.

Pharmacokinetics

Acetaminophen is readily absorbed following oral administration and undergoes wide distribution. Most of an administered dose is metabolized by the liver, and the resultant metabolites are excreted in the urine. The plasma half-life of the drug is approximately 2 hours.

The manner in which acetaminophen is metabolized is dependent on dosage. At low (therapeutic) doses, most of the drug is converted into inactive compounds, while a small fraction is converted into a *toxic substance* that can harm the liver. Fortunately, the toxic product usually undergoes rapid conversion to a nontoxic form. However, when an overdose of acetaminophen is ingested, a large quantity of the toxic metabolite is produced. Under these conditions, the capacity of the liver to detoxify the metabolite is exceeded, and hepatic injury results (see below).

Adverse Effects

Adverse effects are rare at therapeutic doses. As noted above, *acetaminophen does not cause gastric bleeding, does not inhibit platelet aggregation, and does not decrease renal blood flow or cause renal failure.* In addition, *there is no evidence linking acetaminophen with Reye's syndrome.* Individuals who are hypersensitive to aspirin only rarely experience cross-hypersensitivity to acetaminophen.

The risk of *liver injury* is increased in *chronic alcoholics.* Two mechanisms may underlie the increased risk: (1) induction of hepatic drug-metabolizing enzymes (as a result of chronic alcohol consumption) may increase production of the toxic metabolite of acetaminophen, and (2) the alcoholic's liver may have a reduced capacity to convert the toxic metabolite to a nontoxic form.

Therapeutic Uses

Acetaminophen is indicated for relief of pain and fever in patients who cannot tolerate the side ef-fects of aspirin (e.g., patients with bleeding disorders or peptic ulcer disease). Because of its lack of association with Reye's syndrome, acetaminophen is preferred to aspirin for use by children suspected of having chickenpox or influenza. In addition, acetaminophen may be a safe alternative to aspirin for patients who have experienced aspirin hypersensitivity reactions. Because of its weak anti-inflammatory actions, acetaminophen is *not* useful for treating arthritis or rheumatic fever.

Acute Toxicity

Signs and Symptoms. The principal feature of acetaminophen overdosage is *hepatic necrosis.* Severe poisoning can progress to hepatic failure, coma, and death. Early symptoms of poisoning (nausea, vomiting, diarrhea, sweating, abdominal discomfort) belie the severity of intoxication. It is not until 48 to 72 hours after drug ingestion that overt indications of hepatic injury appear.

Treatment. Liver damage can be minimized by administering *acetylcysteine* [Mucomyst], a specific antidote to acetaminophen toxicity. Acetylcysteine reduces injury by promoting inactivation of the toxic metabolite of acetaminophen. Although acetylcysteine is most effective when given shortly after acetaminophen ingestion, the drug can still provide significant protection when administered as long as 24 hours after poisoning has occurred. Acetylcysteine is dispensed in 10% and 20% solutions, and should be diluted to 5% with water, fruit juice, or a cola beverage. The initial dose is 140 mg/kg. Additional doses of 70 mg/kg are administered at 4-hour intervals for the next 72 hours. Acetylcysteine has an extremely unpleasant odor and may induce vomiting. If vomiting interferes with oral treatment, the drug can be administered through an oroduodenal tube.

Preparations, Dosage, and Administration

Acetaminophen is dispensed in a variety of *oral formulations* (standard tablets, chewable tablets, effervescent granules, capsules, liquids, elixirs, solutions) and in *rectal suppositories.* The dosage for adults and children over 12 years is 325 to 650 mg every 4 to 6 hours. Doses for younger children vary with age, progressing from 40 mg (for children aged 3 months or younger) up to 480 mg (for children aged 11 years); these doses may be administered up to five times a day.

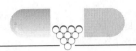 # Summary of Major Nursing Implications

NONSTEROIDAL ANTI-INFLAMMATORY DRUGS

Except where noted, the nursing implications summarized below apply to aspirin and all other NSAIDs.

✓ **Preadministration Assessment**

Therapeutic Goal

Major indications for the NSAIDs are inflammatory disorders (e.g., rheumatoid arthritis), mild-to-moderate pain, fever, primary dysmenorrhea, tendinitis, and bursitis. Applications of individual NSAIDs are summarized in Table 61–2.

Identifying High-Risk Patients

NSAIDs are *contraindicated* for patients with a history of *severe NSAID hypersensitivity.*

NSAIDs should be used with *extreme caution* by *pregnant women* and by patients with *peptic ulcer disease* and *bleeding disorders* (e.g., hemophilia, vitamin K deficiency, hypoprothrombinemia) and by patients taking *oral anticoagulants* or *glucocorticoids. Caution* is also needed when treating *elderly* patients and patients with *congestive heart failure, hypovolemia, hepatic cirrhosis, renal dysfunction, asthma, hay fever, chronic urticaria, nasal polyps,* or a *history of alcoholism* or *heavy cigarette smoking.*

NSAIDs (especially aspirin) should be avoided by children with *chickenpox* or *influenza.*

NSAIDs should be discontinued 1 week prior to *elective surgery* or the anticipated date of *parturition.*

✓ **Implementation: Administration**

Routes

Oral: all NSAIDs.
Intramuscular: *ketorolac.*
Rectal (by suppository): *aspirin* and *indomethacin.*

Administration

Advise patients to take NSAIDs with food, milk, or a glass of water to reduce gastric upset.

Instruct patients not to crush or chew enteric coated or sustained-release formulations.

Advise patients to discard *aspirin* preparations that smell of vinegar.

✓ **Ongoing Evaluation and Interventions**

Minimizing Adverse Effects

Gastrointestinal Effects. NSAIDs frequently cause mild GI reactions (dyspepsia, abdominal pain, nausea). To minimize these effects, advise patients to take NSAIDs with food, milk, or a glass of water.

Long-term, high-dose therapy can cause *gastric ulceration, perforation,* and *hemorrhage.* To reduce the risk of these reactions, avoid NSAIDs in patients with a recent history of peptic ulcer disease and use NSAIDs with caution in patients with other risk factors (advanced age, previous intolerance to NSAIDs, heavy cigarette smoking, history of alcoholism). Warn patients not to consume alcohol.

Instruct patients to notify the physician if gastric irritation is severe or persistent. Switching to a different NSAID (e.g., ibuprofen) may be helpful.

Manage GI ulcers by discontinuing the NSAID and giving an anti-ulcer medication (usually an *H₂-receptor antagonist* or *sucralfate*). Alternatively, it may be possible to continue the NSAID while treating the ulcer with *omeprazole*.

Misoprostol can be given for *prophylaxis* of NSAID-induced ulcers in high-risk patients. Because misoprostol can stimulate uterine contractions, the drug is absolutely contraindicated during pregnancy.

Bleeding. *Aspirin* promotes bleeding by causing *irreversible* suppression of platelet aggregation. Aspirin should be discontinued 1 week prior to elective surgery or parturition. Exercise caution when using aspirin in conjunction with oral anticoagulants. Avoid aspirin in patients with bleeding disorders (e.g., hemophilia, vitamin K deficiency, hypoprothrombinemia).

The nonacetylated salicylates—*sodium salicylate, choline salicylate,* and *magnesium salicylate*—have minimal effects on platelet aggregation. Accordingly, these drugs are preferred for use in surgical patients and patients with bleeding disorders.

All other NSAIDs cause *reversible* suppression of platelet aggregation. As a result, the duration of antiplatelet effects is determined by the plasma half-life of the individual drug.

Renal Impairment. NSAIDs can cause acute renal insufficiency in elderly patients and in patients with congestive heart failure, hypovolemia, hepatic cirrhosis, or pre-existing renal dysfunction. Keep NSAID dosages as low as possible in these patients. Monitor high-risk patients for indications of renal impairment (reduced urine output, weight gain despite diuretic therapy, rapid elevation of serum creatinine and blood urea nitrogen). Discontinue NSAIDs if these signs occur.

Hypersensitivity Reactions. These reactions are most likely in patients with asthma, hay fever, chronic urticaria, or nasal polyps. NSAIDs should be used with caution by these patients. If a severe hypersensitivity reaction occurs, parenteral *epinephrine* is the treatment of choice. Avoid NSAIDs in patients with a history of NSAID hypersensitivity.

Salicylism. *Aspirin* and *other salicylates* can cause salicylism. Educate patients about manifestations of salicylism (tinnitus, sweating, headache, dizziness) and advise them to notify the physician if these occur. Aspirin should be withheld until symptoms subside, after which therapy can resume but at a slightly reduced dosage.

Reye's Syndrome. Use of NSAIDs (especially aspirin) by children with chickenpox or influenza may precipitate Reye's syndrome. Advise parents to consult a physician before administering NSAIDs to children suspected of having these viral infections.

Use in Pregnancy. *Aspirin* can cause *fetal injury*. All other NSAIDs can cause *maternal anemia* and *prolongation of labor and gestation.* NSAIDs should be avoided by expectant mothers unless the potential benefits outweigh the risks. If NSAIDs are employed during pregnancy, they should be discontinued at least 1 week before the anticipated day of delivery.

Minimizing Adverse Interactions

Oral Anticoagulants. NSAIDs can increase the risk of spontaneous bleeding in patients taking oral anticoagulants (e.g., warfarin). Monitor patients for signs of bleeding.

Glucocorticoids. Glucocorticoids increase the risk of gastric ulceration in patients taking NSAIDs. Prophylactic therapy with *misoprostol* can decrease the risk.

Managing Aspirin Toxicity

Aspirin poisoning is an acute medical emergency that requires hospitalization. Treatment is largely supportive and consists of external cooling (e.g., sponging with tepid water), infusion of fluids (to correct dehydration and electrolyte loss), infusion of bicarbonate (to reverse acidosis and promote renal excretion of salicylates), and mechanical ventilation (if respiration is severely depressed). Absorption of aspirin can be reduced by gastric lavage, induction of emesis, and administration of activated charcoal. If necessary, hemodialysis or peritoneal dialysis can accelerate salicylate removal.

ACETAMINOPHEN

Preadministration Assessment

Therapeutic Goal

Acetaminophen is indicated for relief of pain and suppression of fever in patients who are intolerant to aspirin and other NSAIDs. Acetaminophen is preferred to NSAIDs for use in children with chickenpox or influenza.

Identifying High-Risk Patients

Use with caution in chronic alcoholics.

Implementation: Administration

Routes

Oral, rectal.

Administration

Do not exceed recommended doses.

Minimizing Adverse Effects

Acetaminophen is devoid of significant adverse effects at usual therapeutic doses.

Ongoing Evaluation and Interventions

Managing Toxicity

Overdosage can cause hepatic necrosis. *Acetylcysteine* is a specific antidote. Acetylcysteine has an extremely unpleasant odor and may induce vomiting. If vomiting interferes with oral administration, acetylcysteine can be administered through an oroduodenal tube.

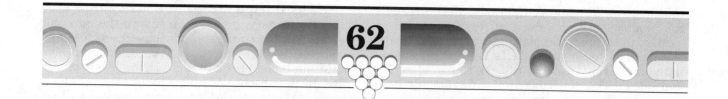

Glucocorticoids in Nonendocrine Diseases

The glucocorticoid drugs (e.g., cortisone, prednisone), which are also known as *corticosteroids*, are nearly identical to the glucose-regulating steroids produced by the adrenal cortex. Accordingly, we can look on the glucocorticoids as having two kinds of effects: physiologic effects and pharmacologic effects. *Physiologic* effects, such as modulation of glucose metabolism, are elicited by *low* doses of glucocorticoids. *Pharmacologic* effects (e.g., suppression of inflammation) occur when the dosage is *high*.

As implied by the chapter title, glucocorticoids have both endocrine and nonendocrine applications. In low (physiologic) doses, glucocorticoids are used to treat endocrine disorders (e.g., adrenocortical insufficiency). In high (pharmacologic) doses, these agents are used to treat inflammatory disorders (e.g., rheumatoid arthritis, asthma) and certain cancers and to suppress immune responses in patients receiving organ transplants. The endocrine applications of the glucocorticoids are discussed in Chapter 53. Nonendocrine uses, which are the most common applications of these drugs, are the subject of this chapter.

Toxicity of the glucocorticoids can be severe and is determined by the pattern of drug use. Glucocorticoids are devoid of toxicity when used in physiologic doses or when taken acutely, even when the dosage is huge. However, when taken in pharmacologic doses for extended periods, glucocorticoids can produce multiple, severe adverse effects.

All of the glucocorticoid drugs can elicit the same spectrum of therapeutic effects. Differences among individual agents pertain to time course of action and side effects. Since the similarities among these drugs are much more striking than the differences, we will forego our practice of focusing on a prototypic agent, and discuss the glucocorticoids as a group. In approaching the glucocorticoids, we will begin with a review of their physiology, after which we will discuss their pharmacology.

REVIEW OF GLUCOCORTICOID PHYSIOLOGY

PHYSIOLOGIC EFFECTS

Physiologic responses can be elicited with low doses of glucocorticoids. When the dosage is high, these effects will simply be more intense. When glucocorticoids are used to treat nonendocrine disorders, physiologic responses will occur as side effects. Physiologic effects of the glucocorticoids are discussed in depth in Chapter 53. The discussion below is intended as a review.

Metabolic Effects. Glucocorticoids influence the metabolism of carbohydrates, proteins, and fats. The principal effect on carbohydrate metabolism is elevation of blood glucose content. This is accomplished by promoting synthesis of glucose from amino acids and by reducing peripheral glucose utilization. Glucocorticoids also promote storage of glucose in the form of glycogen.

Glucocorticoids have an unfavorable impact on protein metabolism. These agents suppress synthesis of proteins from amino acids and divert amino acids for production of glucose. These actions can cause a reduction in muscle mass, thinning of the skin, and a decrease in the protein matrix of bone. Nitrogen balance becomes negative.

The most consistent effect of glucocorticoids on fat metabolism is stimulation of lipolysis (fat breakdown). Long-term, high-dose therapy can cause fat redistribution, resulting in the pot belly, "moon face," and "buffalo hump" that typify Cushing's disease.

Cardiovascular Effects. Glucocorticoids are required to maintain the functional integrity of the vascular system. When levels of endogenous glucocorticoids are low, capillaries become more permeable, vasoconstriction is suppressed, and blood pressure falls. Glucocorticoids increase the number of circulating red blood cells and polymorphonuclear leukocytes. Counts of lymphocytes, eosinophils, basophils, and monocytes are reduced.

Effects During Stress. At times of stress (e.g., anxiety, surgery, infection, trauma), the adrenals secrete large quantities of glucocorticoids and epinephrine. Working together, these compounds help maintain blood pressure and plasma levels of glucose. In the absence of sufficient amounts of glucocorticoids, hypotension and hypoglycemia will occur. If the stress is especially severe, glucocorticoid insufficiency can result in circulatory failure and death.

Effects on Water and Electrolytes. To varying degrees, individual glucocorticoids can exert actions like those of aldosterone, the major mineralocorticoid released by the adrenals. Accordingly, glucocorticoids can act on the kidney to promote retention of sodium and water while increasing urinary excretion of potassium. The net result of these effects is hypernatremia, hypokalemia, and edema. Fortunately, most of the glucocorticoids employed as drugs have very low mineralocorticoid activity (see Table 62–1).

CONTROL OF SYNTHESIS AND SECRETION

Synthesis and release of glucocorticoids are regulated by a negative feedback loop. The principal components of this loop are the hypothalamus, the anterior pituitary, and the adrenal cortex (Fig. 62–1). The loop is turned on when stress or some other stimulus from the central nervous system (CNS) acts on the hypothalamus to cause release of corticotropin releasing factor (CRF). CRF then stimulates the pituitary to release adrenocorticotropic hormone (ACTH), which in turn acts on the adrenal cortex to promote synthesis and release of cortisol (the principal endogenous glucocorticoid). Cortisol then exerts two kinds of effects: (1) it promotes physiologic responses, and (2) it acts on the hypothalamus and pituitary to suppress further release of CRF and ACTH. By inhibiting release of these factors, cortisol suppresses its own production. Hence, this negative feedback system serves to keep glucocorticoid levels within an appropriate range. As discussed later in the chapter, when glucocorticoids are administered chronically in large doses, the feedback loop remains continuously suppressed. This persistent inhibition can be very detrimental.

PHARMACOLOGY OF THE GLUCOCORTICOIDS

PHARMACOLOGIC ACTIONS

When administered in the high doses employed to treat nonendocrine disorders, the glucocorticoids

Table 62–1. Glucocorticoids: Half-Lives, Relative Potencies, and Equivalent Doses

Drug	Biologic Half-Life (hr)	Relative Mineralocorticoid Potency*	Relative Glucocorticoid (Anti-inflammatory) Potency	Equivalent Anti-inflammatory Dose (mg)†
Short-Acting				
Cortisone	8–12	2	0.8	25
Hydrocortisone	8–12	2	1.0	20
Intermediate-Acting				
Prednisone	18–36	1	4	5
Prednisolone	18–36	1	4	5
Methylprednisolone	18–36	0	5	4
Triamcinolone	18–36	0	5	4
Long-Acting				
Betamethasone	36–54	0	20–30	0.75
Dexamethasone	36–54	0	20–30	0.75

*Relative mineralocorticoid activity (sodium and water retention; potassium depletion): 0 = very low; 1 = moderate; 2 = high.
†Approximate *oral* or *intravenous* dose needed to produce equivalent anti-inflammatory effects.

have powerful anti-inflammatory and immunosuppressive actions. These actions do not occur when glucocorticoid doses are physiologic. In addition to these pharmacologic actions, high-dose therapy will intensify the kinds of responses elicited by physiologic doses of glucocorticoids.

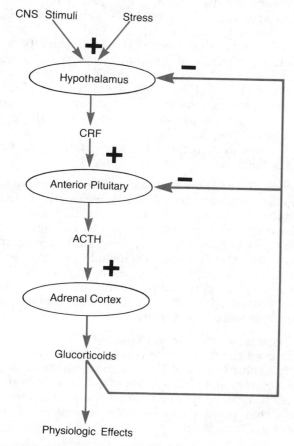

Figure 62–1. Feedback regulation of glucocorticoid synthesis and secretion. (CRF = corticotropin-releasing factor, ACTH = adrenocorticotropic hormone)

Effects on Metabolism and Electrolytes

Qualitatively, the effects of high-dose therapy on metabolism and electrolytes are the same as those that occur at physiologic doses; these responses are simply more intense when the dosage is high. Hence, with pharmacologic doses, glucose levels rise, protein synthesis is suppressed, and fat deposits are mobilized. As noted above, most glucocorticoids have very little mineralocorticoid activity. Accordingly, these drugs do not usually induce significant sodium retention or loss of potassium. However, these effects do occur in some patients and can be hazardous. In addition, high-dose therapy can inhibit intestinal absorption of calcium. This effect is not seen when doses are physiologic.

Anti-inflammatory and Immunosuppressant Effects

The major clinical applications of the glucocorticoids stem from the ability of these drugs to suppress immune responses and inflammation. Since effects on the immune system and inflammation are interrelated, we will consider these effects together.

Before discussing the actions of glucocorticoids, it will be helpful to review the process of inflammation. The characteristic symptoms of inflammation are pain, swelling, redness, and warmth. These effects are initiated by chemical mediators (prostaglandins, histamine, leukotrienes) and are amplified by the actions of lymphocytes and phagocytic cells (neutrophils and macrophages). Prostaglandins and histamine promote several symptoms of inflammation—swelling, redness, and warmth—by causing vasodilation and by increasing capillary permeability. Prostaglandins and histamine also help cause pain: histamine acts by stimulating pain receptors directly; prostaglandins act by sensitizing pain receptors to histamine and other stimuli. Neutrophils and macrophages heighten inflammation by releasing lysosomal enzymes (enzymes that cause direct tissue injury). Lymphocytes, which are important elements of the immune system, intensify inflammation by (1) causing direct cell injury, and (2) promoting formation of antibodies that serve to perpetuate the inflammatory response.

Glucocorticoids act through several mechanisms to interrupt the inflammatory processes. These drugs can inhibit synthesis of chemical mediators (prostaglandins, leukotrienes, histamine) and thereby reduce swelling, warmth, redness, and pain. In addition, these agents suppress infiltration of phagocytes. Hence, damage from release of lysosomal enzymes is averted. Lastly, glucocorticoids suppress proliferation of lymphocytes, and thereby reduce the immune component of inflammation.

On a molecular level, most effects of glucocorticoids can be attributed to promoting the synthesis of specific regulatory proteins. Stimulation of protein synthesis is accomplished as follows: (1) glucocorticoids penetrate the cell membrane and then bind to intracellular receptors; (2) the receptor-steroid complex travels to the cell nucleus where it binds to chromatin in DNA; and (3) the interaction with chromatin triggers transcription of messenger RNA molecules that code for regulatory proteins, thereby increasing synthesis of these regulatory molecules.

It is important to note that the mechanisms by which glucocorticoids suppress inflammation are broader in scope than the mechanisms by which nonsteroidal anti-inflammatory drugs (NSAIDs) act. As discussed in Chapter 61, the anti-inflammatory effects of the NSAIDs can be attributed largely to inhibition of prostaglandin biosynthesis. The glucocorticoids share this mechanism and, as indicated above, act in several other ways as well. It is because of this multiplicity of mechanisms that the anti-inflammatory effects of glucocorticoids are much greater than those of the NSAIDs.

PHARMACOKINETICS

Absorption. The rate of glucocorticoid absorption depends on the route of administration and the particular glucocorticoid derivative being administered. With oral administration, absorption of all glucocorticoids is rapid and nearly complete. Following IM injection, absorption is rapid with two types of glucocorticoid esters (sodium phosphates and sodium succinates) and relatively slow with other derivatives (e.g., acetates, acetonides, tebutates). Absorption from local sites of injection (e.g., intra-articular, intrasynovial) is slower than from IM sites.

Duration of Action. Duration of action is a function of dosage, route of administration, and solubility. For glucocorticoids administered orally or IV, duration of action is determined largely by biologic half-life (see Table 62–1). With IM administration, duration of action is a function of water solubility: highly soluble preparations have a duration of action that is shorter than that of less soluble preparations. For locally ad-

ministered glucocorticoids, duration is determined by solubility and by the specific site of administration.

Metabolism and Excretion. Glucocorticoids are metabolized primarily by the liver. As a rule, metabolites are inactive. Excretion of glucocorticoid metabolites is renal.

THERAPEUTIC USES IN NONENDOCRINE DISORDERS

Glucocorticoids are used to treat endocrine disorders and nonendocrine disorders. Endocrine disorders (e.g., Addison's disease, acute adrenal insufficiency) can be managed with low-dose therapy and are considered in Chapter 53. Nonendocrine applications, which require much higher doses, are discussed below. Because prolonged, high-dose therapy can produce serious adverse effects, the potential benefits of treatment must be weighed carefully against the very real risks.

Rheumatoid Arthritis. Glucocorticoids are indicated for adjunctive treatment of acute exacerbations of rheumatoid arthritis. These drugs can reduce inflammation and pain, but do not alter the course of the disease. Because of the risk of serious complications, prolonged systemic use should be avoided.

When arthritis is limited to just a few joints, intra-articular injections should be employed. Local injections can be highly effective, and cause less toxicity than systemic therapy. Frequently, reductions in pain and inflammation may be so dramatic as to prompt vigorous use of joints that were previously immobile. Since excessive use of diseased joints can cause injury, patients should be warned against overactivity, even though their symptoms may have abated.

The use of glucocorticoids in rheumatoid arthritis is discussed further in Chapter 63.

Systemic Lupus Erythematosus. Systemic lupus erythematosus (SLE) is a chronic disease similar in many ways to rheumatoid arthritis. However, in SLE, inflammation is not limited to joints; rather, inflammation occurs throughout the body. Symptoms frequently include pleuritis, pericarditis, and nephritis. A severe episode of SLE can be fatal. Fortunately, manifestations of SLE can usually be controlled with prompt and aggressive glucocorticoid therapy.

Inflammatory Bowel Disease. Glucocorticoids are used to treat severe cases of ulcerative colitis and Crohn's disease, the two most common forms of inflammatory bowel disease. Administration may be oral, by injection, or by enema. Glucocorticoid therapy of these disorders is considered further in Chapter 68.

Miscellaneous Inflammatory Disorders. Glucocorticoids are useful in treating a variety of inflammatory disorders in addition to those discussed above. Conditions that respond to glucocorticoid therapy include bursitis, tendonitis, synovitis, osteoarthritis, gouty arthritis, and inflammatory disorders of the eye.

Allergic Conditions. Glucocorticoids can control symptoms of allergic reactions. Responsive conditions include bee stings, hay fever (see Chapter 65), and drug-induced allergies. Since responses to glucocorticoids are delayed, these agents have little value as acute therapy for severe allergic reactions (e.g., anaphylaxis). For life-threatening allergic reactions, epinephrine is the treatment of choice.

Asthma. Glucocorticoids are the most effective antiasthmatic agents available. For treatment of asthma, these drugs may be administered orally or by inhalation. Because oral therapy can be associated with serious toxicity, oral glucocorticoids should be reserved for patients who have failed to respond to safer medications (beta$_2$-adrenergic agonists, theophylline, cromolyn sodium). Fortunately, adverse effects are minimal when glucocorticoids are administered by inhalation. The use of glucocorticoids in asthma is discussed further in Chapter 64.

Dermatologic Disorders. Glucocorticoids are beneficial in a wide variety of skin diseases, including pemphigus, psoriasis, mycosis fungoides, seborrheic dermatitis, contact dermatitis, and exfoliative dermatitis. For mild disease, topical administration is usually adequate. Systemic steroids are generally reserved for severe disorders. It should be noted that absorption of topically applied glucocorticoids can be sufficient to produce systemic toxicity. Topical therapy is discussed further in Chapter 70.

Neoplasms. Glucocorticoids are used in conjunction with other anticancer agents to treat acute lymphocytic leukemia, Hodgkin's disease, and non-Hodgkin's lymphomas. Benefits derive from the direct toxicity of glucocorticoids to malignant lymphocytes. Treatment kills lymphoid cells and causes regression of lymphatic tissue. The use of glucocorticoids to treat cancers is discussed further in Chapter 91.

Suppression of Allograft Rejection. Glucocorticoids, together with other immunosuppressant agents, are used to prevent rejection of organ transplants. Treatment with glucocorticoids is initiated at the time of surgery and continued indefinitely. The use of glucocorticoids for immunosuppression is discussed further in Chapter 92.

ADVERSE EFFECTS

The adverse effects discussed below occur in response to *pharmacologic* doses of glucocorticoids.

The intensity of these effects increases with dosage size and duration of treatment. These toxicities are not seen when dosage is physiologic or when treatment is brief (a few days or less). Systemic toxicity can be minimized by topical application of glucocorticoids and use of local injections. Accordingly, these routes should be employed whenever appropriate.

Adrenal Insufficiency. Pharmacologic doses of glucocorticoids can suppress production of glucocorticoids by the adrenals, resulting in adrenal insufficiency. The mechanism, consequences, and management of adrenal insufficiency are discussed in depth later in the chapter.

Infection. By suppressing host defenses (immune responses and phagocytic activity of neutrophils and macrophages), glucocorticoids can increase susceptibility to infection. The risk of acquiring a new infection is increased, as is the risk of reactivating a latent infection (e.g., tuberculosis). In addition, since suppression of the immune system and neutrophils reduces inflammation and other manifestations of infection, a fulminant infection may develop without detection. Hence, not only do glucocorticoids increase susceptibility to infection, they can mask the presence of an infection as it progresses. To minimize acquisition of infection, patients should avoid close contact with individuals who have communicable diseases. If an infection occurs, it should be treated with appropriate antimicrobial drugs. In most cases, glucocorticoid therapy should continue.

Peptic Ulcer Disease. By inhibiting prostaglandin synthesis, glucocorticoids can augment secretion of gastric acid and pepsin, inhibit production of cytoprotective mucus, and reduce gastric mucosal blood flow. These actions predispose the patient to gastrointestinal ulceration. Making matters worse, glucocorticoids can decrease gastric pain, thereby masking ulcer development. As a result, perforation and hemorrhage can occur without warning. The risk of ulceration is increased by concurrent use of other ulcerogenic drugs, such as aspirin and other NSAIDs. To provide early detection of ulcer formation, stools should be periodically checked for occult blood. Patients should be instructed to notify the physician if feces become black and tarry. If gastrointestinal ulceration occurs, glucocorticoids should be slowly withdrawn (unless their continued use is considered essential to support life). Treatment with antiulcer medication (e.g., an H$_2$-receptor antagonist) is indicated.

Fluid and Electrolyte Disturbance. Because of their mineralocorticoid activity, glucocorticoids can cause sodium and water retention and potassium loss. Retention of water and sodium can cause hypertension and edema. Hypokalemia can predispose the patient to dysrhythmias and toxicity from digitalis. Fortunately, most of the glucocorticoids in current use have minimal mineralo-corticoid activity (see Table 62–1). Hence, serious fluid and electrolyte disturbance is rare. The risk of fluid and electrolyte disturbance can be reduced by (1) using glucocorticoids that have low miner-alocorticoid activity, (2) restricting sodium intake, and (3) taking potassium supplements or consuming potassium-rich foods (e.g., bananas, citrus fruits). Patients should be informed about signs of fluid retention (e.g., weight gain, swelling of the lower extremities) and advised to contact the physician if these develop. Patients should also be alert for signs of hypokalemia (e.g., muscle weakness or fatigue, irregular pulses).

Osteoporosis. Osteoporosis is a frequent and serious complication of chronic glucocorticoid therapy. The ribs and vertebrae are affected most, and vertebral compression fractures are common. Patients should be observed for signs of compression fractures (back and neck pain) and for indications of fractures in other bones. If the technology is available, bone status should be evaluated period-ically employing bone densitometry. Development of osteoporosis can be reduced by taking calcium supplements and vitamin D.

Osteoporosis results from a combination of de-creased formation of bone and increased bone re-sorption. Glucocorticoids inhibit the activity of os-teoblasts, the cells responsible for formation of bone. Also, glucocorticoids decrease intestinal ab-sorption of calcium, and thereby promote hypocal-cemia. In response to hypocalcemia, release of parathyroid hormone (PTH) is increased, promot-ing mobilization of calcium from bone.

Glucose Intolerance. Because of their effects on glucose production and utilization, glucocorti-coids can increase plasma glucose levels, causing hyperglycemia and glycosuria. For patients with diabetes, these effects may necessitate an increase in insulin dosage or a reduction in caloric intake. For patients with normal pancreatic function, sig-nificant elevations of blood glucose are unlikely. However, since use of glucocorticoids can unmask latent diabetes, nondiabetics should undergo peri-odic evaluation of glucose levels in blood.

Myopathy. High-dose glucocorticoid therapy can cause myopathy, manifested as muscle weak-ness. The proximal muscles of the arms and legs are affected most. Damage to muscle may be suffi-cient to prevent ambulation. If myopathy develops, glucocorticoid dosage should be reduced. Myopathy then gradually resolves over several months.

Growth Retardation. Glucocorticoids can sup-press growth in children. Growth retardation is probably the result of reduced DNA synthesis and decreased cell division. To assess effects on growth, height and weight should be measured at regular intervals. Growth suppression can be minimized

with alternate-day therapy. This dosing schedule is discussed later in the chapter.

Psychologic Disturbances. Rarely, glucocor-ticoids have caused hallucinations, mood changes (depression, euphoria, mania), and other psycho-logic disturbances. These effects are related more to dosage size than to duration of treatment, and can occur within the first few days of drug use. Previous psychiatric illness does not appear to pre-dispose patients to adverse psychologic effects of glucocorticoids. Conversely, a history of good men-tal health does not guarantee immunity from psy-chologic disturbance.

Cutaneous Atrophy. Prolonged glucocorticoid therapy can cause atrophy of the skin and subcu-taneous tissues. The skin may become thin and shiny, and striations (red or purple lines) may de-velop on the trunk and other regions. The patient may experience unusual bruising, and wounds may heal slowly. Because of subcutaneous fat atro-phy, pitting may develop at sites at glucocorticoid injection.

Cataracts. Cataracts are a common complica-tion of long-term glucocorticoid therapy. Risk fac-tors are in dispute; cataract development may be related to age, dosage, or individual susceptibility. To facilitate early detection, patients should re-ceive an ophthalmologic examination every 6 months. Also, patients should be advised to contact the physician if vision becomes cloudy or blurred.

Negative Nitrogen Balance. This response re-sults from glucocorticoid-induced breakdown of protein. Nitrogen balance can be made more favor-able through liberal protein intake. Accordingly, patients should be advised to consume a high-pro-tein diet. Providing the patient with a diet plan or a list of appropriate foods can be helpful.

Iatrogenic Cushing's Syndrome. Long-term glucocorticoid therapy can induce a cushingoid syndrome whose symptoms are identical to those of naturally occurring Cushing's disease. Promi-nent symptoms are hyperglycemia, glycosuria, fluid and electrolyte disturbances, osteoporosis, muscle weakness, cutaneous striations, and low-ered resistance to infection. Redistribution of fat produces a pot belly, "moon face," and "buffalo hump."

USE IN PREGNANCY AND LACTATION

Pregnancy. Glucocorticoids can cross the pla-centa and affect the developing fetus. Animal stud-ies indicate an increased incidence of cleft palate, spontaneous abortion, and low birth weight. No adequate studies of these effects have been done in humans. Therapy with very large doses can cause fetal adrenal hypoplasia. Hence, when large doses have been employed, the infant should be assessed for adrenal insufficiency and given replacement therapy if indicated. Whenever glucocorticoids are to be used during pregnancy, the benefits must be carefully weighed against the potential risk to the fetus.

Lactation. Glucocorticoids enter breast milk. When physiologic doses or low pharmacologic doses are used, the concentration achieved in milk is probably too low to affect the nursing infant. However, when large pharmacologic doses are employed (e.g., doses greater than 5 mg/day of prednisone or its equivalent) the amount ingested by the infant may be sufficient to cause growth retardation and other adverse effects. Consequently, women receiving high-dose glucocorticoid therapy should be warned against breast-feeding.

DRUG INTERACTIONS

Interactions Related to Potassium Loss. As discussed above, glucocorticoids can increase urinary loss of potassium, and can thereby induce hypokalemia. Consequently, glucocorticoids must be used with caution when combined with *digitalis glycosides* (because hypokalemia increases the risk of digitalis-induced dysrhythmias) and when combined with *thiazide diuretics* or *loop diuretics* (because these potassium-depleting diuretics will increase the risk of hypokalemia). When glucocorticoids are given together with any of the above drugs, it is advisable to monitor plasma potassium levels and be alert for signs of cardiac toxicity.

Insulin and Oral Hypoglycemics. As discussed above, glucocorticoids promote hyperglycemia. To maintain glycemic control, diabetic patients may require increased doses of a glucose-lowering drug (insulin or an oral hypoglycemic agent).

Vaccines. Because of their immunosuppresant actions, glucocorticoids can decrease antibody responses to vaccines. Furthermore, if a live-virus vaccine is employed, there is an increased risk of developing viral disease. Accordingly, attempts at immunization should not be made while glucocorticoids are being used.

Nonsteroidal Anti-inflammatory Drugs (NSAIDs). Since NSAIDs have the same effects on the gastrointestinal tract as do the glucocorticoids, concurrent use of these agents may increase the risk of ulceration. However, if combined use of these drugs permits a reduction in the dosage of both agents, then the risk of ulcer formation may be no greater than when these drugs are taken alone.

SUMMARY OF PRECAUTIONS AND CONTRAINDICATIONS

Contraindications. Glucocorticoids are contraindicated for patients with *systemic fungal infections* and patients receiving *live-virus vaccines*.

Precautions. Glucocorticoids must be used with caution in *pediatric patients* and *women who are pregnant or breast-feeding*. Caution must also be exercised in patients with *hypertension, congestive heart failure, renal impairment, esophagitis, gastritis, peptic ulcer disease, myasthenia gravis, diabetes mellitus, osteoporosis,* and *infections that are resistant to treatment*. In addition, caution is required during concurrent therapy with *potassium-depleting diuretics, digitalis glycosides, insulin, oral hypoglycemics,* and *NSAIDs*.

ADRENAL SUPPRESSION

Development of Adrenal Suppression. Like the naturally occurring glucocorticoids (e.g., cortisol), the glucocorticoids that we administer as drugs suppress release of CRF from the hypothalamus and release of ACTH from the anterior pituitary. By doing so, the glucocorticoid drugs inhibit the synthesis and release of endogenous glucocorticoids by the adrenals. During long-term therapy, the pituitary loses much of its ability to manufacture ACTH and, in response to the prolonged absence of ACTH, the adrenals atrophy and lose their ability to synthesize cortisol and other glucocorticoids. As a result, when prolonged therapy with glucocorticoids is discontinued, there is a period during which the adrenals are unable to produce glucocorticoids. Recovery of adrenal function may take from a few weeks to more than a year. The extent of adrenal suppression and the time required for recovery are determined primarily by the duration of glucocorticoid use; dosage size is of secondary importance. Development of adrenal suppression can be minimized through alternate-day dosing. This procedure is discussed below.

Adrenal Suppression and Stress. As noted above, the adrenals normally secrete large amounts of glucocorticoids at times of stress. When stress is severe (e.g., trauma, surgery) these glucocorticoids are essential for supporting life. Accordingly, *it is imperative that patients receiving long-term glucocorticoid therapy be given increased doses at times of stress* (unless the dosage is already very high). Furthermore, *once glucocorticoid use has ceased, supplemental doses will be required whenever stress occurs until recovery of adrenal function is complete*. Patients should carry an identification card or bracelet informing emergency health care personnel of their glucocorticoid needs. In addition, patients should always have an emergency supply of glucocorticoids on hand.

Glucocorticoid Withdrawal. Withdrawal of glucocorticoids should be done slowly. The withdrawal schedule is determined by the degree of adrenal suppression. A representative schedule is as follows: (1) taper the dosage to a physiologic range over 7 days; (2) switch from multiple daily doses to single doses administered each morning; (3) taper the dosage to 50% of physiologic values over the next month; and (4) monitor for production of endogenous cortisol and, when basal levels have returned to normal, cease routine steroid administration (but be prepared to give supplemental glucocorticoids at times of stress).

In addition to unmasking adrenal insufficiency, cessation of glucocorticoid use may produce a withdrawal syndrome. Symptoms include hypotension, hypoglycemia, myalgia, arthralgia, and fatigue. In patients being treated for arthritis and certain other disorders, these symptoms may be confused with return of the underlying disease. Discomfort of withdrawal can be minimized by gradual dosage reduction and by concurrent treatment with NSAIDs.

PREPARATIONS AND ROUTES OF ADMINISTRATION

Preparations

The glucocorticoids employed clinically include hydrocortisone (cortisol) and synthetic derivatives of this compound. Individual glucocorticoids differ from one another with respect to (1) biologic half-life, (2) mineralocorticoid potency, and (3) glucocorticoid (anti-inflammatory) potency (see Table 62–1).

The term *biologic half-life* refers to the time required for glucocorticoids to leave body tissues. In most cases, these drugs are cleared from tissues more slowly than from the blood. Hence, the biologic half-life is usually longer than the plasma half-life. When glucocorticoids are administered by mouth or by IV injection, it is the biologic half-life, not the plasma half-life, that determines duration of action. Because of differences in their biologic half-lives, individual glucocorticoids can be classified as short-acting, intermediate-acting, or long-acting (see Table 62–1).

Glucocorticoids with high *mineralocorticoid potency* (cortisone, hydrocortisone) can cause significant retention of sodium and water, coupled with depletion of potassium. These mineralocorticoid effects can be especially hazardous for patients with hypertension or congestive heart failure and for patients taking digitalis glycosides. Because of the potential dangers of sodium retention and potassium loss, glucocorticoids with high mineralocorticoid activity should not be administered systemically for long periods.

The differences in *glucocorticoid potency* summarized in Table 62–1 are reflected in the doses required to produce anti-inflammatory effects (and not mineralocorticoid effects). As with other drugs, potency is a relatively unimportant characteristic. However, it *is* important to appreciate that in order to produce equivalent therapeutic effects, dosages for some glucocorticoids must be much larger than for others.

Routes of Administration

Glucocorticoids can be administered *orally*, *parenterally* (IV, IM, SC), *topically*, by *local injection* (e.g., intra-articular, intralesional), and by *inhalation*. Topical application is reserved for dermatologic disorders (see Chapter 70) and inhalational therapy is reserved for treating asthma (see Chapter 64). Since local therapy (topical application, inhalation, local injection) minimizes systemic toxicity, this form of treatment is preferred to systemic therapy (oral, parenteral). When systemic effects are needed, oral administration is preferred to parenteral. It is important to note that even when glucocorticoids are administered for local effects, absorption can be sufficient to produce systemic effects. Accordingly, use of local administration does not eliminate the risk of systemic toxicity.

Individual glucocorticoids are available as various esters (e.g., acetate, sodium phosphate, tebutate). When glucocorticoids are administered by routes other than oral or intravenous, the particular ester being used is a major determinant of duration of action. As indicated in Table 62–2, not all esters can be employed by all routes. Hence, when preparing to administer a glucocorticoid, you should verify that the particular ester to be used is appropriate for the intended route.

DOSAGE

General Guidelines for Dosing

For most patients, the objective of glucocorticoid therapy is to reduce symptoms to an acceptable level. Complete relief of symptoms is usually not an appropriate goal.

Dosage is highly individualized; for any patient with any disease, dosage must be determined empirically (by trial and error). For patients whose disease is not an immediate threat to life, the dosage should be low initially and then increased gradually until symptoms are under control. In the event of life-threatening disease, a large initial dose should be used, and, if a response does not occur rapidly, the dose should be doubled or tripled. When glucocorticoids are used for a prolonged period, the dosage should be reduced until the smallest effective amount has been established. Prolonged treatment with high doses should be done only if the disorder is (1) life-

Table 62–2. Glucocorticoid Routes of Administration

Drug	Systemic				Local				
	PO	IM	IV	SC	IA	IB	IL	IS	ST
Betamethasone	√								
Betamethasone sodium phosphate		√	√		√		√		√
Betamethasone acetate/sodium phosphate		√			√		√	√	√
Cortisone acetate	√	√							
Dexamethasone	√								
Dexamethasone acetate		√			√		√		√
Dexamethasone sodium phosphate		√	√		√		√	√	√
Hydrocortisone	√								
Hydrocortisone acetate					√	√	√	√	√
Hydrocortisone cypionate	√								
Hydrocortisone sodium phosphate		√	√	√					
Hydrocortisone sodium succinate		√	√						
Methylprednisolone	√								
Methylprednisolone acetate		√			√		√		√
Methylprednisolone sodium succinate		√	√						
Prednisolone	√								
Prednisolone acetate		√							
Prednisolone acetate/sodium phosphate		√			√	√		√	√
Prednisolone sodium phosphate		√	√		√		√		√
Prednisolone tebutate					√		√		√
Prednisone	√								
Triamcinolone	√								
Triamcinolone acetonide		√			√	√	√		
Triamcinolone diacetate		√			√		√	√	√
Triamcinolone hexacetonide					√		√		

PO = oral; IM = intramuscular; IV = intravenous; SC = subcutaneous; IA = intra-articular; IB = intrabursal; IL = intralesional; IS = intrasynovial; ST = soft tissue.
Topical preparations are listed in Table 70–1.

threatening, or (2) has the potential to cause permanent disability. During long-term treatment, an increase in dosage will be needed at times of stress (unless the dosage is very high to begin with). If disease status changes, appropriate adjustment of dosage must be made.

As noted above, abrupt termination of long-term therapy may result in harm because of adrenal insufficiency. To minimize the impact of adrenal suppression, withdrawal of glucocorticoids should be gradual. Patients must be warned against abrupt discontinuation of treatment.

Alternate-Day Therapy

In alternate-day therapy, a large dose (of an intermediate-acting agent) is given every other morning. This dosing schedule contrasts with traditional therapy in which multiple smaller doses are administered daily. Benefits of alternate-day therapy are (1) reduced adrenal suppression, (2) reduced risk of growth retardation, and (3) reduced toxicity overall. Adrenal insufficiency is decreased because, over the extended interval between doses, plasma glucocorticoids decline to a level that is low enough to permit some production of ACTH, thereby promoting some synthesis of cortisol by the adrenals. To allow maximal recovery of endocrine function, doses must be administered prior to 9 o'clock in the morning, and long-acting agents must not be used.

Unfortunately, alternate-day therapy does have one drawback: in the long interval between doses, drug levels may fall to a subtherapeutic value, thus permitting a flare-up of symptoms. Symptoms are likely to be most intense late on the second day after each dose is given. If symptoms become intolerable, switching to a single daily dose may be sufficient to provide control. As with alternate-day treatment, patients taking daily doses should administer their medicine before 9 AM.

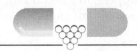

Summary of Major Nursing Implications

GLUCOCORTICOIDS

The nursing implications summarized here apply to all glucocorticoids. These implications apply primarily to the use of glucocorticoids for *nonendocrine diseases*. Implications that apply specifically to use of glucocorticoids for *replacement therapy* are summarized in Chapter 53.

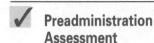
Preadministration Assessment

Therapeutic Goal

Glucocorticoids are used to suppress rejection of organ transplants and to treat a variety of inflammatory, allergic, and neoplastic disorders. When treating inflammatory and allergic disorders, the goal is to suppress signs and symptoms to an acceptable level, and not to eliminate them entirely.

Baseline Data

Make a full assessment of the specific disorder (e.g., rheumatoid arthritis, asthma, psoriasis) to be treated. These data are used to determine the initial dosage and dosage adjustments as treatment proceeds.

Identifying High-Risk Patients

Glucocorticoids are *contraindicated* for patients with *systemic fungal infections* and for individuals receiving *live-virus vaccines*. Use glucocorticoids with *caution* in *pediatric patients* and in *women who are pregnant or breast-feeding*. In addition, exercise *caution* in patients with *hypertension, congestive heart failure, renal impairment, esophagitis, gastritis, peptic ulcer disease, myasthenia gravis, diabetes mellitus, osteoporosis*, and *infections that are resistant to treatment*, and in patients receiving *potassium-depleting diuretics, digitalis glycosides, insulin, oral hypoglycemics*, or *NSAIDs*.

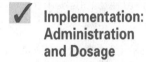
Implementation: Administration and Dosage

Routes and Administration

Glucocorticoids are administered orally, parenterally (IV, IM, SC), topically (to skin and mucous membranes), by inhalation, and by local injection (e.g., intra-articular, intralesional). Routes for specific preparations are summarized in Table 62–2. When preparing to administer a glucocorticoid, verify that the preparation is appropriate for the intended route.

Dosage

Dosage is determined empirically. For patients whose disease does not threaten life, the dosage should be low initially and then gradually increased until the desired response is achieved. For treatment of life-threatening disease, initial doses should be as large as needed to control symptoms. During prolonged therapy, the dosage should be reduced to the smallest effective amount. Supplemental doses will be needed at times of stress (unless the dosage is very high to begin with).

Alternate-Day Therapy

Alternate-day dosing helps minimize adrenal suppression and other toxicities. Instruct patients using this schedule to take their medicine before 9 AM.

Drug Withdrawal

Glucocorticoids must be withdrawn gradually. Warn the patient against abrupt discontinuation of treatment. Following termination, supplemental doses will be needed during times of stress until adrenal function has recovered fully.

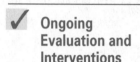 **Ongoing Evaluation and Interventions**

Evaluating Therapeutic Effects

Evaluate therapy by making periodic comparisons of current signs and symptoms with the pretreatment assessment. Dosage is adjusted on the basis of these evaluations.

Minimizing Adverse Effects

General Measures. (1) Keep the dosage as low as possible and the duration of treatment as short as possible. (2) Use alternate-day therapy if possible. (3) When appropriate, administer glucocorticoids topically, by inhalation, or by local injection.

Adrenal Insufficiency. Long-term therapy suppresses the adrenal's ability to make glucocorticoids. Adrenal insufficiency can be minimized through alternate-day dosing and use of glucocorticoids that have an intermediate duration of action. Increase the dosage when stress occurs (e.g., surgery, trauma, infection) unless the dosage is very high to begin with. Following termination of therapy, supplemental doses will be required at times of stress until recovery of adrenal function is complete. Advise the patient to carry some sort of identification (e.g., MedicAlert bracelet) to insure proper dosing in emergencies. Advise the patient to have an emergency supply of glucocorticoids on hand at all times. Expression of adrenal insufficiency will be reduced by withdrawing glucocorticoids gradually.

Infection. Glucocorticoids increase the risk of morbidity from infection. Warn patients against contact with persons who have communicable diseases. Inform patients about early signs of infection (e.g., fever, sore throat) and instruct them to notify the physician if these occur. Treat established infections with appropriate antimicrobial drugs.

Peptic Ulcer Disease. Glucocorticoids increase the risk of ulcer formation and can mask ulcer symptoms. Instruct the patient to notify the physician if feces become black and tarry. Have stools checked periodically for occult blood. If ulcers develop, glucocorticoids should be slowly withdrawn (unless their continued use is considered essential for life) and antiulcer therapy should be instituted.

Fluid and Electrolyte Disturbance. Glucocorticoids can cause sodium and water retention and loss of potassium. These effects can be minimized by (1) using glucocorticoids that have low mineralocorticoid activity, (2) restricting sodium intake, and (3) taking potassium supplements or consuming potassium-rich foods (e.g., bananas, citrus fruits). Educate patients about signs and symptoms of fluid retention (e.g., weight gain, swelling of the lower extremities) and instruct them to notify the physician if these develop.

Osteoporosis. Glucocorticoid-induced osteoporosis can predispose the patient to fractures, especially of the ribs and vertebrae. Monitor patients for signs of compression fractures (neck or back pain) and for indications of other fractures. Ideally, bone status should be evaluated periodically by bone densitometry. Development of osteoporosis can be reduced with calcium supplements and vitamin D.

Glucose Intolerance. Glucocorticoids can cause hyperglycemia and glycosuria. Diabetic patients may need to decrease their caloric intake and increase their dosage of hypoglycemic medication (insulin or oral hypoglycemic).

Growth Retardation. Glucocorticoids can suppress growth in children. Evaluate growth retardation by making periodic measurements of height and weight. Alternate-day therapy will minimize growth suppression.

Cataracts. Cataracts are a common complication of long-term therapy. The patient should receive an ophthalmologic examination every 6 months. Instruct the patient to notify the physician if vision becomes cloudy or blurred.

Negative Nitrogen Balance. Nitrogen loss results from breakdown of protein. Advise patients to consume a high-protein diet and provide them with a diet plan.

Use in Pregnancy and Lactation. Glucocorticoids can induce adrenal hypoplasia in the developing fetus. The benefits of use during pregnancy must be carefully weighed against the risks. When large doses have been employed, the newborn infant should be assessed for adrenal insufficiency, and given replacement therapy if indicated.

During high-dose therapy, the glucocorticoid content of breast milk may become high enough to affect the nursing infant. Warn women who are receiving high-dose therapy not to breast-feed.

Other Adverse Effects. *Psychologic disturbances, cutaneous atrophy, myopathy,* and *Cushing's syndrome* can be minimized only by implementing the general measures noted at the beginning of this section. There are no specific measures to prevent these complications.

Minimizing Adverse Interactions

Interactions Related to Potassium Loss. Glucocorticoid-induced potassium loss can be augmented by *potassium-depleting diuretics* (thiazides, loop diuretics) and can increase the risk of toxicity from *digitalis glycosides.* If glucocorticoids are used concurrently with these drugs, potassium levels should be monitored. Also, be alert for indications of cardiotoxicity.

Insulin and Oral Hypoglycemics. Glucocorticoids can elevate blood levels of glucose. Diabetic patients may need to increase their dosage of insulin or oral hypoglycemic drug.

Vaccines. Glucocorticoids can decrease antibody responses to vaccines and can increase the risk of infection from live-virus vaccines. Attempts at immunization should not be made while glucocorticoids are being used.

Nonsteroidal Anti-inflammatory Drugs (NSAIDs). NSAIDs can increase the risk of gastric ulceration during glucocorticoid therapy. Exercise caution when this combination is employed.

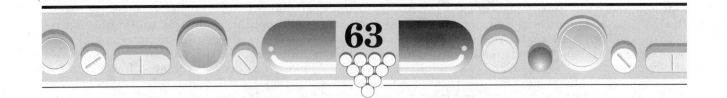

Drug Therapy of Rheumatoid Arthritis and Gout

In this chapter we will focus on the drug therapy of two inflammatory disorders: rheumatoid arthritis and gout. Many of the agents used to treat arthritis have been discussed in the preceding two chapters. Several additional agents are introduced here.

DRUG THERAPY OF RHEUMATOID ARTHRITIS

Rheumatoid arthritis is the most common systemic inflammatory disease, affecting between 5 and 8 million Americans. Although the disease can develop at any age, initial symptoms usually appear during the 30's and 40's. In younger patients, the incidence of arthritis is about 2.5 times greater in females than in males. However, in patients over age 60, the incidence in men and women is equal. Rheumatoid arthritis follows a progressive course, and can eventually cripple its victim. For some patients, drug therapy can halt the advance of the disease. However, for many patients, benefits of treatment may be limited to symptomatic relief.

PATHOPHYSIOLOGY OF ARTHRITIS

Rheumatoid arthritis is an inflammatory disorder whose onset is heralded by symmetric joint

807

stiffness and pain. Symptoms are most intense in the morning and abate as the day advances. Joints become swollen, tender, and warm. For some patients, periods of spontaneous remission occur. For others, injury progresses steadily. In addition to joint injury, rheumatoid arthritis is associated with weakness, fatigue, anorexia, and weight loss. An especially severe manifestation is vasculitis.

The progression of joint deterioration is depicted in Figure 63–1. Inflammation begins in the synovium, the membrane that encloses the joint cavity. The inflammatory process is self-reinforcing and complex; mediators include prostaglandins, immune factors, and other endogenous compounds. As inflammation intensifies, the synovial membrane thickens and begins to envelop the articular cartilage. This overgrowth is referred to as *pannus*. Damage to the cartilage is caused by enzymes released from the pannus and by chemicals and enzymes produced by the inflammatory process raging within the synovial space. Ultimately, the articular cartilage undergoes total destruction, resulting in direct contact between bones of the joint, followed by eventual bone fusion. After this, inflammation subsides. Although it is clear that an autoimmune process is central to the events described, the pathogenesis of rheumatoid arthritis remains incompletely understood.

OVERVIEW OF THERAPY

Treatment has three major objectives: (1) relief of symptoms (pain, inflammation, stiffness), (2) maintenance of joint function and range of motion, and (3) prevention of deformity. To achieve these goals, a combination of pharmacologic and nonpharmacologic measures is employed.

Nondrug Measures

Nondrug measures for management of arthritis include physical therapy, exercise, and surgery. Physical therapy may consist of massage, warm baths, and application of heat to the affected regions. These procedures can enhance mobility and reduce inflammation. A balanced program of rest and exercise can decrease joint stiffness and improve function. However, excessive rest or exercise should be avoided; too much rest will foster stiffness, and too much activity can intensify inflammation.

Orthopedic surgery has made marked advances. For patients with severe disease of the hip or knee, total joint replacement can be performed. When joints of the hands or wrists have been damaged severely, function can be improved through removal of the diseased synovium and repair of ruptured tendons. Plastic implants can help correct deformities.

A complete program of treatment should include patient education and counseling. The patient should be informed about the nature of rheumatoid arthritis, the possible consequences of joint degeneration, management measures, and the benefits and limitations of drug therapy. If loss of mobility limits function at home, on the job, or in school, consultation with a social worker, occupational therapist, or specialist in vocational rehabilitation may be appropriate.

Drug Therapy

Antiarthritic drugs can produce symptomatic relief, and, in some cases, may induce protracted remission. However, remission is rarely complete, and the disease usually advances steadily. As a result, drug therapy is usually chronic. Accordingly, successful treatment requires both motivation and cooperation on the part of the patient.

Classification of Antiarthritic Drugs. As indicated in Table 63–1, the antiarthritic drugs fall into three major categories: (1) *nonsteroidal antiinflammatory drugs* (NSAIDs), (2) *disease-modify-*

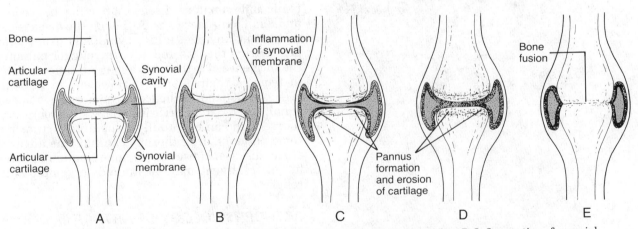

Figure 63–1. Progressive joint degeneration in rheumatoid arthritis. *A,* Healthy joint. *B,* Inflammation of synovial membrane. *C,* Onset of pannus formation and cartilage erosion. *D,* Pannus formation progresses and cartilage deteriorates further. *E,* Complete destruction of joint cavity together with fusion of articulating bones.

Table 63–1. Drugs for Rheumatoid Arthritis

NONSTEROIDAL ANTI-INFLAMMATORY DRUGS (NSAIDs)*

Salicylates
 Aspirin
 Choline salicylate [Arthropan]
 Magnesium salicylate [Magan]
 Sodium salicylate
 Salsalate [Disalcid, Mono-Gesic]

Nonsalicylate NSAIDs
 Diclofenac [Voltaren]
 Diflunisal [Dolobid]
 Etodolac [Lodine]
 Fenoprofen [Nalfon]
 Flurbiprofen [Ansaid]
 Ibuprofen [Motrin, Rufen]
 Indomethacin [Indocin]
 Ketoprofen [Orudis]
 Meclofenamate [Meclomen]
 Nabumetone [Relafen]
 Naproxen [Naprosyn]
 Naproxen sodium [Anaprox]
 Phenylbutazone [Butazolidin]
 Piroxicam [Feldene]
 Sulindac [Clinoril]
 Tolmetin [Tolectin]

DISEASE-MODIFYING ANTIRHEUMATIC DRUGS (DMARDs)†

First-Choice DMARDs
 Hydroxychloroquine [Plaquenil]
 Gold Salts
  Gold sodium thiomalate [Myochrysine]
  Aurothioglucose [Solganal]
  Auranofin [Ridaura]
 Methotrexate [Rheumatrex]
 Sulfasalazine [Azulfidine]

Other DMARDs
 Azathioprine [Imuran]
 Penicillamine [Cuprimine]
 Cyclophosphamide [Cytoxan]

GLUCOCORTICOIDS‡
 Prednisone
 Prednisolone

*NSAIDs relieve symptoms rapidly but do not retard the progression of rheumatoid arthritis. NSAIDs are safer than DMARDs and glucocorticoids and require less vigorous monitoring.

†DMARDs have a delayed onset of action (typically 3 to 5 months) and, hence, are also known as *slow-acting antirheumatic drugs* (SAARDs). DMARDs may retard the progression of rheumatoid arthritis. DMARDs are more toxic than NSAIDs and require more vigorous monitoring.

‡Glucocorticoids relieve symptoms rapidly but do not retard the progression of rheumatoid arthritis. Because of their toxicity, glucocorticoids are generally reserved for short-term therapy.

ing antirheumatic drugs (DMARDs), and (3) *glucocorticoids* (adrenal corticosteroids). The NSAIDs can be subdivided into *salicylates* (e.g., aspirin, choline salicylate) and *nonsalicylates* (e.g., ibuprofen, naproxen). The DMARDs can be subdivided into (1) first-choice DMARDs (e.g., hydroxychloroquine, gold salts), and (2) other DMARDs (e.g., azathioprine).

The three major groups of antiarthritic drugs differ from one another with respect to (1) time course of action, (2) toxicity, and (3) ability to alter

the progression of rheumatoid arthritis. The NSAIDs provide rapid relief of symptoms but do not alter disease progression. These drugs are safer than the DMARDs and the glucocorticoids and, consequently, treatment requires less vigorous monitoring. Like the NSAIDs, glucocorticoids provide rapid relief of symptoms but do not retard disease progression. These drugs can cause serious toxicity with long-term use. Accordingly, treatment is usually restricted to short courses. In contrast to the NSAIDs and glucocorticoids, DMARDs often retard the progression of rheumatoid arthritis. However, the onset of therapeutic effects is delayed, typically for 3 to 5 months. The DMARDs are more toxic than NSAIDs and, therefore, treatment requires vigorous monitoring.

Drug Selection. Drug therapy of arthritis is based on severity of symptoms, the patient's response to treatment, and the patient's ability to tolerate a drug's side effects. A scheme for drug selection is depicted in Figure 63–2. As indicated, NSAIDs are the initial drugs of choice. Because of cost considerations, aspirin or another salicylate is usually chosen first. If side effects of the salicylates are intolerable, one of the newer (nonsalicylate) NSAIDs may be tried. If symptoms cannot be controlled with an NSAID, a DMARD is indicated. Unfortunately, the DMARDs are more toxic than the NSAIDs, and take several months to produce their effects. Since therapeutic effects are delayed, therapy with an NSAID should be continued until the DMARD has produced an adequate response. Of the DMARDs in use, the preferred agents are hydroxychloroquine, gold salts, methotrexate, and sulfasalazine. (Rheumatologists have different opinions as to which of these four is best.) The other DMARDs—azathioprine, penicillamine, and cyclophosphamide—should be employed only if the preferred (safer) DMARDs have been ineffective. Glucocorticoids are generally used on a short-term basis to (1) provide symptomatic relief while responses to DMARDs are developing, and (2) supplement the effects of other drugs if symptoms "flare."

Until recently, patients with mild symptoms were treated with NSAIDs alone; DMARDs were employed only when NSAIDs were ineffective or produced intolerable side effects. Today, many rheumatologists initiate therapy with a DMARD together with an NSAID. This approach is employed in an effort to delay joint degeneration. Recall that NSAIDs only provide symptomatic relief; they do not retard the progression of rheumatoid arthritis. In contrast, DMARDs may be able to arrest the disease process. Accordingly, by instituting DMARD therapy early (rather than waiting until joint degeneration has progressed to the point where NSAIDs can no longer control symptoms), it may be possible to delay or prevent serious joint injury. Since the effects of DMARDs take several months to develop, whereas responses to

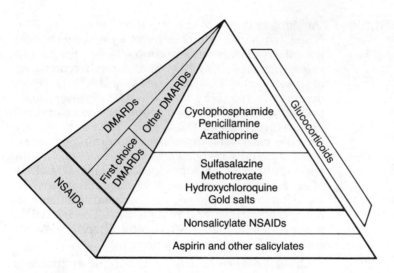

Figure 63–2. Drug-selection pyramid for antiarthritic drugs. Treatment is initiated with agents at the base of the pyramid. As the disease progresses, agents higher up the pyramid are indicated. Glucocorticoids may be used on a short-term basis at any stage of treatment. Drugs high on the pyramid are considerably more toxic than those near the base. (NSAIDs = nonsteroidal anti-inflammatory drugs, DMARDs = disease-modifying antirheumatic drugs)

NSAIDs are immediate, treatment is initiated with an NSAID along with the DMARD; once the DMARD has had time to act, the NSAID can be withdrawn.

PHARMACOLOGY OF THE ANTIARTHRITIC DRUGS

Salicylates

The basic pharmacology of the salicylates is discussed in Chapter 61. Consideration here is limited to the use of these drugs in arthritis.

Role in Arthritis Therapy. For most patients with rheumatoid arthritis, therapy is initiated with aspirin or another salicylate. These drugs are effective, fast acting, and inexpensive. Relief of symptoms is due primarily to anti-inflammatory actions, although analgesic effects are also beneficial. Salicylates only provide symptomatic relief; they do not arrest progression of the disease.

Adverse Effects. Primary adverse effects are *gastrointestinal disturbances* (nausea, gastric distress, ulceration) and *suppression of platelet aggregation*. Use of enteric-coated tablets decreases the risk of gastrointestinal bleeding. Tinnitus and other signs of salicylism usually indicate toxicity. Accordingly, if these signs develop, salicylates should be temporarily withdrawn. Once symptoms have subsided, treatment should resume, but at a slightly reduced dosage. About 0.2% of patients experience hypersensitivity reactions. These reactions are most likely in patients who have nasal polyps, asthma, and hay fever.

Dosage. The dosages employed for anti-inflammatory effects are considerably higher than those required for analgesia or reduction of fever. Patients may need as much as 5.2 gm (16 standard tablets) of aspirin a day. Although there is no precise relationship between plasma salicylate levels and therapeutic responses, levels in the range of 15 to 30 mg/dl are usually effective. Dosages for the salicylates are summarized in Table 63–2.

Achieving Compliance. Because aspirin is such a commonplace drug—advertised on television and available over-the-counter—many patients do not believe in its efficacy. Consequently, if compliance is to be achieved, an effort must be made to convince patients that aspirin really works. In some cases, use of a prescription formulation may help persuade the patient that aspirin is indeed a legitimate and effective medication.

Nonsalicylate NSAIDs

Like the salicylates, the nonsalicylate NSAIDs (e.g., ibuprofen, naproxen) are effective anti-inflammatory drugs and analgesics. Antirheumatic actions are equivalent to those of aspirin. However, for reasons that are not clear, some patients who fail to respond adequately to salicylates may respond more favorably to one of the nonsalicylates. Moreover, a particular patient may respond better to one nonsalicylate NSAID than to another. Consequently, trials with several different nonsalicylates may be needed before an optimal response is achieved. The nonsalicylate NSAIDs differ from the salicylate NSAIDs in two significant ways: (1) nonsalicylate NSAIDs are *more expensive* than the salicylates, and (2) they tend to cause *less gastrointestinal bleeding and tinnitus*. Because of these differences, the nonsalicylates are usually reserved for patients who began therapy with a salicylate but were unable to tolerate its side effects. However, if cost were not a factor, the nonsalicylate NSAIDs would probably replace the salicylates as the drugs of first choice for arthritis therapy. Antiarthritic dosages for the nonsalicylate NSAIDs are summarized in Table 63–2. A more complete discussion of these drugs is presented in Chapter 61.

Table 63–2. Antiarthritic Dosages for Nonsteroidal Anti-inflammatory Drugs		
Generic Name	**Trade Name**	**Daily Dosage**
Salicylates		
Aspirin (extended release)		1.6 gm bid
Choline salicylate	Arthropan	4.8–7.2 gm/day (in divided doses)
Magnesium salicylate	Magan	1090 mg tid or qid
Sodium salicylate		3.6–5.4 gm/day (in divided doses)
Salsalate	Disalcid, Mono-Gesic	3.0–4.0 gm/day (in divided doses)
Nonsalicylate NSAIDs		
Diclofenac	Voltaren	150–200 mg/day (in 3 or 4 doses)
Diflunisal	Dolobid	250–500 mg bid
Etodolac	Lodine	600–1200 mg/day (in 2 to 4 doses)
Fenoprofen	Nalfon	300–600 mg tid or qid
Flurbiprofen	Ansaid	200–300 mg/day (in 2 to 4 doses)
Ibuprofen	Motrin, Rufen	600–800 mg tid or qid
Indomethacin	Indocin	25–50 mg tid
Ketoprofen	Orudis	150–300 mg (in 3 or 4 doses)
Meclofenamate	Meclomen	200–400 mg/day (in 3 or 4 doses)
Nabumetone	Relafen	1.5–2 gm/day (in 1 or 2 doses)
Naproxen	Naprosyn	250–500 mg bid
Naproxen sodium	Anaprox	250–500 mg bid
Phenylbutazone	Butazolidin	300–600 mg/day (in 3 or 4 doses)
Piroxicam	Feldene	5 mg qid
Sulindac	Clinoril	150–200 mg bid
Tolmetin	Tolectin	200–400 mg tid

Glucocorticoids

The glucocorticoids are powerful anti-inflammatory drugs that can *relieve symptoms* of severe rheumatoid arthritis. These drugs do *not* induce remission and they do *not* halt the progression of the disease. For patients with generalized symptoms, *oral* glucocorticoids are indicated. However, if only one or two joints are affected, *intra-articular injections* may be employed. Because long-term, oral therapy can cause serious toxicity (e.g., osteoporosis, gastric ulceration, cataracts), oral glucocorticoids should be restricted to *short-term* use whenever possible. Most often, these drugs are given to provide temporary relief until drugs with a slower onset of action (e.g., gold salts, hydroxychloroquine) can provide control. Long-term therapy should be limited to patients who have failed to respond adequately to all other forms of treatment. The most commonly employed oral glucocorticoids are prednisone and prednisolone. The usual dosage for either drug is 5 to 7.5 mg a day. The pharmacology of the glucocorticoids is discussed at length in Chapter 62 (Glucocorticoids in Nonendocrine Diseases).

Gold Salts

Actions and Uses. The beneficial effects of gold in rheumatoid arthritis have been known since the 1930's. Gold can relieve pain and stiffness and, for some patients, may arrest the progression of joint degeneration. Symptomatic improvement is seen in 60% to 70% of patients. About 15% experience remission. Because the toxicity of gold can be se-

vere, therapy is often reserved for patients who have not responded adequately to salicylates or other NSAIDs. However, since gold salts may prevent joint degeneration, but cannot reverse damage that has already occurred, many rheumatologists initiate treatment with gold early in the course of the disease.

The therapeutic effects of gold take 4 to 6 months to develop. So that expectations can be realistic, patients should be made aware of this latency. Until a response has occurred, concurrent treatment with anti-inflammatory agents is indicated. If remission is less than complete, continued use of NSAIDs will be needed.

Gold preparations are available for intramuscular and oral use. Patients receiving IM therapy require repeated injections over a prolonged period. The oral preparation is more convenient and less toxic than the IM gold salts. Unfortunately, the oral preparation is also less effective.

The exact mechanism by which gold induces remission and relieves symptoms has not been determined. Likely contributory mechanisms are suppression of lysozyme release and suppression of the immune response.

Toxicity. Gold has a number of toxicities that can limit its use. About 15% to 20% of patients must discontinue treatment because of adverse effects. Among the most common reactions are *intense pruritus, rashes,* and *stomatitis* (lesions of the oral mucosa). *Renal toxicity,* manifested as proteinurea, occurs frequently. *Severe blood dyscrasias* (thrombocytopenia, leukopenia, agranulocytosis, aplastic anemia) have developed, but these are rare. Other serious toxicities include encephalitis, hepatitis, peripheral neuritis, pulmonary infiltrates, and profound hypotension. *Oral* gold causes less mucocutaneous and renal toxicity than the intramuscular preparations, but *gastrointestinal reactions* (diarrhea, nausea, abdominal pain) with oral gold are common.

Monitoring. Frequent laboratory tests and clinical evaluations are required to monitor toxicity. At each office visit the patient should be examined for dermatologic reactions and stomatitis. In addition, kidney and liver function must be monitored, and complete blood counts should be performed. The urine should be analyzed for protein. If signs of toxicity are detected, gold therapy should be discontinued immediately. If the adverse reactions are mild, therapy can be resumed 2 to 3 weeks after symptoms have subsided. However, many rheumatologists believe that once *any* toxicity has occurred, further use of gold should be avoided. The chances of severe toxicity can be reduced by initiating treatment at low doses.

Preparation, Dosage, and Administration. *Preparations.* Three gold preparations are available. Two of these— *aurothioglucose* [Solganal] and *gold sodium thiomalate* [Myochrysine]—are administered by IM injection. The third preparation—*auranofin* [Ridaura] – is taken orally.

Intramuscular Dosing. On the first day of treatment, a 10-mg test dose is administered. This is followed on days 7 and 14 by doses of 25 mg. After this, 50-mg doses are injected weekly until a cumulative dose of 1 gm has been administered. If beneficial effects occur, therapy is continued, but the dosing interval is gradually lengthened, first to 2 weeks, then to 3 weeks, and then to 1 month. In the absence of toxicity, monthly maintenance injections can be continued indefinitely.

Oral Dosing. The usual adult dosage is 6 mg/day (administered in one or two doses). If, after 6 months, the response is inadequate, the dosage may be increased to 3 mg three times a day for an additional 3 months. If the response is still insufficient, therapy should be discontinued.

Hydroxychloroquine

Actions and Uses. Hydroxychloroquine [Plaquenil], a drug with antimalarial actions, can produce remission in patients with rheumatoid arthritis. Traditionally, the drug was reserved for patients who had not responded to NSAIDs. Today, the drug may be prescribed earlier in the course of the disease in an effort to delay joint degeneration. Like the gold salts, hydroxychloroquine has a delayed onset of action; full therapeutic effects take 3 to 6 months to develop. Concurrent therapy with anti-inflammatory agents (NSAIDs or glucocorticoids) is indicated during the latency period. The mechanism by which hydroxychloroquine acts is not known.

Toxicity. The most serious toxicity is *retinal damage*. Retinopathy may be irreversible and can produce blindness. Visual loss is directly related to hydroxychloroquine dosage. Low doses may be used in long-term treatment with little risk. When dosage has been excessive, retinal damage may appear after treatment has ceased and may progress in the absence of continued drug use. Patients should receive a thorough ophthalmologic examination prior to treatment and every 6 months thereafter. Hydroxychloroquine should be discontinued at the first sign of retinal injury. Patients should be advised to contact the physician if any visual disturbance is noted.

Preparations, Dosage, and Administration. Hydroxychloroquine [Plaquenil] is dispensed in 200-mg tablets for oral administration. The initial dosage is 200 mg twice daily. Maintenance dosages range from 200 to 400 mg/day. The daily dosage should not exceed 6.4 mg/kg of body weight.

Sulfasalazine

Sulfasalazine [Azulfidine], a drug used for years to treat inflammatory bowel disease (see Chapter 68), is now being used to treat rheumatoid arthritis (although it is not approved by the FDA for this indication). Sulfasalazine can retard progression of joint deterioration and may be superior to hydroxychloroquine in this regard. In one clinical trial, sulfasalazine was as effective as intramuscular gold and caused less toxicity. *Gastrointestinal reactions* (nausea, vomiting, diarrhea, anorexia, abdominal pain) are the most common reason for discontinuing treatment. These reactions can be minimized by using enteric-coated formulations and by dividing the daily dosage. Dermatologic reactions (pruritus, rash, urticaria) are also common. Fortunately, serious adverse effects—hepatitis and bone marrow suppression—are relatively rare. To insure early detection of these reactions, periodic monitoring for hepatitis and bone marrow function (complete blood counts, platelet counts) should be performed. The initial dosage for arthritis is 500 mg/day. This can be gradually increased to a maximum of 2 gm/day (administered in divided doses).

Penicillamine

Penicillamine [Cuprimine, Depen] can induce remission in patients with rheumatoid arthritis. However, treatment may be associated with serious toxicity, especially *bone marrow depression* and *autoimmune disorders*. Consequently, the drug is reserved for patients with severe disease who have failed to respond to more conventional therapy. Therapeutic effects take 2 to 3 months to develop. Arthritic symptoms can be suppressed with NSAIDs or glucocorticoids during this latency period. The initial dosage is 125 mg/day. The daily dosage can be increased by 125-mg increments every 2 to 3 months. Usual maintenance dosages range from 750 to 1000 mg daily. The pharmacology of penicillamine is discussed further in Chapter 93.

Cytotoxic Immunosuppressive Drugs

Three cytotoxic immunosuppressive agents—methotrexate, cyclophosphamide, and azathioprine—can relieve symptoms of severe arthritis. In some cases, prolonged remission may be induced. Two of these drugs—cyclophosphamide and azathioprine—are considerably more toxic than the agents discussed above, and are generally reserved for patients who have not responded to safer medicines.

Methotrexate. Methotrexate [Rheumatrex, others] is the fastest acting of the disease-modifying antiarthritic drugs; therapeutic effects may be seen as early as 3 to 6 weeks. Many rheumatologists consider methotrexate the first-choice drug among the DMARDs. Major toxicities are *hepatic fibrosis, bone marrow suppression, gastrointestinal ulceration,* and *pneumonitis.* Periodic tests of liver and kidney function are mandatory, as are complete blood counts and platelet counts. Methotrexate can cause fetal death and congenital abnormalities. Accordingly, the drug is contraindicated during pregnancy. Methotrexate may be administered once weekly, beginning with a 5-mg dose. The weekly dosage is then gradually increased to a maximum of 15 to 20 mg. The pharmacology of methotrexate is discussed at length in Chapter 91 (Representative Anticancer Drugs).

Azathioprine. The antiarthritic effects of azathioprine [Imuran] are equivalent to those of gold salts and penicillamine. Benefits derive from immunosuppressive and anti-inflammatory actions. Serious toxicities include *hepatitis* and *blood dyscrasias* (leukopenia, thrombocytopenia, anemia). To monitor for these effects, complete blood counts, platelet counts, and tests of liver function are required. Azathioprine is teratogenic in animals and should not be used during pregnancy. The drug may also pose a small risk of malignancy. For treatment of arthritis, the initial dosage is 1 mg/kg/day. The dosage may be gradually increased to a maximum of 2.5 mg/kg/day. In addition to its use in arthritis, azathioprine is employed to prevent organ rejection in patients receiving kidney transplants. This application is discussed in Chapter 92 (Immunosuppressive Drugs).

Cyclophosphamide. Cyclophosphamide [Cytoxan], an anticancer drug, has been used investigationally to treat rheumatoid arthritis. The drug is considerably more toxic than methotrexate or azathioprine. Serious toxicities include *bone marrow suppression, sterility, mucous membrane lesions, hemorrhagic cystitis,* and *induction of cancer.* Because of these effects, cyclophosphamide is reserved for patients with life-threatening complications. The dosage for rheumatoid arthritis is 50 to 100 mg/day. The pharmacology of cyclophosphamide is discussed at length in Chapter 91 (Representative Anticancer Drugs).

DRUG THERAPY OF GOUT

PATHOPHYSIOLOGY OF GOUT

Gout is a recurrent inflammatory disorder characterized by *hyperuricemia* (high blood levels of uric acid) and by episodes of severe joint pain, typically in the large toe. Hyperuricemia can occur through two mechanisms: (1) excessive uric acid production, and (2) impaired renal excretion of uric acid. Acute attacks are precipitated by crystallization of sodium urate (the sodium salt of uric acid) in the synovial space. Deposition of urate crystals promotes inflammation by triggering a complex series of events. A key feature of the inflammatory process is infiltration of leukocytes; once inside the synovial cavity, these cells phagocytize urate crystals and then break down, causing release of destructive lysosomal enzymes. When hyperuricemia is chronic, large and gritty deposits, known as *tophi,* may form in the affected joint. Also, *renal damage* may result from deposition of urate crystals in the kidney. Fortunately, when gout is detected and treated early, the disease can be arrested and these chronic sequelae avoided.

In the absence of treatment, gout progresses through four stages. Stage one consists of *asymptomatic hyperuricemia.* Stage two is characterized by attacks of *acute gouty arthritis.* In stage three, symptoms subside; hence, this phase is known as the *asymptomatic intercritical period.* Stage four—*tophaceous gout*—is distinguished by development of tophi in joints.

OVERVIEW OF THERAPY

Five principal drugs are employed to treat gout. Two of these agents—*colchicine* and *indometha-* cin—relieve inflammation. The other three drugs—*allopurinol, probenecid,* and *sulfinpyrazone*—reduce hyperuricemia. Allopurinol reduces hyperuricemia by inhibiting uric acid formation. In contrast, probenecid and sulfinpyrazone reduce hyperuricemia by promoting uric acid excretion. Because they facilitate urate excretion, probenecid and sulfinpyrazone are called *uricosuric drugs.* In addition to the above agents, *glucocorticoids* and several *nonsteroidal anti-inflammatory drugs* may be employed to treat gout.

Drug selection is determined by the stage of gout being treated. During stage one (asymptomatic hyperuricemia), drugs are rarely employed; treatment is indicated only if symptoms develop or if blood levels of uric acid rise exceptionally high. Stage two (acute gouty arthritis) is treated with colchicine (for the initial episode) and indomethacin (for subsequent attacks). Stage two may also be treated with nonsteroidal anti-inflammatory drugs and, in extreme cases, with glucocorticoids. Allopurinol and the uricosuric drugs should be avoided during stage two. Treatment during stage three (the intercritical period) is variable. Some patients do well on small doses of colchicine, others respond well to antihyperuricemic agents, and still others require no treatment at all. The objective in treating stage four (chronic tophaceous gout) is to promote dissolution of tophi by lowering plasma levels of urate. Allopurinol is the preferred agent for this stage. Drug therapy of gout is summarized in Table 63–3.

PHARMACOLOGY OF THE DRUGS USED TO TREAT GOUT

Colchicine

Colchicine is an anti-inflammatory agent whose effects are specific for gout; the drug is ineffective for other inflammatory disorders. Colchicine is not an analgesic and does not relieve pain in conditions other than gout. The drug's principal adverse effect is gastrointestinal toxicity.

Therapeutic Use. Colchicine has three distinct applications in gout. The drug can be used to (1) treat acute gouty attacks, (2) reduce the incidence of attacks in chronic gout, and (3) abort an impending attack.

Acute Gouty Arthritis. When taken in large doses, colchicine produces dramatic relief of acute gouty attacks. Within hours, patients whose pain had made movement impossible are able to walk. Inflammation disappears completely within 2 to 3 days. Administration may be either intravenous or oral. With intravenous administration, symptoms resolve sooner than with oral administration, and gastrointestinal reactions are minimal. However, if extravasation occurs, intravenous colchicine can cause severe local necrosis.

Table 63–3. Drug Therapy of Gout		
Stage of Gout	**Drug Therapy**	**Comments**
Asymptomatic hyperuricemia	Drugs rarely indicated	
Acute gouty arthritis	Colchicine, indomethacin, and other nonsteroidal anti-inflammatory agents	Colchine is the drug of choice for the first episode. Indomethacin, which has fewer gastrointestinal side effects, is preferred for subsequent attacks.
	Glucocorticoids	Glucocorticoids are reserved for patients who fail to respond to other agents.
Asymptomatic intercritical period	Colchicine Antihyperuricemics: Allopurinol Probenecid Sulfinpyrazone	Allopurinol is indicated if 24-hr urate excretion is high (>800 mg), indicating urate overproduction. A uricosuric agent (sulfinpyrazone, probenecid) is indicated if 24-hour urate excretion is <800 mg, indicating impaired urate excretion.
Chronic tophaceous gout	Allopurinol	The treatment objective is to decrease plasma urate below 7 mg/dl in males and 6 mg/dl in females.

Prophylaxis of Gouty Attacks. When taken during the asymptomatic intercritical period, small doses of colchicine (e.g., 0.5 to 1.0 mg/day) can decrease the frequency and intensity of acute attacks. Colchicine is also given for prophylaxis when therapy with antihyperuricemic agents is initiated, since there is a tendency for gouty episodes to increase at this time.

Abortion of an Impending Attack. During prophylactic therapy with colchicine, patients may experience prodromal signs of a developing gouty attack. If large amounts of colchicine (e.g., 0.5 mg every 2 hours) are taken immediately, the attack may be prevented. Consequently, it is recommended that patients with chronic gout always have colchicine tablets on hand.

Mechanism of Action. We do not fully understand the mechanisms by which colchicine relieves or prevents episodes of gout. It is clear that the drug does not influence either the production or excretion of uric acid. An important contributory action is inhibition of leukocyte infiltration; in the absence of leukocytes, there is no phagocytosis of uric acid and no subsequent release of lysosomal enzymes. Leukocyte migration is inhibited by disruption of microtubules, the structures required for cellular motility. Since microtubules are also required for cell division, colchicine is toxic to any tissue that has a large percentage of proliferating cells. Disruption of cell division underlies the gastrointestinal toxicity of colchicine.

Pharmacokinetics. Colchicine is readily absorbed following oral administration. At therapeutic doses, large amounts re-enter the intestine via the bile and intestinal secretions. The drug is excreted primarily in the feces.

Adverse Effects. The most characteristic signs of colchicine toxicity are *nausea, vomiting, diarrhea,* and *abdominal pain.* These responses, which occur during treatment of acute gouty attacks, result from injury to the rapidly proliferating cells of the gastrointestinal epithelium. If gastrointestinal symptoms develop, colchicine should be discontinued immediately, regardless of the status of joint pain. As noted above, intravenous administration avoids most gastrointestinal toxicity. Diarrhea from colchicine can be managed with opioids.

Precautions. Colchicine should be used with care in elderly and debilitated patients, and in patients with cardiac, renal, and gastrointestinal diseases. Colchicine is classified in FDA Pregnancy Category C (for oral use) and Category D (for IV use). Since the drug can cause fetal harm, it should be avoided during pregnancy unless the perceived benefits are deemed to outweigh the potential risks to the fetus.

Preparations, Dosage, and Administration. Colchicine is dispensed in tablets (0.5 and 0.6 mg) for oral administration and in solution (1 mg/2 ml ampul) for intravenous administration.

Oral. For an acute gouty attack, the dosage is 0.5 to 1.2 mg initially followed by doses of 0.5 to 1.2 mg every 1 to 2 hours. Administration is repeated until pain is relieved or until signs of gastrointestinal toxicity appear. The total dose should not exceed 8 mg. The dosage for prophylaxis is 0.5 to 1.0 mg/day. The dosage for aborting an impending attack is 0.5 mg every 2 hours.

Intravenous. Intravenous administration can be used to treat an acute gouty attack. In many cases, relief can be achieved with a single 2-mg injection. To minimize vascular injury, the contents of 1 ampul (1 mg) should be diluted in 20 ml of sterile 0.9% sodium chloride and then injected slowly (over 5 or more minutes). Extravasation can result in local necrosis with sloughing of skin and subcutaneous tissue. Accordingly, care must be taken to insure that the IV line remains in place.

Indomethacin

Indomethacin [Indocin] is a nonsteroidal anti-inflammatory drug (NSAID) used to treat acute gouty arthritis. For treatment of gout, the drug's efficacy is equivalent to that of colchicine. Like colchicine, indomethacin does not reduce hyperuricemia. Rather, benefits derive from suppressing inflammation. In contrast to colchicine, indomethacin is devoid of severe gastrointestinal effects. Consequently, indomethacin is the drug of choice for treating acute gouty attacks once a diagnosis has been firmly established. The most characteristic side effect of indomethacin is *severe frontal headache*. Like other NSAIDs, indomethacin can promote *gastric ulceration* and should be avoided by patients with a history of peptic ulcer disease. *Probenecid* delays excretion of indomethacin. Accordingly, if probenecid and indomethacin are used together, a reduction in indomethacin dosage may be required. For relief of acute gouty arthritis, the adult dosage is 50 mg initially followed by 25-mg doses three to four times a day. Pain is relieved rapidly (within 2 to 4 hours); swelling subsides in 3 to 5 days. After this time, the dosage should be rapidly reduced, and then treatment should cease entirely. The pharmacology of indomethacin is discussed further in Chapter 61.

Allopurinol

Allopurinol [Zyloprim] is used to reduce blood levels of uric acid. The drug is indicated for primary hyperuricemia of gout and for hyperuricemia occurring secondary to certain blood dyscrasias (e.g., polycythemia vera, leukemia) and to therapy with anticancer drugs.

Mechanism of Action. Allopurinol and its major metabolite—alloxanthine—reduce uric acid levels by inhibiting uric acid production. Allopurinol and alloxanthine are *inhibitors of xanthine oxidase*, an enzyme required for uric acid formation. As indicated in Figure 63–3, xanthine oxidase catalyzes the final two reactions that lead to formation of uric acid from breakdown products of DNA. By inhibiting xanthine oxidase, these compounds can reduce uric acid formation.

Pharmacokinetics. Allopurinol is well absorbed following oral administration. Following absorption, the drug undergoes rapid conversion to alloxanthine, an active metabolite. Since alloxanthine has a prolonged half-life (about 25 hours), therapeutic effects are long lasting. Consequently, allopurinol requires only once-a-day dosing.

Use in Chronic Tophaceous Gout. Allopurinol is the drug of choice for chronic tophaceous gout. By reducing uric acid production and blood levels, the drug prevents tophus formation and promotes regression of tophi that have already formed; joint function is improved. In addition, reversal of hyperuricemia decreases the risk of nephropathy that can occur from deposition of urate crystals in the kidney. During the initial months of treatment, allopurinol may *increase* the incidence of acute gouty arthritis; chances of an attack can be reduced by concurrent treatment with colchicine or indomethacin.

Use in Secondary Hyperuricemia. Hyperuricemia may occur secondary to treatment with anticancer drugs. Uric acid levels are elevated because of the breakdown of DNA that occurs following cell death. To minimize elevations in plasma urate levels, allopurinol should be administered prior to initiation of cancer chemotherapy. Allopurinol is also useful for treating hyperuricemia that may occur secondary to certain blood dyscrasias (e.g., polycythemia vera, myeloid metaplasia, leukemia).

Adverse Effects. Allopurinol is generally well tolerated. The most serious toxicity is a rare but potentially fatal *hypersensitivity syndrome*, characterized by rash, fever, eosinophilia, and dysfunction of the liver and kidneys. If rash or fever develop, allopurinol should be discontinued immediately. Many patients recover spontaneously; others may require hemodialysis or treatment with glucocorticoids. Mild side effects seen occasionally include *gastrointestinal reactions* (nausea, vomiting, diarrhea, abdominal discomfort) and *neurologic effects* (drowsiness, headache, metallic taste). A few patients using allopurinol for prolonged periods have developed *cataracts;* periodic ophthalmic examinations are recommended.

Drug Interactions. Allopurinol can inhibit hepatic drug-metabolizing enzymes, thereby delaying the inactivation of other drugs. This interaction is of particular concern for patients taking *oral anticoagulants* (e.g., warfarin), whose dosage should be reduced. Similarly, if allopurinol is combined with *mercaptopurine* or *azathioprine* (a derivative of mercaptopurine) in the treatment of cancer, dosages of mercaptopurine and azathioprine should be lowered by as much as 75%. The combination of allopurinol plus *ampicillin* is associated with a high incidence of rash. If rash develops, allopurinol should be discontinued immediately.

Preparations, Dosage and Administration. Allopurinol [Zyloprim] is dispensed in 100- and 300-mg tablets for oral use.

For treatment of *chronic tophaceous gout*, the objective is to decrease plasma urate content to 7 mg/dl (or less) in males and 6 mg/dl (or less) in females. Dosages should be individualized to achieve this goal. The usual initial dosage is 100 mg once daily. The dosage is then increased by 100-mg increments at

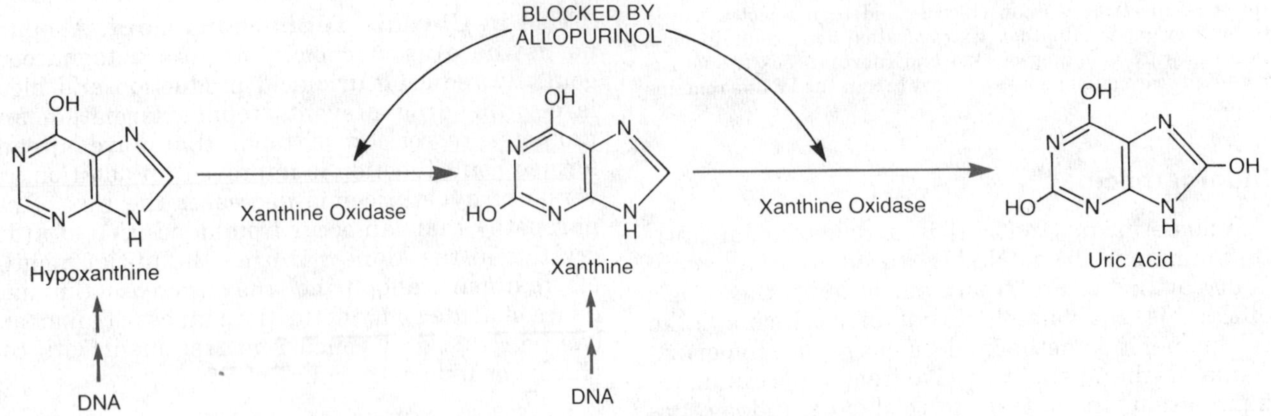

Figure 63–3. Reduction of uric acid formation by allopurinol.

intervals of 1 week until urate has been reduced to an acceptable level, usually at doses of 200 to 300 mg/day. To prevent renal injury, fluid intake should be sufficient to maintain a urine flow of at least 2 L /day.

For *secondary hyperuricemias* in *adults*, dosages range from 100 to 800 mg/day. For *children* aged 6 to 10 years who are undergoing cancer chemotherapy, the recommended dosage is 300 mg daily. The dosage for children under 6 years is 150 mg/day.

Probenecid

Actions and Uses. Probenecid [Benemid, Probalan] acts on the renal tubules to inhibit reabsorption of uric acid. As a result, excretion of uric acid is increased and hyperuricemia is reduced. By lowering plasma urate levels, probenecid prevents formation of new tophi and facilitates regression of tophi that have already formed. The drug may exacerbate acute episodes of gout, and, therefore, treatment should be delayed until the acute attack has been controlled. During the initial months of therapy, probenecid may induce acute attacks of gout. If an attack occurs, colchicine or indomethacin should be added to the regimen. In addition to its use in gout, probenecid may be employed to prolong the effects of penicillins and cephalosporins (by delaying their excretion by the kidneys).

Adverse Effects. Probenecid is well tolerated by most patients. Mild gastrointestinal effects (nausea, vomiting, anorexia) occur occasionally. These responses can be reduced by administering probenecid with food. Hypersensitivity reactions, usually manifested as rash, develop in about 4% of patients. Renal injury may occur from deposition of urate in the kidney. The risk of kidney damage can be minimized by alkalinizing the urine and by consuming 2.5 to 3 L of fluid daily during the first few days of treatment.

Drug Interactions. Aspirin and other salicylates interfere with the uricosuric action of probenecid. Accordingly, probenecid should not be used concurrently with these drugs. Probenecid inhibits the renal excretion of several drugs, including indomethacin and the sulfonamides; dosages of these agents may require reduction.

Preparations, Dosage, and Administration. Probenecid [Benemid, Probalan] is dispensed in 500-mg tablets. The initial dosage for adults is 250 mg twice daily for 1 week. The maintenance dosage is 500 mg twice daily. Administration with food decreases gastrointestinal upset. Therapy should not be initiated during an acute gouty attack.

Sulfinpyrazone

Actions and Uses. Like probenecid, sulfinpyrazone [Anturane] is a uricosuric agent and is employed to reduce hyperuricemia in patients with *chronic* gout. The drug lacks anti-inflammatory and analgesic actions and is of no benefit during an *acute* gouty attack. During the first few months of therapy, sulfinpyrazone may precipitate an acute gouty attack. The risk of an attack can be decreased by concurrent use of colchicine or indomethacin.

Adverse Effects. Gastrointestinal effects (nausea, abdominal pain) are common but rarely necessitate cessation of treatment. These reactions can be reduced by administering sulfinpyrazone with meals. Sulfinpyrazone can exacerbate gastrointestinal ulcers. The drug should be used cautiously in patients with a history of gastric ulcers and is contraindicated in patients with active ulcers. As with probenecid, there is a risk of uric acid deposition in the kidney. This risk can be reduced by alkalinizing the urine and by ingesting large volumes of fluids.

Drug Interactions. *Salicylates* will counteract the uricosuric action of sulfinpyrazone; these drugs should not be taken concurrently. Sulfinpyrazone can inhibit hepatic metabolism of *tolbutamide* (causing hypoglycemia) and *warfarin* (causing bleeding tendencies). If combined with sulfinpyrazone, these drugs may require a reduction in dosage.

Preparations, Dosage, and Administration. Sulfinpyrazone [Anturane] is dispensed in 100-mg tablets and 200-mg capsules. Administration with meals decreases gastrointestinal side effects. The initial adult dosage is 100 to 200 mg twice daily. Maintenance dosages range from 200 to 800 mg/day in divided doses.

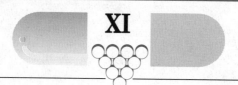

Respiratory Tract Drugs

64

Drug Therapy of Asthma

PATHOPHYSIOLOGY OF ASTHMA

OVERVIEW OF DRUG THERAPY

BETA$_2$-ADRENERGIC AGONISTS

METHYLXANTHINES
    Theophylline
    Aminophylline
    Other Methylxanthines

CROMOLYN SODIUM

NEDOCROMIL SODIUM

GLUCOCORTICOIDS

IPRATROPIUM

DRUG SELECTION IN CHRONIC ASTHMA

Asthma is a very common disorder that affects both children and adults. In the United States, asthma affects between 7 and 20 million people and has an economic cost of about $4 billion. Although rarely fatal, asthma can be both disturbing and disruptive. Unfortunately, there is no cure for asthma; drugs can only provide symptomatic relief.

In approaching the antiasthmatic drugs, we will begin by reviewing the pathophysiology of asthma. After this we will discuss the agents used for treatment. Two classes of antiasthmatic drugs—beta$_2$-adrenergic agonists and glucocorticoids—have been considered at length in previous chapters; accordingly, discussion of these drugs will be brief.

PATHOPHYSIOLOGY OF ASTHMA

Asthma is a complex disease in which a variety of mild stimuli (e.g., inhalation of cold air, exercise) can trigger an episode of bronchospasm, resulting in airway obstruction. These stimuli also promote inflammation, mucosal edema, and plugging of bronchioles with mucus. Central to the disease process is a state referred to as *bronchial hyperreactivity*. It is this hyperreactive state that allows otherwise benign stimuli to have such profound effects. Characteristic signs and symptoms of asthma are a sense of breathlessness and tightness in the chest, together with wheezing, dyspnea, and cough.

819

The events that lead to airway obstruction are summarized in Figure 64–1. As the figure indicates, several factors may contribute to establishing a state of bronchial hyperreactivity. *Chronic inflammation* and *allergens* are of particular importance. The mechanisms by which inflammation, allergens, and other factors induce hyperreactivity are unknown. Once the hyperreactive state exists, trigger factors (re-exposure to allergens, exercise, cold air, intense emotion) are able to cause the release of leukotrienes, histamine, and other substances from mast cells of the lung. These agents intensify inflammation and cause bronchospasm and mucous plugging.

OVERVIEW OF DRUG THERAPY

Drugs Used to Treat Asthma

The principal agents used to treat asthma are (1) beta$_2$-adrenergic agonists, (2) theophylline, (3) glucocorticoids, and (4) cromolyn sodium. The beta$_2$ agonists and theophylline relieve or prevent symptoms by promoting bronchodilation. The glucocorticoids are beneficial because of their power-

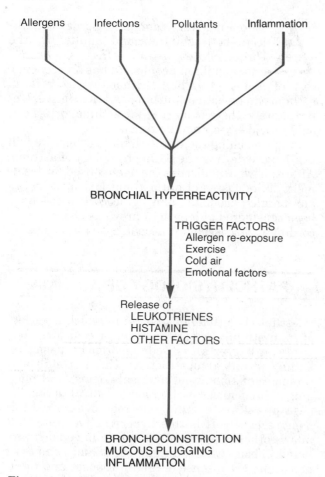

Figure 64–1. **The events that can lead to airway obstruction in asthmatics.**

ful anti-inflammatory actions. Cromolyn prevents the release of leukotrienes and other inflammatory mediators from mast cells. With long-term use, glucocorticoids and cromolyn appear to reduce bronchial hyperreactivity.

Therapeutic Goal

The goal of drug therapy is to prevent life-threatening attacks and permit patients to maintain normal lifestyles. To achieve this goal, drugs are administered with three objectives: (1) relief of acute attacks, (2) prophylaxis of acute attacks, and (3) suppression of chronic inflammation and reduction of bronchial hyperreactivity.

Administration of Antiasthmatic Drugs by Inhalation

Most antiasthmatic drugs can be administered by inhalation, a route with two obvious advantages: (1) therapeutic effects are enhanced (by delivering drugs directly to their site of action), while systemic effects are minimized, and (2) inhalation can produce rapid relief of acute attacks.

Three types of devices are employed to administer antiasthmatic medications by inhalation. These are are (1) metered-dose inhalers, (2) nebulizers, and (3) dry-powder inhalers.

Metered-Dose Inhalers (MDIs). MDIs are small, hand-held, pressurized devices that deliver a measured dose of drug with each activation. Dosing is usually accomplished with 1 or 2 puffs. When two puffs are needed, an interval of at least 1 minute should separate the first puff from the second. When using an MDI, the patient must begin to inhale prior to activating the device. Hence, hand-lung coordination is required. MDIs can be difficult to use correctly and patients will need a demonstration as well as written and verbal instruction. Even with optimal use, only about 10% of the dose reaches the lungs. About 80% impacts the oropharynx and is swallowed, and the remaining 10% is left in the device or exhaled.

Several kinds of *spacers* are available for use with MDIs. All of these devices, which attach directly to the MDI, serve to increase delivery of drug to the lungs and decrease deposition of drug on the oropharyngeal mucosa. In addition, some spacers contain a one-way valve that activates upon inhalation, thereby obviating the need for good hand-lung coordination. The ability of spacers to increase drug delivery appears to be clinically significant primarily for inhaled *glucocorticoids*. In contrast, spacers seem to have little effect on responses to beta$_2$ agonists.

Nebulizers. A nebulizer is a small machine used to convert a drug solution into a mist. The droplets in the mist are much finer than those produced by inhalers. Inhalation of the nebulized mist can be done through a face mask or through a mouthpiece held between the teeth. Nebulizers take several minutes to deliver the same amount of drug contained in one puff from an inhaler. For some patients, a nebulizer may be more effective than an inhaler. Although nebulizers are usually used at home or in a hospital, these devices, which weigh under 10 pounds, are sufficiently portable for use in other locations.

Dry-Powder Inhalers (DPIs). DPIs are used to deliver drugs in the form of a dry, micronized powder directly to the lungs. Currently, only two antiasthmatic drugs—cromolyn sodium and albuterol—are available for administration by DPI. Both drugs are dispensed in single-dose capsules that must be inserted into the DPI before each administration. In contrast to MDIs, DPIs are breath activated. Hence, DPIs don't require the hand-lung coordination needed when using an MDI. When drugs are administered by DPI, up to 20% of the dose can reach the lungs.

BETA₂-ADRENERGIC AGONISTS

Beta₂-adrenergic agonists (e.g., terbutaline, albuterol) are a mainstay of antiasthmatic therapy. These drugs are taken by practically all patients who experience asthma attacks. For treatment of asthma, beta₂ agonists are usually administered by inhalation. However, preparations for oral and parenteral use are also available.

The basic pharmacology of the adrenergic agonists is discussed in Chapter 17. In this chapter, discussion is limited to the use of these drugs in asthma.

Mechanism of Antiasthmatic Action

The beta₂ agonists are sympathomimetic drugs that produce "selective" activation of beta₂-adrenergic receptors. By stimulating beta₂ receptors in the lung, these drugs promote *bronchodilation*, thereby reducing airway resistance. Additional benefits derive from the ability of beta₂ agonists to suppress histamine release in the lung and to increase ciliary motility. The beta₂-selective drugs have largely replaced older, less selective sympathomimetics (e.g., epinephrine, isoproterenol) for asthma therapy.

Antiasthmatic Uses

In treatment of asthma, beta₂ agonists are employed in two ways: they are given *prophylactically* to prevent attacks, and they are taken to *relieve ongoing attacks*. *Inhaled* beta₂ agonists are used to relieve mild-to-moderate attacks and to provide prophylaxis against exercise-induced asthma. Effects generally peak in 30 to 60 minutes and last for 3 to 5 hours. *Oral* administration is used for young children and others who cannot use inhalers. *Parenteral* administration is reserved for emergency treatment.

Adverse Effects

Adverse effects of the beta₂ agonists are determined largely by the route of administration. Side effects associated with oral and parenteral administration are much more intense than those associated with inhalation.

Inhalational Use. When beta₂ agonists are administered by inhalation, undesired effects are minimal. Even when patients self-administer doses that are grossly excessive, severe adverse effects are uncommon.

Oral and Parenteral Use. The selectivity of the beta₂-adrenergic agonists is only relative—not absolute. Accordingly, when these drugs are administered orally and parenterally, they are likely to produce some activation of beta₁ receptors in the heart. If the dosage is excessive, stimulation of cardiac beta₁ receptors can cause *angina pectoris* and *tachydysrhythmias*. Patients should be instructed to report chest pain or changes in heart rate or rhythm. When beta₂ agonists are inhaled, cardiac stimulation can occur but is minimal.

Systemic beta₂ agonists often cause *tremor* by stimulating beta₂ receptors on skeletal muscle. Tremor can be reduced by lowering the dosage. With continued drug use, tremor declines spontaneously.

Drug Interactions

Beta-adrenergic blocking agents (e.g., propranolol) can reduce beneficial responses to beta₂ agonists. This inhibition can be overcome by using larger doses of the beta₂ agonist.

Preparations, Dosage, and Administration

Six beta₂ agonists are available in the United States (Table 64–1). All of these drugs may be administered by inhalation. Three agents—terbutaline, metaproterenol, and albuterol—may also be given orally. One agent—terbutaline—may be given by injection. Dosages are summarized in the table. Note that oral doses are about ten times greater than inhaled doses.

Metered-Dose Inhalers. All of the beta₂ agonists are available in MDIs. The usual dosage is 1 or 2 puffs three or four times a day. When two puffs are needed, an interval of 1 minute or longer should separate puffs. During this interval, some

Table 64-1. Beta₂-Adrenergic Agonists Used in Asthma

Generic Name	Trade Name	Dosage Form	Initial Dosage Adults	Initial Dosage Children
Albuterol	Proventil, Ventolin	MDI (90 µg/puff)	2 puffs q 4–6 hr PRN	2 puffs q 4–6 hr PRN
		DPI (200 µg) [Ventol in Rotocaps]	1–2 caps q 4–6 hr PRN	1–2 caps q 4–6 hr PRN
		Nebulized solution (5 mg/ml)	2.5 mg tid or qid	2.5 mg tid or qid
		Syrup or tablets	2 or 4 mg PO tid or qid	0.1 mg/kg PO q 4–6 hr PRN
		Extended-release tablets [Proventil Repetabs]	4–8 mg PO q 12 hr	0.1 mg/kg PO q 12 hr
Bitolterol	Tornalate	MDI (370 µg/puff)	2–3 puffs q 4–6 hr PRN	2 puffs q 4–6 hr PRN
Isoetharine	Bronkosol, Bronkometer	MDI (340 µg/puff) Nebulized solution	1–2 puffs q 4 hr PRN 2.5–5 ml q 4 hr PRN	
Metaproterenol	Alupent, Metaprel	MDI (650 µg/puff) Nebulized solution (5% solution)	2–3 puffs q 4–6 hr PRN 0.2–0.3 ml q 4–6 hr PRN	2 puffs q 3–4 hr 0.2 ml q 4–6 hr
		Syrup or tablets	20 mg tid or qid PRN	Under 6 years old: 1.3–2.6 mg/kg/day 6 to 9 years old: 10 mg tid or qid Over 9 years old: 20 mg tid or qid
Pirbuterol	Maxair	MDI (200 µg/puff)	2 puffs q 4–6 hr PRN	2 puffs q 4–6 hr PRN
Terbutaline	Brethaire, Brethine, Bricanyl	MDI (200 µg/puff) Tablets Subcutaneous	2–3 puffs q 4–6 hr PRN 2.5–5 mg tid 0.25 mg (repeat after 15–30 min if needed)	2–3 puffs q 4–6 hr PRN 1.25–2.5 mg tid 0.01 mg/kg (repeat after 15–30 min if needed)

MDI = metered-dose inhaler; DPI = dry-powder inhaler

bronchodilation develops, thereby facilitating penetration of the second puff.

Nebulization. Three beta₂ agonists can be administered by nebulization (see Table 64–1). For certain patients, nebulizers can be superior to inhalers. Experience has shown that some patients who have become unresponsive to a beta₂ agonist delivered with an inhaler may be responsive when the same drug is administered by nebulization. This differential effect occurs because the nebulizer delivers the dose slowly (over several minutes); as the bronchi gradually dilate, the drug gains deeper and deeper access to the lungs.

METHYLXANTHINES

We first encountered the methylxanthines (theophylline, caffeine, others) in Chapter 32 (Central Nervous System Stimulants). As discussed in that chapter, the most prominent actions of these drugs are (1) bronchodilation, and (2) CNS excitation. Other actions include cardiac stimulation, vasodilation, and diuresis.

THEOPHYLLINE

Theophylline is the principal methylxanthine employed to treat asthma. Benefits derive primarily from bronchodilation. Theophylline has a narrow therapeutic range, and dosage must be carefully controlled. The drug is usually administered by mouth. Theophylline is not administered by inhalation because the drug is inactive by this route.

Until recently, theophylline was considered a first-line antiasthmatic medication, and nearly all patients with chronic asthma were given the drug. However, over the past few years, use of theophylline has declined—largely because of two factors: (1) development of safer and more effective antiasthmatic medications (inhaled beta₂-selective adrenergic agonists, inhaled glucocorticoids), and (2) an increased appreciation of the role of inflammation in asthma pathology. Because of these developments, theophylline is now considered a second- or third-choice antiasthmatic medication.

Mechanism of Action

Theophylline produces bronchodilation by relaxing smooth muscle of the bronchi. The mechanism of this effect has not been determined. Of the mechanisms that have been proposed, the most probable is blockade of receptors for adenosine.

One frequently discussed mechanism suggests that methylxanthines act by inhibiting an enzyme called *phosphodiesterase*, thereby elevating intracellular levels of cyclic AMP. This mechanism was proposed based on the ability of methylxanthines, in high concentrations, to inhibit phosphodiesterase in the test tube. However, since these high concentrations are not achieved in the body, it seems unlikely that inhibition of phosphodiesterase underlies the effects of methylxanthines in humans.

Use in Asthma

Oral theophylline has been used for maintenance therapy of patients with chronic stable asthma. Although less effective than beta$_2$ agonists, theophylline has a longer duration of action (when administered in sustained-release formulations). When taken on a regular schedule, oral theophylline can decrease the frequency and severity of attacks and can reduce the need for inhaled beta$_2$ agonists and oral glucocorticoids. Because of its prolonged effects, oral theophylline may be most appropriate for patients who experience nocturnal asthma attacks.

Intravenous theophylline has been employed in emergencies. However, the drug is no more effective than beta$_2$ agonists and glucocorticoids, and is clearly more dangerous.

Pharmacokinetics

Absorption. Oral theophylline is available in standard and sustained-release formulations. The standard formulations are rapidly absorbed, but produce wide fluctuations in plasma drug levels. The sustained-release preparations are absorbed more slowly and produce plasma levels that are reasonably stable. Absorption from some sustained-release preparations can be affected by food.

Metabolism. Theophylline is metabolized in the liver. Rates of metabolism are affected by multiple factors—age, disease, drugs—and show wide individual variation. As a result, the plasma half-life of theophylline varies considerably among patients. For example, while the *average* half-life in nonsmoking adults is about 8 hours, the half-life can be as short as 2 hours in some adults and as long as 15 hours in others. Smoking cigarettes (one to two packs per day) accelerates metabolism and decreases the half-life of theophylline by about 50%. The average half-life in children is 4 hours. Metabolism is slowed in patients with certain pathologies (e.g., heart disease, liver disease, prolonged fever). Some drugs (e.g., cimetidine, fluoroquinolone antibiotics) decrease theophylline metabolism. Other drugs (e.g., phenobarbital) accelerate metabolism. Because of these variations in metabolism, individualization of theophylline dosage is essential.

Plasma Drug Levels. Safe and effective therapy requires periodic measurement of theophylline blood levels. Traditionally, dosage has been adjusted to produce theophylline levels between 10 and 20 μg/ml. However, many patients respond well at 5 μg/ml, and, as a rule, there is little benefit to increasing levels above 15 μg/ml. Hence, levels between 5 and 15 μg/ml may be appropriate for many patients. At levels above 20 μg/ml, the risk of significant adverse effects is high.

Toxicity

Symptoms. Toxicity is related to theophylline levels. Adverse effects are uncommon at plasma levels below 20 μg/ml. At levels of 20 to 25 μg/ml, relatively mild reactions occur (e.g., nausea, vomiting, diarrhea, insomnia, restlessness). Serious adverse effects are most likely at levels above 30 μg/ml. These reactions include severe dysrhythmias (e.g., ventricular fibrillation) and convulsions that can be highly resistant to treatment. Death may result from cardiorespiratory collapse.

Treatment. At the first indication of toxicity, administration of theophylline should cease. If a large amount of the drug has been ingested, ipecac should be given to induce vomiting. After this, absorption can be decreased by administering activated charcoal together with a cathartic. Ventricular dysrhythmias respond to lidocaine. Intravenous diazepam may help control seizures.

Drug Interactions

Caffeine. Caffeine is a methylxanthine with pharmacologic properties like those of theophylline (see Chapter 32). Accordingly, caffeine can intensify the adverse effects of theophylline on the CNS and heart. In addition, caffeine can compete with theophylline for drug-metabolizing enzymes, thereby causing theophylline levels to rise. Because of these interactions, individuals taking theophylline should avoid caffeine-containing beverages (e.g., coffee, many soft drinks) and other sources of caffeine.

Drugs That Reduce Theophylline Levels. Several agents—including *phenobarbital, phenytoin,* and *rifampin*—can lower theophylline levels by causing induction of hepatic drug-metabolizing enzymes. Concurrent use of these agents may necessitate an increase in theophylline dosage.

Drugs That Increase Theophylline Levels. Several drugs—including *cimetidine* and the *fluoroquinolone antibiotics* (e.g., ciprofloxacin)—can elevate plasma levels of theophylline, primarily by inhibiting hepatic metabolism. To avoid theophylline toxicity, the dosage of theophylline should be reduced when the drug is combined with these other agents.

Oral Formulations

Oral theophylline is available in standard and sustained-release formulations. The standard formulations are rapidly absorbed, require frequent administration, and produce substantial fluctuations in plasma theophylline levels. Sustained-release formulations are more convenient to use and can produce drug levels that are relatively stable. Accordingly, the sustained-release formulations are preferred for routine therapy. Sustained-release preparations are available in 8-, 12-, and 24-hour forms.

Absorption from sustained-release formulations can be affected markedly by food. For example, absorption from one preparation—Theo-24—is accelerated in the presence of a fatty meal. In contrast, food reduces absorption from a product named Theo-Dur Sprinkle.

Because theophylline has a narrow therapeutic range, and because sustained-release formulations contain large amounts of the drug, accelerated absorption from sustained-release formulations can produce dangerous elevations in theophylline blood levels. Because of this potential hazard, some clinicians avoid the formulations intended for once-a-day administration. These preparations pose the greatest threat because they contain the largest amount of theophylline.

Dosage and Administration

Oral. Dosage must be individualized. Traditionally, dosage has been adjusted to maintain plasma theophylline levels between 10 and 20 μg/ml. However, levels between 5 and 15 μg/ml may be appropriate for many patients. To minimize chances of toxicity, doses should be low initially and then gradually increased. If a dose is missed, the following dose should *not* be doubled, since doing so could produce toxicity. Smokers require higher than average doses; conversely, patients with heart disease, liver dysfunction, or prolonged fever are likely to require relatively low doses. Patients should be instructed not to chew the sustained-release formulations. Product information should be consulted for compatibility with food. Guidelines for maintenance dosing are given below.

Maintenance dosages vary with the age of the patient. A typical maintenance dosage for *adults* is 200 to 300 mg two or three times a day. Guidelines for *pediatric* dosing are as follows: for children aged 1 to 9 years, 22 mg/kg/day; for children aged 9 to 12 years, 20 mg/kg/day; and for children aged 12 to 16 years, 18 mg/kg/day. The number of daily doses depends upon the duration of action of the preparation employed.

Intravenous. Intravenous theophylline is reserved for emergencies. Administration must be done slowly, since rapid injection can cause fatal cardiovascular reactions. Intravenous the-

ophylline is incompatible with many other drugs. Accordingly, compatibility should be verified prior to mixing theophylline with other IV agents. For specific IV dosages, refer to the discussion of *aminophylline* below.

AMINOPHYLLINE

Aminophylline [Truphylline] is a theophylline salt that is considerably more soluble than theophylline itself. In solution, each molecule of aminophylline dissociates to yield two molecules of theophylline. Hence, the pharmacologic properties of aminophylline and theophylline are identical. Aminophylline is available in formulations for oral, intravenous, and rectal administration. Intravenous administration is employed most frequently.

Administration and Dosage

Intravenous. Because of its relatively high solubility, aminophylline is the preferred form of theophylline for intravenous use. Infusions should be done slowly (no faster than 25 mg/minute). Rapid injection can produce severe hypotension and death and must not be done. The usual loading dose is 6 mg/kg. The maintenance infusion rate should be adjusted to provide plasma levels of theophylline that are within the therapeutic range (10 to 20 μg/ml). Aminophylline solutions are incompatible with a number of other drugs. Accordingly, compatibility must be verified before mixing aminophylline with other IV agents.

Oral. Aminophylline is available in tablets and solution for oral administration. Dosing guidelines are the same as for theophylline.

Rectal. Aminophylline is available in *suppositories* and *solution for rectal administration*. Absorption from the suppositories is erratic, and these preparations are not recommended. Rectal solutions provide fast and reliable dosing and are safe for occasional use. Dosages for adults and children are the same as presented above for oral theophylline.

OTHER METHYLXANTHINES

Oxtriphylline. Oxtriphylline [Choledyl] is a salt of theophylline that contains 64% theophylline by weight. The drug is administered by mouth and produces the same effects as pure theophylline. Oxtriphylline offers no therapeutic advantage over theophylline itself. The dose of oxtriphylline equivalent to 100 mg of theophylline is 156 mg.

Dyphylline. Although structurally similar to theophylline, dyphylline is nonetheless a completely distinct compound, and is not converted to theophylline in the body. Dyphylline may be administered orally or IM. The drug has a half-life of 2 hours and is eliminated unchanged in the urine. The maximum adult oral dosage is 15 mg/kg four times a day. The adult IM dosage is 250 to 500 mg every 6 hours.

CROMOLYN SODIUM

Cromolyn sodium [Intal] is a very safe and effective drug for *prophylaxis* of asthma, but is not useful for aborting an ongoing attack. Administration is by inhalation.

Effects on the Lung

Cromolyn acts in part by stabilizing the cytoplasmic membrane of mast cells, thereby preventing the release of histamine and other mediators of allergic responses. In addition, the drug inhibits other inflammatory cells, such as macrophages and eosinophils. Chronic administration decreases inflammation and bronchial hyperreactivity. In contrast to theophylline and the beta$_2$ agonists, cromolyn is not a direct-acting bronchodilator.

Pharmacokinetics

Cromolyn is administered by inhalation. The fraction absorbed from the lungs is small (about 8%) and produces no discernible systemic effects. Absorbed cromolyn is excreted unchanged in the urine. Practically no absorption occurs if the drug is administered orally.

Therapeutic Uses

Chronic Asthma. Cromolyn is a first-line drug for prophylactic therapy of mild-to-moderate chronic asthma. The drug produces adequate control in 60% to 70% of patients. When administered on a regular schedule, cromolyn reduces both the intensity and frequency of attacks. In addition, the drug can decrease the need for other antiasthmatic medications (oral glucocorticoids, beta$_2$ agonists). No tolerance to the drug is seen with long-term use. To be of benefit, cromolyn must be administered *prior* to the onset of an attack; the drug is without effect if taken after an episode has begun. In patients with chronic asthma, maximal effects may take several weeks to develop. Comparative trials indicate that prophylaxis with cromolyn is at least as effective as prophylaxis with theophylline, and is clearly much safer. Cromolyn is especially effective for prophylaxis of seasonal allergic attacks and for acute prophylaxis immediately prior to allergen exposure (e.g., when anticipating mowing the lawn). Because of cromolyn's safety and efficacy, many clinicians feel that cromolyn is the anti-inflammatory drug of first choice for childhood asthma.

Exercise-Induced Asthma. Cromolyn can prevent bronchospasm in patients subject to exercise-induced asthma. For this use, cromolyn should be administered 10 to 15 minutes prior to anticipated exertion (and no more than 1 hour prior).

Allergic Rhinitis. *Intranasal* cromolyn [Nasalcrom] can relieve symptoms of allergic rhinitis. This application is discussed in Chapter 65.

Adverse Effects

Cromolyn sodium is the safest of all antiasthmatic medications. Significant adverse effects occur in fewer than 1 of every 10,000 patients. The most common reactions are wheezing and coughing in response to inhalation of powdered cromolyn.

Preparations, Dosage, and Administration

Cromolyn sodium for inhalation [Intal] can be administered with three different devices: (1) a dry-powder inhaler [Spinhaler], (2) a power-driven nebulizer, and (3) a metered-dose inhaler. Patients will need instruction on how to use these devices. With either the Spinhaler or a nebulizer, the *initial* dosage for adults and children is 20 mg four times a day. With the metered-dose inhaler, the *initial* dosage for adults and children is 2 to 4 puffs (1.6 to 3.2 mg) four times a day. For *maintenance therapy* with any device, the lowest effective dosage should be established. For therapy of chronic asthma, cromolyn must be administered on a regular schedule.

NEDOCROMIL SODIUM

Nedocromil sodium [Tilade] is a new drug with actions and uses like those of cromolyn. Like cromolyn, nedocromil has anti-inflammatory and antiallergic actions that derive in part from suppressing the release of histamine and other substances from mast cells. Nedocromil is administered with a metered-dose inhaler. The drug is indicated for prophylactic therapy only; it is not able to abort an ongoing asthma attack. Like cromolyn, nedocromil can decrease the incidence and severity of attacks and can reduce (but not eliminate) the need for other antiasthmatic medications (oral glucocorticoids, beta$_2$ agonists). The most common adverse effect is an unpleasant taste, which about 5% of patients find intolerable. Otherwise, nedocromil is generally well tolerated. The usual dosage is 2 puffs (3.5 mg) four times a day. Once symptoms are controlled, 2 puffs a day may suffice. Maximal effects may take several weeks to develop.

GLUCOCORTICOIDS

Glucocorticoids (e.g., beclomethasone, prednisone) are the most effective antiasthmatic drugs available. These agents can be administered orally, intravenously, and by inhalation. Adverse reactions to inhaled glucocorticoids and to systemic glucocorticoids taken acutely are minor. However, when glucocorticoids are used on a long-term basis, severe adverse effects may occur. The basic pharmacology of the glucocorticoids is discussed in Chapter 62. Discussion here is limited to the use of glucocorticoids in asthma.

Mechanism of Antiasthmatic Action

Glucocorticoids reduce symptoms of asthma primarily by *suppressing inflammation*. Specific anti-inflammatory effects include (1) decreased synthesis and release of inflammatory mediators (e.g., prostaglandins, leukotrienes, histamine), (2) decreased infiltration and activity of inflammatory cells (e.g., neutrophils, eosinophils), and (3) decreased edema of the airway mucosa (secondary to a decrease in vascular permeability). As a result of suppressing inflammation, glucocorticoids reduce bronchial hyperreactivity. In addition to reducing inflammation, glucocorticoids *decrease airway mucus production and increase the number of bronchial beta$_2$-adrenergic receptors as well as their responsiveness to beta$_2$ agonists.*

Use in Asthma

Glucocorticoids are used for *prophylaxis* in patients with chronic asthma. Since beneficial effects develop slowly, these drugs are not used to abort ongoing attacks. Accordingly, administration must be done on a regular schedule—not on a PRN basis.

Oral Therapy. Oral glucocorticoids are reserved for patients with severe asthma. Because of their potential for toxicity, these drugs are prescribed only when symptoms cannot be controlled with safer medications (beta$_2$ agonists, theophylline, cromolyn sodium). Because the risk of toxicity increases with duration of use, treatment should be as short as possible.

Inhalational Therapy. Inhaled glucocorticoids are now considered a first-line therapy for asthma. Use of these drugs has increased because of two factors: (1) recognition of the role of inflammation in bronchial hyperreactivity and bronchospasm, and (2) the low risk of serious side effects associated with inhalational therapy (as opposed to oral therapy). When administered every day, inhaled glucocorticoids are often more effective than alternate-day therapy with oral glucocorticoids and are considerably safer. To reduce the risks of toxicity, inhaled glucocorticoids should be used in conjunction with bronchodilators (e.g., beta$_2$ agonists), since this permits a reduction in glucocorticoid dosage.

Adverse Effects

Oral Glucocorticoids. When used acutely (less than 10 days), even in very high doses, oral glucocorticoids do not cause significant adverse effects. However, prolonged therapy, even in moderate doses, can be hazardous. Potential adverse effects include *osteoporosis, hyperglycemia, peptic ulcer disease,* and, in young patients, *suppression of growth.*

Adrenal suppression is of particular concern. As discussed in Chapter 62, prolonged use of glucocorticoids can decrease the ability of the adrenal cortex to produce glucocorticoids of its own. Since high levels of glucocorticoids are required to survive severe stress (e.g., surgery, trauma), and since adrenal suppression prevents production of endogenous glucocorticoids, *patients must be given in-creased doses of oral or parenteral glucocorticoids at times of stress. Failure to do so may prove fatal!* It should be noted that *inhaled* glucocorticoids are inadequate as supplements at times of stress. Following withdrawal of oral glucocorticoids, several months are required for recovery of adrenocortical function. Throughout this period, supplemental steroids are required if severe stress occurs.

A complete list of contraindications to oral glucocorticoids is presented in the Summary of Nursing Implications at the end of the chapter.

Inhaled Glucocorticoids. Inhaled glucocorticoids are generally devoid of serious toxicity, even when used in high doses. The most common adverse effects are *oropharyngeal candidiasis* and *dysphonia* (hoarseness, speaking difficulty). Both effects result from local deposition of inhaled glucocorticoids. To minimize these effects, patients should be instructed to (1) gargle after each administration, and (2) employ a spacer device during administration, which will reduce drug deposition in the oropharynx. If candidiasis develops, it can be treated with antifungal medication.

With long-term, high-dose therapy, some adrenal suppression may develop. As a result, patients may require supplemental systemic glucocorticoids to survive severe stress (e.g., surgery, trauma).

Preparations, Dosage, and Administration

Oral Glucocorticoids. *Prednisone* and *prednisolone* are preferred glucocorticoids for oral therapy of asthma. For *acute* therapy, the usual *adult* dosage for either drug is 30 to 40 mg twice daily for 5 to 7 days.

For *long-term* treatment, *alternate-day dosing* is recommended (to minimize adrenal suppression). The *initial adult* dosage is 40 to 60 mg (of prednisone or prednisolone) administered every other morning. The *initial pediatric* dosage is 20 to 40 mg every other morning. After symptoms have been controlled for a month, *adult and pediatric* dosages should be reduced by 5 to 10 mg every 2 weeks to the lowest dosage that keeps the patient free of symptoms. As discussed above, supplemental doses are required at times of stress.

Inhaled Glucocorticoids. Four glucocorticoids are available for administration by inhalation (Table 64–2). All four are dispensed in metered-dose inhalers (MDIs). Patients should be instructed to employ a *spacer device* (holding chamber) with the MDI, since this will (1) increase the amount of glucocorticoid delivered to the lungs (thereby increasing therapeutic effects), and (2) reduce the amount deposited in the oropharynx (thereby reducing adverse effects). Penetration of inhaled glucocorticoids to the lungs can be increased by inhal-

Generic Name	Trade Name	Dose per Puff	Initial Dosage	
			Adults	*Children*
Beclomethasone dipropionate	Beclovent, Vanceril	42 µg	2 puffs tid or qid *or* 4 puffs bid	1 or 2 puffs tid or qid *or* 2–4 puffs bid
Dexamethasone sodium phosphate	Decadron Phosphate Respihaler	84 µg†	3 puffs tid or qid	2 puffs tid or qid
Flunisolide	Aerobid	250 µg	2–4 puffs bid	2 puffs bid
Triamcinolone acetonide	Azmacort	100 µg	2 puffs tid or qid	1 or 2 puffs tid or qid

Table 64–2. Dosages for Inhaled Glucocorticoids*

*All of these drugs are dispensed in metered-dose inhalers. Use of a spacer device with the inhaler can increase therapeutic effects and reduce local adverse effects (dysphonia and candidiasis).
†Each puff releases a dose of dexamethasone phosphate equivalent to 84 µg of dexamethasone.

ing a beta$_2$ agonist 5 minutes prior to inhaling the glucocorticoid.

Inhaled glucocorticoids are administered on a regular schedule—not on a PRN basis. Pediatric and adult dosages for inhaled glucocorticoids are summarized in Table 64–2.

IPRATROPIUM

Ipratropium [Atrovent] is an atropine derivative administered by inhalation to treat chronic asthma. Like atropine itself, ipratropium is a muscarinic antagonist. By blocking muscarinic-cholinergic receptors in the bronchi, ipratropium promotes *bronchodilation*. Therapeutic effects begin within 30 seconds, reach 50% of their maximum in 3 minutes, and persist for about 6 hours. Ipratropium is effective against allergen-induced asthma and exercise-induced asthma—but is less effective than the beta$_2$ agonists. Because ipratropium and the beta$_2$-adrenergic agonists promote bronchodilation by different mechanisms, the beneficial effects of these drugs are additive. Ipratropium is a quaternary ammonium compound and, therefore, always carries a positive charge. As a result, the drug is not readily absorbed from the lungs or from the digestive tract. Accordingly, systemic effects are minimal. The most common adverse reactions are dryness of the oropharynx (5%) and cough or exacerbation of asthma symptoms (3%). Ipratropium is dispensed in a metered-dose inhaler that delivers 18 µg per activation. The recommended adult dosage is 2 to 4 puffs four times a day. The pediatric dosage is 2 puffs four times a day.

DRUG SELECTION IN CHRONIC ASTHMA

Drug therapy of asthma is undergoing significant change. In recent years, use of inhaled glucocorticoids and cromolyn has greatly increased, owing largely to an increased appreciation of the role of inflammation in asthma. In contrast, use of theophylline has sharply declined; once considered a first-line drug for most patients, theophylline is now considered a second- or third-line agent.

The choice of drugs for chronic asthma depends on the frequency and severity of attacks. When attacks are infrequent, PRN therapy with an inhaled beta$_2$-adrenergic agonist is the treatment of choice. For patients who experience frequent attacks, regular use of an inhaled glucocorticoid or cromolyn is indicated; treatment with either agent should be supplemented with an inhaled beta$_2$ agonist as needed. If these measures prove inadequate, regular use of theophylline may be tried. If none of these measures is sufficient, treatment with an oral glucocorticoid (e.g., prednisone) is indicated.

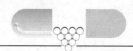

Summary of Major Nursing Implications

BETA₂-ADRENERGIC AGONISTS

Preadministration Assessment

Therapeutic Goal

Inhaled beta₂ agonists are used on a PRN basis for prophylaxis of asthma attacks and to relieve ongoing attacks. *Oral* beta₂ agonists may be used for maintenance therapy.

Baseline Data

Determine the frequency and severity of asthma attacks and attempt to identify trigger factors.

Identifying High-Risk Patients

Systemic (oral, parenteral) beta₂ agonists are *contraindicated* for patients with *tachydysrhythmias* or *tachycardia associated with digitalis toxicity.* Use *systemic* beta₂ agonists with *caution* in patients with *diabetes, hyperthyroidism, organic heart disease, hypertension,* or *angina pectoris.*

Implementation: Administration

Routes

Usual: Inhalation.
Occasional: Oral, subcutaneous.

Administration

Inhalation. Inhaled beta₂ agonists are administered with either a metered-dose inhaler, dry-powder inhaler, or nebulizer. Teach patients how to use these devices. For patients who have difficulty with hand-lung coordination, use of a spacer that has a one-way valve may improve the outcome.

Inform patients who are using metered-dose inhalers or dry-powder inhalers that when two puffs are needed, an interval of at least 1 minute should elapse between puffs.

Inform patients that inhaled beta₂ agonists are intended for PRN use, to be taken several minutes prior to exposure to precipitating factors (exercise, cold, environmental agents), or during an attack to terminate it.

Warn patients against exceeding recommended dosages.

Oral. Instruct patients to take oral beta₂ agonists on a regular schedule—not on a PRN basis.

Instruct patients to swallow sustained-release preparations intact, without crushing or chewing.

Ongoing Evaluation and Interventions

Minimizing Adverse Effects

When administered by *inhalation* at recommended doses, beta₂ agonists are essentially devoid of adverse effects. Cardiac stimulation and tremors are most likely with *systemic* therapy.

Cardiac Stimulation. Excessive dosing with *systemic* beta$_2$ agonists can cause stimulation of beta$_1$ receptors on the heart, resulting in anginal pain and tachydysrhythmias. Instruct the patient to report chest pain and changes in heart rate or rhythm.

Tremor. Tremor is common with systemic beta$_2$ agonists, and usually subsides with continued drug use. If necessary, tremor can be reduced by lowering the dosage.

Minimizing Adverse Interactions

Beta-Adrenergic Blocking Agents. These drugs (e.g., propranolol) can suppress responses to beta$_2$ agonists. If a beta blocker must be used in combination with a beta$_2$ agonist, dosage of the beta$_2$ agonist may need to be increased.

THEOPHYLLINE

 Preadministration Assessment

Therapeutic Goal

Theophylline is a bronchodilator taken on a regular schedule to decrease the intensity and frequency of asthma attacks.

Baseline Data

Determine the frequency and severity of asthma attacks.

Identifying High-Risk Patients

Theophylline is *contraindicated* for patients with *untreated seizure disorders* or *peptic ulcer disease.* Use with *caution* in patients with *heart disease, liver or kidney dysfunction,* or *severe hypertension.*

 Implementation: Administration

Routes

Oral, intravenous.

Administration

Oral. Dosage must be individualized. Doses are low initially and then increased gradually. The dosing objective is to produce plasma theophylline levels in the therapeutic range, which has been defined traditionally as 10 to 20 µg/ml. Warn patients that if a dose is missed, the following dose should *not* be doubled.

Instruct patients to swallow enteric-coated and sustained-release formulations intact, without crushing or chewing.

Warn patients not to switch from one sustained-release formulation to another without consulting the physician.

Consult product information regarding compatibility with food, and advise the patient accordingly.

Intravenous. Administration must be done slowly. Verify compatibility with other IV drugs prior to mixing.

 Ongoing Evaluation and Interventions

Evaluating Therapeutic Effects

Monitor drug levels to insure that they are in the therapeutic range, which has been defined traditionally as 10 to 20 µg/ml. However, many patients respond well to levels of 5 to 15 µg/ml.

Minimizing Adverse Effects

Mild adverse effects (e.g., nausea, vomiting, diarrhea, insomnia, restlessness) develop as plasma drug levels rise above 20 µg/ml. Severe effects (convulsions, ventricular fibrillation) can occur at drug levels above 30 µg/ml. Dosage should be adjusted to keep theophylline levels below 20 µg/ml.

Minimizing Adverse Interactions

Caffeine. Caffeine can intensify the adverse effects of theophylline on the heart and CNS and can decrease theophylline metabolism. Caution patients against consuming caffeine-containing beverages (e.g., coffee, many soft drinks) and other sources of caffeine.

Drugs That Reduce Theophylline Levels. Phenobarbital, phenytoin, rifampin, and other drugs can lower theophylline levels. In the presence of these drugs, the dosage of theophylline may need to be increased.

Drugs That Increase Theophylline Levels. Cimetidine, fluoroquinolone antibiotics, and other drugs can elevate theophylline levels. When combined with these drugs, theophylline should be used in reduced dosage.

Managing Toxicity

Theophylline overdosage can cause severe dysrhythmias and convulsions. Death from cardiorespiratory collapse may occur. Manage toxicity by (1) discontinuing theophylline, (2) administering ipecac (to induce vomiting), and (3) administering activated charcoal (to decrease theophylline absorption) plus a cathartic (to accelerate fecal excretion). Give lidocaine to control ventricular dysrhythmias and IV diazepam to control seizures.

AMINOPHYLLINE

The nursing implications for aminophylline are the same as those for theophylline, except for differences in administration.

Administration

Perform intravenous infusions slowly (no faster than 25 mg/min). Adjust the maintenance infusion rate to provide plasma levels of theophylline between 10 and 20 µg/ml. Verify compatibility with other IV drugs prior to mixing.

CROMOLYN SODIUM

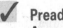 **Preadministration Assessment**

Therapeutic Goal

Cromolyn is used for acute and long-term *prophylaxis* of asthma. The drug will not abort an ongoing asthma attack.

Baseline Data

Determine the frequency and intensity of asthma attacks and attempt to identify trigger factors.

Identifying High-Risk Patients

Cromolyn is *contraindicated* for the rare patient who has experienced an allergic response to cromolyn in the past.

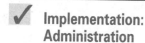

Implementation: Administration

Route

Inhalation.

Administration

Administration Devices. Cromolyn is administered with a dry-powder inhaler [Spinhaler], a nebulizer, or a metered-dose inhaler. Instruct patients on the proper use of these devices.

Acute Prophylaxis. Instruct patients to administer cromolyn 10 to 15 minutes prior to exposure to precipitating factors (e.g., exercise, cold, environmental agents).

Long-Term Prophylaxis. Instruct patients to administer cromolyn on a regular schedule, and inform them that full therapeutic effects may take several weeks to develop.

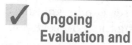

Ongoing Evaluation and Interventions

Evaluating Therapeutic Effects

Beneficial effects are indicated by (1) a reduction in the severity and frequency of asthma attacks, and (2) a reduction in the need for PRN bronchodilators (e.g., beta$_2$-adrenergic agonists).

Minimizing Adverse Effects and Interactions

Cromolyn is devoid of significant adverse effects and drug interactions.

GLUCOCORTICOIDS

The nursing implications summarized below refer specifically to the use of glucocorticoids in asthma. A full summary of nursing implications for glucocorticoids is presented in Chapter 62.

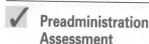

Preadministration Assessment

Therapeutic Goal

Glucocorticoids are used for *prophylaxis* of chronic asthma. They are not used to abort an ongoing attack.

Baseline Data

Determine the severity and frequency of asthma attacks.

Identifying High-Risk Patients

Inhaled Glucocorticoids. These preparations are *contraindicated* for patients with *persistently positive sputum cultures for Candida albicans.*

Oral Glucocorticoids. These preparations are *contraindicated* for patients with *systemic fungal infections* and for individuals receiving *live-virus vaccines*. Use with *caution* in *pediatric patients* and in *women who are pregnant or breast-feeding*. In addition, exercise *caution* in patients with *hyperten-*

sion, congestive heart failure, renal impairment, esophagitis, gastritis, peptic ulcer disease, myasthenia gravis, diabetes mellitus, osteoporosis, or *infections that are resistant to treatment* and in patients receiving *potassium-depleting diuretics, digitalis glycosides, insulin, oral hypoglycemics,* or *nonsteroidal anti-inflammatory drugs.*

Implementation: Administration

Routes

Oral, inhalation.

Administration

Inform patients that glucocorticoids are intended for preventive therapy (not for aborting ongoing attacks), and instruct them to administer glucocorticoids on a regular schedule—not on a PRN basis.

Oral. Alternate-day therapy is recommended to minimize adrenal suppression; instruct the patient to take one dose every other day in the morning. During long-term treatment, supplemental doses must be given at times of severe stress.

Inhalation. Advise patients to employ a *spacer device* with the glucocorticoid metered-dose inhaler, and teach them how to use this device. Inform patients that delivery of glucocorticoids to the bronchial tree can be enhanced by inhaling a beta$_2$ agonist 5 minutes prior to administering the glucocorticoid.

Ongoing Evaluation and Interventions

Evaluating Therapeutic Effects

Beneficial effects are indicated by (1) a reduction in the intensity and severity of asthma attacks, and (2) a reduction in the need for PRN bronchodilators (e.g., beta$_2$-adrenergic agonists).

Minimizing Adverse Effects

Inhaled Glucocorticoids. Advise patients to gargle after each administration and to use a spacer with the metered-dose inhaler. These measures will minimize *dysphonia* and *oropharyngeal candidiasis.* If candidiasis develops, it can be treated with antifungal medication.

Oral Glucocorticoids. Prolonged therapy can cause *adrenal suppression* and other serious adverse effects, including *osteoporosis, hyperglycemia, peptic ulcer disease,* and *growth suppression.* To compensate for adrenal suppression, *patients taking glucocorticoids on a chronic basis must be given supplemental oral or IV doses at times of stress* (e.g., trauma, surgery, infection). Additional nursing implications that apply to adverse effects of long-term glucocorticoid therapy are summarized in Chapter 62.

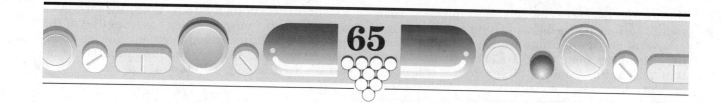

65

Nasal Decongestants, Antitussives, and Related Drugs

The topic of this chapter is drugs used to relieve symptoms of upper respiratory disorders (e.g., allergic rhinitis, colds). Our principal focus will be on nasal decongestants and antitussives (cough suppressants). Other drugs to be considered include antihistamines, intranasal steroids, and intranasal cromolyn.

DRUGS USED TO TREAT RHINITIS

Rhinitis is defined as an inflammation of the nasal mucous membranes. Major symptoms are sneezing, rhinorrhea (runny nose), pruritus (itching), and nasal congestion. (Congestion is caused by dilation and engorgement of nasal blood vessels.)

Rhinitis may be allergic or nonallergic. Allergic rhinitis results from release of histamine in response to specific allergens. Nonallergic rhinitis is a frequent symptom of the common cold.

Allergic rhinitis has two forms: seasonal and perennial. Seasonal rhinitis (hay fever) occurs in the spring and fall in reaction to pollens from weeds, grasses, and trees. Perennial (nonseasonal) rhinitis is triggered by allergens present year round, such as house dust and animal hair.

Several classes of drugs are used to treat rhinitis. Principal among these are (1) nasal decongestants, (2) antihistamines, (3) intranasal cromolyn, and (4) intranasal glucocorticoids. All of these drugs are used to treat allergic rhinitis. In contrast, only the decongestants are used routinely to treat nonallergic rhinitis.

NASAL DECONGESTANTS

Actions and Uses

Nasal decongestants (e.g., phenylephrine, phenylpropanolamine) act by stimulating alpha$_1$-adrenergic receptors on smooth muscle of nasal blood vessels. Stimulation of these receptors causes vasoconstriction, resulting in shrinkage of swollen membranes followed by nasal drainage. With *topical* administration, vasoconstriction is both rapid and intense. In contrast, responses to *oral* decongestants are moderate, delayed, and prolonged. Nasal decongestants can relieve stuffiness associated with allergic rhinitis, sinusitis, and colds.

Adverse Effects

Rebound Congestion. Rebound congestion develops when *topical* decongestants are administered on a regular basis for an extended time. With this pattern of use, as the effects of each application wear off, congestion becomes progressively more severe. To overcome this rebound congestion, the patient must use progressively larger and more frequent doses. Hence, once established, rebound congestion can lead to a cycle of escalating congestion and increased drug use. This cycle can be broken by abrupt decongestant withdrawal. However, this tactic can be extremely uncomfortable. A less drastic approach is to discontinue drug use in one nostril at a time. Rebound congestion can be minimized by limiting use of topical agents to no more than 3 to 5 days. Accordingly, topical decongestants are inappropriate for individuals with chronic rhinitis.

Cardiovascular Effects. By stimulating alpha$_1$-adrenergic receptors on systemic blood vessels, nasal decongestants can cause widespread vasoconstriction. For most patients, effects on systemic vessels are inconsequential. However, for individuals with hypertension or coronary artery disease, decongestant-induced vasoconstriction can be hazardous. Generalized vasoconstriction is most likely with the orally administered decongestants. However, if taken in excess, even the topical agents can cause significant systemic vasoconstriction.

Central Nervous System (CNS) Effects. CNS excitation is the most common adverse effect of the *oral* decongestants. Symptoms include restlessness, irritability, anxiety, and insomnia. These responses are unlikely with topical agents.

Topical Administration

General Considerations. Because of the risk of rebound congestion, topical decongestants should be used for no more than 5 consecutive days. To avoid systemic effects, doses should not exceed those recommended by the manufacturer. The applicator should be cleansed after each use to prevent contamination.

Drops. Drops should be administered with the patient in a lateral, head-low position. This positioning causes the drops to spread slowly over the nasal mucosa, thereby promoting beneficial effects while reducing the amount that is swallowed. Because the number of drops can be precisely controlled, drops allow better control over dosage than sprays. Accordingly, since young children are particularly susceptible to toxicity, drops are preferred to sprays for these patients.

Sprays. Sprays deliver the decongestant in a fine mist. Although convenient, sprays are less effective than an equal volume of properly instilled drops.

Summary of Contrasts Between Oral and Topical Agents

Oral and topical decongestants differ in several important respects. (1) Topical decongestants act faster than the oral agents and are usually more effective. (2) Oral decongestants are longer acting than topical preparations. (3) Systemic effects (e.g., vasoconstriction, CNS stimulation) are more likely with oral decongestants; topical drugs induce these responses only when dosage is excessive. (4) Whereas rebound congestion is common with prolonged use of topical agents, this reaction is rare with the oral agents.

Preparations and Dosage

Properties of Individual Decongestants. *Phenylephrine* is one of the most widely used nasal decongestants. The drug is administered topically (by itself) and orally (as a component of combination preparations). *Phenylpropanolamine* is among the most frequently used oral decongestants. *Ephedrine* causes a high incidence of CNS stimulation. CNS effects are much lower with *pseudoephedrine*, a stereoisomer of ephedrine. *Naphazoline*, one of the newer topical agents, can cause severe rebound congestion.

Dosage and Administration. Dosages and routes of administration for the nasal decongestants are summarized in Table 65–1.

Table 65–1. Nasal Decongestants: Routes and Drugs

Decongestant	Mode of Administration	Frequency of Dosing	Dosage Size†
Ephedrine	Drops	q 8–12 hr	Adults and children over 6 years: 2–3 drops (0.5%) Children under 6 years: Consult physician
Epinephrine	Drops	q 4–6 hr	Adults and children over 6 years: 1–2 drops (0.1%) Children under 6 years: Consult physician
Naphazoline	Drops	q 3 hr	Adults and children over 6 years: 2 drops (0.05%) Children under 6 years: Consult physician
Oxymetazoline	Drops	q 12 hr	Adults and children over 6 years: 2–4 drops (0.05%) Children 2–5 years: 2–3 drops (0.025%)
	Spray	q 12 hr	Adults and children over 6 years: 2–3 sprays (0.05%)
Phenylephrine	Drops	q 2–4 hr	Adults: Several drops (0.25 to 1%) Infants: 1 drop (0.125 to 0.2%)
	Spray	q 3–4 hr	Adults: 1–2 sprays (0.25 to 1%) Children over 6 years: 1–2 sprays (0.25%)
Phenylpropanolamine	Oral	q 4 hr	Adults: 25 mg Children 6–12 years: 12.5 mg
	Oral SR*	q 12 hr	Adults: 75 mg
Propylhexedrine	Inhaler	PRN	Two inhalations: 0.6–0.8 mg
Pseudoephedrine	Oral	q 6–8 hr	Adults: 60 mg Children: 1 mg/kg
	Oral SR*	q 12 hr	Adults: 120 mg
Tetrahydrozoline	Drops	q 3 or more hr	Adults and children over 6 years: 2–4 drops (0.1%) Children: 2–6 years: 2–3 drops (0.05%)
Xylometazoline	Drops	q 8–10 hr	Adults: 2–3 drops (0.1%) Children 2–12 years: 2–3 drops (0.05%)
	Spray	q 8–10 hr	Adults: 2–3 sprays (0.1%)

*Oral SR = sustained release
†For drops and sprays, dosage listed is applied to *each* nostril; numbers in parentheses indicate concentration of solution employed.

ANTIHISTAMINES

The antihistamines are discussed at length in Chapter 60. Consideration here is limited to the use of these agents to treat rhinitis.

Antihistamines (H_1-receptor antagonists) are the drugs prescribed most frequently to treat *allergic* rhinitis. These agents can relieve sneezing, rhinorrhea, and nasal itching. However, antihista-mines do not decrease nasal congestion. Since histamine does not contribute to symptoms of *infectious* rhinitis, antihistamines are of no value in the treatment of colds.

For therapy of allergic rhinitis, antihistamines are most effective when taken *prophylactically*; these drugs are less helpful when taken after symptoms have appeared. Accordingly, antihistamines should be administered on a regular basis throughout the allergy season, even when symptoms are absent.

Adverse effects are usually mild. The most prominent side effect is *sedation*. This response is less prominent with the newer H_1 antagonists (e.g., terfenadine). Anticholinergic effects (e.g., dry mouth, constipation, urinary hesitancy) may also occur.

Doses for H_1 antagonists can be found in Table 60–2.

INTRANASAL CROMOLYN SODIUM

The basic pharmacology of cromolyn sodium is discussed in Chapter 64 (Drugs Used to Treat Asthma). Consideration here is limited to the use of cromolyn to treat rhinitis.

Actions and Uses. Intranasal cromolyn sodium is a safe and effective medication for relieving symptoms of *allergic* rhinitis. In contrast, the drug is of no benefit in the treatment of nonallergic rhinitis. Cromolyn reduces symptoms of allergic rhinitis by acting on mast cells to suppress release of histamine and other mediators of the allergic response. Cromolyn is more beneficial to people with *seasonal* allergic rhinitis than to those with *perennial* rhinitis. For treatment of seasonal allergic rhinitis, cromolyn is equal in efficacy to the antihistamines, but is less effective than intranasal steroids (see below). Like the antihistamines, cromolyn is most effective when taken prior to the onset of symptoms. Beneficial effects may take a week or so to develop; patients should be informed of this delay. Adverse reactions to intranasal cromolyn are minimal.

Dosage and Administration. Intranasal cromolyn sodium [Nasalcrom] is administered with a metered spray device. The usual dosage for adults and children over the age of 6 years is one spray (5.2 mg) per nostril administered three to six times a day. If nasal congestion is present, a topical decongestant should be used prior to administering cromolyn. Like the antihistamines, cromolyn should be administered on a regular schedule throughout the allergy season.

INTRANASAL GLUCOCORTICOIDS

The basic pharmacology of the glucocorticoids is discussed in Chapter 62. Consideration here is limited to the use of these drugs to treat rhinitis.

Actions and Uses. Intranasal glucocorticoids are the most effective drugs for treating both seasonal and perennial rhinitis. Four preparations are available: *dexamethasone, beclomethasone, flunisolide,* and *triamcinolone*. All four are equally effective. Because of their anti-inflammatory ac-

tions, these drugs can prevent or suppress all of the major symptoms of allergic rhinitis (congestion, rhinorrhea, sneezing, nasal itching, erythema). As a rule, intranasal steroids are reserved for patients whose symptoms cannot be controlled with more conventional drugs (decongestants, antihistamines, intranasal cromolyn). Glucocorticoids are not indicated for nonallergic rhinitis.

Adverse Effects. Adverse effects are mild. The most common effects are drying of the nasal mucosa and sensations of burning or itching. These effects seem to be caused by the vehicle employed for administration and not by the steroids themselves.

Because they can suppress host defenses, intranasal glucocorticoids should be employed with caution in patients with tuberculosis or untreated bacterial infection of the lungs.

Systemic effects, including adrenocortical suppression, may occur. However, these responses are rare at recommended doses. Systemic effects are most likely with dexamethasone; reactions can be minimized by limiting use of dexamethasone to no more than 30 days. Since beclomethasone, flunisolide, and triamcinolone undergo rapid deactivation following absorption, these drugs do not achieve significant blood levels. Hence, systemic effects are minimal. Accordingly, these agents are preferred to dexamethasone for intranasal use.

Dosage and Administration. Intranasal glucocorticoids are administered using a metered spray device. Full doses are given initially (Table 65–2). Once symptoms have been controlled, the dosage should be reduced to the lowest effective amount. For patients with seasonal allergic rhinitis, maximal effects may require a week or more to develop. For patients with perennial rhinitis, maximal responses may not be seen for 2 to 3 weeks. If nasal passages are blocked, they should be cleared with a topical decongestant prior to glucocorticoid administration.

DRUGS USED TO TREAT COUGH

Cough is a complex reflex involving the central nervous system, the peripheral nervous system, and the muscles of respiration. The cough reflex can be initiated by irritation of the bronchial mucosa as well as by stimuli arising at sites distant from the respiratory tract. Cough is often beneficial, serving to remove foreign matter and excess secretions from the bronchial tree. Productive cough is characteristic of chronic lung disease (e.g., emphysema, asthma, bronchitis) and should not be suppressed. Not all cough, however, is useful; cough frequently serves only to deprive us of com-

Table 65–2. Intranasal Glucocorticoids			
Generic Name	**Trade Name**	**Dose/Spray (μg)**	**Dosage (Sprays per Nostril)**
Beclomethasone	Beconase, Vancenase	42	Adults: 1 spray 2–4 times/day Children 6–12 years: 1 spray tid
Dexamethasone	Decadron Phosphate Turbinaire	84	Adults: 2 sprays 2–3 times/day Children 6–12 years: 1–2 sprays bid
Flunisolide	Nasalide	50	Adults: 2 sprays bid Children 6–14 years: 1 spray tid or 2 sprays bid
Triamcinolone	Nasacort	55	Adults: 2 sprays 1–2 times/day

fort or sleep. Under these conditions, antitussive medication is appropriate. The most common use of cough medicines is suppression of nonproductive cough associated with the common cold and other upper respiratory infections.

ANTITUSSIVES

Antitussives are drugs that suppress cough. Some of these agents act within the CNS, whereas others act peripherally. The antitussives fall into two major groups: (1) opioid antitussives, and (2) nonopioid antitussives.

Opioid Antitussives

All of the opioid analgesics have the ability to suppress cough. The two opioids used most frequently for cough suppression are *codeine* and *hydrocodone*. Both agents act within the CNS to elevate the cough threshold. Hydrocodone is somewhat more potent than codeine and carries a greater liability for abuse. The basic pharmacology of the opioids is discussed in Chapter 28.

Codeine. Codeine is the most effective cough suppressant available. The drug is active orally and decreases both the frequency and intensity of cough. Doses are low, about one tenth those needed to relieve pain. At these doses, the risk of physical dependence is small.

Like all opioids, codeine can suppress respiration. Accordingly, the drug should be employed with caution in patients with reduced respiratory reserve. In the event of overdosage, respiratory depression may prove fatal; an opioid antagonist (preferably naloxone) should be used to reverse toxicity.

When dispensed by itself, codeine has a significant potential for abuse, and is classified under Schedule II of the Controlled Substances Act. However, the abuse potential of the antitussive mixtures that contain codeine is low. Accordingly, these mixtures are classified under Schedule V.

For treatment of cough, the adult dosage is 10 to 20 mg orally, four to six times a day. Codeine is rarely recommended for children.

Nonopioid Antitussives

Dextromethorphan. Dextromethorphan is the most effective of the nonopioid cough medicines. Except when used for severe acute cough, this drug is just as effective as codeine. Like the opioids, dextromethorphan acts within the CNS. Dextromethorphan is a derivative of the opioids but shares with these agents only the ability to suppress cough; dextromethorphan does not produce analgesia, euphoria, or physical dependence, and lacks any potential for abuse. At therapeutic doses, dextromethorphan does not depress respiration. Adverse effects are mild and rare. Dextromethorphan is the active ingredient in most nonprescription antitussive preparations. The usual adult dosage is 10 to 30 mg every 4 to 8 hours.

Other Nonopioid Antitussives. *Diphenhydramine* is an antihistamine with the ability to suppress cough. The mechanism of antitussive action is unclear. Like other antihistamines, diphenhydramine has sedative and anticholinergic properties. Cough suppression is achieved only at doses that produce prominent sedation. The usual adult dosage is 25 mg every 4 hours.

Benzonatate [Tessalon] is a structural analogue of tetracaine, a local anesthetic. The drug is believed to suppress cough by decreasing the sensitivity of respiratory tract stretch receptors (components of the cough-reflex pathway); CNS mechanisms may also be involved. Adverse effects are usually mild (e.g., sedation, dizziness, constipation). Benzonatate is dispensed in capsules for oral administration. The capsules should be swallowed intact, since chewing produces anesthesia of the mouth and pharynx. The usual adult dosage is 100 mg three times a day. The drug should not be given to infants because anesthesia of the mouth may impair swallowing.

EXPECTORANTS AND MUCOLYTICS

Expectorants. An expectorant is a drug that renders cough more productive by stimulating the flow of respiratory tract secretions. A variety of compounds (e.g., terpin hydrate, ammonium chloride, iodide products) have been promoted for their supposed expectorant actions. However, in almost all cases, efficacy is doubtful. One agent, *guaifenesin* (glyceryl guaiacolate), may be an exception to this rule. However, for this drug to be effective, doses higher than those normally employed may be needed.

Mucolytics. A mucolytic is a drug that reacts directly with mucus to make it more watery. This action should help make cough more productive. Two preparations—*hypertonic saline* and *acetylcysteine*—are employed for their mucolytic actions. Both are administered by inhalation. Unfortunately, both drugs can trigger bronchospasm. Because of its sulfur content, acetylcysteine [Mucomyst] has the additional disadvantage of smelling like rotten eggs.

COLD REMEDIES: COMBINATION PREPARATIONS

The common cold is an acute upper respiratory infection of viral origin. Symptoms include rhinorrhea, sneezing, cough, sore throat, headache, malaise, and myalgia; fever is common in children but rare in adults. The cold is a self-limited disorder and is usually benign. Persistence or worsening of symptoms suggests development of a secondary bacterial infection.

There is no cure for the cold; hence, treatment is purely symptomatic. Since colds are caused by viruses, there is no justification for the routine use of antibacterial drugs. Antibiotics are appropriate only if a bacterial infection arises. There is no evidence that vitamin C can prevent or cure colds.

Because no single drug can relieve all of the symptoms of a cold, the pharmaceutical industry has formulated a vast number of cold remedies that contain a mixture of ingredients. These combination cold remedies should be reserved for patients with multiple symptoms. In addition, the combination chosen should contain only those agents that are appropriate for the symptoms to be treated. Patients who require relief from just a single symptom (e.g., rhinitis, cough, or headache) are best treated with a single-entity preparation.

Combination cold remedies frequently contain two or more of the following: (1) a nasal decongestant, (2) an antitussive, (3) an analgesic, (4) an antihistamine, and (5) caffeine. The purpose of the first three agents is self-evident. In contrast, the roles of antihistamines and caffeine require explanation. Since histamine has nothing to do with the symptoms of a cold, antihistamines are not present to counteract the actions of histamine. Rather, because of their anticholinergic actions, antihistamines are included to suppress secretion of mucus. Caffeine is added to offset the sedative effects of the antihistamine.

Although they can be convenient, combination cold remedies do have disadvantages. As with all fixed-dose combinations, there is the chance that a dosage (e.g., one capsule or one tablet) that produces therapeutic levels of one ingredient may produce levels of other ingredients that are either excessive or subtherapeutic. In addition, the combination may contain ingredients for which the patient has no need. Furthermore, under FDA regulations, a brand-name product can be reformulated and then sold under the same name. Hence, without carefully reading the label, the consumer has no assurance that the brand name product purchased this year contains the same amounts of the same drugs that were present in last year's version of that combination product.

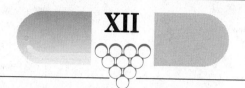

XII

Gastrointestinal Drugs

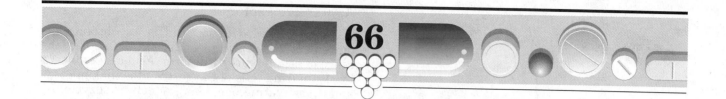

Drugs for Peptic Ulcer Disease

The term *peptic ulcer disease* (PUD) refers to a group of upper gastrointestinal disorders characterized by varying degrees of erosion of the gut wall. Severe ulcers can be complicated by hemorrhage and perforation. Although peptic ulcers can develop in any region exposed to acid and pepsin, ulceration is most common in the lesser curvature of the stomach and in the duodenum. PUD is a very common disorder that affects about 10% of Americans at some time in their lives. Because PUD is so prevalent, antiulcer medications constitute one of our most widely used families of drugs.

PATHOGENESIS OF PEPTIC ULCERS

Peptic ulcers develop when there is an imbalance between mucosal defensive factors and aggressive factors (Fig. 66–1). Major defensive and aggressive factors are discussed below.

Defensive Factors

Defensive factors serve the physiologic role of protecting the stomach and duodenum from self-digestion. Primary defensive factors are mucus, bicarbonate, and submucosal blood flow. When these defenses are intact, generation of ulcers is unlikely. Conversely, when these defenses are compromised, aggressive factors are able to cause in-

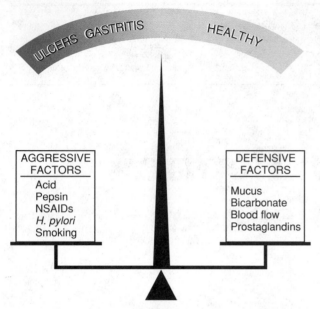

Figure 66–1. The relationship of mucosal defenses and aggressive factors to health and peptic ulcer disease. When aggressive factors outweigh mucosal defenses, gastritis and peptic ulcers result. (NSAIDs = nonsteroidal anti-inflammatory drugs)

jury. Two important factors that can weaken defenses are <u>nonsteroidal anti-inflammatory drugs</u> and gastrointestinal infection with *Helicobacter pylori*.

Mucus. Mucus is secreted continuously by cells of the gastrointestinal mucosa, forming a barrier that protects underlying cells from attack by acid and pepsin.

Bicarbonate. Bicarbonate is secreted by epithelial cells of the stomach and duodenum. Most of this bicarbonate remains trapped in the mucus layer, where it serves to neutralize any hydrogen ions that penetrate the mucus. Bicarbonate produced by the pancreas is secreted into the lumen of the duodenum, where it neutralizes acid delivered from the stomach.

Blood Flow. Blood flow to the cells of the gastrointestinal mucosa is essential for maintaining mucosal integrity. If submucosal blood flow is reduced, the resultant local ischemia can lead to cell injury, thereby increasing vulnerability to attack by acid and pepsin.

Prostaglandins. Prostaglandins play an important role in maintaining defenses. These compounds stimulate secretion of mucus and bicarbonate, and they promote vasodilation, which helps maintain submucosal blood flow. Prostaglandins provide additional protection by suppressing secretion of gastric acid.

Aggressive Factors

Gastric Acid. Gastric acid is an absolute requirement for peptic ulcer formation: in the absence of acid no ulcer will form. Acid causes ulcers by (1) injuring cells of the gastrointestinal mucosa, and (2) activating pepsin, a proteolytic enzyme. In most cases, acid hypersecretion, by itself, is insufficient to generate ulcers. In fact, in most patients with *gastric* ulcers, acid secretion is *normal or reduced*, and, among patients with *duodenal ulcers*, only one third produce excessive amounts of acids. From these observations, we can conclude that in the majority of patients with peptic ulcers, factors in addition to acid must be involved.

Zollinger-Ellison syndrome is the primary disorder in which hypersecretion of acid alone appears to be the sole cause of ulcer formation. The underlying cause of this syndrome is a tumor that secretes gastrin, a hormone that stimulates gastric acid release. In response to high levels of gastrin, gastric acid is produced in huge quantities—quantities that are sufficient to overwhelm mucosal defenses. Zollinger-Ellison syndrome is a rare disorder that accounts for about 0.1% of duodenal ulcers.

Pepsin. Pepsin is a proteolytic enzyme present in gastric juice. Like gastric acid, pepsin can injure unprotected cells of the gastric and duodenal mucosa.

Helicobacter pylori. *H. pylori* is a gram-negative bacterium that can colonize the stomach and duodenum. By taking up residence between epithelial cells and the mucus barrier that protects them, this organism manages to escape destruction by acid and pepsin.

There is a strong association between *H. pylori* infection and peptic ulcers. *H. pylori* is present in 95% of patients with duodenal ulcers and 75% of patients with gastric ulcers. Furthermore, eradication of the bacterium promotes ulcer healing and minimizes recurrences. Although the mechanism by which *H. pylori* promotes ulcers has not been firmly established, likely possibilities are (1) enzymatic degradation of the protective mucus layer, (2) elaboration of a cytotoxin that injures mucosal cells, and (3) infiltration of neutrophils and other inflammatory cells in response to the organism's presence.

Nonsteroidal Anti-inflammatory Drugs (NSAIDs). NSAIDs are the underlying cause of 30% to 40% of gastric ulcers and 10% of duodenal ulcers. As discussed in Chapter 61, aspirin and other NSAIDs inhibit the biosynthesis of prostaglandins. By doing so, these drugs can decrease submucosal blood flow, suppress secretion of mucus and bicarbonate, and promote secretion of gastric acid. In addition, the NSAIDs can irritate the mucosa directly. NSAID-induced ulcers are most likely with long-term high-dose therapy.

Smoking Cigarettes. Smoking increases the risk of PUD, delays ulcer healing, and increases the risk of recurrence. Measurable ulcerogenic effects can be seen with as few as 10 cigarettes a day. The mechanism by which cigarettes promote ulcers has not been established. It is not known whether smoking cigars or pipes affects ulcer formation or healing.

NONDRUG THERAPY

Optimal antiulcer therapy requires implementation of nondrug measures in addition to drug therapy.

Diet. Despite commonly held beliefs, dietary factors play only a minor role in ulcer management. The traditional "ulcer diet," consisting of bland foods together with milk or cream, does not accelerate healing. Furthermore, there is no convincing evidence that caffeine-containing beverages (coffee, tea, colas) promote ulcer formation or interfere with recovery. Alcohol can be harmful, especially when consumed in large amounts on an empty stomach. Changes in *eating patterns* may be beneficial: consumption of five or six small meals a day, rather than three larger ones, can reduce fluctuations in intragastric pH, and may thereby facilitate healing.

Other Nondrug Measures. Smoking cigarettes is associated with an increased incidence of ulcers and retards recovery. Accordingly, cigarettes should be avoided. Because of their ulcerogenic actions, aspirin and other NSAIDs should be avoided. Stress and anxiety may promote ulcer formation and may delay recovery. Conversely, control of emotional factors may encourage healing.

OVERVIEW OF DRUG THERAPY

This section addresses basic considerations in drug therapy of PUD. Individual antiulcer drugs and selection among them are discussed later in the chapter.

Therapeutic Goal. The goal of drug therapy is to (1) alleviate symptoms, (2) promote healing, (3) prevent complications (hemorrhage, perforation, obstruction), and (4) prevent recurrences. With the possible exception of antibiotics (used to eradicate *H. pylori*), antiulcer drugs do not alter the disease process. Rather, drugs simply create conditions conducive to healing. Since drugs do not usually cure ulcers, the relapse rate is very high.

Overview of the Antiulcer Drugs. As shown in Table 66–1, the antiulcer drugs fall into five major classes: (1) antisecretory agents, (2) mucosal protectants, (3) antisecretory agents that enhance mucosal defenses, (4) antacids, and (5) antibiotics. From this classification, we can see that drugs act in three basic ways to promote ulcer healing. First, they can *reduce gastric acidity*; antisecretory agents, antacids, and misoprostol do this. Second, drugs can *enhance mucosal defenses*; sucralfate, bismuth, and misoprostol do this. Third, drugs can *eradicate H. pylori*; antibiotics and bismuth do this.

Duration of Treatment. Duration of therapy depends largely on ulcer location. As a rule, *gastric ulcers* require 8 to 12 weeks of treatment. *Duodenal ulcers* heal more quickly, usually within 4 to 6 weeks. Duration of treatment is similar for all major antiulcer drugs.

Evaluation. Treatment can be evaluated by monitoring for relief of pain and by performing radiologic or endoscopic examination of the ulcer site. Unfortunately, assessment is seldom straightforward. This is because cessation of pain and disappearance of the ulcer rarely coincide: in most cases, pain subsides prior to completion of healing. However, the converse may also be true: pain may persist even though endoscopic or radiologic examination reveals complete healing.

Maintenance Therapy to Prevent Relapse. Following withdrawal of most antiulcer medications, the incidence of recurrence is 50% to 90% within 12 months. When *H. pylori* has been eradicated with antibiotics, the 12-month recurrence rate is much lower (about 20%). The risk of recurrence can be minimized with maintenance therapy.

A Note About the Effects of Drugs on Pepsin. Pepsin is a proteolytic enzyme that can contribute to ulcer formation. This enzyme promotes ulcers by breaking down protein in the gut wall.

Like most enzymes, pepsin is sensitive to alterations in pH. As pH rises from 1.3 (the usual pH of the stomach) to 2, peptic activity increases by a factor of 4. As pH goes even higher, peptic activity begins to decline. At a pH of 5, peptic activity drops below baseline rates. When pH exceeds 6 to 7, pepsin undergoes irreversible inactivation.

Because the activity of pepsin is pH-dependent, drugs that elevate gastric pH (e.g., antacids, histamine$_2$ antagonists) can cause peptic activity to increase, thereby enhancing pepsin's destructive effects. For example, treatment that produces a 99% reduction in gastric acidity will cause pH to rise from a base level of 1.3 up to 3.3. At pH 3.3, peptic activity will be significantly increased. To avoid activation of pepsin, drugs that reduce acidity should be administered in doses sufficient to raise gastric pH above 5.

Table 66–1. Classification of Antiulcer Drugs

Class	Drugs	Mechanism of Action
Antisecretory Agents		
H$_2$-Receptor Antagonists	Cimetidine [Tagamet] Famotidine [Pepcid] Nizatidine [Axid] Ranitidine [Zantac]	Suppression of acid secretion by blocking H$_2$ receptors on parietal cells
Proton Pump Inhibitors	Omeprazole [Prilosec]	Suppression of acid secretion by inhibiting H$^+$, K$^+$-ATPase, the enzyme that makes gastric acid
Muscarinic Antagonists	Pirenzepine [Gastrozepine]	Suppression of acid secretion by blocking muscarinic-cholinergic receptors (on parietal cells?)
Mucosal Protectants	Sucralfate [Carafate]	Forms a barrier over the ulcer crater that protects against acid and pepsin
	Bismuth [Pepto-Bismol]	Forms a barrier over the ulcer crater that protects against acid and pepsin; reduces colonization with *H. pylori*
Antisecretory Agents that Enhance Mucosal Defenses	Misoprostol [Cytotec]	Protects against NSAID-induced ulcers by stimulating secretion of mucus and bicarbonate, maintaining submucosal blood flow, and suppressing secretion of gastric acid
Antacids	Aluminum hydroxide Magnesium hydroxide Calcium carbonate	Conversion of gastric acid to neutral salts
Antibiotics	Metronidazole [Flagyl] Tetracycline Amoxicillin	Eradication of *H. pylori* infection

HISTAMINE$_2$-RECEPTOR ANTAGONISTS

The histamine$_2$-receptor antagonists (H$_2$RAs) are drugs of first choice for treating gastric and duodenal ulcers. These agents promote ulcer healing by suppressing secretion of gastric acid. Four H$_2$RAs are available: cimetidine, ranitidine, famotidine, and nizatidine. All four are equally effective, and with all four the incidence of serious side effects is low.

CIMETIDINE

Cimetidine [Tagamet] was the first H$_2$RA available and will serve as our prototype for the family. At one time, cimetidine was the most frequently prescribed drug in the United States.

Mechanism of Action

As discussed in Chapter 60, histamine acts through two types of receptors, labeled H$_1$ and H$_2$.

Activation of H$_1$ receptors produces symptoms of allergy. In contrast, activation of H$_2$ receptors, which are located on parietal cells of the stomach (Fig. 66–2), promotes secretion of gastric acid. By blocking H$_2$ receptors, cimetidine reduces both the volume of gastric juice as well as its H$^+$ concentration. Cimetidine suppresses basal acid secretion and reduces stimulation of acid secretion by gastrin and acetylcholine. Since cimetidine produces selective blockade of H$_2$ receptors, the drug does not reduce symptoms of allergy.

Pharmacokinetics

Cimetidine is administered orally, intramuscularly, and intravenously. Comparable blood levels are achieved with all three routes. When the drug is taken orally, food decreases the *rate* of absorption but not the *extent*. Hence, if cimetidine is taken with meals, absorption will be slowed and beneficial effects prolonged. Cimetidine crosses the blood-brain barrier—albeit with difficulty—and CNS side effects can occur. Although some hepatic metabolism takes place, most of each dose is elim-

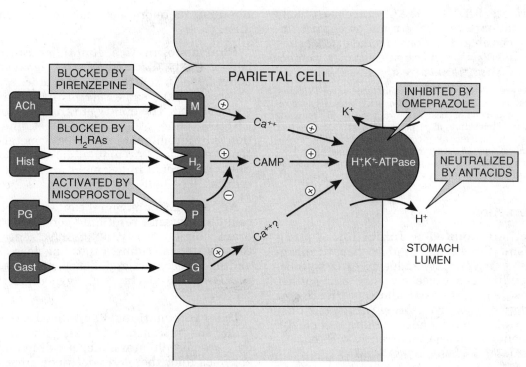

Figure 66–2. A model of the regulation of gastric acid secretion showing the actions of antisecretory drugs and antacids. Production of gastric acid is stimulated by three endogenous compounds: (1) acetylcholine (ACh) acting at muscarinic (M) receptors; (2) histamine (hist) acting at histamine$_2$ (H$_2$) receptors; and (3) gastrin (gast) acting at gastrin (G) receptors. As indicated, all three compounds act through intracellular messengers—either calcium (Ca^{++}) or cyclic AMP (cAMP)—to increase the activity of H$^+$, K$^+$-ATPase, the enzyme that actually produces gastric acid. Prostaglandins (PG) decrease acid production, perhaps by suppressing production of intracellular cAMP. The actions of histamine$_2$-receptor antagonists (H$_2$RAs), other antisecretory drugs, and antacids are indicated.

inated intact in the urine. The half-life of cimetidine is relatively short (about 2 hours), but increases in patients with renal impairment. Dosage should be reduced in these patients.

Therapeutic Uses

Gastric and Duodenal Ulcers. Cimetidine promotes healing of gastric and duodenal ulcers. To heal duodenal ulcers, 4 to 6 weeks of therapy are generally required. To heal gastric ulcers, 8 to 12 weeks may be needed. Long-term therapy with low doses may be given as prophylaxis against recurrence of gastric and duodenal ulcers.

Zollinger-Ellison Syndrome. This syndrome is characterized by hypersecretion of gastric acid and development of peptic ulcers. The underlying cause is secretion of gastrin from a gastrin-producing tumor. Cimetidine can promote healing of ulcers in patients with Zollinger-Ellison syndrome, but only if high doses are employed. These high doses may cause significant adverse effects.

Reflux Esophagitis. Reflux esophagitis is an inflammatory condition caused by reflux of gastric contents back into the esophagus. Cimetidine is a drug of choice for relieving symptoms. However, cimetidine does little to hasten healing.

Stress Ulcers. Ulcers frequently develop in critically ill patients and patients recovering from surgery. The incidence of these ulcers can be reduced by prophylactic use of cimetidine. The dosage should be adjusted to keep gastric pH above 5.

Aspiration Pneumonitis. Anesthesia suppresses the glottal reflex, permitting aspiration of gastric acid. When acid is aspirated, pulmonary injury develops in seconds and can be fatal. Surgical patients at high risk for this disorder include obese patients and women undergoing obstetric procedures. Cimetidine is a drug of choice for preventing aspiration pneumonitis. Gastric acidity can be reduced substantially by administering the drug 60 to 90 minutes prior to anesthesia.

Adverse Effects

The incidence of side effects with cimetidine is low. Furthermore, the effects that do occur are usually benign.

Antiandrogenic Effects. Cimetidine binds to androgen receptors, producing receptor blockade. This action may result in *gynecomastia, reduced libido,* and *impotence.* These effects reverse following termination of treatment.

CNS Effects. Effects on the CNS are most likely in elderly patients who have renal or hepatic impairment. Possible reactions include *confusion*, *hallucinations*, *CNS depression* (lethargy, somnolence), and *CNS excitation* (restlessness, seizures).

Other Adverse Effects. When administered as an IV bolus, cimetidine can cause hypotension and dysrhythmias. These reactions are rare and do not occur with oral therapy. By reducing gastric acidity, cimetidine may permit growth of *Candida* within the stomach. Hematologic effects (neutropenia, leukopenia, thrombocytopenia) occur rarely. Minor side effects include headache, dizziness, myalgia, nausea, diarrhea, constipation, rash, and pruritus.

Drug Interactions

Interactions Related to Inhibition of Drug Metabolism. Cimetidine inhibits hepatic drug-metabolizing enzymes. By reducing drug metabolism, cimetidine can cause levels of many other drugs to rise. Agents of particular concern are *oral anticoagulants, phenytoin, theophylline,* and *lidocaine,* all of which have a narrow margin of safety. If these agents are used concurrently with cimetidine, their dosages should be reduced.

Antacids. Antacids can decrease the absorption of cimetidine. Accordingly, cimetidine and antacids should be administered at least 1 hour apart from each other.

Preparations, Dosage, and Administration

Oral. Cimetidine [Tagamet] is available in tablets (200, 300, 400, and 800 mg) and solution (300 mg/5 ml) for oral administration. For treatment of duodenal and gastric ulcers, the drug may be given once daily (800 mg at bedtime), twice daily (400 mg each dose), or 4 times a day (300 mg with meals and at bedtime). In patients with renal impairment, the dosage should be lowered to 300 mg every 12 hours. For prophylaxis against recurrence of ulcers, a single 400-mg dose at bedtime may be employed. Patients with Zollinger-Ellison syndrome require high doses, but not more than 2.4 gm/day.

Parenteral. Parenteral cimetidine is reserved for patients with hypersecretory conditions (e.g., Zollinger-Ellison syndrome) and ulcers that have failed to respond to oral therapy. The usual dosage (IM or IV) is 300 mg every 6 to 8 hours. Intramuscular injections are made with a concentrated solution (300 mg/2 ml). For IV administration, two concentrations may be employed: (1) the dose may be diluted in a total volume of 20 ml and injected slowly (over 2 minutes), or (2) it may be diluted in 100 ml and infused over 15 minutes.

RANITIDINE

Ranitidine [Zantac] shares many of the properties of cimetidine. However, although similar to cimetidine, ranitidine does differ in three important respects: ranitidine is more potent than cimetidine, produces fewer adverse effects, and causes fewer drug interactions.

Actions. Like cimetidine, ranitidine suppresses secretion of gastric acid by blocking H_2 receptors on parietal cells. The drug does not block H_1 receptors and, therefore, does not reduce symptoms of allergy.

Pharmacokinetics. Ranitidine can be administered orally, IM, and IV. Oral bioavailability is about 50%. In contrast to cimetidine, ranitidine is absorbed at the same rate in the presence or absence of food. The ability of ranitidine to enter the CNS is even less than that of cimetidine. Elimination is by a combination of hepatic metabolism and renal excretion. Accumulation will occur in patients with renal impairment unless the dosage is reduced. The half-life of ranitidine is 2 to 3 hours.

Adverse Effects. Significant side effects are uncommon. Because ranitidine penetrates the blood-brain barrier poorly, CNS effects are rare. In contrast to cimetidine, ranitidine does *not* bind to androgen receptors and, hence, does *not* cause antiandrogenic effects (e.g., gynecomastia, impotence).

Drug Interactions. Ranitidine has few drug interactions. In contrast to cimetidine, ranitidine is only a weak inhibitor of hepatic drug-metabolizing enzymes and, therefore, does not greatly depress metabolism of other drugs. Antacids have only a small effect on ranitidine absorption.

Therapeutic Uses. Ranitidine has the same indications as cimetidine. The drug is approved for (1) short-term treatment of gastric and duodenal ulcers, (2) prophylaxis of recurrent duodenal ulcers, (3) treatment of Zollinger-Ellison syndrome and other hypersecretory states, and (4) treatment of gastroesophageal reflux. Like cimetidine, ranitidine has been used on an investigational basis to relieve symptoms of reflux esophagitis and to prevent aspiration pneumonitis and stress ulcers. Because it produces fewer side effects than cimetidine, and because of its greater potency, ranitidine is preferred to cimetidine for treating hypersecretory states (e.g., Zollinger-Ellison syndrome).

Preparations, Dosage, and Administration. Ranitidine [Zantac] is available in tablets (150 and 300 mg), in a syrup (15 mg/ml), and as an injection (0.5 and 25 mg/ml).

Oral. The usual adult dosage for therapy of gastric and duodenal ulcers is 150 mg twice a day. (Note that this dosage is considerably lower than that for cimetidine.) Alternatively, a 300-mg dose can be given once daily at bedtime. For patients with Zollinger-Ellison syndrome, higher doses may be required. The dosage for preventing recurrence of duodenal ulcers is 150 mg once daily at bedtime. Since its absorption is not affected by food, ranitidine can be administered without regard to meals.

Parenteral. The usual parenteral dosage (IM or IV) is 50 mg every 6 to 8 hours. Intramuscular doses can be injected without dilution. For IV injection, the preparation should be diluted to a volume of 20 ml and administered slowly (over 5 or more minutes). For IV infusion, the drug should be diluted in 100 ml and administered over 15 to 20 minutes.

FAMOTIDINE AND NIZATIDINE

Contrasts with Ranitidine. Famotidine [Pepcid] and nizatidine [Axid] are very similar to ranitidine. Both agents are approved for (1) treatment of duodenal ulcers, (2) treatment of gastroesophageal reflux, and (3) prevention of duodenal ulcer recurrence. In addition, famotidine is approved for treatment of gastric ulcers and hypersecretory states (e.g., Zollinger-Ellison syndrome). Like ranitidine, famotidine and nizatidine do not bind to androgen receptors and, hence, do not have antiandrogenic effects. These two drugs do not inhibit hepatic drug-metabolizing enzymes and, hence, do not suppress the metabolism of other drugs.

Dosage. For *treatment of duodenal and gastric ulcers*, the dosage for *famotidine* is 20 mg twice daily or 40 mg once daily at bedtime; the dosage for *nizatidine* is 150 mg twice daily or 300 mg once daily at bedtime. For *preventing the recurrence of duodenal ulcers*, the dosage for *famotidine* is 20 mg once daily at bedtime and the dosage for *nizatidine* is 150 mg once daily at bedtime.

OTHER ANTIULCER DRUGS

SUCRALFATE

Sucralfate [Carafate] is an effective antiulcer medication notable for its minimal side effects and lack of significant drug interactions. The drug promotes ulcer healing by creating a protective barrier against acid and pepsin. Sucralfate has no acid-neutralizing capacity and does not decrease acid secretion.

Mechanism of Antiulcer Action. Sucralfate is a complex substance composed of sulfated sucrose and aluminum hydroxide. Under mildly acidic conditions (pH less than 4), sucralfate undergoes polymerization and cross-linking reactions. The resultant product is a viscid and very sticky gel that adheres to the ulcer crater, creating a barrier to back diffusion of hydrogen ions, pepsin, and bile salts. Attachment to the ulcer appears to last for up to 6 hours.

Pharmacokinetics. Sucralfate is administered orally, and systemic absorption is minimal (3% to 5%). About 90% of each dose is eliminated in the feces.

Therapeutic Uses. Sucralfate is approved for acute therapy and maintenance therapy of duodenal ulcers. Rates of healing are comparable to those achieved with cimetidine. Controlled trials indicate that sucralfate can also promote healing of gastric ulcers.

Adverse Effects. Sucralfate has no known serious adverse effects. The most significant side effect is *constipation,* and this occurs in only 2% of patients. Since sucralfate is not absorbed, systemic effects are absent.

Drug Interactions. Interactions with other drugs are minimal. By raising gastric pH above 4, *antacids* may interfere with sucralfate's effects. This interaction can be minimized by administering these drugs at least 30 minutes apart from each other.

Sucralfate may impede the absorption of some drugs, including phenytoin, theophylline, digoxin, warfarin, and the fluoroquinolone antibiotics (e.g., ciprofloxacin, norfloxacin). These interactions can be minimized by administering sucralfate at least 2 hours apart from these other drugs.

Preparations, Dosage, and Administration. Sucralfate [Carafate] is dispensed in 1-gm tablets for oral administration. The drug should be taken on an empty stomach. The recommended adult dosage is 1 gm four times a day, administered 1 hour before meals and at bedtime. However, a dosing schedule of 2 gm twice a day appears to be equally effective. Treatment should continue for 4 to 8 weeks.

Sucralfate tablets are large and can be difficult to swallow, especially by the elderly. Although there is no liquid formulation commercially available, one can be prepared by dispersing the tablets in 20 to 30 ml of water.

OMEPRAZOLE

Omeprazole [Prilosec] is the prototype of a new class of antiulcer medications: the *proton pump inhibitors.* The drug is the most effective agent available for suppressing secretion of gastric acid. Side effects from short-term therapy are minimal. With long-term therapy there is some concern about possible carcinogenesis.

Mechanism of Action. Omeprazole is a prodrug that undergoes conversion to its active form within parietal cells of the stomach. The active form causes *irreversible* inhibition of H^+,K^+-ATPase—the enzyme that generates gastric acid (see Fig. 66–2). Because it blocks the final common pathway of gastric acid production, omeprazole can inhibit basal and stimulated acid release. A single 30-mg oral dose produces a 97% reduction in acid secretion within 2 hours. Because inhibition of the ATPase is irreversible, effects will persist until new enzyme can be synthesized. Partial recovery of acid production occurs 3 to 5 days after termination of treatment. Full recovery may take several weeks.

Pharmacokinetics. Administration is oral. Since the drug is acid labile, it is dispensed in capsules that contain protective enteric-coated granules; the capsule dissolves in the stomach, but the granules do not dissolve until they reach the relatively alkaline environment of the duodenum, thereby protecting the drug from destruction by stomach acid. About 50% of each dose reaches the systemic circulation. The drug undergoes hepatic metabolism followed by renal excretion. The plasma half-life of omeprazole is short (about 1 hour). However, since omeprazole acts by irreversible enzyme inhibition, its effects persist long after the drug has been cleared from the blood.

Therapeutic Use. Omeprazole is approved for short-term therapy of duodenal ulcers and gastroesophageal reflux, and for long-term therapy of hypersecretory conditions (e.g., Zollinger-Ellison syndrome). The drug has been used on an investigational basis for short-term therapy of gastric ulcers. Except for therapy of hypersecretory states, treatment should be limited to 4 to 8 weeks.

In clinical trials, duodenal ulcers healed faster with omeprazole (40 mg/day) than with conventional doses of H₂RAs. However, by the end of 8 weeks, the success rate was equivalent with both treatments. Patients who fail to respond to H₂RAs often can benefit from omeprazole. The 6-month relapse rate following discontinuation of omeprazole is equivalent to that seen with H₂RAs.

Adverse Effects. Effects seen with *short-term* therapy are generally inconsequential. Like the H₂RAs, omeprazole can cause headache, diarrhea, nausea, and vomiting. The incidence of these effects is less than 1%.

With *long-term* therapy, there is concern about the risk of *cancer*. Gastric carcinoid tumors have developed in rats given omeprazole daily for 2 years. These tumors are related to hypersecretion of *gastrin*, which occurs in response to omeprazole-induced suppression of gastric acidity. Gastrin has a trophic effect on cells of the gastric epithelium; hyperplasia of these cells may precede development of gastric carcinoid tumors. To date, no gastric tumors have been attributed to omeprazole therapy. However, experience with long-term use of the drug is limited. Accordingly, until more is understood about the consequences of prolonged therapy, use of omeprazole should be limited to 4 to 8 weeks by most patients.

Preparations, Dosage, and Administration. Omeprazole [Prilosec] is dispensed in 20-mg sustained-release capsules for oral administration. For treatment of active *duodenal ulcer* and *gastroesophageal reflux*, the usual dosage is 20 mg once a day for 4 to 8 weeks. For treatment of Zollinger-Ellison syndrome and other hypersecretory states, doses up to 120 mg three times a day may be needed.

MISOPROSTOL

Therapeutic Use. Misoprostol [Cytotec] is an analogue of prostaglandin E₁. In the United States, the drug is approved only for *preventing gastric ulcers caused by long-term therapy with nonsteroidal anti-inflammatory drugs (NSAIDs)*. In other countries, misoprostol is also used to treat peptic ulcers unrelated to NSAIDs.

Mechanism of Action. In normal individuals, prostaglandins help protect the stomach by (1) suppressing secretion of gastric acid, (2) promoting secretion of bicarbonate and cytoprotective mucus, and (3) maintaining submucosal blood flow (by promoting vasodilation). As discussed in Chapter 61, aspirin and other NSAIDs cause gastric ulcers in part by inhibiting prostaglandin biosynthesis. Misoprostol prevents NSAID-induced ulcers by serving as a replacement for endogenous prostaglandins.

Adverse Effects. The most common reactions are dose-related *diarrhea* (13% to 40%) and *abdominal pain* (7% to 20%). Some women experience *spotting* and *dysmenorrhea*.

Misoprostol is contraindicated for use during pregnancy. The drug is classified in FDA Pregnancy Category X: the risk of use by pregnant women clearly outweighs any possible benefits. Prostaglandins stimulate uterine contractions. Administration during pregnancy has caused partial or complete expulsion of the developing fetus. If women of child-bearing age are to use misoprostol, they must (1) be able to comply with birth-control measures, (2) be given oral and written warnings about the dangers of misoprostol, (3) have a negative *serum* pregnancy test result within 2 weeks prior to beginning therapy, and (4) begin therapy only on the second or third day of the next normal menstrual cycle.

Preparations, Dosage, and Administration. Misoprostol [Cytotec] is dispensed in 100- and 200-μg tablets for oral administration. The usual dosage is 200 μg four times a day administered with meals and at bedtime. Patients who cannot tolerate this dosage may try 100 μg four times a day.

ANTACIDS

Antacids are alkaline compounds that neutralize stomach acid. The principal indications for these drugs are peptic ulcer disease and reflux esophagitis.

Beneficial Actions

Antacids react with gastric acid to produce neutral salts or salts of low acidity. By neutralizing acid, these drugs decrease destruction of the gut wall. In addition, if acid neutralization is sufficient to elevate gastric pH above 5, activity of pepsin will decline. In addition to neutralizing acid and inactivating pepsin, antacids may be able to enhance mucosal protection by stimulating production of prostaglandins. Antacids do not coat the ulcer crater to protect it from acid and pepsin. With the exception of sodium bicarbonate, antacids are poorly absorbed and, therefore, do not alter systemic pH.

Therapeutic Uses

Peptic Ulcer Disease. The primary indication for antacids is peptic ulcer disease. Rates of healing are equivalent to those achieved with H₂RAs. At one time, antacids were the mainstay of antiulcer therapy. However, these drugs have been largely replaced by newer medications (H₂RAs, sucralfate, omeprazole) that are equally effective, more convenient to administer, and cause fewer side effects.

Other Uses. Antacids are administered prior to anesthesia to prevent *aspiration pneumonitis*. In addition, these drugs can provide prophylaxis against *stress-induced ulcers*. For patients with *reflux esophagitis*, antacids can produce symptomatic relief, but they do not accelerate healing. Although these drugs are used widely by the general public to relieve functional symptoms (dyspepsia, heartburn, "acid indigestion"), there are no controlled studies that demonstrate efficacy in these conditions.

Potency, Dosage, and Formulations

Potency. Antacid potency is expressed in terms of *acid-neutralizing capacity* (ANC). ANC is defined as the number of mEq of hydrochloric acid that can be neutralized by a given weight or volume of antacid. Individual antacids differ widely in ANC. The ANC of commonly used proprietary preparations is listed in Table 66–2.

Table 66–2. Composition and Acid-Neutralizing Capacity of Commonly Used Over-the-Counter Antacid Suspensions

Product	Acid Neutralizing Capacity (mEq/5 ml)	Active Ingredients (mg/5 ml)				Sodium (mg/5 ml)
		$Al(OH)_3$	$Mg(OH)_2$	Simeth-icone	Other	
AlternaGEL	16	600				<2.5
Aludrox	12	307	103			2.3
Amphojel	10	320				2.3
Basaljel	12				$Al(OH)CO_3$*	2.9
Camalox	18	225	200		$CaCO_3$ 250	1.2
DiGel	—	200	200	20		<5
Gelusil	12	200	200	25		0.7
Gelusil-II	24	400	400	30		1.3
Kudrox DS†	25	565	180			<15
Maalox	15	225	200			1.4
Maalox TC†	27	600	300			0.8
Milk of magnesia	14		390			0.1
Mylanta-II	25	400	400	40		1.1
Riopan	15				Magaldrate 540	<0.1
Riopan XS†	30				Malaldrate 1080	0.3
Riopan Plus	15			20	Magaldrate 540	<0.1
Riopan Plus 2	30			30	Malaldrate 1080	0.3
WinGel	10	180	160			—

*Equivalent to 400 mg $Al(OH)_3$.
†XS = extra strength; TC = therapeutic concentrate; DS = double strength

Dosage. The objective of peptic ulcer therapy is to promote healing, and not simply to relieve pain. Consequently, antacids should be taken on a regular schedule, not just in response to discomfort. In the usual dosing schedule, antacids are administered 7 times a day: 1 and 3 hours after each meal and at bedtime.

Dosage recommendations should be based on ANC and not on weight or volume of antacid. The ANC of a single dose usually ranges from 20 to 80 mEq. Single doses for *gastric ulcers* are relatively low (20 to 40 mEq), whereas single doses for *duodenal ulcers* are higher (40 to 80 mEq). Frequent administration of even larger doses (120 mEq) may be required if ulceration is especially severe.

To provide maximum benefits, treatment should elevate gastric pH above 5. At this pH there is inhibition of pepsin's activity in addition to nearly complete (greater than 99.9%) neutralization of acid.

Antacids are inconvenient and unpleasant to ingest, making compliance difficult to achieve—especially in the absence of pain. Patients should be encouraged to take their medication as prescribed, even after symptoms have subsided.

Formulations. Antacids are available in solid (tablet) and liquid formulations. Antacid tablets should be chewed thoroughly and followed with a glass of water or milk. Liquid preparations should be shaken before dispensing. As a rule, liquids (suspensions) are more effective than tablets.

Adverse Effects

Constipation and Diarrhea. Most antacids affect the bowel. Some (e.g., aluminum hydroxide) promote constipation, whereas others (e.g., magnesium hydroxide) promote diarrhea. Effects on the bowel can be minimized by combining an antacid that promotes constipation with one that promotes diarrhea. Patients should be taught to adjust the dosage of one agent or the other to normalize bowel function.

Sodium Loading. Some antacid preparations contain substantial amounts of sodium (see Table 66–2). Since sodium excess can exacerbate hypertension and heart failure, patients with these disorders should avoid preparations that have a high sodium content.

Drug Interactions

By raising gastric pH *antacids can influence the dissolution and absorption of many other drugs*, including cimetidine and ranitidine. These interactions can be minimized by allowing 1 hour between antacid administration and administration of other drugs.

Antacids can interfere with the actions of *sucralfate*, a locally

Table 66–3. Classification of Antacids

Aluminum Compounds
  Aluminum hydroxide
  Aluminum carbonate
  Aluminum phosphate
  Dihydroxyaluminum sodium carbonate

Magnesium Compounds
  Magnesium hydroxide (milk of magnesia)
  Magnesium oxide

Calcium Compounds
  Calcium carbonate

Sodium Compounds
  Sodium bicarbonate

Other
  Magaldrate (a complex of magnesium and aluminum compounds)

acting antiulcer medication. To minimize this interaction, these drugs should be administered 1 hour apart from each other.

If absorbed in substantial amounts, antacids can alkalinize the urine. This elevation of urinary pH can accelerate excretion of acidic drugs and delay excretion of basic drugs.

Antacid Families

There are four major groups of antacids: (1) *aluminum* compounds, (2) *magnesium* compounds, (3) *calcium* compounds, and (4) *sodium* compounds. Individual agents that belong to these groups are listed in Table 66–3. Representative members of these groups are discussed below.

Representative Antacids

Antacids differ from one another with respect to ANC, onset and duration of action, effects on the bowel, systemic effects, and special applications. In this section, we will discuss the two most commonly used antacids—magnesium hydroxide and aluminum hydroxide—and two less commonly used drugs—calcium carbonate and sodium bicarbonate. The distinguishing properties of these agents are summarized in Table 66–4.

Magnesium Hydroxide. This antacid is rapid acting, has high ANC, and produces effects of long duration. These properties make magnesium hydroxide an antacid of choice. The liquid formulation of magnesium hydroxide is often referred to as *milk of magnesia*.

The most prominent adverse effect is *diarrhea*, which results from retention of water within the intestinal lumen. To compensate for this effect, magnesium hydroxide is usually administered in combination with aluminum hydroxide, an antacid that promotes constipation. However, if the dose of magnesium hydroxide is sufficiently high, no amount of aluminum hydroxide will prevent diarrhea. Since stimulation of the bowel can be hazardous for patients with intestinal obstruction or appendicitis, magnesium hydroxide should be avoided in patients with undiagnosed abdominal pain. Because of its effect on the bowel, magnesium hydroxide is frequently employed as a laxative (see Chapter 67). In patients with renal impairment, magnesium may accumulate to high levels, causing signs of toxicity (e.g., CNS depression).

Aluminum Hydroxide. This drug has relatively low ANC, is slow acting, but produces effects of long duration. Although rarely used alone, this preparation is widely used in combination with magnesium hydroxide (see Table 66–2). Aluminum hydroxide preparations contain significant amounts of sodium and appropriate caution should be exercised. The most common adverse effect is *constipation*.

Aluminum hydroxide adsorbs a variety of compounds. Binding of certain drugs (e.g., tetracyclines, warfarin, digoxin) may reduce their therapeutic effects. Aluminum hydroxide has a high affinity for phosphate. By binding phosphate, the drug can reduce phosphate absorption, and can thereby cause *hypophosphatemia*. Aluminum hydroxide can also bind to pepsin, which may facilitate ulcer healing.

Table 66–4. Representative Antacids: Summary of Distinguishing Properties

Antacid	Effect on the Bowel		Raises Systemic pH	Comments
	Constipation	*Diarrhea*		
Aluminum hydroxide	+	−	−	Can cause hypophosphatemia; can treat hyperphosphatemia.
Magnesium hydroxide	−	+	−	Can cause Mg toxicity (CNS depression) in patients with renal impairment.
Calcium carbonate	+	−	−	May cause acid rebound or milk-alkali syndrome; releases CO_2.
Sodium bicarbonate	−	−	+	Not used routinely to treat ulcers; used to treat acidosis and to alkalinize urine; high risk of sodium loading; releases CO_2.

Calcium Carbonate. Calcium carbonate, like magnesium hydroxide, is rapid acting, has high ANC, and produces effects of long duration. Because of these properties, calcium carbonate was once considered the ideal antacid. However, because of concerns about *acid rebound* (stimulation of acid secretion), use of calcium carbonate has declined. The principal adverse effect is *constipation*. This can be overcome by using the drug in combination with a magnesium-containing antacid (e.g., magnesium hydroxide). Calcium carbonate releases carbon dioxide in the stomach, and can thereby cause eructation (belching) and flatulence. Rarely, systemic absorption is sufficient to produce the *milk-alkali syndrome*, a condition characterized by hypercalcemia, metabolic alkalosis, soft-tissue calcification, and impaired renal function. The palatability of calcium carbonate is low and this can detract from compliance.

Sodium Bicarbonate. Although capable of neutralizing gastric acid, sodium bicarbonate is unfit for treating ulcers. This agent has a rapid onset of action but its effects are short-lasting. Like calcium carbonate, sodium bicarbonate liberates carbon dioxide, thereby increasing intra-abdominal pressure and promoting eructation and flatulence. Absorption of sodium can exacerbate hypertension and heart failure. In patients with renal impairment, sodium bicarbonate can cause systemic alkalosis. (Other antacids rarely alter systemic pH.) Because of its brief duration, high sodium content, and capacity for causing alkalosis, sodium bicarbonate is inappropriate for treating PUD. The drug *is* useful, however, for (1) treating acidosis, and (2) elevating urinary pH to promote excretion of acidic drugs following overdosage.

ANTICHOLINERGICS

Atropine and other classic muscarinic antagonists have a very limited role in treating PUD. This is because the doses required to inhibit acid secretion are so high that they produce muscarinic blockade throughout the body. Hence, when used to treat ulcers, these drugs cause a high incidence of anticholinergic side effects, such as dry mouth, constipation, urinary retention, and disturbance of vision.

Pirenzepine. Pirenzepine [Gastrozepine] is a unique muscarinic antagonist available for treatment of PUD. In contrast to the classic anticholinergic drugs, pirenzepine produces "selective" blockade of the muscarinic receptors that regulate gastric acid secretion (see Fig. 66–2). As a result, the drug can inhibit acid secretion without causing pronounced anticholinergic side effects. For treatment of duodenal ulcers, pirenzepine (50 mg two to three times/day) is about equal to cimetidine (1 gm/day).

Following oral administration, about 20% to 30% of the drug is absorbed. Very little crosses the blood-brain barrier. About 80% is excreted unchanged in the urine. The drug has a half-life of approximately 10 hours.

The most common side effect is dry mouth. In addition, pirenzepine can cause constipation, visual disturbances, nausea, vomiting, and diarrhea.

BISMUTH

Bismuth salts can promote ulcer healing. Proposed mechanisms include (1) formation of a protective coating over the ulcer crater, (2) promoting secretion of bicarbonate and prostaglandins, and (3) suppressing growth of *H. pylori*. In patients with uncomplicated peptic ulcers, bismuth produces healing rates comparable to those seen with H₂RAs and sucralfate—and ulcer recurrence rates are lower with bismuth than with the other two drugs.

Bismuth is generally well tolerated. The drug can impart a harmless black coloration to the stool, and patients should be forewarned of this effect. Stool discoloration may confound interpretation of gastric bleeding. Long-term therapy may carry a risk of neurologic injury. Accordingly, treatment should be limited to 8 weeks.

In the United States, *bismuth subsalicylate* [Pepto-Bismol, others] is the only bismuth preparation available. A dosage of 525 mg (305 mg elemental bismuth) four times a day is proba-

bly effective. *Colloidal bismuth subcitrate* [De-Nol] is used widely in Europe.

ANTIBACTERIAL DRUGS

With increased appreciation of the role of *H. pylori* in ulcerogensis, there may be an expanding role for antibiotics in ulcer therapy. Clinical trials indicate that long-term ulcer recurrence rates are greatly reduced when *H. pylori* has been eradicated. (The 12-month recurrence rate with most antiulcer drugs is 50% to 90%, compared with only 20% when *H. pylori* has been eradicated.) With the most frequently used antibacterial regimen—*bismuth* plus *metronidazole* plus *tetracycline*—*H. pylori* is eliminated from 85% of patients for up to 1 year. Furthermore, healing rates for duodenal ulcer are comparable to those achieved with H₂RAs. Unfortunately, antibiotics present a greater risk than traditional antiulcer medications (e.g., H₂RAs, sucralfate). Diarrhea occurs in 30% of patients, sometimes because of suprainfection with *Clostridium difficile*. In addition, antibiotic therapy may promote emergence of drug-resistant bacteria. Because of questions about safety, efficacy, and bacterial drug resistance, antibiotics are not considered first-line therapy for peptic ulcer disease at this time. Until more clinical trials have been conducted, it is recommended that antimicrobial therapy be limited to patients with complicated duodenal ulcers and to patients with severe ulcers that have not responded to conventional therapy. Three of the regimens employed to eradicate *H. pylori* are presented in Table 66–5.

DRUG SELECTION

Initial Therapy of Uncomplicated Gastric and Duodenal Ulcers

In the United States, H₂RAs are the drugs employed most frequently for initial therapy of uncomplicated PUD. These agents are very safe, and, for many patients, are effective with once-a-day dosing. All of the H₂RAs are equally effective. Duodenal ulcers generally heal within 4 to 6 weeks; gastric ulcers generally heal within 8 to 12 weeks.

Sucralfate is just as effective as the H₂RAs but is less convenient. The drug must be taken four times a day and the tablets are large, making them difficult for some patients to swallow. Furthermore, administration of sucralfate must be separated from meals and from administration of other drugs. Because of these factors, sucralfate is less attractive than the H₂RAs.

Omeprazole is a second-line drug for treating uncomplicated PUD. Rates of healing are faster than with the H₂RAs, but omeprazole is more expensive. In addition, there is some concern about the long-term safety of this drug.

Table 66–5. Multidrug Regimens Used to Eradicate *H. pylori*	
Regimens	**Dosages**
Standard Therapy	
Bismuth subsalicylate	525 mg qid for 14 days
Metronidazole	250 mg qid for 14 days
Tetracycline	500 mg qid for 14 days
Modified Standard Therapy*	
Bismuth subsalicylate	525 mg qid for 14 days
Metronidazole	250 mg qid for 14 days
Amoxicillin	500 mg tid for 14 days
Second Line Therapy†	
Bismuth subsalicylate	525 mg qid for 14 days
Tetracycline	500 mg qid for 14 days
Erythromycin base	500 mg qid for 14 days
Omeprazole	400 mg qd for 14 days

*For patients who cannot tolerate tetracycline in the standard triple therapy.

†For patients infected with metronidazole-resistant strains of *H. pylori*.

Antacids are no longer employed as sole therapy of PUD. Although these drugs are as effective as the H_2RAs, they are much less convenient. Antacids are unpleasant to ingest and must be administered seven times a day. Currently, antacids are employed as adjuncts to other antiulcer medications to provide rapid relief of dyspepsia and pain. *Misoprostol, bismuth,* and *antibiotics* are not recommended for routine therapy of uncomplicated PUD.

Therapy of Ulcer Recurrences

In many patients, ulcers recur within 12 months after discontinuing treatment. If the patient is subject to early or frequent recurrences, continuous maintenance therapy is indicated. The drugs used most frequently are the H_2RAs, administered in low doses once daily at bedtime. If relapse occurs despite low-dose maintenance therapy, the dosage of the H_2RA should be increased; following healing, full-dose therapy should be continued.

Refractory Ulcers

A refractory ulcer is defined as one that persists despite 12 weeks of conventional therapy. Treatment options include (1) use of omeprazole (40 mg/day), (2) use of H_2RAs in supranormal dosages, and (3) multidrug therapy (e.g., omeprazole plus sucralfate). If these measures fail, antimicrobial therapy directed at *H. pylori* may be indicated; the regimen used most frequently is a combination of bismuth, metronidazole, and tetracycline.

NSAID-Induced Ulcers

Therapy with aspirin and other NSAIDs is associated with a relatively high incidence of PUD, especially in elderly patients. Only one drug—*misoprostol*—is approved for prophylaxis of NSAID-induced ulcers. This drug, which is taken along with the NSAID, should be reserved for patients considered at high risk of ulcer development. Since misoprostol stimulates uterine contractions, the drug must never be given to women who are pregnant. If an ulcer develops despite prophylaxis with misoprostol, the NSAID should be discontinued or given in reduced dosage. The ulcer can be treated with conventional doses of omeprazole or an H_2RA.

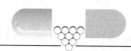

Summary of Major Nursing Implications

H₂-RECEPTOR ANTAGONISTS

Cimetidine	Famotidine
Ranitidine	Nizatidine

Preadministration Assessment

Therapeutic Goal

The objective in treating PUD is to relieve pain, promote healing, prevent ulcer recurrence, and prevent complications.

Baseline Data

Diagnosis requires radiographic or endoscopic visualization of the ulcer.

Identifying High-Risk Patients

Use H₂RAs with caution in patients with renal or hepatic dysfunction.

Implementation: Administration

Routes

Cimetidine and *ranitidine*: Oral, IM, and IV.
Famotidine: Oral and IV.
Nizatidine: Oral only.

Administration

Oral. Inform patients that these drugs may be taken without regard to meals.

Dosing may be done once daily at bedtime, twice daily, or 4 times a day. Make sure the patient knows which dosing schedule has been prescribed.

Intramuscular. *Cimetidine* and *ranitidine*: use concentrated solutions for IM injections.

Intravenous. *Cimetidine, famotidine,* and *ranitidine*: for IV *injection*, dilute in a small volume (e.g., 20 ml) and inject slowly (over 5 or more minutes). For IV *infusion*, dilute in a large volume (100 ml) and infuse over 15 to 20 minutes.

Implementation: Measures to Enhance Therapeutic Effects

Advise patients to avoid cigarettes and ulcerogenic over-the-counter drugs (aspirin and other NSAIDs). Caution patients to consume alcohol only in moderation and only in conjunction with food. Inform patients that five or six small meals per day may be preferable to three larger ones. Advise patients that reducing stress may accelerate ulcer healing.

Ongoing Evaluation and Interventions

Evaluating Therapeutic Effects

Monitor for relief of pain. Radiologic or endoscopic examination of the ulcer site may also be employed. Monitor gastric pH; treatment should increase pH to 5 or above. Educate patients about signs of GI bleeding (e.g., black, tarry stools, "coffee-ground" vomitus) and instruct them to notify the physician if these are observed.

Minimizing Adverse Effects

Antiandrogenic Effects. *Cimetidine* can cause gynecomastia, reduced libido, and impotence. These effects reverse after drug withdrawal.

CNS Effects. *Cimetidine* can cause confusion, hallucinations, lethargy, somnolence, restlessness, and seizures. These responses are most likely in elderly patients who have renal or hepatic impairment. Inform patients about possible CNS effects and instruct them to notify the physician if these occur. CNS effects are less likely with ranitidine, famotidine, and nizatidine.

Minimizing Adverse Interactions

Interactions Secondary to Inhibition of Drug Metabolism. *Cimetidine* inhibits hepatic drug-metabolizing enzymes and can thereby increase levels of other drugs. Drugs of particular concern are *oral anticoagulants*, *phenytoin*, *theophylline*, and *lidocaine*. Dosages of these drugs may need to be reduced.

Ranitidine inhibits drug metabolism, but to a lesser degree than cimetidine. *Famotidine* and *nizatidine* do not inhibit drug metabolism.

Antacids. Antacids can decrease absorption of *cimetidine* and *ranitidine*. At least 1 hour should separate administration of these drugs.

ANTACIDS

Preadministration Assessment

Therapeutic Goal and Baseline Data
See Implications for H$_2$-receptor antagonists.

Identifying High-Risk Patients
Use *all* antacids with *caution* in patients with *hypertension* or *congestive heart failure.* Use *magnesium-containing* antacids with *caution* in patients with *renal* insufficiency.

Implementation: Administration

Route
Oral.

Administration
Instruct patients to administer antacids 7 times a day: 1 and 3 hours after meals and at bedtime.

Instruct patients to take their medication on a regular schedule even after pain has subsided, since relief of pain does not necessarily indicate healing.

Instruct patients to shake liquid preparations before dispensing.

Instruct patients to chew antacid tablets thoroughly and to follow administration with a glass of water or milk.

Ongoing Evaluation and Interventions

Evaluating Therapeutic Effects
See Implications for H$_2$-receptor antagonists.

Minimizing Adverse Effects
Constipation and Diarrhea. To minimize disruption of bowel function, a constipating antacid (aluminum hydroxide, calcium carbonate) is combined

with a laxative antacid (magnesium hydroxide). Teach the patient to adjust the dosage of the constipating agent and laxative agent as needed to normalize bowel function.

Sodium Loading. Sodium in antacids can exacerbate hypertension and congestive heart failure. Patients with these disorders should use a low-sodium preparation.

Minimizing Adverse Interactions

Interactions Caused by Elevation of Gastric pH. By <u>raising</u> gastric pH, antacids can <u>reduce</u> the availability of other drugs, including cimetidine and ranitidine, and can <u>decrease</u> the antiulcer effects of sucralfate. To minimize these interactions, instruct patients to allow <u>1 hour</u> or more between antacid administration and administration of other drugs.

Aluminum Hydroxide. This antacid can bind to a variety of drugs (e.g., tetracyclines, warfarin, digoxin), thereby decreasing their availability. Increased doses of these agents may be needed.

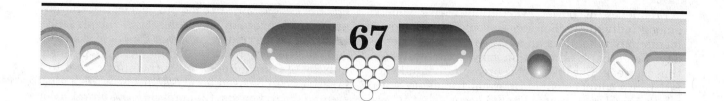

Laxatives

Laxatives are used to ease or stimulate defecation. These agents can soften the stool, increase stool volume, hasten fecal passage through the intestine, and facilitate evacuation from the rectum. When properly employed, laxatives are valuable medications. However, these agents are also subject to widespread abuse. Misuse of laxatives is largely the result of misconceptions about what constitutes normal bowel function.

Before talking about laxatives, it will be helpful to distinguish between two terms: *laxative effect* and *catharsis*. The term *laxative effect* refers to production of a soft, formed stool over a period of 1 or more days. In contrast, the term *catharsis* applies when evacuation of the bowel is fluid and prompt. Hence, a laxative effect is relatively mild, whereas catharsis is more intense.

GENERAL CONSIDERATIONS

Function of the Colon

The principal function of the colon is to absorb water and electrolytes. Absorption of nutrients here is minimal. Normally, about 1500 ml of fluid enters the colon each day. Approximately 90% of this fluid undergoes absorption. When intestinal function is healthy, the extent of fluid absorption is such that the resulting stool is soft (but formed) and capable of elimination without strain. However, when fluid absorption is excessive, as can happen when transport through the intestine is delayed, the resultant stool is dehydrated and hard. Conversely, if insufficient fluid is absorbed, watery stools will result.

Frequency of bowel evacuation varies widely among individuals. For some people, bowel movements may take place an average of three times a day. For others, elimination may occur only two times a week. Because of this broad individual variation, we cannot define a normal frequency with which bowel movements should occur. That is, although a daily bowel movement may be normal for some people, this timing may be abnormal for many others.

Dietary Fiber

Proper function of the bowel is highly dependent on dietary fiber. (Fiber is that component of vegetable matter that escapes digestion in the stomach and small intestine.) Fiber facilitates colonic function in two ways: (1) some types of fiber absorb water, thereby softening the feces and increasing their mass, and (2) other types of fiber are digested by colonic bacteria, whose subsequent growth increases fecal bulk. The best source of fiber is bran. Fiber can also be obtained from fruits and vegetables. Ingestion of 20 to 60 gm of fiber per day should optimize intestinal function.

Constipation

Constipation is determined primarily by stool *consistency* (degree of hardness). Alterations in bowel movement *frequency* are of secondary importance. Hence, if the interval between bowel movements becomes prolonged, but the stool remains soft and hydrated, a diagnosis of constipation would be improper. Conversely, if bowel movements occur with regularity, but the feces are hard and dry, we would consider constipation to be present—despite the regular and frequent passage of stool.

The principal cause of constipation is poor diet—specifically, a diet deficient in fiber and fluid. Certain drugs (e.g., opioids, anticholinergics, some antacids) may also cause constipation.

In most cases, constipation can be readily corrected. Stools will become softer and more easily passed within days of increasing fiber and fluid in the diet. Mild exercise, especially after meals, will also help improve function of the bowel. If necessary, a laxative may be employed—but only briefly and only as an adjunct to diet and exercise.

Indications for Laxative Use

Laxatives can be highly beneficial when employed for valid indications. By softening the stool, laxatives can reduce the painful elimination that can be associated with episiotomy and with hemorrhoids and other anorectal lesions. In patients with cardiovascular diseases (e.g., aneurysm, myocardial infarction, disease of the cerebral or cardiac vasculature), softening of the stool decreases the amount of strain needed to defecate, thereby avoiding dangerous elevations of blood pressure. In geriatric patients, laxatives can help compensate for loss of tone in abdominal and perineal muscle. As an adjunct to anthelmintic therapy, laxatives can be used for (1) obtaining a fresh stool sample for diagnosis, (2) emptying the bowel prior to treatment (so as to increase parasitic exposure to anthelmintic medication), and (3) facilitating export of dead parasites following anthelmintic use. Additional applications of laxatives include (1) emptying of the bowel prior to surgery and diagnostic procedures (e.g., radiologic examination, proctosigmoidoscopy), (2) modification of the effluent from an ileostomy or colostomy, (3) prevention of fecal impaction in bedridden patients, (4) removal of ingested poisons, and (5) correction of constipation associated with pregnancy or use of certain drugs.

Contraindications to Laxative Use

Laxatives are contraindicated for individuals with certain disorders of the bowel. Specifically, laxatives must be avoided by individuals experiencing abdominal pain, nausea, cramps, or other symptoms of appendicitis, regional enteritis, diverticulitis, and ulcerative colitis. Laxatives are also contraindicated for patients with acute surgical abdomen. In addition, laxatives should not be used in the presence of fecal impaction or obstruction of the bowel; under these conditions, increased peristalsis may cause bowel perforation. Lastly, laxatives should not be employed habitually for the treatment of constipation. Reasons for this last prohibition are discussed later in the chapter.

Laxative Classification Schemes

Traditionally, laxatives have been classified according to general mechanism of action. This scheme has four major categories: (1) bulk-forming agents, (2) surfactants, (3) contact laxatives, and (4) saline laxatives. The drugs that belong to these classes are listed in Table 67–1.

From a clinical perspective, it can be helpful to classify laxatives according to therapeutic effect (time of onset and impact on stool consistency). When these properties are considered, most laxatives fall into one of three groups (labeled I, II, and III in this chapter). Group I agents act rapidly (within 2 to 6 hours) to impart a watery consistency to the stool. Laxatives in group I are especially useful when preparing the bowel for diagnostic procedures and surgery. Group II agents have an intermediate latency (6 to 12 hours) and produce a stool that is semifluid in texture. Group II drugs are the agents most frequently abused by the general public. The group III laxatives act slowly (in 1 to 3 days) and produce a soft but formed stool. Uses for this group include treatment

	Table 67–1. Classification of Laxatives by Pharmacologic Category		
Class	**Laxative**	**Site of Action**	**Mechanism of Action**
Bulk-Forming Laxatives	Methylcellulose Psyllium Polycarbophil	Small and large intestine	These absorb water, thereby softening and enlarging the fecal mass; fecal swelling may promote peristalsis.
Surfac-tants	Docusate sodium Docusate calcium Docusate potassium	Small and large intestine	Surfactant action softens stool by facilitating penetration of water; cause secretion of water and electrolytes into intestine.
Contact Laxatives	Bisacodyl Senna Cascara sagrada Phenolphthalein	Colon	These soften feces by (1) causing secretion of water and electrolytes into the intestine, and (2) decreasing water and electrolyte absorption; may also act directly to stimulate peristalsis.
	Castor oil	Small intestine	
Saline Laxatives	Magnesium hydroxide Magnesium sulfate Magnesium citrate Sodium phosphate	Small and large intestine	Osmotic action retains water and thereby softens the feces; fecal swelling may promote peristalsis.
Miscellaneous Laxatives	Mineral oil	Colon	Provides lubrication and reduces absorption of water.
	Glycerin suppository	Colon	Lubricates feces and causes reflex rectal contraction.
	Lactulose	Colon	Similar to saline laxatives.
	Polyethylene glycol-electrolyte solution	Small and large intestine	Similar to saline laxatives.

of constipation and prevention of straining at stool. Laxatives that belong to groups I, II, and III are listed in Table 67–2.

BASIC PHARMACOLOGY OF LAXATIVES

BULK-FORMING AGENTS

The bulk-forming laxatives (e.g., methylcellulose, psyllium) have actions and effects very similar to those of dietary fiber. These agents consist of natural or semisynthetic polysaccharides and celluloses derived from grains and other plant material. With regard to clinical response, the bulk-forming agents belong to category III: these drugs produce a soft, formed stool 1 to 3 days after the onset of treatment.

Mechanism of Action. The effects of bulk-forming agents on bowel function are identical to those of dietary fiber. Following ingestion, these agents, which are nondigestible and nonabsorbable, swell in water to form a viscous solution or gel, thereby softening the fecal mass and increasing its bulk. Fecal volume may be further enlarged by growth of colonic bacteria, which can utilize these materials as nutrients. Transit through the intestine is hastened because swelling of the fecal mass stretches the intestinal wall, thereby stimulating peristalsis.

Indications. Bulk-forming laxatives are the preferred agents for temporary treatment of constipation. Also, these drugs are widely used by patients with diverticulosis and irritable bowel syndrome. In addition, by altering fecal consistency, these agents can provide symptomatic relief of diarrhea and can reduce discomfort and inconvenience for patients with an ileostomy or colostomy.

Adverse Effects. Untoward effects are minimal. Since the bulk-forming agents are not absorbed, systemic reactions are rare. *Esophageal obstruction* can occur if these agents are swallowed in the absence of sufficient fluid. To avoid this effect, bulk-forming laxatives should be adminis-

		Group III
Table 67–2. Classification of Laxatives by Therapeutic Response		

Group I Laxatives: Produce Watery Stool in 2 to 6 Hours	Group II Laxatives: Produce Semifluid Stool in 6 to 12 Hours	Group III Laxatives: Produce Soft Stool in 1 to 3 Days

Saline laxatives (in high doses)
   Magnesium salts
   Sodium salts
	Saline laxatives (in low doses)
	   Magnesium salts
	   Sodium salts
		Bulk-forming agents
		   Methylcellulose
		   Psyllium
		   Polycarbophil

Castor oil
 	
Polyethylene glycol-electrolyte solution
	Contact laxatives (except castor oil)
	   Bisacodyl (PO)*
	   Phenolphthalein
	   Senna
	   Cascara
		Surfactants
		   Docusate salts
		
		Lactulose

*Bisacodyl is also available as a suppository whose onset time is 15 minutes.

tered with a full glass of water or juice. If their passage through the intestine is arrested, the bulk-forming agents may produce *intestinal obstruction* or *impaction*. Accordingly, these agents should be avoided when there is narrowing of the intestinal lumen.

Preparations, Dosage, and Administration. *Psyllium* (prepared from Plantago seed), *methylcellulose*, and *polycarbophil* are the principal bulk-forming laxatives. Dosages for psyllium and methylcellulose are presented in Table 67–3. As noted above, all bulk-forming agents should be administered with a full glass of water or juice.

SURFACTANTS

Actions. The surfactants (e.g., docusate sodium) are group III laxatives: these agents produce a soft stool several days after the onset of treatment. Surfactants alter stool consistency by lowering surface tension, an action that facilitates penetration of water into the feces. The surfactants may also act on the intestinal wall to (1) inhibit fluid absorption, and (2) stimulate secretion of water and electrolytes into the intestinal lumen. In this respect surfactants resemble the contact laxatives (see below).

Preparations, Dosage, and Administration. The surfactant family consists of three *docusate salts*: docusate sodium, docusate potassium, and docusate calcium. Dosage for docusate sodium [Colace], the prototype surfactant, is presented in Table 67–3. Administration of all surfactants should be accompanied by a full glass of water.

CONTACT LAXATIVES

The contact laxatives (e.g., bisacodyl, castor oil) act on the intestinal wall to produce a net increase in the amount of fluid and electrolytes within the intestinal lumen. The contact agents promote fluid and electrolyte accumulation by (1) increasing the secretion of water and ions into the intestine, and (2) reducing water and electrolyte absorption. Most contact laxatives act on the colon, producing a semifluid stool within 6 to 12 hours.

In some texts, the contact laxatives are referred to as *stimulant* laxatives. This older name was coined because these drugs were thought to increase peristalsis by stimulating a nerve plexus within the intestinal wall. However, although this concept has merit, its validity has never been proved. Accordingly, the term *contact laxative* would appear more appropriate.

Contact laxatives are widely used (and abused) by the general public, and are of concern for this reason. These laxatives have few legitimate applications.

Significant differences exist among the various contact laxatives. Properties of individual agents are discussed below.

Bisacodyl. Bisacodyl [Dulcolax, others] is unique among the contact laxatives in that it can be administered by rectal suppository as well as by mouth. *Oral* bisacodyl acts within 6 to 12 hours. Hence, tablets may be given at bedtime to produce a laxative response the following morning. Bisacodyl *suppositories* act rapidly (in 15 to 60 minutes). Dosage for bisacodyl is presented in Table 67–3.

Bisacodyl tablets are enteric coated to prevent gastric irritation. Patients should be advised not to chew or crush the tablets because this will destroy the coating. Since milk and antacids accelerate dissolution of the enteric coating, bisacodyl tablets should be administered no sooner than 1 hour after these substances.

Bisacodyl suppositories may cause a burning sensation. With continued use, proctitis may develop. Accordingly, long-term use of suppositories should be discouraged.

Table 67–3. Representative Laxatives: Trade Names, Dosage Forms, and Dosage

Class	Generic Name	Trade Names	Dosage Forms	Dosage and Administration
Bulk-Forming	Methylcellulose	Citrucel	Powder	Powder: 1 heaping tsp in 8 oz cold water 1–3 times a day
	Psyllium	Effer-Syllium, Konsyl, Metamucil, Naturacil, Perdiem Fiber, others	Granules, powder, effervescent powder	Adults: 1 rounded tsp (or 1 packet) mixed with water or other fluid, taken 1 to 3 times/day Children over 6 years: 1.25–15 g daily
Surfactant	Docusate sodium	Colace, Modane Soft, others	Capsules, tablets, syrup	Adults and children over 12 years: 50–360 mg/day Children 2 to 12 years: 50–150 mg/day (All doses taken with a full glass of water)
Contact	Bisacodyl	Dulcolax, others	Tablets, rectal suppository	Adults: 10-mg tablet or 10-mg suppository Children: 5-mg tablet or 5-mg suppository
	Phenolphthalein	Ex-Lax, Phenolax, others	Tablets, wafers, liquid	Adults: 30–270 mg/day Children: (6 years or older) 30–60 mg/day; (2–5 years) 15–20 mg/day
Saline	Magnesium hydroxide (milk of magnesia)		Liquid	Low dose: 15–30 ml High dose: 30–60 ml
Other	Mineral oil	Nujol, Neo-Cultol, Milkinol, others	Liquid, jelly, emulsion	Adults: 15–45 ml PO bid Children over 6 years: 10–15 ml PO at bedtime

Phenolphthalein. Phenolphthalein is similar in structure and actions to bisacodyl. This agent acts on the colon to produce a semifluid stool in 6 to 8 hours. About 15% of each dose is absorbed and then excreted by the kidney. The drug imparts a harmless pink tint to the urine. Patients should be forewarned of this effect. Phenolphthalein is the active ingredient in many over-the-counter (OTC) laxatives [Ex-Lax, Phenolax, others]. Dosage is presented in Table 67–3.

Anthraquinones. Anthraquinone compounds are the active ingredients in *cascara sagadra* and *senna*, laxatives that are derived from plants. The actions and applications of these laxatives are similar to those of bisacodyl and phenolphthalein. The anthraquinones act on the colon to produce a soft or semifluid stool in 6 to 12 hours. Systemic absorption followed by renal secretion may be sufficient to impart a harmless yellowish-brown or pink color to the urine. Patients should be forewarned of this effect.

Castor Oil. Castor oil is the only contact laxative that acts on the small intestine (see Table 67–1). As a result, this agent acts quickly (in 2 to 6 hours) to produce a stool of watery consistency.

Hence, unlike the other contact laxatives, which are all group II agents, castor oil belongs to therapeutic category I. Use of castor oil is limited to situations in which rapid and thorough evacuation of the bowel is desired (e.g., preparation for radiologic procedures). Castor oil is far too powerful for routine use in the treatment of constipation. Because of its relatively prompt action, castor oil should not be administered at bedtime. Castor oil has an unpleasant taste. Palatability can be improved by chilling and mixing with fruit juice.

SALINE LAXATIVES

Actions and Uses. The saline laxatives (e.g., magnesium hydroxide, sodium phosphate) are poorly absorbed salts whose osmotic action draws water into the intestinal lumen. Accumulation of water causes the fecal mass to soften and swell; swelling, in turn, stretches the intestinal wall and thereby stimulates peristalsis. When administered in low doses, the saline laxatives produce a soft or semifluid stool in 6 to 12 hours. In high doses, these agents act rapidly (in 2 to 6 hours) to cause a fluid evacuation of the bowel. High-dose therapy is employed to empty the bowel in preparation for diagnostic and surgical procedures. High doses are also employed to purge the bowel of ingested poisons, and to evacuate dead parasites following anthelmintic therapy.

Preparations. The saline laxatives include *magnesium salts* (magnesium hydroxide, magnesium citrate, and magnesium sulfate), *sodium salts* (sodium phosphate and sodium biphosphate), and *potassium salts* (potassium bitartrate and potassium phosphate). Dosage for magnesium hydroxide solution (also known as milk of magnesia) is presented in Table 67–3.

Adverse Effects. Saline laxatives can cause substantial loss of water. To avoid dehydration, treatment should be accompanied by augmented intake of fluids. Although the saline laxatives are poorly and slowly absorbed, some absorption does take place. In patients with renal dysfunction, magnesium and potassium can accumulate to toxic levels. Accordingly, saline laxatives that contain these elements are contraindicated in patients with kidney disease. Sodium absorption can cause fluid retention, which in turn can exacerbate heart failure, hypertension, and edema. Accordingly, sodium-containing laxatives are contraindicated for patients with these disorders.

MISCELLANEOUS LAXATIVES

Mineral Oil. Mineral oil is a mixture of indigestible and poorly absorbed hydrocarbons. Laxative action is produced by lubrication. Mineral oil is especially useful when administered rectally to treat fecal impaction.

Mineral oil can produce a variety of adverse effects. Aspiration of oil droplets can cause lipid pneumonia. Anal leakage can cause pruritus and soiling. Systemic absorption can produce deposition of mineral oil in the liver. Excessive dosing can decrease the absorption of fat-soluble vitamins.

Lactulose. Lactulose is a semisynthetic disaccharide composed of galactose and fructose. Lactulose is poorly absorbed and cannot be digested by intestinal enzymes. In the colon, resident bacteria metabolize lactulose to lactic, formic, and acetic acids. These acids exert a mild osmotic action, producing a soft, formed stool in 1 to 3 days. Although lactulose can relieve constipation, this agent is more expensive than therapeutically equivalent agents (bulk-forming laxatives) and also causes unpleasant side effects (flatulence and cramping are common). Accordingly, lactulose should be reserved for patients who do not respond adequately to bulk-forming laxatives. In addition to its laxative action, lactulose can enhance intestinal excretion of ammonia. This property has been exploited to lower blood ammonia in patients with portal hypertension and hepatic encephalopathy occurring secondary to chronic liver disease.

Glycerin. Glycerin, which is administered as a suppository, is an osmotic agent that softens and lubricates inspissated feces. The drug may also stimulate rectal contraction. Evacuation occurs about 30 minutes after suppository insertion. Glycerin suppositories have been useful for re-establishing normal bowel function following termination of chronic laxative use.

Polyethylene Glycol-Electrolyte Solutions. These bowel-cleansing solutions [CoLyte, GoLYTELY, others] contain a mixture of polyethylene glycol (a nonabsorbable osmotic agent) together with potassium chloride, sodium chloride, sodium sulfate, and sodium bicarbonate. The mixture is isosmotic with body fluids, and its composition is such that water and electro-lytes are neither absorbed from nor secreted into the intestinal lumen. Hence, water is not lost and electrolyte balance is preserved. As a result, polyethylene glycol-electrolyte solutions can be used safely in patients who are dehydrated and in those who are especially sensitive to alterations in electrolyte levels (i.e., patients with renal impairment or cardiovascular disease). These preparations are indicated primarily for cleansing the bowel prior to diagnostic procedures. Dosage volume is huge (about 4 L). Patients must ingest 250 to 300 ml every 10 minutes for 2 to 3 hours. Bowel movements commence about 1 hour after initiation of treatment.

LAXATIVE ABUSE

Causes. Many people believe that a daily and bountiful bowel movement is a requisite of good health and that any deviation from this pattern merits correction. Such misconceptions are reinforced by aggressive marketing of over-the-counter laxative preparations, of which there are literally hundreds. Not infrequently, the combination of tradition supported by advertising has led to habitual self-prescribing of laxatives by people for whom these agents are not indicated.

Laxatives can help perpetuate their own use. Strong laxatives can purge the entire bowel. When such overemptying occurs, spontaneous evacuation will be impossible until bowel content has been replenished, which may take 2 to 5 days. During the period of bowel refilling, the laxative user, having experienced no movement of the bowel, often becomes convinced that constipation has returned. In response, he or she takes yet another dose of laxative, thereby purging the bowel once more. In this manner, a vicious cycle of repeated laxative use and purging becomes established.

Consequences. Chronic exposure to laxatives can diminish defecatory reflexes, leading to further reliance on laxatives. Laxative abuse may also cause more serious pathologic changes, including electrolyte imbalance, dehydration, and colitis.

Treatment. The first step in breaking the laxative habit is abrupt cessation of laxative use. Following drug withdrawal, bowel movements will be absent for several days; the patient should be informed of this fact. Any misconceptions that the patient has regarding bowel function should be corrected: the patient should be taught that a once-daily bowel movement may not be normal for him or her and that stool *quality* is more important than frequency and quantity. Instruction on bowel training (heeding the defecatory reflex, establishing a consistent time for bowel movements) should be provided. Increased consumption of fiber (bran, fruits, vegetables) should be stressed. The patient should be encouraged to exercise daily, especially after meals. Finally, the patient should be advised that if a laxative must be used, it should be used only briefly and in the smallest effective dosage. Agents that produce catharsis must be avoided.

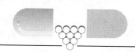

Summary of Major Nursing Implications

LAXATIVES

 Implications That Apply to All Laxatives

Identifying High-Risk Patients

Laxatives are contraindicated for individuals with *abdominal pain, nausea, cramps,* and other symptoms of *appendicitis, regional enteritis, diverticulitis,* and *ulcerative colitis.* Laxatives are also contraindicated for patients with *acute surgical abdomen, fecal impaction,* and *obstruction of the bowel.*

Reducing Laxative Abuse

Patient education is a key factor in reducing laxative abuse. Educate the patient about normal bowel function (to correct misconceptions) and provide instruction on establishing good bowel habits (heeding the defecatory reflex, establishing a consistent time for bowel movements). Advise the patient to exercise (especially after meals) and to increase consumption of fiber (bran, fruits, vegetables). Inform the patient that laxatives should be used only when clearly necessary and then only briefly in the lowest effective dosage. Warn the patient against using cathartics.

 Implications That Apply to Specific Laxatives

Bulk-Forming Laxatives: Psyllium, Methylcellulose, and Polycarbophil

Instruct the patient to take bulk-forming agents with a full glass of water or juice to prevent esophageal obstruction.

Bulk-forming laxatives are contraindicated for individuals with narrowing of the intestinal lumen, a condition that increases the risk of intestinal obstruction and impaction.

Surfactants: Docusate Salts

Instruct the patient to take surfactant agents with a full glass of water.

Contact Laxatives

Contact agents are the laxatives most commonly abused by the general public. Discourage the patient from inappropriate use of these drugs.

Bisacodyl. Administered PO and by rectal suppository. Instruct the patient to take oral bisacodyl no sooner than 1 hour after ingestion of milk or antacids. Instruct the patient to swallow tablets intact, without crushing or chewing.

Suppositories may cause a burning sensation; forewarn the patient. Warn the patient that prolonged use of bisacodyl suppositories can cause proctitis.

Phenolphthalein. Forewarn the patient that phenolphthalein may impart a harmless pink tint to the urine.

Anthraquinones: Cascara Sagadra and Senna. Forewarn the patient that anthraquinones can impart a harmless yellowish-brown or pink color to the urine.

Castor Oil. Castor oil acts rapidly (in 2 to 6 hours); do not administer at bedtime. Advise the patient not to take castor oil late at night. Warn the patient that castor oil is a powerful laxative and should not be used to treat routine constipation. Administer in chilled fruit juice to improve palatability.

Saline Laxatives: Magnesium Salts, Sodium Salts, and Potassium Salts

Effects are dose dependent. Low doses produce a soft or semifluid stool in 6 to 12 hours. Higher doses cause watery evacuation of the bowel in 2 to 6 hours.

To prevent dehydration, increase fluid intake during treatment.

Magnesium salts and *potassium salts* are contraindicated for patients with *renal dysfunction.*

Sodium salts are contraindicated for patients with *heart failure, hypertension,* or *edema.*

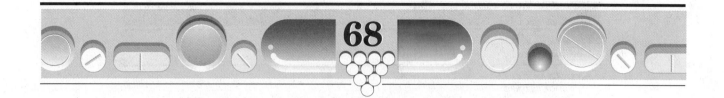

Miscellaneous Gastrointestinal Drugs

ANTIEMETICS

DRUGS FOR MOTION SICKNESS

ANTIDIARRHEAL AGENTS
Nonspecific Antidiarrheal Agents
Management of Infectious Diarrhea

DRUGS FOR INFLAMMATORY BOWEL DISEASE

PANCREATIC ENZYMES

DRUGS USED TO DISSOLVE GALLSTONES

ANORECTAL PREPARATIONS

I n this chapter we will discuss an assortment of gastrointestinal (GI) drugs with indications that range from emesis to colitis to gallstones. Two groups are emphasized: (1) antiemetics, and (2) antidiarrheals.

ANTIEMETICS

Emesis is a complex reflex brought about by activation of the vomiting center, a nucleus of neurons located in the medulla oblongata. Certain stimuli (e.g., gastrointestinal irritation) activate the vomiting center directly. Other stimuli (e.g., drugs, toxins, radiation) act within the medulla to stimulate the chemoreceptor trigger zone (CTZ), which in turn causes activation of the vomiting center. The vomiting center may also be activated by input from the cerebral cortex, as happens in the anticipatory vomiting seen in patients who are undergoing cancer chemotherapy.

A variety of neurotransmitter receptors are involved in the vomiting reflex. Included are receptors that can be influenced by acetylcholine, histamine, serotonin, dopamine, benzodiazepines, and cannabinoids. Presumably, it is by altering the function of these receptors that emetogenic compounds and antiemetic drugs produce their effects.

A major application of the antiemetics is

865

Table 68–1. Antiemetics

Class and Generic Name	Trade Name	Adult Dosage
ANTIDOPAMINERGICS		
Phenothiazines		
Chlorpromazine	Thorazine	10–25 mg (PO, IM, IV) q 4–6 hr PRN
Fluphenazine	Prolixin	1.25–2.5 mg (PO, IM) q 6–8 hr PRN
Perphenazine	Trilafon	8–30 mg/day in divided doses (PO, IM, IV)
Prochlorperazine	Compazine	5–10 mg (PO, IM, IV) 3–4 times a day PRN
Promazine	Sparine	25–50 mg (PO, IM) q 4–6 hr PRN
Thiethylperazine	Torecan	10 mg (PO) 3 times a day
Butyrophenones		
Haloperidol	Haldol	1–5 mg (PO, IM, IV) q 12 hr PRN
Droperidol	Inapsine	2.5–5 mg (IM, IV) q 4–6 hr PRN
Others		
Metoclopramide	Reglan	1–2 mg/kg (IV) q 2 hr × 2, then q 3 hr × 3
Domperidone	Motilium	15 mg (IV), then 7.5 mg 2 q hr × 7
ANTICHOLINERGICS		
Antihistaminics		
Buclizine	Bucladin-S	50 mg (PO) twice daily
Cyclizine	Marezine	50 mg (PO, IM) q 4–6 hr PRN
Dimenhydrinate	Dramamine	50–100 mg (PO, IM, IV) q 4–6 hr PRN
Diphenhydramine	Benadryl	10–50 mg (PO, IM, IV) q 4–6 hr PRN
Hydroxyzine	Vistaril, Atarax	25–100 mg (PO, IM) q 6 hr PRN
Meclizine	Bonine, Antivert	25–50 mg (PO) q 24 hr PRN
Promethazine	Phenergan	12.5–25 mg (PO, IM, IV) q 4–6 hr PRN
Pyrilamine	Nisaval	25–50 mg (PO) 3–4 times a day PRN
Others		
Scopolamine	Transderm Scop	0.5 mg (transdermal) q 72 hr PRN
Trimethobenzamide	Tigan	200–250 mg (PO, IM) 3–4 times a day PRN
GLUCOCORTICOIDS		
Dexamethasone	Decadron	10 mg (IV) before chemotherapy, then 4–8 mg
Methylprednisolone	Solu-Medrol	2 doses of 125–500 mg (IV) 6 hr apart before chemotherapy
CANNABINOIDS		
Dronabinol	Marinol	5–7.5 mg/m^2 (PO) q 2–4 hr PRN
Nabilone	Cesamet	1–2 mg (PO) 3–4 times a day PRN
BENZODIAZEPINES		
Lorazepam	Ativan	0.5–4 mg (IV) before chemotherapy
Diazepam	Valium	2–5 mg (PO) q 3 hr
ANTISEROTONERGIC		
Ondansetron	Zofran	0.15 mg/kg (IV) before chemotherapy, repeat at 4 and 8 hr
MISCELLANEOUS		
Diphenidol	Vontrol	25–50 mg (PO) q 4 hr PRN
Benzquinamide	Emete-Con	25–50 mg (IM, IV) q 3–4 hr PRN
Phosphorated carbohydrate solution	Emetrol	15–30 ml (PO) q 1–3 hr PRN

suppression of nausea and vomiting associated with cancer chemotherapy. These sequelae of chemotherapy can be extremely intense—so intense, in fact, that patients may discontinue chemotherapy rather than endure further discomfort. For patients undergoing chemotherapy, antiemetic therapy offers three major benefits. First, treatment can reduce anticipatory nausea and vomiting. Second, treatment can prevent the malnutrition and dehydration that can be caused by frequent nausea and vomiting. Third, by reducing discomfort, antiemetics can increase compliance with the chemo-

therapeutic program. Frequently, antiemetic combinations are more beneficial than single-drug treatment. The superior efficacy of combination therapy suggests that cancer chemotherapy may cause emesis by multiple mechanisms.

As a rule, antiemetics are more effective when taken prophylactically than when taken to suppress emesis that has already begun. For prophylaxis, antiemetics are usually administered by mouth. For suppression of active emesis, parenteral or rectal administration may be required.

Many different antiemetics are available. Their

classification, trade names, and dosages are summarized in Table 68–1. Properties of the principal agents are discussed below.

Phenothiazines

The phenothiazines (e.g., prochlorperazine) suppress emesis by blockade of dopamine receptors in the CTZ. These drugs can be used to suppress emesis associated with surgery, cancer chemotherapy, radiation therapy, and toxins. The phenothiazines can produce a variety of serious side effects. These include extrapyramidal reactions, anticholinergic effects, hypotension, and sedation. The basic pharmacology of the phenothiazines is discussed in Chapter 24 (Antipsychotic Agents and Their Use in Schizophrenia).

Butyrophenones

Two butyrophenones—*haloperidol* [Haldol] and *droperidol* [Inapsine]—are used as antiemetics. Like the phenothiazines, the butyrophenones suppress emesis by blocking dopamine receptors in the CTZ. The butyrophenones are useful for postoperative nausea and vomiting, and for emesis caused by cancer chemotherapy, radiation therapy, and toxins. Potential side effects are similar to those of the phenothiazines: extrapyramidal reactions, sedation, and hypotension. The pharmacology of the butyrophenones is discussed in Chapter 24.

Cannabinoids

Antiemetic Applications. Two cannabinoids—*dronabinol* [Marinol] and *nabilone* [Cesamet]—have been approved for treating nausea and vomiting associated with cancer chemotherapy. Dronabinol (delta-9-tetrahydrocannabinol, THC) is the principal psychoactive agent in *Cannabis sativa* (marijuana). Nabilone is a synthetic derivative of dronabinol. Clinical experience indicates that for certain cancer patients, the cannabinoids are superior to traditional antiemetics (e.g., prochlorperazine, metoclopramide). The mechanism by which cannabinoids suppress emesis is not known. The basic pharmacology of the cannabinoids is discussed in Chapter 34 (Drugs of Abuse).

Appetite Stimulation. *Dronabinol* was recently approved for stimulating appetite in patients with AIDS. The goal is to reduce AIDS-induced anorexia and prevent or reverse weight loss.

Adverse Effects. When cannabinoids are used to prevent emesis or stimulate appetite, they can produce subjective effects identical to those elicited by smoking marijuana. Patients may experience temporal disintegration, dissociation, depersonalization, and dysphoria. Many people find these re-

actions intolerable. Because of their central nervous system (CNS) effects, cannabinoids are contraindicated for patients with psychiatric disorders. Dronabinol and nabilone have a high potential for abuse and are classified under Schedule II of the Controlled Substances Act. In addition to their subjective effects, cannabinoids can cause tachycardia and hypotension and, therefore, must be used with caution in patients with cardiovascular disease.

Preparations, Dosage, and Administration. Dronabinol [Marinol] and nabilone [Cesamet] are both dispensed in capsules for oral use. To *prevent emesis*, the dosage for dronabinol is 5 to 7.5 mg/m² every 2 hours as needed; the dosage for nabilone is 1 to 2 mg three or four times daily as needed.

Only *dronabinol* is approved for *stimulating appetite in patients with AIDS*. The recommended initial dosage is 2.5 mg twice daily, before lunch and supper. If this dosage is intolerable, 2.5 mg once daily may be tried. The maximum recommended daily dosage is 20 mg in divided doses.

Benzodiazepines

Two benzodiazepines—*diazepam* [Valium] and *lorazepam* [Ativan]—are used to alleviate nausea and vomiting associated with cancer chemotherapy. Antiemetic effects of diazepam derive primarily from suppression of anxiety. Lorazepam is beneficial because of its ability to produce antegrade amnesia. When given to alleviate nausea and vomiting, lorazepam is usually combined with metoclopramide and dexamethasone. The benzodiazepines are discussed at length in Chapter 27.

Glucocorticoids

Two glucocorticoids—*methylprednisolone* and *dexamethasone*—have been employed investigationally to treat emesis brought on by cancer chemotherapy. Clinical experience has shown these drugs to be effective alone and in combination with other antiemetics. The mechanism by which glucocorticoids suppress emesis is not known. Both dexamethasone and methylprednisolone are administered intravenously. Optimal dosage has not been determined. Since antiemetic use is intermittent and short-term, serious side effects do not occur. The pharmacology of the glucocorticoids is discussed in Chapter 62.

Metoclopramide

Actions. Metoclopramide [Reglan] has two beneficial actions: (1) it blocks dopamine receptors in the CTZ, thereby suppressing emesis, and (2) it increases upper GI motility (by enhancing the actions of acetylcholine).

Therapeutic Uses. Metoclopramide is a drug of choice for suppressing nausea and vomiting caused by highly emetic anticancer agents (e.g., cisplatin, dacarbazine). In addition, metoclopramide is given to suppress postoperative emesis and emesis caused by radiation therapy, toxins, and opioids. Other applications include relief of diabetic gastroparesis and suppression of gastroesophageal reflux.

Adverse Effects. With high-dose therapy, sedation and diarrhea are common. Like other dopamine antagonists, metoclopramide may cause extrapyramidal reactions, especially in children. These reactions can often be controlled by injection of diphenhydramine (a drug with prominent anticholinergic actions). Because of its ability to increase gastric and intestinal motility, metoclopramide is contraindicated in the presence of obstruction, hemorrhage, and perforation of the GI tract.

Preparations, Dosage, and Administration. Metoclopramide [Reglan] is available in tablets (10 mg), syrup (5 mg/ml), and as an injection (5 mg/ml). Oral preparations are used for diabetic gastroparesis and gastroesophageal reflux.

For prophylaxis of chemotherapy-induced emesis, treatment is intravenous. Dosing is begun 30 minutes prior to chemotherapy. The initial dose is 1 to 2 mg/kg infused over 15 minutes or more. Additional doses of 1 to 2 mg/kg are administered 2, 4, 7, 10, and 13 hours after the first dose.

Ondansetron

Ondansetron [Zofran] is a new drug used to suppress nausea and vomiting associated with cancer chemotherapy. This drug acts by blocking serotonin receptors (specifically, 5-HT$_3$ receptors) in the CTZ and on afferent vagal neurons in the upper GI tract. Clinical trials have shown that ondansetron alone is more effective than metoclopramide alone. Ondansetron is even more effective when combined with dexamethasone. The most common side effects are headache and diarrhea. Since ondansetron does not block dopamine receptors, it does not cause extrapyramidal effects (e.g., akathisia, acute dystonia).

Administration is intravenous or oral. The initial IV dose is 0.15 mg/kg infused slowly (over 15 minutes) beginning 30 minutes before chemotherapy. This dose is repeated 4 and 8 hours later. Oral ondansetron is available in 4- and 8-mg tablets. The usual dosage is 8 µg three times a day.

DRUGS FOR MOTION SICKNESS

Motion sickness can be caused by sea, air, automobile, and space travel. Symptoms are nausea, vomiting, pallor, and cold sweating. The drugs used to treat motion sickness are most effective when given prophylactically, rather than after symptoms have begun.

Scopolamine

Scopolamine, a muscarinic antagonist, is the most effective drug for prophylaxis and treatment of motion sickness. Benefits derive from suppression of nerve traffic within the labyrinth of the inner ear. The most common side effects are dry mouth, blurred vision, and drowsiness. More severe but less common effects are urinary retention, constipation, and disorientation.

Scopolamine is available for oral, subcutaneous, and trans-

dermal administration. The transdermal system [Transderm Scop], an adhesive patch that contains scopolamine, is applied behind the ear. Claims that the transdermal formulation produces fewer anticholinergic side effects than the oral formulation do not seem to be true.

Antihistamines

The antihistamines used to treat motion sickness are listed in Table 68–1. Because these drugs block receptors for acetylcholine in addition to receptors for histamine, they appear in the table as a subclass under *Anticholinergics*. There is no correlation between the ability of antihistamines to prevent motion sickness and their potency as blockers of cholinergic and histaminic receptors. Hence, the mechanism by which they suppress motion sickness is unclear. The most important side effect of antihistamines is sedation. In addition, these drugs can cause typical anticholinergic effects, including dry mouth, blurred vision, and urinary retention. Promethazine is the most effective antihistamine for prophylaxis of motion sickness. Unfortunately, sedation limits its utility. For treatment of motion sickness, the antihistamines are less effective than scopolamine.

ANTIDIARRHEAL AGENTS

Diarrhea is characterized by stools of excessive volume and fluidity, and by increased frequency of defecation. Diarrhea is a symptom of gastrointestinal disease and not a disease per se. Causes include infection, maldigestion, inflammation, and functional disorders of the bowel. The most serious complications of diarrhea are dehydration and depletion of electrolytes. Management is directed at the following: (1) diagnosis and treatment of the underlying disease, (2) replacement of lost water and salts, (3) relief of cramping, and (4) reducing the passage of unformed stools.

Antidiarrheal drugs fall into two major groups: (1) specific antidiarrheal drugs, and (2) nonspecific antidiarrheal drugs. The specific agents are drugs that treat the underlying cause of diarrhea. Included in this group are anti-infective drugs and drugs used to correct malabsorption syndromes. Nonspecific antidiarrheals are agents that act on or within the bowel to provide symptomatic relief; these drugs do not influence the actual cause of diarrhea.

NONSPECIFIC ANTIDIARRHEAL AGENTS

Opioids

Opioids are the most effective antidiarrheal drugs. By stimulating opioid receptors in the GI tract, these agents suppress peristalsis, thereby facilitating absorption of water and electrolytes. As a result, the fluidity and volume of stools are reduced, as is the frequency of defecation. At the doses employed to relieve diarrhea, subjective effects and dependence do not occur. However, excessive doses can elicit typical morphine-like subjective effects. If severe overdosage occurs, it should be treated with naloxone. In patients with inflammatory bowel disease, opioids may cause toxic megacolon.

Several opioid preparations—diphenoxylate, difenoxin, loperamide, paregoric, and opium tincture—are approved for treatment of diarrhea. Of these, diphenoxylate [Lomotil, others] and loperamide [Imodium] are the most frequently employed. Pharmacologic properties of these agents are discussed below. Dosages for diarrhea are summarized in Table 68–2.

Diphenoxylate. Diphenoxylate is an opioid whose only indication is diarrhea. The drug is insoluble in water and, hence, cannot be abused by parenteral routes. When taken orally in antidiarrheal doses, diphenoxylate has no significant effect on the CNS. However, if taken in high doses, the drug can elicit typical morphine-like subjective responses.

Diphenoxylate is dispensed only in combination with atropine. The combination, whose trade name is *Lomotil*, is available in tablets and an oral liquid. Each tablet or 5 ml of liquid contains 2.5 mg of diphenoxylate and 25 µg of atropine sulfate. The atropine is present to discourage diphenoxylate abuse: doses of the combination that are sufficiently high to produce euphoria from the diphenoxylate would produce unpleasant side effects from the correspondingly high dose of atropine. Accordingly, the combination has a very low potential for abuse and is classified as a Schedule V preparation.

Difenoxin. Difenoxin is the major active metabolite of diphenoxylate. Like diphenoxylate, difenoxin can elicit morphine-like subjective effects if taken in high doses. To discourage excessive dosing, difenoxin, like diphenoxylate, is dispensed only in combination with atropine. The trade name for the combination is *Motofen*. Because its abuse potential is somewhat greater than that of diphenoxylate plus atropine, Motofen is classified as a Schedule IV preparation.

Loperamide. Loperamide [Imodium] is a structural analogue of meperidine. The drug is employed to treat diarrhea and to reduce the volume of discharge from ileostomies. Beneficial effects result from suppression of bowel motility, and perhaps from suppression of fluid secretion into the intestinal lumen. The drug is poorly absorbed and does not readily cross the blood-brain barrier. Very large oral doses fail to elicit morphine-like subjective effects. Loperamide has little or no potential for abuse, and is not classified under the Controlled Substances Act. The drug is dispensed in 2-mg capsules and in a liquid formulation (1 mg/5 ml).

Paregoric. Paregoric (camphorated tincture of opium) is a dilute solution of powdered opium, containing 0.4% opium by weight. Paregoric contains morphine (0.4 mg/ml) as its principal active ingredient. The primary application for paregoric is diarrhea, although the preparation is approved for the same indications as morphine. Antidiarrheal doses cause neither euphoria nor analgesia. Very high doses can cause typical morphine-like responses. Paregoric has a moderate potential for abuse and is classified as a Schedule III preparation.

Opium Tincture. Opium tincture is an alcohol-based solution that contains 10% opium by weight. The principal active ingredient—morphine—is present in a concentration of 10 mg/ml (25 times higher than the concentration of morphine in paregoric). The primary indication for opium tincture is diarrhea. In addition, the preparation (in dilute form) may be given to suppress symptoms of withdrawal in opioid-dependent neonates. When administered in antidiarrheal doses, opium tincture does not produce analgesia or euphoria. However, high doses can cause typical opioid-agonist effects. Opium tincture has a high potential for abuse and is classified as a Schedule II preparation.

Other Nonspecific Antidiarrheals

Bulk-Forming Agents. Paradoxically, methylcellulose, polycarbophil, and other bulk-forming laxatives are useful in the management of diarrhea. Benefits derive from giving the stool a more firm, less watery consistency. Stool volume is not decreased. The bulk-forming laxatives are discussed in Chapter 67.

Anticholinergic Antispasmodics. Muscarinic antagonists (e.g., atropine) can relieve cramping associated with diarrhea; these drugs do not alter fecal consistency or volume. Because of undesirable side effects (e.g., blurred vision, photophobia, dry

Table 68–2. Opioids Used to Treat Diarrhea

Generic Name	Trade Name	CSA* Schedule	Antidiarrheal Dosage
Diphenoxylate (plus atropine)†	Lomotil, others	V	Adults: 5 mg, 4 times/day Children (initial dosage): age 2 to 5 years—1 mg, 4 times/day age 5 to 8 years—1–2 mg, 4 times/day age 8 to 12 years—1–2 mg, 4 times/day
Difenoxin (plus atropine)†	Motofen	IV	Adults: 2 mg initially, then 1 mg after each loose stool
Loperamide	Imodium	NR‡	Adults (initial dose): 4 mg Children (initial dosage): age 2–5 years—1 mg, 3 times/day age 5–8 years—2 mg, 2 times/day age 8–12 years—2 mg, 3 times/day
Paregoric (camphorated tincture of opium; contains 0.4 mg morphine/ml)		III	Adults: 5 to 10 ml, 1–4 times/day Children: 0.25 to 0.5 ml/kg, 1–4 times/day
Opium tincture (opioid content equivalent to 10 mg morphine/ml)		II	0.6 ml 4 times/day

*Controlled Substances Act
†Diphenoxylate and difenoxin are dispensed only in combination with atropine. The atropine dose is subtherapeutic and is present to discourage abuse.
‡Not regulated under the CSA.

mouth, urinary retention, tachycardia), anticholinergic drugs are of limited use. The pharmacology of the muscarinic blockers is discussed in Chapter 13.

Adsorbents. Several substances (bismuth salts, kaolin, pectin) are said to adsorb toxins, bacteria, and viruses. However, definitive proof of such claims is lacking. Side effects of the adsorbents are minimal, although these preparations can interfere with the absorption of other drugs.

MANAGEMENT OF INFECTIOUS DIARRHEA

General Considerations. Infectious diarrhea may be produced by enteric infection with a variety of bacteria and protozoa. These infections are usually self-limited. Mild diarrhea can be managed with nonspecific antidiarrheals. However, in many cases, no treatment at all is required. Antibiotics should be administered only when clearly indicated. Indiscriminate use of antibiotics is undesirable in that it can promote emergence of antibiotic-resistant organisms, and can produce an asymptomatic carrier state by killing most, but not all, of the infectious agents. Conditions that do merit antibiotic treatment include severe infections with *Salmonella, Shigella, Campylobacter*, or *Clostridium*.

Traveler's Diarrhea. Tourists are often plagued by infectious diarrhea. This condition is known variously as Montezuma's revenge, the Aztec two-step, and Rangoon runs. In most cases, the causative organism is *Escherichia coli*. As a rule, treatment is unnecessary: infection with *E. coli* is self-limited and will run its course in 1 to 2 days. Symptomatic relief can be achieved with nonspecific antidiarrheals. However, by slowing peristalsis, these agents may delay export of the offending organism, and may thereby prolong the infection. Prophylaxis is possible with *doxycycline, trimethoprim-sulfamethoxazole*, and other antibiotics. However, since these drugs can cause serious side effects, prophylaxis is not recommended. The risk of traveler's diarrhea can be greatly reduced by avoiding local drinking water and carefully washing foods.

DRUGS FOR INFLAMMATORY BOWEL DISEASE

Inflammatory bowel disease (IBD) has two principal forms: *Crohn's disease* and *ulcerative colitis*. Crohn's disease is characterized by transmural inflammation. The disease usually affects the terminal ileum, but can also affect any other part of the gastrointestinal tract. Ulcerative colitis is characterized by inflammation of the mucosa and submucosa of the colon and rectum. Both diseases produce abdominal cramps and diarrhea. Ulcerative colitis may produce rectal bleeding as well. In the United States, IBD afflicts about 1 million people.

Treatment of IBD depends upon its severity. When the condition is mild to moderate, it can often be managed with dietary measures and drugs. When inflammation is severe, surgery may be indicated. The principal medications employed are *sulfasalazine* and *glucocorticoids* (e.g., hydrocortisone). These

agents may be used alone or in combination. None of these drugs is curative; at best, they may control the disease process.

Sulfasalazine

Sulfasalazine [Azulfidine] belongs to the same chemical family as the sulfonamide antibiotics. However, although similar to the sulfonamides, sulfasalazine is not employed to treat infectious diseases. Rather, the drug is approved only for treatment of IBD. In addition, the drug has been used on an investigational basis to treat rheumatoid arthritis (see Chapter 63).

Actions. Sulfasalazine is metabolized by intestinal bacteria into two compounds: 5-aminosalicylic acid (5-ASA) and sulfapyridine. 5-ASA is the component responsible for reducing inflammation in IBD. In contrast, sulfapyridine is responsible for the adverse effects of treatment. Possible mechanisms by which 5-ASA reduces inflammation include suppression of prostaglandin synthesis and suppression of the migration of inflammatory cells into the affected region.

Therapeutic Uses. Sulfasalazine is most effective in the treatment of acute episodes of mild-to-moderate ulcerative colitis. Responses are less satisfactory when symptoms are severe. Sulfasalazine may also benefit patients with acute Crohn's disease.

Adverse Effects. Nausea, fever, rash, and arthralgia are common. Hematologic disorders (e.g., agranulocytosis, hemolytic anemia, macrocytic anemia) may also occur. Accordingly, complete blood counts should be obtained periodically. Sulfasalazine appears safe for use during pregnancy and lactation.

Preparations, Dosage, and Administration. Sulfasalazine [Azulfidine] is available in 500-mg tablets (plain and enteric coated) and in a suspension (250 mg/5 ml). The *initial* adult dosage is 500 mg/day. *Maintenance* dosages range from 2 to 4 gm/day in divided doses.

Glucocorticoids

The basic pharmacology of the glucocorticoids is discussed in Chapters 53 and 62; discussion here is limited to application of these drugs in IBD. Glucocorticoids can relieve symptoms of ulcerative colitis and Crohn's disease. Benefits derive from the anti-inflammatory actions of these drugs. As discussed in Chapter 62, long-term use of glucocorticoids can cause severe adverse effects, including adrenal suppression, osteoporosis, increased susceptibility to infection, and a cushingoid syndrome. When used to treat IBD, glucocorticoids may be administered orally or by injection. In addition, one agent—hydrocortisone—can be administered as a retention enema. Use of this route minimizes systemic absorption, thereby reducing the risk of adverse effects.

Mesalamine

Mesalamine is the generic name for 5-aminosalicylic acid (5-ASA), the active agent in sulfasalazine. Mesalamine is approved for treatment of mild-to-moderate ulcerative colitis. The drug is not approved for maintenance therapy. Mesalamine can be administered by retention enema, by rectal suppository, and by mouth (in tablets that dissolve when they reach the terminal ileum). The most common side effects of oral therapy are headache and gastrointestinal upset. The adult dosage for oral mesalamine [Asacol] is 800 mg three times a day. The 60-mg rectal suppositories [Rowasa] are administered twice daily. The retention enema [Rowasa] is administered once daily (4 gm in 60 ml).

Olsalazine

Olsalazine [Dipentum] is a dimer composed of two molecules of 5-aminosalicylic acid (5-ASA), the active component of sulfasalazine. Olsalazine is approved for maintenance therapy of ulcerative colitis in patients unable to tolerate sulfasalazine. The drug's most common adverse effect is watery diarrhea, which occurs in 17% of those treated. Other side effects include abdominal pain, cramps, acne, rash, and joint pain. Olsalazine is dispensed in tablets for oral administration. The adult dosage is 500 mg twice daily with food.

PANCREATIC ENZYMES

The pancreas produces four digestive enzymes: *lipase, amylase, chymotrypsin,* and *trypsin.* These enzymes are secreted into the duodenum, where they help digest fats, carbohydrates, and proteins. To protect these enzymes from stomach acid and pepsin, the pancreas secretes bicarbonate. The bicarbonate neutralizes acid in the duodenum, and the resulting elevation in pH inactivates pepsin.

Deficiency of pancreatic enzymes can compromise digestion, especially the digestion of fats. Fatty stools are characteristic of the deficiency. When availability of pancreatic enzymes is reduced, replacement therapy is needed. Causes of deficiency include pancreatectomy, cystic fibrosis, pancreatitis, and obstruction of the pancreatic duct.

Pancreatic enzymes are available as two basic preparations: *pancreatin* and *pancrelipase.* Pancreatin is made from hog or beef pancreas. Pancrelipase is made from hog pancreas. Pancrelipase has enzyme activity far greater than that of pancreatin. As a result, pancrelipase is the preferred preparation. Trade names for pancrelipase include Viokase, Entolase, Cotazym, and Pancrease MT.

Both pancreatin and pancrelipase are available in capsules that contain enteric-coated microspheres. The microsphere-containing preparations are preferred to conventional formulations (tablets, capsules) because the conventional formulations frequently fail to dissolve within the appropriate region of the intestine (i.e., the duodenum and upper jejunum).

Antacids and histamine$_2$-receptor blockers may be employed as adjuvants to pancreatic enzyme therapy. The purpose of these adjuvants is to reduce gastric pH, thereby protecting the enzymes from inactivation. However, these adjuvants are beneficial only when secretion of gastric acid is excessive.

Adverse reactions to pancreatic enzymes are rare. Allergic reactions occur occasionally. Large doses can cause diarrhea, nausea, and cramping.

Dosage is adjusted on an individual basis. Determining factors include the extent of enzyme deficiency, dietary fat content, and enzyme activity of the preparation selected. The efficacy of therapy can be evaluated by measuring the reduction in 24-hour fat excretion. Pancreatic enzymes should be taken with every meal and snack.

DRUGS USED TO DISSOLVE GALLSTONES

The gallbladder serves as a repository for bile, a fluid composed of cholesterol, bile acids, and other substances. Following its production in the liver, bile may be secreted directly into the small intestine or it may be transferred to the gallbladder, where it is concentrated and stored.

Bile has two principal functions: (1) it aids in the digestion of fats, and (2) it serves as the only medium by which cholesterol is excreted from the body. The acids present in bile facilitate the absorption of fats. In addition, bile acids help solubilize cholesterol.

Cholelithiasis (development of gallstones) is the most common form of gallbladder disease. Most stones are formed from cholesterol. Stones made of cholesterol alone cannot be detected with x-rays, and, hence, are said to be *radiolucent.* In contrast, stones that contain calcium (in addition to cholesterol) are *radiopaque* (i.e., they absorb x-rays and therefore can be seen in a radiograph). Risk factors for cholelithiasis include obesity and high blood levels of cholesterol.

For many people, gallstones can be present for years without causing symptoms. When symptoms do develop, they can be much like those of indigestion (bloating, abdominal discomfort, gassiness). If a stone should lodge in the bile duct, severe pain and jaundice may result.

Cholelithiasis may be treated surgically (by excision of the gallbladder) or with drugs. In general, when intervention is required, surgery is the preferred modality. In asymptomatic patients, more conservative measures (weight loss and reduced fat intake) may be indicated. Medications employed to dissolve gallstones are discussed below.

Chenodiol (Chenodeoxycholic Acid)

Actions. Chenodiol [Chenix] is a naturally occurring bile acid that reduces hepatic production of cholesterol. Reduced cholesterol production lowers the cholesterol content of bile, which in turn facilitates the gradual dissolution of cholesterol gallstones. Chenodiol may also increase the amount of bile acid in bile, an effect that may enhance cholesterol solubility. It should be noted that chenodiol is useful only in dissolving *radiolucent* stones. *Radiopaque* stones (stones with significant calcium content) are not affected.

Therapeutic Use. Chenodiol is given to promote dissolution of cholesterol gallstones, but only in carefully selected patients. Success is most likely in women who have low cholesterol levels, stones of small size, and the ability to tolerate high doses of the drug. Complete disappearance of stones occurs in only 20% to 40% of patients. Therapy is usually prolonged; 2 years is common.

Adverse Effects. Diarrhea occurs in 30% to 40% of patients; dosage reduction will decrease this response. Of much greater concern, chenodiol can damage the liver. Hence, patients must undergo periodic testing of liver function. Because of its hepatotoxic effects, chenodiol is contraindicated for patients with pre-existing liver impairment. Chenodiol is also contraindicated during pregnancy (FDA Pregnancy Category X) because serious hepatic, renal, and adrenal lesions have occurred in monkeys exposed to the drug *in utero.*

Preparations, Dosage, and Administration. Chenodiol [Chenix] is dispensed in 250-mg tablets for oral administration. Initial dosage is 250 mg twice daily. The dosage is then gradually increased to 15 mg/kg/day (administered in two divided doses).

Ursodiol (Ursodeoxycholic Acid)

Ursodiol [Actigall] is an analogue of chenodiol. Like chenodiol, ursodiol reduces the cholesterol content of bile, thereby facilitating the gradual dissolution of cholesterol gallstones. In contrast to chenodiol, ursodiol does not increase production of bile acids. Like chenodiol, ursodiol promotes dissolution of *radiolucent* gallstones but not *radiopaque* gallstones. Ursodiol is indicated for dissolution of cholesterol gallstones in carefully selected patients.

Ursodiol is well tolerated. Significant adverse effects are rare. The drug is classified in FDA Pregnancy Category B.

Ursodiol is dispensed in 300-mg capsules for oral administration. The usual adult dosage is 4 to 5 mg/kg twice daily (1 capsule in the morning and 1 in the evening). Treatment lasts for months.

Monoctanoin

Monoctanoin [Moctanin] is a semisynthetic vegetable oil that can dissolve *cholesterol* gallstones; extended direct contact with the gallstones is required. The only use for monoctanoin is removal of stones that remain in the common bile duct following cholecystectomy (surgical removal of the gallbladder). Administration is by continuous perfusion through a catheter placed directly in the common bile duct. Duration of perfusion is 1 to 3 weeks. Complete dissolution of stones occurs in approximately one third of those treated. Partial dissolution occurs in about 30% more. The most common side effects are gastrointestinal disturbances (abdominal pain, nausea, vomiting).

ANORECTAL PREPARATIONS

Anorectal preparations can provide symptomatic relief from the discomfort of hemorrhoids and other anorectal disorders.

The composition of these preparations varies widely. *Local anesthetics* (e.g., benzocaine, dibucaine) and *hydrocortisone* (a glucocorticoid) are common ingredients. Hydrocortisone suppresses inflammation, itching, and swelling. Local anaesthetics reduce itching and pain. Anorectal preparations may also contain *emollients* (e.g., mineral oil, lanolin), whose lubricant properties reduce irritation, and *astringents* (e.g., bismuth subgallate, witch hazel, zinc oxide), which serve to reduce irritation and inflammation. Anorectal preparations are available in multiple formulations: suppositories, creams, ointments, and foams.

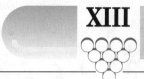

XIII

Ophthalmic Drugs

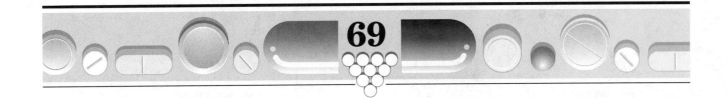

Drugs for Disorders
of the Eye

The drugs addressed in this chapter are used to diagnose and treat ophthalmic disorders. Our primary focus will be on glaucoma. Many of the drugs considered in this chapter have been discussed at length in previous chapters; for these drugs, discussion here is limited to applications that pertain to the eye.

GLAUCOMA AND ITS TREATMENT

PATHOPHYSIOLOGY AND OVERVIEW OF TREATMENT

The term *glaucoma* refers to a group of diseases characterized by elevation of intraocular pressure (IOP) with resultant damage to the optic nerve; blindness can occur. Glaucoma has two principal forms: *open-angle glaucoma* and *closed-angle glaucoma*. In both disorders, the cause of abnormally high IOP is impairment of aqueous humor outflow from the anterior chamber of the eye. As indicated in Figure 69–1, aqueous humor, which is produced by the ciliary body, is secreted into the posterior chamber of the eye, circulates around the iris into the anterior chamber, and then exits the anterior chamber via the trabecular meshwork and canal of Schlemm. When the exit routes become constricted or blocked, aqueous humor accumulates within the anterior and posterior chambers, causing IOP to rise. In both open- and closed-angle glaucoma, impairment (or loss) of vision results from injury to

875

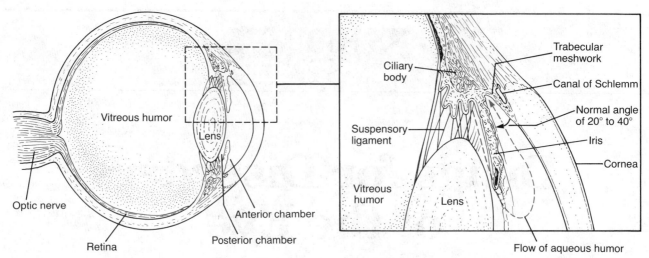

Figure 69–1. Anatomy of the normal eye.

the optic nerve: the increase in IOP causes compression of the blood vessels that supply the optic nerve; the resultant reduction in local blood flow is responsible for optic nerve injury.

Closed-Angle Glaucoma

Closed-angle glaucoma is precipitated by displacement of the iris such that it covers the trabecular meshwork, thereby preventing exit of aqueous humor from the anterior chamber. This disorder is referred to as *closed-angle* or *narrow-angle* glaucoma because the angle between the cornea and the iris is greatly reduced (Fig. 69–2). Closed-angle glaucoma is sudden in onset and extremely painful. In the absence of treatment, irreversible loss of vision occurs in 1 to 2 days. This disorder is much less common than open-angle glaucoma.

Treatment consists of *drug therapy* (to control the acute attack) followed by *corrective surgery*. A combination of drugs (osmotic agents, short-acting miotics, carbonic anhydrase inhibitors, topical beta-adrenergic blocking agents) is employed to suppress symptoms. Once IOP has been reduced with drugs, definitive treatment can be rendered with surgery. Two surgical procedures are employed: *laser iridotomy* and *iridectomy* performed by conventional surgery. Both procedures alter the iris to permit unimpeded outflow of aqueous humor.

Open-Angle Glaucoma

Open-angle glaucoma is by far the most common cause of increased IOP. Approximately 90% to 95% of individuals with glaucoma have this form of the disease. Elevation of IOP is caused by abnormalities in the trabecular meshwork and canal of Schlemm that produce resistance to the outflow of aqueous humor; there is no closure of the filtration angle. Open-angle glaucoma is a painless, insidi-

ous disease in which injury to the eye develops over a period of years. Symptoms are absent until extensive visual damage has been produced. The disease usually has a genetic basis and is most common in those over the age of 40.

Open-angle glaucoma is managed primarily by chronic drug therapy. Drugs decrease IOP by either (1) promoting outflow of aqueous humor, or (2) decreasing aqueous humor production. The principal agents employed are *pilocarpine* (a muscarinic cholinergic agonist) and *beta-adrenergic blocking drugs* (e.g., timolol). Other medications include epinephrine, cholinesterase inhibitors, and carbonic anhydrase inhibitors. With one exception—carbonic anhydrase inhibitors—the drugs employed to treat open-angle glaucoma are administered topically. Because most antiglaucoma agents are applied locally, systemic effects are rare. However, serious systemic reactions can occur if sufficient absorption from the eye takes place. In the event that drug therapy is unable to reduce IOP to an acceptable level, surgery is indicated to facilitate aqueous humor outflow. The drugs employed in open-angle glaucoma are summarized in Table 69–1.

DRUGS USED TO TREAT GLAUCOMA

Pilocarpine

Pilocarpine is a direct-acting muscarinic agonist (parasympathomimetic agent). The basic pharmacology of the muscarinic agonists is discussed in Chapter 13. Consideration here is limited to the use of pilocarpine in glaucoma.

Effects on the Eye. By stimulating cholinergic receptors in the eye, pilocarpine produces two direct effects: (1) *miosis* (constriction of the pupil caused by contraction of the iris sphincter), and (2) *contraction of the ciliary muscle* (an action that

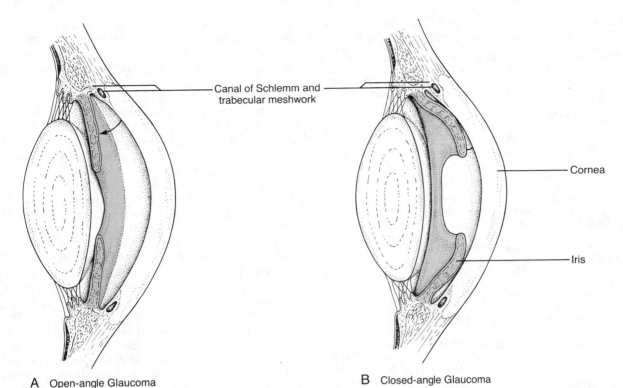

A Open-angle Glaucoma

B Closed-angle Glaucoma

Figure 69–2. Comparative anatomy of the eye in open-angle and closed-angle glaucoma. *A,* Note that the angle between the iris and cornea is open, permitting unimpeded outflow of aqueous humor through the canal of Schlemm and the trabecular meshwork. *B,* Note that the angle between the iris and cornea is constricted, thereby blocking outflow of aqueous humor through the canal of Schlemm and the trabecular meshwork.

focuses the lens for near vision). IOP is lowered indirectly. In patients with *open-angle glaucoma,* IOP is reduced because the tension generated by contraction of the ciliary muscle promotes widening of the spaces within the trabecular meshwork, thereby facilitating outflow of aqueous humor. In

Table 69–1. Drugs Used in Open-Angle Glaucoma

Beta-Adrenergic Blocking Agents
Betaxolol
Carteolol
Levobunolol
Metipranolol
Timolol

Miotics: Direct Acting
Pilocarpine
Carbachol

Miotics: Cholinesterase Inhibitors
Demecarium
Echothiophate
Isoflurophate

Sympathomimetics
Epinephrine
Dipivefrin

Carbonic Anhydrase Inhibitors
Acetazolamide
Dichlorphenamide
Methazolamide

closed-angle glaucoma, contraction of the iris sphincter pulls the iris away from the pores of the trabecular meshwork, thereby removing the impediment to aqueous humor outflow.

Therapeutic Uses. Pilocarpine is a first-line drug for initial and maintenance therapy of open-angle glaucoma. Although cholinesterase inhibitors act in much the same manner as pilocarpine (see below), pilocarpine is preferred to these drugs. In addition to its applications in open-angle glaucoma, pilocarpine can be used for emergency treatment of acute angle-closure glaucoma.

Adverse Effects. The major side effects of pilocarpine concern the eye. Contraction of the ciliary muscle focuses the lens for near vision; corrective lenses can provide partial compensation for this problem. Occasionally, sustained contraction of the ciliary muscle causes retinal detachment. Constriction of the pupil, caused by contraction of the iris sphincter, may decrease visual acuity. Pilocarpine may also produce local irritation, eye pain, and brow ache.

Rarely, pilocarpine is absorbed in amounts sufficient to cause systemic effects. Stimulation of muscarinic receptors throughout the body can produce a variety of responses, including bradycardia, bronchospasm, hypotension, urinary urgency, diarrhea, hypersalivation, and sweating. Caution should be exercised in patients with asthma or bradycardia. Systemic toxicity can be reversed with a muscarinic antagonist (e.g., atropine).

Preparations, Dosage, and Administration. Pilocarpine is available in solution, a gel, and an "ocular system." With all three formulations, administration is topical. Pilocarpine solutions have a relatively short duration of action and must be administered more frequently than the gel or ocular system.

Pilocarpine Solutions. Pilocarpine hydrochloride [Adsorbocarpine, Akarpine, Isopto Carpine, Pilocar, Piloptic, Pilostat] and *pilocarpine nitrate* [Pilagan] are dispensed in solution for topical application to the conjunctiva. Concentrations range from 0.25% to 10%. For maintenance therapy of open-angle glaucoma, the usual dosage is 1 drop of solution (0.5% to 4%) applied four times a day. For patients with acute angle-closure glaucoma, the drug is applied much more frequently (e.g., every 5 to 10 minutes for 3 to 6 doses, then 1 drop every 1 to 3 hours).

Pilocarpine Gel. Pilocarpine ophthalmic gel [Pilopine HS] consists of 4% pilocarpine hydrochloride in an aqueous gel base. The preparation has a long duration of action, making once-a-day dosing sufficient. For chronic open-angle glaucoma, the usual dosage is one-half inch of gel applied to the conjunctiva at bedtime.

Pilocarpine Ocular System. The pilocarpine ocular system [Ocusert Pilo-20, Ocusert Pilo-40] consists of a bilayered membrane surrounding a reservoir of pilocarpine solution. The tiny unit is placed in the conjunctival sac, after which pilocarpine is slowly released. A replacement unit should be installed once a week. The ocular system is indicated for chronic open-angle glaucoma. Since the unit may fall out during sleep, patients should be advised to check each morning for its presence. Occasionally, the ocular system may migrate to the cornea, causing discomfort and disturbance of vision. Conjunctival irritation may also occur.

Beta-Adrenergic Blocking Agents

Five beta-adrenergic antagonists—*betaxolol, carteolol, metipranolol, levobunolol,* and *timolol*—are approved for treatment of glaucoma. These agents cause less disturbance of vision than pilocarpine and are first-line drugs for glaucoma. The basic pharmacology of the beta-blocking drugs is discussed in Chapter 18. Consideration here is limited to the use of these agents in glaucoma.

Mechanism of Action. The beta-adrenergic blockers lower IOP by decreasing production of aqueous humor. Reductions in IOP occur with "nonselective" beta blockers (drugs that block beta$_1$ *and* beta$_2$ receptors) as well as with "cardioselective" beta blockers (drugs that block beta$_1$ receptors only). It is not certain that the beneficial effects of the beta-receptor antagonists are actually due to beta-receptor blockade. This uncertainty stems from the observation that beta-adrenergic *agonists* (e.g., isoproterenol) can also lower IOP.

Use in Glaucoma. Beta blockers are used primarily for open-angle glaucoma. These drugs are suitable for initial therapy and maintenance therapy. Efficacy of the beta blockers is equivalent to that of pilocarpine. In addition to their use in open-angle glaucoma, beta-receptor antagonists may be employed in combination with other drugs for emergency management of acute closed-angle glaucoma.

Adverse Effects. Local effects are generally minimal, although patients commonly complain of transient ocular stinging. Occasionally, the beta blockers cause conjunctivitis, blurred vision, photophobia, and dry eyes.

Beta blockers can be absorbed in amounts sufficient to cause *systemic effects*. These reactions are more important than local effects. Effects on the heart and lung are of greatest concern.

Blockade of cardiac beta$_1$ receptors can produce bradycardia and A-V heart block. Pulse rate should be monitored. Because of their ability to depress cardiac function, beta blockers are contraindicated for patients with heart failure, A-V heart block, sinus bradycardia, and cardiogenic shock. The risk of cardiac effects is about equal with all of the ophthalmic beta blockers.

Blockade of beta$_2$ receptors in the lung can cause bronchospasm. Constriction of the bronchi can occur with "beta$_1$-selective" antagonists as well as with "nonselective" beta-adrenergic blockers. However, the risk is greatest with the nonselective agents. Only one ophthalmic beta blocker is beta$_1$ selective. This agent—*betaxolol*—would seem to be the best drug for patients with asthma or chronic obstructive pulmonary disease.

Preparations, Dosage, and Administration. The ophthalmic beta blockers are listed in Table 69–2. As shown in the table, these drugs differ from one another in two important ways: (1) receptor selectivity, and (2) frequency of dosing.

Sympathomimetics: Epinephrine and Dipivefrin

Epinephrine is an adrenergic agonist that acts at alpha- and beta-adrenergic receptors. The basic pharmacology of epinephrine is discussed in Chapter 17. Consideration here is limited to the use of this drug in glaucoma.

Dipivefrin is a prodrug form of epinephrine. Because of its high lipid solubility, dipivefrin penetrates the cornea more readily than epinephrine. Once in the eye, dipivefrin is converted to its active form—epinephrine—by ocular enzymes.

Actions and Uses in Glaucoma. Epinephrine is used to treat open-angle glaucoma. The drug reduces IOP apparently by increasing aqueous humor outflow. The mechanism by which outflow is enhanced is not understood. Epinephrine may be used alone and in combination with beta blockers, carbonic anhydrase inhibitors, osmotic agents, and miotics (pilocarpine, cholinesterase inhibitors).

Adverse Effects. Mild reactions—headache, brow ache, blurred vision, ocular irritation—are relatively common. In the patient whose lens has been removed, epinephrine can cause an unusual edema of the retina. This reaction is reversible upon discontinuation of treatment. Epinephrine can dilate the pupil and thereby aggravate closed-angle glaucoma. Accordingly, epinephrine is contraindicated for patients with this disorder. Systemic absorption can cause tachycardia and elevation of blood

Table 69–2. Beta-Adrenergic Blocking Agents Used in Glaucoma

Drug	Receptor Specificity	Formulation	Usual Dosage
Betaxolol [Betoptic]	beta$_1$	0.25% suspension 0.5% solution	1 drop twice a day 1 drop twice a day
Carteolol [Ocupress]	beta$_1$, beta$_2$	1% solution	1 drop twice a day
Levobunolol [Betagan Liquifilm]	beta$_1$, beta$_2$	0.25% solution 0.5% solution	1 drop twice a day 1 drop once or twice a day
Metipranolol [OptiPranolol]	beta$_1$, beta$_2$	0.3% solution	1 drop twice a day
Timolol [Timoptic]	beta$_1$, beta$_2$	0.25% solution 0.5% solution	1 drop once or twice a day 1 drop once or twice a day

pressure; caution should be exercised in patients with hypertension, dysrhythmias, and hyperthyroidism (hyperthyroidism sensitizes the heart to stimulation by catecholamines).

Preparations, Dosage, and Administration. Ophthalmic solutions of epinephrine contain one of two salts: *epinephrine hydrochloride* [Epifrin, Glaucon] or *epinephrine borate* [Epinal, Eppy/N]. For treatment of open-angle glaucoma, 1 drop of solution (0.25% to 2%) is instilled into the conjunctival sac once or twice daily.

Dipivefrin [Propine] is dispensed in a 0.1% solution. For treatment of open-angle glaucoma, 1 drop is instilled into the conjunctival sac every 12 hours.

Long-Acting Cholinesterase Inhibitors: Demecarium, Echothiophate, and Isoflurophate

The basic pharmacology of the cholinesterase inhibitors is discussed in Chapter 16. Consideration here is limited to the use of these drugs in glaucoma.

Effects on the Eye. The cholinesterase inhibitors inhibit breakdown of acetylcholine (ACh), thereby promoting accumulation of ACh at muscarinic receptors. By doing so, cholinesterase can produce the same ocular effects as pilocarpine (i.e., miosis, focusing of the lens for near vision, reduction of IOP).

Use in Glaucoma. The cholinesterase inhibitors are indicated for chronic open-angle glaucoma. However, because of concerns about adverse effects (see below), these agents are not drugs of first choice. Rather, they should be reserved for patients who have responded poorly to preferred medications (pilocarpine, epinephrine, beta-adrenergic antagonists).

Adverse Effects. Like pilocarpine, cholinesterase inhibitors can cause *myopia* (secondary to contraction of the ciliary muscle) and *excessive pupillary constriction*. However, of much greater concern is the association between long-acting cholinesterase inhibitors and development of *cataracts*. Absorption of cholinesterase inhibitors into the systemic circulation can produce typical parasympathomimetic responses, including bradycardia, bronchospasm, sweating, salivation, urinary urgency, and diarrhea.

Preparations, Dosage, and Administration. Demecarium bromide [Humorsol] is dispensed in sterile solution (0.125%, 0.25%) for topical application to the eye. For initial treatment of open-angle glaucoma, 1 drop is instilled into the conjunctival sac every 12 to 48 hours.

Echothiophate iodide [Phospholine Iodide] is dispensed as a powder for reconstitution to solutions that range in strength from 0.03% to 0.25%. For initial treatment of open-angle glaucoma, 1 drop of 0.03% or 0.06% solution is instilled into the conjunctival sac every 12 to 48 hours.

Isoflurophate [Floropryl] is dispensed in an ointment (0.025%) for topical use. For treatment of open-angle glaucoma, one-quarter inch of ointment is applied to the eye every 8 to 72 hours.

Physostigmine [Eserine, Isopto Eserine] is dispensed in solution (0.25%, 0.5%) and an ointment (0.25%) for topical use. Dosage for the solution is 1 or 2 drops applied to the eye up to four times a day. The ointment is applied to the lower fornix up to three times a day. Chronic treatment with physostigmine is associated with a high incidence of conjunctivitis.

Carbonic Anhydrase Inhibitors

Three carbonic anhydrase inhibitors—*acetazolamide, dichlorphenamide,* and *methazolamide*—are used to treat glaucoma. Acetazolamide is the most frequently employed.

Actions and Uses in Glaucoma. The carbonic anhydrase inhibitors lower IOP by decreasing production of aqueous humor. Maximally effective doses reduce flow of aqueous humor by 50%. Administration is *oral*.

Carbonic anhydrase inhibitors are employed primarily for long-term treatment of open-angle glaucoma. These agents are not drugs of first choice. Rather, they should be reserved for patients who have been refractory to treatment with preferred medications (pilocarpine, beta-blocking drugs, epinephrine, cholinesterase inhibitors). Carbonic anhydrase inhibitors may also be given (in combination with other antiglaucoma drugs) to produce rapid lowering of IOP in patients with angle-closure glaucoma.

Adverse Effects. Carbonic anhydrase inhibitors can produce a variety of adverse effects. Effects on the nervous system are relatively common and include malaise, anorexia, fatigue, and paresthesias. The sense of malaise causes many patients to discontinue drug use. Reduced appetite, coupled with gastrointestinal disturbances (nausea, vomiting, diarrhea) may result in weight loss. Carbonic anhydrase inhibitors are teratogenic in animals and should be avoided by women who are pregnant, especially during the first trimester. Additional concerns are hypokalemia and formation of renal calculi.

Preparations, Dosage, and Administration. Acetazolamide [Diamox, Dazamide] is dispensed in tablets (125 and 250 mg) and sustained-release capsules (500 mg) for oral use, and as an injection (500 mg/vial) for IM and IV administration. The usual dosage range is 250 mg to 1 gm per day in divided doses.

Dichlorphenamide [Daranide] and *methazolamide* [Neptazane] are available in 50-mg tablets for oral use. The usual dosage for dichlorphenamide is 25 to 50 mg one to three times a day. The usual dosage for methazolamide is 50 to 100 mg two or three times a day.

Osmotic Agents

Four osmotic agents—*mannitol, urea, glycerin,* and *isosorbide*—are employed in the treatment of glaucoma. These preparations render the plasma hypertonic to intraocular fluid and thereby draw water from the eye. This action results in a rapid and marked reduction of IOP. The principal indication for osmotic agents is emergency treatment of acute closed-angle glaucoma. Use in open-angle glaucoma is limited to the perioperative period. Two of the osmotic agents (glycerin and isosorbide) are administered orally; the other two (mannitol and urea) are administered by IV infusion. Doses for these drugs range from 0.5 to 2 gm/kg. Common side effects are headache, nausea, and vomiting. The use of mannitol for osmotic diuresis is discussed in Chapter 35.

CYCLOPLEGICS AND MYDRIATICS

Cycloplegics are drugs that cause paralysis of the ciliary muscle, whereas *mydriatics* are drugs that dilate the pupil. Cycloplegics and mydriatics are employed primarily to facilitate diagnosis and surgery of ophthalmic disorders. Agents used to produce cycloplegia, mydriasis, or both fall into two classes: (1) *anticholinergic agents* (muscarinic antagonists), and (2) *adrenergic agonists*.

ANTICHOLINERGIC AGENTS

Several muscarinic antagonists (Table 69–3) are employed topically for diagnosis and treatment of ophthalmic disorders. The basic pharmacology of the anticholinergic drugs is discussed in Chapter 13. Consideration here is limited to the ophthalmic applications of these drugs.

Effects on the Eye

The anticholinergic drugs produce mydriasis and cycloplegia. Mydriasis results from blockade of the muscarinic receptors that promote contraction of the iris sphincter; cycloplegia is caused by blockade of the muscarinic receptors that promote contraction of the ciliary muscle. As discussed below, relaxation of the iris can lead to elevation of IOP.

Ophthalmic Applications

Adjunct to Measurement of Refraction. The term *refraction* refers to the bending of light by the cornea and lens. When ocular refraction is proper, incoming light is bent such that a sharp image is formed on the retina. Errors in refraction can produce nearsightedness, farsightedness, and astigmatism (a visual disturbance caused by irregularities in the curvature of the cornea).

Both the mydriatic and cycloplegic properties of the muscarinic antagonists can be of use in evaluating errors of refraction. Mydriasis (widening of the pupil) facilitates observation of the eye's interior. Cycloplegia (paralysis of the ciliary muscle) prevents the lens from undergoing changes in configuration during the assessment.

Intraocular Examination. Dilatation of the pupil with an anticholinergic agent facilitates observation of the inside of the eye. In addition, by paralyzing the iris sphincter, muscarinic antagonists prevent reflexive constriction of the pupil in response to the light from an ophthalmoscope (the hand-held device used to view the eye's interior). Since adrenergic agonists (e.g., phenylephrine) also dilate the pupil—but by a mechanism different from that of the anticholinergic drugs—an adrenergic agonist can be combined with a muscarinic antagonist to increase the degree of mydriasis.

Intraocular Surgery. Anticholinergic agents may be employed to facilitate ocular surgery and reduce postoperative complications. Mydriasis in-

			Time Course of Effects			
			Mydriasis		Cycloplegia	
Generic Name	**Trade Name(s)**	**Strength of Solution (%)**	*Peak (min)*	*Recovery (days)*	*Peak (min)*	*Recovery (days)*
Atropine	Atropisol Isopto Atropine Atropine Care	1	30–40	7–12	60–180	6–12
Cyclopentolate	AK-Pentolate Cyclogyl I-Pentolate	0.5–1	30–60	1	25–75	0.25–1
Homatropine	Isopto Homatropine	1	40–60	1–3	30–60	1–3
Scopolamine	Isopto Hyoscine	0.5	20–30	3–7	30–60	3–7
Tropicamide	Mydriacyl Tropicacyl Opticyl	0.5–1	20–40	0.25	20–35	0.25

Table 69–3. Muscarinic Antagonists Used for Mydriasis and Cycloplegia

duced by these drugs can aid in cataract extraction and in procedures to correct retinal detachment. For these operations, the muscarinic antagonist may be combined with an adrenergic agonist to maximize pupillary dilatation. In certain postoperative patients, mydriatics are employed to prevent development of synechiae (adhesions of the iris to neighboring structures in the eye).

Treatment of Anterior Uveitis. Uveitis is an inflammation of the uvea (the vascular layer of the eye). Symptoms include ocular pain and photophobia. Uveitis is treated with a glucocorticoid (to reduce inflammation) plus an anticholinergic agent. By promoting relaxation of the ciliary muscle and the iris sphincter, anticholinergic drugs help relieve pain and prevent adhesion of the iris to the lens.

Adverse Effects

Blurred Vision and Photophobia. The most common side effects of topical anticholinergic drugs are photophobia and blurred vision. Photophobia occurs because paralysis of the iris sphincter prevents the pupil from constricting in response to bright light. Vision is blurred because paralysis of the ciliary muscle prevents focusing for near vision.

Precipitation of Angle-Closure Glaucoma. By relaxing the iris sphincter, anticholinergic drugs can induce closure of the filtration angle in individuals whose eyes have a narrow angle to begin with. Angle closure occurs as follows: (1) partial dilatation of the pupil maximizes contact between the iris and the lens, thereby impeding exit of aqueous humor from the posterior chamber, and (2) the resultant increase in pressure within the posterior chamber pushes the iris forward, causing blockage of the trabecular meshwork. Caution must be exercised in patients predisposed to angle closure.

Systemic Effects. Topically applied anticholinergic drugs can be absorbed in amounts sufficient to produce systemic toxicity. Symptoms include dry mouth, blurred vision, photophobia, constipation, fever, tachycardia, and CNS effects (confusion, hallucinations, delirium, coma); death can occur. Muscarinic poisoning can be treated with physostigmine (see Chapter 16).

ADRENERGIC AGONISTS

Adrenergic agonists are mydriatic agents; pupillary dilatation results from stimulation of alpha-adrenergic receptors located on the radial (dilator) muscle of the iris. The adrenergic agonists do not cause cycloplegia. Of the adrenergic agents given to induce mydriasis, *phenylephrine* is the most fre-

quently employed. The adrenergic agonists are considered at length in Chapter 17. The discussion here is limited to the mydriatic use of *phenylephrine*.

Therapeutic and Diagnostic Applications

The mydriatic applications of phenylephrine are much like those of the anticholinergic drugs. Phenylephrine-induced mydriasis is used as an aid to intraocular surgery, measurement of refraction, and ophthalmoscopic examination. In patients with anterior uveitis, phenylephrine is given to dilate the pupil as part of an overall program of treatment.

Adverse Effects

Effects on the Eye. Like the anticholinergic drugs, phenylephrine can precipitate angle-closure glaucoma secondary to production of mydriasis; caution must be exercised in patients whose filtration angle is naturally narrow. Contraction of the dilator muscle may dislodge pigment granules from degenerating cells of the iris; these granules, which appear as "floaters" in the anterior chamber, are usually cleared from the eye within a day. Phenylephrine may also cause ocular pain, corneal clouding, and brow ache.

Systemic Effects. Rarely, topically applied phenylephrine is absorbed in amounts sufficient to produce systemic toxicity. Cardiovascular responses (e.g., hypertension, ventricular dysrhythmias, cardiac arrest) are of greatest concern. Other systemic reactions include sweating, blanching, tremor, agitation, and confusion.

MISCELLANEOUS OPHTHALMIC DRUGS

Demulcents (Artificial Tears)

Ophthalmic demulcents are isotonic solutions employed as substitutes for natural tears. Most preparations contain *polyvinyl alcohol, cellulose esters,* or both. Artificial tears are indicated for treatment of dry-eye syndromes and for relief of discomfort and dryness caused by irritants, wind, and sun. In addition, demulcents may be used to lubricate artificial eyes. Artificial tears are devoid of adverse effects and, hence, may be administered as frequently and for as long as desired.

Ocular Decongestants

Ocular decongestants are weak solutions of adrenergic agonists applied topically to produce constriction of dilated conjunctival blood vessels. These preparations are used to reduce redness of the eye caused by minor irritation. The adrenergic agents employed as decongestants are *phenylephrine, naphazoline,* and *tetrahydrozoline.* When applied to the eye in the low concentrations present in decongestant products, adrenergic agonists rarely cause adverse effects. Local reactions (stinging, burning, reactive hyperemia) may occur with overuse. The adrenergic agonists are discussed at length in Chapter 17.

Glucocorticoids

Glucocorticoids (corticosteroids) are used for inflammatory disorders of the eye (e.g., uveitis, iritis, conjunctivitis). Administration may be topical or by local injection. Short-term therapy is generally devoid of adverse effects. In contrast, prolonged therapy may cause cataracts, reduced visual acuity, and glaucoma. In addition, there is an increased risk of infection secondary to corticosteroid-induced suppression of host defenses. The glucocorticoids are discussed at length in Chapter 62.

Dyes

Fluorescein is a water-soluble dye that produces an intense green color. This agent is applied to the surface of the eye to detect lesions of the corneal epithelium: intact areas of the cornea remain uncolored while abrasions and other defects turn bright green. Intravenous fluorescein is used to facilitate visualization of retinal blood vessels; IV fluorescein has been employed as an aid for evaluating diabetic retinopathy and other abnormalities of the retinal vasculature. Fluorescein can also be used topically and IV to assess flow of aqueous humor. Adverse effects from systemic administration include nausea, vomiting, paresthesias, and pruritus; severe reactions (anaphylaxis, pulmonary edema, cardiac arrest) are rare.

Rose bengal is applied topically to visualize abrasions of the corneal and conjunctival epithelium. Injured tissue appears rose colored when viewed with a slit lamp. The dye is employed for diagnosis of superficial injury to corneal and conjunctival tissue.

Corneal Dehydrating Agents

Anhydrous glycerin [Ophthalgan], *hypertonic sodium chloride* [Adsorbonac, AK-NaCl, Muro–128], and *hypertonic glucose* [Glucose-40] are used topically to reduce edema of the cornea. When applied to the surface of the eye, these agents create a hypertonic film that extracts water from the corneal epithelium. Topical glycerin is painful and therefore unsuited for long-term use. Hypertonic sodium chloride may cause transient stinging and burning.

Chymotrypsin

Chymotrypsin [Catarase, Zolyse] is a proteolytic enzyme employed during surgery of intracapsular cataracts; the enzyme is given to dissolve the ciliary zonules (i.e., the suspensory structures that support the lens). Chymotrypsin is administered by injection behind the iris into the posterior chamber. Adverse effects include elevation of intraocular pressure, corneal edema, and uveitis; healing of incisions may be delayed.

Antiviral Agents

Three drugs—trifluridine, vidarabine, and idoxuridine—are used topically to treat viral infections of the eye. The pharmacology and applications of these drugs are discussed in Chapter 84 (Antiviral Agents).

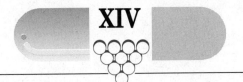

Dermatologic Drugs

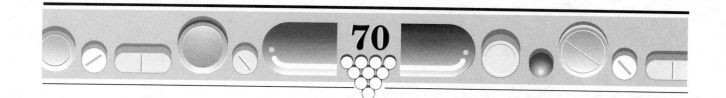

Drugs for Dermatologic Disorders

O ur objective in this chapter is to discuss some of the more frequently encountered dermatologic drugs. Most are employed topically; some require systemic administration. Before discussing the dermatologic drugs, we will review the anatomy of the skin.

ANATOMY OF THE SKIN

The skin is composed of three distinct layers: the epidermis, the dermis, and a layer of subcutaneous fat. These layers and other features of the skin are depicted in Figure 70–1.

Epidermis. The epidermis is the outermost layer of the skin and is composed almost entirely of closely packed cells. As indicated in Figure 70–1B, the epidermis itself consists of several layers. The deepest layer, known as the *basal cell layer* or *stratum germinativum*, contains the only epidermal cells that are mitotically active. All cells of the epidermis arise from this layer. Production of new cells within the basal layer pushes older cells outward. During their migration, these cells become smaller and flatter. As epidermal cells near the surface of the skin, they die and their cytoplasm becomes converted to keratin, a hard proteinaceous material. Because of its high content of ker-

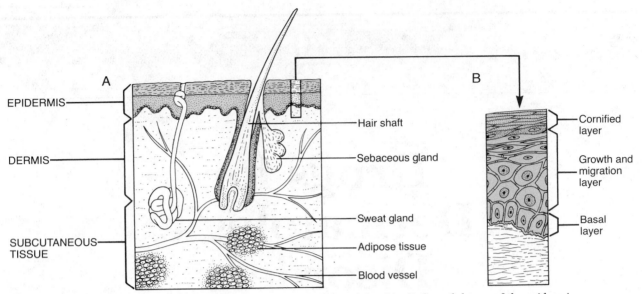

Figure 70–1. Anatomy of the skin. *A,* Major structures of the skin. *B,* Growth layers of the epidermis.

atin, the outer layer of the epidermis has a rough, horny texture. Because of its texture, this layer is referred to as the *cornified layer* or *stratum corneum.* By a process that is not fully understood, the surface of the stratum corneum undergoes continuous exfoliation (shedding). This shedding completes the growth cycle of the epidermis.

In addition to germinal cells, the basal layer of the epidermis contains *melanocytes.* These cells, which are few in number, serve to produce *melanin,* the pigment that determines skin color. Following its synthesis within melanocytes, melanin is transferred to other cells of the epidermis. Melanin protects the skin against ultraviolet radiation, which is the principal stimulus for melanin production.

Dermis. The dermis underlies the epidermis and is composed largely of connective tissue, primarily *collagen.* A major function of the dermis is to provide support and nourishment for the epidermis. Structures found in the dermis include blood vessels, nerves, and muscle. The dermis also contains *sweat glands, sebaceous glands,* and *hair follicles,* structures that are unique to the skin. The sebaceous glands secrete an oily composite known as *sebum.* Almost all sebaceous glands are found in association with hair follicles (see Figure 70–1).

Subcutaneous Tissue. Subcutaneous tissue consists in large part of fat. This fatty layer provides protection and insulation. In addition, the stored fat constitutes a reserve source of calories.

TOPICAL GLUCOCORTICOIDS

The basic pharmacology of the anti-inflammatory corticosteroids is discussed in Chapter 62.

Consideration here is limited to the use of glucocorticoids to treat disorders of the skin.

Actions and Uses. Topical glucocorticoids are employed to relieve inflammation and itching associated with a variety of dermatologic disorders (e.g., insect bites, minor burns, seborrheic dermatitis, psoriasis, eczema, pemphigus). The mechanisms by which glucocorticoids suppress inflammation and other symptoms are discussed in Chapter 62.

The vehicle in which a glucocorticoid is dispersed (e.g., cream, ointment, gel) can enhance the therapeutic response by facilitating penetration of the glucocorticoid to its site of action. The vehicle may provide additional benefits by acting as a drying agent or an emollient.

Relative Potency. Glucocorticoid preparations vary widely in potency. As indicated in Table 70–1, steroid preparations can be assigned to five groups based on their relative potency. Preparations within each group are of approximately equal potency.

It is important to note that the intensity of the response to topical glucocorticoids depends not only on the concentration and inherent activity of the glucocorticoid, but also on the vehicle employed and the method of application. Occlusive dressings can enhance percutaneous absorption by as much as tenfold, thereby greatly increasing pharmacologic effects.

Absorption. Topical glucocorticoids can be absorbed into the systemic circulation. The extent of absorption is proportional to the duration of use and the area over which the preparation has been applied. Absorption is higher from regions where the skin is especially permeable (scalp, axilla, face, eyelids, neck, perineum, genitalia) and lower from

Table 70–1. Relative Potency of Topical Glucocorticoid Preparations

Potency Class and Drug	Formulation	Concentration
Super-High Potency		
Betamethasone dipropionate [Diprolene]	Cream, ointment, lotion	0.05%
Clobetasol propionate [Temovate]	Cream, ointment	0.05%
Diflorasone diacetate [Psorcon]	Ointment	0.05%
Halobetasol propionate [Ultravate]	Cream, ointment	0.05%
High Potency		
Amcinonide [Cyclocort]	Cream, ointment, lotion	0.1%
Betamethasone dipropionate [Diprosone]	Cream, ointment, lotion	0.05%
Diflorasone diacetate [Florone, Maxiflor]	Cream, ointment	0.05%
Fluocinolone acetonide [Synalar]	Cream	0.2%
Fluocinonide [Lidex]	Cream, ointment	0.05%
Halcinonide [Halog]	Cream, ointment, solution	0.1%
Triamcinolone acetonide [Aristocort]	Cream, ointment	0.5%
Medium Potency		
Betamethasone benzoate [Uticort]	Lotion	0.025%
Betamethasone valerate [Valisone]	Cream, ointment, lotion	0.1%
Desoximetasone [Topicort]	Cream	0.05%
Fluocinolone acetonide [Flurosyn, Synalar]	Cream, ointment	0.025%
Hydrocortisone valerate [Westcort]	Cream, ointment	0.2%
Mometasone furoate [Elocon]	Cream, ointment, lotion	0.1%
Flurandrenolide [Cordran]	Cream, ointment, lotion	0.05%
Halcinonide [Halog]	Cream	0.025%
Triamcinolone acetonide [Aristocort, Kenalog]	Cream, ointment, lotion	0.1%
Fluticasone propionate [Cutivate]	Ointment	0.005%
	Cream	0.05%
Low Potency		
Betamethasone valerate [Valisone]	Cream	0.01%
Clocortolone [Cloderm]	Cream	0.1%
Desonide [DesOwen, Tridesilon]	Cream, ointment	0.05%
Fluocinolone acetonide [Flurosyn, Synalar]	Cream	0.01%
Flurandrenolide [Cordran]	Cream, ointment	0.025%
Triamcinolone acetonide [Aristocort, Kenalog]	Cream, ointment, lotion	0.025%
Lowest Potency		
Dexamethasone [Decadron Phosphate]	Cream	0.1%
Hydrocortisone [Cort-Dome]	Cream, ointment, lotion	1%
Hydrocortisone [Hydrocort]	Cream, ointment	2.5%

regions where penetrability is poor (back, palms, soles). Absorption through intact skin is less than through inflamed skin. As noted above, absorption is influenced by the vehicle employed, and can be greatly increased by use of an occlusive dressing.

Adverse Effects. Adverse effects may be local or systemic. Factors that increase the risk of adverse effects include use of high-potency glucocorticoids, use of occlusive dressings, prolonged therapy, and application over a large surface area.

Local Reactions. Glucocorticoids increase the risk of local infection, and may also produce irritation. With prolonged use, glucocorticoids can cause atrophy of the dermis and epidermis, resulting in thinning of the skin, striae (stretch marks), purpura (red spots caused by local hemorrhage), and telangiectasia (red, wart-like lesions caused by capillary dilation). Long-term therapy may induce acne and hypertrichosis (excessive growth of hair, especially on the face).

Systemic Toxicity. Topical glucocorticoids can be absorbed in amounts sufficient to produce systemic toxicity. Principal concerns are growth retardation (in children) and adrenal suppression (in patients of all ages). Systemic toxicity is more likely under extreme conditions of use (prolonged therapy in which extensive surfaces are treated with large doses of high-potency agents in conjunction with occlusive dressings). When these conditions are present, monitoring of the hypothalamic-pituitary-adrenal axis is indicated. Systemic toxicity of the glucocorticoids is discussed at length in Chapter 62.

Administration. Topical glucocorticoids should be applied in a thin film and gently rubbed into the skin. Patients should be advised not to use occlusive dressings (bandages, plastic wraps) unless directed to do so by the physician. Tight-fitting diapers and plastic pants can act as occlusive dressings and should not be worn when glucocorticoids are applied to the diaper region of infants.

KERATOLYTIC AGENTS

Keratolytic agents are drugs that promote shedding of the horny layer of the skin. Effects range from peeling to extensive desquamation of the stratum corneum. Three keratolytic compounds—*salicylic acid, resorcinol,* and *sulfur*—are considered below. A fourth agent—*benzoyl peroxide*—is discussed in the context of drugs used to treat acne.

Salicylic Acid. Salicylic acid promotes desquamation by dissolving the intracellular cement that binds scales to the stratum corneum. Keratolytic effects are achieved with drug concentrations ranging from 3% to 6%. At concentrations above 6%, tissue injury is likely. Low (3% to 6%) concentrations are used to treat dandruff, seborrheic dermatitis, acne, and psoriasis. Higher concentrations (up to 40%) are used to remove warts and corns.

Salicylic acid is readily absorbed through the skin; systemic toxicity (salicylism) can result. Symptoms include tinnitus, hyperpnea, and psychologic disturbances. Systemic effects can be minimized by avoiding prolonged use of high concentrations over a large surface.

Resorcinol. Resorcinol has mild keratolytic and antimicrobial activity. The drug is used to treat acne, eczema, psoriasis, and seborrheic dermatitis. Resorcinol is available in a variety of formulations, including shampoos, ointments, lotions, and creams. Usual concentrations range from 1% to 10%.

Sulfur. Sulfur promotes peeling and drying. The compound has been used to treat acne, dandruff, psoriasis, and seborrheic dermatitis. Sulfur is available in lotions, gels, and shampoos. Concentrations range from 2% to 10%.

ACNE AND ITS TREATMENT

PATHOPHYSIOLOGY

Acne is a skin disorder common in adolescents and young adults. Lesions usually develop on the face, neck, chest, shoulders, and back. In mild acne, *open comedones* (blackheads) are the most common lesion. A comedo forms when sebum combines with keratin to form a plug within a pore (oxidation of the sebum causes the exposed surface of the plug to turn black). *Closed comedones* (whiteheads) develop when pores become stuffed with sebum and scales below the skin surface. In its most severe form, acne is characterized by abscesses and inflammatory cysts.

Onset of acne is initiated by increased production of androgens during adolescence. Under the influence of these hormones, sebum production and turnover of follicular epithelial cells are increased, leading to plugging of pores. Symptoms are intensified by the activity of *Propionibacterium acnes*, an organism that converts sebum into irritant fatty acids. This bacterium also releases chemotactic factors that promote inflammation. Oily skin and a genetic predisposition are additional contributing factors.

OVERVIEW OF TREATMENT

Nondrug Therapy

Nondrug measures can help minimize lesions, especially in patients with milder forms of acne.

Surface oiliness should be reduced by gentle cleansing two to three times daily. Care should be taken to avoid irritation from vigorous scrubbing and use of abrasives. Oil-based moisturizing products should be avoided. Additional nondrug measures (e.g., comedo extraction, dermabrasion, collagen injection) may be indicated for some individuals. Dietary measures are devoid of beneficial effects.

Drug Therapy

Drug selection is based on severity of symptoms. *Mild* acne can be managed with cleansers, drying agents (acetone, alcohol), and keratolytics (sulfur, resorcinol, salicylic acid, and 2.5% or 5% benzoyl peroxide). Topical agents for *moderate* acne include 10% benzoyl peroxide, tretinoin, and antibiotics (clindamycin, erythromycin, meclocycline, tetracycline). Oral tetracycline may also be used. Drugs for *severe* acne include systemic antibiotics (usually tetracycline), isotretinoin, and intralesional glucocorticoids.

DRUGS USED TO TREAT ACNE

Benzoyl Peroxide

Actions and Uses. Benzoyl peroxide is employed topically to treat mild-to-moderate acne. The drug decreases symptoms by (1) promoting keratolysis (peeling of the horny layer of the epidermis) and (2) suppressing growth of *P. acnes*. (Antibacterial effects result from release of active oxygen.)

Adverse Effects. Benzoyl peroxide may produce drying and peeling of the skin. If signs of severe local irritation occur (e.g., burning, blistering, scaling, swelling), the frequency of application should be reduced. The drug is absorbed through the skin, but systemic toxicity has not been reported.

Preparations, Dosage, and Administration. Benzoyl peroxide is available in a variety of formulations (e.g., lotions, creams, gels) for topical use. Concentrations range from 2.5% to 10%. For initial therapy, once-a-day application is recommended. Later, the frequency of administration can be increased to four times per day as tolerance permits. Patients should be advised to avoid application to the eyes, mouth, and mucous membranes, and to inflamed or denuded skin.

Antibiotics

Topical. Topical antibiotics are indicated for moderate acne. Agents approved for this use are *clindamycin, tetracycline, meclocycline,* and *erythromycin*. Clindamycin is employed most frequently. Although tetracycline is the most frequently used *oral* antibiotic for acne, it is the least frequently used *topical* antibiotic. The low use of topical tetracycline is based on its relatively low efficacy when used topically and the fact that it gives a yellow color to the skin.

Oral. When acne is severe enough to warrant systemic antibiotic therapy, oral *tetracycline* is the treatment of choice. Tetracycline is effective, inexpensive, and has low toxicity. Treatment reduces the population of *P. acnes*, the amount of keratin in sebaceous follicles, and the percentage of free fatty acids in surface lipids. A satisfactory alternative to tetracycline is *erythromycin*. Oral *clindamycin* is effective in acne, but the risk of severe toxicity (pseudomembranous colitis) limits the drug's utility.

Tretinoin

Therapeutic Use. Tretinoin, a derivative of vitamin A, is indicated for *topical* treatment of *mild-to-moderate* acne. Therapeutic effects can be enhanced by using tretinoin in combination with benzoyl peroxide and oral antibiotics. Tretinoin should not be confused with isotretinoin, an antiacne medication that is administered orally (see below).

In recent years, topical tretinoin has been used in attempts to improve the appearance of photodamaged skin. Clinical trials suggest a possible modest reduction in roughness, wrinkling, and hyperpigmented macules ("liver spots").

Mechanism of Action. Although the precise mechanism of action is not known, tretinoin is thought to produce its beneficial effects at least in part by increasing the turnover and reducing the cohesiveness of epithelial cells within hair follicles. These actions may promote removal of existing comedones and may suppress the formation of new plugs. By reducing the thickness of the stratum corneum, tretinoin can enhance penetration of other antiacne drugs.

Adverse Effects. Tretinoin can cause localized reactions, but absorption is insufficient to produce systemic toxicity. In patients with sensitive skin, tretinoin may induce blistering, peeling, crusting, burning, and edema. These effects can be intensified by concurrent use of abrasive soaps and keratolytic agents (e.g., sulfur, resorcinol, benzoyl peroxide, salicylic acid). Accordingly, these preparations should be discontinued prior to tretinoin therapy. Tretinoin can aggravate symptoms of eczema and sunburn.

Preparations, Dosage, and Administration. Tretinoin [Retin-A] is available in three formulations: cream (0.05%, 0.1%), gel (0.01%, 0.025%), and liquid (0.05%). Administration is topical, usually once daily at bedtime. Before application, the skin should be washed, toweled dry, and then allowed to dry fully for 15 to 30 minutes. The drug should not be applied to open wounds or to areas of sunburn or windburn. Contact with the eyes, nose, and mouth should be avoided.

Isotretinoin

Actions and Use. Isotretinoin, a derivative of vitamin A, is used to treat *severe* acne vulgaris, a condition for which the drug is highly effective. For most patients, a single course of therapy can produce complete and prolonged remission. However, because the risk of serious side effects is high, isotretinoin should be reserved for patients who have failed to respond to more conventional agents, including oral antibiotics.

Isotretinoin has several actions that may contribute to its antiacne effects. The drug decreases sebum production and sebaceous gland size. In addition, it reduces inflammation and keratinization. Lastly, by decreasing availability of sebum, a nutrient for *P. acnes*, isotretinoin lowers the skin population of this microbe.

Pharmacokinetics. Absorption from the gastrointestinal tract is rapid but incomplete. In the blood, isotretinoin is nearly 100% bound to plasma albumin. The drug undergoes metabolism in the liver and possibly in cells of the intestinal wall. Excretion is by a combination of renal and biliary processes. The drug's half-life is 10 to 20 hours.

Adverse Effects. The most common reactions are nosebleeds (80%), inflammation of the lips (90%), inflammation of the eyes (40%), and dryness or itching of the skin, nose, and mouth (80%). About 15% of patients experience pain, tenderness, or stiffness in muscles, bones, and joints. Less common reactions include skin rash, headache, hair loss, and peeling of skin from the palms and soles. Reductions in night vision have occurred, sometimes with sudden onset. The skin may become sensitized to ultraviolet light; patients should be advised to wear protective clothing or a sunscreen if responses to sunlight become exaggerated. Rarely, isotretinoin may cause optic neuritis, cataracts, papilledema (edema of the optic disk), and pseudotumor cerebri (benign elevation of intracranial pressure).

Triglyceride levels may become elevated. Blood triglyceride content should be measured prior to treatment and periodically during therapy until effects on triglycerides have been evaluated. Alcohol can potentiate hypertriglyceridemia and should be avoided.

Although adverse effects occur frequently, most reverse upon discontinuing the drug. Teratogenic effects are the major and obvious exception to this rule.

Contraindication: Pregnancy. *Isotretinoin is teratogenic and must not be used during pregnancy.* The drug is classified in FDA Pregnancy Category X: the risks of use during pregnancy clearly outweigh any possible benefits. Major fetal abnormalities that have occurred include hydrocephalus, microcephaly, facial malformation, cleft palate, cardiovascular defects, and abnormal formation of the outer ear.

Before isotretinoin is given to women of childbearing age, pregnancy should be ruled out and a method of contraception implemented. Contraception should be initiated at least 1 month prior to the onset of treatment and should continue for at least 1 month after treatment has ceased. Women should be thoroughly counseled about the potential for fetal harm if pregnancy should occur. If pregnancy does occur, isotretinoin should be discontinued immediately, and possible termination of the pregnancy should be discussed.

Drug Interactions. Adverse effects of isotretinoin can be increased by *tetracyclines* and *vitamin A.* Tetracyclines increase the risk of pseudotumor cerebri and papilledema. Vitamin A, being a relative of isotretinoin, can produce generalized intensification of isotretinoin toxicity. Because of the potential for increased toxicity, tetracyclines and vitamin A supplements should be discontinued prior to isotretinoin therapy.

Preparations, Dosage, and Administration. Isotretinoin [Accutane] is dispensed in capsules (10, 20, and 40 mg) for oral administration. The usual course of treatment is 0.5 to 1 mg/ kg/day (in two divided doses) for 15 to 20 weeks. If needed, a second course may be given, but not until 2 months have elapsed after completing the first course.

PSORIASIS AND ITS TREATMENT

PATHOPHYSIOLOGY

Psoriasis is a chronic disorder that follows an erratic course. The initial episode usually develops in early adulthood. Subsequent attacks may occur spontaneously or may be triggered by emotional stress, streptococcal pharyngitis (sore throat), and certain drugs (e.g., propranolol, indomethacin). There is no cure for psoriasis, but symptoms can usually be controlled with medication. Drug-induced remission is common and may last for a few weeks to many years.

Psoriasis has varying degrees of severity. Mild disease manifests as red patches covered with silvery scales; lesions typically appear on the scalp, elbows, knees, palms, and soles. Severe disease may involve the entire skin surface and mucous membranes. In addition, patients may develop superficial pustules, high fever, leukocytosis, and painful fissuring of the skin. The primary defect underlying symptoms is accelerated maturation of the epidermis: in people with psoriasis, epidermal cells complete their growth cycle in 3 to 4 days, rather than the 26 to 28 days required for maturation in healthy skin.

OVERVIEW OF DRUG THERAPY

Drug selection is based on the severity of symptoms. For mild psoriasis, topical glucocorticoids are usually adequate; keratolytic agents (e.g., sulfur, salicylic acid) may be useful adjuncts to steroid therapy. For patients with moderate symptoms, coal tar or anthralin may be added to the regimen. Topical therapy with tar and anthralin can be enhanced by exposing the skin to ultraviolet light. Severe psoriasis may require treatment with systemic methotrexate or with photochemotherapy. Vitamin A derivatives—etretinate, tretinoin, isotretinoin—may also be employed.

DRUGS USED TO TREAT PSORIASIS

Anthralin

Actions and Uses. Anthralin is indicated only for topical treatment of psoriasis. The drug inhibits DNA synthesis and thereby suppresses proliferation of hyperplastic epidermal cells.

Adverse Effects. Anthralin may cause local irritation, especially when applied in concentrations exceeding 1%. Erythema (redness) may develop in normal skin adjacent to areas of treatment. Severe conjunctivitis can develop following contact with the eyes. Systemic toxicity has not been documented. Anthralin preparations can stain clothing, skin, and hair.

Preparations, Dosage, and Administration. Anthralin is dispensed in ointments and creams, with concentrations ranging from 0.1% to 1%. In conventional therapy, the drug is applied to lesions at bedtime and allowed to remain in place overnight. Stains can be avoided by wearing old clothing and by covering treated areas with a dressing. Trade names for anthralin products are Anthra-Derm, Lasan, Drithocreme, and Dritho-Scalp.

Tars

Tars suppress DNA synthesis, mitotic activity, and cell proliferation. Coal tar is the tar employed most frequently. Preparations that contain juniper tar, birch tar, and pine tar are also available. Tar-containing products (e.g., shampoos, lotions, creams) are used to treat psoriasis and other chronic disorders of the skin. Tars have an unpleasant odor and can cause irritation, smarting, and burning. They may also stain the skin and hair. Systemic toxicity does not occur.

Methotrexate

The basic pharmacology of methotrexate [Folex, Mexate] is discussed in Chapter 91 (Representative Anticancer Drugs). Consideration here is limited to the use of methotrexate for psoriasis.

Actions and Use in Psoriasis. Methotrexate is a cytotoxic agent that shows some selectivity for tissues with a high growth fraction (i.e., tissues with a large percentage of actively dividing cells). Benefits in psoriasis result from reduced proliferation of epidermal cells. The biochemical mechanisms underlying suppression of cell growth and division are discussed in Chapter 91. Methotrexate is highly toxic (see below) and should be used only in patients with severe, debilitating psoriasis that has not responded to safer therapy.

Adverse Effects. Methotrexate is administered systemically, and toxicity can be severe. Death has occurred. Patients should be fully informed of the risks of treatment. Close medical supervision is required. Gastrointestinal effects (diarrhea, ulcerative stomatitis) are the most frequent causes for interruption of therapy. Blood dyscrasias (anemia, leukopenia, thrombocytopenia) from bone marrow depression are an additional major concern. With prolonged use, even at relatively low doses, methotrexate can cause significant harm to the liver; hepatic function should be monitored. The drug can cause congenital anomalies and fetal death. Accordingly, methotrexate is contraindicated during pregnancy.

Dosage and Administration. Methotrexate may be administered PO, IM, or IV. Various dosing schedules have been developed. In one schedule, the drug is administered once a week as a single large dose (10 to 25 mg). In an alternative schedule, three smaller doses (2.5 to 5 mg) are administered at 12-hour intervals; this dosing sequence is repeated weekly. Regardless of the schedule chosen, dosages must be individualized.

Photochemotherapy (PUVA Therapy)

Photochemotherapy combines the use of long-wave ultraviolet radiation (ultraviolet A, UVA) with *methoxsalen*, an orally administered photosensitive drug. Methoxsalen belongs to a chemical family known as psoralens. In response to UVA light shined on the skin, methoxsalen is thought to undergo a photochemical reaction with DNA, resulting in the formation of a DNA-psoralen complex. This alteration in DNA structure is thought to underlie the ability of photochemotherapy to decrease proliferation of epidermal cells. Adverse effects associated with the procedure include pruritus, nausea, and erythema. In addition, the process may accelerate aging of the skin and may increase the risk of skin cancer. Photochemotherapy is indicated for patients with extensive, active psoriasis who have not responded adequately to more conventional therapy. An alternative name for photochemotherapy is *PUVA therapy*; PUVA is an acronym derived from *psoralen* and *ultraviolet A*.

Etretinate

Therapeutic Use. Oral etretinate is indicated for severe pustular and erythrodermic psoriasis. Side effects can be severe. Hence, the drug should be reserved for patients who have not responded to safer treatments. Initial responses develop in many patients after 4 to 6 weeks of treatment. However, other patients may require 6 months of treatment before a clinical response is evident. Long-term maintenance therapy is sometimes required.

Mechanism of Action. Etretinate acts on epithelial cells to inhibit keratinization, proliferation, and differentiation. These actions probably contribute to the drug's beneficial effects in psoriasis. Benefits may also derive from the drug's anti-inflammatory and immunomodulatory actions.

Adverse Effects. Adverse effects are extremely common. Dermatologic effects (hair loss; peeling of palms, soles, and fingertips) occur in 75% of patients. Mucous membranes are affected, causing dry nose (75%), thirst and sore mouth (50-75%), and nose bleed (25%). Other very common reactions include bone and joint pain (50-75%), muscle cramps (25-50%), fatigue (50-75%), headache (25-50%), and eye irritation (50-75%). In addition, etretinate can elevate plasma concentrations of cholesterol and triglycerides, and can reduce levels of high-density lipoproteins.

Contraindication: Pregnancy. *Etretinate can cause severe fetal malformations and must not be used during pregnancy.* The drug is classified in FDA Pregnancy Category X: the risks to the developing fetus outweigh any possible benefits of treatment. Pregnancy must be ruled out before etretinate is given. Women of child-bearing age should be instructed to use some form of contraception before starting treatment, during treatment, and for an indefinite period after treatment has stopped (etretinate can be measured in the blood up to 3 years after terminating treatment). If pregnancy occurs during treatment, etretinate should be discontinued immediately, and termination of pregnancy should be considered.

Preparations, Dosage, and Administration. Etretinate [Tegison] is dispensed in capsules (10 and 25 mg) for oral administration. The usual initial adult dosage is 0.75 to 1 mg/kg/day in divided doses. The maximum dosage is 1.5 mg/kg/day.

MISCELLANEOUS DERMATOLOGIC DRUGS

AGENTS USED TO REMOVE WARTS

The common wart (verruca vulgaris) is a virally induced skin disease that manifests as a hard, horny nodule. Warts may appear anywhere on the body but are most common on the hands and feet. It should be noted that warts are benign lesions and their presence is no threat to health.

Warts may be removed by physical procedures and by application of drugs. The nondrug methods of wart removal are freezing, electrodesiccation (destruction with an electric current), and curettage (surgical removal with a loop-shaped cutting tool). The principal pharmacologic agents employed are *salicylic acid, podophyllum resin, podofilox,* and *cantharidin.* Salicylic acid was discussed earlier in the chapter; podophyllum, podofilox, and cantharidin are discussed below.

Podophyllum Resin

Actions and Uses. Podophyllum resin is indicated primarily for condylomata acuminata (venereal warts). The drug is not very effective against common warts. The major active component of podophyllum resin is *podophyllotoxin,* a compound that inhibits synthesis of DNA and mitosis. These actions eventually lead to cell death and erosion of warty tissue.

Adverse Effects. Podophyllum can be absorbed in amounts sufficient to cause systemic toxicity. Systemic effects are most likely when the drug is applied to large areas and in excessive amounts. Potential systemic reactions include central and peripheral neuropathy, kidney damage, and blood dyscrasias. Podophyllum is teratogenic and must not be used during pregnancy.

Preparations and Administration. Podophyllum resin [Pod-Ben-25, Podocon-25, Podofin] is available in a 25% solution for topical use. Application should be limited to small areas. The drug should not be applied to moles or birthmarks, nor should it be applied to warts that are bleeding or friable (easily crumbled) or that have undergone recent biopsy. When used to remove venereal warts, podophyllum resin should be washed off 1 to 6 hours after application. Treatment may be repeated at weekly intervals for up to 4 weeks.

Cantharidin

Cantharidin [Cantharone, Verr-Canth] is a topical agent used to remove common warts and the nodules associated with molluscum contagiosum, a benign, virally induced skin disease. Clearance of these growths results from acantholysis (dissolution of intercellular bridges within the epidermis). Lower layers of the skin are not affected. For treatment of common warts, cantharidin is applied to the lesion, allowed to dry, and covered with nonporous tape. The tape should be removed in 24 hours. If needed, this procedure may be repeated in 1 to 2 weeks. Cantharidin is harmful to normal skin. In the event of accidental exposure, the affected area should be cleansed immediately with acetone or alcohol.

ANTIPERSPIRANTS AND DEODORANTS

Perspiration is produced by two types of sweat glands: *eccrine* glands and *apocrine* glands. The eccrine glands secrete profuse, watery perspiration. The output of apocrine glands is low in volume and rich in organic compounds. The unpleasant odor associated with sweating results from chemical and bacterial degradation of the compounds in apocrine sweat. Eccrine glands contribute to odor formation by creating a moist environment that favors growth of bacteria. Perspiration odor can be reduced with *antiperspirants* (agents that decrease flow of eccrine sweat) and *deodorants* (antiseptics that suppress growth of skin-dwelling bacteria).

Antiperspirants. The principal compounds employed as antiperspirants are *aluminum chlorohydrate, aluminum zirconium chlorohydrate, aluminum chloride,* and *buffered aluminum sulfate.* These agents can decrease flow of eccrine sweat by 20% to 50%. The reduction in flow is thought to result from inhibition of sweat production and from partial occlusion of sweat glands. Topical antiperspirants can cause stinging, burning, itching, and irritation; dermatitis and ulceration occur rarely.

Deodorants. Deodorants inhibit growth of the surface bacteria that degrade components of apocrine sweat into malodorous products; deodorants do not suppress sweat formation.

Agents employed as deodorants include *carbanilide, triclocarban,* and *triclosan.* These antiseptics are the active ingredients in deodorant soaps, such as Dial, Lifebuoy, Safeguard, and Zest.

DRUGS FOR SEBORRHEIC DERMATITIS AND DANDRUFF

Seborrheic dermatitis is characterized by inflammation and scaling of the scalp and face. Skin of the underarms, chest, and anogenital region may also be affected. The disorder is associated with increased rates of maturation and proliferation of epidermal cells. Activity of *Pityrosporum ovale,* a microbe belonging to the yeast family, may also contribute to symptoms. Dandruff results from a mild form of seborrheic dermatitis involving the scalp.

A variety of compounds are used to treat seborrheic dermatitis and dandruff. *Topical corticosteroids* are often the most effective form of therapy; benefits derive from the ability of these drugs to suppress proliferation of epidermal cells. Several compounds, including *pyrithione zinc, selenium sulfide, chloroxine, salicylic acid,* and *sulfur,* are employed in antidandruff-antiseborrheic shampoos. Pyrithione zinc, selenium sulfide, and chloroxine possess cytotoxic and modest antifungal activity; hence, these agents can decrease epidermal cell proliferation and may also suppress growth of *P. ovale.* Beneficial effects of salicylic acid and sulfur derive from keratolytic actions.

TOPICAL MINOXIDIL FOR BALDNESS

Minoxidil is a direct-acting vasodilator used primarily for severe hypertension. The basic pharmacology of minoxidil is discussed in Chapter 39. Consideration here is limited to the use of minoxidil to promote hair growth.

Actions, Uses, and Dosage. A 2% minoxidil solution [Rogaine] is approved for topical treatment of male-pattern baldness. The usual dosage is 1 ml applied 2 times/day. Topical minoxidil increases cutaneous blood flow (by inducing vasodilation), and may also stimulate resting hair follicles to enter a state of active growth. These actions may explain the ability of minoxidil to promote hair growth.

Clinical Response. Minoxidil can retard loss of hair and stimulate hair growth. Beneficial effects take several months to develop. Unfortunately, response rates have been somewhat disappointing: only about one third of patients experience significant restoration of hair to regions of baldness. Hair regrowth is most likely when baldness has developed recently and has been limited to a small area. Upon discontinuation of minoxidil, newly gained hair is lost in 3 to 4 months, and the natural progression of hair loss resumes. In some cases, beneficial effects may decline even with uninterrupted treatment.

Adverse Effects. Topical minoxidil is generally devoid of adverse effects. A few patients have experienced pruritus and local allergic responses (e.g., rash, swelling, burning sensation). Absorption is low (about 1.5%), and systemic reactions (e.g., hypotension, headache, flushing) are rare.

DEBRIDING ENZYMES

Topical enzymes can be applied to burns and wounds to facilitate debridement (removal of foreign material and necrotic tissue). Three such debriding preparations—*collagenase, sutilains,* and a *fibrinolysin-desoxyribonuclease combination*—are discussed below.

Collagenase. Collagenase [Santyl] digests native and denatured collagen, the compound that composes 75% of the dry weight of skin. By dissolving collagen, the enzyme can facilitate loosening and removal of tissue debris. Collagenase is used to promote debridement of dermal lesions and severe burns. The enzyme is inactivated by detergents, certain antiseptics (hexachlorophene, nitrofurazone, benzalkonium chloride, iodine), and heavy metals (e.g., mercury, silver). Accordingly, these compounds must be removed by careful washing prior to collagenase use. Collagenase ointment is applied once daily and covered with a sterile dressing. Side effects are limited to transient erythema in surrounding tissue. Allergic and toxic reactions have not been reported.

Sutilains. Sutilains [Travase] is a proteolytic enzyme that digests necrotic material but has no effect on viable tissue. The enzyme is used as an aid to debridement of decubitus ulcers, second- or third-degree burns, and other skin lesions. Like collagenase, sutilains can be inactivated by detergents and certain antiseptics (e.g., hexachlorophene, nitrofurazone, benzalkonium chloride, iodine); hence, these agents must be removed by washing prior to sutilains application. Sutilains ointment should be applied to the site of injury and to adjacent healthy skin, and the treated area should then be covered with a wet dressing. Application may be repeated three or four times each day. Mild local reactions (transient pain, paresthesias) are benign. In the event of more serious local toxicity (hemorrhage, dermatitis), sutilains should be discontinued. Systemic toxicity has not been reported.

Fibrinolysin plus Desoxyribonuclease. Fibrinolysin is an enzyme that digests fibrin, a major component of clots; desoxyribonuclease digests desoxyribonucleic acid (DNA). The rationale for the combined use of these enzymes derives from the observation that purulent exudates are composed largely of fibrin and nucleic acids. The enzyme combination is indicated for debridement of surgical wounds, ulcerative lesions, and second- or third-degree burns. Side effects include local irritation and erythema. The combination of fibrinolysin plus desoxyribonuclease is dispensed in two forms: an ointment, and a powder for reconstitution to solution. These products are marketed under the trade name Elase.

FLUOROURACIL

The basic pharmacology of fluorouracil is discussed in Chapter 91 (Representative Anticancer Drugs). Discussion here is limited to the use of fluorouracil for dermatologic disorders.

Actions and Uses in Dermatology. Fluorouracil is indicated for topical treatment of *multiple actinic keratoses* and *superficial basal cell carcinoma*. Cytotoxic effects result from disruption of DNA and RNA synthesis. A course of topical treatment elicits the following sequence of responses: (1) mild inflammation; (2) severe inflammation, often with burning, stinging, and vesicle formation; (3) tissue disintegration, characterized by erosion, ulceration, and necrosis; and (4) healing. Although fluorouracil is only applied for 2 to 6 weeks, the process just described may require 3 or more months for completion.

Adverse Effects. Among the more frequent reactions to fluorouracil are itching, burning, rash, inflammation, and increased sensitivity to sunlight. Intense, burning pain develops occasionally. Darkening of the skin is rare. Absorption is insufficient to cause systemic toxicity.

Preparations and Administration. Fluorouracil [Efudex, Fluoroplex] is dispensed in a cream (1% and 5%) and solution (1%, 2%, and 5%) for topical use. For treatment of actinic keratoses, the drug is applied twice daily until a stage-three response (tissue disintegration) develops, usually within 2 to 6 weeks. Complete healing may not occur for another 1 to 2 months.

SUNSCREENS

Sunlight has multiple effects on the skin. In addition to promoting tanning, solar radiation can cause burns, premature aging of the skin, and skin cancer. Sun exposure can also cause photosensitivity reactions to drugs. All of these effects are due to ultraviolet light. Sunburn, carcinogenesis, and premature aging of the skin are caused primarily by ultraviolet (UV) radiation in the B range (wavelengths of 290 to 320 nm). In contrast, tanning and most drug-related photosensitivity reactions are triggered by UV light in the A range (wavelengths of 320 to 400 nm).

Therapeutic Uses of Sunscreens. Sunscreens impede penetration of solar radiation to viable cells of the skin. These preparations are used primarily to prevent sunburn. Sunscreens are also used to prevent skin cancer, delay premature aging of the skin, and prevent photosensitivity reactions to certain drugs (e.g., tricyclic antidepressants, phenothiazines, sulfonamides, sulfonylureas).

Compounds Employed as Sunscreens. Most compounds employed as sunscreens act by absorbing UV light. The agents used to absorb UV radiation fall into five major groups: (1) para-aminobenzoic acid (PABA) and its esters, (2) cinnamates, (3) salicylates, (4) benzophenones, and (5) anthranilates. All of these compounds absorb UV radiation in the B range; only the benzophenones and anthranilates have the additional ability to absorb some UVA light.

Two new sunscreen formulations—Photoplex and Shade UVA Guard—offer extended protection against UVA radiation. Photoplex has two active ingredients: padimate O, which provides UVB protection, and avobenzone, which provides extended UVA protection. Shade UVA Guard has three active ingredients: octyl methoxycinnamate, which provides UVB protection, and avobenzone and oxybenzone, which provide extended UVA protection. Because they protect against UVA, Photoplex and Shade UVA Guard may be superior to other sunscreens for preventing photosensitivity reactions to drugs.

Some sunscreens act as physical barriers to the sun's rays. Hence, rather than absorbing solar radiation, these compounds reflect and scatter sunlight, thereby preventing its penetration to the skin. The agents employed as physical sunblocks include *titanium dioxide, zinc oxide,* and *talc.* Preparations containing these compounds are especially useful for protecting limited areas (e.g., nose, lips, tips of ears).

Sun Protection Factor. Commercial sunscreen products are labeled with a sun protection factor (SPF). The SPF is determined by shining UV light on adjacent regions of protected and unprotected skin and recording the time required for erythema (redness) to develop in both areas. The SPF is calculated by dividing the time required for erythema to develop in the protected region by the time required for erythema to develop in the unprotected region. For example, if the unprotected region developed erythema in 15 minutes, whereas 150 minutes were required for burn to appear in the protected region, the sunscreen would have an SPF of 10 (150 divided by 15). The SPF for most sunscreens lies between 2 (low protection) and 15 (high protection). It should be noted that the methods for determining the SPF are not highly precise; hence, all products labeled with the same SPF may not provide an equal degree of protection.

Using Sunscreens to Prevent Sunburn. Sunscreens must be used properly to achieve maximum benefit. Individuals who have skin that burns easily should choose a preparation with a high SPF. For all people, protection is greatest when a sunscreen has been allowed to penetrate the skin in advance of exposure to the sun. Accordingly, it is recommended that sunscreens be applied 30 minutes to 1 hour prior to going outdoors. The amount applied is an important determinant of protection; 2 mg/cm^2 is considered adequate. Sunscreens should be reapplied after swimming and profuse sweating; failure to do so reduces the duration of protection. However, it is important to note that reapplication will not extend the period of protection beyond that indicated by the SPF. That is, if treated skin can be expected to burn when sun exposure exceeds 2 hours, no amount of reapplication can prevent burning if the duration of exposure exceeds this limit.

Environmental factors play a part in sunscreen use. The intensity of UVB radiation is greatest between the hours of 10 AM and 3 PM. Accordingly, the need for a sunscreen is correspondingly high during this time. Ultraviolet radiation can be reflected by painted surfaces, white sand, and snow, thereby augmenting total UV exposure; the contribution of reflected radiation should be considered when choosing a sunscreen. Clouds can filter out UV radiation. However, it should be appreciated that the amount of UV light reaching the ground on a bright day with thin cloud cover can be as much as 80% of that reaching the ground on days that are sunny and clear. Ultraviolet radiation can penetrate at least several centimeters of clear water; swimmers should be made aware of this fact.

Adverse Effects of Sunscreens. Sunscreens are generally well tolerated. Contact sensitivity and photosensitivity reactions occur in a few individuals. These reactions can be elicited by almost all sunscreen products. However, for most people, a nonsensitizing preparation can be found.

LOCAL ANESTHETICS

Local anesthetics (e.g., benzocaine, dibucaine) can be applied topically to relieve pain and itching associated with various skin disorders, including sunburn, plant poisoning, fungal infections, diaper rash, and eczema. Selection of a topical anesthetic is based on required duration of action, desired vehicle (cream, ointment, solution, gel), and prior history of hypersensitivity reactions. The pharmacology of the local anesthetics is discussed in Chapter 31. Table 31–2 lists the agents available for application to the skin.

ANTI-INFECTIVE AGENTS

The skin is subject to fungal, viral, and bacterial infections. Some of these infections respond to topical treatment, whereas others require systemic therapy. *Antibacterial* drugs are discussed in Chapters 73 through 85. *Antifungal* and *antiviral* drugs are discussed in Chapters 83 and 84, respectively. Topical drugs for prophylaxis against infection (antiseptics) are discussed in Chapter 85.

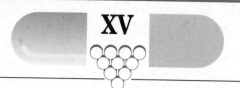

XV

Nutrients

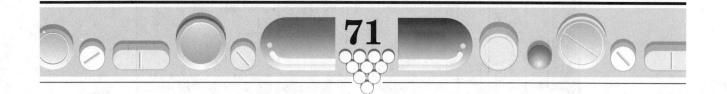

Vitamins

Vitamins have the following defining characteristics: (1) they are *organic* compounds, (2) they are required in *minute* amounts for growth and maintenance of health, and (3) they do not serve as sources of energy (in contrast to fats, carbohydrates, and proteins), but rather are *essential for energy transformation and for the regulation of metabolic processes.* Several vitamins are inactive in their native form and must be converted into active compounds within the body.

GENERAL CONSIDERATIONS

VITAMIN ALLOWANCES

Recommended Dietary Allowances

Recommended dietary allowances (RDAs) for vitamins are listed in Table 71–1. These values are established by the Food and Nutrition Board of the National Academy of Sciences and are intended to provide a standard for good nutrition. RDAs are revised periodically as new information becomes available. The values in Table 71–1 were released in 1989. It is important to note that RDAs apply only to individuals in good health. Vitamin requirements can be increased by illness. Hence, the allowances recommended in the table may not be appropriate for people who are sick. With the possible exception of the RDA for vitamin D, the values in the table represent a 100% *excess* of the vitamin intake considered necessary to avoid deficiency. Hence, RDAs should not be looked upon as *minimum* daily requirements. Also, RDAs should

Table 71–1. Recommended Daily Dietary Allowances[a]

	Age (years)	Fat-Soluble Vitamins				Water-Soluble Vitamins						
		A (μg RE)[b]	D (μg)[c]	E (mg αTE)[d]	K (μg)	C (mg)	Thiamine (mg)	Riboflavin (mg)	Niacin (mg NE)[e]	B_6 (mg)	Folacin (μg)	B_{12} (μg)
Infants	0.0–0.5	375	7.5	3	5	30	0.3	0.4	5	0.3	25	0.3
	0.5–1.0	375	10	4	10	35	0.4	0.5	6	0.6	35	0.5
Children	1–3	400	10	6	15	40	0.7	0.8	9	1.0	50	0.7
	4–6	500	10	7	20	45	0.9	1.1	12	1.1	75	1.0
	7–10	700	10	7	30	45	1.0	1.2	13	1.4	100	1.4
Males	11–14	1000	10	10	45	50	1.3	1.5	17	1.7	150	2.0
	15–18	1000	10	10	65	60	1.5	1.8	20	2.0	200	2.0
	19–24	1000	10	10	70	60	1.5	1.7	19	2.0	200	2.0
	25–50	1000	5	10	80	60	1.5	1.7	19	2.0	200	2.0
	51+	1000	5	10	80	60	1.2	1.4	15	2.0	200	2.0
Females	11–14	800	10	8	45	50	1.1	1.3	15	1.4	150	2.0
	15–18	800	10	8	55	60	1.1	1.3	15	1.5	180[f]	2.0
	19–24	800	10	8	60	60	1.1	1.3	15	1.6	180[f]	2.0
	25–50	800	5	8	65	60	1.0	1.3	15	1.6	180[f]	2.0
	51+	800	5	8	65	60	1.0	1.2	13	1.6	180[f]	2.0
Pregnant		800	10	10	65	70	1.5	1.6	17	2.2	400	2.2
Breast-feeding	1st 6 months	1300	10	12	65	95	1.6	1.8	20	2.1	280	2.6
	2nd 6 months	1200	10	11	65	90	1.6	1.7	20	2.1	260	2.6

[a]The allowances are intended to provide for individual variations among most normal persons as they live in the United States under usual environmental stresses.
[b]Retinol equivalents (1 RE = 1 μg retinol or 6 μg beta-carotene)
[c]As cholecalciferol (10 μg cholecalciferol = 400 IU vitamin D)
[d]Alpha-tocopherol equivalents (1 alpha-TE = 1 mg d-alpha-tocopherol)
[e]1 NE (niacin equivalent) is equal to 1 mg of niacin or 60 mg of dietary tryptophan.
[f]The Centers for Disease Control and Prevention recommends that all women who may become pregnant ingest 400 μg of folic acid each day.
Adapted with permission from Recommended Dietary Allowances, 10th ed. Copyright 1992 by the National Academy of Sciences. Courtesy of the National Academy Press, Washington, DC.

not be confused with official United States Recommended Daily Allowances (see below).

For the vast majority of healthy people, diet alone can be relied upon to provide RDAs of all vitamins. Consequently, although consumption of vitamin supplements is widespread, the practice is generally unnecessary and, in some cases, may even be harmful.

In the case of two vitamins—biotin and pantothenic acid—no RDAs have been set because of a lack of sufficient data. In lieu of RDAs, the Food and Nutrition Board has set established ranges of Estimated Safe and Adequate Daily Dietary Intakes for these vitamins. These values do not appear in Table 71–1, but they *are* given in the text.

United States Recommended Daily Allowances

Official United States Recommended Daily Allowances (U.S. RDAs), which are designated by the United States Food and Drug Administration, serve as a legal standard for labeling foods with respect to their nutritional content. U.S. RDAs are also used for labeling over-the-counter vitamin supplements. The U.S. RDAs are derived from RDAs established by the Food and Nutrition Board in 1968, and are similar to the RDAs presented in Table 71–1.

CLASSIFICATION OF VITAMINS

The vitamins are divided into two major groups: fat-soluble vitamins and water-soluble vitamins. In the fat-soluble group are vitamins A, D, E, and K. The water-soluble group consists of vitamin C and members of the vitamin B complex (thiamine, riboflavin, niacin, pyridoxine, pantothenic acid, biotin, folic acid, cyanocobalamin).

FAT-SOLUBLE VITAMINS

VITAMIN A (RETINOL)

Actions. Vitamin A, also known as retinol, has multiple functions. In the eyes, vitamin A plays an important role in adaptation to dim light. The vitamin is also needed to maintain the structural and functional integrity of the skin and mucous membranes.

Sources. Requirements for vitamin A can be met by (1) consuming foods that contain preformed vitamin A (retinol), and (2) consuming foods that contain beta-carotene, a compound that is converted to retinol by cells of the intestinal mucosa. Preformed vitamin A is present only in foods of animal origin. Good sources are butter, eggs, whole milk, and liver. Beta-carotene is a pigment found in many plants. Especially rich sources are carrots, spinach, tomatoes, and pumpkins.

Units. The unit employed to measure vitamin A activity is called the *retinol equivalent*. By definition, 1 retinol equivalent equals 1 μg of retinol or 6 μg of beta-carotene. The 1:6 ratio between retinol and beta-carotene reflects the fact that dietary beta-carotene is poorly absorbed and incompletely converted into retinol. Hence, 6 μg of dietary beta-carotene is required to produce the nutritional effect of 1 μg of retinol.

In the past, vitamin A activity was measured in International Units (IU). One IU is equal to 0.3 retinol equivalents.

Pharmacokinetics. Under normal conditions, dietary vitamin A is readily absorbed and then stored in the liver. As a rule, liver reserves of the vitamin are large and will last for months if intake of retinol ceases. Normal plasma levels for retinol range from 30 to 70 μg/dl. In the absence of vitamin A intake, these levels will be maintained through mobilization of liver reserves. As liver stores approach depletion, plasma levels will begin to decline. Signs and symptoms of deficiency appear when plasma levels fall below 20 μg/dl.

Deficiency. Because of the role of vitamin A in dark adaptation, night blindness is often the first indication of deficiency. With time, vitamin A deficiency may lead to *xerophthalmia* (a dry, thickened condition of the conjunctiva) and *keratomalacia* (degeneration of the cornea with keratinization of the corneal epithelium). When vitamin A deficiency is severe, blindness may occur. In addition to effects on the eye, deficiency can produce skin lesions and dysfunction of mucous membranes.

Toxicity. Excessive doses of vitamin A can cause toxicity (hypervitaminosis A). Chronic intoxication affects multiple organ systems, especially the liver. Symptoms of toxicity are diverse and may include vomiting, jaundice, hepatosplenomegaly, skin changes, hypomenorrhea, and elevation of intracranial pressure. Most symptoms disappear following vitamin A withdrawal. To avoid toxicity, it is recommended that routine consumption of vitamin A not exceed 7500 retinol equivalents per day.

Therapeutic Uses. The only indication for vitamin A is prevention or correction of vitamin A deficiency. Certain derivatives of vitamin A (tretinoin, isotretinoin, etretinate) are used to treat acne and other dermatologic disorders (see Chapter 70).

Preparations, Dosage, and Administration. Vitamin A (retinol) is dispensed in the form of drops and capsules for oral administration and as an injection for intramuscular use. Oral administration is generally preferred. For *prevention* of deficiency, dietary plus medicinal vitamin A should add up to the

RDA (see Table 71–1). For *treatment* of deficiency, doses as high as 100 times the RDA may be required.

VITAMIN D

Vitamin D plays a critical role in the regulation of calcium and phosphorus metabolism. In children, vitamin D deficiency causes *rickets*. In adults, deficiency causes *osteomalacia*. Excessive amounts of the vitamin are toxic. Symptoms result primarily from hypercalcemia. The pharmacology and physiology of vitamin D are discussed at length in Chapter 52 (Drugs Affecting Calcium Levels and Utilization).

VITAMIN E (ALPHA-TOCOPHEROL)

Vitamin E (alpha-tocopherol) is essential to the health of many species, but has no established role in the nutrition of humans. The vitamin has antioxidant properties and these may help protect essential cellular components from oxidation. It may also protect red blood cells from hemolysis. In laboratory animals, vitamin E deficiency produces a variety of symptoms, some of which are severe. In humans, vitamin E deprivation has no discernible effect. The vitamin is also devoid of toxicity to humans. Since the nutritional role of vitamin E is uncertain, it is difficult to determine dietary requirements. The RDAs given in Table 71–1 are sufficient to maintain plasma content of the vitamin within the normal range. Although numerous uses for vitamin E have been proposed, the only established indication is the prevention or correction of deficiency. However, recent studies suggest that *high* doses of vitamin E (e.g., 250 alpha-tocopherol equivalents/day) may protect against heart disease; clinical studies designed to provide a definitive answer to this question are in progress. Vitamin E is present in fresh greens and many other vegetables. Vegetable oils are especially rich sources.

VITAMIN K

Action. Vitamin K is required for the synthesis of prothrombin and three other clotting factors (factors VII, IX, and X). All of these vitamin K–dependent factors are needed for coagulation of blood.

Forms and Sources of Vitamin K. Vitamin K occurs in nature as vitamin K_1 (phytonadione) and vitamin K_2. Phytonadione is present in a wide variety of foods. Vitamin K_2 is synthesized by the normal flora of the gut. Two other forms of the vitamin—vitamin K_3 (menadione) and vitamin K_4 (menadiol)—have been produced synthetically. Phytonadione, menadione, and menadiol are available for therapeutic use. There are no commercial preparations of vitamin K_2.

Requirements. Human requirements for vitamin K have not been precisely defined. The values established by the Food and Nutrition Board approximate 1 µg/kg of body weight. For most individuals, vitamin K requirements are readily met through dietary sources and through vitamin K synthesized by intestinal bacteria. Since bacterial colonization of the gut is not complete until several days after birth, levels of vitamin K may be low during the immediate postnatal period.

Pharmacokinetics. Intestinal absorption of the natural forms of vitamin K (phytonadione and vitamin K_2) is adequate only in the presence of *bile salts*. Menadione and menadiol do not require bile salts for absorption. Following absorption, vitamin K is concentrated in the liver. Metabolism and excretion occur rapidly, and very little storage in tissues occurs.

Deficiency. Vitamin K deficiency produces bleeding tendencies. If the deficiency is severe, spontaneous hemorrhage may occur. In newborns, intracranial hemorrhage is of particular concern.

An important cause of deficiency is reduced absorption. Since the natural forms of vitamin K require bile salts for their uptake, any condition that decreases availability of these salts (e.g., obstructive jaundice) can lead to deficiency. Malabsorption syndromes (sprue, celiac disease, cystic fibrosis of the pancreas) can also decrease vitamin K uptake. Other potential causes of impaired absorption are ulcerative colitis, regional enteritis, and surgical resection of the intestine.

Disruption of intestinal flora may result in deficiency by eliminating vitamin K–synthesizing bacteria. Hence, deficiency may occur secondary to use of antibiotics. In infants, diarrhea may cause bacterial losses sufficient to result in deficiency.

The normal infant is born vitamin K deficient. Consequently, in order to rapidly elevate prothrombin levels, and thereby reduce the risk of neonatal hemorrhage, it is recommended that all infants receive a single injection of phytonadione (vitamin K_1) immediately after delivery.

As discussed in Chapter 46, oral anticoagulants (e.g., warfarin) act as antagonists of vitamin K, and thereby decrease synthesis of vitamin K–dependent clotting factors. As a result, oral anticoagulants produce a state that is the functional equivalent of vitamin K deficiency. If the dosage of an oral anticoagulant is excessive, hemorrhage can occur secondary to lack of prothrombin.

Adverse Effects. As discussed below, menadione and menadiol present special risks to newborns and infants. Accordingly, these agents should be reserved for older children and adults, and should not be given during the last weeks of pregnancy.

Severe Hypersensitivity Reactions. *Intravenous* administration of *phytonadione* has caused serious reactions (shock, respiratory arrest, cardiac arrest) that resemble anaphylaxis or hypersensitivity reactions. Death has occurred. Consequently, phytonadione should be administered intravenously only when other routes are not feasible and only if the potential benefits clearly outweigh the risks.

Hyperbilirubinemia. When administered *parenterally* to newborns, vitamin K derivatives can elevate plasma levels of bilirubin, thereby posing a risk of kernicterus. The incidence of hyperbilirubinemia is greater among premature infants than full-term infants. Although all forms of vitamin K can elevate bilirubin levels, the risk is higher with menadione and menadiol than with phytonadione.

Hemolytic Anemia. Menadione and menadiol can promote hemolysis of red blood cells; phytonadione does not share this property. The risk of hemolytic anemia is highest among infants and individuals whose red cells have a genetic deficiency in glucose-6-phosphate dehydrogenase.

Therapeutic Uses and Dosage. Vitamin K derivatives have two major applications: (1) correction or prevention of hypoprothrombinemia and bleeding caused by vitamin K deficiency, and (2) control of hemorrhage caused by overdosage with oral anticoagulants.

Vitamin K Deficiency. As discussed above, vitamin K deficiency can result from impaired absorption and from insufficient synthesis of the vitamin by intestinal flora. Rarely, deficiency may be caused by inadequate diet. For children and adults, the usual dosage for correction of vitamin K deficiency ranges from 5 to 15 mg/day.

As noted above, infants are born vitamin K deficient. To prevent hemorrhagic disease in neonates, it is recommended that all newborns be given an injection of *phytonadione* (0.5 to 1 mg) immediately after delivery.

Oral Anticoagulant Overdosage. Vitamin K will reverse hypoprothrombinemia and bleeding caused by excessive dosing with oral anticoagulants. Phytonadione is the only form of the vitamin effective for this use. Bleeding is controlled within hours of drug administration. (See Chapter 46 for dosage.)

Preparations and Routes of Administration. *Menadione* (vitamin K_3) is available in 5-mg tablets for oral use.

Menadiol sodium diphosphate (vitamin K_4), marketed under the trade name Synkayvite, is available in 5-mg tablets for oral use and as an injection for parenteral (SC, IM, and IV) administration.

Phytonadione (vitamin K_1) is available in 5-mg tablets, marketed under the trade name Mephyton, and in two parenteral formulations. Proprietary names for the parenteral products are AquaMEPHYTON and Konakion. AquaMEPHYTON may be administered IM, SC, and IV. However, since IV administration is dangerous, this route should be used only when other routes are not feasible, and only if the perceived benefits outweigh the substantial risks. Konakion is intended for IM use only.

WATER-SOLUBLE VITAMINS

The group of water-soluble vitamins consists of vitamin C and members of the vitamin B complex (thiamine, riboflavin, niacin, pyridoxine, pantothenic acid, biotin, folic acid, cyanocobalamin). The B vitamins differ widely from one another both in structure and function. They are grouped together because they were first isolated from the same sources (yeast and liver). Vitamin C is not found in the same foods as the B vitamins and, hence, is classified by itself.

Two compounds—pangamic acid and laetrile—have been falsely promoted as B vitamins. Pangamic acid has been marketed as "vitamin B_{15}" and laetrile as "vitamin B_{17}." There is no proof that these compounds act as vitamins or that they have any other role in human nutrition.

VITAMIN C (ASCORBIC ACID)

Actions. Vitamin C participates in multiple biochemical reactions. These include synthesis of adrenal steroids, conversion of folic acid to folinic acid, and regulation of the respiratory cycle in mitochondria. At the tissue level, vitamin C is required for production of collagen and other compounds that compose the intercellular matrix that binds cells together.

Sources and Requirements. The main dietary sources of ascorbic acid are citrus fruits and juices, tomatoes, potatoes, and other fruits and vegetables. Orange juice and lemon juice are especially rich sources.

The RDA for adults is 60 mg. For women, the RDA increases to 70 mg during pregnancy and to 95 mg during lactation. RDAs for children are given in Table 71–1.

Deficiency. Deficiency of vitamin C can lead to *scurvy*, a disease that is rare in the United States. Symptoms include faulty bone and tooth development, loosening of the teeth, gingivitis, bleeding gums, poor wound healing, hemorrhage into muscles and joints, and ecchymoses (skin discoloration caused by leakage of blood into subcutaneous tissues). Many of these symptoms result from disruption of the intercellular matrix of capillaries and other tissues.

Adverse Effects. Ascorbic acid rarely causes adverse effects, even when taken in huge doses. Very large amounts can induce diarrhea through direct irritation of the intestinal mucosa. Excessive doses may also promote formation of kidney stones by inducing excretion of large quantities of oxalic acid.

Therapeutic Use. The only established indication for vitamin C is prevention and treatment of scurvy. For severe, acute deficiency, parenteral administration is recommended. The usual adult dosage for scurvy is 0.3 to 1 gm/day.

Vitamin C has been advocated for therapy of many conditions unrelated to deficiency, including cancers, asthma, osteoporosis, and the common cold. Claims of efficacy for several of these conditions have been definitively disproved. Other claims remain unproven. Studies have shown that large doses of the vitamin do not reduce the incidence of colds, although the intensity or duration of illness may be reduced slightly. Research has failed to show any benefit of vitamin C therapy for patients with advanced cancer, atherosclerosis, or schizophrenia. Vitamin C does not promote healing of wounds.

Preparations and Routes of Administration. Vitamin C is available in formulations for oral and parenteral administration. Oral products include tablets (ranging from 25 to 1500 mg), timed-release capsules (500 mg), and syrups (20 and 100 mg/ml). For parenteral use, vitamin C is available as ascorbic acid, sodium ascorbate, and calcium ascorbate. Administration may be SC, IM, or IV.

NIACIN (NICOTINIC ACID)

Nicotinic acid is a vitamin and also has a role as a medicine. In its medicinal role, nicotinic acid is used to treat hyperlipidemias; the doses required are *much* higher than those used to correct or prevent nutritional deficiency. Discussion in this chapter focuses on nicotinic acid as a vitamin. Use of this agent for control of lipoprotein levels is discussed in Chapter 45.

Physiologic Actions. Before it can exert physiologic effects, niacin must first be converted into NAD (nicotinamide-adenine dinucleotide) or into NADP (nicotinamide-adenine dinucleotide phosphate). NAD and NADP then act as coenzymes in oxidation-reduction reactions essential for cellular respiration.

Sources. Nicotinic acid (or its nutritional equivalent, nicotinamide) is present in many foods of plant and animal origin. Particularly rich sources are liver, chicken, yeast, peanuts, and cereal bran or germ.

In humans, the amino acid *tryptophan* can be converted to nicotinic acid; hence, proteins can be a source of the vitamin. It is estimated that about 60 mg of dietary tryptophan is required to produce 1 mg of nicotinic acid.

Requirements. RDAs for nicotinic acid are stated as *niacin equivalents*. By definition, 1 niacin equivalent is equal to 1 mg of niacin (nicotinic

acid) or to 60 mg of tryptophan. RDAs are summarized in Table 71–1.

Deficiency. The syndrome caused by niacin deficiency is called *pellagra*, a term that is a condensation of the Italian words *pelle agra*, meaning "rough skin." As suggested by this name, a prominent symptom of pellagra is dermatitis, characterized by scaling and cracking of the skin in areas exposed to the sun. Other symptoms involve the gastrointestinal tract (abdominal pain, diarrhea, soreness of the tongue and mouth) and central nervous system (irritability, insomnia, memory loss, anxiety, dementia). All symptoms are readily reversed with niacin replacement therapy.

Adverse Effects. Nicotinic acid has very low toxicity, and small doses are completely devoid of adverse effects. When taken in the large amounts that are sometimes required to treat pellagra, nicotinic acid can cause vasodilation with resultant flushing, dizziness, and nausea. These reactions are temporary and harmless. Toxicity associated with high-dose therapy is discussed further in Chapter 45.

Nicotinamide, a compound that can substitute for nicotinic acid in the treatment of pellagra, is not a vasodilator and, hence, does not produce the adverse effects associated with large doses of nicotinic acid. Accordingly, nicotinamide is often preferred to nicotinic acid for treating pellagra.

Therapeutic Uses. In its capacity as a vitamin, nicotinic acid is indicated only for the prevention or treatment of niacin deficiency. As noted, if given in large doses, nicotinic acid may also be used for hyperlipidemias (see Chapter 45).

Preparations, Dosage, and Administration. *Nicotinic acid* (niacin) is available in tablets (20 to 500 mg), capsules (125 to 500 mg), and as an elixir (10 mg/ml) for oral use. Niacin is also dispensed as an injection (100 mg/ml) for parenteral (SC, IM, and IV) administration. Dosages for mild deficiency range from 10 to 20 mg/day. For treatment of pellagra, daily doses may be as high as 500 mg. Dosages for treatment of hyperlipidemia are given in Chapter 45.

Nicotinamide (niacinamide) is dispensed in tablets (50 to 1000 mg) for oral administration and as an injection (100 mg/ml) for parenteral use. For treatment or prevention of pellagra, dosages range from 150 to 500 mg/day. Unlike nicotinic acid, nicotinamide has no effect on plasma lipoproteins and, hence, is not used to treat hyperlipidemias.

RIBOFLAVIN

Actions. In order to exert its physiologic effects, riboflavin must first be converted into one of two active forms: flavin-adenine dinucleotide (FAD) or flavin mononucleotide (FMN). In the form of FAD and FMN, riboflavin acts as a coenzyme for a variety of oxidative reactions.

Sources and Requirements. Riboflavin is present in a variety of foods of animal and vegetable origin. Good sources are meats, chicken, eggs, and milk. Liver has an especially high riboflavin content. RDAs for riboflavin are summarized in Table 71–1.

Deficiency. In its early state, riboflavin deficiency manifests as *sore throat* and *angular stomatitis* (cracks in the skin at the corners of the mouth). Symptoms that may appear later include *cheilosis* (painful cracks in the lips), *glossitis* (inflammation of the tongue), *vascularization of the cornea,* and *itchy dermatitis of the scrotum or vulva.* Riboflavin deficiency rarely occurs alone. Rather, deficiency is usually observed in conjunction with insufficiency of other B vitamins.

Toxicity. Riboflavin appears to have no toxic effects in humans. When large doses are administered, the excess is rapidly excreted in the urine.

Therapeutic Use. Riboflavin is indicated only for prevention and correction of riboflavin deficiency.

Preparations, Dosage, and Administration. Riboflavin is dispensed in tablets (5 to 100 mg) for oral administration. Daily doses for deficiency states range from 5 to 10 mg.

THIAMINE (VITAMIN B₁)

Actions and Requirements. The active form of thiamine (thiamine pyrophosphate) is an essential coenzyme for carbohydrate metabolism. Thiamine requirements are related to caloric intake, and are greatest when carbohydrates are the primary source of calories. For maintenance of good health, thiamine consumption should be at least 0.3 mg per 1000 kcal in the diet. The RDAs in Table 71–1 represent approximately 0.5 mg of thiamine per 1000 kcal. Hence, these values allow about a twofold margin of safety. As indicated in Table 71–1, thiamine requirements increase markedly during pregnancy and lactation.

Sources. Thiamine is present in a variety of foods of plant and animal origin. Pork products are especially rich in the vitamin. Other good sources include peanuts, asparagus, and cereals (whole-grain and enriched).

Deficiency. Severe thiamine deficiency produces *beriberi,* a disorder having two distinct forms: *wet beriberi* and *dry beriberi. Wet beriberi* is so named because its primary symptom is fluid accumulation in the legs. Cardiovascular complications (palpitations, EKG abnormalities, high-output heart failure) are common and may progress rapidly to circulatory collapse and death. *Dry beriberi* is characterized by neurologic and motor deficits (e.g., anesthesia of the feet, ataxic gait, foot drop, and wrist drop). Edema and cardiovascular symptoms are absent. Wet beriberi responds rapidly and dramatically to replacement therapy. In contrast, recovery from dry beriberi is often very slow.

In the United States, thiamine deficiency occurs most commonly in alcoholics. In this population, deficiency manifests as *Wernicke's syndrome* rather than as frank beriberi. This syndrome is a serious disorder of the central nervous system having neurologic and psychologic manifestations. Symptoms include nystagmus, diplopia, ataxia, and an inability to remember the recent past. Failure to correct the thiamine deficit may result in irreversible damage to the brain. Accordingly, if Wernicke's syndrome is suspected, parenteral thiamine should be administered immediately.

Adverse Effects. When administered orally, thiamine is devoid of adverse effects. Very rarely, parenteral administration has produced anaphylactic reactions. These reactions probably reflect hypersensitivity to thiamine.

Therapeutic Use. The only indication for thiamine is treatment and prevention of thiamine deficiency.

Preparations, Dosage, and Administration. Thiamine is dispensed in tablets (5 to 500 mg) for oral use and as an injection (100 and 200 mg/ml) for IM or IV administration. Dosages range from 5 to 30 mg daily. For mild deficiency, oral thiamine is preferred. Parenteral administration should be reserved for severe deficiency states (wet or dry beriberi, Wernicke's syndrome).

PYRIDOXINE (VITAMIN B₆)

Actions. Before it can influence biologic processes, pyridoxine must first be converted to its active form: pyridoxal phosphate. As pyridoxal phosphate, the vitamin participates in the metabolism of amino acids and proteins.

Requirements. Pyridoxine requirements parallel intake of protein: as protein consumption increases, the need for pyridoxine increases as well. For the average adult male, 2.0 mg of pyridoxine daily will maintain good nutrition. The RDA for adult females is 1.6 mg per day. Pyridoxine requirements increase during pregnancy and lactation.

Sources. Pyridoxine is found in a variety of foods of animal and vegetable origin. Good sources include milk, meats (especially liver and kidney), soybeans, and whole-grain cereals.

Deficiency. Pyridoxine deficiency may result from poor diet, certain medications (especially isoniazid), and inborn errors of metabolism. Symptoms of deficiency include peripheral neuritis, seizures, glossitis, and skin lesions on the face.

In the United States, dietary deficiency of vitamin B₆ is rare, except among alcoholics. Within the alcoholic population, vitamin B₆ deficiency has an incidence of about 20% to 30% and occurs in combination with deficiency of other B vitamins.

Isoniazid (an antituberculosis drug) prevents

conversion of vitamin B_6 to its active form, and may thereby induce symptoms of deficiency (peripheral neuritis). Patients taking isoniazid who are predisposed to this neuropathy (e.g., alcoholics, diabetics) should receive daily pyridoxine supplements.

Inborn errors of metabolism can prevent efficient utilization of vitamin B_6, resulting in greatly increased pyridoxine requirements. In the infant with such an inherited disorder, prominent symptoms are irritability, convulsions, and anemia. Unless treatment with vitamin B_6 is initiated early, permanent retardation may result.

Adverse Effects. At low doses, pyridoxine is devoid of adverse effects. However, if extremely large doses are taken (250 to 1000 times the RDA), neurologic injury may result. Symptoms include ataxia and numbness of the feet and hands.

Drug Interactions. Vitamin B_6 interferes with the utilization of levodopa by patients taking this drug for parkinsonism. Accordingly, patients receiving levodopa should be advised against taking vitamin B_6.

Therapeutic Uses. Pyridoxine is indicated for the prevention and treatment of all vitamin B_6 deficiency states (dietary deficiency, isoniazid-induced deficiency, pyridoxine-dependency syndrome).

Preparations, Dosage, and Administration. Pyridoxine is dispensed in tablets (10 to 500 mg) for oral use and as an injection (100 mg/ml) for IM or IV administration. The dosage for correcting dietary deficiency is 10 to 20 mg/day for 3 weeks followed by daily doses of 1.5 to 2.5 mg. For treatment of deficiency induced by isoniazid, the daily dosage is 50 to 200 mg. For prophylaxis against isoniazid-induced deficiency, the dosage is 25 to 50 mg/day. Pyridoxine dependency syndrome may require initial doses up to 600 mg/day followed by daily doses of 25 to 50 mg for life.

PANTOTHENIC ACID

The active form of pantothenic acid (coenzyme A) is an essential factor in a variety of biochemical processes. These include gluconeogenesis, intermediary metabolism of carbohydrates, and synthesis of steroid hormones, porphyrins, and acetylcholine. Pantothenic acid is present in numerous foods, and spontaneous deficiency has not been reported. No official RDA has been established. However, the Food and Nutrition Board has published "estimated safe and adequate daily dietary intake" levels: 2 to 3 mg for infants, 3 to 7 mg for children, and 4 to 7 mg for adults. Aside from minor gastrointestinal discomfort, no toxicity has been noted with doses 1000 times greater than these in adults. Pantothenic acid is available in single-ingredient tablets and in many multivitamin preparations. However, because deficiency does not occur, there is no indication for taking this vitamin.

BIOTIN

Biotin is a cofactor for several reactions involved in the metabolism of carbohydrates and fats. This vitamin is present in a variety of foods. In addition, biotin is synthesized by intestinal bacteria in amounts sufficient to meet human nutritional needs. Consequently, biotin deficiency is extremely rare. When deficiency has been induced experimentally in volunteers, symptoms have included fatigue, depression, anorexia, muscle pain, and dermatitis. Biotin appears to be devoid of toxicity: subjects given large doses experienced no apparent ill effects. Because the amount of biotin produced by intestinal flora has not been quantified, the Food and Nutrition Board has been unable to establish an RDA for this vitamin. However, as with pantothenic acid, the Board has published "estimated safe and adequate daily dietary intake" levels. These are: 10 to 15 µg for infants, 20 to 30 µg for children aged 1 to 10 years, and 30 to 100 µg for children over 11 years and for adults.

CYANOCOBALAMIN AND FOLIC ACID

Cyanocobalamin (vitamin B_{12}) and folic acid (folacin) are essential factors in the synthesis of DNA. Deficiency of either vitamin manifests as megaloblastic anemia. Cyanocobalamin deficiency produces neurologic damage as well. Because deficiency presents as anemia, folic acid and cyanocobalamin are discussed in Chapter 47 (Drugs for Deficiency Anemias). The RDAs for these compounds are given in Table 71–1.

Folic Acid Deficiency and Fetal Development. Deficiency of folic acid during pregnancy can impair development of the central nervous system, resulting in *anencephaly* and *spina bifida*. Anencephaly (failure of the brain to develop) is uniformly fatal. Spina bifida, a condition characterized by defective development of the bony encasement of the spinal cord, can result in nerve damage, paralysis, and other complications. Since the central nervous system develops early in pregnancy, it is essential that adequate levels of folic acid be present when pregnancy begins; if women wait until pregnancy is confirmed before increasing folic acid intake, it may be too late to prevent these disorders. Accordingly, the federal Centers for Disease Control and Prevention now recommends that *all women who may become pregnant consume 400 µg of folic acid each day*. Since pregnancy can occur despite birth control measures, this recommendation applies even to women who don't *intend* to become pregnant.

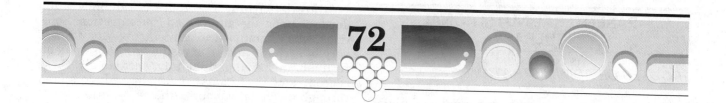

Parenteral and Enteral Nutrition

Good nutrition is required to maintain health and to permit healing at times of illness. As a rule, required nutrients—amino acids, carbohydrates, fats, vitamins, and minerals—can be obtained simply by ingestion of appropriate foods. However, this is not always the case: circumstances frequently arise in which nutritional needs cannot be fulfilled by eating. Under these conditions, nutritional support is required. Specific indications for nutritional support include (1) malnutrition, (2) coma, (3) bowel obstruction, (4) cancer chemotherapy (because of associated nausea and vomiting), and (5) trauma, major burns, and severe infection (because these disorders cause a hypermetabolic state). Nutritional support is also indicated to permit bowel rest for patients with inflammatory bowel disease and for those recovering from bowel surgery.

There are two major categories of nutritional support: *enteral* (via the gastrointestinal tract) and *parenteral* (intravenous). *Enteral* nutritional therapy is indicated for (1) patients who have a healthy digestive tract but are unable or unwilling to eat sufficient food, and (2) patients who have a digestive or absorptive disorder that cannot be overcome by modification of diet. *Parenteral* nutritional support is indicated when nutrition cannot be maintained by eating or by enteral therapy.

905

PARENTERAL NUTRITIONAL THERAPY

ROUTES OF ADMINISTRATION

Parenteral nutritional therapy may be administered through a *peripheral* vein or through a *central venous catheter* (which delivers nutrient solution directly into the superior vena cava). Peripheral infusion is indicated only for *short-term therapy* with relatively *dilute* nutrient solutions. If therapy is to be *prolonged* (i.e., lasting more than 10 to 12 days) or if *strongly hypertonic* solutions are to be given, central administration is required.

COMPONENTS OF A PARENTERAL NUTRITIONAL REGIMEN

The principal component of a parenteral nutritional regimen is a solution of amino acids. To this may be added dextrose, fats, vitamins, and minerals as required.

Amino Acids

Nutritional Role. Amino acids serve two purposes: (1) they foster conservation of existing lean body mass, and (2) they promote wound healing and restoration of lean body mass. For healthy adults, the recommended dietary allowance (RDA) for amino acids is 0.9 gm/kg. The RDA for healthy infants and children ranges from 1.4 to 2.2 gm/kg. RDA values increase significantly in the presence of malnutrition, trauma, burns, or infection.

Complications of Therapy. Blood urea nitrogen (BUN) may rise to dangerous levels, especially in patients with kidney dysfunction. If elevation of BUN exceeds normal limits, amino acid administration should be discontinued. In patients with liver disease, amino acid infusion may result in hepatic coma due to accumulation of nitrogenous compounds. Caution must be exercised in patients with cirrhosis, viral hepatitis, or cancer involving the liver.

Formulations. Amino acid solutions are available in general and specialized formulations. The general formulations consist of essential and nonessential amino acids; total amino acid concentrations range from 3.0% to 11.4%. Some mixtures also contain electrolytes. The general formulations will satisfy the nutritional requirements of most patients. Specialized products have been formulated to meet the unique needs of certain patients—specifically, patients in a state of high metabolic stress and patients experiencing liver failure or severe renal impairment. Special formulations are also available for pediatric patients.

Administration. The route of administration depends upon the amino acid concentration. Solutions whose amino acid content exceeds 4% are very hypertonic and, as a result, will cause phlebitis if administered peripherally. Accordingly, these concentrated solutions must be administered through a central venous catheter. Solutions composed of less than 4% amino acids may be administered peripherally.

Dextrose

Nutritional Role. In order to utilize amino acids for conservation and synthesis of protein, the body requires a source of nonprotein calories. Dextrose (*D*-glucose) can provide these calories. For the average adult, daily requirements range from 30 to 50 kcal/kg (the equivalent of 9 to 15 gm of dextrose/kg).

Complications of Therapy. *Glucose intolerance* (hyperglycemia, glycosuria, osmotic diuresis) can occur. This response is most likely during the first few days of treatment. Glucose intolerance can be minimized by initiating therapy with low doses (300 to 350 gm/day) followed by gradual dosage elevation. This progressive dosing schedule permits the body to produce the extra amounts of insulin needed to process the abnormal glucose load. Glucose content of blood and urine should be measured every 6 hours until glucose tolerance has been demonstrated (usually within 2 to 3 days). If tolerance fails to develop, insulin can be added to the infusion mixture to control hyperglycemia. This IV insulin can be supplemented with subcutaneous insulin as needed. Special care must be exercised with the diabetic patient.

Hypertonic solutions of dextrose may cause *thrombosis* if administered via a peripheral vein. Consequently, solutions in excess of 10% dextrose should be infused via a central venous catheter.

Since insulin levels are elevated during dextrose therapy, and since insulin promotes cellular uptake of potassium, infusion of dextrose may be accompanied by *hypokalemia*. Hypokalemia can be avoided by monitoring plasma potassium content and administering potassium as required.

If dextrose is abruptly discontinued, *hypoglycemia* may develop (because of continued release of endogenous insulin). Accordingly, dextrose should be withdrawn slowly: when infusion of hypertonic dextrose is stopped, infusion of 10% dextrose should be instituted and maintained for 1 to 2 hours.

Administration. Depending on their concentrations, dextrose solutions may be administered through a peripheral vein or centrally. Hypertonic solutions (i.e., solutions containing more than 10% dextrose) can be administered safely only through a central venous catheter. More dilute solutions may be given by peripheral infusion. Dextrose solutions may be mixed with amino acid solutions prior to administration.

Fat

Nutritional Role. Intravenous fat emulsions can serve two functions: (1) they can prevent or reverse essential fatty acid deficiency (EFAD), and (2) they can serve as a source of nonprotein calories. When the objective of administration is avoidance or reversal of EFAD, fat emulsions are given in relatively small amounts (3% to 8% of total caloric intake). Much larger doses (up to 60% of total caloric intake) are used when fats are intended as a source of energy. When fats are administered for their caloric content, dextrose dosage must be adjusted downward to keep total caloric intake constant. Most fat emulsions are prepared from soybean oil. The principal components of these emulsions are linoleic, oleic, palmitic, linolenic, and stearic acids.

Complications of Therapy. Although fat emulsions are generally very safe, *death has occurred following administration to preterm infants.* Autopsy findings indicate fat accumulation within the vasculature of the lungs. Intravenous fats should be administered slowly to preterm infants, and then only if the potential benefits of treatment clearly outweigh the risks.

The most common adverse effect of fat infusion is *hyperlipidemia.* This is especially likely in patients whose capacity to metabolize fats is impaired. Hyperlipidemia may also occur in patients with normal fat-metabolizing capacity if administration is too rapid or if too much dextrose is administered concurrently. Blood should be monitored for fat content to insure that lipemia clears between infusions.

Administration. Fat emulsions are isotonic with plasma and, therefore, may be administered safely through a peripheral vein. Central administration may be performed as well. Some preparations may be mixed with amino acid and dextrose solutions. Others must be administered separately. Fat emulsions may be infused in the same vein as dextrose-amino acid solutions. When this is done, the Y-connector through which the fat will flow should be placed *below* any in-line filter that may be present. This placement is needed because particles in fat emulsions are too large to pass through bacterial and particulate filters. Infusion of fat emulsion should be slow (0.5 to 1 ml/min) for the first 15 to 30 minutes. In the absence of adverse reactions (e.g., dyspnea, cyanosis, allergic responses), the infusion rate may then be increased.

Electrolytes, Vitamins, and Trace Elements

In addition to amino acids, carbohydrates, and fats, patients receiving parenteral nutrition must be supplied with vitamins, electrolytes (sodium, potassium, calcium, magnesium, phosphate), and trace elements (copper, chromium, iodine, manganese, molybdenum, selenium, zinc). These nutrients should be incorporated into the regimen from the onset of treatment. The pharmacology of vitamins is discussed in Chapter 71. Electrolytes are discussed in Chapter 36.

PREPARATION OF PARENTERAL NUTRIENT SOLUTIONS

Parenteral nutrient solutions are prepared by mixing hypertonic dextrose with an amino acid solution. Vitamins, minerals, and electrolytes are then added as indicated. Although a fat emulsion may also be added to this mixture, the usual practice is to administer fats separately. To prevent bacterial contamination, parenteral solutions should be prepared aseptically under a laminar-flow hood. Solutions should be stored under refrigeration and administered within 24 hours. Preparations that have become cloudy or darkened should be discarded. Drugs should not be added to solutions unless compatibility has been established.

MONITORING TREATMENT

Nutritional therapy is assessed through bedside examination, determination of blood and urine chemistries, and daily monitoring of weight, intake, and output. Weight measurement provides the best overall index of the efficacy of treatment. However, although weight gain can be a measure of success, be aware that large increases in weight (greater than 0.5 kg/day) may indicate excessive fluid retention. This possibility should be evaluated.

Blood and urine chemistries should be determined prior to treatment and throughout the period of nutritional support. Serum should be measured frequently for BUN, electrolytes, triglycerides, and glucose. Prothrombin time, platelet counts, and serum osmolarity should be determined weekly. Blood for laboratory tests should not be drawn from the vein being used to infuse nutrients.

COMPLICATIONS OF TREATMENT

The principal complications of parenteral nutritional therapy are infection and metabolic disturbances. Mechanical complications related to the catheter may also occur.

Infection. Patients receiving parenteral nutritional support are at constant risk of infection. This risk can be minimized by employing aseptic technique during catheter insertion and during preparation and administration of solutions. Use of a 0.22-micron filter can provide partial protection. A filter will hold back bacteria present in the feeding solution, but will not hold back bacterial endotoxins. Also, the filter can only retain bacteria that have entered the line at a site above the filter. In the event of fever, sepsis should be suspected. To assess for sepsis, blood for culture should be drawn from the tip of the intravenous line as well as from a separate venous site. If temperature remains elevated and no cause can be found, the catheter and nutrient solution should be replaced and the tip of the catheter should be cultured for bacterial contamination. If the fever does not drop rapidly, antibiotic therapy should be instituted.

Metabolic Disturbances. The principal metabolic complications of parenteral nutritional therapy have been discussed. These complications include hyperglycemia, hypoglycemia, hyperlipidemia, and elevation of BUN. In addition, the patient may experience overhydration, dehydration, acid-base imbalance, electrolyte imbalance, and deficiencies in trace elements and vitamins.

Catheter-Related Complications. Infusion into a peripheral vein may produce phlebitis at or near the site of catheter insertion. If this occurs, the catheter should be moved. The risk of phlebitis can be reduced by selecting a large peripheral vein and by infusing the nutrient solution slowly. Other catheter-related complications include pneumothorax (caused by insertion of a central catheter) and central venous thrombosis.

ENTERAL NUTRITIONAL THERAPY

Enteral nutritional therapy is defined as the provision of nutrients by way of the gastrointestinal tract. Administration may be oral or through a tube. Enteral therapy is indicated for two groups: (1) patients with a healthy digestive tract but who cannot or will not ingest sufficient food (e.g., anorectic patients, patients with an impaired ability to chew or swallow), and (2) patients with a digestive or absorptive disorder that cannot be compensated for by modification of diet. Depending on patient status, enteral therapy may be used as a supplement to oral feeding or to meet all nutritional needs. Contraindications to enteral therapy include total bowel obstruction, uncontrollable vomiting, and a predisposition to aspiration.

METHODS OF DELIVERY

Oral. Oral nutritional support is indicated for patients with an intact digestive system who re-

quire supplemental feeding to meet increased nutritional needs. Patients for whom oral therapy may be appropriate include those with trauma, malignancy, or protein-calorie malnutrition. Oral therapy may also be given to patients with digestive and absorptive disturbances that are mild enough not to require enteral feeding by tube.

Tube Feeding. Candidates for tube feeding include anorectic and comatose patients, patients unable to chew or swallow, and certain infants. For short-term therapy, a *nasogastric* tube is commonly used. When intragastric administration is contraindicated or when aspiration is a concern, a *nasoduodenal* or *nasojejunal* tube may be employed. For prolonged therapy, feeding tubes may be surgically implanted directly into the esophagus, stomach, or jejunum. Tube feeding is more effective and better tolerated when performed by slow infusion (over a period of hours) than when periodic bolus administrations are performed. Use of an infusion pump is recommended.

COMPONENTS OF AN ENTERAL NUTRITIONAL REGIMEN

Amino Acids. All patients require an adequate supply of amino acids in order to conserve or rebuild lean body mass. Enteral solutions provide amino acids in various forms: intact proteins, hydrolyzed proteins, and free amino acids. Specialized products are available to meet the unique amino acid needs of patients who have renal failure or severe hepatic dysfunction.

Carbohydrates. Carbohydrates—in the form of dextrose, sucrose, lactose, starch, dextrin, and glucose oligosaccharides—are the primary source of calories in most enteral regimens. The simple sugars (dextrose, sucrose, and lactose) are absorbed more readily than complex carbohydrates (e.g., dextrin, starch). Hence, for patients with limited absorptive capacity, the simple sugars may be preferred. Because of their high osmolality, simple sugars can retain water in the intestinal lumen and can thereby promote diarrhea. Lactose intolerance (an inability to digest and absorb lactose) is common. For patients who are unable to process lactose, a lactose-free formulation should be employed.

Fat. Fats serve as a source of calories and are required to prevent and correct essential fatty acid deficiency. Most enteral formulations contain a high percentage of fat (in the form of polyunsaturated fats). However, the fat content of some formulas is quite low. The fats most frequently employed are corn oil, soybean oil, and safflower oil.

Other Components. Enteral nutritional solutions should supply sufficient *water* to maintain hydration. Also, the formulation should provide required *electrolytes*, *vitamins*, and *trace elements*. Many oral formulations contain flavoring agents; the patient should be consulted regarding taste preference.

COMPLICATIONS OF TREATMENT

The most dangerous complication of enteral therapy is *aspiration pneumonitis*, a condition that can be fatal. To reduce the risk of aspiration, the upper body should be elevated (by raising the head of the bed to a 30-degree angle) during the infusion and for at least 1 hour after. High-risk patients (e.g., those prone to vomiting and those that lack a gag reflex) must not be given bolus feeding. For these people, feeding should be done by slow drip, and then only if the tip of the feeding tube has been placed into the duodenum or jejunum. If these tube placements are not possible, enteral therapy should be replaced with parenteral nutritional support.

About 10% of patients who are fed through a nasogastric tube experience adverse effects (e.g., diarrhea, vomiting, insufficient gastric emptying, gastrointestinal bleeding). To minimize these effects, initial therapy should be delivered at a slow rate using a dilute nutrient solution. As the patient adjusts to therapy, the infusion rate and nutrient concentration can be increased.

Like parenteral nutritional therapy, enteral therapy may be associated with metabolic disturbances (e.g., hyperglycemia, fluid and electrolyte imbalance, fatty acid deficiency). Monitoring serum glucose and electrolyte levels will help minimize metabolic disorders.

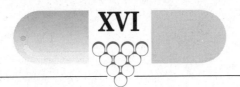

XVI

Chemotherapy of Infectious Diseases

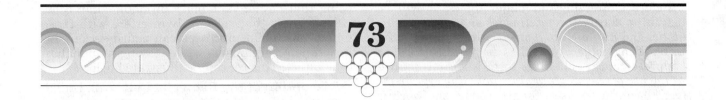

73

Basic Considerations in the Chemotherapy of Infectious Diseases

With this chapter we begin our study of drugs used to treat infectious diseases. These agents, which are given to approximately 30% of all hospitalized patients, constitute one of our most widely used families of drugs.

Modern antimicrobial agents had their debut in the 1930's and 1940's, and have greatly reduced morbidity and mortality from infection. As newer drugs are introduced, our ability to fight infections increases even more. However, despite impressive advances, continued progress is needed: there are organisms that respond poorly to available drugs; there are effective drugs whose use is limited by toxicity; and there is, because of evolving microbial resistance, the constant threat that currently effective antibiotics may be rendered useless.

In this introductory chapter, our discussion focuses on two principal themes. The first is microbial susceptibility to drugs, and includes special emphasis on microbial drug resistance. The second major theme considers how to use antimicrobial agents properly; this discussion includes criteria for drug selection, host factors that modify drug use, therapy with antimicrobial combinations, and use of antimicrobial agents for prophylaxis.

913

Before addressing our major topics, it will be helpful to clarify three terms: *chemotherapy*, *antibiotic*, and *antimicrobial agent*. Although we often think of *chemotherapy* as the use of drugs to kill or suppress cancer cells, this term was first defined as *the use of chemicals against invading organisms* (e.g., bacteria, viruses, fungi). Today, the word is applied to the treatment of cancer *and* to the treatment of infection. Hence, not only do we speak of cancer chemotherapy, we also speak of chemotherapy of infectious diseases.

It has become common practice to use the terms *antibiotic* and *antimicrobial drug* interchangeably. We will follow that practice here. However, you should be aware that the formal definitions of these words are not identical. Strictly speaking, an *antibiotic* is a chemical that is produced by one microorganism and has the ability to harm other microbes. Under this definition, only those compounds that are actually made by microorganisms qualify as antibiotics; drugs such as the sulfonamides, which are produced in the laboratory, would not be considered antibiotics under the strict definition. In contrast, an *antimicrobial drug* is defined as any agent, natural or synthetic, that has the ability to kill or suppress microorganisms. Under this definition, no distinction is made between compounds produced by microbes and those made by chemists. From the perspective of therapeutics, there is no benefit to be gained from distinguishing between drugs made by microorganisms and drugs made by people; hence, the current practice of using the terms antibiotics and antimicrobial drugs as synonyms.

SELECTIVE TOXICITY

What Is Selective Toxicity?

The term *selective toxicity* is defined as the ability of a drug to harm a target cell or target organism without injuring other cells or organisms with which the target is in intimate contact. As applied to antimicrobial drugs, selective toxicity indicates the ability of an antibiotic to kill or suppress infecting microbes without causing injury to the host. It is this property of selective toxicity that makes antibiotics the valuable drugs that they are: if it weren't for their selective toxicity, that is, if antibiotics were as harmful to the host as they are to infecting organisms, these drugs would have no therapeutic utility.

How Is Selective Toxicity Achieved?

How is it that a drug can be highly toxic to microbes but benign to cells of the host? The answer to this question lies with differences in the cellular chemistry of mammals and microbes. There are biochemical processes critical to microbial well-

being that do not take place in mammalian cells. Hence, drugs that selectively interfere with these unique microbial processes can cause serious injury to microorganisms while leaving mammalian cells intact. This concept is illustrated below.

Disruption of the Bacterial Cell Wall. Unlike mammalian cells, bacteria are encased in a rigid cell wall. The protoplasm within this wall has a high concentration of solutes, making osmotic pressure within the bacterium high. If it were not for the cell wall, bacteria would absorb water, swell, and then burst. Several kinds of drugs (penicillins, cephalosporins, others) act to weaken the cell wall and thereby promote bacterial lysis. Since mammalian cells have no cell wall, drugs directed at this structure do not affect the host.

Inhibition of an Enzyme Unique to Bacteria. The sulfonamides provide an excellent example of drugs whose selective toxicity derives from inhibition of an enzyme that is essential for bacterial growth but is not present in cells of the host. The enzyme that the sulfonamides inhibit is needed by bacteria for production of folic acid, a compound required by all cells (mammalian and bacterial) for synthesis of essential molecules (DNA, RNA, proteins). The folic acid used by mammalian cells is acquired directly from dietary sources. In contrast, bacteria lack the ability to take up folic acid from their environment. Hence, to meet their needs for this compound, bacteria first take up para-aminobenzoic acid (PABA), which is a precursor of folic acid, and then use the PABA to form folic acid. The sulfonamide drugs suppress bacterial growth by inhibiting an enzyme required to produce folic acid from PABA. Since mammalian cells do not synthesize folic acid, toxicity of sulfonamides is selective for microbes.

Disruption of Bacterial Protein Synthesis. In bacteria as well as in mammalian cells, synthesis of proteins employs cellular components called ribosomes. However, although both cell types employ ribosomes, bacteria have ribosomes that differ in structure from those of mammals. Because of this structural difference, it is possible for drugs to disrupt the function of bacterial ribosomes while having little or no effect on ribosomes of the host. By doing so, drugs can alter protein synthesis in bacteria while leaving mammalian protein synthesis untouched. Hence, once again we see that biochemical differences between microbes and host cells can be exploited to produce selectively toxic effects.

CLASSIFICATION OF ANTIMICROBIAL DRUGS

Various schemes are employed for classification of antimicrobial drugs. The two schemes most suited to our objectives are considered below.

Classification by Susceptible Organism

Antibiotics differ widely in their antimicrobial activity. Some agents, called *narrow-spectrum* drugs, are active against only a few microorganisms. In contrast, *broad-spectrum* antibiotics are active against a wide variety of microbes. As we will see, narrow-spectrum drugs are generally preferred to broad-spectrum agents. Because of differences in antimicrobial spectra, not all drugs are appropriate for all patients: if therapy is to be successful, we must choose an antibiotic that is active against the specific organism responsible for the infection to be treated.

Table 73–1 classifies the major antimicrobial drugs according to susceptible organisms. The table shows three major groups: *antibacterial drugs*, *antifungal drugs*, and *antiviral drugs*. In addition, the table subdivides the antibacterial drugs into *narrow-spectrum* and *broad-spectrum* agents, and indicates the principal classes of bacteria against which these drugs are active.

Classification by Mechanism of Action

The antimicrobial drugs fall into seven major groups based on their mechanisms of action. This classification scheme is summarized in Table 73–2. Properties of the seven major classes are discussed briefly below.

1. *Drugs that inhibit bacterial cell wall synthesis or activate enzymes that disrupt the cell wall.* These drugs (e.g., penicillins, cephalosporins) weaken the cell wall and thereby promote bacterial lysis and death.
2. *Drugs that increase cell membrane permeability.* Drugs in this group (e.g., amphotericin B) increase the permeability of cell membranes, causing leakage of intracellular material.
3. *Drugs that cause lethal inhibition of bacterial protein synthesis.* The aminoglycosides (e.g., gentamicin) are the only drugs in this group. It is not known why inhibition of protein synthesis by these agents results in cell death.
4. *Drugs that cause nonlethal inhibition of protein synthesis.* Like the aminoglycosides, the drugs

---

Table 73–1. Classification of Antimicrobial Drugs by Susceptible Organisms*

ANTIBACTERIAL

Narrow Spectrum
Gram-positive cocci and gram-positive bacilli
  Penicillin G and V
  Penicillinase-resistant penicillins: methicillin, nafcillin
  Vancomycin
  Erythromycin
  Clindamycin
Gram-negative aerobes
  Aminoglycosides: gentamicin, others
  Cephalosporins (first and second generations)
Mycobacterium tuberculosis
  Isoniazid
  Rifampin
  Ethambutol
  Pyrazinamide

Broad Spectrum
Gram-positive cocci and gram-negative bacilli
  Broad-spectrum penicillins: ampicillin, others
  Extended-spectrum penicillins: carbenicillin, others
  Cephalosporins (third generation)
  Tetracyclines
  Imipenem
  Trimethoprim
  Sulfonamides: sulfisoxazole, sulfamethoxazole, others
  Fluoroquinolones: ciprofloxacin, norfloxacin, others

ANTIVIRAL
  Acyclovir
  Azidothymidine
  Amantadine

ANTIFUNGAL
  Amphotericin B
  Ketoconazole
  Itraconazole

*The classification in this table is simplified. Table 73–3 presents a more comprehensive list of microorganisms and the drugs active against them.

Table 73–2. Classification of Antimicrobial Drugs by Mechanism of Action

Drug Class	Antibiotics
Inhibitors of cell wall synthesis	Penicillins Cephalosporins Imipenem Vancomycin
Drugs that disrupt the cell membrane	Amphotericin B Ketoconazole
Bacter*icidal* inhibitors of protein synthesis	Aminoglycosides
Bacterio*static* inhibitors of protein synthesis	Clindamycin Erythromycin Tetracyclines
Drugs that interfere with synthesis of DNA or RNA	Fluoroquinolones Rifampin
Antimetabolites	Flucytosine Sulfonamides Trimethoprim
Drugs that inhibit viral replication of DNA	Acyclovir Vidarabine Zidovudine
Inhibitor of mycolic acid synthesis	Isoniazid
Drugs whose mechanism is unknown	Amantadine Ethambutol Pyrazinamide

in this group (e.g., tetracyclines) inhibit bacterial protein synthesis. However, in contrast to the aminoglycosides, these agents only slow microbial growth; they do not kill bacteria at clinically achievable concentrations.

5. *Drugs that inhibit synthesis of nucleic acids.* These drugs inhibit synthesis of DNA or RNA by binding directly to nucleic acids or by interacting with enzymes required for nucleic acid synthesis. Members of this group include rifampin and the fluoroquinolones (e.g., ciprofloxacin).

6. *Antimetabolites.* These drugs disrupt specific biochemical reactions. The result is either a decrease in the synthesis of essential cell constituents or synthesis of nonfunctional analogues of normal metabolites. Examples of antimetabolites include trimethoprim and the sulfonamides.

7. *Inhibitors of viral DNA synthesis.* These drugs (e.g., acyclovir, zidovudine) inhibit viral enzymes responsible for DNA synthesis, thereby preventing viral replication.

When considering the *antibacterial* drugs, it is useful to distinguish between agents that are *bactericidal* and those that are *bacteriostatic*. A *bactericidal* drug is one that is directly lethal to bacteria at clinically achievable concentrations. In contrast, *bacteriostatic* drugs are agents that can slow microbial growth but do not cause cell death. When a bacteriostatic drug is used, elimination of bacteria

must ultimately be accomplished by host defenses (the immune system working in concert with phagocytic cells).

ACQUIRED RESISTANCE TO ANTIMICROBIAL DRUGS

Over time, an organism that had once been highly responsive to an antibiotic may become less susceptible, or it may lose sensitivity to the drug entirely. In some cases, resistance to multiple drugs develops. Acquired resistance is of great concern in that it can render currently effective drugs useless, thereby creating a clinical crisis and a constant need for new antimicrobial agents. In the discussion that follows, we will examine the mechanisms by which microbial drug resistance is acquired, and we will discuss methods by which emergence of resistance can be delayed. Please note that it is the *microbe* that becomes drug resistant and not the patient.

Mechanisms of Microbial Drug Resistance

Microorganisms become drug resistant because of alterations in their function or structure. Four such microbial alterations are described below.

Microbes may elaborate drug-metabolizing enzymes. For example, many bacteria are now resistant to penicillin G because of increased production of penicillinase, an enzyme that converts penicillin into an inactive product. Through production of enzymes, some microorganisms are able to inactivate several different kinds of antibiotics.

Microbes may cease active uptake of certain drugs. Since the site of action of many antibiotics is intracellular, reduced drug uptake will result in resistance. This mechanism is responsible for some cases of resistance to tetracyclines.

Microbial drug receptors may undergo change, resulting in decreased antibiotic binding and action. For example, some bacteria are now resistant to streptomycin because of structural changes in bacterial ribosomes, the sites at which streptomycin acts to inhibit protein synthesis.

Microbes may synthesize compounds that antagonize drug actions. For example, by acquiring the ability to synthesize increased quantities of PABA, some bacteria have developed resistance to sulfonamides.

Mechanisms by Which Resistance Is Acquired

The alterations in structure and function discussed above are brought about by changes in the microbial genome. These genetic changes may result from spontaneous mutation or by acquisition of DNA from an external source. The most important mechanism by which bacteria obtain external DNA is conjugation with other bacteria.

Spontaneous Mutation. Spontaneous mutation results in random changes in a microbe's DNA. As a rule, such mutations confer resistance to *only one drug*. Development of multiple drug resistance would require multiple mutations, a phenomenon that is rare.

Conjugation. Conjugation is a process by which extrachromosomal DNA is transferred from one bacterium to another. In order to transfer resistance by conjugation, the donor organism must possess two unique DNA segments, one that codes for the mechanisms of drug resistance and one that codes for the "sexual" apparatus required for DNA transfer. Together, these two DNA segments constitute an *R factor* (resistance factor).

Conjugation takes place primarily between *gram-negative* bacteria. Genetic material may be transferred between members of the same species or between bacteria of different species. Because transfer of R factors is not species specific, it is possible for pathogenic bacteria to acquire R factors from the normal flora of the body. Since R factors are becoming common in normal flora, the possibility of transferring resistance from normal flora to pathogens is of real clinical concern.

In contrast to spontaneous mutation, conjugation frequently results in *multiple drug resistance*. This can be achieved, for example, by transfer of DNA that codes for several different drug-metabolizing enzymes. Hence, in a single event, a drug-sensitive bacterium can be changed into one that is highly drug resistant.

Relationships Between Antibiotic Use and The Emergence of Drug-Resistant Microbes

Use of antibiotics promotes the emergence of drug-resistant microbes. It should be emphasized, however, that although antibiotics promote drug resistance, these agents are not mutagenic and do not directly cause the genetic changes that underlie reduced drug sensitivity; spontaneous mutation and conjugation are random events whose incidence is independent of drug use. Drugs simply serve to make conditions favorable for overgrowth of those microbes that possess mechanisms of drug resistance.

How Do Antibiotics Promote Resistance? To answer this question, we need to recall two aspects of microbial ecology: (1) microbes secrete compounds that are toxic to other microbes, and (2) microbes within a given ecologic niche (e.g., large intestine, urogenital tract, skin) compete with one another for available nutrients. Under drug-free conditions, the various microbes in a given location keep one another in check. Furthermore, if none of these organisms is drug resistant, introduction of antibiotics will be equally detrimental to all members of the population, and, therefore, will not promote the growth of any individual. However, *if a drug-resistant organism is present, antibiotics will create selection pressure favoring the growth of that microbe*: by killing off the sensitive organisms, the drug will eliminate toxins produced by those microbes, and thereby facilitate survival of the microbe that is drug resistant. Also, elimination of sensitive organisms will remove competition for available nutrients, thereby making conditions even more favorable for the drug-resistant microbe to flourish. Hence, although drug resistance is of no benefit to an organism when there are no antibiotics around, when antibiotics are used, these agents create selection pressure favoring overgrowth of those microbes that are resistant.

Which Antibiotics Promote Resistance? *All* antimicrobial drugs promote the emergence of drug-resistant organisms. However, some agents are more likely to promote resistance than others. Since *broad-spectrum* antibiotics kill off more competing organisms than do narrow-spectrum drugs, emergence of resistance is facilitated most by the broad-spectrum drugs.

Does the Amount of Antibiotic Use Influence the Emergence of Resistance? You bet! The more that antibiotics are used, the faster drug-resistant organisms will emerge. Not only do antibiotics promote emergence of resistant pathogens, these drugs also promote overgrowth of normal flora that possess mechanisms for resistance. Since drug use can increase resistance in normal flora, and since these organisms can transfer resistance to pathogens, every effort should be made to avoid use of antibiotics by individuals who don't actually need them (i.e., individuals who are free of a treatable infection). Because all use of antibiotics will further the emergence of resistance, there can be no excuse for casual or indiscriminate dispensing of antimicrobial medications.

Since hospitals are sites of intensive antibiotic use, resident organisms can be extremely drug resistant. As a result, *nosocomial* infections (infections acquired in hospitals) are among the most difficult to treat.

Suprainfection

Suprainfection is simply a special example of the emergence of drug resistance. A suprainfection is defined as a *new* infection that appears during the course of treatment for a primary infection. A new infection can develop because antibiotic use can eliminate the inhibitory influence of normal flora, thereby allowing a second infectious agent to flourish. Because broad-spectrum antibiotics kill off more normal flora than do narrow-spectrum drugs, suprainfections are more likely during use of broad-spectrum agents. Suprainfections can be difficult to treat, since they are, by definition, caused by microbes that are drug resistant. It should be noted that in some texts, suprainfections are referred to as *superinfections*; this name may have been chosen to reflect the difficulties of treatment.

Delaying the Emergence of Resistance

Several measures can help delay the emergence of resistance. First, antimicrobial agents should be used only when actually needed. (It is estimated that in some settings, as much as 95% of antibiotic use is unnecessary.) Second, narrow-spectrum agents should be employed whenever possible; routine use of broad-spectrum drugs to compensate for diagnostic imprecision should be discouraged. Third, newer antibiotics should be reserved for situations in which older drugs are dangerous or no longer effective. Widespread use of the newer drugs will only serve to hasten their obsolescence.

SELECTION OF ANTIBIOTICS

The therapeutic objective when treating infection is to produce maximal antimicrobial effects while causing minimal harm to the host. Achieving this goal requires selection of the antibiotic that is most appropriate for the individual patient. When choosing this antibiotic, three principal factors must be considered: (1) the identity of the infecting organism, (2) drug sensitivity of the infecting organism, and (3) host factors, such as the site of infection and the status of host defenses.

For any given infection, several drugs may be effective. However, for most infections, there is usually one drug that is superior to the alternatives (Table 73–3). This drug of first choice may be preferred for several reasons, such as greater efficacy, lower toxicity, or narrower spectrum. Whenever possible, the drug of first choice should be employed. Alternative agents should be used only when the first-choice drug is inappropriate. Conditions that might rule out use of a first-choice agent include (1) allergy to the drug of choice, (2) inability of the drug of choice to penetrate to the site of infection, and (3) unusual susceptibility of the patient to a toxicity of the first-choice drug.

Empiric Therapy Prior to Completion of Laboratory Tests

Optimal antimicrobial therapy requires identification of the infecting organism and determination of its drug sensitivity. However, when the patient has a severe infection, it may be necessary to begin treatment before test results are available. Under these conditions, drug selection must be based on clinical evaluation and knowledge of which microbes are most likely to cause infection at a particular site in a given patient. If necessary, a broad-spectrum agent can be used for initial treatment. Then, once the identity and drug sensitivity of the infecting organism have been determined, the patient can be switched to a more selective antibiotic. When conditions demand that we start therapy in the absence of laboratory data, it is essential that samples of exudates and body fluids be obtained for culture *prior to initiation of treatment*; if antibiotics are present at the time of sampling, these agents can suppress microbial growth in culture, thereby impeding identification.

Identification of the Infecting Organism

The first rule of antimicrobial therapy is to *match the drug with the bug*. Hence, whenever possible, the infecting organism should be identified prior to initiation of therapy. If treatment is begun in the absence of a definitive diagnosis, positive identification should be established as soon as possible, since this will permit adjustment of the regimen to better conform with the drug sensitivity of the infecting organism.

The quickest, simplest, and most versatile technique for identifying microorganisms is microscopic examination of a *gram-stained* preparation. Samples for examination can be obtained from pus, sputum, urine, blood, and other body fluids. The most useful samples are direct aspirates from the site of infection.

In some cases, only a small number of infecting organisms will be present. Under these conditions, positive identification may require that the microbes be grown out in culture. As stressed above, material for culture should be obtained prior to initiating treatment. Furthermore, these samples should be taken in a fashion that minimizes contamination with normal body flora. Identification will be facilitated by avoiding exposure of samples to low temperature, antiseptics, and oxygen.

Determination of Drug Susceptibility

Because of the emergence of drug-resistant organisms, testing for drug sensitivity is common. However, sensitivity testing is not always needed. Rather, testing is indicated only when the infecting organism is one in which resistance is likely. Hence, for microbes such as the group A streptococci, which have remained highly susceptible to penicillin, sensitivity testing is unnecessary. In contrast, when resistance is common, as it is with *Staphylococcus aureus* and the gram-negative bacilli, tests for drug sensitivity should be performed.

Table 73–3. Antimicrobial Drugs of Choice

Organism	Drug of First Choice	Alternative Drugs
Gram-Positive Cocci		
Staphylococcus aureus		
Nonpenicillinase-producing	Penicillin G or V	Cefazolin, vancomycin, imipenem
Penicillinase-producing	Nafcillin	Cefazolin, vancomycin, amoxicillin-clavulanic acid
Methicillin-resistant	Vancomycin, with or without rifampin and/or gentamicin	Trimethoprim-sulfamethoxazole, minocycline
Streptococcus pyogenes (Group A) and groups C and G	Penicillin G or V	Cefazolin, vancomycin, erythromycin
Streptococcus, Group B	Penicillin G or ampicillin	Cefazolin, vancomycin, erythromycin
Streptococcus viridans group	Penicillin G with or without gentamicin	Cefazolin, vancomycin
Streptococcus bovis	Penicillin G	Cefazolin, vancomycin
Streptococcus faecalis (enterococcus)		
Endocarditis and other severe infections	Penicillin G or ampicillin with gentamicin	Vancomycin with gentamicin
Uncomplicated urinary tract infection	Ampicillin or amoxicillin	Nitrofurantoin, a fluoroquinolone
Streptococcus, anaeorbic	Penicillin G	Clindamycin, cefazolin, vancomycin
Streptococcus pneumoniae (pneumococcus)	Penicillin G or V	Erythromycin, cefazolin, vancomycin, chloramphenicol
Gram-Negative Cocci		
Neisseria gonorrhoeae (gonococcus)	Ceftriaxone	Penicillin G, amoxicillin, spectinomycin, cefoxitin, trimethoprim-sulfamethoxazole, chloramphenicol, a fluoroquinolone
Neisseria meningitidis (meningococcus)	Penicillin G	Cefuroxime, chloramphenicol
Gram-Positive Bacilli		
Bacillus anthracis	Penicillin G	Erythromycin, a tetracycline
Clostridium difficile	Vancomycin or metronidazole	Bacitracin
Clostridium perfringens	Penicillin G	Metronidazole, chloramphenicol
Clostridium tetani	Penicillin G	A tetracycline
Corynebacterium diphtheriae	Erythromycin	Penicillin G
Listeria monocytogenes	Ampicillin with or without gentamicin	Trimethoprim-sulfamethoxazole
Enteric Gram-Negative Bacilli		
Bacteroides		
Oropharyngeal strains (not *B. fragilis* group)	Penicillin G	Metronidazole, clindamycin, cefoxitin
Gastrointestinal strains (*B. fragilis* group)	Metronidazole	Clindamycin, imipenem, ticarcillin-clavulanic acid
Campylobacter jejuni	A fluoroquinolone or ciprofloxacin	A tetracycline, gentamicin
Escherichia coli	A first-generation cephalosporin	Ampicillin with or without gentamicin, ticarcillin–clavulanic acid, trimethoprim-sulfamethoxazole
Enterobacter species	Imipenem	Ciprofloxacin, trimethoprim-sulfamethoxazole, a third-generation cephalosporin
Helicobacter pylori	A tetracycline plus metronidazole plus bismuth subsalicylate	
Klebsiella pneumoniae	Cefotaxime	Gentamicin, tobramycin, amikacin
Proteus, indole positive (including *Providencia rettgeri* and *Morganella morganii*)	Cefotaxime, ceftizoxime, or ceftriaxone	Gentamicin, a fluoroquinolone, trimethoprim-sulfamethoxazole
Proteus mirabilis	Ampicillin	A first-generation cephalosporin, trimethoprim-sulfamethoxazole
Salmonella typhi	Ceftriaxone	Trimethoprim-sulfamethoxazole, ampicillin, amoxicillin, chloramphenicol
Other *Salmonella*	Ceftriaxone or cefotaxime	Trimethoprim-sulfamethoxazole, ciprofloxacin, chloramphenicol, ampicillin
Serratia	Cefotaxime, ceftizoxime, or ceftriaxone	Gentamicin, amikacin, imipenem
Shigella	A fluoroquinolone	Trimethoprim-sulfamethoxazole, ciprofloxacin, ampicillin, ceftriaxone
Yersinia enterocolitica	Trimethoprim-sulfamethoxazole	A fluoroquinolone, gentamicin, tobramycin

Table continued on following page

Table 73–3. Antimicrobial Drugs of Choice *Continued*		
Organism	**Drug of First Choice**	**Alternative Drugs**
Other Gram-Negative Bacilli		
Acinetobacter	Imipenem	Trimethoprim-sulfamethoxazole, tobramycin, gentamicin
Bordetella pertussis (whooping cough)	Erythromycin	Trimethoprim-sulfamethoxazole, ampicillin
Brucella (brucellosis)	A tetracycline plus gentamicin	Rifampin plus a tetracycline, trimethoprim-sulfamethoxazole, chloramphenicol with or without streptomycin
Calymmatobacterium granulomatis	A tetracycline	Streptomycin
Francisella tularensis (tularemia)	Streptomycin or gentamicin	A tetracycline, chloramphenicol
Gardnerella (Haemophilus) vaginalis	Metronidazole	Ampicillin
Haemophilus ducreyi (chancroid)	Ceftriaxone or erythromycin	Trimethoprim-sulfamethoxazole
Haemophilus influenzae		
Meningitis, epiglottitis, arthritis, and other serious infections	Cefotaxime or ceftriaxone	Cefuroxime, chloramphenicol
Upper respiratory infection and bronchitis	Trimethoprim-sulfamethoxazole	Ampicillin or amoxicillin
Legionella micdadei	Erythromycin with or without rifampin	Trimethoprim-sulfamethoxazole
Legionella pneumophila (legionnaires' disease)	Erythromycin plus rifampin	Trimethoprim-sulfamethoxazole
Pasteurella multocida	Penicillin G	A tetracycline, a cephalosporin
Pseudomonas aeruginosa		
Urinary tract infection	Ciprofloxacin	Piperacillin, ceftazidime, imipenem, carbenicillin, ticarcillin
Other infections	Ticarcillin, mezlocillin, or piperacillin plus tobramycin, gentamicin or amikacin	Tobramycin, gentamicin or amikacin plus ceftazidime, imipenem or aztreonam
Pseudomonas mallei (glanders)	Streptomycin with a tetracycline	Streptomycin plus chloramphenicol
Pseudomonas pseudomallei (melioidosis)	Ceftazidime	Chloramphenicol plus doxycycline plus trimethoprim-sulfamethoxazole
Pseudomonas cepacia	Trimethoprim-sulfamethoxazole	Chloramphenicol, ceftazidime
Spirillum minus (rat bite fever)	Penicillin G	A tetracycline, streptomycin
Streptobacillus moniliformis (rat bite fever)	Penicillin G	A tetracycline, streptomycin
Vibrio cholerae (cholera)	A tetracycline	Trimethoprim-sulfamethoxazole, a fluoroquinolone
Yersinia pestis (plague)	Streptomycin	A tetracycline, chloramphenicol, gentamicin
Mycobacteria		
Mycobacterium tuberculosis	Isoniazid plus rifampin plus pyrazinamide with or without ethambutol	Ethambutol, streptomycin, cycloserine, ethionamide, kanamycin, capreomycin, ciprofloxacin, ofloxacin
Mycobacterium leprae (leprosy)	Dapsone plus rifampin	Clofazimine
Mycobacterium avium complex	Clarithromycin ± rifampin ± ethambutol ± clofazimine	Rifampin with ethambutol, ciprofloxacin, and clofazimine ± amikacin, capreomycin
Actinomycetes		
Actinomycetes israelii	Penicillin G	A tetracycline
Nocardia	Trimethoprim-sulfamethoxazole	Sulfisoxazole, imipenem, amikacin, minocycline
Chlamydiae		
Chlamydia psittaci	A tetracycline	Chloramphenicol
Chlamydia trachomatis		
Trachoma	A tetracycline (oral plus topical)	A sulfonamide (oral plus topical)
Inclusion conjunctivitis	Erythromycin (oral or IV)	A sulfonamide
Pneumonia	Erythromycin	A sulfonamide
Urethritis, cervicitis	Erythromycin or doxycycline	Azithromycin, ofloxacin, sulfisoxazole
Lymphogranuloma venereum	Doxycycline	Erythromycin
Mycoplasma		
Mycoplasma pneumoniae	Erythromycin or a tetracycline	Clarithromycin
Ureaplasma urealyticum	Erythromycin	A tetracycline, clarithromycin
Rickettsiae		
Rocky Mountain spotted fever, endemic typhus (murine), trench fever, typhus, scrub typhus, Q fever	A tetracycline	Chloramphenicol, a fluoroquinolone

Table 73–3. Antimicrobial Drugs of Choice *Continued*

Organism	Drug of First Choice	Alternative Drugs
Spirochetes		
Borrelia burgdorferi (Lyme disease)	Doxycycline	Amoxicillin, ceftriaxone
Borrelia recurrentis (relapsing fever)	A tetracycline	Penicillin G
Leptospira	Penicillin G	A tetracycline
Treponema pallidum (syphilis)	Penicillin G	A tetracycline, ceftriaxone
Treponema pertenue (yaws)	Penicillin G	A tetracycline
Fungi		
Aspergillus species	Amphotericin B	Itraconazole
Blastomyces dermatitidis	Amphotericin B or ketoconazole	Itraconazole
Candida species (systemic)	Amphotericin B ± flucytosine	Fluconazole
Coccidioides immitis	Amphotericin B or ketoconazole	Itraconazole, fluconazole
Cryptococcus neoformans	Amphotericin B ± flucytosine	Itraconazole, fluconazole
Histoplasma capsulatum	Amphotericin B or ketoconazole	Itraconazole
Mucor	Amphotericin B	
Paracoccidioides brasiliensis	Amphotericin B or ketoconazole	Itraconazole
Sporothrix schenckii	Amphotericin B	Itraconazole
Viruses		
Cytomegalovirus	Ganciclovir	Foscarnet
Herpes simplex virus		
Keratitis	Trifluridine	Vidarabine, idoxuridine
Genital	Acyclovir	
Encephalitis	Acyclovir	Vidarabine
Neonatal	Acyclovir	Vidarabine
Disseminated, adult	Acyclovir	Vidarabine
Human immunodeficiency virus	Zidovudine (azidothymidine)	Didanosine
Influenza A	Amantadine	Ribavirin
Respiratory syncytial virus	Ribavirin	
Varicella-zoster virus	Acyclovir	Foscarnet

Disk-Diffusion Test. The most widely used method for assessing drug sensitivity is the disk-diffusion test, also known as the Kirby-Bauer test. This test is performed by inoculating an agar plate with the infecting organism and then placing on that plate several small disks, each of which is impregnated with a different antibiotic. Because of diffusion, an antibiotic-containing zone becomes established around each of the disks. As the bacteria proliferate, growth will be inhibited around those disks that contain an antibiotic to which the bacteria are sensitive. The degree of drug sensitivity is proportional to the size of the bacteria-free zones. Hence, by measuring the diameter of these zones, we can determine the drugs to which the organism is more susceptible, as well as those to which it is highly resistant.

Broth Dilution Procedure. An alternative method for assessing drug sensitivity is known as the broth dilution procedure. In this procedure, bacteria are grown in a series of tubes containing different concentrations of an antibiotic, thereby permitting assessment of antibacterial effects at specific drug concentrations. The advantage of this method over the disk-diffusion test is that it provides a more precise measure of drug sensitivity. By using the broth dilution procedure, we can es-

tablish close estimates of two clinically useful values: (1) the *minimum inhibitory concentration* or *MIC* (defined as the lowest concentration of antibiotic that produces complete inhibition of bacterial growth), and (2) the *minimum bactericidal concentration* or *MBC* (defined as the lowest concentration of drug that produces a 99.9% decline in the number of bacterial colonies). Because of the quantitative information provided, broth dilution procedures are especially useful for guiding therapy of infections that are especially difficult to treat.

HOST FACTORS THAT MODIFY DRUG CHOICE, ROUTE OF ADMINISTRATION, OR DOSAGE

In addition to matching the drug with the bug and determining the drug sensitivity of an infecting organism, we must consider host factors when prescribing an antimicrobial drug. Two host factors—host defenses and the site of infection—are unique to the selection of antibiotics. Other host factors, such as age, pregnancy, and previous drug reactions, are the same factors that must be considered when choosing any other medication.

Host Defenses

Host defenses consist primarily of the immune system and phagocytic cells (macrophages, neutrophils). Without the contribution of these defenses, successful antimicrobial therapy would be rare. In most cases, the drugs we use to treat infection do not produce cure on their own. Rather, these agents work in concert with host defense systems to subdue infection. Accordingly, the usual objective of antibiotic treatment is not outright kill of infecting organisms. Rather, the goal is to suppress microbial growth to the point at which the balance is tipped in favor of the host. Underscoring the critical role of host defenses is the grim fact that people whose defenses are impaired, such as those with acquired immunodeficiency syndrome (AIDS) and those undergoing cancer chemotherapy, frequently die from infections that drugs alone are unable to control. When treating the immunocompromised host, our only hope lies with the use of drugs that are rapidly bactericidal, and even these agents may prove inadequate.

Site of Infection

To be effective, an antibiotic must be present at the site of infection in a concentration greater than the MIC. At some sites, drug penetration may be hampered, making it difficult to achieve the MIC. For example, drug access can be impeded in meningitis (because of the blood-brain barrier), endocarditis (because bacterial vegetations in the heart are difficult to penetrate), and infected abscesses (because of poor vascularity and the presence of pus and other material). When treating meningitis, two approaches may be used to achieve the MIC: (1) we can select a drug that can readily cross the blood-brain barrier, and (2) we can inject an antibiotic directly into the subarachnoid space. When pus and other fluids hinder drug access, surgical drainage is indicated.

Foreign materials (e.g., cardiac pacemakers, prosthetic joints and heart valves, synthetic vascular shunts) present a special local problem. Phagocytes react to these objects and attempt to destroy them. Because of this behavior, the phagocytes are less able to attack bacteria, thereby allowing microbes to flourish at the site. When attempts are made to treat these infections, relapse and failure are common. In many cases, the infection can be eliminated only by removing the foreign material.

Other Host Factors

Age. Infants and the elderly are highly vulnerable to drug toxicity. In the elderly, heightened drug sensitivity is due in large part to reduced rates of drug metabolism and drug excretion, which can result in accumulation of antibiotics to toxic levels.

Multiple factors contribute to antibiotic sensitivity in infants. Because of poorly developed kidney and liver function, neonates eliminate drugs slowly. To avoid drug accumulation, many antibiotics must be used in low dosage. The very young are also subject to special toxicities. For example, use of sulfonamides in newborns can produce kernicterus, a severe neurologic disorder caused by displacement of bilirubin from plasma proteins (see Chapter 78). The tetracyclines provide another example of a drug toxicity unique to the young: these antibiotics bind to developing teeth, causing discoloration.

Pregnancy and Lactation. Antimicrobial drugs can cross the placenta, posing a risk to the developing fetus. As noted above, tetracyclines can stain immature teeth. When gentamicin is used during pregnancy, irreversible hearing loss may result.

Antibiotic use during pregnancy may also pose a risk to the expectant mother. It has been shown, for example, that during pregnancy there is an increased incidence of toxicity from tetracycline, characterized by hepatic necrosis, pancreatitis, renal damage, and, in extreme cases, death.

Antibiotics can enter breast milk, possibly affecting the nursing infant. Sulfonamides, for example, can reach levels in milk that are sufficient to cause kernicterus in nursing newborns. As a general guideline, antibiotics and all other drugs should be avoided by women who are breast-feeding.

Previous Allergic Reaction. Severe allergic reactions are more common with the *penicillins* than with any other family of drugs. As a rule, patients with a history of allergy to the penicillins should not receive them again. The exception to this rule is treatment of a life-threatening infection for which no suitable alternative is available. In addition to the penicillins, other antibiotics (sulfonamides, trimethoprim, erythromycin) are associated with a high incidence of allergic responses. However, *severe* reactions to these agents are relatively rare.

Genetic Factors. As with other drugs, responses to antibiotics can be influenced by the patient's genetic heritage. For example, some antibiotics (e.g., sulfonamides, nalidixic acid) can cause hemolysis in patients who, because of their genetic makeup, have red blood cells that are deficient in an enzyme called glucose-6-phosphate dehydrogenase. Clearly, people with this deficiency should not be given antibiotics that are likely to induce red cell lysis.

Genetic factors can also affect rates of metabolism. For example, hepatic inactivation of isoniazid is rapid in some people and slow in others. If the dosage is not adjusted accordingly, isoniazid may accumulate to toxic levels in the slow metabolizers, whereas drug levels may remain subtherapeutic in the rapid metabolizers.

DOSAGE SIZE AND DURATION OF TREATMENT

Successful therapy requires that the antibiotic be present at the site of infection in an effective concentration for a sufficient time. Dosages should be adjusted to produce drug concentrations that are equal to or greater than the MIC for the infection being treated. Drug levels four to eight times the MIC are often desirable.

Duration of therapy depends on a number of variables, including the status of host defenses, the site of the infection, and the identity of the infecting organism. *It is imperative that antibiotics not be discontinued prematurely. Patients should be instructed to take their medication for the entire prescribed course, even though symptoms may subside before the full course has been completed.* Early withdrawal is a common cause of recurrent infection, and the organisms responsible for relapse are likely to be more drug resistant than those that were present when therapy began.

THERAPY WITH ANTIBIOTIC COMBINATIONS

Therapy with a combination of antimicrobial agents is indicated *only in specific situations*. Under these well-defined conditions, use of multiple drugs may be life-saving. However, it should be stressed that although antibiotic combinations do have a valuable therapeutic role, routine use of two or more antibiotics should be discouraged. When an infection is caused by a single, identified microbe, treatment with just one drug is usually most appropriate.

Antimicrobial Effects of Antibiotic Combinations

When two antibiotics are used together, the result may be *additive*, *potentiative*, or, in certain cases, *antagonistic*. An *additive* response is one in which the antimicrobial effect of the combination is equal to the sum of the effects of the two drugs alone. A *potentiative* interaction is one in which the effect of the combination is greater than the sum of the effects of the individual agents. A classic example of potentiation is produced by the combination of trimethoprim plus sulfamethoxazole, drugs that inhibit sequential steps in the synthesis of tetrahydrofolic acid (see Chapter 78).

In certain cases, a combination of two antibiotics may be *less* effective than one of the agents by itself. Such reduced responses indicate antagonism between the drugs. Antagonism is most likely when a *bacteriostatic* agent (e.g., tetracycline) is combined with a *bactericidal* drug (e.g., penicillin). Antagonism occurs because bactericidal drugs are usually effective only against organisms that are actively growing. Hence, when bacterial growth has been suppressed by a bacteriostatic drug, the effects of a bactericidal agent can be reduced. If host defenses are intact, antagonism between two antibiotics may be of little clinical significance. However, if host defenses are compromised, the consequences of antagonism can be dire.

Indications for Antibiotic Combinations

Initial Therapy of Severe Infection. The most common indication for use of multiple antibiotics is initial therapy of severe infection of unknown etiology, especially in the neutropenic host. Until the infecting organism has been identified, wide antimicrobial coverage will be needed. Just how broad the coverage is will depend on the clinician's skill in narrowing the field of potential causative organisms. Once the identity of the infecting microbe is known, drug selection can be adjusted accordingly. As discussed above, samples for culture should be obtained before drug therapy has begun.

Mixed Infections. An infection may be caused by more than one microbe. Multiple infecting organisms are common in brain abscesses, pelvic infections, and infections resulting from perforation of abdominal organs. When the infecting microbes differ from one another in drug susceptibility, treatment with more than one antibiotic is required.

Prevention of Resistance. Although use of multiple antibiotics is usually associated with *promotion* of drug resistance, there is one disease—*tuberculosis*—in which drug combinations are employed for the specific purpose of *suppressing* the emergence of resistant bacteria. Just why tuberculosis differs from other infections in this regard is discussed in Chapter 81.

Decreased Toxicity. In some situations, an antibiotic combination can reduce the risk of toxicity to the host. For example, by combining flucytosine with amphotericin B in the treatment of fungal meningitis, the dosage of amphotericin B can be reduced, thereby decreasing the risk of amphotericin-induced damage to the kidneys.

Enhanced Antibacterial Action. In specific infections, a combination of antibiotics can have greater antibacterial action than a single agent. This is true of the combined use of penicillin plus an aminoglycoside in the treatment of enterococcal endocarditis. Penicillin acts to weaken the bacterial cell wall; the aminoglycoside acts to suppress protein synthesis. The combination has enhanced antibacterial action because, by weakening the cell wall, penicillin facilitates penetration of the aminoglycoside to its intracellular site of action, thereby increasing the effects of the aminoglycoside.

Disadvantages of Antibiotic Combinations

Use of multiple antibiotics has several drawbacks, including (1) increased risk of toxic and allergic reactions, (2) possible antagonism of antimicrobial effects, (3) increased risk of suprainfection, (4) selection of drug-resistant bacteria, and (5) increased cost. Because of these detriments, antimicrobial combinations should be employed only when clearly indicated.

PROPHYLACTIC USE OF ANTIMICROBIAL DRUGS

It is estimated that between 30% and 50% of the antibiotics used in the United States are administered for prophylaxis. That is, these agents are given to prevent an infection from occurring rather than to treat an infection that is already established. Much of the prophylactic use of antibiotics is uncalled for. However, in certain situations, antimicrobial prophylaxis is both appropriate and effective. Whenever prophylaxis is attempted, the benefits must be weighed against the risks of toxicity, allergic reactions, suprainfection, and selection of drug-resistant organisms. Generally approved indications for prophylaxis are discussed below.

Surgery. Prophylactic use of antibiotics can decrease the incidence of infection in certain kinds of surgery. Procedures in which prophylactic efficacy has been documented include cardiac surgery, peripheral vascular surgery, orthopedic surgery, and surgery on the gastrointestinal tract (stomach, duodenum, colon, rectum, appendix). Prophylaxis is also beneficial for women undergoing a hysterectomy or an emergency cesarean section. In "dirty" surgery (operations performed on perforated abdominal organs, compound fractures, or lacerations from animal bites), the risk of infection is nearly 100%. For these operations, use of antibiotics is considered *treatment,* not prophylaxis. When antibiotics are given for prophylaxis, they should be administered before surgery has begun. If the procedure is unusually long, readministration during surgery may be indicated. As a rule, postoperative antibiotics are unnecessary. For most operations, a first-generation cephalosporin (e.g., cefazolin, cephalothin) will provide the needed protection.

Bacterial Endocarditis. Individuals with congenital or valvular heart disease and those with prosthetic heart valves are unusually susceptible to bacterial endocarditis. For these people, endocarditis can develop following surgery, dental procedures, and other procedures that may dislodge bacteria into the bloodstream. Hence, prior to undergoing such procedures, these patients should receive prophylactic antimicrobial medication.

Neutropenia. Severe neutropenia puts individuals at high risk of infection. There is some evidence that the incidence of bacterial infection may be reduced through antibiotic prophylaxis. However, prophylaxis may increase the risk of infection with fungi: by killing normal flora, whose presence helps suppress fungal growth, antibiotics can encourage fungal invasion.

Other Indications for Antimicrobial Prophylaxis. For young women with recurrent urinary tract infection, prophylaxis with trimethoprim-sulfamethoxazole may be helpful. Amantadine (an antiviral agent) may be employed for prophylaxis against type A influenza. For individuals who have had severe rheumatic carditis, lifelong prophylaxis with penicillin may be needed. Antimicrobial prophylaxis is indicated following exposure to organisms responsible for sexually transmitted diseases (e.g., syphilis, gonorrhea).

MISUSES OF ANTIMICROBIAL DRUGS

Throughout this chapter, we have focused on the proper use of antimicrobial medications. In this concluding section, we will examine important ways in which antibiotics are misused.

Attempted Treatment of Untreatable Infection. The majority of viral infections, including mumps, chickenpox, and most upper respiratory infections, do not respond to currently available drugs. Hence, when drug therapy of these disorders is attempted, patients are exposed to all the risks of drug use without receiving any benefits.

Treatment of Fever of Unknown Origin. Although fever can be a sign of infection, it can also signify other diseases, including hepatitis, arthritis, and cancer. Unless the cause of a fever has been shown to be infection, antibiotics should not be employed. Reasons for this prohibition are the following: (1) if the fever is *not* due to an infection, antibiotics would not only be inappropriate but would also expose the patient to unnecessary toxicity and would delay correct diagnosis of the fever's cause, and (2) if the fever *is* caused by infection, antibiotics could hamper later attempts to identify the infecting organism.

There is one situation in which fever, by itself,

does constitute an indication for antibiotic use. That situation is fever in the neutropenic host. Since fever may indicate infection, and since infection can be lethal to the neutropenic patient, these patients should be given antibiotics when fever occurs—even if fever is the only indication that an infection may be present.

Improper Dosage. Like all other medications, antibiotics must be used in appropriate dosages. If the dosage is too low, the patient will be exposed to a risk of adverse effects without benefit of antibacterial effects. If the dosage is too high, the risks of suprainfection and adverse effects become unnecessarily high.

Treatment in the Absence of Adequate Bacteriologic Information. As stressed earlier, proper antimicrobial therapy requires information on the identity and drug sensitivity of the infecting organism. Except in life-threatening situations, therapy should not be undertaken in the absence of bacteriologic information. This important guideline is often ignored.

Omission of Surgical Drainage. Antibiotics may have limited efficacy in the presence of foreign material, necrotic tissue, or pus. Hence, when appropriate, surgical drainage and cleansing should be performed to promote antimicrobial effects.

MONITORING ANTIMICROBIAL THERAPY

Antimicrobial therapy is assessed by monitoring clinical responses and laboratory results. The frequency of monitoring is directly proportional to the severity of infection. Important clinical indicators of success are reduction of fever and resolution of signs and symptoms related to the affected organ system (e.g., improvement of breath sounds in patients with pneumonia).

Various laboratory tests are used to monitor treatment. Serum drug levels may be monitored for two reasons: (1) to insure that levels are sufficient for antimicrobial effects, and (2) to avoid toxicity from excessive levels. Success of therapy is indicated by the disappearance of infectious organisms from post-treatment cultures; these cultures may become sterile within hours of the onset of treatment (as may happen with urinary tract infections) or they may not become sterile for weeks (as may happen with tuberculosis).

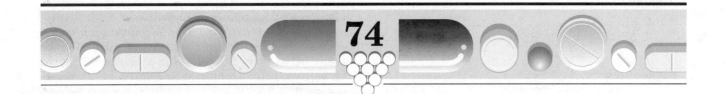

74

Drugs That Weaken the Bacterial Cell Wall I: Penicillins

INTRODUCTION TO THE PENICILLINS

The penicillins are nearly ideal antibiotics. These drugs are active against a variety of bacteria and their direct toxicity is low. Allergic reactions constitute their principal adverse effects. Owing to their safety and effectiveness, the penicillins are widely prescribed.

Because they have a beta-lactam ring in their structure (see Figure 74–1), the penicillins are referred to as *beta-lactam antibiotics*. The beta-lactam family also includes the cephalosporins, aztreonam, and imipenem; these drugs are discussed in Chapter 75. All of the beta-lactam antibiotics share the same mechanism of action: disruption of the bacterial cell wall.

MECHANISM OF ACTION

To understand the actions of the penicillins, we must first understand the structure and function of the bacterial cell wall. The cell wall is a rigid, permeable, meshlike structure that lies outside the cytoplasmic membrane. Within the cytoplasmic membrane, osmotic pressure is very high, creating a strong tendency for the bacterium to take up

927

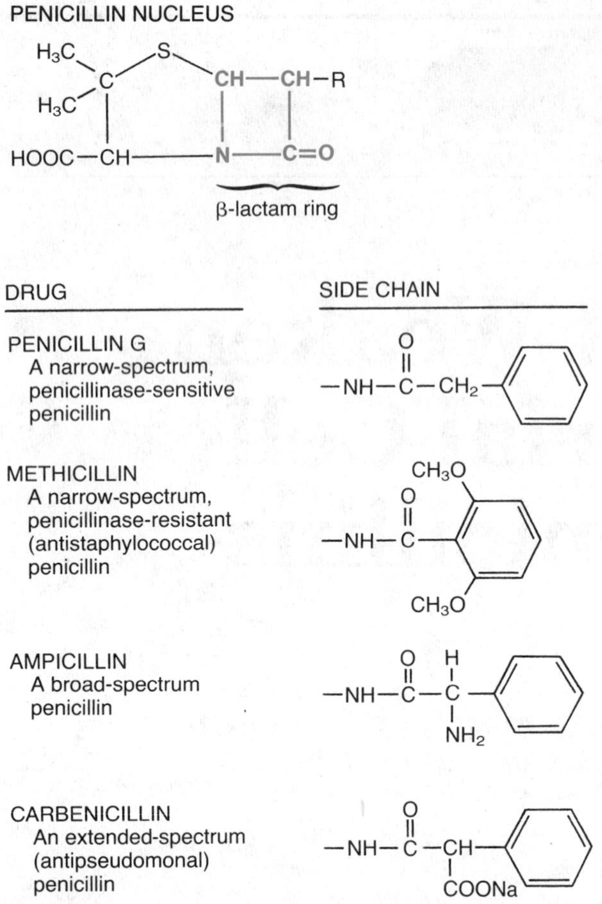

PENICILLIN NUCLEUS

β-lactam ring

DRUG	SIDE CHAIN
PENICILLIN G A narrow-spectrum, penicillinase-sensitive penicillin	
METHICILLIN A narrow-spectrum, penicillinase-resistant (antistaphylococcal) penicillin	
AMPICILLIN A broad-spectrum penicillin	
CARBENICILLIN An extended-spectrum (antipseudomonal) penicillin	

Figure 74–1. Structural formulas of representative penicillins. The unique structure of individual penicillins is determined by the side chain coupled to the penicillin nucleus at the position labeled R. This side chain influences acid stability, pharmacokinetic properties, penicillinase resistance, and ability to bind specific penicillin-binding proteins.

water and swell. If it were not for the rigid cell wall, which prevents the bacterium from expanding, water would be absorbed to such an extent that the bacterium would eventually burst.

The penicillins weaken the cell wall, causing the bacterium to take up excessive amounts of water and then rupture. Hence, the penicillins are usually bactericidal. For reasons that are not understood, penicillins are lethal only to bacteria that are undergoing active growth and division.

Penicillins weaken the cell wall by two actions: (1) *inhibition of transpeptidases* and (2) *disinhibi-*

tion (activation) of autolysins. *Transpeptidases* are enzymes critical to cell wall synthesis. Specifically, these enzymes catalyze the formation of *cross-bridges* between the peptidoglycan polymer strands that form the cell wall; these bridges give the cell wall its strength (see Figure 74–2). *Autolysins* are bacterial enzymes that cleave bonds in the cell wall. Bacteria employ these enzymes to break down segments of the cell wall to permit growth and division. By simultaneously inhibiting transpeptidases and activating autolysins, the penicillins disrupt synthesis of the cell wall and promote its active destruction; these combined actions result in cell lysis and death.

The molecular targets of the penicillins (transpeptidases, autolysins, other bacterial enzymes) are known collectively as *penicillin-binding proteins* (PBPs). These molecules are called PBPs because penicillins must bind to them to produce antibacterial effects. More than eight different PBPs have been identified. The PBPs that are most important in mediating the bactericidal actions of the penicillins are named PBP1 and PBP3. As indicated in Figure 74–3, PBPs are located on the *outer* surface of the cytoplasmic membrane.

Since mammalian cells lack a cell wall, and since penicillins act specifically on enzymes that affect cell wall integrity, the penicillins have virtually no *direct* effects on cells of the host. As a result, the penicillins are among our safest antibiotics.

MECHANISMS OF BACTERIAL RESISTANCE

Bacterial resistance to penicillins is determined primarily by two factors: (1) inability of penicillins to reach their targets (PBPs) and (2) inactivation of penicillins by bacterial enzymes.

The Gram-Negative Cell Envelope

All bacteria are surrounded by a cell envelope. However, the cell envelope of gram-negative organisms differs from that of gram-positive organisms. Because of this difference, most penicillins are inactive against gram-negative bacteria.

As indicated in Figure 74–3, the cell envelope of *gram-positive* bacteria has only two layers: the cy-

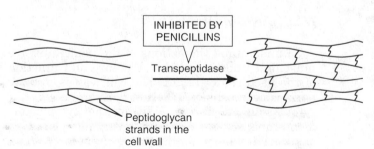

Figure 74–2. Inhibition of transpeptidase by penicillins. The bacterial cell wall is composed of long strands of a peptidoglycan polymer. As depicted, transpeptidase enzymes create cross-bridges between the peptidoglycan strands, giving the cell wall its strength. By inhibiting transpeptidases, penicillins prevent cross-bridge synthesis and thereby weaken the cell wall.

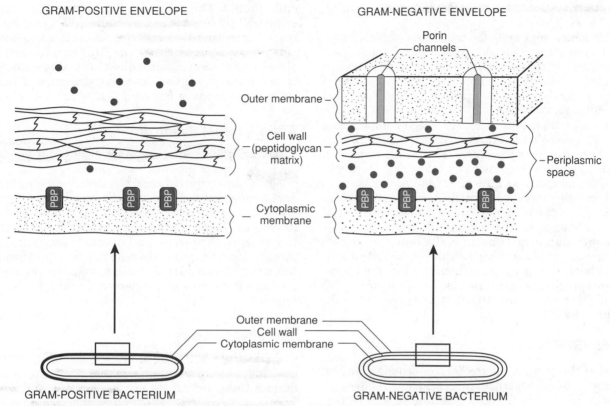

Figure 74–3. The bacterial cell envelope. Note that the gram-positive cell envelope lacks an outer membrane. The outer membrane of the gram-negative cell envelope prevents certain penicillins from reaching their target molecules. (PBP = penicillin-binding protein [transpeptidases and other penicillin target molecules]. Filled circles [●] represent beta-lactamases.)

toplasmic membrane plus a relatively thick cell wall. Despite its thickness, the cell wall can be readily penetrated by penicillins, giving them easy access to PBPs on the cytoplasmic membrane. As a result, penicillins are generally very active against gram-positive organisms.

The *gram-negative* cell envelope has *three* layers: the cytoplasmic membrane, a relatively thin cell wall, and an additional, *outer membrane* (Fig. 74–3). Like the gram-positive cell wall, the gram-negative cell wall can be easily penetrated by penicillins. The outer membrane, in contrast, is difficult to penetrate: only those penicillins that can pass through the small pores in the outer membrane are able to cross and reach PBPs on the cytoplasmic membrane. Since most penicillins cannot pass through the outer membrane, most penicillins are inactive against gram-negative bacteria.

Penicillinases (Beta-Lactamases)

Beta-lactamases are enzymes that cleave the beta-lactam ring, and thereby render penicillins and other beta-lactam antibiotics inactive (Fig. 74–4). Bacteria produce a variety of beta-lactamases; some are specific for penicillins, some are specific for other beta-lactam antibiotics (e.g., cephalosporins), and some act on several kinds of beta-lactam antibiotics. Those beta-lactamases

that act selectively on penicillins are referred to as *penicillinases*.

Penicillinases are synthesized by gram-positive and gram-negative bacteria. Gram-positive organisms produce large amounts of these enzymes, and then release them into the surrounding medium. In contrast, gram-negative bacteria produce penicillinases in relatively small amounts, and, rather than exporting them to the environment,

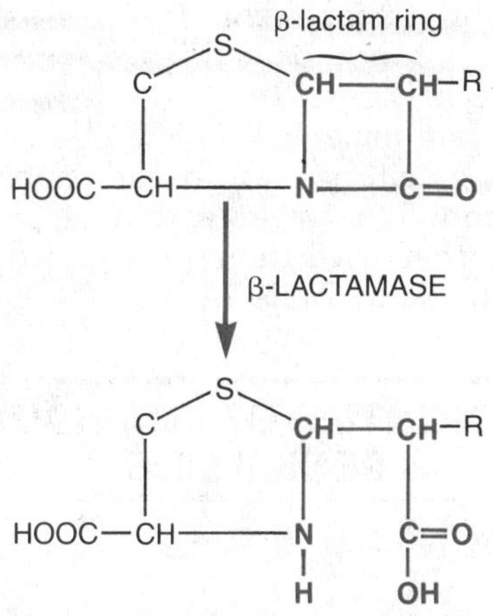

Figure 74–4. The effect of beta-lactamase on the penicillin nucleus.

secrete them into the periplasmic space (see Figure 74–3).

The genes that code for synthesis of beta-lactamases are located on plasmids (extrachromosomal DNA) and chromosomes. Genes that are present on plasmids may be transferred from one bacterium to another, thereby promoting the spread of penicillin resistance.

Transfer of resistance is of special importance with *Staphylococcus aureus*. When penicillin was first introduced in the early 1940's, all strains of *Staph. aureus* were sensitive to the drug. However, by 1960, as many as 80% of *Staph. aureus* isolates in hospitals displayed penicillin resistance. Fortunately, a penicillin derivative (methicillin) that has resistance to the actions of beta-lactamases was introduced at this time. To date, no known strains of *Staph. aureus* produce beta-lactamases capable of inactivating methicillin or related penicillinase-resistant penicillins (although some strains of this organism are resistant to these drugs for other reasons).

CHEMISTRY

All of the penicillins are derived from a common nucleus: 6-aminopenicillanic acid. As shown in Figure 74–1, this nucleus contains a beta-lactam ring joined to a second ring. The beta-lactam ring is essential for antibacterial actions. Properties of individual penicillins are determined by additions made to the basic nucleus, primarily at the site labeled R. These modifications determine (1) affinity for PBPs, (2) resistance to penicillinases, (3) ability to penetrate the gram-negative cell envelope, (4) resistance to stomach acid, and (5) pharmacokinetic properties.

CLASSIFICATION

The most useful classification of penicillins is based on antimicrobial spectrum. When classified according to spectrum, the penicillins fall into four major groups: (1) narrow-spectrum penicillins that are penicillinase-sensitive, (2) narrow-spectrum penicillins that are penicillinase-resistant (antistaphylococcal penicillins), (3) broad-spectrum penicillins (aminopenicillins), and (4) extended-spectrum penicillins (antipseudomonal penicillins). The individual agents that belong to these groups, together with their principal target organisms, are listed in Table 74–1.

PROPERTIES OF INDIVIDUAL PENICILLINS

PENICILLIN G

Penicillin G (benzylpenicillin) was the first penicillin available and is the prototype for the penicillin family. This agent is often referred to simply as *penicillin*. Penicillin G is bactericidal to a number of gram-positive bacteria as well as to some gram-negative organisms. Despite the introduction of newer antibiotics, penicillin G remains a drug of choice for many infections. The structure of penicillin G is shown in Figure 74–1.

Antimicrobial Spectrum

Penicillin G is active against *most gram-positive bacteria* (except penicillinase-producing staphylococci), gram-negative cocci (*Neisseria meningitidis* and nonpenicillinase-producing strains of *N. gonorrhoeae*), anaerobic bacteria, and spirochetes (including *Treponema pallidum*). With few exceptions, gram-negative bacilli are resistant. Although many organisms respond to penicillin G, the drug is considered a narrow-spectrum agent (as compared with other members of the penicillin family).

Therapeutic Uses

Penicillin G is a drug of first choice for infections caused by sensitive gram-positive cocci. Important among these infections are pneumonia and meningitis caused by *Streptococcus pneumoniae* (pneumococcus), pharyngitis caused by *Streptococcus pyogenes*, and infectious endocarditis caused by *Streptococcus viridans*. Penicillin is also the preferred drug for use against those few strains of *Staphylococcus aureus* that are not producers of penicillinase.

Penicillin is a preferred agent for infections caused by several gram-positive bacilli. These infections are gas gangrene (caused by *Clostridium perfringens*), tetanus (caused by *Clostridium tetani*), and anthrax (caused by *Bacillus anthracis*).

Penicillin is the drug of first choice for meningitis caused by *Neisseria meningitidis* (meningococcus). Although once the drug of choice for gonorrhea (caused by *Neisseria gonorrhoeae*), penicillin has been replaced by ceftriaxone as the primary treatment for this infection; penicillin is now limited to treating infections caused by nonpenicillinase-producing strains of *N. gonorrhoeae*.

Penicillin is the drug of choice for syphilis, an infection caused by the spirochete *Treponema pallidum*.

In addition to treatment of active infections, penicillin G has important *prophylactic* applications. The drug is used to prevent *syphilis* in sexual partners of individuals known to have this infection. Benzathine penicillin G (administered monthly for life) is employed for prophylaxis against recurrent attacks of *rheumatic fever*; treatment is recommended for patients with a history of recurrent rheumatic fever and for those with clear evidence of rheumatic heart disease. Penicil-

Table 74–1. Classification of the Penicillins		
Penicillin Class	**Drug**	**Clinically Useful Antimicrobial Spectrum**
Narrow-spectrum penicillins: penicillinase sensitive	Penicillin G Penicillin V	*Streptococcus* species, *Neisseria* species, many anaerobes, spirochetes, others
Narrow-spectrum penicillins: penicillinase resistant (antistaphylococcal penicillins)	Methicillin Nafcillin Oxacillin Cloxacillin Dicloxacillin	*Staphylococcus aureus*
Broad-spectrum penicillins (aminopenicillins)	Ampicillin Amoxicillin Bacampicillin	*Haemophilus influenzae, Escherichia coli, Proteus mirabilis,* enterococci, *Neisseria gonorrhoeae*
Extended-spectrum penicillins (antipseudomonal penicillins)	Carbenicillin indanyl Ticarcillin Mezlocillin Piperacillin	Same as broad-spectrum penicillins plus *Pseudomonas aeruginosa, Enterobacter* species, *Proteus* (indole positive), *Bacteroides fragilis,* many *Klebsiella*

lin is also employed for *prophylaxis of bacterial endocarditis*; candidates for therapy include individuals with (1) prosthetic heart valves, (2) most congenital heart diseases, (3) acquired heart valvular disease, (4) mitral valve prolapse, and (5) previous history of bacterial endocarditis. For prevention of endocarditis, penicillin is administered prior to dental procedures and other procedures that are likely to produce temporary bacteremia.

Pharmacokinetics

Absorption. Penicillin G is available as four different salts: (1) *sodium* penicillin G, (2) *potassium* penicillin G, (3) *procaine* penicillin G, and (4) *benzathine* penicillin G. These salts differ with respect to route of administration and time course of action. With all four preparations, the salt dissociates to release penicillin G, the active form of these preparations.

Oral Use. Oral administration is rare. Penicillin G is unstable in acid, and the majority of an oral dose is destroyed in the stomach. Food delays gastric emptying and prolongs exposure of penicillin to gastric acid. Accordingly, to maximize oral absorption, penicillin G should be administered at least 1 hour before meals or 2 hours after. To produce equivalent blood levels, oral doses must be four to five times greater than parenteral doses.

Intravenous Use. When high blood levels are needed rapidly, penicillin can be administered IV. Only the sodium and potassium salts should be given by this route. The procaine and benzathine salts must never be administered IV.

Intramuscular Use. All forms of penicillin may be administered IM. However, it is important to note that the different salts are absorbed at very different rates. As indicated in Figure 74–5, absorption of *sodium* and *potassium* penicillin G is rapid; peak blood levels are achieved about 15 min-

utes after injection. In contrast, the *procaine* and *benzathine* salts are absorbed slowly. Because of their delayed absorption, these salts are referred to as *repository* forms of penicillin. When benzathine penicillin is injected, penicillin G is absorbed into the blood for weeks, but serum levels remain very low (see Fig. 74–5). Consequently, this preparation is useful only against highly sensitive organisms (e.g., *Treponema pallidum*, the bacterium that causes syphilis).

Distribution. Penicillin distributes well to most tissues and body fluids. In the *absence* of inflammation, penetration of the meninges and into fluids of joints and the eyes is poor. However, in the *presence* of inflammation, entry into cerebrospinal fluid, joints, and the eyes is enhanced, permitting treatment of infections caused by susceptible organisms.

Elimination. Penicillin is eliminated by the kidneys, primarily as the unchanged drug. Renal excretion of penicillin is accomplished mainly (90%) by active tubular secretion; the remaining 10% results from glomerular filtration. In older children and adults, the half-life of penicillin is very short (about 30 minutes). Kidney dysfunction causes the half-life to increase dramatically, and may necessitate a reduction in dosage. In patients at high risk of toxicity (patients with renal impairment, acutely ill patients, the elderly, the very young) kidney function should be monitored.

Renal excretion of penicillin can be delayed with *probenecid*, a compound that competes with penicillin for active tubular transport. Formerly, when penicillin was both scarce and expensive, probenecid was employed routinely to prolong the effects of the drug. Since penicillin is now available in abundance and at low cost, concurrent use of probenecid is rarely indicated.

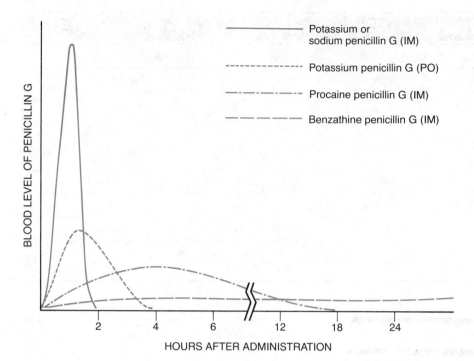

Figure 74–5. Penicillin G blood levels following the administration of oral and intramuscular formulations of penicillin G. (Adapted from Pratt, W.B. and Fekety, R. The Antimicrobial Drugs. New York, Oxford University Press, 1986.)

Side Effects and Toxicities

Penicillin G is the least toxic of all antibiotics, and is among the safest of all medications. *Allergic reactions* are the principal concern; these reactions are discussed separately below. In addition to allergic reactions, penicillin G may cause *pain at sites of IM injection*, prolonged (but reversible) *sensory and motor dysfunction* following accidental injection into a peripheral nerve, and *neurotoxicity* (seizures, confusion, hallucinations) if blood levels are allowed to climb too high. Inadvertent *intraarterial* injection can produce severe reactions (gangrene, necrosis, sloughing of tissue) and must be avoided.

Certain adverse effects may be caused by compounds coadministered with penicillin, and not by penicillin itself. For example, the procaine component of procaine penicillin G may cause bizarre behavioral effects when procaine penicillin is given in large doses. When large IV doses of potassium penicillin G are administered rapidly, hyperkalemia can result, possibly causing dysrhythmias and even cardiac arrest. Large intravenous doses of sodium penicillin G can cause sodium overload; exercise caution in patients with hypertension or cardiac disease.

Penicillin Allergy

General Considerations. *Penicillins are the most common cause of drug allergy;* between 1% and 10% of patients who receive penicillins experience an allergic response. Reactions vary in severity from minor rashes to life-threatening anaphylaxis. Although allergic reactions can occur following administration of penicillins by any route, severe reactions are most likely with parenteral use. As with most allergic reactions, there is no direct relationship between the size of the dose and the intensity of the allergic response. Although prior exposure to penicillins is required for an allergic reaction to occur, responses may occur in the absence of prior penicillin use, since patients may have been exposed to penicillins produced by fungi or to penicillins present in foods of animal origin.

Because of cross-sensitivity, patients allergic to one penicillin should be considered allergic to all penicillins. In addition, about 5% to 10% of individuals allergic to penicillins display cross-sensitivity to *cephalosporins*. If at all possible, patients with penicillin allergy should not be treated with any member of the penicillin family; cephalosporins may be used cautiously in some patients.

Individuals allergic to penicillin should be encouraged to wear a Medic-Alert bracelet or some other form of identification to alert health care personnel to their condition.

Types of Allergic Reactions. Penicillin reactions are classified as *immediate, accelerated,* and *late.* Immediate reactions occur 2 to 30 minutes after drug administration; accelerated reactions occur within 1 to 72 hours; and late reactions may take days or even weeks to develop.

Anaphylaxis (laryngeal edema, bronchoconstriction, severe hypotension) is an immediate hypersensitivity reaction, and is the reaction of greatest concern. Anaphylactic reactions occur more frequently with penicillins than with any other drugs. Fortunately, even with penicillins, the incidence of anaphylaxis is only about 0.02%. However, when these reactions occur, the risk of mortality is high (approximately 10%). The primary treatment for anaphylaxis is *epinephrine* (SC, IM, or IV) plus respiratory support. To insure prompt treatment if anaphylaxis should develop, patients receiving parenteral penicillins should remain in the physician's office for at least 30 minutes after drug injection (i.e., until the risk of an anaphylactic reaction has passed).

Development of Penicillin Allergy. Before discussing penicillin allergy itself, we need to review development of allergy to small molecules as a class. Drugs and other small molecules are unable to induce antibody formation directly. Therefore, in order to promote antibody formation, the small molecule must first bond covalently to a larger molecule (usually a protein). In these combinations, the small molecule is referred to as a *hapten*. The hapten-protein combination constitutes the complete *antigen* that stimulates antibody formation.

The hapten involved in development of penicillin antibodies is rarely intact penicillin itself. Rather, compounds formed from the degradation of penicillin are the actual haptens. As a result, most "penicillin antibodies" are not directed at penicillin itself. Instead, these antibodies are directed at various penicillin degradation products.

Skin Tests for Penicillin Allergy. Allergy to penicillin can decrease over time. Hence, an intense allergic reaction in the past does not necessarily indicate that such a reaction will occur again. In patients with a history of penicillin allergy, skin tests can be employed to assess the current risk of a severe reaction. These tests are performed by injecting a tiny amount of allergen intradermally and observing for an allergic response.

Two reagents can be employed to assess penicillin allergy. One of these, *benzylpenicilloyl-polylysine* (BPO-PL), tests primarily for *delayed* hypersensitivity. This reagent is referred to as a *major antigenic determinant*, a term indicating that the antibodies for which this reagent tests are relatively common. BPO-PL is a large polymeric molecule that is poorly absorbed. Hence, even in patients with severe penicillin allergy, a skin test with this compound carries little risk of a systemic reaction.

The second skin-test reagent, known as the *minor determinant mixture* (MDM), detects antibodies that mediate *immediate* allergic responses (e.g., anaphylaxis). The term *minor* indicates that the antibodies being tested for are relatively uncommon and not that the allergic response mediated by these antibodies is of minor significance. It is important to note that skin testing with MDM can be dangerous: in patients with severe penicillin allergy, the skin test itself can precipitate an anaphylactic reaction. Accordingly, the test should be performed only if epinephrine and facilities for respiratory support are immediately available.

For two reasons, penicillin itself is rarely employed for skin tests. First, skin testing with penicillin can elicit an anaphylactic reaction in highly sensitized individuals. Second, use of penicillin can produce a false-negative result. This second point is paradoxical and requires explanation. Recall that most antibodies that mediate penicillin allergy are directed against degradation products of penicillin, and not against penicillin itself. Nonetheless, intact penicillin is able to bind to the active site of these antibodies—but that binding will not trigger an immune response. As a result, when small amounts of degradation products are formed following intradermal injection of penicillin, the presence of large amounts of intact penicillin can compete with those products for antibody-binding sites, thereby preventing the degradation products from triggering an allergic reaction.

Management of Patients with a History of Penicillin Allergy. All patients who are candidates for penicillin therapy should be asked if they have ever experienced an allergic reaction to penicillin. For patients who indicate a history of penicillin allergy, the general rule is to avoid penicillins entirely. If the allergy is mild, a *cephalosporin* is often an appropriate alternative. However, if there is a history of anaphylaxis or some other severe allergic reaction, it is prudent to avoid cephalosporins as well (since there is a 5% to 10% risk of cross-sensitivity to cephalosporins). When a cephalosporin is indicated, an oral cephalosporin is preferred to a parenteral cephalosporin, since, as with the penicillins, the risk of severe allergic responses is lower with oral therapy. For many infections, *vancomycin* and *erythromycin* are effective and safe alternatives for patients with penicillin allergy.

Rarely, a patient with a history of anaphylaxis may have a life-threatening infection (e.g., enterococcal endocarditis) for which the alternatives to penicillins are ineffective. In these cases, the potential benefits of penicillin therapy outweigh the risks, and treatment should be instituted. To minimize the chances of an anaphylactic reaction, penicillin should be administered according to a desensitization schedule. In this procedure, an initial small dose is followed at 15-minute intervals by progressively larger doses until the full therapeutic dose has been achieved (in about 4 hours). It should be noted that the desensitization procedure is not without risk. Accordingly, epinephrine and facilities for respiratory support should be immediately available.

Drug Interactions

Aminoglycosides. For some infections, penicillins are used in combination with an aminoglycoside (e.g., gentamicin). By weakening the cell wall, the penicillin facilitates access of the aminoglycoside to its intracellular site of action, thereby increasing bactericidal effects. Unfortunately, when penicillins are present in high concentrations, they interact chemically with aminoglycosides to cause inactivation of the aminoglycoside. Accordingly, *penicillins and aminoglycosides should not be mixed in the same intravenous solution.* Rather, these drugs should be administered separately. Once penicillins have been diluted in body fluids, the potential for inactivation of aminoglycosides is minimal.

Probenecid. As noted in the discussion of penicillin elimination, probenecid can delay renal excretion of penicillin, thereby prolonging antibacterial effects.

Bacteriostatic Antibiotics. Since penicillins are most effective against actively growing bacteria, concurrent use of a bacteriostatic antibiotic (e.g., tetracycline) could, in theory, reduce the bactericidal effects of the penicillin. However, the clinical significance of such interactions is not known. Moreover, there are infections for which combined therapy with a bacteriostatic agent and a penicillin is indicated. When such combined chemotherapy is employed, the penicillin should be administered a few hours before the bacteriostatic drug to minimize any reduction of penicillin's effects.

Preparations, Dosage, and Administration

Preparations and Routes of Administration. Penicillin G is available as four different salts (sodium, potassium, procaine, and benzathine). These salts differ with respect to routes of administration: *potassium* penicillin G is administered PO, IM, and IV; *sodium* penicillin G is administered IM and IV; *benzathine* penicillin G [Bicillin] is administered IM and PO; and *procaine* penicillin G is administered IM. You should check to insure that the penicillin salt to be administered is appropriate for the intended route.

Dosage. Dosage of penicillin G is prescribed in units (1 unit equals 0.6 μg). Dosage ranges are summarized in Table 74–2. For any particular patient, the specific dosage will depend on the type and severity of infection. The dosage should be reduced in patients with severe renal dysfunction.

Administration. Oral penicillin G should be taken with a full glass of water at least 1 hour before meals or 2 hours after. Solutions for parenteral administration should be prepared according to the manufacturer's instructions. During IM injection, care should be taken to avoid inadvertent injection into an artery or peripheral nerve.

PENICILLIN V

Penicillin V is similar to penicillin G in most respects. These drugs differ primarily in their acid stability: penicillin V is stable in stomach acid, whereas penicillin G is not. As a result, when these two agents are administered orally in comparable doses, penicillin V achieves serum levels that are two to five times those of penicillin G. Accordingly, penicillin V is preferred to penicillin G for oral therapy. Penicillin V may be taken with meals. Dosages are summarized in Table 74–2. Trade names include Ledercillin VK, Pen-Vee K, and Veetids.

PENICILLINASE-RESISTANT PENICILLINS (ANTISTAPHYLOCOCCAL PENICILLINS)

By altering the penicillin side chain, pharmaceutical chemists have created a group of penicillins

that are highly resistant to inactivation by beta-lactamases. In the United States, five such drugs are available: *methicillin, nafcillin, oxacillin, cloxacillin,* and *dicloxacillin.* These agents have a very narrow antimicrobial spectrum and are used only against penicillinase-producing strains of staphylococcus (*Staphylococcus aureus* and *Staphylococcus epidermidis*). Since most strains of staphylococci produce penicillinase, the penicillinase-resistant penicillins are drugs of choice for the majority of staphylococcal infections. It should be noted that these agents should not be used against infections caused by nonpenicillinase-producing staphylococci, since these drugs are less active than penicillin G against these bacteria.

An increasing clinical problem is the emergence of staphylococcal strains referred to as *methicillin-resistant,* a term used to indicate *lack of susceptibility to methicillin and all other penicillinase-resistant penicillins.* This resistance to methicillin appears to result from production of altered PBPs to which the penicillinase-resistant penicillins are unable to bind. Currently, vancomycin is the drug of choice for infections caused by methicillin-resistant staphylococci.

Methicillin

Methicillin [Staphcillin] is the oldest of the penicillinase-resistant penicillins and is no longer widely employed. In addition to causing allergic reactions typical of all penicillins, methicillin may produce interstitial nephritis, an adverse effect that is usually reversible, but sometimes progresses to complete renal failure. Methicillin may be administered IM and IV, but, because of acid lability, cannot be taken by mouth. The structure of methicillin is shown in Figure 74–1. Dosages are summarized in Table 74–2.

Nafcillin

Nafcillin is usually administered IM or IV. The drug is available in a formulation for oral use, but absorption from the gastrointestinal tract is incomplete and erratic; consequently, oral administration is not recommended. Trade names are Nafcil, Nallpen, and Unipen. Dosages are summarized in Table 74–2.

Oxacillin, Cloxacillin, and Dicloxacillin

These three drugs are similar in structure and pharmacokinetic properties. All are acid stable and available for oral administration; oxacillin may also be administered parenterally (IM and IV). Oral administration of all three drugs may be done with meals. Dosages and trade names are summarized in Table 74–2.

BROAD-SPECTRUM PENICILLINS (AMINOPENICILLINS)

The family of broad-spectrum penicillins consists of *ampicillin, amoxicillin,* and *bacampicillin.* These drugs have the same antimicrobial spectrum as penicillin G, *plus* increased activity against certain gram-negative bacilli, including *Haemophilus influenzae, Escherichia coli, Salmonella,* and *Shigella.* This broadened spectrum is due in large part to an increased ability to pene-

Table 74–2. Dosages for Penicillins

Generic Name	Trade Name	Route	Dosing Interval (hr)	Total Daily Dosage[a] Adults	Total Daily Dosage[a] Children
Narrow-Spectrum Penicillins: Penicillinase-Sensitive					
Penicillin G	Many trade names	PO	6	1.6–3.2 million units[b]	40,000–80,000 units/kg[b]
		IM, IV	4	1.2–2.4 million units[b]	100,000–250,000 units/kg[b]
Penicillin V	Ledercillin VK, Veetids, Pen-Vee K	PO	4–6	0.5–2 g	25–50 mg/kg
Narrow-Spectrum Penicillins: Penicillinase-Resistant (Antistaphylococcal Penicillins)					
Methicillin	Staphcillin	IM, IV	4–6	4–12 gm	100–200 mg/kg
Nafcillin	Nafcil, Nallpen, Unipen	PO	6	2–4 gm	50–100 mg/kg
		IM, IV	4–6	2–9 gm	100–200 mg/kg
Oxacillin	Bactocill, Prostaphlin	PO	6	2–4 gm	50–100 mg/kg
		IM, IV	4–6	2–12 gm	100–200 mg/kg
Cloxacillin	Cloxapen, Tegopen	PO	6	2–4 gm	50–100 mg/kg
Dicloxacillin	Dycill, Dynapen, Pathocil	PO	6	1–2 gm	12.5–25 mg/kg
Broad-Spectrum Penicillins (Aminopenicillins)					
Ampicillin	Amcill, Omnipen, Principen, Polycillin, Totacillin	PO	6–8	2–4 gm	50–100 mg/kg
		IM, IV	6–8	2–12 gm	10–200 mg/kg
Ampicillin + sulbactam	Unasyn	IM, IV	6	4–8 gm[c]	—
Amoxicillin	Amoxil, Larotid, Trimox, Polymox, others	PO	8	0.75–1.5 gm	20–40 mg/kg
Amoxicillin + clavulanate	Augmentin	PO	8	250–500 mg[d]	20–40 mg/kg[d]
Bacampicillin	Spectrobid	PO	12	0.8–1.6 gm	25–50 mg/kg
Extended-Spectrum Penicillins (Antipseudomonal Penicillins)					
Carbenicillin Indanyl	Geocillin	PO	4–6	1.5–3 gm	—
		IM	6	4–8 gm	50–200 mg/kg
		IV	4–6	30–40 gm	100–600 mg/kg
Ticarcillin	Ticar	IM	6	4 gm	50–100 mg/kg
		IV	4–6	200–300 mg/kg	200–300 mg/kg
Ticarcillin + clavulanate	Timentin	IV	4–6	200–300 mg/kg[e]	—
Mezlocillin	Mezlin	IM	6	4–8 gm	—
		IV	r4–6	6–18 gm	300 mg/kg
Piperacillin	Pipracil	IM	6–12	6–8 gm	—
		IV	4–6	12–24 gm	200–300 mg/kg

[a]Doses vary widely, depending upon the type and severity of infection; doses and dosing intervals presented here may not be appropriate for all patients.
[b]10,000 units = 6 mg.
[c]Dose based on ampicillin content.
[d]Dose based on amoxicillin content.
[e]Dose based on ticarcillin content.

trate the gram-negative cell envelope. All of the broad-spectrum penicillins are readily inactivated by beta-lactamases. Hence, these drugs are ineffective against most infections caused by *Staphylococcus aureus*.

Properties of individual broad-spectrum penicillins are discussed below. Dosages are summarized in Table 74–2.

Ampicillin

Ampicillin was the first broad-spectrum penicillin available for clinical use. The agent is a pre-ferred or alternative drug for infections caused by *Streptococcus faecalis*, *Bordetella pertussis*, *Proteus mirabilis*, *E. coli*, *Salmonella*, *Shigella*, and *Haemophilus influenzae*. The drug's most common side effects are rashes and diarrhea; both reactions occur more frequently with ampicillin than with any other penicillin. Administration may be parenteral or by mouth. It should be noted, however, that for oral therapy, amoxicillin is generally preferred (see below). Trade names are Amcill, Omnipen, Polycillin, Principen, and Totacillin.

Ampicillin is also available in a fixed-dose combination with clavulanic acid, an inhibitor of bacterial beta-lactamases. The combination is marketed under the trade name Unasyn. Routes and usual dosages are summarized in Table 74–2. Dosages must be reduced in patients with renal impairment.

Amoxicillin

Amoxicillin is similar to ampicillin in structure and actions. These drugs differ primarily in acid stability, amoxicillin being the more acid resistant. Hence, when the two drugs are administered orally in equivalent doses, blood levels of amoxicillin are greater than those of ampicillin. Accordingly, when oral therapy is indicated, amoxicillin is usually preferred. Oral amoxicillin may be administered with meals. Amoxicillin produces less diarrhea than ampicillin, perhaps because less amoxicillin remains unabsorbed in the intestine. Trade names include Amoxil, Larotid, Polymox, and Trimox. As discussed later in the chapter, amoxicillin is available in a fixed-dose combination with sulbactam, an inhibitor of bacterial beta-lactamases.

Bacampicillin

Bacampicillin [Spectrobid] is a prodrug form of ampicillin; once in the body, bacampicillin is rapidly converted to ampicillin, its active form. Bacampicillin is acid stable and administration is oral. The drug may be taken with meals. Because of its resistance to acid, bacampicillin produces blood levels of ampicillin that are two times greater than those achieved with equivalent oral doses of ampicillin itself. Despite this difference, bacampicillin offers no clinical advantage over ampicillin or amoxicillin, and is usually more expensive.

EXTENDED-SPECTRUM PENICILLINS (ANTIPSEUDOMONAL PENICILLINS)

The family of extended-spectrum penicillins consists of four drugs: *ticarcillin, carbenicillin indanyl, mezlocillin,* and *piperacillin.* The antimicrobial spectrum of these drugs includes organisms that are susceptible to the aminopenicillins plus *Pseudomonas aeruginosa, Enterobacter* species, *Proteus* (indole-positive), *Bacteroides fragilis,* and many *Klebsiella.* All of the extended-spectrum penicillins are susceptible to beta-lactamases, and, hence, are ineffective against most strains of *Staphylococcus aureus.*

The extended-spectrum penicillins are used primarily for infections with *Pseudomonas aeruginosa.* These infections often occur in the immunocompromised host and can be very difficult to eradicate. To increase killing of *Pseudomonas,* an antipseudomonal aminoglycoside (gentamicin, tobramycin, amikacin, netilmicin) is almost always added to the regimen. When these combinations are employed, the penicillin and the aminoglycoside should not be mixed in the same IV solution,

since high concentrations of penicillins can inactivate aminoglycosides.

Properties of individual extended-spectrum penicillins are discussed below. Dosages are summarized in Table 74–2.

Ticarcillin

Antimicrobial Spectrum and Therapeutic Use. Ticarcillin [Ticar] has one of the broadest antimicrobial spectra of all penicillins. However, like other extended-spectrum penicillins, the drug is susceptible to destruction by penicillinase.

The primary indication for ticarcillin is infection caused by *Pseudomonas aeruginosa.* When used against *Pseudomonas,* the drug is usually employed in combination with an aminoglycoside.

Adverse Effects. In addition to promoting the allergic reactions typical of all penicillins, ticarcillin can cause unique adverse effects. Since the drug is administered as the *disodium salt,* and since large intravenous doses are often required, symptoms of *sodium overload* (e.g., congestive heart failure) may develop. Also, ticarcillin interferes with platelet function and can thereby promote *bleeding.*

Preparations and Administration. Ticarcillin is unstable in acid and, therefore, must be administered parenterally (IM or IV). When ticarcillin is used in combination with an aminoglycoside, the two drugs should be administered separately.

As discussed later in the chapter, ticarcillin is available in a fixed-dose combination with clavulanic acid, a beta-lactamase inhibitor. The combination [Timentin] is administered intravenously.

Dosages for patients with normal kidney function are summarized in Table 74–2. Dosages must be reduced in patients with renal impairment.

Carbenicillin Indanyl

Carbenicillin indanyl [Geocillin] is acid stable and administered orally. Following absorption, the drug is converted to carbenicillin, its active form. Excretion is renal, and the drug becomes concentrated in urine. Carbenicillin indanyl is indicated only for urinary tract infections caused by *Pseudomonas aeruginosa* or indole-positive *Proteus.* Drug levels at sites outside the urinary tract are too low for clinically significant antibacterial effects. Oral carbenicillin should not be taken with meals.

Newer Antipseudomonal Penicillins: Mezlocillin and Piperacillin

Mezlocillin [Mezlin] and piperacillin [Pipracil] have broad antimicrobial spectra. However, like other extended-spectrum penicillins, these drugs are penicillinase sensitive. Both drugs are highly active against *Pseudomonas aeruginosa,* and their principal indication is infection with this organism. Like ticarcillin, mezlocillin and piperacillin can cause bleeding tendencies secondary to disruption of platelet function. Both drugs are acid labile and must be administered parenterally (IM or IV). The risk of sodium overload with IV mezlocillin or IV piperacillin is much less than with IV ticarcillin. When these drugs are used in combination with an aminoglycoside, they should not be mixed in the same IV solution. Dosages of mezlocillin and piperacillin for patients with normal kidney function are shown in Table 74–2. Dosages of both drugs should be reduced in patients with renal dysfunction.

PENICILLINS COMBINED WITH A BETA-LACTAMASE INHIBITOR

As their name indicates, beta-lactamase inhibitors are drugs that inhibit bacterial beta-lactamases. By combining a beta-lactamase inhibitor with a penicillinase-sensitive penicillin, we can extend the antimicrobial spectrum of the penicillin. In the United States, three beta-lactamase inhibitors are used: *clavulanic acid, tazobactam,* and *sul-*

bactam. These agents are not dispensed alone. Rather, they are dispensed in fixed-dose combinations with a penicillin. Four such combination products are available:

Ampicillin + sulbactam [Unasyn]
Amoxicillin + clavulanic acid [Augmentin]
Ticarcillin + clavulanic acid [Timentin]
Piperacillin + tazobactam [Zosyn]

Since beta-lactamase inhibitors have minimal toxicity, adverse effects seen with the combination products are those caused by the penicillin. Routes of administration and dosages for these combination products are summarized in Table 74–2.

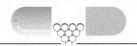

Summary of Major Nursing Implications

PENICILLINS

Except where indicated otherwise, the implications summarized below apply to all members of the penicillin family.

**Preadministration
Assessment**

Therapeutic Goal

Treatment of infections caused by sensitive bacteria.

Baseline Data

The physician may order tests to identify the infecting organism and its drug sensitivity. Take samples for microbiologic culture prior to initiation of treatment.

In patients with a history of penicillin allergy, a skin test may be performed to determine current allergic status.

Identifying High-Risk Patients

Penicillins are *contraindicated* for patients with a *history of severe allergic reactions to penicillins, cephalosporins, or imipenem.*

**Implementation:
Administration**

Routes

Penicillins are administered orally, IV, and IM. Routes for individual agents are summarized in Table 74–2. Before giving a penicillin, check to insure that the preparation is appropriate for the intended route.

Dosage

Doses for penicillin G are prescribed in units (1 unit equals 0.6 μg). Doses for all other penicillins are prescribed by weight.

Dosages for individual penicillins are summarized in Table 74–2.

Administration

During IM injection, aspirate to avoid injection into an artery. Take care to avoid injection into a nerve.

Instruct the patient to take oral penicillins with a full glass of water 1 hour before meals or 2 hours after. *Penicillin V, amoxicillin, amoxicillin/ clavulanate,* and *bacampicillin* may be taken with meals.

Instruct the patient to complete the prescribed course of treatment, even though symptoms may abate before the full course is over.

Probenecid may be administered with penicillins to delay penicillin excretion.

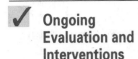

**Ongoing
Evaluation and
Interventions**

Evaluating Therapeutic Effects

Monitor the patient for indications of antimicrobial effects (e.g., reduction in fever, pain, or inflammation; improved appetite or sense of well-being).

Monitoring Kidney Function

Renal impairment can cause penicillins to accumulate to toxic levels; monitoring kidney function can help avoid injury. Measurement of intake and output is of particular value in patients with kidney disease, in acutely ill patients, and in the very old and very young. Notify the physician if a significant change in intake-output ratio develops.

Minimizing Adverse Effects

Allergic Reactions. Penicillin allergy is common; rarely, life-threatening anaphylaxis occurs. Interview the patient for a history of penicillin allergy.

For patients with prior allergic responses, a skin test may be ordered to assess current allergic status. Exercise caution: the skin test itself can cause a severe reaction. Accordingly, when skin tests are performed, epinephrine and facilities for respiratory support should be immediately available.

Advise the patient with penicillin allergy to wear some form of identification (e.g., MedicAlert bracelet) to inform emergency health care personnel of the allergy.

Instruct outpatients to report any signs of an allergic response (e.g., skin rash, itching, hives).

Whenever a parenteral penicillin is used, keep the patient under observation for at least 30 minutes (i.e., until the risk of anaphylaxis has passed). If anaphylaxis occurs, treatment consists of *epinephrine* (SC, IM, or IV) plus respiratory support.

As a rule, patients with a history of penicillin allergy should not receive penicillins again. If previous reactions have been mild, a cephalosporin (preferably oral) may be an appropriate alternative. However, if severe immediate reactions have occurred, cephalosporins should be avoided.

Rarely, a patient with a history of anaphylaxis may nonetheless require penicillin therapy. To minimize the risk of a severe reaction, administer penicillin according to a desensitization schedule. Be aware, however, that the procedure does not guarantee that anaphylaxis will not occur. Accordingly, epinephrine and facilities for respiratory support must be immediately available.

Sodium Loading. High intravenous doses of *sodium penicillin G, carbenicillin,* or *ticarcillin* can produce sodium overload. Exercise caution in patients under sodium restriction (e.g., cardiac patients, those with hypertension). Electrolytes should be measured periodically. Monitor cardiac status.

Hyperkalemia. High doses of intravenous *potassium penicillin G* may cause hyperkalemia, possibly resulting in dysrhythmias or cardiac arrest. Electrolyte and cardiac status should be monitored.

Effects Resulting from Incorrect Injection. Serious adverse reactions have occurred because of intra-arterial injections and injections made into peripheral nerves. Take care to avoid inadvertent injection into these sites.

Minimizing Adverse Interactions

Aminoglycosides. When present in high concentration, penicillins can inactivate aminoglycosides (e.g., gentamicin). Do not mix penicillins and aminoglycosides in the same IV solution.

Bacteriostatic Antibiotics. Suppression of bacterial growth with a bacteriostatic agent can, in theory, decrease the effectiveness of penicillins. When a bacteriostatic drug is combined with a penicillin, administer the penicillin a few hours before the bacteriostatic drug.

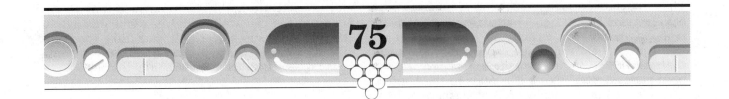

75

Drugs That Weaken the Bacterial Cell Wall II: Cephalosporins, Imipenem, Aztreonam, and Vancomycin

CEPHALOSPORINS

OTHER INHIBITORS OF CELL WALL SYNTHESIS
Imipenem
Aztreonam
Vancomycin

Like the penicillins, the drugs discussed in this chapter are inhibitors of cell wall synthesis. By disrupting the cell wall, these drugs produce bacterial lysis and death. Most of the chapter focuses on the cephalosporins, our most extensively used antibacterial drugs. With only one exception—vancomycin—the drugs addressed in this chapter belong to the beta-lactam family of antibiotics.

CEPHALOSPORINS

The cephalosporins are beta-lactam antibiotics similar in structure and actions to the penicillins.

These drugs are bactericidal, often resistant to beta-lactamases, and active against a broad spectrum of pathogens. Toxicity is low. Because of these properties, the cephalosporins are popular therapeutic agents and constitute our most widely used group of antibiotics. Hospitals in the United States spend more money on cephalosporins than on all other antibiotics combined.

Chemistry

All of the cephalosporins are derived from the same nucleus. As shown in Figure 75–1, this nucleus contains a *beta-lactam ring* fused to a second ring. The beta-lactam ring is required for antibacterial activity. Unique properties of individual cephalosporins are determined by additions made to the nucleus at the sites labeled R_1, R_2, and R_3. Structures of three representative cephalosporins are shown.

Mechanism of Action

The cephalosporins are bactericidal drugs with a mechanism of action like that of the penicillins. These agents bind to penicillin-binding proteins (PBPs) and thereby (1) disrupt cell wall synthesis,

and (2) activate autolysins (enzymes that cleave bonds in the cell wall). The resultant damage to the cell wall causes death by lysis. Like the penicillins, cephalosporins are most effective against cells undergoing active growth and division.

Resistance

The principal cause of cephalosporin resistance is production of beta-lactamases, enzymes that cleave the beta-lactam ring of cephalosporins, and thereby render these drugs inactive. The beta-lactamases that act on cephalosporins are sometimes referred to as *cephalosporinases*. Some of the beta-lactamases that act on cephalosporins can also cleave the beta-lactam ring of penicillins.

Not all cephalosporins are equally susceptible to beta-lactamases. Most *first-generation* cephalosporins are destroyed by beta-lactamases; *second-generation* cephalosporins are less sensitive to destruction; and most *third-generation* cephalosporins are highly resistant to beta-lactamases.

In some cases, bacterial resistance results from production of altered PBPs that have a low affinity for cephalosporins. Methicillin-resistant staphylococci produce these unusual PBPs and are resistant to cephalosporins as a result.

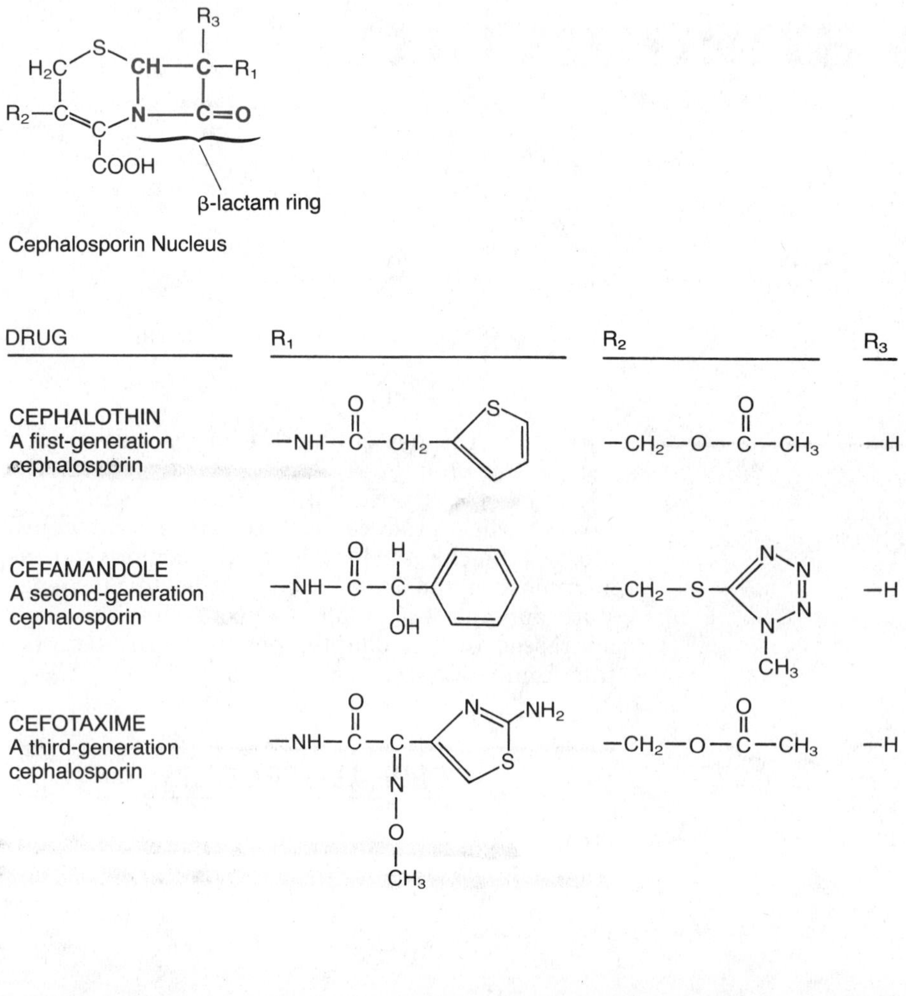

Cephalosporin Nucleus

Figure 75–1. Structural formulas of representative cephalosporins. The unique structure and pharmacologic properties of individual cephalosporins are determined by additions made to the cephalosporin nucleus at the positions labeled R_1, R_2, and R_3.

Classification and Antimicrobial Spectra

The cephalosporins have been grouped into three "generations" based on the order of their introduction to clinical use. The generations differ significantly with respect to antimicrobial spectra. In general, *as we progress from first-generation agents to third-generation agents, there is (1) increasing activity against gram-negative bacteria and anaerobes, (2) increasing resistance to destruction by beta-lactamases, and (3) increasing ability to reach the cerebrospinal fluid* (CSF). These differences are summarized in Table 75–1.

First-generation cephalosporins, represented by cephalothin, are highly active against gram-positive bacteria. These drugs are the most active of all cephalosporins against staphylococci and nonenterococcal streptococci. However, those staphylococci that are resistant to methicillin are also resistant to first-generation cephalosporins (and to most other cephalosporins as well). The first-generation drugs have only modest activity against gram-negative bacteria. These drugs do not reach effective concentrations in CSF.

Second-generation cephalosporins (e.g., cefamandole) have enhanced activity against gram-negative bacteria. The increase is due to a combination of factors: (1) increased affinity for PBPs of gram-negative bacteria, (2) increased ability to penetrate the gram-negative cell envelope, and (3) increased resistance to beta-lactamases produced by gram-negative organisms. None of the second-generation agents is active against *Pseudomonas aeruginosa*. These drugs do not reach effective concentrations in CSF.

Third-generation cephalosporins (e.g., cefotaxime) have a very broad spectrum of antimicrobial activity. Because of increased resistance to beta-lactamases, these agents are considerably more active against gram-negative aerobes than are the first- and second-generation drugs. Some third-generation cephalosporins (e.g., ceftazidime) have important activity against *Pseudomonas aeruginosa*. Others (e.g., cefixime) lack such activity. In contrast to first- and second-generation cephalosporins, the third-generation agents are able to reach clinically effective concentrations in CSF.

Pharmacokinetics

Absorption. Because of poor absorption from the gastrointestinal tract, *most cephalosporins must be administered parenterally* (IM or IV). Of the 24 cephalosporins used in the United States, only 8 can be administered by mouth (see Table 75–2). Of these, only two (cephradine and cefuroxime) can be administered orally *and* by injection.

Distribution. Cephalosporins distribute well to most body fluids and tissues. Therapeutic concentrations are achieved in pleural, pericardial, and peritoneal fluids. Concentrations in ocular fluids are generally low. Penetration to the CSF by first- and second-generation drugs is unreliable, and these drugs should not be used to treat bacterial meningitis. In contrast, CSF levels achieved with third-generation drugs are generally sufficient for bactericidal effects.

Elimination. Practically all cephalosporins are eliminated by the kidneys; excretion is by a combination of glomerular filtration and active tubular secretion. Probenecid can decrease tubular secretion of some cephalosporins, thereby prolonging their effects. In patients with renal insufficiency, dosages of most cephalosporins must be reduced to prevent accumulation to toxic levels. Two cephalosporins—*cefoperazone* and *ceftriaxone*—are eliminated largely by nonrenal routes. Consequently, there is no need to reduce the dosage of these drugs in patients with kidney dysfunction.

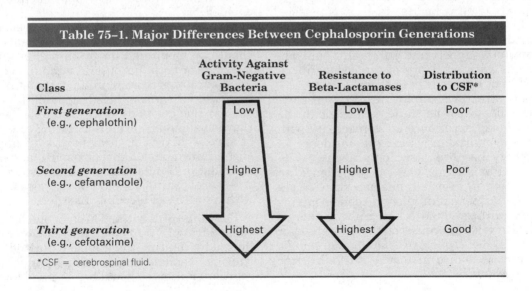

Table 75–1. Major Differences Between Cephalosporin Generations

Class	Activity Against Gram-Negative Bacteria	Resistance to Beta-Lactamases	Distribution to CSF*
First generation (e.g., cephalothin)	Low	Low	Poor
Second generation (e.g., cefamandole)	Higher	Higher	Poor
Third generation (e.g., cefotaxime)	Highest	Highest	Good

*CSF = cerebrospinal fluid.

Table 75–2. Pharmacokinetic Properties of the Cephalosporins

Class	Drug	Routes of Administration	Major Route of Elimination	Half-life (hours) Normal Renal Function	Half-life (hours) Severe Renal Impairment
First Generation	Cefadroxil	PO	Renal	1.2–1.3	20–25
	Cephalexin	PO	Renal	0.4–1.0	10–20
	Cephradine	PO, IM, IV	Renal	0.8–2.0	8–15
	Cefazolin	IM, IV	Renal	1.5–2.2	24–50
	Cephalothin	IM, IV	Renal	0.4–1.0	3–18
	Cephapirin	IM, IV	Renal	0.3–0.7	2.4
Second Generation	Cefaclor	PO	Renal	0.6–0.9	2–3
	Cefamandole	IM, IV	Renal	0.5–1.0	8–14
	Cefmetazole	IV	Renal	1.2	—
	Cefprozil	PO	Renal	1.3	5–6
	Cefpodoxime	PO	Renal	2–3	9.8
	Cefonicid	IM, IV	Renal	3.5–4.9	17–56
	Ceforanide	IM, IV	Renal	2.5–3.5	25–30
	Cefotetan	IM, IV	Renal	3.0–4.5	13–35
	Cefoxitin	IM, IV	Renal	0.7–1.0	13–22
	Cefuroxime	IM, IV	Renal	1.0–1.9	15–22
	Loracarbef	PO	Renal	1	32
Third Generation	Cefixime	PO	Renal	3–4	11.5
	Cefoperazone	IM, IV	Biliary	1.7–2.6	2.2
	Cefotaxime	IM, IV	Renal	0.9–1.4	3–11
	Ceftazidime	IM, IV	Renal	1.9–2.0	—
	Ceftizoxime	IM, IV	Renal	1.1–2.3	30
	Ceftriaxone	IM, IV	Hepatic	5.8–8.7	15.7
	Moxalactam	IM, IV	Renal	1.9–3.5	19–30

Adverse Effects

The cephalosporins are generally well tolerated and constitute one of our safest groups of antimicrobial drugs. Serious adverse effects are rare.

Allergic Reactions. Hypersensitivity reactions are the most frequent adverse effects. Maculopapular rash that develops several days after the onset of treatment is most common. Severe, immediate reactions (e.g., bronchospasm, anaphylaxis) are rare. If, during the course of treatment, signs of allergy appear (e.g., urticaria, rash, hypotension, difficulty in breathing), administration should be discontinued immediately. Anaphylaxis is treated with respiratory support and parenteral epinephrine. Patients with a history of cephalosporin allergy should not be given these drugs.

Because of structural similarities between penicillins and cephalosporins, patients allergic to one type of drug may experience cross-reactivity with the other. In clinical practice, the incidence of cross-reactivity has been low: only about 5% to 10% of penicillin-allergic patients experience an allergic reaction if given a cephalosporin. For patients with *mild* penicillin allergy, cephalosporins can be used with minimal concern about allergic responses. However, because of the potential for fatal anaphylaxis, *cephalosporins should not be given to patients with a history of severe allergic reactions to penicillins.*

Bleeding. Four cephalosporins—*cefamandole, cefoperazone, cefotetan,* and *moxalactam*—cause bleeding tendencies. Two mechanisms are involved: (1) reduction of prothrombin levels (through interference with vitamin K metabolism), and (2) impairment of platelet aggregation. All four drugs share the first mechanism; only *moxalactam* damages platelets. Because moxalactam suppresses hemostasis in two ways, bleeding can be considerably more severe than with the other three drugs. Consequently, moxalactam should be avoided.

Several measures can reduce the risk of hemorrhage. During prolonged treatment, patients should be monitored for prothrombin time, bleeding time, or both. Parenteral vitamin K can correct an abnormal prothrombin time. Patients should be observed for signs of bleeding, and, if bleeding develops, the cephalosporin should be withdrawn. Caution should be exercised during concurrent use of anticoagulants or thrombolytic agents. Because of their antiplatelet effects, aspirin and other nonsteroidal anti-inflammatory drugs should be used with care. Caution should be exercised in patients with a history of bleeding disorders.

Thrombophlebitis. Thrombophlebitis may develop during IV infusion. This reaction can be minimized by rotating the infusion site and by administering cephalosporins slowly and in dilute solution. Patients should be observed for phlebitis;

if the reaction develops, the infusion site should be changed.

Other Adverse Effects. Cephalosporins may cause *pain at sites of IM injection*; patients should be forewarned of this possibility. Rarely, cephalosporins may be the cause of *antibiotic-associated (pseudomembranous) colitis* due to overgrowth with *Clostridium difficile*. If this suprainfection develops, the cephalosporin should be discontinued and, if necessary, oral vancomycin or metronidazole should be given. *Nephrotoxicity* has been associated with cephalothin.

Drug Interactions

Probenecid. Probenecid delays renal excretion of some cephalosporins and can thereby prolong their effects. This is the same interaction that occurs between probenecid and the penicillins.

Alcohol. Four cephalosporins—*cefamandole, cefoperazone, cefotetan,* and *moxalactam*—induce a state of alcohol intolerance. If a patient receiving one of these drugs were to ingest alcohol, a *disulfiram-like reaction* could occur. As discussed in Chapter 33, the disulfiram effect is brought on by accumulation of acetaldehyde, and can be extremely dangerous. Accordingly, patients taking these cephalosporins must not consume alcohol in any form.

Drugs That Promote Bleeding. As noted above, four cephalosporins—*cefamandole, cefoperazone, cefotetan,* and *moxalactam*—promote bleeding tendencies. Caution should be exercised if these drugs are used in combination with other drugs that promote bleeding (nonsteroidal anti-inflammatory drugs, anticoagulants, and thrombolytics).

Therapeutic Uses

The therapeutic role of the cephalosporins is continually evolving as new agents are introduced and as more experience is gained with older drugs. Only general recommendations are considered here.

The cephalosporins are broad-spectrum, bactericidal drugs with a high therapeutic index. These agents have been employed widely and successfully against a variety of infections. Cephalosporins can be useful alternatives for patients with mild penicillin allergy.

The three generations of cephalosporins differ significantly in their applications. *The first- and second-generation cephalosporins are rarely drugs of choice for active infections.* In most cases, equally effective and less expensive alternatives are available. In contrast, *the third-generation agents have qualities that make them the preferred therapy for several infections.*

First-Generation Cephalosporins. When a cephalosporin is indicated for a *gram-positive infection*, a first-generation drug should be used;

these agents are the most active of the cephalosporins against gram-positive organisms and are less expensive than other cephalosporins. First-generation agents are frequently employed as alternatives to penicillins to treat infections caused by staphylococci or streptococci (except enterococci) in patients with penicillin allergy. However, it is important to note that cephalosporins should be given only to patients with a history of *mild* penicillin allergy, and not to those who have experienced severe, immediate hypersensitivity reactions.

The first-generation agents have been employed widely for *prophylaxis against infection in surgical patients.* First-generation agents are preferred to second- or third-generation cephalosporins for surgical prophylaxis because they are as effective as the newer drugs, less expensive, and have a narrower antimicrobial spectrum.

Second-Generation Cephalosporins. Specific indications for second-generation cephalosporins are limited. *Cefuroxime*, a prototype for the group, has been used with success against pneumonia caused by *Haemophilus influenzae, Klebsiella,* pneumococci, and staphylococci. Oral cefuroxime is useful for otitis, sinusitis, and respiratory tract infections. Cefoxitin is useful for abdominal and pelvic infections.

Third-Generation Cephalosporins. Because of their high activity against gram-negative organisms, and because of their ability to penetrate to the CSF, third-generation cephalosporins are drugs of choice for meningitis caused by enteric, gram-negative bacilli. *Ceftazidime* is of special utility for treating meningitis caused by *Pseudomonas aeruginosa. Nosocomial infections* caused by gram-negative bacilli are often resistant to first- and second-generation cephalosporins and to most other commonly used antibiotics; these infections are appropriate indications for the third-generation drugs. Two third-generation agents—*ceftriaxone* and *cefotaxime*—are drugs of choice for infections caused by *Neisseria gonorrhoeae* (gonorrhea), *Haemophilus influenzae, Proteus, Salmonella, Klebsiella,* and *Serratia.*

The third-generation cephalosporins should not be used routinely. Rather, these agents should be given only when conditions demand, since in this way emergence of organisms resistant to these drugs will be delayed.

Drug Selection

Two dozen cephalosporins are currently employed in the United States, and selection among them can be a challenge. Within each generation, the similarities among cephalosporins are more pronounced than the differences. Hence, aside from cost, there is frequently no rational basis for choosing one drug over another. However, there *are* some differences between cephalosporins, and these differences may render one agent preferable to another for treating a specific infection in a specific patient. The differences that do exist can be grouped into three main categories: (1) antimicrobial spectrum, (2) adverse effects, and (3) pharmacokinetics (e.g., route of administration, penetration to the CSF, time course, mode of elimination). Drug selection based on consideration of these differences is discussed below.

Antimicrobial Spectrum. A prime rule of antimicrobial therapy is to match the drug with the bug: the drug should be active against known or suspected pathogens, but its spectrum should be no broader than actually required. When a cephalosporin is appropriate, we should select from among those drugs shown to have good activity against the causative pathogen. The third-generation agents, with their very broad antimicrobial spectra, should be avoided in situations where a narrower spectrum, first- or second-generation drug would be sufficient.

For some infections, one cephalosporin may be decidedly more effective than all others, and should be selected on this basis. For example, *ceftazidime* (a third-generation drug) is the most effective of all cephalosporins against *Pseudomonas aeruginosa* and is clearly the preferred cephalosporin for treating infections caused by this microbe.

Adverse Effects. Although most cephalosporins produce the same spectrum of adverse effects, a few agents can cause unique reactions. In particular, four cephalosporins—*cefamandole, cefoperazone, cefotetan,* and *moxalactam*—produce bleeding tendencies and intolerance to alcohol. When an equally effective alternative is available, it would be prudent to avoid these four drugs.

Pharmacokinetics. Four pharmacokinetic properties are of particular interest: (1) route of administration, (2) duration of action, (3) distribution to CSF, and (4) route of elimination. The relationship of these properties to drug selection is discussed below.

Route of Administration. Eight cephalosporins can be administered orally. These oral cephalosporins may be preferred agents for treating mild-to-moderate infections in patients who cannot tolerate parenteral agents.

Duration of Action. In patients with normal renal function, the half-lives of the cephalosporins range from about 30 minutes to 9 hours (see Table 75–2). Because they require fewer administrations per day, drugs with a long half-life are frequently preferred to those with a short half-life. The drugs with the longest half-lives in each generation are as follows: first generation, *cefazolin* (1.5 to 2 hours); second generation, *cefonicid* (4.5 hours); and third generation, *ceftriaxone* (6 to 9 hours).

Distribution to Cerebrospinal Fluid. Only the third-generation agents produce CSF levels sufficient for bactericidal effects. Hence, for treatment of meningitis caused by susceptible organisms, third-generation agents are preferred over other cephalosporins. Only one third-generation drug (cefoperazone)

Drug	Trade Name(s)	Route	Dosing Interval (hrs)	Total Daily Dosage* Adults (gm)	Total Daily Dosage* Children (mg/kg)
First Generation					
Cefadroxil	Duricef, Ultracef	PO	12, 24	1–2	30
Cephalexin	Keflex, Keflet, Keftab	PO	6	1–4	25–50
Cephradine	Velosef	IM, IV	4, 6	2–12	50–100
		PO	6	1–4	25–50
Cefazolin	Ancef, Kefzol	IM, IV	6, 8	2–12	80–160
Cephalothin	Keflin	IM, IV	4, 6	2–12	80–160
Cephapirin	Cefadyl	IM, IV	4, 6	2–12	40–80
Second Generation					
Cefaclor	Ceclor	PO	8	0.75–1.5	20–40
Cefamandole	Mandol	IM, IV	4, 8	1.5–12	50–150
Cefmetazole	Zefazone	IV	6, 12	4–8	—
Cefprozil	Cefzil	PO	12, 24	0.5–1	30
Cefpodoxime	Vantin	PO	12	0.2–0.4	10
Cefonicid	Monocid	IM, IV	24	0.5–2	—
Ceforanide	Precef	IM, IV	12	1–2	20–40
Cefotetan	Cefotan	IM, IV	12	2–6	—
Cefoxitin	Mefoxin	IM, IV	4, 8	3–12	80–160
Cefuroxime	Ceftin, Kefurox, Zinacef	IM, IV	8	2.25–9	50–100
		PO	12	0.5–1	250–500
Loracarbef	Lorabid	PO	12, 24	0.5–1	30
Third Generation					
Cefixime	Suprax	PO	24	0.4	8
Cefoperazone	Cefobid	IM, IV	6, 8	2–12	100–150
Cefotaxime	Claforan	IM, IV	4, 8	2–12	100–200
Ceftazidime	Fortaz, Tazidime, Tazicef	IM, IV	8, 12	0.5–6	90–150
Ceftizoxime	Cefizox	IM, IV	6, 12	2–12	150–200
Ceftriaxone	Rocephin	IM, IV	12, 24	1–4	50–100
Moxalactam	Moxam	IM, IV	8	2–12	150–200

Table 75–3. Cephalosporin Dosages

*With the exceptions of cefoperazone and ceftriaxone, cephalosporins require a reduction of dosage for patients with severe kidney dysfunction.

is notable for its *inability* to achieve therapeutic concentrations in the CSF.

Route of Elimination. Most cephalosporins are eliminated by the kidneys and, if dosage is not carefully adjusted, may accumulate to toxic levels in patients with kidney dysfunction. Only two agents—*cefoperazone* and *ceftriaxone*—are eliminated in significant amounts by nonrenal routes, and, hence, can be used with relative safety in patients with significant renal impairment.

Dosage and Administration

Routes of Administration. Most cephalosporins cannot be absorbed from the gastrointestinal tract and must therefore be administered parenterally (IM or IV). As shown in Table 75–3, only eight cephalosporins can be given orally. Two drugs—*cephradine* and *cefuroxime*—can be administered both orally and by injection.

Dosage. Dosages are summarized in Table 75–3. For most cephalosporins (*cefoperazone* and *ceftriaxone* excepted), the dosage should be reduced in patients with significant renal impairment.

Oral Administration. If oral cephalosporins produce nausea, administration with food can reduce the response. Oral suspensions should be stored under refrigeration.

Intramuscular Administration. Intramuscular injections should be made deep into a large muscle. Intramuscular injection of cephalosporins is frequently painful; the patient should be forewarned. The injection site should be checked for induration, tenderness, and redness; the physician should be informed if these reactions occur.

Intravenous Administration. For intravenous therapy, cephalosporins may be administered by three techniques: (1) bolus injection, (2) slow injection (over a 3- to 5-minute period), and (3) continuous infusion. The physician's order should state which method is to be used. If there is uncertainty as to method of administration, clarification should be requested. Solutions for parenteral administration should be prepared according to the manufacturer's recommendations.

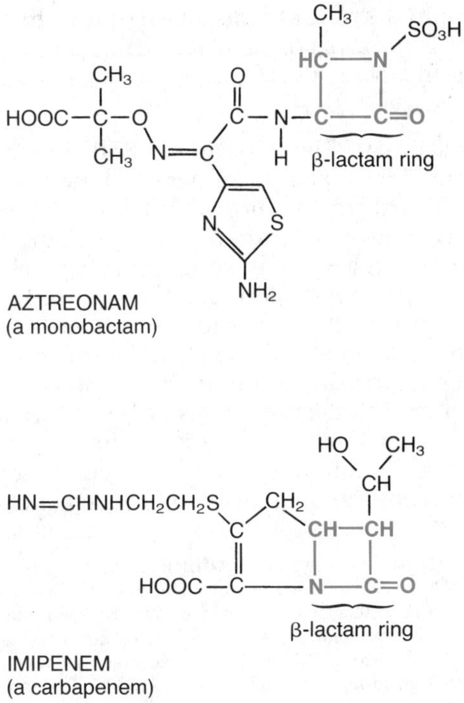

OTHER INHIBITORS OF CELL WALL SYNTHESIS

IMIPENEM

Imipenem [Primaxin], a new beta-lactam antibiotic, has the broadest antimicrobial spectrum of any drug. Because of its broad spectrum, imipenem may be of special use for treating mixed infections in which anaerobes, *Staphylococcus aureus*, and gram-negative bacilli may all be involved. Imipenem is dispensed in fixed-dose combination with cilastatin, a compound that inhibits destruction of imipenem by renal enzymes.

Chemistry. Imipenem belongs to a new class of beta-lactam antibiotics known as *carbapenems*. At this time, imipenem is the only carbapenem employed clinically. The structure of imipenem is shown in Figure 75–2.

Mechanism of Action. Imipenem binds to two penicillin-binding proteins (PBP1 and PBP2), causing weakening of the bacterial cell wall with

AZTREONAM
(a monobactam)

IMIPENEM
(a carbapenem)

Figure 75–2. Miscellaneous beta-lactam antibiotics.

subsequent lysis and death. Antimicrobial effects are enhanced by the drug's resistance to practically all beta-lactamases, and by its ability to penetrate the gram-negative cell envelope.

Antimicrobial Spectrum. Imipenem is active against most bacterial pathogens, including organisms resistant to other antibiotics. The drug is highly active against gram-positive cocci and most gram-negative cocci and bacilli. In addition, imipenem is the most effective beta-lactam antibiotic for use against anaerobic bacteria.

Pharmacokinetics. Imipenem is not absorbed from the gastrointestinal tract and must therefore be given parenterally (IV or IM). The drug is well distributed to tissues and body fluids. Imipenem penetrates the meninges, and therapeutic concentrations can be achieved in the CSF.

Elimination is primarily renal. When employed alone, imipenem is inactivated by an enzyme (dipeptidase) present in the kidney; as a result, drug levels in urine are low. To increase urinary concentrations, imipenem is administered in combination with *cilastatin*, a dipeptidase inhibitor. When the combination is used, about 70% of an administered dose of imipenem is excreted unchanged in the urine.

Adverse Effects. Imipenem is generally well tolerated. *Gastrointestinal effects* (nausea, vomiting, diarrhea) are most common. *Hypersensitivity reactions* (rashes, pruritus, drug fever) have occurred; patients allergic to other beta-lactam antibiotics may have an allergic reaction if given imipenem. *Suprainfections* with bacteria or fungi develop in about 4% of patients. Rarely, seizures have occurred.

Therapeutic Use. Because of its broad spectrum and low toxicity, imipenem has been used widely. The drug has proved effective for serious infections caused by gram-positive cocci, gram-negative cocci and bacilli, and anaerobic bacteria. This broad antimicrobial spectrum gives imipenem special utility for chemotherapy of mixed infections (e.g., simultaneous infection with aerobic and anaerobic bacteria). When imipenem has been given alone to treat infections caused by *Pseudomonas aeruginosa*, resistant organisms have emerged. Consequently, imipenem should be combined with another antipseudomonal drug for use against this microbe.

Preparations, Dosage, and Administration. Imipenem is dispensed in 1:1 fixed-dose combinations with cilastatin. The combination products are marketed under the trade name Primaxin. Two formulations are available: Primaxin I.V. and Primaxin I.M., for intravenous and intramuscular use, respectively. These products are dispensed in powder form and must be reconstituted in accord with the manufacturer's instructions. The usual adult dosage (based on imipenem content) is 250 to 500 mg every 6 hours. Dosage should be reduced in patients with renal impairment.

AZTREONAM

Chemistry. Aztreonam [Azactam] belongs to a new class of beta-lactam antibiotics known as *monobactams*. These agents contain a beta-lactam ring, but this ring is not fused with a second ring. The structure of aztreonam is shown in Figure 75–2.

Mechanism of Action. Aztreonam binds to PBP3. Hence, like most beta-lactam antibiotics, the drug inhibits bacterial cell wall synthesis, ultimately causing the cell to rupture and die. The drug does not bind to PBPs produced by anaerobes or gram-positive bacteria.

Antimicrobial Spectrum and Therapeutic Use. Aztreonam has a narrow antimicrobial spectrum: the drug is active only against gram-negative aerobic bacteria. Susceptible organisms include *Neisseria* species, *Haemophilus influenzae*, *Pseudomonas aeruginosa*, and Enterobacteriaceae (e.g., *E. coli*, *Klebsiella*, *Proteus*, *Serratia*, *Salmonella*, *Shigella*). Aztreonam is highly resistant to beta-lactamases and, therefore, is active against many gram-negative aerobes that produce these enzymes. The drug is not active against gram-positive bacteria and anaerobes.

Aztreonam has been useful against serious infections with gram-negative aerobic bacteria. Clinical experience with aztreonam is still limited, and the drug's therapeutic niche has not been completely defined.

Pharmacokinetics. Aztreonam is not absorbed from the gastrointestinal tract and must therefore be administered parenterally (IM or IV). Once in the bloodstream, the drug distributes widely to most tissues and body fluids. Therapeutic concentrations can be achieved in the CSF. Aztreonam is eliminated by the kidneys, primarily as the unchanged drug.

Adverse Effects. Aztreonam is generally well tolerated. Adverse effects are like those of other beta-lactam antibiotics. The most common side effects are pain and thrombophlebitis at sites of injection. Because aztreonam differs greatly in structure from penicillins and cephalosporins, there is little cross-allergenicity between these drugs. Hence, it appears that az-

treonam is safe for patients with allergies to other beta-lactam antibiotics.

Preparations, Dosage, and Administration. Aztreonam [Azactam] is dispensed in powdered form to be reconstituted for IM or IV administration. The usual adult dosage is 1 to 2 gm every 8 to 12 hours. Dosage should be reduced in patients with kidney dysfunction.

VANCOMYCIN

Vancomycin [Vancoled, Vancocin] is a potentially toxic drug used only for serious infections. Principal indications are antibiotic-associated colitis (caused by *Clostridium difficile*), infection with methicillin-resistant *Staphylococcus aureus*, and treatment of serious infections by susceptible organisms in patients allergic to penicillins. Vancomycin is the only drug considered in this chapter whose structure does not contain a beta-lactam ring.

Mechanism of Action. Like the other drugs discussed in this chapter, vancomycin inhibits cell wall synthesis and thereby promotes bacterial lysis and death. However, in contrast to the beta-lactam antibiotics, vancomycin does not interact with penicillin-binding proteins. Instead, vancomycin disrupts the cell wall by binding to molecules that serve as precursors for cell wall biosynthesis.

Antimicrobial Spectrum. Vancomycin is active primarily against gram-positive bacteria. The drug is especially active against *Staphylococcus aureus* and *Staph. epidermidis*, including strains of both species that are methicillin resistant. Other susceptible organisms include streptococci and *Clostridium difficile*.

Pharmacokinetics. Absorption from the gastrointestinal tract is poor. Hence, for most infections, vancomycin is given parenterally (by slow intravenous infusion). Oral administration is employed only for infections of the intestine.

Vancomycin is well distributed to most tissues and body fluids. Although the drug enters the CSF, levels may be insufficient to treat meningitis. Hence, if meningeal infection fails to respond to IV therapy, concurrent intrathecal administration may be required.

Vancomycin is eliminated unchanged by the kidneys. In patients with kidney dysfunction, dosage must be reduced.

Therapeutic Use. Vancomycin should be reserved for treatment of serious infections. This agent is the drug of choice for infections caused by methicillin-resistant *Staph. aureus* or *Staph. epidermidis*; most strains of these bacteria remain vancomycin sensitive. Oral vancomycin is the treatment of choice for antibiotic-associated colitis caused by suprainfection with *Clostridium difficile*. The drug is also employed as an alternative to penicillins and cephalosporins to treat severe infections (e.g., staphylococcal and streptococcal endocarditis) in patients allergic to the beta-lactam antibiotics.

Adverse Effects. The most serious adverse effect is *ototoxicity*. Although hearing loss is often reversible, permanent impairment of hearing can occur. Ototoxicity is most likely when plasma levels of vancomycin exceed 30 μg/ml. The risk of hearing loss is increased by high dosage, prolonged treatment, renal impairment, and concurrent use of other ototoxic drugs (e.g., aminoglycosides, ethacrynic acid).

Rapid infusion of vancomycin can cause a variety of disturbing effects, including rashes, flushing, tachycardia, and hypotension. These effects, which are thought to result from release of histamine, can be avoided by infusing vancomycin slowly (over 60 minutes or more).

Thrombophlebitis is common. This reaction can be minimized by administering vancomycin in dilute solution and by changing the infusion site frequently.

Patients who are allergic to penicillins are not cross-allergic to vancomycin. Accordingly, vancomycin is an alternative to these beta-lactam antibiotics in patients allergic to them.

Preparations, Dosage, and Administration. For treatment of *systemic infection*, vancomycin [Vancoled] is administered by intermittent infusion over 60 minutes or more. The usual adult dosage is 2 gm/day administered in divided doses at 6- or 12-hour intervals. The dosage for children is 44 mg/kg/day administered in divided doses at 6- or 12-hour intervals. In patients with renal impairment, dosages must be reduced. Serum drug levels should be monitored to insure that dosage is appropriate. Blood for measuring drug levels should be drawn 1.5 to 2.5 hours after completing the IV infusion. Peak levels of 30 to 40 µg/ml are generally acceptable.

For treatment of *antibiotic-associated colitis*, vancomycin [Vancocin] is given orally. The adult dosage is 125 to 500 mg every 6 hours. The dosage for children is 11 mg/kg every 6 hours. Since vancomycin is not absorbed from the gastrointestinal tract, there is no need to decrease oral doses in patients with renal impairment.

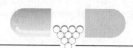

Summary of Major Nursing Implications

CEPHALOSPORINS

Except where indicated, the implications summarized below apply to all members of the cephalosporin family.

 Preadministration Assessment

Therapeutic Goal

Treatment of infections caused by susceptible organisms.

Baseline Data

The physician may order tests to determine the identity and drug sensitivity of the infecting organism. Take samples for culture prior to initiation of treatment.

Identifying High-Risk Patients

Cephalosporins are *contraindicated* for patients with *a history of allergic reactions to cephalosporins or severe allergic reactions to penicillins.*

 Implementation: Administration

Routes

Most cephalosporins are administered parenterally (IM or IV). Eight are administered orally; of these, two—cephradine and cefuroxime—can also be administered parenterally. Routes for individual cephalosporins are given in Table 75–3.

Dosage

Dosages are summarized in Table 75–3. Dosages for all cephalosporins except *cefoperazone* and *ceftriaxone* should be reduced in patients with significant renal impairment.

Administration

Oral. Advise the patient to take oral cephalosporins with food if gastric upset occurs. Instruct the patient to refrigerate oral suspensions.

Instruct the patient to complete the prescribed course of therapy even though symptoms may abate before the full course is over.

Intramuscular. Make IM injections deep into a large muscle. These injections are frequently painful; forewarn the patient. Check the injection site for induration, tenderness, and redness; notify the physician if these occur.

Intravenous. Techniques for IV administration include bolus injection, slow injection (over 3 to 5 minutes), and continuous infusion. The physician's order should specify which method to use; request clarification if the order is unclear.

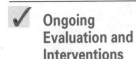

**Ongoing
Evaluation and
Interventions**

Evaluating Therapeutic Effects

Monitor the patient for indications of antimicrobial effects (e.g., reduction in fever, pain, or inflammation; improved appetite or sense of well-being).

Minimizing Adverse Effects

Allergic Reactions. Hypersensitivity reactions are relatively common; life-threatening anaphylaxis has occurred. Avoid cephalosporins in patients with a history of cephalosporin allergy or *severe* penicillin allergy; if penicillin allergy is *mild*, cephalosporins can be used with relative safety. Instruct the patient to report any signs of allergy (e.g., skin rash, itching, hives). If anaphylaxis occurs, administer parenteral epinephrine and provide respiratory support.

Bleeding. Cefamandole, cefoperazone, cefotetan, and moxalactam can promote bleeding. Severe bleeding is most likely with moxalactam; this drug should be avoided. Monitor prothrombin time, bleeding time, or both. Parenteral vitamin K can correct abnormal prothrombin time. Observe patients for signs of bleeding; if bleeding develops, discontinue drug use. Exercise caution in patients with a history of bleeding disorders and in patients receiving drugs that can interfere with hemostasis (aspirin and other nonsteroidal anti-inflammatory drugs, anticoagulants, thrombolytics).

Thrombophlebitis. Intravenous cephalosporins may cause thrombophlebitis. To minimize this reaction, rotate the injection site and inject cephalosporins slowly and in dilute solution. Observe the patient for phlebitis; change the infusion site if phlebitis develops.

Antibiotic-Associated Colitis. Colitis may develop, especially with use of broad-spectrum cephalosporins. Notify the physician if diarrhea develops (a possible indication of colitis). If antibiotic-associated colitis is diagnosed, discontinue the cephalosporin. Oral vancomycin or metronidazole may be needed.

Minimizing Adverse Interactions

Alcohol. Cefamandole, cefoperazone, cefotetan, and moxalactam can cause alcohol intolerance; ingestion of alcohol can result in a serious disulfiram-like reaction. Inform patients about alcohol intolerance and warn them not to consume alcoholic beverages.

Drugs That Promote Bleeding. Drugs that interfere with hemostasis (*aspirin and other nonsteroidal anti-inflammatory drugs, anticoagulants, thrombolytics*) can intensify bleeding tendencies caused by *cefamandole, cefoperazone, cefotetan*, and *moxalactam*. These drugs should not be used in combination.

76

Bacteriostatic Inhibitors of Protein Synthesis: Tetracyclines, Macrolides, Clindamycin, Chloramphenicol, and Spectinomycin

TETRACYCLINES

MACROLIDES
Erythromycin
Clarithromycin
Azithromycin

CLINDAMYCIN

CHLORAMPHENICOL

SPECTINOMYCIN

All of the drugs discussed in this chapter are inhibitors of bacterial protein synthesis. Unlike the aminoglycosides, whose effects on protein synthesis produce microbial death, the drugs considered here are bacteriostatic. That is, these agents suppress bacterial growth and replication but do not produce outright kill.

TETRACYCLINES

The tetracyclines are *broad-spectrum* antibiotics. Six members of the family are available in the

953

United States. All six—tetracycline, oxytetracycline, demeclocycline, methacycline, doxycycline, and minocycline—are similar in structure, antimicrobial actions, and adverse effects. Principal differences among the tetracyclines are pharmacokinetic. Since the similarities among these drugs are more pronounced than the differences, we will discuss the tetracyclines as a group, rather than focusing on a prototype. Unique properties of individual tetracyclines are indicated where appropriate.

Mechanism of Action

The tetracyclines suppress bacterial growth by inhibiting protein synthesis. These drugs block protein synthesis by binding to the 30S ribosomal subunit, thereby inhibiting binding of transfer RNA to the messenger RNA–ribosome complex. As a result, addition of amino acids to the growing peptide chain is prevented. At the concentrations achieved clinically, the tetracyclines are bacteriostatic.

Selective toxicity of the tetracyclines is determined in large part by the relative inability of these drugs to cross mammalian cell membranes. In order to influence protein synthesis, tetracyclines must first gain access to the cell interior. Entry into bacteria is accomplished by way of an energy-dependent transport process. Mammalian cells lack such a transport system, and, therefore, do not actively accumulate the drug. Consequently, although tetracyclines are inherently capable of inhibiting protein synthesis in mammalian cells, drug levels within host cells remain too low to suppress protein production.

Microbial Resistance

Bacterial resistance to the tetracyclines results from reduced drug accumulation. Two mechanisms are responsible: (1) decreased drug uptake, and (2) acquisition of the ability to actively extrude tetracyclines. Tetracycline resistance is an inducible trait. That is, exposure to tetracyclines acts as a stimulus to cause an increase in resistance.

Antimicrobial Spectrum

The tetracyclines are broad-spectrum antibiotics. These agents are active against a wide variety of gram-positive and gram-negative bacteria. Sensitive organisms include *Rickettsia*, spirochetes, *Brucella*, *Chlamydia*, *Mycoplasma*, and *Vibrio cholerae*.

Therapeutic Uses

Treatment of Infectious Diseases. Extensive use of tetracyclines has resulted in increasing bacterial resistance. Because of microbial resistance, and because antibiotics with greater selectivity and less toxicity are now available, use of tetracyclines has declined. Today, tetracyclines are rarely drugs of first choice for *common* bacterial diseases. However, these agents *are* valuable for treating several *uncommon* infections. Disorders for which

tetracyclines are considered first-line drugs include (1) rickettsial diseases (e.g., Rocky Mountain spotted fever, typhus fever, Q fever), (2) infections caused by *Chlamydia trachomatis* (trachoma, lymphogranuloma venereum, urethritis, cervicitis), (3) brucellosis, (4) cholera, (5) pneumonia caused by *Mycoplasma pneumoniae*, (6) Lyme disease, and (7) gastric infection with *Helicobacter pylori*.

Treatment of Acne. Tetracyclines are used topically and orally for severe acne vulgaris. Beneficial effects derive from suppressing the growth and metabolic activity of *Propionibacterium acnes*, causing the organism to reduce secretion of inflammatory chemicals. Oral doses of tetracyclines employed in acne are relatively low. As a result, adverse effects are minimal. Treatment of acne is discussed further in Chapter 70 (Drugs for Dermatologic Disorders).

Peptic Ulcer Disease. There is increasing evidence that a bacterium—*Helicobacter pylori*—is a major contributing factor to peptic ulcer disease. Tetracyclines, in combination with metronidazole and bismuth subsalicylate, are the current treatment of choice for eradicating this organism. The role of *H. pylori* in ulcer formation is discussed in Chapter 66 (Drugs for Peptic Ulcer Disease).

Pharmacokinetics

Individual tetracyclines differ significantly in their pharmacokinetic properties. Of particular significance are differences in half-life and route of elimination. Also of clinical importance are differences in the extent to which food decreases absorption. The pharmacokinetic properties of individual tetracyclines are summarized in Table 76–1.

Duration of Action. The tetracyclines can be divided into three groups: short acting, intermediate acting, and long acting (see Table 76–1). These differences in time course are related to differences in lipid solubility: the short-acting tetracyclines (tetracycline, oxytetracycline) have relatively low lipid solubility, whereas the long-acting agents (doxycycline, minocycline) have relatively high lipid solubility.

Absorption. All of the tetracyclines are orally effective, although the extent of absorption differs among individual agents (see Table 76–1). Absorption of the short-acting and intermediate-acting tetracyclines is reduced in the presence of food. In contrast, food does not reduce absorption of the long-acting agents.

The tetracyclines form insoluble chelates with calcium, iron, magnesium, aluminum, and zinc. Formation of such chelates decreases absorption. Accordingly, *tetracyclines should not be administered together with* (1) *calcium supplements*, (2) *milk products* (because they contain calcium), (3)

Table 76–1. Pharmacokinetic Properties of the Tetracyclines

Class	Drug	Lipid Solubility	Percent of Oral Dose Absorbed	Effect of Food on Absorption	Principal Route of Elimination	Half-life Normal (hours)	Half-life Anuric (hours)
Short Acting	Tetracycline	Low	76	Decrease	Renal	8	57–108*
	Oxytetracycline	Low	58	Decrease	Renal	9	47–66*
Intermediate Acting	Demeclocycline	Moderate	66	Decrease	Renal	12	40–60*
	Methacycline	Moderate	58	Decrease	Renal	14	44*
Long Acting	Doxycycline	High	93	No change	Hepatic	18	12–22
	Minocycline	High	95	No change	Hepatic	16	11–23

*Because of greatly prolonged half-life and potential for accumulation to toxic levels, this drug should not be employed in patients with kidney dysfunction.

iron supplements, (4) *magnesium-containing laxatives*, and (5) *most antacids* (because they contain magnesium, aluminum, or both).

Distribution. Tetracyclines are widely distributed to most tissues and body fluids. However, penetration to the cerebrospinal fluid (CSF) is poor and levels achieved in the CSF are inadequate for treating meningeal infections. Tetracyclines readily cross the placenta and enter the fetal circulation.

Elimination. Tetracyclines are eliminated via renal and hepatic routes. All tetracyclines are excreted by the liver into the bile. After the bile enters the intestine, most tetracyclines are reabsorbed.

Ultimate elimination of short-acting and intermediate-acting tetracyclines is in the urine, largely as the unchanged drug (see Table 76–1). Because these agents undergo renal excretion, they can accumulate to toxic levels if kidney function fails. Consequently, *short-acting and intermediate-acting tetracyclines should not be administered to patients with renal failure.*

The long-acting tetracyclines are eliminated by the liver, primarily as metabolites. Because these agents are excreted by the liver, their half-lives are unaffected by kidney dysfunction. Accordingly, *the long-acting agents are drugs of choice for tetracycline-responsive infections in patients with renal impairment.*

Adverse Effects

Gastrointestinal Irritation. Tetracyclines irritate the gastrointestinal tract. As a result, oral therapy is frequently associated with epigastric burning, cramps, nausea, vomiting, and diarrhea. These reactions can be reduced by giving tetracyclines with meals, although food may decrease absorption. Occasionally, tetracyclines have caused esophageal ulceration. This reaction can be minimized by avoiding administration at bedtime.

Since diarrhea may result from suprainfection of the bowel (in addition to nonspecific irritation), it is important that the cause of diarrhea be determined.

Effects on Bones and Teeth. Tetracyclines bind to calcium in developing teeth, resulting in yellow or brown discoloration; hypoplasia of the enamel may also occur. The intensity of tooth discoloration is related to the total cumulative dose; staining is darker with prolonged and repeated treatment. When taken after the fourth month of gestation, tetracyclines can cause staining of *deciduous* teeth. However, use of these drugs during pregnancy will not affect the *permanent teeth*. Discoloration of permanent teeth occurs when tetracyclines are taken by patients aged 4 months to 8 years, the interval during which tooth enamel is being formed. Accordingly, these drugs should be avoided if at all possible by children under the age of 8 years. The risk of tooth discoloration with *doxycycline* and *oxytetracycline* may be less than with other tetracyclines.

Tetracyclines can suppress long-bone growth in premature infants. This effect is reversible upon discontinuation of treatment.

Suprainfection. As discussed in Chapter 73, a suprainfection is an overgrowth with drug-resistant microbes. This overgrowth occurs secondary to suppression of drug-sensitive organisms. Because the tetracyclines are broad-spectrum agents, and, therefore, can decrease viability of a wide variety of microbes, the risk of suprainfection is greater than with antibiotics that have a more narrow antimicrobial spectrum.

Suprainfection of the bowel with staphylococci or with *Clostridium difficile* produces severe diarrhea and can be life-threatening. The infection caused by *C. difficile* is known as *antibiotic-associated colitis* or *pseudomembranous colitis*. Patients should be instructed to notify the physician if significant diarrhea occurs so that the possibility of bacterial suprainfection can be evaluated. If a diagnosis of suprainfection with staphylococci or *C. difficile* is made, tetracyclines should be discontinued immediately. Treatment consists of oral *vancomycin* or *metronidazole* plus vigorous fluid and electrolyte replacement therapy.

Overgrowth with fungi (commonly *Candida albicans*) may occur in the mouth, pharynx, vagina, and bowel. Symptoms include vaginal or anal itching; inflammatory lesions of the anogenital region; and a black, furry appearance of the tongue. Suprainfection with *Candida* can be managed by discontinuing tetracycline use. When this is not possible, treatment with an antifungal drug is indicated.

Hepatotoxicity. Tetracyclines can cause fatty infiltration of the liver. Hepatotoxicity manifests clinically as lethargy and jaundice. Rarely, the condition progresses to massive liver failure. Liver damage is most likely when tetracyclines are administered intravenously in high dosage (greater than 2 gm/day). Pregnant and postpartum women who have kidney disease are at particularly high risk of liver damage.

Renal Toxicity. Tetracyclines may exacerbate renal dysfunction in patients with pre-existing kidney disease. Since most tetracyclines are excreted by the kidneys, these agents should not be given to patients with renal impairment. Exceptions to this rule are *doxycycline* and perhaps *minocycline*. Since these two agents are eliminated primarily by the liver, decreased kidney function does not cause them to accumulate.

Photosensitivity. All of the tetracyclines can increase the sensitivity of the skin to ultraviolet light. The most common result is exaggerated sunburn. Patients should be advised to avoid prolonged exposure to sunlight, wear protective clothing, and apply a sunscreen to exposed skin.

Other Adverse Effects. *Vestibular toxicity*, manifesting as dizziness, lightheadedness, and unsteadiness, has occurred with *minocycline*. Rarely, tetracyclines have produced *pseudotumor cerebri* (a benign elevation in intracranial pressure). In a few patients, *demeclocycline* has produced *nephrogenic diabetes insipidus*, a syndrome characterized by thirst, increased frequency of urination, and unusual weakness or tiredness. Because of their irritant properties, tetracyclines can cause *pain at sites of IM injection* and *thrombophlebitis when administered IV*.

Drug and Food Interactions

As noted above, tetracyclines can form nonabsorbable chelates with certain metal ions (calcium, iron, magnesium, aluminum, zinc). Substances that contain these ions include *milk products, calcium supplements, iron supplements, magnesium-containing laxatives*, and *most antacids*. If a tetracycline is administered with these agents, absorption of the tetracycline will be decreased. To minimize interference with tetracycline absorption, *tetracyclines should be administered at least 2 hours before or 2 hours after ingestion of chelating agents.*

Dosage and Administration

Administration. Tetracyclines may be administered orally, intravenously, and by intramuscular injection. Oral administration is preferred, and all tetracyclines are available in oral formulations. As a rule, oral tetracyclines should be taken on an empty stomach (1 hour before or 2 hours after meals) and with a full glass of water. An interval of at least 2 hours should separate administration of oral tetracyclines and ingestion of products capable of chelating these drugs (e.g., milk, calcium or iron supplements, antacids). Several tetracyclines can be given intravenously (Table 76–2), but this route should be employed only when oral therapy cannot be tolerated or has proved inadequate. Intramuscular injection is extremely painful and used only rarely.

Dosage. Dosage is determined by the nature and intensity of the infection being treated. Typical doses for adults and children over the age of 8 years are summarized in Table 76–2.

Summary of Major Precautions

With the exceptions of doxycycline and minocycline, the tetracyclines are eliminated primarily in the urine, and will accumulate to toxic levels in the presence of kidney disease; accordingly, most tetracyclines should not be administered to patients with renal failure. Tetracyclines can cause discoloration of deciduous and permanent teeth; tooth discoloration can be avoided by withholding these drugs from pregnant women and from children under the age of 8 years. Diarrhea may indicate a potentially life-threatening suprainfection of the bowel; advise patients to notify the physician if diarrhea occurs. High-dose intravenous therapy has been associated with severe liver damage, particularly in pregnant and postpartum women who have kidney disease; as a rule, women in these categories should not receive tetracyclines.

Summary of Unique Properties of Individual Tetracyclines

Tetracycline. Tetracycline hydrochloride [Achromycin, Sumycin, others] is the least expensive and most widely used member of the tetracycline family. This drug has the indications, pharmacokinetics, adverse effects, and drug interactions described above for the tetracyclines as a group. Like most tetracyclines, tetracycline hydrochloride should not be administered with food, and is contraindicated for patients with kidney dysfunction. This agent and all other tetracyclines should not be given to pregnant women or children under the age of 8 years.

Oxytetracycline. Oxytetracycline [Terramycin, others] is a short-acting agent and is similar to tetracycline in most respects. The principal difference between these drugs is cost: brand name preparations of oxytetracycline are more expensive than brand name preparations of tetracycline.

Demeclocycline. Demeclocycline [Declomycin] shares the actions, indications, and adverse effects described above for the tetracyclines as a group. Because of its intermediate duration

Table 76-2. Tetracyclines: Routes of Administration, Dosage Interval, and Dosage

Class	Drug	Trade Names	Route	Usual Dosing Interval (hours)	Total Daily Dose Adult (mg)	Total Daily Dose Pediatric[a] (mg/kg)
Short Acting	Tetracycline	Achromycin, Sumycin, others	PO	6	1000–2000	25–50
			IV[b]	12	500–1000	10–20
			IM[c]	12	300	15–25
	Oxytetracycline	Terramycin, Uri-Tet	PO	6	1000–2000	25–50
			IM[c]	12	300	15–25
Intermediate Acting	Demeclocycline	Declomycin	PO	12	600	6–12
	Methacycline	Rondomycin	PO	12	600	6–12
Long Acting	Doxycycline	Vibramycin, others	PO	24	100[d]	2.2[e]
			IV[b]	24	100–200[f]	2.2–4.4[g]
	Minocycline	Minocin	PO	12	200[h]	4[i]
			IV[b]	12	200[h]	4[i]

[a]Doses presented are for children over the age of 8 years; use in children below this age may cause permanent staining of teeth.
[b]The intravenous route is used only if oral therapy cannot be tolerated or is inadequate.
[c]Intramuscular injection is extremely painful and used only rarely.
[d]First-day regimen is 100 mg initially followed by 100 mg 12 hours later.
[e]First-day regimen is 2.2 mg/kg initially followed by 2.2 mg/kg 12 hours later.
[f]First-day regimen is 200 mg in 1 or 2 slow infusions (1 to 4 hours).
[g]First-day regimen is 4.4 mg/kg in 1 or 2 slow infusions (1 to 4 hours).
[h]First-day regimen is 200 mg initially followed by 100 mg 12 hours later.
[i]First-day regimen is 4 mg/kg initially followed by 2 mg/kg 12 hours later.

of action, demeclocycline can be administered at dosing intervals that are longer than those used for tetracycline. Demeclocycline is a relatively new drug, and treatment can be expensive.

Demeclocycline is unique among the tetracyclines in its ability to stimulate urine flow. This side effect can lead to excessive urination, thirst, and tiredness. Because of its effect on renal function, demeclocycline has been employed therapeutically to promote urine production in patients suffering from the syndrome of inappropriate (excessive) secretion of antidiuretic hormone.

Methacycline. Methacycline [Rondomycin] shares the actions, indications, and adverse effects described above for the tetracyclines as a group. Like demeclocycline, methacycline is an intermediate-acting agent and, hence, administration can be less frequent than with tetracycline. The cost of methacycline is even greater than that of demeclocycline.

Doxycycline. Doxycycline [Vibramycin, others] is a long-acting agent and shares the actions and adverse effects described above for the tetracyclines as a group. Because of its prolonged half-life, doxycycline can be administered once daily. Absorption of oral doxycycline is greater than that of tetracycline and is not diminished by food or milk; thus, the drug may be administered with meals. Doxycycline is eliminated primarily by nonrenal mechanisms. As a result, this agent is safe for patients with renal failure. Doxycycline is a first-line drug for Lyme disease and chlamydial infections (urethritis, cervicitis, lymphogranuloma venereum).

Minocycline. Minocycline [Minocin] is a long-acting agent similar in most respects to doxycycline. Like doxycycline, minocycline can be taken with food. Minocycline is safe for patients with kidney disease. Minocycline is unique among the tetracyclines in that it can damage the vestibular system, causing unsteadiness, lightheadedness, and dizziness; vestibular toxicity limits the use of this drug. Minocycline is expensive; a course of treatment costs significantly more than therapy with tetracycline.

MACROLIDES

The macrolides are broad-spectrum antibiotics that act by inhibiting bacterial protein synthesis. These drugs are called macrolides because of their large size. Erythromycin is the oldest member of the family. Azithromycin and clarithromycin, the newest macrolides, are derivatives of erythromycin. All of the macrolides are devoid of serious toxicity.

ERYTHROMYCIN

Erythromycin has a relatively broad spectrum of antimicrobial action and is a preferred or alternative treatment for a number of infectious diseases. The drug is one of our safest antibiotics. Erythromycin will serve as our prototype for the macrolide family.

Mechanism of Action

Antibacterial effects result from inhibition of protein synthesis: erythromycin binds to the 50S ribosomal subunit and thereby blocks addition of new amino acids to the growing peptide chain. Erythromycin is usually bacteriostatic, but can be bactericidal against highly susceptible organisms or when present at high concentrations. The drug is selectively toxic to bacteria because ribosomes in the cytoplasm of mammalian cells do not bind the drug. Also, in contrast to chloramphenicol (see below), erythromycin cannot cross the mitochondrial membrane, and, therefore, does not inhibit protein synthesis in host mitochondria.

Antimicrobial Spectrum

Erythromycin's antibacterial spectrum is *similar to that of penicillin*. The drug is active against most gram-positive bacteria as well as some gram-negative microbes. Bacterial sensitivity is determined in large part by the ability of erythromycin to gain access to the cell interior.

Therapeutic Uses

Erythromycin is a commonly used antimicrobial agent. *This drug is the treatment of first choice for several infections and is employed as an alternative to penicillin G in patients allergic to penicillins.*

Erythromycin is the preferred treatment for pneumonia caused by *Legionella pneumophila* (*legionnaires' disease*). The regimen for this infection also includes rifampin.

Erythromycin is considered the drug of first choice for individuals infected with *Bordetella pertussis*, the causative agent of *whooping cough*. Since symptoms are caused by a toxin, erythromycin does little to alter the course of the disease. However, by eliminating *B. pertussis* from the nasopharynx, treatment does lower infectivity.

Corynebacterium diphtheriae is highly sensitive to erythromycin. Accordingly, erythromycin is the treatment of choice for *acute diphtheria* and eliminating the diphtheria carrier state.

Several infections respond equally well to erythromycin and to tetracyclines. Both agents are drugs of first choice for certain chlamydial infections (urethritis, cervicitis) and for pneumonia caused by *Mycoplasma pneumoniae*.

Erythromycin is commonly employed as an alternative to penicillin G in patients with penicillin allergy. The drug is used most frequently as a substitute for penicillin to treat respiratory tract infections caused by *Streptococcus pneumoniae* and by group A *Strep. pyogenes*. Erythromycin can also be employed as an alternative to penicillin for preventing recurrences of rheumatic fever and bacterial endocarditis.

Pharmacokinetics

Absorption and Bioavailability. Erythromycin for oral administration is available in four forms: *erythromycin base* and three derivatives of the base: *erythromycin estolate, erythromycin stearate,* and *erythromycin ethylsuccinate*. The base is unstable in stomach acid, and absorption can be variable; the derivatives were synthesized to improve bioavailability. Bioavailability has also been enhanced by use of acid-resistant coatings. These coatings protect erythromycin while it is in the stomach and then dissolve in the duodenum, thereby permitting absorption of erythromycin from the small intestine. As a rule, *food decreases the absorption of erythromycin base and erythromycin stearate,* whereas absorption of the estolate and ethylsuccinate forms is not affected. Only erythromycin base is biologically active; the derivatives must be converted to the base (either in the intestine or following absorption) in order to exert antibacterial effects. When used properly (i.e., when dosage is correct and the effects of food are accounted for), all of the oral erythromycins produce equivalent therapeutic effects.

In addition to its oral forms, erythromycin is available as *erythromycin lactobionate* for intravenous use. This IV preparation produces plasma drug levels that are higher than those achieved with oral erythromycins.

Distribution. Erythromycin is readily distributed to most tissues and body fluids. Penetration to the CSF, however, is poor. Erythromycin crosses the placenta, but adverse effects on the fetus have not been observed.

Elimination. Erythromycin is eliminated primarily by hepatic mechanisms. The drug is concentrated in the liver and then excreted in the bile. A small amount (10% to 15%) is excreted unchanged in the urine. Since elimination is primarily hepatic, the dosage need not be reduced in patients with renal dysfunction.

Adverse Effects

Erythromycin is generally free of serious toxicity and is one of the safest antibiotics available. The toxicity of principal concern is occasional production of liver injury with erythromycin *estolate*.

Gastrointestinal Effects. Gastrointestinal disturbances (epigastric pain, nausea, vomiting, diarrhea) are the most common adverse effects. These can be reduced by administering erythromycin with meals. However, this should be done only when using those forms of erythromycin whose absorption is unaffected by food (erythromycin estolate, erythromycin ethylsuccinate, certain enteric-coated formulations of erythromycin base). Patients who experience persistent or severe gastrointestinal reactions should notify the physician.

Liver Injury. The most serious toxicity of erythromycin is *cholestatic hepatitis*. This reaction, which occurs almost exclusively in adults, is caused by *erythromycin estolate* and not by other forms of the drug. Symptoms include nausea, vomiting, abdominal pain, jaundice, and elevations in plasma levels of bilirubin and liver transaminases. Hepatic injury usually develops 10 to 20 days after initiation of treatment. However, the reaction can occur within hours if erythromycin is administered to patients who have experienced hepatotoxicity in the past. Because of its capacity for injuring the liver, erythromycin estolate should be avoided by patients with pre-existing hepatic disease. Patients should be instructed to report signs of liver injury (e.g., severe abdominal pain, yellow discoloration of the skin or eyes, darkened urine, pale stools). Symptoms reverse following drug withdrawal.

Other Adverse Effects. By killing off sensitive gut flora, erythromycin can promote *suprainfection of the bowel. Thrombophlebitis* can occur with intravenous administration; this reaction can be minimized by slow infusion of dilute drug solution. Rarely, high-dose therapy has caused *transient loss of hearing.*

Drug Interactions

Erythromycin can increase the plasma levels and half-lives of several drugs. Important among these are *theophylline* (used to treat asthma), *carbamazepine* (an anticonvulsant), and *warfarin* (an anticoagulant). The mechanism by which erythromycin increases levels of these drugs appears to be inhibition of hepatic metabolism. When these agents are combined with erythromycin, the patient should be monitored closely for signs of toxicity.

Erythromycin prevents binding of *chloramphenicol* and *clindamycin* to bacterial ribosomes, thereby antagonizing the effects of these antibiotics. Accordingly, concurrent use of erythromycin with these other drugs is not recommended.

Erythromycin increases the risk of severe ventricular dysrhythmias in patients receiving *astemizole* or *terfenadine*, both of which are antihistamines. Accordingly, these drugs should not be used concurrently.

Preparations, Dosage, and Administration

Preparations. Erythromycin is available in formulations for oral and intravenous administration. All preparations have the same antimicrobial spectrum and indications. Adverse effects are also similar, except that cholestatic hepatitis occurs only with erythromycin estolate.

Oral Dosage and Administration. Oral erythromycins should be administered on an empty stomach and with a full glass of water. If necessary, some preparations (erythromycin estolate, erythromycin ethylsuccinate, certain enteric-coated preparations of erythromycin base) can be administered with food to decrease gastrointestinal reactions. The usual *adult* dosage for *erythromycin base, estolate,* and *stearate* is 250 to 500 mg every 6 hours; the adult dosage for *erythromycin ethylsuccinate* is 400 to 800 mg every 6 hours. The usual *pediatric* dosage for all oral erythromycins is 7.5 to 12.5 mg/kg every 6 hours.

Trade names for oral erythromycins include E-Mycin, ERYC, and PCE Dispertab (for erythromycin base); Ilosone (for eryth-

romycin estolate); E.E.S. and EryPed (for erythromycin ethylsuccinate); and Eramycin, Erythrocin, and Wyamycin S (for erythromycin stearate).

Intravenous Dosage and Administration. Intravenous administration is reserved for severe infections and is used only rarely. Continuous infusion is preferred to intermittent administration. Only *erythromycin lactobionate* is given IV. The usual *adult* dosage is 1 to 4 gm daily. The usual *pediatric* dosage is 15 to 50 mg/kg/day. Erythromycin should be infused slowly and in dilute solution to minimize the risk of thrombophlebitis. For instruction on preparation and storage of IV solutions, consult the manufacturer's literature.

CLARITHROMYCIN

Actions and Therapeutic Uses. Like erythromycin, clarithromycin [Biaxin Filmtabs] binds the 50S subunit of bacterial ribosomes, causing inhibition of protein synthesis. The drug is approved for respiratory tract infections and uncomplicated infections of the skin and skin structures. It is under investigation for treatment of disseminated *Mycobacterium avium* infections and other infections associated with AIDS.

Pharmacokinetics. Clarithromycin is well absorbed following oral administration, regardless of the presence of food. The drug is widely distributed and readily penetrates cells. Elimination is by hepatic metabolism and renal excretion. A reduction in dosage may be needed in patients with severe renal dysfunction.

Adverse Effects and Interactions. Clarithromycin is well tolerated and does not produce the intense nausea seen with erythromycin. The most common reactions (3%) have been diarrhea, nausea, and distorted taste; all have been described as mild-to-moderate. In clinical trials, only 3% of patients withdrew because of side effects, compared with 20% who withdrew when taking erythromycin. High doses of clarithromycin have caused fetal abnormalities in laboratory animals; possible effects on the human fetus are unknown. Like erythromycin, clarithromycin can elevate blood levels of *carbamazepine* and *theophylline*; dosages of these drugs may need to be reduced.

Preparations, Dosage, and Administration. Clarithromycin [Biaxin Filmtabs] is dispensed in tablets (250 and 500 mg) for oral administration. The recommended dosage is 250 or 500 mg every 12 hours for 7 to 14 days; the exact dosage size and duration depend on the infection being treated. The drug may be taken without regard to meals.

AZITHROMYCIN

Actions and Therapeutic Uses. Like erythromycin, azithromycin [Zithromax] binds the 50S subunit of bacterial ribosomes, causing inhibition of protein synthesis. The drug is approved for respiratory tract infections, uncomplicated infections of the skin and skin structures, and nongonococcal urethritis caused by *Chlamydia trachomatis*. Like clarithromycin, azithromycin is being investigated as treatment for disseminated *Mycobacterium avium* infections and other infections associated with AIDS.

Pharmacokinetics. Absorption of azithromycin is reduced by 50% in the presence of food. Accordingly, the drug should not be administered with meals. Following absorption, azithromycin is widely distributed to tissues and becomes concentrated in cells. The drug is eliminated in the bile, both as metabolites and parent drug.

Adverse Effects and Interactions. Like clarithromycin, azithromycin is well tolerated and does not produce the intense nausea seen with erythromycin. The most common reactions have been diarrhea (5%) and nausea and abdominal pain (3%). In one clinical trial, only 0.7% of patients withdrew because of drug-induced side effects. Aluminum- and magnesium-containing antacids reduce the rate (but not the extent) of azithromycin absorption.

Preparations, Dosage, and Administration. Azithromycin [Zithromax] is dispensed in 250-mg capsules for oral administration. The usual dosing schedule is 500 mg once on the first day, followed by 250 mg once daily on the following 4 days. The drug should be taken 1 hour before meals or 2 hours after. It must not be taken with food or with aluminum- or magnesium-containing antacids.

CLINDAMYCIN

Clindamycin [Cleocin] can promote severe antibiotic-associated colitis, a condition that can be fatal. Because of the risk of colitis, indications for clindamycin are limited. Currently, the drug is indicated only for certain anaerobic infections located outside the CNS.

Mechanism of Action

Clindamycin binds to the 50S subunit of bacterial ribosomes and thereby inhibits protein synthesis. The ribosomal site at which clindamycin binds overlaps the binding sites for erythromycin and chloramphenicol. As a result, these agents may antagonize one another's effects. Accordingly, there are no indications for concurrent use of clindamycin with these other antibiotics.

Antimicrobial Spectrum

Clindamycin is active against most anaerobic bacteria (gram-positive and gram-negative) and most gram-positive aerobes. Gram-negative aerobes are generally resistant. Susceptible anaerobes include *Bacteroides fragilis*, *Fusobacterium*, *Clostridium perfringens*, and anaerobic streptococci. Clindamycin is usually bacteriostatic; however, bactericidal effects may occur if the target organism is especially sensitive. Resistance can be a significant clinical problem with *B. fragilis*.

Therapeutic Use

Because of its efficacy against gram-positive cocci, clindamycin was once used widely as an alternative to penicillin. However, following the discovery that clindamycin can promote pseudomembranous colitis (see below), use of this drug has declined. Today, clindamycin is employed primarily for anaerobic infections outside the CNS (the drug does not cross the blood-brain barrier). Clindamycin is a preferred drug for abdominal and pelvic infections caused by *Bacteroides fragilis*. In addition, it can be used as a substitute for penicillin G to treat severe infections with other anaerobes (e.g., *Clostridium perfringens*, *Fusobacterium nucleatum*, anaerobic streptococci).

Pharmacokinetics

Absorption and Distribution. Clindamycin may be administered orally, IM, and IV. Absorption from the gastrointestinal tract is nearly complete and is not affected by food. The drug is widely distributed to most body fluids and tissues, including

synovial fluid and bone. Penetration to the cerebrospinal fluid is poor.

Elimination. Clindamycin undergoes hepatic metabolism to active and inactive products. These metabolites are excreted in the urine and bile. Only 10% of the drug is eliminated unchanged by the kidneys. In normal individuals, the half-life of clindamycin is approximately 3 hours; this value is increased only slightly in patients with substantial reductions in liver or kidney function. Hence, dosage need not be reduced in such patients. However, the drug may accumulate to toxic levels in the presence of *combined* renal and hepatic disease. Under these conditions, a reduction in dosage is indicated.

Adverse Effects

Antibiotic-Associated Colitis. The most severe toxicity associated with clindamycin is a condition known as *antibiotic-associated colitis,* formerly called *pseudomembranous colitis*. The cause is suprainfection of the bowel with *Clostridium difficile*, an anaerobic gram-positive bacillus. Antibiotic-associated colitis is characterized by profuse, watery diarrhea (10 to 20 stools per day), abdominal pain, fever, and leukocytosis. Stools often contain mucus and blood. Symptoms usually begin during the first week of treatment; however, they may also develop as much as 4 to 6 weeks after clindamycin withdrawal. Left untreated, the condition can be fatal. Antibiotic-associated colitis occurs with parenteral and oral therapy. Because of the risk of colitis, patients should be instructed to report significant diarrhea (more than 5 watery stools per day). If suprainfection with *C. difficile* is diagnosed, clindamycin should be discontinued and the patient should be given oral vancomycin or metronidazole, which are drugs of choice for eliminating *C. difficile* from the bowel. Diarrhea usually ceases 3 to 5 days after initiation of vancomycin treatment. Vigorous replacement therapy with fluids and electrolytes is usually indicated. Drugs that decrease bowel motility (e.g., opioids, anticholinergics) may worsen symptoms and should not be used.

Other Adverse Effects. *Diarrhea* (unrelated to pseudomembranous colitis) is relatively common. *Hypersensitivity reactions* (especially rashes) occur frequently. *Hepatotoxicity* and *blood dyscrasias* (agranulocytosis, leukopenia, thrombocytopenia) develop rarely. Rapid intravenous administration can cause *EKG changes, hypotension,* and *cardiac arrest*.

Preparations, Dosage, and Administration

Preparations. Clindamycin is available as *clindamycin hydrochloride* and *clindamycin palmitate hydrochloride* for *oral* use and as *clindamycin phosphate* for IM or IV use. Clindamycin hydrochloride [Cleocin] is dispensed in capsules (75, 150, and 300 mg). Clindamycin palmitate hydrochloride [Cleocin Pediatric] is dispensed as flavored granules; these are reconstituted with fluid to make an oral solution containing 15 mg of clindamycin per ml. Clindamycin phosphate [Cleocin Phosphate] is dispensed in solution (150 mg/ml).

Oral Dosage and Administration. For *clindamycin hydrochloride,* the adult dosage ranges from 150 to 450 mg every 6 hours; the pediatric dosage ranges from 8 to 20 mg/kg daily in three or four divided doses. For *clindamycin palmitate hydrochloride,* adult and pediatric dosages range from 8 to 25 mg/kg/day administered in three or four divided doses. Oral clindamycin should be taken with a full glass of water. The drug may be administered with meals.

Parenteral Dosage and Administration. For parenteral (IM or IV) therapy, *clindamycin phosphate* is employed. Intramuscular and IV dosages are the same. The usual adult dosage is 0.6 to 3.6 gm/day administered in three or four divided doses. The usual pediatric dosage is 15 to 40 mg/kg/day in three or four divided doses.

CHLORAMPHENICOL

Chloramphenicol [Chloromycetin] is a broad-spectrum antibiotic with the potential for causing fatal aplastic anemia. Because of the risk of severe blood disorders, use of chloramphenicol is limited to treatment of serious infections for which less toxic drugs are ineffective.

Mechanism of Action

The antibacterial effects of chloramphenicol result from inhibition of protein synthesis. The drug binds reversibly to the 50S subunit of bacterial ribosomes and thereby prevents addition of new amino acids to the growing peptide chain. Chloramphenicol is usually bacteriostatic, but can be bactericidal against highly susceptible organisms or if drug concentrations are high.

Since most protein synthesis in mammalian cells is carried out in the cytoplasm employing ribosomes that are insensitive to chloramphenicol, toxic effects of chloramphenicol are restricted largely to bacteria. However, since the ribosomes of mammalian *mitochondria* are very similar to the ribosomes of bacteria, chloramphenicol is capable of decreasing mitochondrial protein synthesis in the host. This action may underlie certain adverse effects of the drug (e.g., dose-dependent bone marrow depression, gray syndrome in infants).

Antimicrobial Spectrum

Chloramphenicol is active against a broad spectrum of bacteria. A large number of gram-positive and gram-negative aerobic organisms are sensitive. Included in this group are *Salmonella typhi*, *Haemophilus influenzae*, *Neisseria meningitidis*, and *Streptococcus pneumoniae*. Most anaerobic bacteria (e.g., *Bacteroides fragilis*) are also susceptible. In addition, chloramphenicol is active against rickettsiae, chlamydiae, mycoplasmas, and treponemas.

Resistance

Resistance among gram-negative bacteria results from acquisition of an R factor that codes for acetyltransferase, an enzyme that can inactivate chloramphenicol. This same R factor also codes for resistance to tetracyclines, and frequently confers resistance to penicillins as well.

Pharmacokinetics

Chloramphenicol is available in three forms: chloramphenicol *base*, chloramphenicol *palmitate*, and chloramphenicol *succinate*. The base and palmitate are administered orally, whereas the succinate is administered IV. The palmitate and succinate esters are prodrugs that must be hydrolyzed to free chloramphenicol before they can act.

Absorption. Chloramphenicol *base* is readily absorbed following oral administration. For absorption of the *palmitate* to take place, the molecule must first be hydrolyzed to chloramphenicol base by pancreatic lipases in the duodenum. When the palmitate is administered to newborns, blood levels of chloramphenicol are highly variable.

Following IV administration, chloramphenicol *succinate* must be hydrolyzed to chloramphenicol before it can exert antibacterial effects. This conversion is variable and incomplete. Production of active drug is especially erratic in newborns, infants, and young children.

Distribution. Chloramphenicol is highly lipid soluble and widely distributed to body tissues and fluids. Therapeutic concentrations are readily achieved in the CSF, and drug levels in the brain may be as much as nine times those in plasma. As a result, chloramphenicol can be of special value for treating meningitis and brain abscesses caused by susceptible bacteria. The drug crosses the placenta and is secreted in breast milk.

Metabolism and Excretion. Chloramphenicol is eliminated primarily by hepatic metabolism. Inactive metabolites are excreted in the urine. In patients with liver dysfunction, the half-life of chloramphenicol is prolonged and drug accumulation can occur. Accordingly, the dosage should be reduced in the presence of liver disease. Because the kidneys serve only to excrete inactive metabolites, there is no need for dosage reduction in patients with renal dysfunction. In neonates, hepatic metabolism is not fully developed and the half-life of chloramphenicol is prolonged.

Monitoring Chloramphenicol Serum Levels. Because chloramphenicol has a low therapeutic index, and because serum levels of the drug can vary substantially among patients, monitoring of chloramphenicol blood levels is frequently indicated. Monitoring is especially important for neonates, infants, and young children, since chloramphenicol levels in these patients can be especially variable. Monitoring is also important for patients with liver disease and for those receiving certain drugs (e.g., phenytoin, phenobarbital, rifampin) that can alter the rate of chloramphenicol metabolism. For most infections, effective therapy is achieved with peak serum drug levels of 10 to 20 μg/ml and trough levels of 5 to 10 μg/ml. The risk of dose-dependent bone marrow depression is significantly increased when peak levels rise above 25 μg/ml.

Therapeutic Use

Chloramphenicol was once employed widely; however, awareness that the drug can cause fatal aplastic anemia has led to sharp restrictions in its use. Currently, chloramphenicol is indicated only for severe (life-threatening) infections for which safer drugs are either ineffective or contraindicated.

Chloramphenicol is a drug of choice for acute typhoid fever caused by sensitive strains of *Salmonella typhi*. However, chloramphenicol is not recommended for routine therapy of the typhoid carrier state.

Chloramphenicol is lethal to *Haemophilus influenzae*, an organism that can infect the meninges and other sites. At one time, chloramphenicol plus ampicillin was considered the regimen of choice for initial treatment of meningitis caused by this microbe. However, the development of third-generation cephalosporins that readily penetrate the meninges has reduced the use of chloramphenicol for this infection.

Adverse Effects

The most important adverse effects of chloramphenicol are gray syndrome and toxicities related to the blood. It is because of these adverse effects that indications for chloramphenicol are limited.

Gray Syndrome. Gray syndrome is a potentially fatal toxicity observed most commonly in newborns. Initial symptoms are vomiting, abdominal distention, cyanosis, and gray discoloration of the skin. These may be followed by vasomotor collapse and death. The syndrome results from accumulation of chloramphenicol to high levels. Newborns are especially vulnerable to the gray syndrome because (1) hepatic function is insufficient to detoxify chloramphenicol, and (2) renal function is insufficient to excrete active drug. Although the gray syndrome is usually observed in neonates, it can occur in older children and adults if dosage is excessive. If drug use is discontinued immediately upon appearance of early symptoms, the syndrome is usually reversible. The risk of gray syndrome in infants can be reduced by using appropriately low doses and monitoring chloramphenicol levels in serum.

Reversible Bone Marrow Depression. Chloramphenicol can produce dose-related depression of the bone marrow, resulting in anemia and sometimes leukopenia and thrombocytopenia as well. This effect is a toxic reaction to chloramphenicol and occurs most commonly when plasma drug levels exceed 25 μg/

ml. The cause of bone marrow depression appears to be inhibition of protein synthesis in host mitochondria. To promote early detection of bone marrow depression, complete blood counts should be performed prior to therapy and every 2 days during the period of treatment. Patients should be advised to notify the physician if signs of blood disorders develop (e.g., sore throat, fever, unusual bleeding or bruising). Chloramphenicol should be withdrawn if evidence of bone marrow depression is detected. Depression of bone marrow usually reverses within 1 to 3 weeks following discontinuation of drug use. The anemia associated with toxic bone marrow depression is not related to aplastic anemia (see below).

Aplastic Anemia. Rarely, chloramphenicol produces aplastic anemia, a condition characterized by pancytopenia and bone marrow aplasia. This reaction is usually fatal. Aplastic anemia occurs with an incidence of approximately 1 in 35,000 and is not related to chloramphenicol dosage. As a rule, the reaction develops weeks or months after termination of treatment. Aplastic anemia can occur with oral, intravenous, or even topical (ophthalmic) use of the drug. The mechanism underlying aplastic anemia has not been determined, but toxicity may result from a genetic predisposition. Unfortunately, aplastic anemia cannot be predicted by monitoring the blood.

Other Adverse Effects. *Gastrointestinal effects* (vomiting, diarrhea, glossitis) occur occasionally. *Herxheimer reactions* have occurred during treatment of typhoid fever. *Neurologic effects* (peripheral neuropathy, optic neuritis, confusion, delirium) develop rarely, usually in association with prolonged treatment. Other rare toxicities include *suprainfection of the bowel, allergic reactions,* and *fever.*

Drug Interactions

Chloramphenicol can inhibit hepatic drug-metabolizing enzymes, thereby prolonging the half-lives of a variety of drugs. Agents whose metabolism may be affected include *phenytoin* (an anticonvulsant), *warfarin* (an anticoagulant), and two oral hypoglycemics, *tolbutamide* and *chlorpropamide*. If these drugs are taken concurrently with chloramphenicol, their dosages should be reduced to avoid accumulation to toxic levels.

Preparations, Dosage, and Administration

General Considerations Regarding Route of Administration and Dosage. For treatment of systemic infections, chloramphenicol may be administered orally or IV. For initial therapy of serious infections, the intravenous route is generally preferred; oral therapy may be substituted later if conditions warrant.

As a rule, the dosing objective is to produce plasma levels of chloramphenicol within the range of 10 to 20 $\mu g/ml$. This objective can be achieved by monitoring serum levels of the drug.

Monitoring is especially important in newborns, patients with liver disease, and patients receiving drugs that can alter chloramphenicol disposition (e.g., phenytoin).

Preparations. *Chloramphenicol base* [Chloromycetin] is dispensed in 250-mg capsules for oral administration. *Chloramphenicol palmitate* [Chloromycetin Palmitate] is available as an oral suspension (30 mg/ml). *Chloramphenicol sodium succinate* [Chloromycetin Sodium Succinate] is dispensed as a powder to be reconstituted for IV infusion.

Dosage and Administration. Recommended dosages for oral and intravenous administration are the same. As a rule, oral doses should be taken on an empty stomach at least 1 hour before meals or 2 hours after. If gastric upset occurs, discomfort may be reduced by taking chloramphenicol with food. The usual dosage for adults and children is 12.5 to 25 mg/kg every 6 hours. For infants 7 days old or less, the usual dosage is 25 mg/kg once a day. For infants more than 7 days old, the recommended dosage is 25 mg/kg every 12 hours. The dosage should be reduced for patients with liver dysfunction.

SPECTINOMYCIN

Mechanism of Action and Antimicrobial Spectrum. Spectinomycin [Trobicin] binds to the 30S ribosomal subunit and thereby suppresses bacterial protein synthesis. The drug is active against a number of gram-negative bacteria. Resistance develops frequently.

Therapeutic Use. Because resistant organisms emerge rapidly, use of spectinomycin is limited. The principal indication for the drug is anogenital *gonorrhea* in patients who cannot tolerate ceftriaxone, the drug of choice for this infection.

Pharmacokinetics. Spectinomycin is administered only by IM injection; the drug is not absorbed from the gastrointestinal tract and cannot be used orally. Most of an administered dose is excreted unchanged in the urine. The plasma half-life is approximately 2 hours.

Adverse Effects. Spectinomycin is generally well tolerated. Adverse effects seen occasionally include soreness at the site of injection, dizziness, nausea, urticaria, pruritus, chills, fever, and insomnia.

Preparations, Dosage, and Administration. Spectinomycin [Trobicin] is dispensed as a sterile powder together with sufficient diluent to produce a 400 mg/ml solution upon reconstitution. For treatment of uncomplicated gonorrhea of the rectum or genitalia, the usual adult dose is 2 gm administered as a single IM (intragluteal) injection. For children weighing less than 45 kg, a single injection of 40 mg/kg is given. For disseminated gonococcal infection, the adult dosage is 2 gm twice a day for 3 days.

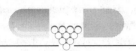

Summary of Major Nursing Implications

TETRACYCLINES

Except where stated otherwise, the implications summarized below pertain to all members of the tetracycline family.

Therapeutic Goal

Treatment of tetracycline-sensitive infections and acne.

Identifying High-Risk Patients

Tetracyclines should not be used during *pregnancy* or by *children under the age of 8 years.* Except for *doxycycline* and *minocycline*, tetracyclines must be used with great *caution* in patients with *significant renal impairment*.

Routes

Oral, IM, IV. For routes applicable to specific agents, see Table 76-2.

Administration

Oral. Advise patients to take oral tetracyclines on an empty stomach (1 hour before meals or 2 hours after) and with a full glass of water. *Doxycycline* and *minocycline* may be taken with food.

Absorption of tetracyclines will be reduced by certain chelating agents: *milk products, calcium supplements, iron supplements, magnesium-containing laxatives,* and most *antacids.* Instruct the patient to separate ingestion of tetracyclines and these chelators by at least 2 hours.

Instruct the patient to complete the prescribed course of treatment, even though symptoms may abate before the full course is over.

Parenteral. *Intravenous* administration is performed only when oral administration is ineffective or cannot be tolerated. *Intramuscular* injection is painful and used only rarely.

Minimizing Adverse Effects

Gastrointestinal Irritation. Inform the patient that GI distress (epigastric burning, cramps, nausea, vomiting, diarrhea) can be reduced by taking tetracyclines with meals.

Effects on Teeth. Tetracyclines can discolor developing teeth. To prevent this effect, avoid use of tetracyclines by pregnant women and by children under the age of 8 years.

Suprainfection. Tetracyclines can promote bacterial suprainfection of the bowel, resulting in severe diarrhea. Instruct the patient to notify the physician if significant diarrhea develops. If suprainfection is diagnosed, discontinue tetracyclines immediately; treatment consists of oral vancomycin or metronidazole plus vigorous fluid and electrolyte replacement therapy.

Preadministration Assessment

Implementation: Administration

Ongoing Evaluation and Interventions

Fungal overgrowth may occur in the mouth, pharynx, vagina, and bowel. Inform patients about symptoms of fungal infection (vaginal or anal itching; inflammatory lesions of the anogenital region; black, furry appearance of the tongue), and advise them to notify the physician if these occur. Suprainfection caused by *Candida* can be managed by discontinuing the tetracycline or by giving an antifungal drug.

Hepatotoxicity. Tetracyclines can cause fatty infiltration of the liver, resulting in jaundice and, rarely, massive liver failure. The risk of liver injury can be reduced by (1) avoiding high-dose intravenous therapy, and (2) withholding tetracyclines from pregnant and postpartum women who have kidney disease.

Renal Toxicity. Tetracyclines can exacerbate pre-existing renal impairment. With the exception of *doxycycline* and perhaps *minocycline*, tetracyclines should not be used by patients with kidney disease.

Photosensitivity. Tetracyclines can increase the sensitivity of the skin to ultraviolet light, thereby increasing the risk of sunburn. Advise the patient to avoid prolonged exposure to sunlight, wear protective clothing, and apply a sunscreen to exposed skin.

ERYTHROMYCIN

The implications summarized below pertain to all forms of erythromycin except where noted otherwise.

 Preadministration Assessment

Therapeutic Goal

Erythromycin is indicated for legionnaires' disease, whooping cough, diphtheria, urethritis and cervicitis caused by *Chlamydia trachomatis*, and other infections caused by erythromycin-sensitive organisms. The drug is also used as a substitute for penicillin G in penicillin-allergic patients.

Identifying High-Risk Patients

All erythromycins are contraindicated in patients taking astemizole or terfenadine. Erythromycin estolate is contraindicated for patients with *liver disease.*

 Implementation: Administration

Routes

Oral: *Erythromycin base, erythromycin estolate, erythromycin ethylsuccinate,* and *erythromycin stearate.*
Intravenous: *Erythromycin lactobionate.*

Administration

Oral. Advise the patient to take oral preparations on an empty stomach (1 hour before meals or 2 hours after) and with a full glass of water. However, if GI upset occurs, administration may be done with meals.

Inform patients using *erythromycin estolate, erythromycin ethylsuccinate,* and *enteric-coated formulations of erythromycin base* that these preparations may be taken without regard to meals.

Instruct the patient to complete the prescribed course of treatment, even though symptoms may abate before the full course is over.

Intravenous. Administer by slow infusion and in dilute solution to minimize thrombophlebitis.

 Ongoing Evaluation and Interventions

Minimizing Adverse Effects

Gastrointestinal Effects. Gastrointestinal disturbances (epigastric pain, nausea, vomiting, diarrhea) can be reduced by administering erythromycin with meals. Advise the patient to notify the physician if gastrointestinal reactions are severe or persistent.

Liver Injury. *Erythromycin estolate* may cause *cholestatic hepatitis.* Inform patients about signs of liver injury (e.g., severe abdominal pain, yellow discoloration of skin or eyes, darkened urine, pale stools), and advise them to notify the physician if these develop. If cholestatic hepatitis occurs, erythromycin estolate should be withdrawn. Erythromycin estolate should not be given to patients with liver dysfunction.

Minimizing Adverse Interactions

Erythromycin can increase the half-lives and plasma levels of several drugs, including *theophylline, carbamazepine,* and *warfarin.* When these agents are combined with erythromycin, monitor the patient closely for toxicity.

Erythromycin can antagonize the antibacterial actions of *clindamycin* and *chloramphenicol.* Concurrent use of erythromycin with these agents is not recommended.

Erythromycin increases the risk of severe ventricular dysrhythmias in patients receiving *astemizole* or *terfenadine,* both of which are antihistamines. Accordingly, these drugs should not be used concurrently.

CLINDAMYCIN

✓ **Preadministration Assessment**

Therapeutic Goal
Treatment of anaerobic infections outside the CNS.

✓ **Implementation: Administration**

Routes
Oral, IM, IV.

Administration
Instruct the patient to take oral clindamycin with a full glass of water.

Instruct the patient to complete the prescribed course of treatment, even though symptoms may abate before the full course is over.

 Ongoing Evaluation and Interventions

Minimizing Adverse Effects
Antibiotic-Associated Colitis. Clindamycin can promote antibiotic-associated colitis, a potentially fatal suprainfection. Prominent symptoms are profuse watery diarrhea, abdominal pain, fever, and leukocytosis. Stools often contain mucus and blood. Instruct the patient to report significant diarrhea (more than five watery stools per day). If antibiotic-associated colitis is diag-

nosed, discontinue clindamycin. Treatment consists of oral vancomycin or metronidazole and vigorous replacement therapy with fluids and electrolytes. Drugs that decrease bowel motility (e.g., opioids, anticholinergics) may worsen symptoms and should be avoided.

CHLORAMPHENICOL

Preadministration Assessment

Therapeutic Use

Treatment of severe (life-threatening) infections for which safer drugs are ineffective or contraindicated.

Baseline Data

Obtain blood cell counts.

Identifying High-Risk Patients

Chloramphenicol is *contraindicated* for patients with a *history of toxic reactions to chloramphenicol.* The drug should be used *cautiously* in patients with *liver disease* and during *pregnancy* and *lactation.*

Implementation: Administration

Routes

Oral, intravenous. Dosage is the same by both routes.

Administration

Instruct patients to take chloramphenicol on an empty stomach at least 1 hour before meals or 2 hours after. If GI upset occurs, the drug may be taken *with* meals.

Instruct the patient to complete the prescribed course of treatment, even though symptoms may abate before the full course is over.

Ongoing Evaluation and Interventions

Monitoring Drug Levels

Knowledge of plasma drug levels is particularly valuable in patients with liver disease, the young (newborns, infants, young children), and patients receiving drugs that can alter chloramphenicol disposition (e.g., phenobarbital, phenytoin, rifampin). The dosage is usually adjusted to produce peak plasma drug levels of 10 to 20 μg/ml and trough levels of 5 to 10 μg/ml.

Minimizing Adverse Effects

Gray Syndrome. The gray syndrome usually occurs in newborns. Manifestations include vomiting, abdominal distention, cyanosis, and gray discoloration of the skin; vasomotor collapse and death can occur. Observe the patient for symptoms and terminate therapy if they occur. The risk of gray syndrome can be reduced by use of appropriately low doses and monitoring chloramphenicol levels in blood.

Reversible Bone Marrow Depression. Chloramphenicol can produce reversible dose-related depression of bone marrow, manifesting as anemia, leukopenia, and thrombocytopenia. Blood cell counts should be done prior to therapy and every 2 days during therapy. Inform patients about early signs of hematologic toxicity (e.g., sore throat, fever, unusual bleeding or bruising), and instruct them to notify the physician if these occur. If bone marrow depression is diagnosed, chloramphenicol should be withdrawn immediately. The risk of bone marrow depression can be minimized by keeping peak plasma drug levels below 25 μg/ml.

Aplastic Anemia. Very rarely, chloramphenicol causes aplastic anemia, a condition with a high rate of mortality. The risk of aplastic anemia can be minimized by using chloramphenicol only when clearly indicated.

Minimizing Adverse Interactions

Chloramphenicol can prolong the half-lives of a variety of drugs, including *phenytoin, warfarin,* and *oral hypoglycemics.* If these drugs are combined with chloramphenicol, their dosages should be reduced.

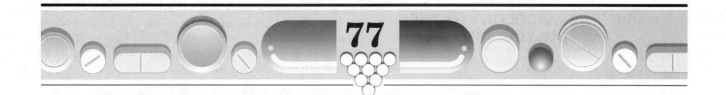

77

Bactericidal Inhibitors of Protein Synthesis: The Aminoglycosides

BASIC PHARMACOLOGY OF THE AMINOGLYCOSIDES

PROPERTIES OF INDIVIDUAL AMINOGLYCOSIDES

Gentamicin
Tobramycin
Amikacin
Other Aminoglycosides

The aminoglycosides are narrow-spectrum antibiotics, used primarily against aerobic gram-negative bacilli. These drugs inhibit protein synthesis and cause bacterial death. The aminoglycosides can cause serious injury to the kidney and inner ear. Because of these toxicities, indications for the aminoglycosides are limited. All of the aminoglycosides carry multiple positive charges. As a result, these agents are not absorbed from the gastrointestinal tract and, hence, must be administered parenterally to treat systemic infections. In the United States, eight aminoglycosides are approved for clinical use. The agents employed most commonly are *gentamicin*, *tobramycin*, and *amikacin*. In approaching the aminoglycosides, we will first discuss the properties shared by these drugs as a group. After this, we will consider the unique characteristics of individual aminoglycosides.

969

BASIC PHARMACOLOGY OF THE AMINOGLYCOSIDES

Chemistry

The aminoglycosides are composed of two or more amino sugars connected by a glycoside linkage, hence the family name. At physiologic pH, these drugs are polycations (i.e., they carry several positive charges) and, therefore, cannot readily cross membranes. As a result, aminoglycosides are not absorbed from the gastrointestinal tract, do not enter the cerebrospinal fluid, and are rapidly excreted by the kidneys. Structural formulas for the three major aminoglycosides are shown in Figure 77–1.

Mechanism of Action

The aminoglycosides disrupt bacterial protein synthesis. These drugs bind to the 30S ribosomal subunit, causing inhibition of protein synthesis and misreading of the genetic code. The aminoglycosides are rapidly *bactericidal*. Although the bactericidal effects of the aminoglycosides are correlated with blockade of protein synthesis, we do not understand just why these drugs cause bacterial death. That is, it is not known why disruption of protein synthesis by aminoglycosides is lethal,

since complete blockade of protein synthesis by other antibiotics (e.g., tetracyclines, chloramphenicol) is usually only bacteriostatic. Misreading of the genetic code does not explain the ability of the aminoglycosides to kill.

Microbial Resistance

The principal cause for bacterial resistance is production of enzymes that can inactivate aminoglycosides. Among gram-negative bacteria, the genetic information needed to synthesize these enzymes is acquired by transfer of R factors. To date, more than 20 different aminoglycoside-inactivating enzymes have been identified. Since each of the aminoglycosides can be modified by more than one of these enzymes, and since each enzyme can act on more than one aminoglycoside, patterns of bacterial resistance to the aminoglycosides can be complex.

Of all the aminoglycosides, *amikacin* is least susceptible to inactivation by bacterial enzymes. As a result, resistance to amikacin is uncommon. To minimize emergence of bacteria resistant to this drug, it is recommended that amikacin be reserved for infections that are unresponsive to other aminoglycoside drugs.

Antimicrobial Spectrum

Bactericidal effects of the aminoglycosides are limited almost exclusively to *aerobic gram-nega-*

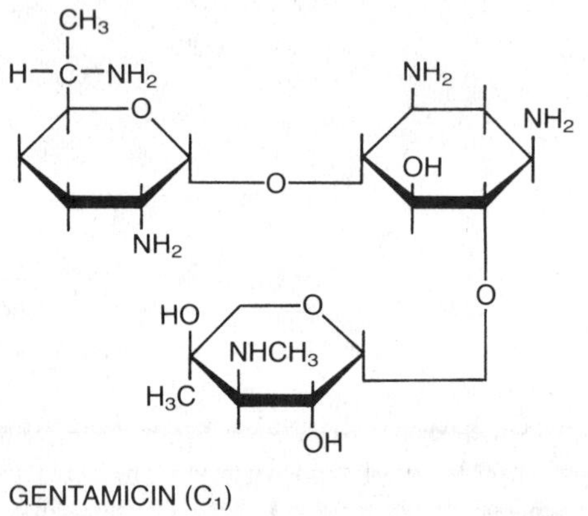

GENTAMICIN (C₁)

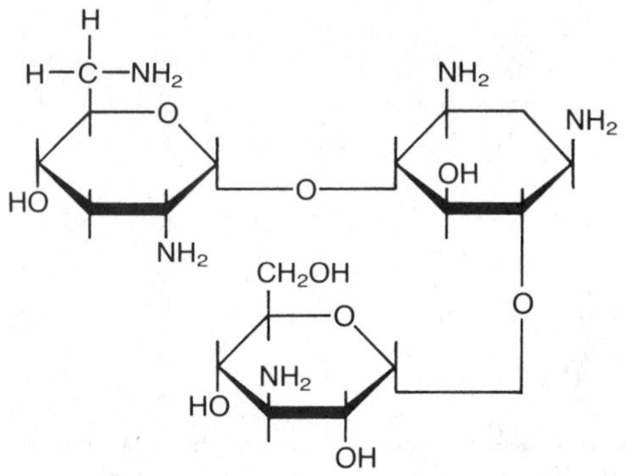

TOBRAMYCIN

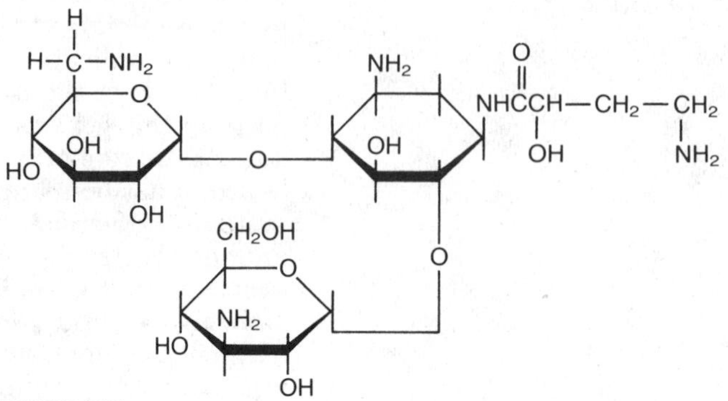

AMIKACIN

Figure 77–1. Structural formulas of the major aminoglycosides.

tive bacilli. Sensitive organisms include *Escherichia coli, Klebsiella pneumoniae, Serratia marcescens, Proteus mirabilis,* and *Pseudomonas aeruginosa.* Aminoglycosides are inactive against most gram-positive bacteria.

Aminoglycosides are *ineffective* against *anaerobes.* To produce their antibacterial effects, aminoglycosides must be transported across the bacterial cell membrane, a process that is oxygen dependent. Since, by definition, anaerobic organisms live in the absence of oxygen, these microbes cannot take up the aminoglycosides and, therefore, are drug resistant. For the same reason, aminoglycosides are inactive against facultative bacteria when these organisms are living under anaerobic conditions.

Therapeutic Use

Parenteral Therapy. The principal use for parenteral aminoglycosides is treatment of *serious infections due to aerobic gram-negative bacilli.* Primary target organisms are *Pseudomonas aeruginosa* and the Enterobacteriaceae (e.g., *E. coli, Klebsiella, Serratia, Proteus mirabilis*). The aminoglycosides used most often against these infections are gentamicin, tobramycin, and amikacin. Selection among these three drugs depends in large part on patterns of resistance in a given community or hospital. In settings where resistance to aminoglycosides is uncommon, either gentamicin or tobramycin is usually preferred. Of these two drugs, gentamicin is less costly and may be selected on this basis. Organisms resistant to both gentamicin and tobramycin are usually sensitive to amikacin. Accordingly, in settings where resistance to gentamicin and tobramycin is common, amikacin may be preferred for initial therapy.

Oral Therapy. Aminoglycosides are not absorbed from the gastrointestinal tract; hence, oral administration is used only for local effects within the intestine. In patients anticipating elective colorectal surgery, oral aminoglycosides have been given prophylactically to suppress bacterial growth in the bowel. One aminoglycoside (paromomycin) is used to treat intestinal amebiasis and tapeworm infestation.

Topical Therapy. *Neomycin* is available in formulations for application to the eyes, ears, and skin. Topical preparations of *gentamicin* and *tobramycin* are used to treat conjunctivitis caused by susceptible gram-negative bacilli. *Gentamicin* is also available in a formulation intended for application to the skin. However, because gentamicin-resistant organisms emerge rapidly, this preparation is not recommended.

Pharmacokinetics

All of the aminoglycosides have similar pharmacokinetic profiles. Pharmacokinetic properties of the principal aminoglycosides are summarized in Table 77–1.

Absorption. Because they are polycations, the aminoglycosides cross membranes poorly. As a result, very little (about 1%) of an oral dose is absorbed. Hence, for treatment of systemic infections, aminoglycosides must be given parenterally (IM or IV). Absorption following application to the intact skin is minimal. However, when used for wound irrigation, aminoglycosides may be absorbed in amounts sufficient to produce systemic toxicity.

Distribution. Distribution of aminoglycosides is limited largely to extracellular fluid. Entry into the cerebrospinal fluid is insufficient to treat meningitis in adults. Aminoglycosides bind tightly to renal tissue, achieving levels in the kidney up to 50 times higher than levels in serum. These high levels correlate with production of nephrotoxicity (see below). Aminoglycosides penetrate readily to the perilymph and endolymph of the inner ear, and there is a direct relationship between levels achieved in these fluids and production of ototoxicity (see below). Aminoglycosides can cross the placenta and may have toxic effects on the fetus.

Elimination. The aminoglycosides are eliminated primarily by the kidneys. These drugs are not metabolized. In patients with normal renal function, the half-lives of the aminoglycosides range from 2 to 3 hours. However, since elimination is almost exclusively renal, half-lives increase dramatically in patients with kidney dysfunction (see Table 77–1). *Accordingly, if serious toxicity is to be avoided, it is essential to reduce the dosage or increase the dosing interval in patients with kidney disease.*

Interpatient Variation. Different patients receiving the same aminoglycoside dosage (in mg/kg of body weight) can achieve widely different serum levels of drug. This interpatient variation is caused by a number of factors, including age, percent body fat, and pathophysiology (e.g., kidney dysfunction, fever, edema, dehydration). Because of variability among patients, aminoglycoside dosage must be individualized. As dramatic evidence of this need, in one clinical study it was observed that in order to produce equivalent serum drug levels, the required doses of aminoglycosides ranged from as little as 0.5 mg/kg in one patient to a high of 25.8 mg/kg in another—a difference in dosage of more than 50-fold.

Maintaining Appropriate Serum Drug Levels

For therapy with aminoglycosides to be both safe and effective, serum drug levels should be maintained within a narrow range. This is necessary because the levels that cause toxicity are only slightly greater than those required for antibacterial effects. In order to keep aminoglycoside levels within an acceptable range, dosage must be carefully adjusted for each patient.

Monitoring of serum drug levels provides the

		Total Daily Dosage (mg/kg)*		Normal Dosing Interval (hours)	Half-life in Adults (hrs)		Target Serum Drug Levels (μg/ml)	
Drug	Routes of Adminis- tration	Adults	Children		Normal	Anuric	Peak	Trough
Amikacin	IM, IV	15	15	8 or 12	2–2.5	24–60	20–30	4–8
Gentamicin	IM, IV	3–5	6–7.5	8	2–3	24–60	6–10	1–2
Tobramycin	IM, IV	3–5	6–7.5	8	2	24–60	6–10	1–2
Netilmicin	IM, IV	4–6.5	5.5–8	8	2–2.7	40	6–10	1–2

Table 77–1. Dosages and Pharmacokinetic Properties of the Major Aminoglycosides

*Because of interpatient variability, standard doses cannot be relied upon to produce appropriate serum drug levels; dosage should be adjusted on the basis of serum drug measurements.

best basis for adjustment of aminoglycoside dosage. To produce bacterial kill while minimizing the risk of toxicity, it is necessary to keep peak and trough levels within an appropriate range. Dosage should be adjusted so that peak levels are high enough to kill bacteria but not so high as to be toxic. Since excessive trough levels correlate with increased toxicity, high trough levels must be avoided. When using gentamicin, for example, the dosage should be adjusted so that peak serum levels range from 6 to 10 μg/ml while trough levels range from 1 to 2 μg/ml. Peak and trough levels for other aminoglycosides are summarized in Table 77–1.

When drawing blood samples for determination of aminoglycoside levels, timing is important. Samples for measurement of peak levels should be taken 1 hour after IM injection and 30 minutes after completion of an IV infusion. Blood for trough measurements should be taken just prior to the next dose.

Adverse Effects

The aminoglycosides can produce serious toxicity, especially to the inner ear and kidney. These toxicities limit the clinical utility of these drugs.

Ototoxicity. All of the aminoglycosides can damage the inner ear, thereby impairing balance and hearing. Hearing loss results from damage to hair cells within the cochlea; disruption of balance results from damage to hair cells of the vestibular apparatus. The biochemical basis of these effects is not known. Factors that increase the risk of ototoxicity include (1) kidney dysfunction, (2) concurrent use of ethacrynic acid (a drug that has ototoxic properties of its own), and (3) administration of aminoglycosides in excessive doses or for more than 10 days.

Patients should be monitored for ototoxicity. Hearing loss begins with decreased acuity in the high-frequency range. This initial effect can be detected only through audiometric testing. Auditory toxicity may also manifest as tinnitus or a sense of fullness in the ears. Symptoms of vestibular damage include nausea, unsteadiness, dizziness, and vertigo. Patients should be informed about the symptoms of ototoxicity and instructed to notify the physician if they occur.

If ototoxicity is detected, aminoglycosides should be withdrawn or given in reduced dosage. If impairment of hearing or balance is only moderate, symptoms usually reverse following discontinuation of drug use. However, if ototoxicity is extensive, the patient may suffer permanent hearing impairment or even complete hearing loss.

The risk of ototoxicity can be minimized in several ways. Dosages should be adjusted so that *trough* serum drug levels do not exceed recommended values. (Aminoglycosides diffuse out of the endolymph and perilymph during the trough time, thereby decreasing exposure of sensitive cells to these drugs.) Special care should be exercised to insure safe levels in patients with kidney dysfunction. When possible, aminoglycosides should be used for no more than 10 days. Concurrent use of ethacrynic acid should be avoided. Patients should be monitored for early signs of cochlear and vestibular damage.

Nephrotoxicity. Aminoglycosides can injure cells of the proximal renal tubules. These drugs are taken up by tubular cells and achieve high intracellular concentrations. There is a direct correlation between intracellular levels and renal injury. Aminoglycoside-induced nephrotoxicity usually manifests as acute tubular necrosis. Prominent symptoms are proteinuria, casts in the urine, production of dilute urine, and elevations in serum creatinine and blood urea nitrogen (BUN). Serum creatinine and BUN should be monitored. The risk of nephrotoxicity is especially high in the elderly, in patients with pre-existing kidney disease, and in patients receiving other nephrotoxic drugs (e.g., amphotericin B, cephalothin). Fortunately, cells of the proximal tubule regenerate readily. As a result, injury to the kidney usually reverses following cessation of aminoglycoside use.

Neuromuscular Blockade. Aminoglycosides can inhibit neuromuscular transmission, causing flaccid paralysis and potentially fatal depression of respiration. Most episodes of neuromuscular blockade have occurred following intraperitoneal or intrapleural instillation of aminoglycosides. However, neuromuscular blockade has also occurred following intravenous and intramuscular administration. The risk of paralysis is increased by concurrent use of neuromuscular blocking agents and general anesthetics. Myasthenia gravis constitutes an additional risk. Neuromuscular blockade can be reversed by calcium; IV infusion of a calcium salt (e.g., calcium gluconate) is the treatment of choice. Because of increased physician awareness, aminoglycoside-induced neuromuscular blockade is now a clinical rarity.

Other Adverse Effects. Hypersensitivity reactions (e.g., rash, pruritus, urticaria) occur occasionally. Blood dyscrasias (neutropenia, agranulocytosis, aplastic anemia) are rare. Streptomycin has been associated with neurologic disorders (optic nerve dysfunction, peripheral neuritis, paresthesias of the face and hands). Oral neomycin has caused suprainfection of the bowel and intestinal malabsorption; topical neomycin may cause contact dermatitis.

Drug Interactions

Penicillins. Penicillins and aminoglycosides are frequently employed in combination to enhance bacterial kill. (By disrupting the cell wall, penicillins facilitate access of aminoglycosides to their site of action.) When present in high concentrations, penicillins can inactivate aminoglycosides by direct chemical interaction. Accordingly, *penicillins and aminoglycosides should not be mixed together in the same intravenous solution.* (Inactivation is not likely to occur within the body, since drug concentrations are usually too low for significant chemical interaction.)

Ototoxic Drugs. The risk of injury to the inner ear is significantly increased by concurrent use of *ethacrynic acid*, a loop diuretic that has ototoxic actions of its own. The combination of an aminoglycoside with two other loop diuretics, furosemide and bumetanide, appears to cause no more ototoxicity than the aminoglycoside alone.

Nephrotoxic Drugs. The risk of renal damage is increased by concurrent therapy with other nephrotoxic agents. Additive or potentiative nephrotoxicity has been observed with *methoxyflurane, amphotericin B, cephalosporins, polymyxins,* and *vancomycin.*

Skeletal Muscle Relaxants. Aminoglycosides can intensify neuromuscular blockade induced by tubocurarine, pancuronium, and other skeletal muscle relaxants. If aminoglycosides are used with these agents, caution must be exercised to avoid respiratory arrest.

PROPERTIES OF INDIVIDUAL AMINOGLYCOSIDES

GENTAMICIN

Therapeutic Use. Gentamicin [Garamycin, Jenamicin] is used to treat serious infections caused by aerobic gram-negative bacilli. Primary target organisms are *Pseudomonas aeruginosa* and the Enterobacteriaceae (e.g., *E. coli, Klebsiella, Serratia, Proteus mirabilis*). In hospitals where resistance is not a problem, gentamicin is often the preferred aminoglycoside for use against these bacteria. The principal advantage of gentamicin over the other major aminoglycosides (tobramycin and amikacin) is low cost. Unfortunately, resistance to gentamicin is increasing, and cross-resistance to tobramycin is common. For infections that are resistant to gentamicin and tobramycin, amikacin is usually effective. In addition to its use against gram-negative bacilli, gentamicin can be combined with ampicillin or penicillin to treat enterococcal endocarditis.

Adverse Effects and Interactions. Like all other aminoglycosides, gentamicin is toxic to the kidney and inner ear. Caution must be exercised when combining gentamicin with other nephrotoxic and ototoxic drugs. Gentamicin is inactivated by penicillins and should not be mixed with these drugs in the same IV solution.

Preparations, Dosage, and Administration. Gentamicin sulfate [Garamycin, Jenamicin] is dispensed in several concentrations for IM and IV administration. The usual adult dosage is 1 to 1.7 mg/kg every 8 hours. The usual pediatric dosage is 2 to 2.5 mg/kg every 8 hours. Because of substantial interpatient variation, it is desirable to monitor serum drug levels and to adjust dosage accordingly: peak levels should range from 6 to 10 µg/ml and trough levels should range from 1 to 2 µg/ml. In patients with renal dysfunction, the dosage should be reduced or the dosing interval increased. For intravenous administration, the drug should be diluted in either sodium chloride for injection or 5% dextrose and infused over 30 minutes or more. Gentamicin should not be mixed with penicillins in the same IV solution. Duration of treatment is usually 7 to 10 days.

TOBRAMYCIN

Uses, Adverse Effects, and Interactions. Tobramycin [Nebcin] is similar to gentamicin in its uses, adverse effects, and interactions. The drug is more active than gentamicin against *Pseudomonas aeruginosa*, but less active against enterococci and *Serratia*. Like all other aminoglycosides, tobramycin can injure the inner ear and kidney. If possible, concurrent therapy with other ototoxic or nephrotoxic drugs should be avoided.

Preparations, Dosage, and Administration. Tobramycin sulfate [Nebcin] is dispensed in solution (10 and 40 mg/ml) and as a powder (30 mg/ml after reconstitution) for IM and IV administration. The usual adult dosage is 1 to 1.7 mg/kg every 8 hours. The usual pediatric dosage is 2 to 2.5 mg/kg every 8 hours. Ideally, dosages should be individualized to produce peak and trough levels within the ranges indicated in Table 77–1. In patients with renal dysfunction, dosage should be reduced or the dosing interval increased. For intravenous administration, the drug should be diluted in either sodium chloride for injection or 5% dextrose and infused over 30 minutes or more. Tobramycin should not be mixed with penicillins in the same IV solution. Duration of treatment is usually 7 to 10 days.

AMIKACIN

Uses, Adverse Effects, and Interactions. Amikacin [Amikin] has two outstanding features: (1) of all the aminoglycosides, amikacin has the broadest spectrum of action against gram-negative bacilli, and (2) of all the aminoglycosides, amikacin is the least vulnerable to inactivation by bacterial enzymes. Because most aminoglycoside-inactivating enzymes do not affect amikacin, the incidence of bacterial resistance to this agent is lower than with other aminoglycosides. As a result, amikacin is often effective against bacteria that are resistant to the other major aminoglycosides (gentamicin and tobramycin). In hospitals where resistance to gentamicin and tobramycin is common, amikacin is the preferred agent for initial treatment of infections caused by aerobic gram-negative bacilli. However, in settings where resistance to the other aminoglycosides is infrequent, amikacin should be reserved for infections of proven aminoglycoside resistance; this practice will delay emergence of organisms resistant to amikacin. Like all other aminoglycosides, amikacin is toxic to the kidney and inner ear. Caution should be exercised if amikacin is used in combination with other ototoxic or nephrotoxic drugs.

Preparations, Dosage, and Administration. Amikacin sulfate [Amikin] is available in solution (50 and 250 mg/ml) for parenteral (IM and IV) administration. For intravenous use, amikacin should be diluted in sodium chloride or 5% dextrose for injection; infusion time should be 30 to 60 minutes in adults, and 1 to 2 hours in infants. The recommended dosage for adults and children is 15 mg/kg/day administered in equally divided doses at 8- or 12-hour intervals. In patients with kidney dysfunction, dosage should be reduced or the dosing interval increased; dosage adjustments should be based on measurements of serum drug levels. As a rule, duration of treatment should not exceed 10 days.

OTHER AMINOGLYCOSIDES

Netilmicin

Netilmicin [Netromycin] has an antibacterial spectrum similar to that of gentamicin. Netilmicin has some resistance to the bacterial enzymes that inactivate gentamicin and tobramycin. However, netilmicin is more vulnerable to inactivation than amikacin. Like other aminoglycosides, netilmicin is ototoxic and nephrotoxic, although ototoxicity may be less than with other aminoglycosides. Administration is IM or IV. The dosage for adults is 1.3 to 2.2 mg/kg every 8 hours; the dosage for children is 1.8 to 2.7 mg/kg every 8 hours. Duration of treatment ranges from 7 to 14 days.

Neomycin

Neomycin is the most toxic of the aminoglycosides; the drug can cause severe damage to the kidneys and inner ear. Because of its toxicity, neomycin is not administered parenterally. Neomycin is employed primarily for topical treatment of infections of the eye, ear, and skin. The drug is also administered orally to suppress bowel flora prior to surgery of the intestine. Since aminoglycosides are not absorbed from the gastrointestinal tract, oral administration constitutes a local (nonsystemic) use of the drug. Oral neomycin can cause suprainfection of the bowel as well as an intestinal malabsorption syndrome.

Kanamycin

Kanamycin [Kantrex] is an older aminoglycoside to which bacterial resistance is common. The drug is still active against some gram-negative bacilli, but *Serratia* and *Pseudomonas aeruginosa* are resistant. Because of resistance, systemic use of the drug has sharply declined; for treatment of systemic infections, gentamicin, tobramycin, and amikacin are preferred. Like neomycin, kanamycin is employed to suppress bacterial flora of the bowel prior to elective colorectal surgery. Kanamycin is dispensed in capsules for oral use and as an injection for IM and IV administration.

Streptomycin

Streptomycin, discovered in 1943, was the first aminoglycoside drug. Although once employed widely, streptomycin has been largely replaced by safer or more effective medications. As discussed in Chapter 81, streptomycin can be used in combination with other drugs to treat tuberculosis, but newer and safer agents (rifampin, isoniazid, ethambutol) are generally preferred. Streptomycin is also indicated for several uncommon infections (plague, tularemia, glanders, brucellosis). When combined with ampicillin or penicillin G, streptomycin may be used for enterococcal endocarditis.

Paromomycin

Paromomycin [Humatin] is an aminoglycoside employed only for local effects within the intestine. The drug is administered orally to treat intestinal amebiasis and tapeworm infestations. The dosage for both indications is 8 to 12 mg/kg three times daily for 5 to 10 days. Principal adverse effects are nausea, cramps, and diarrhea. Paromomycin is dispensed in 250-mg capsules.

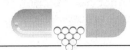

Summary of Major Nursing Implications

AMINOGLYCOSIDES

Amikacin	Kanamycin
Gentamicin	Neomycin
Tobramycin	Paromomycin
Netilmicin	

Except where noted, the implications summarized below apply to all of the aminoglycosides.

Preadministration Assessment

Therapeutic Goal

Parenteral Therapy. Treatment of serious infections caused by gram-negative aerobic bacilli.

Oral Therapy. Suppression of bowel flora prior to elective colorectal surgery.

Topical Therapy. Treatment of local infections of the eyes, ears, and skin.

Identifying High-Risk Patients

Aminoglycosides must be used with *caution* in patients with *renal impairment, pre-existing hearing impairment*, and *myasthenia gravis*, and in patients receiving *ototoxic drugs* (especially *ethacrynic acid*), *nephrotoxic drugs* (e.g., *amphotericin B, cephalosporins, vancomycin*), and *neuromuscular blocking agents*.

Implementation: Administration

Routes

Intramuscular and intravenous: *gentamicin, tobramycin, amikacin, netilmicin, kanamycin.*
Oral: *neomycin, kanamycin, paromomycin.*
Topical: *neomycin, gentamicin, tobramycin.*

Administration

Aminoglycosides must be given parenterally (IV, IM) to treat systemic infections. Intravenous infusions should be done slowly (over 30 minutes or more). Do not mix aminoglycosides and penicillins in the same IV solution.

When possible, adjust the dosage on the basis of plasma drug levels. Draw blood samples for measurement of peak levels 1 hour after IM injection and 30 minutes after completion of an IV infusion; draw samples for trough levels just prior to the next dose.

In patients with renal dysfunction, the dosage should be reduced or the dosing interval increased.

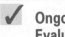 **Ongoing Evaluation and Interventions**

Monitoring Summary

Monitor peak and trough aminoglycoside levels, inner ear function (hearing and balance), creatinine clearance, BUN, and urine output.

Minimizing Adverse Effects

Ototoxicity. Aminoglycosides can damage the inner ear, impairing hearing and balance. Monitor for ototoxicity; use audiometry in high-risk patients. Inform patients about symptoms of ototoxicity (hearing loss, tinnitus, nausea, unsteadiness, dizziness, vertigo) and instruct them to notify the physician if these occur. If ototoxicity is detected, aminoglycosides should be discontinued or used in reduced dosage.

Nephrotoxicity. Aminoglycosides can cause acute tubular necrosis. To evaluate renal injury, monitor serum creatinine and BUN. If oliguria or anuria develop, withhold the aminoglycoside and notify the physician.

Neuromuscular Blockade. Aminoglycosides can inhibit neuromuscular transmission, causing potentially fatal respiratory depression. Carefully observe patients with myasthenia gravis and patients receiving skeletal muscle relaxants or general anesthetics. Aminoglycoside-induced neuromuscular blockade can be reversed with intravenous *calcium gluconate.*

Minimizing Adverse Interactions

Penicillins. Aminoglycosides can be inactivated by high concentrations of penicillins. Never mix penicillins and aminoglycosides in the same intravenous solution.

Ototoxic and Nephrotoxic Drugs. Exercise caution when using aminoglycosides in combination with other nephrotoxic or ototoxic drugs. Increased nephrotoxicity has been observed with *methoxyflurane, amphotericin B, cephalosporins, polymyxins,* and *vancomycin.* The risk of ototoxicity is increased by *ethacrynic acid.*

Skeletal Muscle Relaxants. Aminoglycosides can intensify neuromuscular blockade induced by tubocurarine, pancuronium, and other skeletal muscle relaxants. When aminoglycosides are used concurrently with these agents, exercise caution to avoid respiratory arrest.

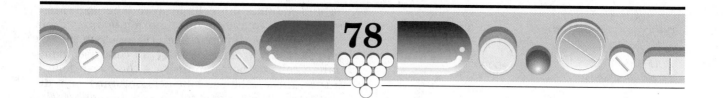

78

Sulfonamides and Trimethoprim

SULFONAMIDES
    Basic Pharmacology
    Sulfonamide Preparations

TRIMETHOPRIM

TRIMETHOPRIM-SULFAMETHOXAZOLE

The sulfonamides and trimethoprim are broad-spectrum antimicrobial drugs that have closely related mechanisms of action: interference with the synthesis of tetrahydrofolic acid. In approaching these drugs, we will discuss the sulfonamides first and then trimethoprim. We will conclude with a discussion of trimethoprim-sulfamethoxazole, an important fixed-dose combination product.

SULFONAMIDES

The sulfonamides were the first drugs available for systemic treatment of bacterial infections. The introduction and subsequent widespread use of these drugs produced a sharp decline in morbidity and mortality from susceptible infections. Until the penicillins became generally available, sulfonamides remained the mainstay of antibacterial chemotherapy. With the advent of newer antimicrobial drugs, use of the sulfonamides has greatly declined. However, the sulfonamides still have an important therapeutic role, primarily in the treatment of urinary tract infections. With the introduction of trimethoprim-sulfamethoxazole in the 1970's, indications for the sulfonamides have expanded.

BASIC PHARMACOLOGY

Similarities among the sulfonamides are more striking than differences. Accordingly, rather than

977

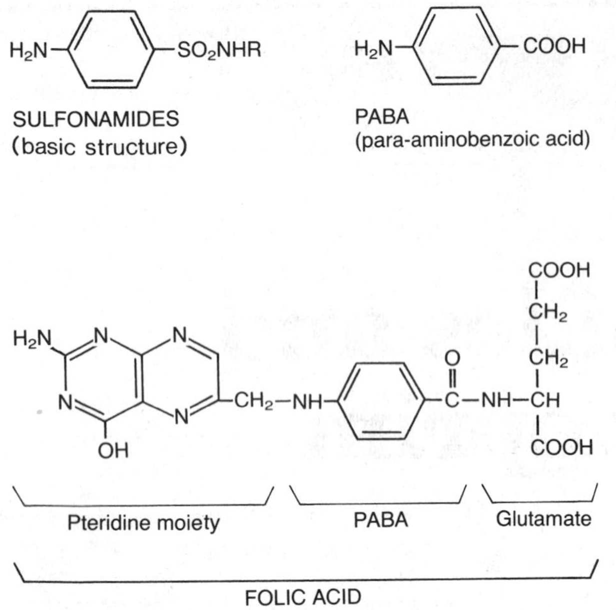

Figure 78–1. Structural relationships among sulfonamides, PABA, and folic acid.

focusing on a representative prototype, we will discuss the sulfonamides as a group.

Chemistry

The general structural formula for the sulfonamides is shown in Figure 78–1. As you can see, sulfonamides are structural analogues of para-aminobenzoic acid (PABA). The antimicrobial actions of the sulfonamides are based on this structural similarity.

Individual sulfonamides vary greatly with respect to solubility in water. The older sulfonamides have low solubility. As a result, these agents often crystallized out in the urine, causing injury to the kidneys. The sulfonamides in current use have relatively high water solubility. Hence, the risk of renal damage is now low.

Mechanism of Action

Sulfonamides suppress bacterial growth by inhibiting synthesis of folic acid (folate), a compound required by all cells for biosynthesis of DNA, RNA, and proteins. The steps in folate synthesis are shown in Figure 78–2. As indicated, sulfonamides block the step in which PABA is combined with pteridine to form dihydropteroic acid. Because of their structural similarity to PABA, sulfonamides act as competitive inhibitors of this reaction. Sulfonamides are usually bacteriostatic. Hence, host defenses are essential for complete elimination of infection.

If all cells require folate, why do sulfonamides not harm the host? The answer to this question is based on differences between the ways that bacte-

ria and mammalian cells acquire folic acid. Most bacteria are unable to take up folate from their environment. As a result, bacteria must synthesize their folic acid from precursors. In contrast, mammalian cells do not manufacture their own folate. Rather, these cells use folic acid obtained from dietary sources. Uptake of folate by mammalian cells is accomplished using a specialized transport system. Since mammalian cells use preformed folic acid rather than synthesizing it, sulfonamides are harmless to the host.

Microbial Resistance

Many bacterial species have developed resistance to sulfonamides, thereby decreasing the utility of these drugs. Resistance is especially high among gonococci, meningococci, staphylococci, streptococci, and shigellae. Resistance may be acquired by spontaneous mutation or by transfer of R factors. Principal mechanisms of resistance are (1) synthesis of PABA in amounts sufficient to overcome sulfonamide-mediated inhibition of dihydropteroate synthetase, (2) alteration in the structure of di-

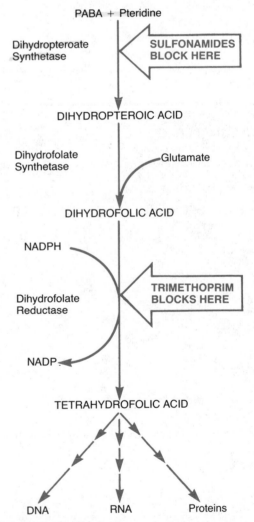

Figure 78–2. Sites of action of sulfonamides and trimethoprim. Sulfonamides and trimethoprim inhibit sequential steps in the synthesis of tetrahydrofolic acid (FAH_4). In the absence of FAH_4, bacteria are unable to synthesize nucleic acids and proteins.

hydropteroate synthetase such that binding and inhibition by sulfonamides is reduced, and (3) reduced sulfonamide uptake.

Antimicrobial Spectrum

The sulfonamides are active against a broad spectrum of microbes. Susceptible organisms include gram-positive cocci, gram-negative bacilli, actinomycetes (e.g., *Nocardia*), chlamydiae (e.g., *Chlamydia trachomatis*), and some protozoa (e.g., *Toxoplasma*, plasmodia).

Therapeutic Uses

Although the sulfonamides were once employed widely, applications are now limited. Sulfonamide use has declined for two reasons: (1) introduction of bactericidal antibiotics that have less toxicity than sulfonamides, and (2) development of bacterial resistance to sulfonamides. Today, urinary tract infection is the principal indication for sulfonamides. In addition, sulfonamides are drugs of choice for nocardiosis.

Urinary Tract Infection. Sulfonamides are often preferred drugs for acute infections of the urinary tract. About 90% of these infections are due to *Escherichia coli*, a bacterium that is usually sulfonamide sensitive. Of the sulfonamides available, *sulfisoxazole* is generally favored. This drug has high solubility in urine, achieves effective concentrations within the urinary tract, and is less expensive than other sulfonamide preparations. When infection is recurrent, or when urinary tract obstruction is present, treatment with a sulfonamide alone may not be sufficient. Treatment of urinary tract infections is discussed further in Chapter 79.

Other Uses. Sulfonamides are drugs of choice for nocardiosis (infection with *Nocardia asteroides*). In addition, sulfonamides are alternatives to doxycycline and erythromycin for infections caused by *Chlamydia trachomatis* (trachoma, inclusion conjunctivitis, urethritis, lymphogranuloma venereum). Sulfonamides may be combined with erythromycin or penicillin to treat otitis media caused by amoxicillin-resistant strains of *H. influenzae*. For patients allergic to penicillin, sulfonamides are alternative drugs for prophylaxis of rheumatic fever. Sulfonamides are used in conjunction with pyrimethamine to treat two protozoal infections: toxoplasmosis and malaria caused by chloroquine-resistant *Plasmodium falciparum*.

One sulfonamide preparation—sulfasalazine—is used to treat ulcerative colitis. The benefits of sulfasalazine in this disorder are not due to suppression of microbial growth. Treatment of ulcerative colitis is considered in Chapter 68.

Pharmacokinetics

Absorption. Sulfonamides are well absorbed following oral administration. When applied topically to the skin or mucous membranes, sulfonamides may be absorbed in amounts sufficient to cause systemic effects.

Distribution. Sulfonamides are well distributed to all tissues. Concentrations in pleural, peritoneal, ocular, and similar body fluids may be as much as 80% of the concentration in blood. Sulfonamides readily cross the placenta, and levels achieved in the fetus are sufficient to produce antimicrobial effects and toxicity.

Metabolism. Sulfonamides are metabolized in the liver; the principal reaction is acetylation. Acetylated derivatives of sulfonamides lack antimicrobial activity, but are just as toxic as the parent compounds. Acetylation may decrease sulfonamide solubility, thereby increasing the risk of renal damage from crystal formation.

Excretion. Sulfonamides are excreted primarily by the kidneys. Hence, the rate of renal excretion is the principal determinant of sulfonamide half-life. Sulfonamides that are excreted slowly have a longer duration of action than those that are excreted rapidly.

Adverse Effects

Sulfonamides can cause multiple adverse effects. Prominent among these are hypersensitivity reactions, blood dyscrasias, and kernicterus (in newborn infants). Renal damage from crystalluria had been a problem with older sulfonamides but is of minimal concern with the drugs available today.

Hypersensitivity Reactions. Sulfonamides can induce a variety of hypersensitivity reactions. Mild reactions (rash, drug fever, photosensitivity) are relatively common. To minimize photosensitivity reactions, patients should avoid prolonged exposure to sunlight, wear protective clothing, and apply a sunscreen to exposed skin. Hypersensitivity reactions are especially frequent with topical sulfonamides. As a result, these preparations are no longer employed routinely. Rather, their use is restricted to ophthalmic infections, burns, and vaginitis caused by *Gardnerella vaginalis*.

The most severe hypersensitivity response to sulfonamides is *Stevens-Johnson syndrome,* a rare reaction that has a mortality rate of about 25%. Symptoms include widespread lesions of the skin and mucous membranes, together with fever, malaise, and toxemia. The reaction is most likely with long-acting sulfonamides, agents that have been banned in the United States. Shorter-acting sulfonamides may also induce the syndrome, but the incidence with these drugs is low. To minimize the risk of severe reactions, sulfonamides should be discontinued as soon as skin rash of any sort is observed. In addition, sulfonamides should not be given to patients with a history of hypersensitivity to the sulfonamides or to chemically related drugs, including sulfonylureas (oral hypoglycemic drugs), thiazide diuretics, and loop diuretics.

Hematologic Effects. Sulfonamides can cause *hemolytic anemia* in patients whose red blood cells have a genetically determined deficiency in glucose-6-phosphate dehydrogenase (G-6-PD). This inherited trait is most common among African Americans and people of Mediterranean origin. Rarely, hemolysis occurs in the absence of G-6-PD deficiency. Red cell lysis can produce fever, pallor, and jaundice; patients should be observed for these signs. In addition to hemolytic anemia, sulfonamides can cause agranulocytosis, leukopenia, thrombocytopenia, and, very rarely, aplastic anemia. When sulfonamides are used for a long time, periodic blood tests should be obtained.

Kernicterus. Kernicterus is a disorder in newborns caused by deposition of bilirubin in the brain. Bilirubin is neurotoxic and can cause severe neurologic deficits and even death. Under normal conditions, infants are not vulnerable to kernicterus, because any bilirubin present in the blood is tightly bound to plasma proteins, and, therefore, is not free to enter the central nervous system (CNS). Sulfonamides promote kernicterus by displacing bilirubin from plasma proteins. Since the blood-brain barrier of infants is poorly developed, the newly freed bilirubin has easy access to sites within the brain. *Because of the risk of kernicterus, sulfonamides should not be administered to infants under the age of 2 months. In addition, sulfonamides should not be given to pregnant women near term or to mothers who are breast-feeding.*

Renal Damage from Crystalluria. Because of their low solubility, older sulfonamides tended to come out of solution in the urine, forming crystalline aggregates in the kidneys, ureters, and bladder. These aggregates caused irritation and obstruction, sometimes resulting in anuria and even death. Renal damage is uncommon with today's sulfonamides because their solubility is relatively high. To minimize the risk of renal damage, adults should maintain a daily urine output of 1200 ml. This can be accomplished by consuming 8 to 10 glasses of water each day. Since the solubility of sulfonamides is highest at elevated pH, alkalinization of the urine (e.g., with sodium bicarbonate) can further decrease the chances of crystalluria.

Drug Interactions

Sulfonamides can intensify the effects of warfarin, phenytoin, and oral hypoglycemics (e.g., tolbutamide). The principal mechanism of potentiation is inhibition of hepatic metabolism. When combined with sulfonamides, these drugs may require a reduction in dosage to prevent toxic effects.

SULFONAMIDE PREPARATIONS

The sulfonamides fall into two major categories: (1) systemic sulfonamides, and (2) sulfonamides used for local effects. The sulfonamides employed for systemic therapy are more widely used.

Systemic Sulfonamides

The systemic sulfonamides can be subdivided based on duration of action. As indicated in Table 78–1, two groups are available in the United States: (1) short-acting agents, and (2) intermediate-acting agents. Long-acting sulfonamides produce a high incidence of Stevens-Johnson syndrome and have been withdrawn from the American market. The short-acting sulfonamides are used primarily to treat infections of the urinary tract. Except where noted below, the adverse effects and drug interactions of individual sulfonamides are the same as those discussed above. Dosages and trade names for systemic sulfonamides are summarized in Table 78–1.

Sulfisoxazole. Sulfisoxazole [Gantrisin], a short-acting sulfonamide, can be considered the prototype of the sulfonamide family. This drug is the preferred sulfonamide for chemotherapy of urinary tract infections. Sulfisoxazole is just as effective as other sulfonamides and less expensive. Moreover, because of its high water solubility, sulfisoxazole poses a minimal risk of crystalluria. Since high plasma concentrations of sulfisoxazole can be achieved, the drug is useful against a variety of systemic infections (e.g., nocardiosis, melioidosis, chancroid). In addition, sulfisoxazole can be combined with penicillin or erythromycin to treat otitis media caused by amoxicillin-resistant *H. influenzae*. The drug is also used for prophylaxis of rheumatic fever in patients allergic to penicillin. Sulfisoxazole may be administered orally and by injection (IV, SC, IM). Oral administration is preferred.

Sulfamethoxazole. Sulfamethoxazole [Gantanol, Urobak] is the only intermediate-acting sulfonamide available. Indications for this drug are the same as for sulfisoxazole. Because of its prolonged duration of action, sulfamethoxazole can be administered less frequently than the short-acting sulfonamides. This drug has lower water solubility than sulfisoxazole, and, hence, presents a greater risk of injury to the kidneys. The risk of renal damage can be minimized by maintaining adequate hydration. Sulfamethoxazole is employed primarily in fixed-dose combination with trimethoprim. This combination is discussed later in the chapter. Administration is oral.

Sulfadiazine. Sulfadiazine is a short-acting sulfonamide. The drug is less soluble than other short-acting agents. Hence, if renal damage is to be avoided, high urine flow must be maintained. Sulfadiazine crosses the blood-brain barrier with ease, and, therefore, is the best sulfonamide for prophylaxis of meningitis. Sulfadiazine is also a preferred agent for chemotherapy of nocardiosis. When combined with pyrimethamine, sulfadiazine is useful against toxoplasmosis. The drug is dispensed in tablets for oral administration.

Sulfacytine. Sulfacytine [Renoquid] is a newer sulfonamide. The drug is short acting and has high water solubility. The only indication for this agent is acute infection of the urinary tract. Sulfacytine is more expensive than the older sulfonamides. Administration is oral.

Sulfamethizole. Sulfamethizole [Thiosulfil Forte] is a short-acting sulfonamide. The drug is used only for urinary tract infections. Sulfamethizole is dispensed in tablets for oral administration.

Trisulfapyrimidines. Trisulfapyrimidines is a preparation containing relatively low amounts of three poorly soluble sulfonamides: sulfadiazine, sulfamerazine, and sulfamethazine. Before the more soluble sulfonamides became available, combination preparations such as trisulfapyrimidines were employed in efforts to decrease sulfonamide-induced damage to the kid-

Class*	Generic Name	Trade Name	Usual Adult Oral Dosage
Short Acting	Sulfisoxazole	Gantrisin	1 gm every 4 to 6 hours
	Sulfacytine	Renoquid	250 mg every 6 hours
	Sulfadiazine	—	1 gm every 4 to 6 hours
	Sulfamethizole	Thiosulfil Forte	0.5 to 1 gm every 6 hours
	Trisulfapyrimidines: Sulfadiazine plus Sulfamerazine plus Sulfamethazine	Triple Sulfa No. 2	1 gm every 6 hours
Intermediate Acting	Sulfamethoxazole	Gantanol, Urobak	1 gm every 12 hours

*Long-acting sulfonamides (e.g., sulfamethoxypyridazine, sulfameter) are no longer available in the United States.

neys. The rationale for these combinations is as follows. First, by combining three sulfonamides in low dosage, powerful antibacterial action can be achieved because the effects of the individual drugs are additive. Second, since the presence of one sulfonamide does not influence the solubility of the others, it is possible for the total urinary concentration of sulfonamide to be high without risking formation of crystals, provided the concentration of the individual agents remains below each drug's level of saturation. With the advent of more soluble sulfonamides, multiple sulfonamide preparations have become obsolete. Trisulfapyrimidines is the only such combination that remains on the market.

Topical Sulfonamides

Topical sulfonamides have been associated with a high incidence of hypersensitivity reactions and are not used routinely. The preparations discussed below have proven utility, and they present a relatively low risk of hypersensitivity.

Sulfacetamide. Sulfacetamide is widely used for superficial infections of the eye (e.g., conjunctivitis, corneal ulcer). The drug may cause blurred vision, sensitivity to bright light, headache, browache, and local irritation. Hypersensitivity is rare, but severe reactions have occurred. Accordingly, sulfacetamide should not be used by patients with a history of hypersensitivity to sulfonamides, sulfonylureas, or thiazide or loop diuretics. Sulfacetamide is available in solution and ointment formulations for local application to the eye. Trade names include Isopto Cetamide and Sodium Sulamyd.

Silver Sulfadiazine and Mafenide. Both of these sulfonamides are employed to prevent bacterial colonization in patients with second- and third-degree burns. Mafenide acts by the same mechanism as other sulfonamides. In contrast, antibacterial effects of silver sulfadiazine are due primarily to release of free silver—and not to the sulfonamide portion of the molecule. Local application of mafenide is frequently painful. In contrast, application of silver sulfadiazine is usually pain free. Following topical application, both agents can be absorbed in amounts sufficient to produce systemic effects. Mafenide, but not silver sulfadiazine, is metabolized to a compound that can suppress renal excretion of acid, thereby causing acidosis. Accordingly, patients receiving mafenide should be monitored for acid-base status. If acidosis becomes severe, mafenide should be discontinued for 1 to 2 days. Mafenide is marketed under the trade name Sulfamylon. The trade name for silver sulfadiazine is Silvadene.

TRIMETHOPRIM

Like the sulfonamides, trimethoprim [Proloprim, Trimpex] interferes with microbial produc-

tion of tetrahydrofolic acid. Trimethoprim is active against a broad spectrum of microbes.

Mechanism of Action

As indicated in Figure 78–2, trimethoprim is an *inhibitor of dihydrofolate reductase*, the enzyme that converts dihydrofolic acid to its active form (tetrahydrofolic acid). Hence, like the sulfonamides, trimethoprim suppresses bacterial synthesis of DNA, RNA, and proteins. Depending upon conditions at the site of infection, trimethoprim may be bactericidal or bacteriostatic.

Although mammalian cells also contain dihydrofolate reductase, trimethoprim is selectively toxic to bacteria. This selectivity is based on structural differences between bacterial dihydrofolate reductase and the enzyme found in mammalian cells. Because of these structural differences, trimethoprim inhibits the bacterial enzyme at concentrations about 40,000 times lower than those required to inhibit mammalian dihydrofolate reductase. As a result, we can suppress bacterial growth with doses of trimethoprim that have essentially no effect on the host.

Microbial Resistance

Bacteria acquire resistance to trimethoprim by three mechanisms: (1) synthesis of increased amounts of dihydrofolate reductase, (2) production of an altered dihydrofolate reductase that has a low affinity for trimethoprim, and (3) reduced cellular permeability to trimethoprim. Resistance has resulted from spontaneous mutation and transfer of R factors. In the United States, bacterial resistance is uncommon.

Antimicrobial Spectrum

Trimethoprim is active against many gram-positive bacilli and some gram-negative bacilli (e.g., *Corynebacterium diphtheriae*, *Listeria monocytogenes*). Most aerobic gram-negative bacilli of clinical importance are also sensitive, including *E. coli*, *Klebsiella*, *Proteus mirabilis*, *Serratia marcescens*, *Salmonella*, *Shigella*, and *H. influenzae*. In addition, trimethoprim is active against some pathogenic protozoa (e.g., *Pneumocystis carinii*, *Toxoplasma gondii*, and the protozoa responsible for malaria).

Therapeutic Uses

Trimethoprim is approved only for initial therapy of acute, uncomplicated urinary tract infections due to susceptible organisms (e.g., *E. coli*, *Proteus mirabilis*, *Enterobacter* species, and *Staphylococcus saprophyticus*). When combined with sulfamethoxazole, trimethoprim has considerably more applications; these are discussed later in the chapter.

Pharmacokinetics

Trimethoprim is absorbed rapidly and completely from the gastrointestinal tract. The drug is quite lipid soluble and, hence, undergoes wide distribution to body fluids and tissues. Trimethoprim readily crosses the placenta. Most of an administered dose is excreted unchanged by the kidneys. Hence, in the presence of renal dysfunction, the half-life of trimethoprim is prolonged. The concentration of trimethoprim achieved in urine is considerably higher than the concurrent concentration in blood.

Adverse Effects

Trimethoprim is generally well tolerated. The most frequent adverse effects are itching and rash. Gastrointestinal reactions (e.g., epigastric distress, nausea, vomiting, glossitis, stomatitis) occur occasionally.

Hematologic Effects. Since mammalian dihydrofolate reductase is relatively insensitive to trimethoprim, toxicities related to suppression of tetrahydrofolate production are rare. These rare effects—*megaloblastic anemia*, *thrombocytopenia*, *neutropenia*—occur only in individuals with pre-existing folic acid deficiency. Accordingly, caution should be exercised when administering trimethoprim to patients in whom folate deficiency might be likely (e.g., alcoholics, pregnant women, debilitated patients). If early signs of bone marrow suppression occur (e.g., sore throat, fever, pallor), complete blood counts should be performed. If a significant reduction in blood cell counts is observed, trimethoprim should be discontinued. Administration of folinic acid (leucovorin) will restore normal hematopoiesis.

Use in Pregnancy and Lactation. Large doses of trimethoprim have caused fetal malformations in animals. To date, no developmental abnormalities have been observed in humans. However, since trimethoprim readily crosses the placenta, prudence dictates that the drug not be used routinely during pregnancy. The risk of exacerbating pregnancy-related folate deficiency is an additional reason not to use the drug at this time.

Trimethoprim is excreted in breast milk and may interfere with folic acid utilization by the nursing infant. The drug should be administered with caution to women who are breast-feeding.

Preparations, Dosage, and Administration

Trimethoprim [Proloprim, Trimpex] is dispensed in 100- and 200-mg tablets for oral use. For urinary tract infections, the usual dosage is 100 mg every 12 hours or 200 mg every 24 hours. Duration of treatment is 10 days. Dosage should be reduced in patients with renal dysfunction.

TRIMETHOPRIM-SULFAMETHOXAZOLE

Trimethoprim (TMP) and sulfamethoxazole (SMZ) are marketed together in a fixed-dose combination product. This combination (TMP-SMZ) is a powerful antimicrobial preparation whose components act in concert to inhibit sequential steps in the synthesis of tetrahydrofolic acid. Trade names for TMP-SMZ include Bactrim and Septra. In many countries, the combination is known as co-trimoxazole.

Mechanism of Action

The antimicrobial effects of TMP-SMZ result from inhibiting consecutive steps in the synthesis of tetrahydrofolic acid: SMZ acts first to inhibit incorporation of PABA into folic acid; TMP then inhibits dihydrofolate reductase, the enzyme that converts dihydrofolic acid into tetrahydrofolate (see Figure 78–2). As a result of these actions, the ability of the target organism to produce nucleic acids and proteins is suppressed. By inhibiting two reactions required for synthesis of tetrahydrofolate, TMP and SMZ potentiate each other's effects. That is, the antimicrobial effect of the combination is more powerful than the sum of the effects of TMP and SMZ used alone. TMP-SMZ is selectively toxic to microbes because (1) mammalian cells use preformed folic acid and, therefore, are not affected by SMZ, and (2) dihydrofolate reductases of mammalian cells are relatively insensitive to inhibition by TMP.

Microbial Resistance

Resistance to the combination of TMP plus SMZ appears to be less than to either drug alone. This is logical since the chances of an organism acquiring resistance to both drugs are less than its chances of developing resistance to just one drug or the other. Specific mechanisms of resistance to sulfonamides and TMP are discussed earlier in the chapter.

Antimicrobial Spectrum

TMP-SMZ is active against a wide range of gram-positive and gram-negative bacteria. This should be no surprise since TMP and SMZ by themselves are broad-spectrum antimicrobial drugs. Most urinary tract pathogens are susceptible. Specific bacteria against which TMP-SMZ is consistently effective include *E. coli*, *Proteus mirabilis*, *Salmonella typhi*, *Shigella* species, *Vibrio cholerae*, *Haemophilus influenzae*, and *Yersinia pestis*. TMP-SMZ is also active against *Nocardia* and certain protozoa (*Pneumocystis carinii* and *Plasmodium* species).

Therapeutic Uses

TMP-SMZ is a preferred or alternative medication for a variety of infectious diseases. The combination is especially valuable for urinary tract infections, otitis media, bronchitis, shigellosis, and pneumonia caused by *Pneumocystis carinii*.

Urinary Tract Infection. TMP-SMZ is indicated for chemotherapy of uncomplicated urinary tract infection caused by susceptible strains of *E. coli*, *Klebsiella*, *Enterobacter*, *Proteus mirabilis*, *P. vulgaris*, and *Morganella morganii*. The combination is particularly useful for chronic and recurrent infections.

***Pneumocystis carinii* Pneumonia.** TMP-SMZ is a treatment of choice for *Pneumocystis carinii* pneumonia (PCP), an infection that is common in the immunocompromised host (e.g., cancer patients, organ transplant recipients, individuals with AIDS). When given to AIDS patients, TMP-SMZ produces a high incidence of adverse effects. The dosage for treating PCP in AIDS patients is given in Chapter 88.

Gastrointestinal Infections. TMP-SMZ is a treatment of choice for shigellosis caused by susceptible strains of *Shigella flexneri* and *S. sonnei*. In addition, the combination is an alternative to chloramphenicol and ampicillin for typhoid fever.

Other Infections. TMP-SMZ can be used for otitis media and acute exacerbations of chronic bronchitis when these infections are due to susceptible strains of *Haemophilus influenzae* or *Streptococcus pneumoniae*. The preparation is also useful against urethritis and pharyngeal infection caused by penicillinase-producing *Neisseria gonorrhoeae*. Other infections that can be treated with TMP-SMZ include whooping cough, nocardiosis, brucellosis, melioidosis, and chancroid.

Pharmacokinetics

Absorption and Distribution. TMP-SMZ may be administered orally and by IV infusion. Both components of TMP-SMZ are well distributed throughout the body. Therapeutic concentrations are achieved in tissues and body fluids (e.g., vaginal secretions, cerebrospinal fluid, pleural effusions, bile, aqueous humor). Both TMP and SMZ readily cross the placenta and both enter breast milk.

Plasma Drug Levels. Optimal antibacterial effects are produced when the ratio of TMP to SMZ is 1:20. To achieve this 1:20 ratio in *plasma*, TMP and SMZ must be administered in a ratio of 1:5. Hence, standard tablets contain 80 mg of TMP and 400 mg of SMZ. Because the plasma half-lives of TMP and SMZ are similar (10 hours for TMP and 11 hours for SMZ), levels of both drugs decline in parallel, and the 1:20 ratio is maintained as the drugs undergo elimination.

Elimination. Both TMP and SMZ are excreted primarily by the kidneys. About 70% of urinary SMZ is present as inactive metabolites. In contrast, TMP undergoes little hepatic metabolism prior to excretion in the urine. Both agents are concentrated in the urine. Hence, levels of active drug are higher in the urine than in plasma, despite some conversion to inactive products.

Adverse Effects

TMP-SMZ is generally well tolerated; toxicity from routine use is rare. The most common ad-verse effects are nausea, vomiting, and rash. However, although infrequent, all of the serious toxicities associated with sulfonamides can occur with TMP-SMZ. That is, the combination can cause hypersensitivity reactions (including Stevens-Johnson syndrome), blood dyscrasias (hemolytic anemia, agranulocytosis, leukopenia, thrombocytopenia, aplastic anemia), kernicterus, and renal damage. Primarily because of its TMP component, TMP-SMZ can induce megaloblastic anemia, but only in patients who are folate deficient. TMP-SMZ may also cause adverse CNS effects (headache, depression, hallucinations). Patients suffering from AIDS are unusually susceptible to TMP-SMZ toxicity. In this group, the incidence of adverse effects (rash, recurrent fever, leukopenia) is about 55%.

Several measures can reduce the incidence and severity of adverse effects. Crystalluria can be avoided by maintaining adequate hydration. Periodic blood tests permit early detection of hematologic disorders. To avoid kernicterus, TMP-SMZ should be withheld from pregnant women near term, nursing mothers, and infants under the age of 2 months. The risk of megaloblastic anemia can be reduced by withholding sulfonamides from individuals with a probability of folate deficiency (e.g., debilitated patients, pregnant women, alcoholics). Hypersensitivity reactions can be minimized by avoiding TMP-SMZ in patients with a history of hypersensitivity to sulfonamides or chemically related drugs, including thiazide diuretics, loop diuretics, and oral hypoglycemics (sulfonylureas).

Drug Interactions

Interactions of TMP-SMZ with other drugs are due primarily to the presence of SMZ. Hence, like sulfonamides used alone, SMZ in the combination can intensify the effects of warfarin, phenytoin, and oral hypoglycemics (e.g., tolbutamide). Accordingly, when these drugs are combined with TMP-SMZ, a reduction in their dosage may be needed.

Preparations, Dosage, and Administration

Preparations. Trimethoprim-sulfamethoxazole [Bactrim, Septra, others] is dispensed in tablets and a suspension for oral use, and in solution for IV infusion. The ratio of TMP to SMZ in all preparations is 1:5. Two strengths of tablets are available: standard tablets contain 80 mg TMP and 400 mg SMZ; double-strength tablets contain 160 mg TMP and 800 mg SMZ. Each ml of the oral suspension contains 8 mg TMP and 40 mg SMZ. Each ml of the IV infusion solution contains 16 mg TMP and 80 mg SMZ.

Oral Dosing. For management of most infections, the usual *adult* dosage is 160 mg TMP plus 800 mg SMZ administered every 12 hours for 10 to 14 days. To treat shigellosis or traveler's diarrhea, the same dose is administered every 12 hours for 5 days. In the presence of renal impairment (creatinine clearance 15 to 30 ml/min), the dosage should be reduced by 50%. If creatinine clearance is below 15 ml/minute, TMP-SMZ should not be used.

To treat urinary tract infections and acute otitis media in *children*, the usual dosage is 4 mg/kg TMP plus 20 mg/kg SMZ administered every 12 hours for 10 days. For treatment of shigellosis, the same dose is administered every 12 hours for 5 days. As in adults, the dosage should be reduced in patients with renal dysfunction.

Intravenous Dosing. Intravenous TMP-SMZ is used for severe infections. The following dosages are for adults and children, and are based on the TMP component of TMP-SMZ. For urinary tract infection or shigellosis, the total daily dose is 8 to 10 mg/kg. This total dose is administered in two to four divided doses given at equally spaced intervals. Duration of treatment is 14 days for urinary tract infection and 5 days for shigellosis. For treatment of *Pneumocystis carinii* pneumonia, the total daily dose is 15 to 20 mg/kg. This dose is administered in three or four divided doses given at equally spaced intervals. Duration of treatment is 2 weeks or less. Dosage for all indications should be reduced in patients with renal impairment.

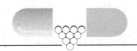

Summary of Major Nursing Implications

SULFONAMIDES

The nursing implications summarized here apply to *systemic* sulfonamides. Implications specific to topical sulfonamides are not summarized.

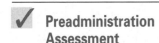

✓ **Preadministration Assessment**

Therapeutic Goal

Sulfonamides are used primarily for *urinary tract infections* caused by *E. coli* and other susceptible organisms.

Identifying High-Risk Patients

Sulfonamides are *contraindicated* during *pregnancy and lactation*, for *infants under the age of 2 months*, and for patients with a *history of hypersensitivity to sulfonamides and chemically related drugs, including thiazide diuretics, loop diuretics, and oral hypoglycemics (sulfonylureas)*. Exercise *caution* in patients with *renal impairment*.

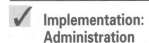

✓ **Implementation: Administration**

Routes

All systemic sulfonamides can be administered orally. *Sulfisoxazole* can also be administered parenterally (IV, SC, IM).

Administration

Advise patients to take oral sulfonamides on an empty stomach and with a full glass of water.

Instruct patients to complete the prescribed course of treatment, even though symptoms may abate before the full course is over.

Administer IV sulfisoxazole by slow injection or IV drip.

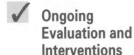

✓ **Ongoing Evaluation and Interventions**

Minimizing Adverse Effects

Hypersensitivity Reactions. Sulfonamides can induce *severe hypersensitivity reactions* (e.g., Stevens-Johnson syndrome). Do not give sulfonamides to patients with a history of hypersensitivity to sulfonamides or chemically related drugs, including sulfonylureas, thiazide diuretics, and loop diuretics. Instruct the patient to discontinue drug use immediately at the first sign of hypersensitivity (e.g., rash).

Photosensitivity reactions may occur. Advise the patient to avoid prolonged exposure to sunlight, wear protective clothing, and apply a sunscreen to exposed skin.

Hematologic Effects. Sulfonamides can cause hemolytic anemia and other blood dyscrasias (agranulocytosis, leukopenia, thrombocytopenia, aplastic anemia). Observe patients for signs of hemolysis (fever, pallor, jaundice). When sulfonamide therapy is prolonged, periodic blood cell counts should be made.

Kernicterus. Sulfonamides can cause kernicterus in newborns. Do not give these drugs to pregnant women near term, nursing mothers, or infants under the age of 2 months.

Renal Damage. Deposition of sulfonamide crystals can injure the kidney. To minimize crystalluria, maintain hydration sufficient to produce a daily urine flow of 1200 ml in adults. Alkalinization of urine (e.g., with sodium bicarbonate) can also be beneficial. Advise outpatients to consume 8 to 10 glasses of water per day.

Minimizing Adverse Interactions

Sulfonamides can intensify the effects of *warfarin, phenytoin,* and *oral hypoglycemics* (e.g., tolbutamide). When combined with sulfonamides, these drugs may require a reduction in dosage.

TRIMETHOPRIM

Preadministration Assessment

Therapeutic Goal

Initial treatment of uncomplicated urinary tract infections caused by *E. coli* and other susceptible organisms.

Identifying High-Risk Patients

Trimethoprim is *contraindicated* in *patients with folate deficiency* (manifested as megaloblastic anemia). When possible, the drug should be avoided during *pregnancy and lactation.*

Implementation: Administration

Route

Oral.

Dosage and Administration

Instruct patients to complete the prescribed course of treatment, even though symptoms may abate before the full course is over.
Reduce the dosage in patients with renal dysfunction.

Ongoing Evaluation and Interventions

Minimizing Adverse Effects

Hematologic Effects. Trimethoprim can cause blood dyscrasias (megaloblastic anemia, thrombocytopenia, neutropenia) by exacerbating pre-existing folic acid deficiency. Avoid trimethoprim when folate deficiency is likely (e.g., in alcoholics, pregnant women, debilitated patients). Inform patients about early signs of blood disorders (e.g., sore throat, fever, pallor), and instruct them to notify the physician if these occur. Complete blood counts should be performed. If a significant reduction in counts is observed, discontinue trimethoprim. Normal hematopoiesis can be restored with folinic acid (leucovorin).

Use in Pregnancy and Lactation. Trimethoprim should be avoided during pregnancy and lactation. The drug can exacerbate folate deficiency in pregnant women and cause folate deficiency in the nursing infant whose mother is taking trimethoprim.

TRIMETHOPRIM-SULFAMETHOXAZOLE

Preadministration Assessment

Therapeutic Goal

Indications include urinary tract infections caused by *E. coli* and other susceptible organisms; shigellosis; *Pneumocystis carinii* pneumonia; and otitis media caused by susceptible strains of *H. influenzae*.

Identifying High-Risk Patients

TMP-SMZ is *contraindicated* during *pregnancy and lactation*, for *infants under the age of 2 months*, in patients with *folate deficiency* (manifested as megaloblastic anemia), and for patients with a *history of hypersensitivity to sulfonamides and chemically related drugs, including thiazide diuretics, loop diuretics, and oral hypoglycemics (sulfonylureas)*.

Implementation: Administration

Routes

Oral, intravenous (for severe infections).

Dosage Adjustment

In patients with renal impairment (creatinine clearance 15 to 30 ml/min) decrease dosage by 50%. If creatinine clearance falls below 15 ml/min, discontinue drug use.

Administration

Instruct the patient to complete the prescribed course of treatment, even though symptoms may abate before the full course is over.

Ongoing Evaluation and Interventions

Minimizing Adverse Effects

Although serious adverse reactions are rare, TMP-SMZ can nonetheless cause all of the toxicities associated with sulfonamides and trimethoprim used alone. Hence, the nursing implications summarized above regarding adverse effects of the sulfonamides alone and trimethoprim alone apply to the combination of TMP-SMZ as well.

Minimizing Adverse Interactions

TMP-SMZ has the same drug interactions as sulfonamides used alone. That is, TMP-SMZ can increase the effects of *warfarin, phenytoin,* and *oral hypoglycemics*. When combined with TMP-SMZ, these drugs may require a reduction in dosage.

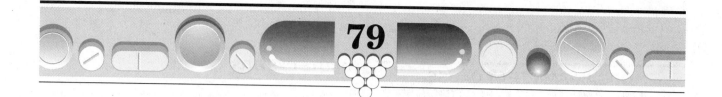

79

Drug Therapy of Urinary Tract Infections

79

79

ORGANISMS THAT CAUSE URINARY
TRACT INFECTIONS

OVERVIEW OF THE DRUGS USED TO
TREAT URINARY TRACT INFECTIONS

SPECIFIC URINARY TRACT INFECTIONS
AND THEIR TREATMENT
    Acute Cystitis
    Acute Urethral Syndrome
    Recurrent Urinary Tract Infections
    Acute Pyelonephritis
    Acute Bacterial Prostatitis

URINARY TRACT ANTISEPTICS
    Nitrofurantoin
    Methenamine
    Nalidixic acid
    Cinoxacin

Urinary tract infections (UTIs) are the most common infections encountered today. Estimates indicate that between 10% and 20% of all females experience at least one UTI, and many experience recurrent infections. UTIs occur much less frequently in males than in females, but are more likely to be associated with complications (e.g., septicemia, pyelonephritis).

Infections may be limited to bacterial colonization of the urine, or bacteria may invade tissues of the urinary tract. When bacteria invade tissues, characteristic inflammatory syndromes result: *urethritis* (inflammation of the urethra), *cystitis* (inflammation of the urinary bladder), *pyelonephritis* (inflammation of the kidney and its pelvis), and *prostatitis* (inflammation of the prostate).

UTIs may be classified according to their location—in either the lower urinary tract or the upper urinary tract. Within this classification scheme, *cystitis* and *urethritis* are considered *lower tract infections*, whereas *pyelonephritis* is considered an *upper tract infection*.

UTIs are referred to as being *complicated* or *uncomplicated*. *Complicated* UTIs occur in males or females and are associated with some *predisposing factor*, such as calculi (stones), prostatic hypertrophy, an indwelling catheter, or an impediment to the flow of urine (e.g., physical obstruction). *Uncomplicated* UTIs occur primarily in women of

79

989

child-bearing age and are not associated with any particular predisposing factor.

ORGANISMS THAT CAUSE URINARY TRACT INFECTIONS

The bacteria that cause UTIs differ between community-acquired infections and hospital-acquired (nosocomial) infections. The majority (80%) of uncomplicated, community-acquired UTIs are caused by *Escherichia coli*. Rarely, other gram-negative bacilli—*Klebsiella, Enterobacter, Proteus, Providencia, Pseudomonas*— are the cause. Gram-positive cocci, especially *Staphylococcus saprophyticus*, account for 10% to 15% of community-acquired infections. Hospital-acquired UTIs are frequently caused by *Klebsiella, Proteus, Enterobacter, Pseudomonas*, staphylococci, and enterococci; *E. coli* is responsible for less than 50% of nosocomial infections. Although most UTIs involve only one organism, infection with multiple organisms may occur, especially in patients with an indwelling urinary catheter, renal stones, or chronic renal abscesses.

OVERVIEW OF THE DRUGS USED TO TREAT URINARY TRACT INFECTIONS

Several classes of antibiotics are used to treat UTIs. These include the sulfonamides, trimethoprim, penicillins, aminoglycosides, cephalosporins, tetracyclines, and fluoroquinolones. The drugs employed for *oral* therapy of UTIs are summarized in Table 79–1. Those employed for *parenteral* therapy are summarized in Table 79–2. With the exception of the urinary tract antiseptics noted in Table 79–1, all of these antibiotics are discussed at length in other chapters. The basic pharmacology of the urinary tract antiseptics is presented at the end of this chapter.

SPECIFIC URINARY TRACT INFECTIONS AND THEIR TREATMENT

In this section, we consider the characteristics and treatment of the major UTIs: acute cystitis, acute urethral syndrome, acute pyelonephritis, acute bacterial prostatitis, and recurrent UTIs. Most of these infections can be treated with oral therapy on an outpatient basis. The principal exception to this rule is severe pyelonephritis, which requires intravenous therapy in a hospital setting.

Drugs and dosages for outpatient therapy are summarized in Table 79–3.

ACUTE CYSTITIS

Acute cystitis is a lower urinary tract infection that occurs most often in women of child-bearing age. Clinical manifestations are dysuria, urinary urgency, urinary frequency, suprapubic discomfort, pyuria, and bacteriuria (more than 100,000 bacteria/ml of urine). It is important to note that many women (30% or more) with symptoms of acute cystitis also have asymptomatic upper urinary tract infection (subclinical pyelonephritis). In uncomplicated, community-acquired cystitis, the principal causative organisms are *Escherichia coli* (80%), *Staphylococcus saprophyticus* (11%), and *Streptococcus faecalis*.

For community-acquired infections, three types of oral therapy can be employed: (1) single-dose therapy, (2) short-course therapy (3 to 5 days), and (3) conventional therapy (7 to 14 days). *Single-dose* therapy and *short-course* therapy are recommended only for uncomplicated, community-acquired infections in women who are not pregnant and whose symptoms began less than 7 days before treatment is to be given. Short-course therapy is more effective than single-dose therapy and is preferred. Advantages of short-course therapy over conventional therapy are lower cost, greater compliance, fewer side effects, and less potential for causing bacterial resistance. *Conventional* therapy is indicated for all patients who do not meet the criteria for short-course therapy; these include males, children, pregnant women, and women with suspected upper tract involvement. Drugs and dosing regimens for oral therapy of acute cystitis are summarized in Table 79–3.

ACUTE URETHRAL SYNDROME

Acute urethral syndrome occurs in females. Clinical manifestations are dysuria, urinary frequency, urinary urgency, and pyuria. There is no significant bacteriuria (i.e., bacterial counts are less than 100,000/ml). The syndrome is usually caused by *E. coli, Staphylococcus saprophyticus*, or *Chlamydia trachomatis*. It may also be caused by *Neisseria gonorrhoeae, Gardnerella vaginalis*, and *Ureaplasma urealyticum*.

Treatment depends on the causative organisms. For infections caused by *E. coli* or staphylococci, a single dose of two double-strength tablets of trimethoprim-sulfamethoxazole is often curative. If this is ineffective, or if the infection is due to *Chlamydia, Ureaplasma*, or *Trichomonas*, doxycycline should be used (100 mg twice daily for 10 to 14 days). Doxycycline is also effective against gonococcal urethritis, but ceftriaxone is preferred.

Table 79–1. Drugs for Oral Therapy of Urinary Tract Infections	
Drugs	**Comments**
Sulfonamides	Sulfonamides are useful for the first episodes of infection. They have generally been replaced by more active agents due to development of bacterial resistance. Their only advantage is low cost.
Trimethoprim-sulfamethoxazole	This combination is highly effective against most aerobic enteric bacteria, except *Pseudomonas*. High urinary tract tissue levels and urine levels are achieved, which may be important in treatment of complicated infections. Also effective as prophylaxis for recurrent infection.

Penicillins
  Ampicillin
  Amoxicillin
  Amoxicillin-clavulanate
  Carbenicillin indanyl
	Ampicillin, the standard broad-spectrum penicillin, is active against most enteric bacteria that cause UTI, but reports of *E. coli* resistance are increasing. Amoxicillin is better absorbed and has fewer side effects. Amoxicillin-clavulanate is preferred for resistance problems. Carbenicillin indanyl is indicated only for UTI, and is active against *Pseudomonas*.

Cephalosporins
  Cephalexin
  Cephradine
  Cefaclor
  Cefuroxime
  Cefixime
	These drugs offer no major advantages over other drugs for UTI and are more expensive. They may be useful in cases of resistance to amoxicillin and trimethoprim-sulfamethoxazole. These drugs are not as effective for single-dose therapy.

Tetracyclines
  Tetracycline
  Doxycycline
  Oxytetracycline
  Minocycline
	These drugs are effective for initial episodes of UTI. However, resistance develops rapidly, and, therefore, treatment should be guided by sensitivity testing. Use can result in candidal overgrowth. Tetracyclines are useful primarily for chlamydial infections.

Fluoroquinolones
  Ciprofloxacin
  Norfloxacin
  Ofloxacin
  Enoxacin
  Lomefloxacin
	These broad-spectrum antibiotics are active against most organisms that cause UTI, including *Proteus, E. coli,* and other Enterobacteriaceae. Ciprofloxacin and ofloxacin are used parenterally as well as orally.

Urinary Tract Antiseptics
  Methenamine
  Nalidixic acid
  Cinoxacin
  Nitrofurantoin
	Methenamine is reserved for prophylactic therapy and suppressive use between episodes of infection. Nalidixic acid and cinoxacin are effective for initial episodes of infection due to *E. coli* and other Enterobacteriaceae, but not *Proteus*. Nitrofurantoin is effective both as a therapeutic and prophylactic agent in patients with recurrent urinary tract infections; the drug's main advantage is lack of resistance, even after prolonged therapy.

Adapted from DiPiro, J. T. (ed.). Pharmacotherapy: A Pathophysiologic Approach, 2nd ed. Norwalk, CT, Appleton & Lange, 1992.

RECURRENT URINARY TRACT INFECTIONS

Recurrent urinary tract infections result from *relapse* or from *reinfection. Relapse* is caused by recolonization with the same organism responsible for the initial infection, whereas *reinfection* is caused by colonization with a new organism.

Reinfection. More than 80% of recurrent UTIs in females are due to reinfection. These usually involve the lower urinary tract and may be related to sexual intercourse or use of a contraceptive diaphragm. If reinfections are *infrequent* (only one or two a year), each episode should be treated as a separate infection. Single-dose or short-course therapy can be used.

When reinfections are *frequent* (three or more a year), long-term prophylaxis may be indicated. Prophylaxis can be achieved with low daily doses of trimethoprim (100 mg), nitrofurantoin (50 or 100 mg), or trimethoprim-sulfamethoxazole (one-half of a single-strength tablet). Prophylaxis should continue for 6 to 12 months. During this time, periodic urine cultures should be obtained. If a symptomatic episode occurs, standard therapy for acute cystitis should be given. If reinfection is associated with sexual intercourse, the risk can be decreased by voiding after intercourse and by single-dose prophylaxis (e.g., 2 double-strength tab-

Table 79–2. Drugs for Parenteral Therapy of Urinary Tract Infections	
Drugs	**Comments**
Aminoglycosides Gentamicin Tobramycin Amikacin Netilmicin	Gentamicin and tobramycin are equally effective, and gentamicin is less expensive. Tobramycin is more active against *Pseudomonas,* which may be important in serious systemic infections. Amikacin is generally reserved for multiresistant bacteria.
Penicillins Ampicillin Carbenicillin Ticarcillin Mezlocillin Piperacillin	These agents are generally equally effective for susceptible bacteria. The extended spectrum penicillins are more active against *Pseudomonas* and enterococci, and are often preferred over cephalosporins. Penicillins are very useful in renally impaired patients or when an aminoglycoside is to be avoided.
Cephalosporins	Second- and third-generation cephalosporins have a broad spectrum of activity against gram-negative bacteria but are not active against enterococci and have limited activity against *Pseudomonas.* They are useful for nosocomial infections and urosepsis due to susceptible pathogens.
Imipenem-cilastatin	This combination has a very broad spectrum of activity, including gram-positive, gram-negative, and anaerobic bacteria. It is active against enterococci and *Pseudomonas,* but may be associated with candidal suprainfection.
Aztreonam	This monobactam is active only against gram-negative bacteria, including *Pseudomonas.* Generally useful for nosocomial infections when aminoglycosides are to be avoided and in penicillin-allergic patients.
Fluoroquinolones Ciprofloxacin Ofloxacin	These broad-spectrum antibiotics are active against most organisms that cause UTI, including *Proteus, E. coli,* and other Enterobacteriaceae.

Adapted from DiPiro, J. T. (ed.). Pharmacotherapy: A Pathophysiologic Approach, 2nd ed. Norwalk, CT, Appleton & Lange, 1992.

lets of trimethoprim-sulfamethoxazole taken after intercourse).

Relapse. Recolonization with the original infecting organism accounts for 20% of recurrent UTIs. Symptoms that reappear shortly after completion of a course of therapy suggest either a structural abnormality of the urinary tract, involvement of the kidneys, or chronic bacterial prostatitis (the most common cause of recurrent UTIs in males). If obstruction of the urinary tract is present, it should be corrected surgically. If renal calculi are the cause of relapse, they should be removed.

Drug therapy is progressive. When relapse occurs in women after short-course therapy, a 2-week course of therapy should be tried. If this fails, an additional 4 to 6 weeks of therapy should be tried. If this too is unsuccessful, long-term therapy (6 months) may be indicated. Drugs employed for long-term therapy of relapse include trimethoprim-sulfamethoxazole, norfloxacin, and ciprofloxacin.

ACUTE PYELONEPHRITIS

Acute pyelonephritis is an infection of the kidney. This disorder is common in young children,

women of child-bearing age, and the elderly. Clinical manifestations include fever, chills, severe flank pain, dysuria, urinary frequency, urinary urgency, pyuria, and usually bacteriuria (more than 100,000 bacteria/ml of urine). *E. coli* is the causative organism in 90% of initial, community-acquired infections. *Mild-to-moderate infection* can be treated on an outpatient basis with oral trimethoprim-sulfamethoxazole (one double-strength tablet twice daily for 2 weeks or longer). *Severe infection* requires hospitalization and intravenous antibiotics; the preferred therapy is an aminoglycoside (e.g., gentamicin, amikacin) combined with ampicillin. Once the infection has been controlled with IV antibiotics, therapy with oral antibiotics can be instituted.

ACUTE BACTERIAL PROSTATITIS

Acute bacterial prostatitis is defined as inflammation of the prostate caused by local bacterial infection. Clinical manifestations include high fever, chills, malaise, myalgia, localized pain, and various urinary tract symptoms (dysuria, nocturia, urinary urgency, urinary frequency, urinary retention). In most cases (80%), *E. coli* is the causative organism. Infection is frequently associated with

Table 79–3. Oral Therapy of Urinary Tract Infections in Adults

Acute Cystitis	
Trimethoprim-sulfamethoxazole (double-strength tablets)	2 tablets once *or* 1 tablet twice daily for 3 days *or* 1 tablet twice daily for 10–14 days
Trimethoprim	400 mg once *or* 200 mg twice daily for 3 days *or* 100 mg twice daily for 10–14 days
Sulfisoxazole	2 gm once *or* 1 gm every 6 hours for 10–14 days
Amoxicillin	3 gm once *Or* 250 mg twice daily for 10–14 days
Norfloxacin	400 mg twice daily for 10–14 days
Ciprofloxacin	500 mg twice daily for 10–14 days
Ofloxacin	200 mg twice daily for 7–10 days
Enoxacin	400 mg twice daily for 10–14 days
Lomefloxacin	400 mg once daily for 10–14 days
Nitrofurantoin	200 mg once *or* 100 mg every 6 hours for 3 days
Acute Urethral Syndrome: Initial Therapy	
Trimethoprim-sulfamethoxazole	2 double-strength tablets once
Amoxicilliln	3 gm once
Acute Urethral Syndrome: If Initial Therapy Fails	
Doxycycline	100 mg twice daily for 10–14 days
Long-Term Prophylaxis of Recurrent Infection	
Trimethoprim-sulfamethoxazole	1/2 single-strength tablet daily for 6 months
Nitrofurantoin	50 mg once daily for 6 months
Trimethoprim	100 mg once daily for 6 months
Acute Pyelonephritis (mild)	
Trimethoprim-sulfamethoxazole	One double-strength tablet twice daily for 2 weeks or longer
Acute Bacterial Prostatitis	
Trimethoprim-sulfamethoxazole	One double-strength tablet twice daily for 30 days

an indwelling urethral catheter, urethral instrumentation, or transurethral prostatic resection. However, in many patients, the infection has no obvious cause. Bacterial prostatitis responds well to antimicrobial therapy. Drugs for oral therapy include trimethoprim-sulfamethoxazole and the fluoroquinolones (e.g., ciprofloxacin, norfloxacin). Aminoglycosides (e.g., gentamicin, amikacin) are used for parenteral therapy.

URINARY TRACT ANTISEPTICS

The urinary tract antiseptics are drugs whose use is restricted to the treatment of urinary tract infections (UTIs). The major urinary tract antiseptics are *nitrofurantoin, methenamine, nalidixic acid,* and *cinoxacin.* All four drugs become concentrated in the urine, and are active against the common urinary tract pathogens. These drugs do not achieve effective antibacterial concentrations in blood or tissues, and, therefore, cannot be used for infections at sites outside the urinary tract. As a rule, the urinary tract antiseptics are second-choice drugs for treatment and prophylaxis of UTIs.

NITROFURANTOIN

Nitrofurantoin [Furadantin, Macrodantin, others] is a broad-spectrum antimicrobial drug. The agent is bacteriostatic in low concentrations and bactericidal in high concentrations. Therapeutic levels are achieved only in the urine. Hence, the drug is useful only against infections of the urinary tract. The mechanism of action of nitrofurantoin is unknown, as is the basis for its selective toxicity to microorganisms.

Antimicrobial Spectrum

Nitrofurantoin is active against a large number of gram-positive and gram-negative bacteria. Susceptible organisms include staphylococci, streptococci, *Neisseria, Bacteroides,* and most strains of *Escherichia coli.* These sensitive bacteria rarely acquire resistance. Organisms that are frequently insensitive include *Proteus, Pseudomonas, Enterobacter,* and *Klebsiella.*

Therapeutic Use

Nitrofurantoin is indicated for acute infections of the lower urinary tract that are caused by susceptible organisms. In addition, nitrofurantoin can be used for prophylaxis of recurrent lower UTI. The drug is not recommended for infections of the upper urinary tract.

Pharmacokinetics

Absorption and Distribution. Nitrofurantoin is available in two oral formulations: *macrocrystalline* and *microcrystalline*. The macrocrystalline preparation is absorbed relatively slowly, and produces less gastrointestinal distress than the microcrystalline form. Both formulations produce equivalent therapeutic effects. Nitrofurantoin is distributed to tissues but only in small amounts. Therapeutic concentrations are achieved only in the urine.

Metabolism and Excretion. About two thirds of a dose undergoes metabolic degradation, primarily in the liver; the remaining one third is excreted intact by the kidneys. Nitrofurantoin achieves a urinary concentration of about 200 μg/ml (compared with less than 2 μg/ml in the plasma). The drug imparts a harmless brown color to the urine; patients should be forewarned of this effect.

For two reasons, the drug should not be administered to individuals with kidney impairment (creatinine clearance less than 40 ml/minute). First, in the absence of proper renal function, levels of nitrofurantoin in the urine are too low to be effective. Second, renal dysfunction reduces nitrofurantoin excretion, causing plasma drug levels to rise, thereby presenting a risk of systemic toxicity.

Adverse Effects

Gastrointestinal Effects. The most frequent adverse reactions are gastrointestinal disturbances (e.g., anorexia, nausea, vomiting, diarrhea). These can be minimized by administering nitrofurantoin with milk or meals, reducing the dosage, and using the macrocrystalline formulation.

Pulmonary Reactions. Nitrofurantoin can induce two kinds of pulmonary reactions: acute and subacute. Acute reactions, which are most common, are manifested by dyspnea, chest pain, chills, fever, cough, and alveolar infiltrates. These symptoms resolve in 2 to 4 days following cessation of nitrofurantoin use. Acute pulmonary responses are thought to be hypersensitivity reactions. Patients with a history of such responses should not receive nitrofurantoin again. Subacute reactions are rare and occur during prolonged treatment. Symptoms (e.g., dyspnea, cough, malaise) usually regress over weeks to months after nitrofurantoin withdrawal. However, in some patients permanent lung damage may occur.

Hematologic Effects. Nitrofurantoin can cause a variety of hematologic reactions, including agranulocytosis, leukopenia, thrombocytopenia, and megaloblastic anemia. In addition, hemolytic anemia may occur in infants and patients whose red blood cells have an inherited deficiency in glucose-6-phosphate dehydrogenase. Because of the potential for hemolytic anemia in newborns, nitrofurantoin is contraindicated for pregnant women near term and for infants under the age of 1 month.

Peripheral Neuropathy. Damage to sensory and motor nerves is a serious concern. Demyelinization and nerve degeneration can occur and may be irreversible. Early symptoms include muscle weakness, tingling sensations, and numbness. The patient should be informed of these symptoms and instructed to report them. Neuropathy is most likely in patients with renal impairment and those taking nitrofurantoin chronically.

Other Adverse Effects. Nitrofurantoin can cause multiple neurologic effects (e.g., headache, vertigo, drowsiness, nystagmus); all are readily reversible. Hepatotoxicity (cholestatic jaundice, chronic hepatitis, hepatocellular damage) occurs rarely.

Preparations, Dosage, and Administration

Preparations. Microcrystalline nitrofurantoin [Furadantin, others] is dispensed in tablets (50 and 100 mg), capsules (50 and 100 mg), and an oral suspension (5 mg/ml). Macrocrystalline nitrofurantoin [Macrodantin] is dispensed in capsules (25, 50, and 100 mg).

Dosage and Administration. For *treatment* of acute UTI, the *adult* dosage is 50 mg three to four times a day; the *pediatric* dosage is 5 to 7 mg/kg/day administered in four divided doses. For *prophylaxis* of recurrent UTI, low doses are employed (e.g., 50 to 100 mg at bedtime for adults and 1 mg/kg/day in one or two doses for children). Nitrofurantoin can be administered with meals and milk to reduce gastrointestinal distress.

METHENAMINE

Mechanism of Action

Under acidic conditions, methenamine slowly decomposes into ammonia and formaldehyde. The formaldehyde denatures bacterial proteins, causing death. For formaldehyde to be released, the urine must be acidic (pH 5.5 or less). Since formaldehyde is not formed at physiologic systemic pH, methenamine is devoid of systemic toxicity.

Antimicrobial Spectrum

Virtually all bacteria are susceptible to formaldehyde; resistance does not exist. Certain bacteria (e.g., *Proteus* species) can elevate urinary pH (by splitting urea to form ammonia). Since formaldehyde is not released under alkaline conditions, infections with these urea-splitting organisms are often unresponsive to methenamine.

Therapeutic Uses

Methenamine is used for *chronic* UTI, but is not recommended for *acute* infection. The drug can suppress recurrent UTI in females, but trimethoprim-sulfamethoxazole is preferred for this indication. Methenamine is not active against infections of the upper urinary tract, since there is insufficient time for formaldehyde to be formed as the drug traverses the kidney. Methenamine does not prevent UTIs associated with catheters.

Pharmacokinetics

Absorption and Distribution. Methenamine is rapidly absorbed after oral administration. However, approximately 30% of each dose may be converted to ammonia and formaldehyde in the acidic environment of the stomach. This reaction can be minimized by use of enteric-coated preparations. The drug is distributed throughout total body water.

Excretion. Methenamine is eliminated by the kidneys. Within the urinary tract, about 20% of the drug decomposes to form formaldehyde. Levels of formaldehyde are highest within the bladder. Since formaldehyde generation takes place slowly, and since transit time through the kidney is brief, formaldehyde levels in the *kidney* remain subtherapeutic. Ingestion of large amounts of fluid will reduce antibacterial effects by diluting methenamine and raising urinary pH. Poorly metabolized acids (e.g., hippuric acid, mandelic acid, ascorbic acid) have been administered with methenamine in attempts to acidify the urine, and thereby increase formaldehyde formation; however, there is no evidence that these acids enhance therapeutic effects.

Adverse Effects and Precautions

Methenamine is relatively safe and generally well tolerated. Gastric distress occurs occasionally, presumably from formaldehyde release in the stomach. Use of enteric-coated preparations may reduce this response. Chronic high-dose therapy can cause bladder irritation, manifested as dysuria, frequent voiding, urinary urgency, proteinuria, and hematuria. Since decomposition of methenamine generates ammonia (in addition to formaldehyde), the drug is contraindicated for patients with liver dysfunction. Methenamine salts (methenamine mandelate, methenamine hippurate) should not be used by patients with renal impairment, since crystalluria may be caused by precipitation of the mandelate or hippurate moiety.

Drug Interactions

Urinary Alkalinizers. Drugs that elevate urinary pH (e.g., acetazolamide, sodium bicarbonate) will inhibit formaldehyde production, and will thereby reduce the antibacterial effects of methenamine. Patients should not be given alkalinizing agents.

Sulfonamides. Methenamine should not be combined with sulfonamides: formaldehyde forms an insoluble complex with sulfonamides, thereby posing a risk of urinary tract injury from crystalluria.

Preparations, Dosage, and Administration

Methenamine is dispensed in tablets for oral administration. The usual adult dosage is 1 gm four times a day. The dosage for children aged 6 to 12 years is 500 mg four times a day. For children under the age of 6 years, the usual dosage is 50 mg/kg/day in three divided doses.

Methenamine mandelate [Mandelamine, Mandameth] is dispensed in tablets (plain and enteric coated), a suspension, and granules—all for oral use. Dosages are the same as for methenamine.

Methenamine hippurate [Hiprex, Urex] is dispensed in 1-gm tablets for oral administration. The dosage for adults and children over the age of 12 years is 1 gm two times a day. For children aged 6 to 12 years, the dosage is 500 mg to 1 gm twice a day.

NALIDIXIC ACID

Mechanism of Action

Nalidixic acid [NegGram], a chemical relative of the fluoroquinolones, inhibits replication of bacterial DNA, thereby causing DNA degradation and cell death. The precise target of nalidixic acid is *DNA gyrase*, the bacterial enzyme that converts closed-circular DNA into a supercoiled configuration; if supercoiling does not occur, DNA replication cannot take place.

Microbial Resistance

Resistant bacteria often emerge during treatment. Two mechanisms for resistance have been described: (1) production of an altered DNA gyrase with reduced sensitivity to nalidixic acid, and (2) reduced bacterial uptake of nalidixic acid. Cross-resistance with cinoxacin is common. A frequent factor in resistance is treatment with suboptimal doses. (Low levels of nalidixic acid favor overgrowth with drug-resistant organisms.) Fortunately, resistance to nalidixic acid is not carried on R factors, and, therefore, is not transferable.

Antimicrobial Spectrum

Nalidixic acid is active against most gram-negative urinary tract pathogens, including *E. coli*, *Klebsiella*, *Enterobacter*, and *Proteus species*. *Pseudomonas aeruginosa* is resistant, as are most gram-positive aerobic cocci.

Therapeutic Uses

Nalidixic acid is approved only for treatment of UTIs. This drug has been used to control acute infection and for prophy-laxis against recurrent UTI. However, for both applications, other drugs are preferred. Nalidixic acid is not useful against infections outside the urinary tract.

Pharmacokinetics

Nalidixic acid is well absorbed from the gastrointestinal tract, and then undergoes rapid hepatic metabolism. Only one metabolite—hydroxynalidixic acid—has antibacterial actions. Nalidixic acid and its metabolites are excreted in the urine. The concentration of active drug in urine is about ten times greater than in plasma. Therapeutic levels are achieved in urine even in patients with moderate-to-severe renal impairment. Drug concentrations outside the urinary tract are too low for antibacterial effects.

Adverse Effects

Although nalidixic acid can cause multiple untoward effects, the incidence of severe reactions is low. The most common effects are gastrointestinal disturbances (nausea, vomiting, abdominal discomfort), rash, and visual disturbances (blurred vision, diplopia, poor accommodation, photophobia, altered color perception). Patients experiencing altered visual acuity should exercise appropriate caution. Photosensitivity reactions can occur; patients should be advised to avoid excessive exposure to sunlight, wear protective clothing, and apply a sunscreen to exposed skin. Convulsions have occurred on occasion; accordingly, nalidixic acid is contraindicated for individuals with a history of convulsive disorders. Nalidixic acid may produce intracranial hypertension in pediatric patients; the drug should not be administered to children under the age of 3 months. Blood dyscrasias (thrombocytopenia, leukopenia, hemolytic anemia) and jaundice are rare; however, when nalidixic acid is used for more than 2 weeks, blood cell counts and liver function tests should be performed.

Drug Interactions

Nalidixic acid can intensify the effects of oral anticoagulants (e.g., warfarin) by displacing these agents from binding sites on plasma proteins. Accordingly, when an oral anticoagulant is combined with nalidixic acid, a reduction in anticoagulant dosage may be needed.

Preparations, Dosage, and Administration

Nalidixic acid [NegGram] is dispensed in tablets (250 mg, 500 mg, 1 gm) and in suspension (50 mg/ml) for oral use. The adult dosage is 1 gm four times a day for 1 week. For children under the age of 12 years, the dosage is 55 mg/kg/day in four divided doses. Nalidixic acid should not be given to children less than 3 months old.

CINOXACIN

Cinoxacin [Cinobac] is a close chemical relative of nalidixic acid. Both drugs have the same mechanism of action, antimicrobial spectrum, and indications. Furthermore, organisms that are resistant to nalidixic acid are often resistant to cinoxacin. As with other urinary tract antiseptics, therapeutic levels of cinoxacin are achieved only in the urine. Adverse effects are like those of nalidixic acid, but their incidence is relatively low. Cinoxacin is excreted by the kidneys, primarily as the unchanged drug. The drug is dispensed in 250- and 500-mg capsules for oral use. The usual adult dosage is 1 gm/day administered in two or four divided doses. The dosage should be reduced in patients with renal impairment; failure to do so could result in accumulation of cinoxacin to toxic levels.

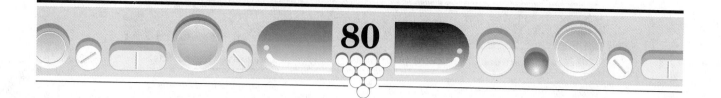
Drugs for Sexually Transmitted Diseases

CHLAMYDIA TRACHOMATIS INFECTIONS

GONOCOCCAL INFECTIONS

NONGONOCOCCAL URETHRITIS

PELVIC INFLAMMATORY DISEASE

ACUTE EPIDIDYMITIS

SYPHILIS

ACQUIRED IMMUNODEFICIENCY SYNDROME

CHANCROID

TRICHOMONIASIS

BACTERIAL VAGINOSIS

HERPES SIMPLEX INFECTIONS

GENITAL AND ANAL WARTS (CONDYLOMA ACUMINATUM)

PEDICULOSIS PUBIS AND SCABIES

Sexually transmitted diseases (STDs) are defined as infectious or parasitic diseases that are transmitted primarily through sexual contact. STDs are common in the United States and constitute a major public health problem. Our objective in this chapter is to describe the principal STDs and provide an overview of their drug therapy. Table 80–1 presents a summary of the common STDs, their causative organisms, and the drugs of choice for treatment.

CHLAMYDIA TRACHOMATIS INFECTIONS

Chlamydia trachomatis is the most common cause of bacterial STD in the United States. The various strains of this organism can cause genital tract infections, proctitis, conjunctivitis, neonatal ophthalmia and pneumonia, and lymphogranuloma venereum. Drugs of choice for these infections are summarized in Table 80–1.

Genital Tract Infections. Genital tract infections (e.g., urethritis, cervicitis, epididymitis) with *C. trachomatis* are common. About 3 million new cases develop each year. One reason for this explosive spread is the mild nature of symptoms, especially in women. Unfortunately, although symp-

997

Table 80–1. Sexually Transmitted Diseases: Causative Organisms and Drugs of Choice

Disease or Syndrome	Drug(s) of Choice	Causative Organism(s)
Chlamydia trachomatis Infections		*Chlamydia trachomatis*
Urethritis Cervicitis Proctitis Conjunctivitis	Doxycycline (PO)	
Infection in pregnancy	Erythromycin (PO)	

Neonatal infections:
  Ophthalmia
  Pneumonia
	Erythromycin (PO or IV)	

Lymphogranuloma venereum	Doxycycline (PO)	
Gonococcal Infections (Gonorrhea)		*Neisseria gonorrhoeae*
Urethral Cervical Rectal Pharyngeal Ophthalmia (adults)	Ceftriaxone (IM)	
Bacteremia Arthritis Meningitis	Ceftriaxone (IM or IV) *or* cefotaxime (IV)	
Neonatal ophthalmia	Ceftriaxone (IM) *or* cefotaxime (IM or IV)	
Nongonococcal Urethritis	Doxycycline (PO)	*Chlamydia trachomatis, Ureaplasma urealyticum, Trichomonas vaginalis*
Pelvic Inflammatory Disease (PID)		*Neisseria gonorrhoeae, Chlamydia trachomatis*

Inpatients	Initial therapy:
	  Doxycycline (IV) *plus either* cefoxitin (IV) *or* cefotetan (IV)
	Followed by:
	  Doxycycline (PO)	

Outpatients	Initial therapy:
	  Ceftriaxone (IM) *or* cefoxitin (IM) combined with probenecid (PO)
	Followed by:
	  Doxycycline (PO)	

Sexually Acquired Epididymitis	Ceftriaxone (IM) followed by doxycycline (PO)	*Chlamydia trachomatis, Neisseria gonorrhoeae*
Syphilis		*Treponema pallidum*
Early stage (primary, secondary, or latent syphilis of less than 1 year's duration) Late stage (syphilis of more than 1 year's duration)	Benzathine penicillin G (IM)	
Neurosyphilis	Penicillin G (IV)	
Congenital syphilis	Penicillin G (IV) *or* procaine penicillin G (IM)	

Table 80–1. Sexually Transmitted Diseases: Causative Organisms and Drugs of Choice *Continued*

Disease or Syndrome	Drug(s) of Choice	Causative Organism(s)
Acquired Immunodeficiency Syndrome (AIDS)	Zidovudine (PO)	*Human immunodeficiency virus*
Bacterial Vaginosis	Metronidazole (PO)	*Gardnerella vaginalis, Mycoplasma hominis, various anaerobes*
Trichomoniasis	Metronidazole (PO)	*Trichomonas vaginalis*
Chancroid	Erythromycin (PO) *or* ceftriaxone (IM)	*Haemophilus ducreyi*
Herpes simplex	Acyclovir (PO or IV)	*Herpes simplex virus*
Genital and Anal Warts	Preferred treatment: Cryotherapy Alternative treatments: Podophyllum resin *or* trichloroacetic acid (both topical)	*Human papillomavirus*
Pediculosis Pubis	Lindane *or* 1% permethrin (both topical)	*Phthirus pubis* (pubic lice)
Scabies	Lindane *or* 5% permethrin (both topical)	*Sarcoptes scabiei*

toms are mild, infection is not benign: the Centers for Disease Control and Prevention (CDC) estimates that these infections cause sterility in up to 50,000 women each year, primarily from fallopian tube scarring.

For uncomplicated urethral, cervical, or rectal infections in adults, the recommended treatment is 100 mg of oral *doxycycline* twice daily for 7 days. For patients who cannot take tetracyclines, *erythromycin* or *ofloxacin* may be used.

Infection in Pregnancy. The drug of choice for *C. trachomatis* infections during pregnancy is *erythromycin*. Either of three preparations may be used: erythromycin base, erythromycin stearate, or erythromycin ethylsuccinate. Erythromycin *estolate* is contraindicated during pregnancy because of the risk of maternal liver injury. For women who cannot take erythromycin, *amoxicillin* can be used as a substitute. Although doxycycline and other tetracyclines are active against *C. trachomatis*, these drugs are contraindicated because they can damage fetal teeth and bones. Similarly, sulfisoxazole and other sulfonamides are active, but these drugs are contraindicated near term because they can cause kernicterus in the infant. When attempting to control *C. trachomatis* infection in pregnancy, simultaneous therapy of the male sexual partner is essential.

Neonatal Ophthalmia and Pneumonia. About half the infants born to women with cervical *C. trachomatis* acquire the infection during the birth process. These infants are at risk for conjunctivitis and pneumonia. Pneumonia is generally not severe and lasts about 6 weeks. Conjunctivitis does not result in blindness and spontaneously resolves in 6 months. The preferred treatment for both infections is systemic *erythromycin*, 12.5 mg/kg (PO or IV) four times daily for 1 week. Although topical erythromycin, tetracycline, or silver nitrate may be given to prevent conjunctivitis, none of these treatments is completely effective.

Lymphogranuloma Venereum. Lymphogranuloma venereum (LGV) is caused by a unique strain of *C. trachomatis*. Transmission is strictly by sexual contact. LGV is most common in tropical countries, but does occur in the United States, especially in the South. Infection begins as a small erosion or papule in the genital region. From this site, the organism migrates to regional lymph nodes, causing swelling, tenderness, and blockage of lymphatic flow. Tremendous enlargement of the genitalia may result. The enlarged nodes, called buboes, may break open and drain. The treatment of choice for genital, inguinal, and anorectal LGV is *doxycycline*, 100 mg PO twice daily for 3 weeks. *Erythromycin* may be used as a substitute.

GONOCOCCAL INFECTIONS

Gonorrhea. This infection is caused by *Neisseria gonorrhoeae*, a gram-negative diplococcus frequently referred to as the gonococcus. The incidence of gonorrhea is high: about 700,000 cases are reported annually, and we can assume that many more go unreported. Gonorrhea is transmitted primarily by sexual contact, although it can also be transmitted by contact with infected exudates.

The intensity of symptoms differs between men and women. In men, the main symptoms are a burning sensation while urinating and a puslike discharge from the penis. In contrast, gonorrhea in women is commonly asymptomatic. However, serious infection of female reproductive structures (vagina, urethra, cervix, ovaries, fallopian tubes) can occur, ultimately resulting in sterility. Among people who engage in oral sex, the mouth and throat can become infected, causing a sore throat and tonsillitis. Among people who engage in receptive anal sex, the rectum can become infected, causing a purulent discharge and constant urge to move the bowels. Bacteremia can develop in both sexes, causing cutaneous lesions, arthritis, and, rarely, meningitis and endocarditis.

Because of antibiotic resistance, treatment of gonorrhea has changed over the years—and undoubtedly will continue to evolve. In the 1930's, virtually all strains of the gonococcus were sensitive to sulfonamides. However, within a decade, sulfonamide resistance had become common. Fortunately, by this time penicillin had become available, and the drug was active against all gonococcal strains. However, in 1976, organisms resistant to penicillin began to emerge. Currently, about 10% of gonococci in the United States are penicillin resistant. Tetracycline resistance has also been noted.

At this time, the drug of choice for uncomplicated gonorrhea is *ceftriaxone*, administered as a single IM dose (125 to 250 mg). For patients who cannot use ceftriaxone, alternatives are cefixime, ciprofloxacin, and ofloxacin. Since patients infected with *N. gonorrhoeae* very frequently are co-infected with *C. trachomatis*, treatment should always include a course of oral doxycycline (or erythromycin if doxycycline cannot be used).

For disseminated gonorrhea (bacteremia, arthritis, meningitis), parenteral therapy is required. Cefotaxime (IV) or ceftriaxone (IV or IM) is recommended.

Gonococcal Neonatal Ophthalmia. This infection is acquired from an infected mother during the birthing process. The initial symptom is conjunctivitis. Over time, other structures of the eye become involved. Blindness can result. Gonococcal ophthalmia is prevented by applying a topical drug to the conjunctival sac immediately postpartum.

Any of three agents is effective: *0.5% erythromycin, 1% tetracycline,* or *1% silver nitrate.* For infants with active ophthalmia, parenteral therapy with ceftriaxone (IM) or cefotaxime (IM or IV) is indicated.

NONGONOCOCCAL URETHRITIS

Nongonococcal urethritis (NGU) is defined as urethritis caused by any organism other than *Neisseria gonorrhoeae*, the gonococcus. The most common infectious agents are *Chlamydia trachomatis* (25% to 40%), *Ureaplasma urealyticum* (about 20%), and *Trichomonas vaginalis* (<5%). NGU is diagnosed by the presence of polymorphonuclear leukocytes and a negative culture for *N. gonorrhoeae*. The infection is especially prevalent among sexually active adolescent girls. The drug of choice for NGU is *doxycycline*. Dosage is 100 mg twice daily for 7 days. In patients for whom doxycycline is contraindicated (pregnant women, young children), *erythromycin* can be used instead.

PELVIC INFLAMMATORY DISEASE

Acute pelvic inflammatory disease (PID) is a syndrome that includes endometritis, pelvic peritonitis, tubo-ovarian abscess, and inflammation of the fallopian tubes. Infertility can result. Prominent symptoms are abdominal pain, vaginal discharge, and fever. Most frequently, PID is caused by *Neisseria gonorrhoeae* and/or *Chlamydia trachomatis*. However, *Mycoplasma hominis* as well as assorted anaerobic and facultative bacteria may also be involved.

Because multiple organisms are likely to be involved, drug therapy must provide broad coverage. Since no single drug can do this, combination therapy is required. For the hospitalized patient, treatment can be initiated with IV *doxycycline* plus either *IV cefoxitin* or *IV cefotetan*. This IV therapy is followed by oral therapy with *doxycycline*. The entire course of treatment takes 10 to 14 days. For the outpatient, treatment can be initiated with either *ceftriaxone* (IM) or *cefoxitin* (IM) combined with probenecid (PO). This IM therapy is followed by oral therapy with *doxycycline* for 10 to 14 days. Since PID can be difficult to treat, and since the consequences of failure can be severe (e.g., sterility), many experts recommend that all patients receive intravenous antibiotics in a hospital.

ACUTE EPIDIDYMITIS

Epididymitis may be acquired by sexual contact or nonsexually. Sexually acquired epididymitis is usually caused by *Neisseria gonorrhoeae* and/or *Chlamydia trachomatis*. This syndrome occurs primarily in young adults (under 35 years) and may be associated with urethritis. Primary symptoms are fever accompanied by pain in the back of the testicles that develops over the course of several hours. The infection can be treated with a single IM dose of *ceftriaxone* (250 mg) followed by 10 days of treatment with oral *doxycycline* (300 mg twice daily). Testicular pain can be managed with analgesics, bed rest, and ice packs.

Nonsexually transmitted epididymitis generally occurs in older men and men who have had urinary tract instrumentation. Causative organisms are gram-negative enteric bacilli and *Pseudomonas*. Ciprofloxacin can be used for treatment.

SYPHILIS

Syphilis is caused by the spirochete *Treponema pallidum*. The incidence of syphilis has increased steadily over the past decade to reach its highest rate in 40 years. Fortunately, *T. pallidum* has remained highly responsive to penicillin, the drug of choice for treatment.

Characteristics. Syphilis develops in three stages, termed primary, secondary, and tertiary. *T. pallidum* enters the body by penetrating the mucous membranes of the mouth, vagina, or urethra of the penis. After an incubation period of 1 to 4 weeks, a primary lesion, called a chancre, develops at the site of entry. The chancre is a hard, red, protruding, painless sore. Nearby lymph nodes may become swollen. Within a few weeks the chancre heals spontaneously, although *T. pallidum* is still present.

Two to six weeks after the chancre heals, secondary syphilis develops. Symptoms result from spread of *T. pallidum* via the bloodstream. Skin lesions and flulike symptoms (fever, headache, reduced appetite, general malaise) are typical. Enlarged lymph nodes and joint pain may also be present. The symptoms of secondary syphilis resolve in 4 to 8 weeks—but then may recur episodically over the next 3 to 4 years.

Tertiary syphilis develops 5 to 40 years after the initial infection. Almost any organ can be involved. Infection of the brain—neurosyphilis—is common, and can cause senility, paralysis, and severe psychiatric symptoms. The heart valves and aorta may be damaged. Lesions may also occur in the skin, bones, joints, and eyes. The risk of neurosyphilis is increased in individuals who are infected with the human immunodeficiency virus (HIV).

Infants exposed to *T. pallidum in utero* can be born with syphilis. Signs of congenital syphilis include sores, rhinitis, severe tenderness over bones, and deafness.

Treatment. *Penicillin G* is the drug of choice for all stages of syphilis. The form and dosage of penicillin G depend on the disease stage. *Early syphilis* (primary, secondary, or latent syphilis of less than 1 year's duration) is treated with a single IM dose (2.4 million units) of benzathine penicillin G . *Late syphilis* (more than 1 year's duration) is also treated with IM benzathine penicillin G, but the dosage is increased (2.4 million units once a week for 3 weeks). *Neurosyphilis* requires more aggressive therapy. The recommended treatment is 2 to 4 million units of *intravenous* penicillin G every 4 hours for 10 to 14 days. For *congenital syphilis*, two regimens have been recommended: (1) IV penicillin G, 50,000 units/kg every 8 to 12 hours for 10 to 14 days, or (2) IM procaine penicillin G, 50,000 units/kg once daily for 10 to 14 days. *Syphilis in pregnancy* should be treated with penicillin G, using a dosage appropriate to the stage of the disease. If a pregnant woman is allergic to penicillins, the U.S Public Health Service recommends that she go through a penicillin-allergy desensitization protocol to permit penicillin use, rather than substituting another drug for penicillin.

ACQUIRED IMMUNODEFICIENCY SYNDROME

Characteristics. Acquired immunodeficiency syndrome (AIDS) is caused by the human immunodeficiency virus (HIV). Since its identification as a new disease in 1981, AIDS has become a worldwide epidemic. Millions of people are infected. The costs of caring for AIDS patients are staggering—about 10.3 billion dollars in 1992 in the United States alone. The personal and social costs are incalculable.

AIDS is transmitted sexually and by other means. HIV is present in all body fluids of infected individuals. Transmission can be via intimate contact with blood, semen, and vaginal secretions. The disease can be transmitted by sexual contact, transfusion, and accidental needle sticks. In addition, it can be transmitted to the developing fetus by an infected mother. Initially, HIV infection was limited largely to homosexual males, intravenous drug abusers, and hemophiliacs. However, the disease can now be found routinely in the population at large. The risk of contracting HIV can be greatly reduced by use of condoms and by screening blood supplies for the virus.

HIV can damage many cell types—especially those of the immune and nervous systems. By attacking cells of the nervous system, the virus can cause dementia and peripheral neuropathies. By attacking cells of the immune system, the virus can greatly compromise the ability to mount an immune response. Immune suppression predisposes the patient to neoplasms (e.g., Kaposi's sarcoma, a rare form of skin cancer) and to opportunistic infections, such as those caused by *Pneumocystis carinii, Candida albicans*, cytomegalovirus, herpes simplex virus, *Treponema pallidum*, and *Mycobacterium tuberculosis*. The drugs used to treat these AIDS-associated infections are summarized in Table 80–2. It should be noted that because HIV has a long and highly variable incubation period, neurologic and immunodeficiency symptoms may not appear until years after the infection was actually acquired.

Symptoms of immune deficiency result primarily from depletion of T-helper lymphocytes. In particular, the virus attacks T_4 lymphocytes that carry the CD4 protein—a protein that acts as a receptor for HIV. Since T cells play a central role in the immune response, it is no wonder that their depletion has such devastating effects. In addition to infecting T cells, HIV can infect monocytes and macrophages, both of which carry the CD4 receptor. Infected monocytes are not killed by HIV and, hence, can act as a reservoir for the virus. Infected

Table 80–2. Drugs of Choice for AIDS-Associated Infections

AIDS-Associated Infection	Drugs of Choice	Alternative Drugs
Pneumocystis carinii Pneumonia		
Active infection	Trimethoprim + sulfamethoxazole **or** Pentamidine	Trimethoprim + dapsone **or** clindamycin + primaquine **or** Trimetrexate + folinic acid
Prophylaxis	Trimethoprim + sulfamethoxazole	Dapsone **or** Pentamidine aerosol
Toxoplasmosis	Pyrimethamine + sulfadiazine	Pyrimethamine + clindamycin
Candidiasis		
Oral	Nystatin solution or tablets **or** Clotrimazole troches	Ketoconazole **or** Fluconazole
Esophageal	Fluconazole **or** Ketoconazole	Amphotericin B
Coccidioidomycosis		
Active infection	Amphotericin B	Fluconazole
Suppressive therapy	Amphotericin B	Ketoconazole
Cryptococcosis		
Active infection	Amphotericin B ± flucytosine	Fluconazole **or** itraconazole
Suppressive therapy	Fluconazole	Amphotericin B
Histoplasmosis	Amphotericin B	Itraconazole
Cytomegalovirus	Ganciclovir	Foscarnet
Herpes Simplex Virus	Acyclovir	Foscarnet
Varicella Zoster	Acyclovir	Foscarnet
Dermatomal Zoster	Acyclovir	Foscarnet
Syphilis		
Early stage	Benzathine penicillin G **or** Doxycycline **or** Erythromycin	For all stages: Amoxicillin + probenecid **or** Doxycycline **or** Ceftriaxone **or** Benzathine penicillin G + doxycycline
Late stage	Benzathine penicillin G **or** Doxycycline	
Neurosyphilis	Aqueous penicillin G **or** procaine penicillin G + probenecid	
Tuberculosis		
Active infection	Isoniazid + pyrazinamide + rifampin + ethambutol	
Prophylaxis	Isoniazid	
Disseminated Mycobacterium Avium Complex	Clarithromycin or azithromycin, either one combined with one or more of the following: ethambutol, clofazimine, ciprofloxacin, amikacin	

macrophages are the major cell type that harbors HIV in the brain, perhaps contributing to neurologic symptoms.

Treatment. *Zidovudine* (azidothymidine, AZT) is the current drug of choice for HIV-infected people. The drug suppresses viral replication, but does not kill the virus. Accordingly, AZT does not offer cure, but it can (1) delay onset of symptoms, (2) reduce severity of symptoms, and (3) significantly prolong life. When taken early in the course of HIV infection, AZT can delay progression of early AIDS-related complex (ARC) to advanced ARC and full-blown AIDS. Also, treatment can increase CD4 T-lymphocyte counts, reduce the incidence of opportunistic infections, and reduce titers of p24 antigen (a marker protein for HIV). Additional benefits include weight gain and, perhaps, improvement in neurologic status. Since AZT does not eradicate the virus, patients should be warned that treatment will not prevent transmission of HIV by sexual contact. The major adverse effects of AZT are hematologic: anemia, neutropenia, and thrombocytopenia. The basic pharmacology of AZT is discussed in Chapter 84 (Antiviral Agents).

Two newer drugs—*didanosine* (dideoxyinosine, ddI) and *zalcitabine* (dideoxycytidine, ddC)—may be used as alternatives to AZT in patients unresponsive to or intolerant of AZT. Like AZT, both ddI and ddC act by suppressing viral replication. The basic pharmacology of these drugs is discussed in Chapter 84. In addition to these agents, more than 50 other drugs are currently under investigation as possible treatments for HIV infection.

CHANCROID

Chancroid, also known as soft chancre, is caused by *Haemophilus ducreyi*. Transmission is primarily by sexual contact. The infection is characterized by a painful, ragged ulcer at the site of inoculation, usually the external genitalia. Regional lymph nodes may be swollen. Multiple secondary lesions may develop. Although primarily a tropical disease, chancroid has become an important STD in the United States. Recommended treatments are (1) *ceftriaxone*, 250 mg IM as a single injection, and (2) *erythromycin*, 500 mg PO four times daily for 7 days.

TRICHOMONIASIS

Trichomoniasis is an STD caused by *Trichomonas vaginalis*. In women, the infection may be asymptomatic or may cause a thin, watery vaginal discharge, along with burning and itching sensations. In men, the infection is usually symptom-

free. Most infections can be eliminated with a single, 2-gram dose of *metronidazole*. This dose can be repeated in the event of treatment failure. Metronidazole is contraindicated during the first trimester of pregnancy, but can be taken during the second and third trimesters. Although they may be asymptomatic, male partners of infected women may also be infected and should be treated.

BACTERIAL VAGINOSIS

Bacterial vaginosis results from an alteration in vaginal microflora. Organisms responsible for the syndrome include *Gardnerella vaginalis* (also known as *Haemophilus vaginalis*), *Mycoplasma hominis*, and various anaerobes. The syndrome occurs most commonly in sexually active women, but may not actually be transmitted sexually. Bacterial vaginosis is characterized by a malodorous vaginal discharge, elevation of vaginal pH (above 4.5), and generation of a fishy odor when vaginal secretions are mixed with 10% potassium hydroxide. The recommended treatment is oral *metronidazole*, 500 mg twice a day for 7 days.

HERPES SIMPLEX INFECTIONS

Characteristics. Most genital herpes infections are caused by herpes simplex virus type 2 (HSV-2). A few genital infections are caused by herpes simplex virus type 1, the herpesvirus that causes cold sores. Genital herpes is transmitted primarily by sexual contact. In the United States, the infection has reached epidemic proportions, afflicting some 20 million people. There is no cure.

Symptoms of primary infection develop 6 to 8 days after contact. In females, blisters or vesicles can appear on the perianal skin, labia, vagina, cervix, and foreskin of the clitoris. In males, vesicles develop on the penis and occasionally on the testicles. Painful urination and a watery discharge can occur in both sexes. Also, the patient may experience systemic symptoms: fever, headache, myalgia, and tender, swollen lymph nodes in the affected region. Within days, the original blisters can evolve into large, painful, ulcer-like sores. Over the next 2 to 3 weeks, all symptoms resolve spontaneously. However, this does not indicate cure: the virus remains present in a latent state and can cause recurrence. Since we can't eliminate the virus, symptoms may recur for life. Fortunately, subsequent episodes become progressively shorter and less severe, and in some cases cease entirely. Transmission of HSV-2 can occur during the symptomatic period and for one week after. Infected individuals should avoid sexual contact during this time. Use of a condom reduces the risk of transmission.

Neonatal Infection. Genital herpes in pregnant women can be transmitted to the infant. The infant can acquire the virus *in utero* or during delivery. Infection acquired *in utero* can result in spontaneous abortion or fetal malformation. Infection acquired during delivery can cause severe neurologic damage and even death. To protect the infant during delivery, birth should be accomplished by cesarean section if the mother has an active infection.

Treatment. *Acyclovir* is the drug of choice for genital herpes. Although this drug cannot eliminate the virus, it can reduce systemic symptoms and shorten the duration of pain and viral shedding. When taken continuously, it can decrease the rate of recurrence. Depending on the intensity of symptoms, administration may be oral or intravenous. Topical administration may also be used, but is not very effective. Patients should be warned that acyclovir will not protect against transmission of HSV-2 when infections are active and that sexual intimacy should be avoided at these times. The pharmacology of acyclovir is discussed in Chapter 84.

GENITAL AND ANAL WARTS (CONDYLOMA ACUMINATUM)

Genital and perianal warts are caused by human papillomaviruses (HPVs), of which there are 40 different types. Although warts caused by most types of HPV are benign, warts caused by a few types have been strongly associated with genital carcinoma. Accordingly, a wart biopsy may be appropriate.

HPV can be transmitted by sexual contact. Individuals with anogenital warts should be warned that they can transmit the infection to sexual partners. Partners of infected individuals should be examined for warts. Use of a condom can minimize the risk of transmission.

Several forms of therapy are used to remove venereal warts. However, no form of therapy has been shown to eradicate the virus. Hence, even after successful wart removal, the virus is likely to still be present.

For most patients with external genital or perianal warts, cryotherapy (freezing) is the treatment of choice. This can be done with liquid nitrogen or a cryoprobe. Alternatives to cryotherapy include topical drugs, electrodesiccation, electrocautery, laser surgery, and conventional surgery.

Of the drugs used to treat venereal warts, *podophyllum resin* (podophyllin) is employed most widely. Podophyllum resin is a mixture of resins from the May apple or mandrake (*Podophyllum peltatum Linne*). The active ingredient in the resin is podophyllotoxin. Formulations used to remove warts contain 25% podophyllum resin. These formulations are highly caustic and should be applied only by a trained physician. To minimize the risk of toxicity from systemic absorption, the resin should be washed off with alcohol or with soap and water within 1 to 4 hours of its application. Each treatment should be limited to a small surface area and to a small number of warts. A similar but less caustic preparation (0.5% podofilox), marketed under the trade name Condylox, is available for use at home. Topical *trichloroacetic acid* is an alternative to podophyllin.

PEDICULOSIS PUBIS AND SCABIES

Pediculosis pubis and scabies are skin infestations caused by lice and mites, respectively. Both infestations produce intense itching, and both can be transmitted by sexual contact. Topical *lindane* or *permethrin* can eliminate both organisms. Pediculosis, scabies, and the drugs used for treatment are discussed in Chapter 88 (Ectoparasiticides).

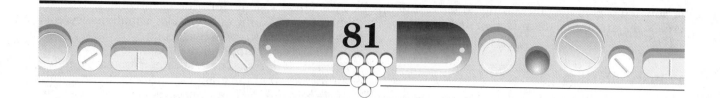
Antimycobacterial Agents: Drugs for Tuberculosis and Leprosy

O ur focus in this chapter is on tuberculosis and leprosy, diseases caused by mycobacteria. The mycobacteria are slow-growing microbes, and the infections they cause require prolonged treatment. Because therapy is prolonged, drug toxicity and poor patient compliance can be significant clinical problems. In addition, prolonged treatment presents a high risk of causing the emergence of drug-resistant bacteria.

PATHOGENESIS OF TUBERCULOSIS

Tuberculosis is an infectious disease caused by *Mycobacterium tuberculosis*, an organism also known as the tubercle bacillus. Infections may be limited to the lungs or may be disseminated. In the United States, approximately 10 million people harbor tubercle bacilli. In most cases, the bacteria are quiescent, and the infected individual is free of symptoms. However, when the disease is active, morbidity can be significant; about 2000 Americans die from tuberculosis annually. After years of being on the decline, the number of reported cases of tuberculosis is now increasing. Much of this increase is attributed to infection in people with AIDS.

Primary Infection

Infection with *M. tuberculosis* is acquired by inhaling infected sputum that has been aerosolized by coughing or sneezing. Hence, initial infection is in the lung. Once in the lung, tubercle bacilli are taken up by phagocytic cells (macrophages and neutrophils). Initially, these organisms are resistant to the destructive activity of phagocytes and they multiply freely within them. Infection can spread from the lungs to other organs via the lymphatic and circulatory systems.

In most cases, immunity to *M. tuberculosis* develops within a few weeks, and the infection is brought under complete control. The immune system facilitates control by increasing the ability of phagocytes to suppress multiplication of tubercle bacilli. Because of this rapid response by the immune system, most individuals with primary infection never develop clinical or radiologic evidence of disease. However, even though symptoms are absent and the progression of infection is halted, the infected individual is likely to harbor tubercle bacilli lifelong (unless drugs are given to eliminate quiescent bacilli). Hence, in the absence of treatment, the threat of reactivation of the infection is ever present.

Reactivation

In the United States, most cases of active tuberculosis are thought to result from reactivation of latent tubercle bacilli. That is, active infection is caused by multiplication of tubercle bacilli that had been dormant following control of a primary infection by host defenses. Reactivation often produces necrosis and cavitation of lung tissue. Lung tissue may also become caseous (cheeselike in appearance). Since phagocytes do not function at sites of necrosis, cellular immunity is unable to suppress the active infection. In the absence of treatment, progressive tissue destruction may result in death.

DIAGNOSIS OF TUBERCULOSIS

Screening of Asymptomatic Individuals

In order to eliminate tuberculosis, it is essential that we detect and treat individuals with asymptomatic infection. Detection is accomplished by screen testing. It is recommended that all high-risk persons be screened. In this group are those with HIV infection, health care workers, and those with other risk factors for tuberculosis, such as chronic renal failure, hematologic malignancy, and use of immunosuppressive drugs.

The screen employed most commonly is the *tuberculin skin test*. The test is performed by giving an intradermal injection of a protein derived from *M. tuberculosis*. (The protein is referred to as *purified protein derivative*, or *PPD*.) The test is read 48 to 72 hours after injection. In people harboring tubercle bacilli, injection of PPD can elicit a local hypersensitivity reaction. A positive reaction is indicated by the size of the zone of induration (hardness)—not the zone of erythema (redness). It should be noted that false-negative results are common, and can be as high as 70% in patients with AIDS.

Diagnosis

If an individual has a positive tuberculin skin test or clinical manifestations that suggest tuberculosis, diagnostic testing for tuberculosis should be done. A definitive diagnosis is made with chest x-rays and microbiologic evaluation of sputum. A chest x-ray should be ordered for all persons suspected of active infection.

Sputum is evaluated in two ways: (1) by microscopic examination of sputum smears, and (2) by culturing sputum samples. Microscopic examination cannot provide a definitive diagnosis. This is because direct observation cannot distinguish between *Mycobacterium tuberculosis* and other mycobacteria. Furthermore, microscopic examination is much less sensitive than culturing. Accordingly, sputum cultures are required for definitive diagnosis. Because *M. tuberculosis* grows very slowly, results of sputum cultures are often delayed (by as long as 3 to 6 weeks). However, with newer culturing techniques, results have been obtained in less than 1 week. In addition to providing positive identification of *M. tuberculosis*, cultures are necessary to determine drug sensitivity.

OVERVIEW OF ANTITUBERCULOUS THERAPY

BASIC PRINCIPLES OF TREATMENT

The availability of modern chemotherapeutic agents has dramatically altered the treatment of tuberculosis. Whereas patients once faced lengthy hospitalization, therapy can now be performed on an outpatient basis. Prolonged bed rest is not required, nor is it recommended.

The objective of antituberculous therapy is to eliminate symptoms of active disease and prevent relapse. To accomplish this goal, treatment must kill those tubercle bacilli that are actively dividing as well as those that are "resting." Success is indicated by an absence of observable mycobacteria in sputum and by the failure of sputum cultures to yield any colonies of tubercle bacilli. Once sputum tests have become negative (usually in 3 to 6 months), therapy should continue for an additional 3 to 6 months.

Antituberculous regimens must always contain two or more drugs. Because treatment is prolonged, there is a high risk that drug-resistant bacilli will emerge if only one antituberculous agent is employed. Since the chances of a bacterium developing resistance to two drugs is very low, treatment with two or more antibiotics minimizes the risk of drug resistance. Not only do drug combinations decrease the risk of resistance, combination therapy can reduce the incidence of relapse: since some drugs (e.g., isoniazid, rifampin) are especially effective against actively dividing bacilli, whereas other drugs (e.g., pyrazinamide) are most active against intracellular (quiescent) bacilli, by using certain combinations of antituberculous agents we can increase the chances of killing all tubercle bacilli present, whether they are actively multiplying or resting. Hence, the risk of relapse is lowered.

In Chapter 73 (Basic Considerations in the Chemotherapy of Infectious Diseases), we noted that therapy with multiple antibiotics broadens the spectrum of antimicrobial coverage, thereby increasing the risk of suprainfection. This is not the case with multiple drug therapy of tuberculosis. Most of the drugs used against *M. tuberculosis* are selective for this organism. As a result, these drugs, even when used in combination, do not kill off other microorganisms, and, therefore, do not create the conditions that lead to suprainfection.

CHEMOTHERAPY OF ACTIVE TUBERCULOSIS

A variety of regimens have been employed to treat active tuberculosis. Drug selection is based largely on drug susceptibility of the infecting organism and on the immunocompetency of the host. Most regimens contain isoniazid plus rifampin. In the event of suspected or proved resistance to these agents, additional drugs are added.

Standard Therapy. The two regimens used most frequently for initial therapy of uncomplicated tuberculosis are summarized in Table 81–1. The first regimen, named the *6-month short course,* has two phases. The initial phase consists of daily therapy with *isoniazid, rifampin,* and *pyrazinamide.* The second (and longer) phase consists of daily or biweekly therapy with *isoniazid* and *rifampin.* The goal of the initial phase is to eliminate actively dividing extracellular tubercle bacilli, thereby rendering the sputum noninfectious. The goal of the second phase is to eliminate intracellular "persisters." The *9-month short*

course, an alternative to the 6-month short course, consists of just two drugs: *isoniazid* and *rifampin.* These are taken daily for 1 month and then either daily or biweekly for another 8 months. Note that both regimens are prolonged, making compliance a significant problem.

Therapy in Patients with AIDS. Between 2% and 20% of patients with AIDS develop active tuberculosis. Because of their reduced ability to fight infection, these patients require more aggressive therapy than immunocompetent patients. The regimen employed has two phases (Table 81–2). The initial phase consists of daily therapy with four drugs: *isoniazid, rifampin, pyrazinamide,* and *ethambutol.* (Ethambutol is added to the regimen in patients with CNS involvement, disseminated tuberculosis, or suspected isoniazid resistance.) The second (and longer) phase consists of daily therapy with *isoniazid* and *rifampin.* In addition to patients with AIDS, this regimen is employed for (1) immunocompetent patients with severe disease (e.g., disseminated tuberculosis, tuberculous meningitis), (2) patients exposed to drug-resistant tubercle bacilli, and (3) patients who have emigrated from countries in which drug resistance is common.

EVALUATING THERAPY OF ACTIVE TUBERCULOSIS

Three modes are employed to evaluate therapy: chest x-rays, bacteriologic evaluation of sputum, and clinical evaluation.

In patients with positive pretreatment sputum tests, sputum should be evaluated monthly for tubercle bacilli. With proper drug selection and good compliance, nearly 100% of patients should have negative cultures after 6 months of treatment. Treatment failures should be evaluated for drug resistance and patient compliance. In the absence of demonstrated drug resistance, treatment with the same regimen should continue, using direct observation of drug administration to assure that medication is being taken as prescribed. In patients with drug-resistant tuberculosis, *two* effective drugs should be added to the regimen.

In patients with negative pretreatment sputum tests, treatment is monitored by chest x-rays and clinical evaluation. In most patients, clinical manifestations (e.g., fever, malaise, anorexia, cough) should decrease markedly within 2 weeks. The x-ray should show improvement within 3 months.

After completion of therapy, patients should be examined every 3 to 6 months for signs and symptoms of relapse.

PROPHYLAXIS WITH ISONIAZID

People who have been exposed to tuberculosis but have not developed active disease can be given

Table 81–1. Regimens for Initial Therapy of Uncomplicated Tuberculosis

Regimen	Dosages
6-Month Short Course	
Initial Phase (2 months)	ISONIAZID (if taken daily)
ISONIAZID *plus*	Adults: 5 mg/kg (max 300 mg)
RIFAMPIN *plus*	Children: 10–20 mg/kg (max 300 mg)
PYRAZINAMIDE	ISONIAZID (if taken biweekly)
All three drugs are taken *daily*	Adults: 15 mg/kg (max 900 mg)
	Children: 20–40 mg/kg (max 900 mg)
Second Phase (4 months)	RIFAMPIN (daily or biweekly)
ISONIAZID *plus*	Adults: 10 mg/kg (max 600 mg)
RIFAMPIN	Children: 10–20 mg/kg (max 600 mg)
Both drugs are taken *daily or biweekly*	PYRAZINAMIDE (daily)
	Adults: 20–30 mg/kg (max 2 gm)
	Children: same as adults
9-Month Short Course	
ISONIAZID *plus*	ISONIAZID (if taken daily)
RIFAMPIN	Adults: 300 mg
Both drugs are taken *daily for 9 months*	Children: 10 mg/kg (max 300 mg)
or	ISONIAZID (if taken biweekly)
after *1 month of daily therapy*, both may	Adults: 15 mg/kg (usually 900 mg)
be taken *biweekly*	Children: 20 mg/kg
	RIFAMPIN (daily or biweekly)
	Adults: 600 mg
	Children: 15 mg/kg (max 600 mg)

isoniazid for prophylaxis. The benefits of prophylaxis are twofold: (1) prevention of active tuberculosis in the person receiving treatment, and (2) prevention of the spread of infection to others. When used for prophylaxis, isoniazid is administered daily for 6 to 12 months. Isoniazid is the only drug shown to be effective for preventive therapy.

Candidates for prophylaxis include (1) HIV-infected individuals with significant reactions to a tuberculin test, (2) individuals in close contact with tuberculosis patients, and (3) newly infected individuals. Since the chance of developing serious disease is especially high among infants, adolescents, and patients undergoing immunosuppressive therapy, these people should almost always be treated. A comprehensive list of candidates for isoniazid prophylaxis is given in Table 81–3.

As a rule, the potential benefits of preventive therapy outweigh the risks of liver damage, the principal toxicity of isoniazid. However, because prophylaxis does carry some risk (hepatotoxicity), not everyone who has been exposed to tuberculosis is a candidate. Prophylaxis is contraindicated for individuals with liver disease and for those who have had serious adverse reactions to isoniazid in the past. Since the risk of isoniazid-induced liver

Table 81–2. Therapy of Tuberculosis in Patients with AIDS

Regimen	Dosage
Initial Phase (2 months)	
ISONIAZID *plus*	ISONIAZID
RIFAMPIN *plus*	Adults: 5 mg/kg (max 300 mg)
PYRAZINAMIDE *plus*	Children: 10–20 mg/kg (max 300 mg)
ETHAMBUTOL*	
All drugs are taken *daily*	RIFAMPIN
	Adults: 10 mg/kg (max 600 mg)
Second Phase	Children: 10–20 mg/kg (max 600 mg)
	PYRAZINAMIDE
ISONIAZID *plus*	Adults: 20–30 mg/kg (max 2 gm)
RIFAMPIN	Children: same as adults
Both drugs are taken *daily* for at least 7	ETHAMBUTOL
more months or for at least 6 months after	Adults: 15–25 mg/kg (max 2.5 gm)
sputum cultures become negative	Children: same as adults

*Ethambutol is added to the regimen in patients with CNS involvement, disseminated tuberculosis, or suspected isoniazid resistance.

Table 81–3. Individuals for Whom Isoniazid Prophylaxis Is Recommended (In Order of Priority)

1. HIV-infected persons with a significant reaction to a tuberculin test

2. Household members and other close contacts of patients with active pulmonary tuberculosis

3. Newly infected persons (i.e., those who have had a tuberculin skin test conversion during the previous 2 years)

4. Persons with a history of tuberculosis and inadequate chemotherapy

5. Persons with a positive tuberculin skin test and an abnormal chest x-ray consistent with previous (nonprogressive) tuberculous disease. These patients have a negative bacteriology and stable parenchymal lesions

6. Persons with significant reactions to a tuberculin skin test and who are at special risk of developing active tuberculosis. These include patients with:

—Silicosis
—Diabetes mellitus
—Certain hematologic and reticuloendothelial diseases (leukemia, Hodgkin's disease)
—End-stage renal disease
—Clinical conditions associated with substantial weight loss or chronic undernutrition, including the postgastrectomy state, intestinal bypass surgery, chronic peptic ulcer disease, chronic malabsorption syndromes, and carcinomas of the oropharynx and upper gastrointestinal tract that inhibit adequate nutritional intake

and patients undergoing:

—Prolonged therapy with glucocorticoids
—Immunosuppressive therapy

7. All tuberculin skin test reactors under age 35

Adapted from Drug Evaluations Annual 1993, p. 1600, Table 4. Chicago, American Medical Association, 1992.

damage increases significantly with advancing age, people over the age of 35 should not be treated routinely; rather, preventive therapy should be reserved for tuberculin-positive patients in whom other risk factors are present, such as diabetes, leukemia, or drug-induced immunosuppression. In the event of pregnancy, prophylaxis should be postponed until after delivery.

PHARMACOLOGY OF INDIVIDUAL ANTITUBERCULOUS AGENTS

Based on their clinical utility, the antituberculous drugs can be divided into two groups: first-line drugs and second-line drugs. The first-line drugs are *isoniazid, rifampin, pyrazinamide, ethambutol,* and *streptomycin.* Of these, isoniazid and rifampin are the most important. The second-line drugs—*para-aminosalicylic acid (PAS), kanamycin, capreomycin, ethionamide,* and *cycloserine*—are generally more toxic and less effective than the primary drugs. The second-line agents are used in combination with the primary drugs to treat disseminated tuberculosis and tuberculosis caused by organisms resistant to the first-line drugs. Dosages and applications of the first-line drugs are summarized in Tables 81–1 and 81–2. Toxicities of all the antituberculous drugs are summarized in Table 81–4.

ISONIAZID

Isoniazid [Laniazid, Nydrazid] is the primary agent for treatment and prophylaxis of tuberculosis. This drug is superior to alternative drugs with regard to efficacy, toxicity, ease of use, patient acceptance, and affordability. With the exception of those patients who cannot tolerate the drug, isoniazid should be taken by all individuals infected with isoniazid-sensitive strains of *M. tuberculosis.*

Antimicrobial Spectrum and Mechanism of Action

Isoniazid is highly selective for mycobacteria. The drug can kill tubercle bacilli at concentrations 10,000 times lower than those needed to affect gram-positive and gram-negative bacteria. Isoniazid is bactericidal to mycobacteria that are actively dividing but is only bacteriostatic to "resting" organisms.

Although the mechanism by which isoniazid acts is not known with certainty, available data suggest that the drug suppresses bacterial growth by inhibiting synthesis of mycolic acid, a component of the mycobacterial cell wall. Since mycolic acid is not produced by other bacteria or by cells of the host, this mechanism would explain the selective action of isoniazid against mycobacteria.

Table 81–4. Major Toxicities of the Antituberculous Drugs	
Primary Drugs	
Isoniazid	Hepatotoxicity, peripheral neuritis
Rifampin	Hepatotoxicity
Pyrazinamide	Hepatotoxicity
Ethambutol	Optic neuritis
Streptomycin	Eighth nerve damage, nephrotoxicity
Second-Line Drugs	
Para-aminosalicylic acid	GI intolerance
Ethionamide	GI intolerance, hepatotoxicity
Cycloserine	Psychoses, seizures, rash
Capreomycin	Eighth nerve damage, nephrotoxicity
Kanamycin	Eighth nerve damage, nephrotoxicity

Resistance

Mycobacteria can develop resistance to isoniazid during treatment. Acquired resistance results from spontaneous mutation—not from transfer of R factors. The mechanism underlying resistance appears to be failure of the drug to enter bacteria. Development of resistance can be decreased through multiple-drug therapy.

Pharmacokinetics

Absorption and Distribution. Isoniazid is administered orally and by IM injection. The drug is well absorbed following administration by either route. Once in the blood, isoniazid is widely distributed to tissues and body fluids. Concentrations in cerebrospinal fluid (CSF) are about 20% of those in plasma.

Metabolism. Isoniazid is inactivated in the liver, primarily by *acetylation*. The ability to acetylate isoniazid is genetically determined: about 50% of people in the United States are *rapid* acetylators and the other 50% are *slow* acetylators. The half-life of isoniazid in rapid acetylators is approximately 1 hour. The half-life in slow acetylators is about 3 hours. It is important to note that differences in rates of acetylation generally have little impact on the *efficacy* of isoniazid, provided patients are taking the drug daily. However, *nonhepatic toxicities* may be more likely in slow acetylators, since drug accumulation is greater in these patients.

Excretion. Isoniazid is excreted in the urine, primarily as inactive metabolites. In patients who are slow acetylators and who also have renal insufficiency, the drug may accumulate to toxic levels.

Therapeutic Use

Isoniazid is indicated only for treatment and prophylaxis of tuberculosis. When taken for prophylaxis, isoniazid is administered alone. When employed for treatment, the drug must be taken in combination with at least one other antituberculous agent (e.g., rifampin).

Adverse Effects

Peripheral Neuropathy. Dose-related peripheral neuropathy is the drug's most common adverse effect. Principal symptoms are symmetric paresthesias (tingling, numbness, burning, pain) of the hands and feet. Clumsiness, unsteadiness, and muscle aches may also develop. Peripheral neuropathy results from isoniazid-induced deficiency in pyridoxine (vitamin B_6). If peripheral neuropathy develops, it can be reversed by administering pyridoxine (50 to 200 mg daily). In patients predisposed to neuropathy (e.g., alcoholics, diabetics) small doses of pyridoxine (6 to 50 mg/day) can be administered with isoniazid as prophylaxis against peripheral neuritis. This practice reduces the risk of neuropathy from 20% down to less than 1%.

Hepatotoxicity. Isoniazid can cause hepatocellular injury and multilobular necrosis. Death has occurred. Liver injury is probably due to production of a toxic isoniazid metabolite. The greatest risk factor for liver damage is advancing age: the incidence of hepatotoxicity is nil in patients under 20 years; 1.2% in those aged 35 to 49; 2.3% in those aged 50 to 64; and 8% in those over 65. Patients should be informed about signs of hepatitis (anorexia, malaise, fatigue, nausea, yellowing of the skin or eyes) and instructed to notify the physician if these develop. Patients should also undergo monthly evaluation for these signs. Some clinicians perform monthly determinations of serum aspartate aminotransferase (AST) activity, since elevation of AST activity is indicative of liver injury. However, since AST levels may rise and then return to normal, despite continued isoniazid use, increases in AST may not be predictive of clinical hepatitis. It is recommended that isoniazid be withdrawn if signs of hepatitis develop or if AST activity rises to a level three times greater than the pretreatment baseline. Caution should be exercised when giving isoniazid to alcoholics and individuals with pre-existing disorders of the liver.

Other Adverse Effects. A variety of *CNS effects* can occur, including optic neuritis, seizures, dizziness, ataxia, and psychologic disturbances (depression, agitation, impairment of memory, hallucinations, toxic psychosis). *Anemia* may result from isoniazid-induced deficiency in pyridoxine. *Gastrointestinal distress, dry mouth,* and *urinary retention* occur on occasion. *Allergy* to isoniazid can produce fever, rashes, and a syndrome resembling lupus erythematosus.

Drug Interactions

Phenytoin. Isoniazid can interfere with the metabolism of phenytoin, thereby causing the anticonvulsant to accumulate to toxic levels. Signs of phenytoin excess include ataxia and incoordination. Plasma levels of phenytoin should be monitored, and phenytoin dosage should be reduced as appropriate. Dosage of isoniazid should not be changed.

Alcohol, Rifampin, and Pyrazinamide. Daily ingestion of alcohol and concurrent therapy with rifampin or pyrazinamide increase the risk of hepatotoxicity. Patients should be encouraged to reduce or eliminate consumption of alcohol.

Preparations, Dosage, and Administration

Preparations. Isoniazid [Laniazid, Nydrazid] is dispensed in tablets (50, 100, and 300 mg) and a syrup (10 mg/ml) for oral use, and in solution (100 mg/ml in 10 ml vials) for IM injection. Isoniazid is also available in fixed-dose combination with rifampin. Capsules of this combination contain 150 mg of isoniazid plus 300 mg of rifampin and are marketed under the trade name *Rifamate.*

Dosage and Administration

Oral. For treatment of active tuberculosis, the usual adult dosage is 300 mg/day. Alternatively, a dosage of 15 mg/kg twice a week can be employed. The pediatric dosage for active tuberculosis is 10 to 20 mg/kg/day. For prophylaxis of tuberculosis, the adult dosage is 300 mg/day and the pediatric dosage is 10 mg/kg/day.

Intramuscular. Parenteral therapy is administered in critical situations when oral treatment is not possible. The dosage is 300 mg daily.

RIFAMPIN

Rifampin [Rifadin, Rimactane] is equal to isoniazid in importance as an antituberculous drug. The combination of rifampin plus isoniazid constitutes the most frequently prescribed regimen for treatment of uncomplicated pulmonary tuberculosis.

Antimicrobial Spectrum

Rifampin is a broad-spectrum antibiotic. The drug is active against most gram-positive bacteria as well as many gram-negative organisms. The drug is bactericidal to *Mycobacterium tuberculosis* and *M. leprae.* Other bacteria that are highly sensitive include *Neisseria meningitidis, Haemophilus influenzae, Staphylococcus aureus,* and *Legionella* species.

Mechanism of Action, Resistance

Rifampin inhibits bacterial DNA-dependent RNA polymerase, causing suppression of RNA synthesis and, therefore, protein synthesis. The results are bactericidal. Since mammalian RNA polymerases are not affected by the drug, rifampin is selectively toxic to microbes. Bacterial resistance to rifampin results from production of an altered form of RNA polymerase.

Pharmacokinetics

Absorption and Distribution. Rifampin is well absorbed if taken on an empty stomach. However, if the drug is taken with or shortly after a meal, both the rate and extent of absorption can be significantly reduced. Rifampin is distributed widely to tissues and body fluids, including the cerebrospinal fluid. The drug is lipid soluble and, hence, has ready access to intracellular bacteria.

Elimination. Rifampin is eliminated primarily by hepatic metabolism. Only about 20% of the drug leaves the body in the urine. Rifampin induces hepatic drug-metabolizing enzymes, including those responsible for its own inactivation. As a result, the rate at which rifampin is metabolized increases over the first weeks of therapy, causing the half-life of the drug to decrease from an initial value of about 4 hours down to 2 hours at the end of 2 weeks. Because rifampin is eliminated by hepatic metabolism, patients with liver dysfunction require a reduction in dosage. No change in dosage is needed in patients with kidney disease.

Therapeutic Use

Tuberculosis. Rifampin is one of our most effective antituberculous drugs. This agent is bactericidal to tubercle bacilli at extracellular and intracellular sites. Rifampin is a drug of choice for treating pulmonary tuberculosis and disseminated disease. Because resistance can develop rapidly when rifampin is employed alone, the drug is always employed in combination with at least one other antituberculous agent. Despite the capacity of rifampin to produce a variety of adverse effects, toxicity rarely requires discontinuation of treatment.

Leprosy. Rifampin is bactericidal to *Mycobacterium leprae* and has become an important agent for the treatment of leprosy.

Meningococcus Carriers. Rifampin is highly active against *Neisseria meningitidis* and is indicated for short-term (4-day) therapy to eliminate this bacterium from the nasopharynx of asymptomatic carriers. Because resistant organisms emerge rapidly, rifampin should not be used to treat active meningococcal disease.

Adverse Effects

Rifampin is generally well tolerated. When employed at recommended dosages, the drug rarely causes significant toxicity. The most common adverse effect of concern is hepatitis.

Hepatotoxicity. Rifampin is toxic to the liver and may cause jaundice and even hepatitis. Asymptomatic elevation of liver enzymes occurs in about 14% of patients. The incidence of hepatitis is less than 1%. Hepatotoxicity is most likely in alcoholics and patients with pre-existing liver disease. These individuals should be monitored closely for signs of liver dysfunction. Tests of liver function (serum transaminase levels) should be made prior to treatment and every 2 to 4 weeks thereafter. Patients should be informed about signs of hepatitis (jaundice, anorexia, malaise, fatigue, nausea) and instructed to notify the physician if these develop.

Discoloration of Body Fluids. Rifampin frequently imparts a red-orange color to urine, sweat, saliva, and tears. Patients should be forewarned of this harmless effect. Permanent staining of soft contact lenses has occurred on occasion; the patient should consult an ophthalmologist regarding the advisability of contact lens use.

Other Adverse Effects. *Gastrointestinal disturbances* (anorexia, nausea, abdominal discomfort) and *cutaneous reactions* (flushing, itching, rash) occur occasionally. Rarely, intermittent high-dose therapy has produced a *flulike syndrome*, characterized by fever, chills, muscle aches, headache, and dizziness. This reaction appears to have an immunologic basis. In some patients, high-dose therapy has been associated with *shortness of breath, hemolytic anemia, shock,* and *acute renal failure.*

Drug Interactions

Accelerated Metabolism of Other Drugs. Because of its ability to induce hepatic drug-metabolizing enzymes, rifampin can increase the rate at which many drugs are metabolized. This action can reduce the effects of a variety of medicines, including *oral contraceptives, coumarin anticoagulants, glucocorticoids,* and *methadone.* When these drugs are used in conjunction with rifampin, an increase in their dosages may be required.

Isoniazid and Pyrazinamide. Rifampin, isoniazid, and pyrazinamide are all hepatotoxic. Hence, when these drugs are used in combination, as they often are, the risk of liver injury may be greater than when they are used alone.

Preparations, Dosage, and Administration

Preparations. Rifampin [Rifadin, Rimactane] is dispensed in capsules (150 and 300 mg) for oral administration. A fixed-dose oral combination (300 mg rifampin plus 150 mg isoniazid) is available under the trade name *Rifamate*. Rifampin [Rifadin] is also available in powder form to be reconstituted for IV infusion.

Oral Dosage and Administration. For treatment of tuberculosis, the usual adult dosage is 600 mg (or 10 mg/kg) daily. The pediatric dosage is 10 to 20 mg/kg/day. Rifampin is administered in single daily doses 1 hour before a meal or 2 hours after. The dosage should be reduced in the presence of liver dysfunction.

Intravenous Administration. Dissolve 600 mg of powdered rifampin in 10 ml of sterile water for injection to make a concentrated solution (60 mg/ml). Dilute an appropriate dose of the concentrate in 500 ml of 5% dextrose and infuse over 3 hours.

PYRAZINAMIDE

Antimicrobial Activity and Therapeutic Use

Pyrazinamide is bactericidal to *Mycobacterium tuberculosis*. The mechanism of antibacterial action is not known. Currently, the combination of pyrazinamide with rifampin and isoniazid is considered the antituberculous regimen of choice. In this regimen, pyrazinamide is discontinued after 2 months, while the other two agents are continued for an additional 4 months (see *6-Month Short Course* in Table 81–1).

Pharmacokinetics

Pyrazinamide is well absorbed following oral administration and is widely distributed to tissues and body fluids. In the liver, the drug is converted to pyrazinoic acid, an active metabolite, and then to 5-hydroxypyrazinoic acid, which is inactive. Excretion is renal, primarily as inactive metabolites.

Adverse Effects

Hepatotoxicity. Liver injury is the principal adverse effect of pyrazinamide. High-dose therapy has caused hepatitis, and, rarely, fatal hepatic necrosis. Fortunately, these reactions are relatively uncommon with the low-dose, short-term therapy employed currently. The earliest manifestations of liver damage are elevations in serum levels of transaminases (aspartate aminotransferase [AST] and alanine aminotransferase [ALT]). Levels of these enzymes should be measured prior to treatment and every 2 to 4 weeks during the course of therapy. Patients should be informed about signs of hepatitis (e.g., malaise, anorexia, nausea, vomiting, yellowish discoloration of the skin and eyes) and instructed to notify the physician if these develop. Pyrazinamide should be discontinued if significant injury to the liver occurs. The drug should not be used by patients with pre-existing liver dysfunction. The risk of liver injury is increased by concurrent therapy with isoniazid and rifampin, both of which are hepatotoxic.

Other Adverse Effects. Pyrazinamide and its metabolites can inhibit renal excretion of uric acid, thereby causing *hyperuricemia*; although usually asymptomatic, pyrazinamide-induced hyperuricemia has resulted in *gouty arthritis* rarely. Additional adverse effects include *arthralgia, gastrointestinal disturbances* (nausea, vomiting, diarrhea), *rashes,* and *photosensitivity.*

Preparations, Dosage, and Administration

Pyrazinamide is dispensed in 500-mg tablets for oral administration. The usual adult dosage is 20 to 30 mg/kg administered once a day. The maximum daily dosage should not exceed 2 gm.

ETHAMBUTOL

Antimicrobial Action

Ethambutol [Myambutol] is active only against mycobacteria; nearly all strains of *M. tuberculosis* are sensitive. The drug is bacteriostatic, not bactericidal. Ethambutol is usually active against tubercle bacilli that are resistant to isoniazid and rifampin. The mechanism by which ethambutol acts is not known.

Therapeutic Use

Ethambutol is an important antituberculous drug. This agent is employed for initial treatment of tuberculosis and for retreatment of patients who have received therapy previously. Like other drugs for tuberculosis, ethambutol is always employed as part of a multidrug regimen.

Pharmacokinetics

Ethambutol is readily absorbed following oral administration. The drug is widely distributed to most tissues and body fluids; levels in cerebrospinal fluid, however, remain low. Ethambutol undergoes little hepatic metabolism and is excreted primarily in the urine. In patients with normal kidney function, the drug's half-life is 3 to 4 hours; the half-life increases to 8 hours in patients with renal impairment.

Adverse Effects

Ethambutol is generally well tolerated. The only significant adverse effect is optic neuritis.

Optic Neuritis. Ethambutol can produce dose-related optic neuritis, resulting in blurred vision, constriction of the visual field, and disturbance of color discrimination. The mechanism underlying these effects is not known. Symptoms usually resolve upon discontinuation of treatment; however, for some patients, visual disturbance has persisted. Fortunately, ocular toxicity is rare at currently recommended doses. Baseline testing of vision should be performed prior to ethambutol use. Patients should be advised to report any alteration in vision. Since symptoms (blurring of vision, reduced color discrimination) often precede visual

changes that can be measured objectively, routine testing during treatment is rarely helpful. If ocular toxicity develops, ethambutol should be withdrawn immediately. Because visual changes can be difficult to monitor in pediatric patients, ethambutol is not recommended for children under 13 years of age.

Other Adverse Effects. Ethambutol can produce *allergic reactions* (dermatitis, pruritus), *gastrointestinal upset,* and *confusion.* The drug inhibits renal excretion of uric acid, causing *asymptomatic hyperuricemia* in about 50% of patients; occasionally, elevation of uric acid levels results in *acute gouty arthritis.* Rare adverse effects include *peripheral neuropathy, renal damage,* and *thrombocytopenia.*

Preparations, Dosage, and Administration

Ethambutol [Myambutol] is dispensed in 100- and 400-mg tablets for oral administration. For *initial* therapy of tuberculosis, the usual dosage for adults and children is 15 mg/kg once a day. For retreatment therapy, the usual dosage is 25 mg/kg/day for 60 days, and 15 mg/kg/day thereafter; all doses are given once a day. Ethambutol may be taken with food if GI upset occurs.

STREPTOMYCIN

Streptomycin, an aminoglycoside antibiotic, was our first effective antituberculous drug. The basic pharmacology of streptomycin and the other aminoglycosides is discussed in Chapter 77. Discussion here is limited to the use of streptomycin for tuberculosis.

Antibacterial Activity. Streptomycin is bactericidal to tubercle bacilli *in vitro*; however, the drug has relatively low sterilizing activity *in vivo.* This discrepancy is explained by the inability of streptomycin to penetrate mammalian cells: since tubercle bacilli are frequently present at intracellular sites, many escape exposure to the drug.

Adverse Effects. The most characteristic toxicity is *injury to the eighth cranial nerve, resulting in hearing loss and disturbance of balance.* However, when the drug is prescribed properly, effects on auditory and vestibular function are rare. The risk of eighth nerve toxicity is increased by advanced age and kidney dysfunction. Tests of hearing and balance should be performed periodically during the course of treatment. Special care should be taken to adjust the dosage in patients with renal impairment. Additional adverse effects include *nephrotoxicity, facial paresthesias,* and *rash.*

Therapeutic Status, Dosage, and Administration. Streptomycin must be administered by IM injection. Because it cannot be used orally, and because of its potential for eighth nerve toxicity, streptomycin is considerably less attractive than the newer antituberculous drugs (rifampin, isoniazid, pyrazinamide) for initial treatment. Accordingly, use of this once-popular agent has sharply declined. Today, streptomycin is employed primarily in three-drug regimens for chemotherapy of severe mycobacterial infection. The usual adult dosage is 15 mg/kg 5 days a week. The recommended dosage for children is 20 to 40 mg/kg/day.

SECOND-LINE ANTITUBERCULOUS DRUGS

The group of second-line antituberculous drugs consists of *para-aminosalicylic acid (PAS), kanamycin, capreomycin, ethionamide,* and *cycloserine.* In general, these drugs are more toxic and less effective than the first-line antituberculous drugs. As a result, the principal use of second-line drugs is treatment of tuberculosis caused by organisms that have proved resistant to the first-line agents. In addition, the second-line drugs are used to treat severe pulmonary tuberculosis as well as disseminated (extrapulmonary) infection. The second-line drugs are always employed in conjunction with a major antituberculous drug. Principal toxicities are summarized in Table 81–4.

Para-Aminosalicylic Acid (PAS)

Actions and Uses. PAS is similar in structure and actions to the sulfonamides. Like the sulfonamides, PAS exerts its antibacterial effects by inhibiting synthesis of folic acid. However, in contrast to the sulfonamides, which are broad-spectrum antibiotics, PAS is active only against mycobacteria. In the United States, PAS has been employed primarily as a substitute for ethambutol in regimens for pediatric patients. The drug is always used in combination with other antituberculous agents.

Pharmacokinetics. PAS is administered orally and is well absorbed from the gastrointestinal tract. The drug is distributed widely to most tissues and body fluids; however, levels in CSF remain low. PAS undergoes extensive hepatic metabolism. Metabolites and parent drug are excreted in the urine.

Adverse Effects. PAS is poorly tolerated by adults; children accept the drug somewhat better. The most frequent adverse effects are gastrointestinal disturbances (nausea, vomiting, diarrhea). Because PAS is administered in large doses as a sodium salt, substantial sodium loading may occur. Additional adverse effects are allergic reactions, hepatotoxicity, and goiter.

Preparations, Dosage, and Administration. Aminosalicylate sodium [Sodium P.A.S.] is dispensed in 500-mg tablets for oral administration. Tablets that are discolored (brown, purple) should not be used. The drug loses its effectiveness if exposed to sunlight, extreme heat, or moisture. Accordingly, it should not be stored in kitchen or bathroom cabinets. If stomach upset occurs, the drug may be administered with food. The daily dosage for adults is 14 to 16 gm in two or three divided doses. The daily dosage for children is 275 to 420 mg/kg in three to four divided doses.

Ethionamide

Actions and Uses. Ethionamide, a relative of isoniazid, is active against mycobacteria, but less so than isoniazid. Ethionamide is administered with other antituberculous drugs to treat tuberculosis that is resistant to first-line agents. Gastrointestinal disturbances limit patient acceptance of the drug.

Pharmacokinetics. Ethionamide is readily absorbed following oral administration. The drug is widely distributed to tissues and body fluids, including the CSF. Ethionamide undergoes extensive metabolism and is excreted in the urine, primarily as metabolites.

Adverse Effects. Gastrointestinal effects (anorexia, nausea, vomiting, diarrhea, metallic taste) occur often; intolerance of these effects frequently leads to discontinuation of the drug. Ethionamide is toxic to the liver. Hepatotoxicity is assessed by measuring serum transaminases (AST, ALT) prior to treatment and periodically thereafter. Additional adverse effects include peripheral neuropathy, CNS effects (convulsions, mental disturbance), and allergic reactions.

Preparations, Dosage, and Administration. Ethionamide [Trecator-SC] is dispensed in 250-mg tablets for oral administration. The usual adult dosage is 0.5 to 1 gm/day in divided doses. The recommended pediatric dosage is 15 to 20 mg/kg/day (maximum of 1 gm).

Cycloserine

Actions and Uses. Cycloserine is an antibiotic produced by a species of *Streptomyces*. The drug is bacteriostatic and acts by inhibiting synthesis of the cell wall. Cycloserine is used to treat tuberculosis that is resistant to first-line drugs. When employed against tuberculosis, cycloserine is always combined with other drugs.

Pharmacokinetics. Cycloserine is rapidly absorbed following oral administration. The drug is widely distributed to tissues and body fluids, including the CSF. Elimination is by hepatic metabolism and renal excretion; about 50% of the drug leaves the body unchanged in the urine. Cycloserine may accumulate to toxic levels in patients with renal impairment.

Adverse Effects. CNS effects occur frequently and can be severe. Possible reactions include anxiety, depression, confusion, hallucinations, paranoia, hyperreflexia, and seizures. Psychotic episodes occur in approximately 10% of those treated; symptoms usually subside within 2 weeks following drug withdrawal. Pyridoxine may prevent neurotoxic effects. Other adverse effects include peripheral neuropathy, hepatotoxicity, and folate deficiency.

Preparations, Dosage, and Administration. Cycloserine [Seromycin Pulvules] is dispensed in 250-mg capsules for oral administration. The initial dosage for adults is 250 mg twice daily for 2 weeks; the maintenance dosage is 500 mg to 1 gm daily in divided doses. The dosage for children is 10 to 20 mg/kg/day.

Capreomycin

Capreomycin [Capastat Sulfate] is an antibiotic derived from a species of *Streptomyces*. Antibacterial effects are probably due to inhibition of protein synthesis. The drug is bacteriostatic to *Mycobacterium tuberculosis*. Capreomycin is used only for tuberculosis resistant to primary agents. The drug's principal toxicity is renal damage; the drug should not be taken by patients with kidney disease. Capreomycin may also cause eighth nerve damage, resulting in hearing loss, tinnitus, and disturbance of balance. Administration is by deep IM injection (the drug is not absorbed from the GI tract and cannot be administered orally). The usual dosage for adults is 1 gm/day for 60 to 120 days, followed by 1-gm doses two to three times weekly. The dosage for children is 15 mg/kg/day (to a maximum of 1 gm).

Kanamycin

Kanamycin is an aminoglycoside antibiotic that is highly active against *M. tuberculosis*. Like streptomycin and other aminoglycosides, kanamycin is nephrotoxic and may damage the eighth cranial nerve. Kanamycin is not absorbed from the GI tract. Administration is by IM injection. The usual adult dosage is 15 mg/kg once daily. Kanamycin is not recommended for children. The pharmacology of kanamycin and other aminoglycosides is discussed in Chapter 77.

DRUGS USED TO TREAT LEPROSY

Leprosy (Hansen's disease) is caused by *Mycobacterium leprae*. Worldwide, leprosy constitutes a major public health problem; about 12 million people are estimated to have the disease. In the United States, the number of cases is approximately 4000.

Leprosy is acquired through exposure to individuals who have the infection. Bacilli are transmitted from the respiratory tract of the infected person to the respiratory tract of the noninfected person. Fortunately, when leprosy is properly treated, infectivity is essentially nil. Accordingly, for patients who are receiving adequate chemotherapy, isolation is not required.

Treatment of leprosy has three major objectives: (1) conversion of the patient to a noninfectious state, (2) prevention of bacterial multiplication, and (3) avoidance or reduction of complications of leprosy. To achieve these objectives, the World Health Organization recommends that all patients receive treatment with multiple drugs. *Dapsone* has been and remains a mainstay of therapy. Other important agents are *rifampin*, *clofazimine*, and *ethionamide*. Therapy is prolonged, lasting from several months to many years.

DAPSONE

Actions and Uses. Dapsone is a primary drug for treatment of leprosy. This agent is effective, low in toxicity, and inexpensive. Dapsone is chemically related to the sulfonamides and probably acts by the same mechanism as those drugs (i.e., inhibition of folic acid synthesis). Depending on its concentration, dapsone can be bactericidal or bacteriostatic. Although once employed alone to treat leprosy, dapsone is now employed in combination with other antileprosy drugs (usually rifampin and clofazimine).

Pharmacokinetics. Dapsone is absorbed slowly but completely from the GI tract. Once in the blood, the drug is widely distributed to tissues and body fluids. Dapsone is acetylated in the liver and has a plasma half-life of 10 to 50 hours. Excretion is renal, primarily as metabolites.

Adverse Effects. Dapsone is generally well tolerated; the drug may be taken for years without causing significant untoward effects. The most common adverse effects are gastrointestinal disturbances, headache, rash, and a syndrome that resembles mononucleosis. Hemolysis occurs occasionally; severe reactions are usually limited to patients with glucose-6-phosphate dehydrogenase deficiency. Death has occurred from agranulocytosis and aplastic anemia; hence, complete blood counts should be performed periodically.

Preparations, Dosage, and Administration. Dapsone is dispensed in 25- and 100-mg tablets for oral administration. The usual dosage for adults and children is 100 mg daily. As a rule, dapsone is administered in combination with other antileprosy drugs (usually rifampin and clofazimine).

CLOFAZIMINE

Actions and Uses. Clofazimine is weakly bactericidal to *Mycobacterium leprae*. The mechanism of antibacterial effects has not been determined. Clofazimine is given with rifampin to treat leprosy that is dapsone resistant. In addition to its antibacterial action, clofazimine has anti-inflammatory actions.

Pharmacokinetics. Clofazimine is administered orally and undergoes partial absorption. Absorbed drug is retained in tissues. Because of tissue retention, the half-life of clofazimine is extremely long (about 70 days).

Adverse Effects. Dangerous reactions are uncommon. However, clofazimine frequently imparts a red-brown color to the skin and conjunctiva. The drug may also discolor urine, sweat, saliva, and tears. Because of these effects on pigmentation, patients with light-colored skin often find clofazimine unacceptable. Deposition of clofazimine in the small intestine produces the drug's most serious effects: intestinal obstruction, pain, and bleeding.

Preparations, Dosage, and Administration. Clofazimine [Lamprene] is dispensed in 50- and 100-mg capsules for oral use. The recommended dosage is 50 mg every day together with a 300-mg dose once a month.

ETHIONAMIDE AND RIFAMPIN

Rifampin and ethionamide are bactericidal to *Mycobacterium leprae*. Both agents are employed in combination with other antileprosy drugs (most commonly dapsone and clofazimine) for initial therapy of the disease. The adult dosage of rifampin is 600 mg daily. The adult dosage of ethionamide ranges from 250 to 375 mg daily. The basic pharmacology of both drugs and their use against tuberculosis are discussed above.

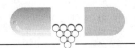

Summary of Major Nursing Implications

The nursing implications summarized below are limited to the drug therapy of *tuberculosis*.

IMPLICATIONS THAT APPLY TO ALL ANTITUBERCULOUS DRUGS

Promoting Compliance

Treatment of active tuberculosis is prolonged (usually 6 to 12 months) and demands concurrent use of two or more drugs. As a result, compliance can be a significant problem. To promote compliance, educate the patient about the rationale for multiple-drug therapy and the need for long-term treatment. Encourage patients to take their medication exactly as prescribed, and to continue treatment until the infection has resolved.

Evaluating Treatment

Success is indicated by (1) reductions in fever, malaise, anorexia, cough, and other clinical manifestations of tuberculosis (usually within weeks), (2) radiographic evidence of improvement (usually in 3 months), and (3) an absence of *M. tuberculosis* in sputum cultures (usually after 3 to 6 months).

ISONIAZID

In addition to the implications summarized below, see above for implications on *promoting compliance* and *evaluating treatment* that apply to all antituberculous drugs.

 Preadministration Assessment

Therapeutic Goal

Treatment or prophylaxis of infection with *Mycobacterium tuberculosis*.

Baseline Data

Obtain a chest x-ray, microbiologic tests of sputum, and baseline tests of liver function.

Identifying High-Risk Patients

Isoniazid is *contraindicated* for patients with *acute liver disease* or a *history of isoniazid-induced hepatotoxicity*. Use the drug with *caution in alcoholics, diabetics, patients with vitamin B_6 deficiency, patients over the age of 50,* and *patients who are taking phenytoin, rifampin, or pyrazinamide.*

 Implementation: Administration

Routes

Oral (usually) and IM (for critical situations when oral treatment is not possible).

Administration

Advise the patient to take isoniazid on an empty stomach, either 1 hour before meals or 2 hours after. Advise the patient to take the drug with meals if GI upset occurs.

Minimizing Adverse Effects

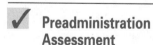 **Ongoing Evaluation and Interventions**

Peripheral Neuropathy. Inform patients about symptoms of peripheral neuropathy (tingling, numbing, burning, or pain in the hands or feet) and instruct them to notify the physician if these occur. Peripheral neuritis can be reversed with small daily doses of pyridoxine (vitamin B₆). In patients at high risk of neuropathy (e.g., alcoholics, diabetics), pyridoxine should be given prophylactically.

Hepatotoxicity. Isoniazid can cause hepatocellular damage and multi-lobular hepatic necrosis. Inform patients about signs of hepatitis (jaundice, anorexia, malaise, fatigue, nausea) and instruct them to notify the physician if these develop. Evaluate patients monthly for signs of hepatitis. Monthly determinations of AST activity may be ordered. If clinical signs of hepatitis appear, or if AST activity exceeds three times the pretreatment baseline, isoniazid should be withdrawn. Daily ingestion of alcohol increases the risk of liver injury; urge the patient to minimize or eliminate alcohol consumption.

Minimizing Adverse Interactions

Isoniazid can suppress the metabolism of *phenytoin*, thereby causing phenytoin levels to rise. Plasma content of phenytoin should be monitored. If necessary, phenytoin dosage should be reduced.

RIFAMPIN

In addition to the implications summarized below, see above for implications on *promoting compliance* and *evaluating treatment* that apply to all antituberculous drugs.

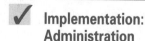 **Preadministration Assessment**

Therapeutic Goal

Treatment of tuberculosis or leprosy.

Baseline Data

Obtain a chest x-ray, microbiologic tests of sputum, and baseline tests of liver function.

Identifying High-Risk Patients

Use with *caution* in patients with *liver disease* and in *alcoholics*.

Implementation: Administration

Routes

Oral, IV.

Dosage

Reduce the dosage in patients with liver dysfunction.

Administration

Instruct the patient to take oral rifampin once a day, either 1 hour before a meal or 2 hours after.

Administer IV rifampin by slow infusion (over 3 hours).

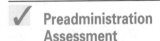

Ongoing Evaluation and Interventions

Minimizing Adverse Effects

Hepatotoxicity. Rifampin may cause jaundice or hepatitis. Inform patients about signs of liver dysfunction (anorexia, darkened urine, pale stools, yellow discoloration of eyes or skin) and instruct them to notify the physician if these develop. Monitor patients for signs of liver dysfunction. Tests of liver function should be made prior to treatment and every 2 to 4 weeks thereafter.

Discoloration of Body Fluids. Forewarn patients that rifampin may impart a harmless red-orange color to urine, sweat, saliva, and tears. Warn patients that soft contact lenses may undergo permanent staining; advise them to consult an ophthalmologist about continued use of these lenses.

Minimizing Adverse Interactions

Accelerated Metabolism of Other Drugs. Rifampin can accelerate the metabolism of many drugs, thereby reducing their therapeutic effects. This action is of particular concern with *oral contraceptives, warfarin, glucocorticoids,* and *methadone.* When these agents are used in conjunction with rifampin, an increase in their dosage may be required.

Pyrazinamide and Rifampin. These hepatotoxic antituberculous drugs can increase the risk of liver injury when used with rifampin.

PYRAZINAMIDE

In addition to the implications summarized below, see above for implications on *promoting compliance* and *evaluating treatment* that apply to all antituberculous drugs.

Preadministration Assessment

Therapeutic Goal

Treatment of tuberculosis.

Baseline Data

Obtain a chest x-ray, microbiologic tests of sputum, and baseline tests of liver function.

Identifying High-Risk Patients

Pyrazinamide is *contraindicated* for patients with *severe liver dysfunction* or *acute gout.* Use with *caution* in *alcoholics.*

Implementation: Administration

Route

Oral.

Administration

Administration is usually done once a day.

**Ongoing
Evaluation and
Interventions**

Minimizing Adverse Effects

Hepatotoxicity. Inform patients about symptoms of hepatitis (e.g., malaise, anorexia, nausea, vomiting, yellowish discoloration of the skin and eyes) and instruct them to notify the physician if these develop. Levels of AST and ALT should be measured prior to treatment and every 2 to 4 weeks thereafter. If severe liver injury occurs, pyrazinamide should be withdrawn. The risk of liver injury is increased by concurrent therapy with isoniazid and rifampin, both of which are hepatotoxic.

ETHAMBUTOL

In addition to the implications summarized below, see above for implications on *promoting compliance* and *evaluating treatment* that apply to all antituberculous drugs.

 **Preadministration
Assessment**

Therapeutic Goal

Treatment of tuberculosis.

Baseline Data

Obtain a chest x-ray, microbiologic tests of sputum, and baseline vision tests.

Identifying High-Risk Patients

Ethambutol is *contraindicated* for patients with known *optic neuritis.*

 **Implementation:
Administration**

Route

Oral.

Administration

Dosing is usually done once a day. Advise the patient to take ethambutol with food if GI upset occurs.

 **Ongoing
Evaluation and
Interventions**

Minimizing Adverse Effects

Optic Neuritis. Ethambutol can cause dose-related optic neuritis. Symptoms include blurred vision, altered color discrimination, and constriction of visual fields. Baseline vision tests are required. Instruct the patient to report any alteration in vision (e.g., blurring of vision, reduced color discrimination). If ocular toxicity develops, ethambutol should be withdrawn at once.

Miscellaneous Antibacterial Drugs

FLUOROQUINOLONES
Ciprofloxacin
Norfloxacin
Newer Fluoroquinolones

ADDITIONAL ANTIBACTERIAL DRUGS
Metronidazole
Rifampin
Bacitracin
Polymyxin B

FLUOROQUINOLONES

The fluoroquinolones are related chemically to nalidixic acid, a narrow-spectrum antibiotic used only for urinary tract infections. In contrast to nalidixic acid, the fluoroquinolones are active against a relatively broad spectrum of bacteria, and have a wide variety of clinical applications.

New fluoroquinolones are being developed rapidly. When the first edition of this text was published, only two fluoroquinolones (ciprofloxacin, norfloxacin) were available in the United States. Now, a total of five have received FDA approval, and more are in clinical trials.

CIPROFLOXACIN

Ciprofloxacin [Cipro] was among the first fluoroquinolones available and will serve as our prototype for the family. This drug can be administered orally and is active against a broad spectrum of bacterial pathogens. The drug has been used as an alternative to parenteral antibiotics for treatment of several serious infections. Because it can be administered by mouth, ciprofloxacin has made it possible to treat many patients on an outpatient basis who would otherwise have required hospitalization for parenteral therapy.

1021

Mechanism of Action

Like nalidixic acid, ciprofloxacin inhibits bacterial DNA gyrase, an enzyme that converts closed circular DNA into a supercoiled configuration. In the absence of supercoiling, DNA replication cannot take place. The drug is rapidly bactericidal. However, the precise mechanism of cell death is not understood.

Antimicrobial Spectrum

Ciprofloxacin is active against a broad spectrum of bacteria, including most aerobic gram-negative bacteria and some gram-positive bacteria. Most urinary tract pathogens, including *Escherichia coli* and *Klebsiella*, are sensitive. The drug is also highly active against most bacteria that cause enteritis (e.g., *Salmonella, Shigella, Campylobacter jejuni, E. coli*). Other sensitive organisms include *Pseudomonas aeruginosa, Haemophilus influenzae*, gonococci, meningococci, and many streptococci. Activity against anaerobes is fair to poor. *Clostridium difficile* is resistant.

Bacterial Resistance

Resistance to fluoroquinolones has developed during treatment of infections with *Staphylococcus aureus, Serratia marcescens, Campylobacter jejuni,* and *Pseudomonas aeruginosa*. Two mechanisms appear to underlie resistance: (1) alterations in DNA gyrase, and (2) reduced ability of the drug to cross bacterial membranes. There have been no reports of transfer of resistance via R factors. It is not yet clear whether resistance to ciprofloxacin will be as serious a clinical problem as resistance to nalidixic acid (see Chapter 79).

Pharmacokinetics

Ciprofloxacin may be administered orally or IV. Following oral administration, the drug is rapidly but incompletely absorbed. High concentrations are achieved in urine, stool, bile, saliva, bone, and prostate tissue. Drug levels in cerebrospinal fluid remain low. Ciprofloxacin has a plasma half-life of about 4 hours. Elimination is by a combination of hepatic metabolism and renal excretion.

Therapeutic Uses

Ciprofloxacin is approved for a wide variety of infections. These include infections of the respiratory tract, urinary tract, gastrointestinal tract, bones, joints, skin, and soft tissues. Because it is active against a variety of pathogens and can be given orally, ciprofloxacin represents an alternative to parenteral treatment for many serious infections. The drug is not useful against infections caused by anaerobes.

Adverse Effects

Ciprofloxacin can induce a variety of mild adverse effects, including gastrointestinal reactions (nausea, vomiting, diarrhea, abdominal pain) and CNS effects (dizziness, headache, restlessness, confusion). *Candida* infections of the pharynx and vagina may develop as a result of treatment. Very rarely, seizures have occurred.

Ciprofloxacin has caused cartilage deterioration in immature animals. Although similar effects have not been observed in humans, *ciprofloxacin is not recommended for use by children under 18 years of age or by women who are pregnant or breast-feeding.*

Drug Interactions

Drugs That Reduce Absorption. Absorption of ciprofloxacin can be reduced by (1) aluminum- or magnesium-containing antacids, (2) iron salts, (3) zinc salts, and (4) sucralfate. These agents should be administered at least 4 hours before or 2 hours after ciprofloxacin.

Theophylline. Ciprofloxacin can increase plasma levels of theophylline, a drug for asthma. Theophylline levels should be monitored and the dosage adjusted accordingly.

Warfarin. Ciprofloxacin can elevate levels of warfarin. Prothrombin time should be monitored and the dosage of warfarin reduced as appropriate.

Preparations, Dosage, and Administration

Oral. Ciprofloxacin [Cipro] is dispensed in tablets (250, 500, and 700 mg) for oral administration. The dosage for urinary tract infections is 250 or 500 mg two times a day, usually for 7 to 14 days. For other infections, dosages range from 500 to 750 mg two times a day. Dosage should be reduced for patients with renal impairment.

Intravenous. Ciprofloxacin [Cipro I.V.] is dispensed in solution (10 and 2 mg/ml) for IV administration. The infusion should be done slowly (over 60 minutes). Intravenous dosages range from from 200 to 400 mg every 12 hours.

NORFLOXACIN

Norfloxacin [Noroxin] is a fluoroquinolone antibiotic with a spectrum of antimicrobial effects like that of ciprofloxacin. The drug is used orally and labeled only for urinary tract infections (UTIs). However, despite the limits of the labeling, norfloxacin has proved useful for bacterial gastroenteritis, gonorrhea, and gonococcal urethritis.

Pharmacokinetics. Norfloxacin undergoes rapid but incomplete absorption following oral administration. The drug is widely distributed to body tissues and fluids. Excretion is primarily renal, and high concentrations are achieved in the urine. About 30% of the drug is eliminated in the bile and feces. In patients with normal kidney function, the half-life of norfloxacin is approximately 4 hours; this value doubles in patients with renal impairment.

Therapeutic Uses. Norfloxacin is labeled only for treatment of UTIs caused by susceptible organisms. The drug has proved effective against UTIs caused by *Pseudomonas aeruginosa* and other gram-negative bacteria that can display multiple drug resistance. In addition to this labeled use, norfloxacin is employed to treat bacterial gastroenteritis (caused by *Escherichia coli, Shigella, Salmonella*, and other pathogens) and gonorrhea and gonococcal urethritis caused by penicillinase-producing *Neisseria gonorrhoeae*.

Adverse Effects. Norfloxacin is generally well tolerated. Gastrointestinal effects (nausea, vomiting, anorexia) have been most frequent. The drug has produced a variety of CNS reactions, including headache, dizziness, drowsiness, lightheadedness, depression, and disturbance of vision. Skin rash develops occasionally. Like ciprofloxacin, norfloxacin has caused deterioration of cartilage in immature animals. Hence, like ciprofloxacin, norfloxacin is not recommended for children under 18 years of age or for women who are pregnant or breast-feeding.

Drug Interactions. Norfloxacin shares the same drug interactions as ciprofloxacin. Absorption is suppressed by antacids (aluminum- and magnesium-containing), iron and zinc salts, and sucralfate. The drug can elevate levels of theophylline and intensify effects of warfarin.

Preparations, Dosage, and Administration. Norfloxacin [Noroxin] is dispensed in 400-mg tablets for oral administration. The drug should be taken on an empty stomach with a full glass of water. For uncomplicated urinary tract infections, the usual dosage is 400 mg twice daily for 3 days. Prolonged treatment (10 days to 3 weeks) is employed for patients with complicated infections of the urinary tract. Dosage should be reduced in the presence of kidney dysfunction.

NEWER FLUOROQUINOLONES

Ofloxacin

Basic Pharmacology. Ofloxacin [Floxin] is similar to ciprofloxacin in mechanism of action, antimicrobial spectrum, therapeutic applications, and adverse effects. Like ciprofloxacin, the drug may be administered orally or IV. In the absence of food, bioavailability of oral ofloxacin is 90%; food greatly reduces availability. Ofloxacin is widely distributed to tissues and excreted in the urine. Like ciprofloxacin, ofloxacin can cause a variety of mild adverse effects, including nausea, vomiting, headache, and dizziness. Serious reactions are rare. Like other fluoroquinolones, ofloxacin can cause cartilage erosion in young laboratory animals and should not be used by children under 18 years or women who are pregnant or breast-feeding. Ofloxacin elevates plasma levels of warfarin, but, in contrast to ciprofloxacin, does not elevate levels of theophylline. Absorption of oral ofloxacin is reduced by antacids (magnesium- and aluminum-containing), sucralfate, and iron and zinc salts.

Preparations, Dosage, and Administration. Ofloxacin is available in tablets (200, 300, and 400 mg) for oral administration and in solution (4, 10, and 20 mg/ml) for slow IV infusion; concentrated solutions must be diluted prior to infusion. The usual *oral* dosage is 200 to 400 mg every 12 hours; duration of treatment may last 1 day to 6 weeks. Dosage should be reduced in patients with renal impairment. Oral ofloxacin should not be taken with food.

Lomefloxacin

Basic Pharmacology. Lomefloxacin [Maxaquin] is similar to ciprofloxacin with regard to mechanism of action, antimicrobial spectrum, and adverse effects. Approved indications are limited to urinary and respiratory tract infections caused by *Haemophilus influenzae* or *Moraxella catarrhalis*. Administration is oral and bioavailability is high (98%), even in the presence of food. The drug is widely distributed to tissues and eliminated by the kidney. Lomefloxacin has a prolonged half-life that permits once-a-day dosing. Like ciprofloxacin, lomefloxacin can cause various mild adverse effects, including nausea, vomiting, headache, and dizziness. Serious reactions are rare. Like other fluoroquinolones, lomefloxacin can cause cartilage erosion in laboratory animals and should not be used by children under the age of 18 or by women who are pregnant or breast-feeding. Absorption of lomefloxacin is reduced by antacids (magnesium- and aluminum-containing), iron and zinc salts, and sucralfate.

In contrast to ciprofloxacin, lomefloxacin does not elevate plasma levels of theophylline.

Preparations, Dosage, and Administration. Lomefloxacin is available in 400-mg tablets for oral administration. The drug may be taken without regard to meals. The usual dosage is 400 mg once a day for 10 to 14 days. Dosage should be reduced in patients with renal impairment.

Enoxacin

Basic Pharmacology. Enoxacin [Penetrex] is similar to ciprofloxacin in mechanism of action and adverse effects. The drug's antimicrobial spectrum is narrower than that of ciprofloxacin. Approved indications are limited to urinary tract infections and uncomplicated urethral and cervical gonorrhea. Administration is oral and bioavailability is high (90%); food reduces availability. The drug is widely distributed to tissues and is eliminated by the kidney. Like ciprofloxacin, enoxacin can cause a variety of mild adverse effects, including nausea, vomiting, headache, and dizziness. Serious reactions are rare. Like other fluoroquinolones, enoxacin can cause cartilage erosion in laboratory animals and should not be used by children under the age of 18 or by women who are pregnant or nursing. Absorption of enoxacin is reduced by antacids (magnesium- and aluminum-containing), iron and zinc salts, and sucralfate. Like ciprofloxacin, enoxacin can elevate plasma levels of theophylline and warfarin.

Preparations, Dosage, and Administration. Enoxacin is available in tablets (200 and 400 mg) for oral administration. The drug should be taken 1 hour before meals or 2 hours after. The dosage for urinary tract infections is 200 or 400 mg every 12 hours for 7 to 14 days. The dosage for uncomplicated gonorrhea is 400 mg once. Doses should be reduced in patients with renal impairment.

ADDITIONAL ANTIBACTERIAL DRUGS

METRONIDAZOLE

Metronidazole [Flagyl, others] is used for protozoal infections and infections caused by obligate anaerobic bacteria. The basic pharmacology of metronidazole is discussed in Chapter 88, as is the use of this drug against protozoal infections. Only the antibacterial applications of metronidazole are considered here.

Mechanism of Antibacterial Action. Metronidazole is lethal to anaerobic organisms only. To exert its bactericidal effects, metronidazole must first be taken up by cells and then converted into its active form; only anaerobes are capable of performing the conversion. The active form of metronidazole interacts with DNA to cause strand breakage and loss of helical structure, effects that result in inhibition of nucleic acid synthesis and cell death. Since aerobic bacteria are unable to activate metronidazole, these organisms are insensitive to the drug.

Antibacterial Spectrum. Metronidazole is active against obligate anaerobes only. Sensitive bacterial pathogens include *Bacteroides fragilis* (and other *Bacteroides* species), *Clostridium difficile* (and other *Clostridium* species), *Fusobacterium* species, *Gardnerella vaginalis*, *Peptococcus* species, and *Peptostreptococcus* species.

Therapeutic Uses. Metronidazole is active against a variety of *anaerobic* bacterial infections, including infections of the central nervous system, abdominal organs, bones and joints, skin and soft tissues, and genitourinary tract. Frequently, such infections also involve aerobic bacteria, and therapy must include a drug that is active against them. Metronidazole is employed for prophylaxis in surgical procedures associated with a high risk of infection by anaerobes (e.g., colorectal surgery, abdominal surgery, vaginal surgery). In addition, the drug is used in combination with a tetracycline and bismuth subsalicylate to eradicate *Helicobacter pylori* in people with peptic ulcer disease. Development of resistance to metronidazole is rare.

Preparations, Dosage, and Administration. For initial treatment of serious bacterial infections, metronidazole is administered by IV infusion. Under appropriate conditions, the patient may be transferred to oral therapy.

Intravenous Formulations. Metronidazole is available in two formulations—powder and solution—for IV use. The powdered form [Flagyl IV] is dispensed in 500-mg vials and must be reconstituted prior to use (see below). The IV solution [Flagyl I.V. RTU, Metronidazole Redi-Infusion, Metro I.V.] contains 5 mg of the drug per ml and is ready to use.

Preparation of Powdered Metronidazole for IV Infusion. The powder is readied for infusion in three steps: (1) reconstitution, (2) dilution in IV solution, and (3) neutralization. These steps must be performed in the order indicated. The powder is reconstituted using 4.4 ml of any of the following liquids: Sterile Water for Injection, Bacteriostatic Water for Injection, 0.9% Sodium Chloride Injection, or Bacteriostatic 0.9% Sodium Chloride Injection. The resulting concentrated solution contains approximately 100 mg of metronidazole per ml. This solution is then diluted to a concentration of 8 mg/ml (or less) using any of the following IV solutions: 0.9% Sodium Chloride Injection, 5% Dextrose Injection, or Lactated Ringer's Injection. Neutralization of the diluted solution is accomplished by adding 5 mEq of sodium bicarbonate injection for each 500 mg of metronidazole present; this procedure should elevate pH to a value between 6.0 and 7.0. Neutralized solutions should not be refrigerated, since cooling may cause metronidazole to precipitate.

Intravenous Dosage and Administration. Infusions must be done slowly (over a 1-hour interval). Therapy of anaerobic infections in adults is initiated with a loading dose of 15 mg/kg. After this, maintenance doses of 7.5 mg/kg are administered every 6 to 8 hours. Duration of treatment is usually 1 to 2 weeks. Patients who have kidney dysfunction and are receiving prolonged treatment may need a reduction in dosage to avoid accumulation of the drug to toxic levels.

Oral Preparations and Dosage. Metronidazole is dispensed in tablets (250 and 500 mg) for oral administration. Trade names are Femazole, Flagyl, Metryl, Metizole, Protostat, and Satric.

The adult dosage for anaerobic infections is 7.5 mg/kg every 6 hours. For bacterial vaginosis in adults, a dosage of 500 mg twice daily for 7 days is effective. Pseudomembranous colitis caused by *Clostridium difficile* is treated with 500 mg three times a day for 7 to 15 days.

RIFAMPIN

Rifampin [Rifadin, Rimactane] is a broad-spectrum antibacterial drug employed primarily for chemotherapy of tuberculosis (see Chapter 81). However, the drug is also used for several nontuberculous infections. Rifampin is useful for treating *asymptomatic carriers* of *Neisseria meningitidis*, but is not given to treat active meningococcal infection. Unlabeled uses include treatment of leprosy, gram-negative bacteremia in infancy, and infections caused by *Staphylococcus aureus* and *S. epidermidis* (e.g., endocarditis, osteomyelitis, prostatitis). Rifampin has also been employed for prophylaxis of meningitis due to *Haemophilus influenzae*. Because resistance can develop rapidly, established bacterial infections should not be treated with rifampin alone. The basic pharmacology of rifampin and the use of this agent in tuberculosis are presented in Chapter 81.

BACITRACIN

Bacitracin is a polypeptide antibiotic produced by a strain of *Bacillus subtilis*. The drug is almost always employed topically. Since parenteral administration can cause serious toxicity, bacitracin is rarely used for systemic infections.

Mechanism of Action and Antimicrobial Spectrum. Bacitracin inhibits synthesis of the bacterial cell wall, thereby causing cell lysis and death. The drug is active against most gram-positive bacteria, including staphylococci, streptococci, and *Clostridium difficile*. *Neisseria* species and *Haemophilus influenzae* are also susceptible, but most other gram-negative bacteria are resistant. Acquisition of resistance by sensitive organisms is uncommon.

Adverse Effects. Rarely, topical bacitracin causes local hypersensitivity reactions. Parenteral (IM) administration can produce severe nephrotoxicity.

Therapeutic Uses. The principal use of bacitracin is topical treatment of bacterial infections. The drug is very active against staphylococci and group A streptococci, the pathogens that cause most acute infections of the skin. Because of this activity, bacitracin has been marketed in a variety of topical preparations for treatment of skin infections. Many of these preparations contain additional antibiotics, usually polymyxin B, neomycin, or both.

Oral bacitracin has been employed investigationally to treat pseudomembranous colitis caused by *Clostridium difficile*. However, vancomycin and metronidazole are preferred for this indication. Bacitracin is not absorbed following oral administration; hence, oral bacitracin does cause systemic toxicity.

Rarely, bacitracin is administered IM to treat life-threatening infections. Because of the risk of nephrotoxicity, parenteral use is reserved for severe infections that cannot be managed with safer drugs.

POLYMYXIN B

Polymyxin B is a bactericidal drug employed primarily for local effects. Because of serious systemic toxicity, parenteral administration is rare.

Antibacterial Spectrum and Mechanism of Action. Polymyxin B is bactericidal to a broad spectrum of aerobic, gram-negative bacilli. Gram-positive bacteria and most anaerobes are resistant.

Bactericidal effects result from binding of polymyxin B to the bacterial cell membrane, an action that disrupts membrane structure and thereby increases membrane permeability. The increase in permeability leads to inhibition of cellular respiration and cell death. The resistance displayed by gram-positive bacteria has been attributed to the thick gram-positive cell wall, a structure that may prevent access of polymyxin B to the cell membrane.

Therapeutic Uses. Polymyxin B is used most commonly for topical treatment of the eyes, ears, and skin. Frequently, preparations designed for application to the skin contain other antibiotics, such as bacitracin and neomycin. In addition to its topical uses, polymyxin B (together with neomycin) has been employed as a bladder irrigant to prevent infection in patients with indwelling catheters.

Parenteral use is extremely limited; polymyxin B is not a drug of choice for any systemic infection. The primary indica-

tion for parenteral polymyxin B is serious infection caused by *Pseudomonas aeruginosa*. Polymyxin may be given when preferred drugs have been ineffective or intolerable.

Adverse Effects. The major adverse effects associated with parenteral therapy are neurotoxicity and nephrotoxicity. Both occur frequently and limit the systemic use of this drug. Polymyxin B is not absorbed from sites of topical application; hence, topical use does not cause systemic effects. Rarely, topical polymyxin B produces hypersensitivity.

Antifungal Agents

The antifungal agents fall into two major groups: (1) drugs used to treat *superficial* mycoses (superficial fungal infections) and (2) drugs used to treat *systemic* mycoses. Systemic infections occur much less frequently than superficial infections, but are considerably more dangerous. Therapy of systemic mycoses is the primary focus of this chapter.

DRUGS FOR SYSTEMIC MYCOSES

Systemic mycoses can be subdivided into two categories: (1) *opportunistic* infections, and (2) *nonopportunistic* infections. The opportunistic mycoses—*candidiasis, aspergillosis, cryptococcosis,* and *mucormycosis*—are seen primarily in the debilitated or immunocompromised host. Nonopportunistic infections can occur in any host. These latter mycoses, which are relatively uncommon, include *sporotrichosis, blastomycosis, histoplasmosis,* and *coccidioidomycosis.*

Therapy of the systemic mycoses can be a significant clinical problem. These infections often resist treatment, and, as a result, the patient may require prolonged therapy with drugs that frequently prove toxic. The principal drugs used for systemic mycoses are discussed below.

AMPHOTERICIN B

Amphotericin B [Fungizone] is an important but dangerous drug. This agent is active against a broad spectrum of pathogenic fungi and is the drug of choice for most systemic mycoses (see Table 83–1). Unfortunately, amphotericin B is highly toxic; renal damage is of particular concern. Because of its potential for harm, amphotericin B should be employed only against infections that are progressive and potentially fatal. For treatment of systemic mycoses, amphotericin B is almost always administered by IV infusion. Intrathecal injection has been used for fungal meningitis. For most systemic infections, administration must be performed daily or every other day for several months.

Chemistry

Amphotericin B belongs to a group of drugs known as *polyene antibiotics,* agents that are so named because their structures contain a series of conjugated double bonds. Nystatin, another antifungal drug, also belongs to this family.

Mechanism of Action

Amphotericin B binds to components of the fungal cell membrane, thereby increasing membrane permeability. This increase in permeability reduces fungal viability by permitting leakage of intracellular cations (especially potassium). Depending on the concentration of amphotericin B and the susceptibility of the fungus, the drug may be fungicidal or fungistatic.

The component of the fungal membrane to which amphotericin B binds is called *ergosterol,* a member of the *sterol* family of compounds. For a cell to be susceptible to amphotericin, its cytoplasmic membrane must contain sterols. Since bacteria have no sterols in their membranes, bacteria are not affected by amphotericin.

Much of the toxicity of amphotericin is attributable to the presence of sterols (principally cholesterol) in mammalian cell membranes. By binding to cholesterol in mammalian membranes, amphotericin is thought to affect host cells in much the same way that it affects fungi. There is some selective toxicity for fungi because amphotericin binds more strongly to ergosterol (the major sterol in fungal membranes) than it does to cholesterol (the principal sterol of mammalian cell membranes).

Microbial Susceptibility and Resistance

Amphotericin B is active against a broad spectrum of fungi. Some protozoa (e.g., *Leishmania braziliensis*) are also susceptible. As noted, all bacteria are resistant to the drug.

Emergence of resistant fungi during therapy with amphotericin is extremely rare. On occasion, resistance has been observed during long-term use of the drug. In all cases in which resistance has developed, the resistant fungi had membranes whose ergosterol content was either reduced or absent.

Therapeutic Uses

Amphotericin B is the drug of choice for most systemic mycoses (see Table 83–1). Prior to the availability of this agent, systemic fungal infections usually proved fatal. Treatment is prolonged. Six to eight weeks is common. In some cases, treatment may last for 3 or 4 months. In addition to its systemic use, amphotericin may be employed topically.

Table 83–1. Drugs of Choice for Systemic Mycoses

Infection	Causative Organism	Drugs of Choice	Alternative Drugs
Aspergillosis	*Aspergillus* species	Amphotericin B	Itraconazole
Blastomycosis	*Blastomyces dermatitidis*	Amphotericin B *or* ketoconazole	Itraconazole
Candidiasis	*Candida* species	Amphotericin B ± flucytosine	Fluconazole
Coccidioidomycosis	*Coccidioides immitis*	Amphotericin B *or* ketoconazole	Itraconazole, fluconazole
Cryptococcosis	*Cryptococcus neoformans*	Amphotericin B ± flucytosine	Itraconazole, fluconazole
Histoplasmosis	*Histoplasma capsulatum*	Amphotericin B *or* ketoconazole	Itraconazole
Mucormycosis	*Mucor*	Amphotericin B	No dependable alternative
Paracoccidioidomycosis	*Paracoccidioides brasiliensis*	Amphotericin B *or* ketoconazole	Itraconazole
Sporotrichosis	*Sporothrix schenckii*	Amphotericin B	Itraconazole

Pharmacokinetics

Absorption and Distribution. Absorption of amphotericin B from the gastrointestinal tract is poor, and oral therapy of systemic infection is not effective. Hence, for treatment of deep mycoses, the drug must be administered IV. Most of the amphotericin present in the body is bound to sterol-containing membranes in various tissues. Levels about half those in the plasma are achieved in aqueous humor and in peritoneal, pleural, and joint fluids. The drug does not readily penetrate to the cerebrospinal fluid.

Metabolism and Excretion. Little is known about the elimination of amphotericin B. We do not know whether the drug is metabolized or how the majority of this compound is removed from the body. Renal excretion of unchanged drug is minimal. Accordingly, there is no need to reduce the dosage in patients with pre-existing kidney dysfunction. Complete elimination of amphotericin takes a long time; the drug has been detected in tissues more than a year after cessation of treatment.

Adverse Effects

Amphotericin can induce a variety of serious adverse effects. Patients should be under close supervision, preferably in a hospital.

Effects Associated with Intravenous Infusion. Intravenous infusion of amphotericin frequently produces chills, rigors, nausea, and headache. Mild reactions can be reduced by pretreatment with aspirin or acetaminophen. Meperidine can be administered if chills and fever are severe. If other measures fail, hydrocortisone (a glucocorticoid) can be used to decrease fever and chills. However, since glucocorticoids can reduce the patient's ability to fight infection, routine use of hydrocortisone should be avoided. In addition to the above effects, infusion of amphotericin is associated with a high incidence of thrombophlebitis; heparin can decrease this reaction.

Nephrotoxicity. Amphotericin exerts direct toxicity on cells of the kidney; renal impairment occurs in practically all patients. The extent of kidney damage is related to the total dose administered during the full course of treatment. In most cases, renal function returns to normal following cessation of drug use. However, if the total dose exceeds 4 gm, residual impairment is likely. Damage to the kidneys can be reduced by maintaining adequate hydration. Other nephrotoxic drugs (e.g., aminoglycosides) should be avoided. To evaluate renal injury, tests of kidney function should be performed weekly; intake and output should be monitored.

Damage to the kidneys may cause nausea and vomiting (secondary to uremia) and hypokalemia. To minimize nausea and vomiting, amphotericin dosage should be reduced if plasma creatinine content rises above 3.5 mg/dl. Potassium supplements may be needed to correct hypokalemia. Patients should undergo frequent determinations of potassium levels and serum creatinine content.

Effects Associated with Intrathecal Injection. Intrathecal administration may cause nausea, vomiting, headache, and pain in the back, legs, and abdomen. Rare reactions include visual disturbances, impairment of hearing, and paresthesias (tingling, numbness, or pain in the hands and feet).

Other Adverse Effects. Infusion of amphotericin may be associated with delirium, hypotension, hypertension, wheezing, and hypoxia. Bone marrow depression has occurred, resulting in normocytic, normochromic anemia; for evaluation, hematocrit determinations should be performed. Rarely, amphotericin has caused rash, convulsions, anaphylaxis, dysrhythmias, acute liver failure, and nephrogenic diabetes insipidus.

Drug Interactions

Nephrotoxic Drugs. Use of amphotericin with other nephrotoxic drugs (e.g., aminoglycosides, cyclosporine) increases the risk of injury to the kidneys. Accordingly, these combinations should be avoided if at all possible.

Flucytosine. Amphotericin potentiates the antifungal actions of flucytosine, apparently by promoting entry of flucytosine into fungal cells. Because of this potentiative interaction, the combination of flucytosine with a relatively low dose of amphotericin can produce antifungal effects equivalent to those of a high dose of amphotericin alone. By allowing a reduction in amphotericin dosage, the combination decreases the risk of amphotericin-induced toxicity.

Dosage and Administration

Intravenous. For treatment of systemic mycoses, amphotericin B is almost always administered by IV infusion. Infusions should be performed slowly (over 2 to 4 hours) to minimize thrombophlebitis and cardiovascular reactions. Alternate-day dosing can reduce adverse effects. As a rule, several months of therapy are required.

Preparation of Solutions for IV Use. Amphotericin B [Fungizone Intravenous] is dispensed as a powder in 50-mg vials. This powder is reconstituted to a concentration of 5 mg/ml using 10 ml of sterile water. This concentrated preparation is then diluted to 0.1 mg/ml with 5% dextrose for injection prior to infusion. Diluents other than those just mentioned will cause amphotericin to precipitate and should not be employed. Since no preservatives or bacteriostatic agents are used, aseptic technique is essential.

IV Dosage and Administration. Dosage is individualized and based on the severity of the disease and the patient's ability to tolerate the drug. Optimal dosage has not been established. A small (1 mg) test dose is often given to assess patient reaction. After this, therapy is initiated with a dosage of 0.25 mg/kg/day. Maintenance dosages range from 0.4 to 0.6 mg/kg/day. The infusion solution should be checked periodically for a precipitate and, if a precipitate is seen, administration should be discontinued immediately. The manufacturer recommends that IV solutions be protected from light; this practice is unnecessary. Because the treatment period is prolonged, it is advisable to rotate sites of administration (to insure continued availability of a vein suitable for infusion).

Intrathecal. Since amphotericin does not readily enter the cerebrospinal fluid, intrathecal injection has been employed to treat fungal meningitis. This route is considered investigational.

FLUCYTOSINE

Flucytosine [Ancobon] is employed to treat serious infections caused by *Candida* species and *Cryptococcus neoformans*. Because development of resistance is common, flucytosine is almost always used in combination with amphotericin B. Caution must be exercised in patients with renal impairment and hematologic disorders.

Mechanism of Action

The antifungal effects of flucytosine derive from disruption of DNA and RNA synthesis. Flucytosine is taken up by fungal cells and converted to 5-fluorouracil, the active form of the drug. The enzyme responsible for this conversion is cytosine deaminase, and fungi that lack cytosine deaminase are not susceptible to the drug. Since mammalian cells lack cytosine deaminase, flucytosine has relatively low toxicity to the host.

Fungal Resistance

Development of resistance to flucytosine during therapy is common and constitutes a serious clinical problem. Several mechanisms of resistance have been described, including (1) a reduction in fungal cytosine permease, the enzyme required for uptake of flucytosine, and (2) loss of cytosine deaminase, the enzyme required to convert flucytosine to its active form.

Antifungal Spectrum and Therapeutic Uses

Flucytosine has a narrow antifungal spectrum. Fungicidal activity is highest against *Candida* species and *Cryptococcus neoformans*. Most other fungi are resistant. Because of this narrow spectrum, flucytosine is indicated only for candidiasis and cryptococcosis. For treatment of serious infections (e.g., cryptococcal meningitis, systemic candidiasis), flucytosine should be combined with amphotericin B. This combination offers two advantages over the use of flucytosine alone: (1) antifungal activity is enhanced, and (2) emergence of resistant fungi is reduced.

Pharmacokinetics

Flucytosine is readily absorbed from the gastrointestinal tract and is well distributed through-

out the body. The drug has good access to the central nervous system; levels in cerebrospinal fluid are about 80% of those in plasma. Flucytosine is eliminated by the kidneys, principally as the unchanged drug. The half-life of flucytosine is about 4 hours in patients with normal renal function. However, in the presence of renal insufficiency, the half-life is greatly prolonged. Accordingly, dosages must be reduced in patients with kidney dysfunction.

Adverse Effects

Hematologic Effects. Bone marrow depression is the most serious complication of treatment. Marrow depression usually manifests as reversible neutropenia or thrombocytopenia. Rarely, fatal agranulocytosis has developed. Platelet and leukocyte counts should be made weekly. Adverse hematologic effects are most likely when plasma levels of flucytosine exceed 100 μg/ml; the dosage should be adjusted to keep drug levels below this value. Flucytosine should be used with caution in patients with pre-existing bone marrow depression.

Hepatotoxicity. Mild and reversible liver dysfunction occurs frequently, but severe hepatic injury is rare. Effects on liver function should be monitored by making weekly determinations of serum transaminase and alkaline phosphatase levels.

Drug Interactions

Flucytosine is often combined with *amphotericin B*. As noted above, this combination offers several advantages. However, use of the combination can also be detrimental. Since amphotericin B is nephrotoxic, and since flucytosine is eliminated by the kidneys, amphotericin B–induced kidney damage may suppress flucytosine excretion and thereby promote flucytosine toxicity. Accordingly, *it is important to monitor renal function and flucytosine levels when amphotericin B and flucytosine are employed concurrently.*

Preparations, Dosage, and Administration

Flucytosine [Ancobon] is dispensed in 250- and 500-mg capsules for oral administration. The usual dosage for patients with normal kidney function is 50 to 150 mg/kg every 6 hours. At this dosage, many patients must ingest 20 or more capsules four times each day. Dosages must be reduced for patients with renal insufficiency. Nausea and vomiting associated with drug administration can be decreased by taking flucytosine capsules a few at a time over a 15-minute interval.

KETOCONAZOLE

Ketoconazole [Nizoral] is an oral alternative to amphotericin B for treatment of less severe systemic mycoses. The drug is safer than amphotericin B and has the additional advantage of being orally usable.

Ketoconazole belongs to the azole family of antifungal agents, for which it can be considered the prototype. Other family members include fluconazole, itraconazole, miconazole, clotrimazole, and econazole. All are active against a broad spectrum of fungi. Some are used for systemic mycoses, some for superficial mycoses, and some for both types of infections.

Mechanism of Action

Ketoconazole inhibits the synthesis of ergosterol, an essential component of the fungal cytoplasmic membrane. This results in increased membrane permeability and leakage of cellular components. Accumulation of ergosterol precursors may also contribute to antifungal actions. Ketoconazole is fungistatic at lower concentrations and fungicidal at higher concentrations.

Antifungal Spectrum

Most of the fungi that cause systemic mycoses are susceptible. Ketoconazole is also active against the fungi that cause superficial infections (dermatophytes and *Candida* species). Emergence of resistance is rare.

Therapeutic Uses

Ketoconazole is an alternative to amphotericin B for treatment of systemic mycoses. The drug is much less toxic than amphotericin but is also less effective. Specific indications are listed in Table 83–1. Responses to ketoconazole are slow. Accordingly, the drug is less useful for treating severe, acute infections than for long-term suppression of chronic mycoses. Ketoconazole is also a valuable drug for treating superficial mycoses; these applications are considered later in the chapter.

Pharmacokinetics

Absorption. Ketoconazole is a weak base and requires an acidic environment for dissolution and absorption. Oral ketoconazole is well absorbed from the gastrointestinal tract, provided that levels of gastric acid are normal. In patients with achlorhydria (absence of gastric acid), absorption is low. Drugs that reduce gastric acidity (e.g., antacids, H_2 blocking agents, omeprazole) decrease ketoconazole absorption.

Distribution. Most of the ketoconazole present in the blood is bound to plasma proteins. The drug crosses the blood-brain barrier poorly and concentrations in cerebrospinal fluid remain low. In contrast, high levels of ketoconazole are achieved in the skin, making oral ketoconazole useful against superficial mycoses.

Elimination. Ketoconazole is eliminated by hepatic metabolism. Its half-life is approximately 3 hours. In the presence of liver dysfunction, the half-life can be substantially prolonged. Since elimination is hepatic, renal impairment does not influence the intensity or duration of action. Hence, no dosage adjustment is needed in patients with kidney disease.

Adverse Effects

Ketoconazole is generally well tolerated. The most common adverse reactions—nausea and vomiting—can be reduced by giving the drug with food. The most serious effects involve the liver.

Hepatotoxicity. Effects of ketoconazole on the liver are rare but potentially severe; fatal hepatic necrosis has occurred. Liver function should be evaluated prior to treatment and at intervals of 1 month or less thereafter. Ketoconazole should be discontinued at the first sign of liver injury. The drug should be employed with caution in patients with a history of hepatic disease. Patients should be advised to notify the physician if symptoms suggesting liver dysfunction develop (e.g., unusual fatigue, anorexia, nausea, vomiting, jaundice, dark urine, pale stools).

Other Adverse Effects. Ketoconazole can produce a variety of relatively mild adverse effects, including rash, itching, dizziness, fever, chills, constipation, diarrhea, photophobia, and headache. The drug can reduce testosterone synthesis and, in males, has caused gynecomastia, oligospermia, and reduced potency. Menstrual irregularities have occurred in females. Rarely, ketoconazole has caused anaphylaxis, severe epigastric pain, and altered function of the adrenals.

Drug Interactions

Drugs That Raise Gastric pH. Drugs that decrease gastric acidity—antacids, H_2 antagonists, omeprazole, anticholinergic drugs—can greatly reduce ketoconazole absorption. To minimize reductions in absorption, these agents should be administered no sooner than 2 hours after ingestion of ketoconazole.

Rifampin. Rifampin reduces plasma levels of ketoconazole, apparently by enhancing hepatic metabolism. If these drugs are used concurrently, ketoconazole dosage should be increased—and even then it may be impossible to achieve therapeutic levels of the drug.

Terfenadine and Astemizole. Ketoconazole increases the risk of potentially fatal cardiac dysrhythmias in patients taking terfenadine or astemizole (nonsedative antihistamines). Accordingly, concurrent use of these drugs is contraindicated.

Preparations, Dosage, and Administration

Ketoconazole [Nizoral] is dispensed in 200-mg tablets for oral administration. The recommended *adult* dosage is 200 mg once a day. For chemotherapy of severe infection, daily doses of 400 to 800 mg may be required. The dosage for *children* over 2 years of age is 3.3 to 6.6 mg/kg/day in a single dose. Duration of treatment is 6 months or longer. Since an acidic environment is needed for ketoconazole absorption, patients with achlorhydria should dissolve the tablets in 4 ml of 0.2 N hydrochloric acid; the solution should be sipped through a plastic or glass straw to avoid damage to the teeth.

FLUCONAZOLE

Actions and Uses. Fluconazole [Diflucan] belongs to the azole group of antifungal agents. The drug has the same mechanism of action as ketoconazole: inhibition of ergosterol synthesis with resultant damage to the cytoplasmic membrane and accumulation of ergosterol precursors. The drug is primarily fungistatic. Fluconazole is used to treat oropharyngeal and esophageal *Candida* infections and meningitis caused by *Cryptococcus neoformans* and *Coccidioides immitis*.

Pharmacokinetics. Fluconazole is well absorbed (90%) following oral administration. The drug is widely distributed to tissues and body fluids, including the cerebrospinal fluid (CSF). Most of the drug is eliminated unchanged in the urine. Fluconazole has a half-life of 30 hours, making once-a-day dosing sufficient.

Adverse Effects and Interactions. Fluconazole is less toxic than ketoconazole and is generally well tolerated. The most common reactions are nausea (3.7%), headache (1.9%), rash (1.8%), vomiting (1.7%), abdominal pain (1.7%), and diarrhea (1.5%). Rarely, treatment has been associated with hepatic necrosis, Stevens-Johnson syndrome, and anaphylaxis. Fluconazole can inhibit hepatic drug-metabolizing enzymes, thereby increasing the levels of other drugs, including oral anticoagulants, phenytoin, and cyclosporine.

Preparations, Dosage, and Administration. Fluconazole [Diflucan] is dispensed in tablets (50, 100, and 200 mg) for oral administration and in solution (2 mg/ml) for intravenous infusion. Since oral absorption is rapid and nearly complete, oral and IV dosages are the same. For treatment of *oropharyngeal and esophageal candidiasis*, the usual dosage is 200 mg on the first day, followed by 100 mg once daily thereafter. For treatment of *systemic candidiasis* and *cryptococcal meningitis*, the usual dosage is 400 mg on the first day, followed by 200 mg once daily thereafter. Duration of treatment ranges from 3 weeks to more than 3 months, depending on the infection being treated.

ITRACONAZOLE

Actions and Uses. Itraconazole [Sporanox], a member of the azole family of antifungal agents, is active against a broad spectrum of fungal pathogens. Like ketoconazole, the drug inhibits synthesis of ergosterol, causing the fungal cell membrane to leak. Approved indications are *blastomycosis* (pulmonary and extrapulmonary) and *histoplasmosis*. However, because of its broad antifungal spectrum, the drug has been used for other systemic fungal infections (*aspergillosis, coccidioidomycosis, cryptococcosis, paracoccidioidomycosis, sporotrichosis*) and also for *superficial fungal infections*.

Pharmacokinetics. Itraconazole is administered orally, and absorption is greatly *enhanced* by the presence of food. The drug is widely distributed to lipophilic tissues. In contrast, concentrations in aqueous fluids (e.g., saliva, CSF) are negligible. The drug undergoes extensive hepatic metabolism. About 40% of an administered dose is excreted in the urine as inactive metabolites.

Adverse Effects. Itraconazole is well tolerated in usual doses. Gastrointestinal reactions (nausea, vomiting, diarrhea) are most common, occurring in about 10% of those treated. Other common reactions include rash (8.6%), headache (3.8%), abdominal pain (3.3%), and edema (3.5%). Hepatitis has occurred rarely, and the involvement of itraconazole is not clear. Liver function should be monitored in patients with pre-existing liver disease.

Drug Interactions. Itraconazole can elevate plasma levels of several drugs, including *cyclosporine, digoxin, sulfonylureas, warfarin,* and *terfenadine*. In patients taking *cyclosporine* or *digoxin*, levels of these drugs should be monitored; in patients taking *sulfonylureas*, blood glucose levels should be monitored; in patients taking *warfarin*, prothrombin time should be monitored. Since the combination of itraconazole with *terfenadine* or *astemizole* can result in potentially fatal cardiac dysrhythmias, these drugs should not be used concurrently.

Phenytoin, isoniazid, and *rifampin* can reduce plasma levels of itraconazole. The dosage of itraconazole may need to be increased.

Preparations, Dosage, and Administration. Itraconazole [Sporanox] is dispensed in 100-mg capsules for oral administration. The drug should be taken with food to increase absorption. The recommended dosage is 200 mg once a day. If needed, the daily dosage may be increased to 400 mg (administered in two divided doses).

MICONAZOLE

Miconazole, like ketoconazole, belongs to the azole family of compounds. The antifungal actions of both drugs are similar. Miconazole is employed primarily for *topical* treatment of *superficial* mycoses. Because of toxicity, miconazole is rarely employed to treat systemic fungal infection. When used for systemic therapy, the drug must be given IV. Administration by this route is associated with a high incidence of adverse effects, including phlebitis, thrombocytosis, nausea, vomiting, pruritus, rash, and fever. Miconazole enhances the actions of oral anticoagulants (e.g., warfarin), and dosages of these drugs must be lowered to avoid hemorrhage. Miconazole can antagonize the effects of amphotericin B in the treatment of candidiasis.

Miconazole for *intravenous* use [Monistat i.v.] is dispensed as a 10 mg/ml solution in 20 ml ampuls. The drug is diluted in 0.9% saline plus 5% dextrose and infused slowly (over 30 to 60 minutes). The *daily* dosage for *adults* is 200 mg to 3.6 gm administered in three or four divided doses at equally spaced intervals. Duration of treatment is 2 to 20 weeks.

DRUGS FOR SUPERFICIAL MYCOSES

The superficial mycoses are caused by two groups of organisms: (1) *Candida* species, and (2) dermatophytes (species of *Epidermophyton, Trichophyton,* and *Microsporum*). Candidal infections usually occur in mucous membranes and moist skin; chronic infections may involve the scalp, skin, and nails. Dermatophytoses are generally confined to the skin, hair, and nails. Superficial infections with dermatophytes are more common than with *Candida*.

Superficial mycoses can be treated with a variety of *topical* agents and with two *oral* drugs: griseofulvin and ketoconazole. For mild-to-moderate infections, topical agents are generally preferred. Specific indications for the drugs used against superficial mycoses are summarized in Table 83–2. Three of these drugs—amphotericin B, ketoconazole, and miconazole—are also used to treat systemic fungal infections.

Vaginal candidiasis is very common and deserves special comment. Approximately 25% of women of child-bearing age develop this infection. Predisposing factors include pregnancy, obesity, diabetes, debilitation, HIV infection, and use of certain drugs, including oral contraceptives, systemic glucocorticoids, anticancer agents, immuno-

Table 83–2. Drugs for Superficial Mycoses

Drug	Route	Dermatophytic (Tinea) Infections			Candida Infections		
		Body, Perineum, Foot, Hand	Scalp, Nails, Beard	Pityriasis (Tinea) Versicolor	Skin	Mouth	Vagina*
Azoles							
Butoconazole	Topical						√
Clotrimazole	Topical	√		√	√	√	√
Econazole	Topical	√		√	√		
Ketoconazole	Topical	√		√	√		
	Oral	√	√	√	√	√	√
Miconazole	Topical	√		√	√		√
Oxiconazole	Topical	√		√			
Sulconazole	Topical	√		√			
Terconazole	Topical						√
Tioconazole	Topical						√
Polyene Antibiotics							
Amphotericin B	Topical				√		
Nystatin	Topical				√	√	√
Others							
Ciclopirox	Topical	√		√	√		
Clioquinol	Topical	√					
Griseofulvin	Oral	√	√				
Haloprogin	Topical	√		√	√		
Naftifine	Topical	√					
Tolnaftate	Topical	√					
Undecylenic acid	Topical	√					

*An expanded summary of drugs for vaginal candidiasis is presented in Table 83–3.

suppressants, and systemic antibiotics. Traditionally, vaginal candidiasis has been treated with topical antifungal drugs applied once daily for 7 to 14 days. When higher doses of our newer drugs are employed, the infection can often be eliminated with just 1 to 3 days of topical therapy. Furthermore, European studies have shown that a single oral dose of fluconazole (150 mg) can be curative. The drugs currently employed for topical treatment of vaginal candidiasis are summarized in Table 83–3; trade names, formulations, and dosing schedules are included. All of these drugs appear to be equally effective. The longer regimens have no demonstrated advantage over the shorter regimens.

The basic pharmacology of the drugs employed for superficial mycoses is discussed below.

AZOLES: CLOTRIMAZOLE, KETOCONAZOLE, OTHERS

Nine members of the azole family are employed to treat superficial mycoses (see Table 83–2). All nine can be administered topically, and one—ketoconazole—may also be administered orally. Two of these azoles—ketoconazole and miconazole—are used to treat systemic mycoses in addition to superficial mycoses.

The azoles are active against a broad spectrum of pathogenic fungi, including dermatophytes and *Candida* species. Antifungal effects result from inhibiting the biosynthesis of ergosterol, an essential component of the fungal cytoplasmic membrane.

Clotrimazole

Therapeutic Uses. Topical clotrimazole is a drug of choice for dermatophytic infections and candidiasis of the skin, mouth, and vagina.

Adverse Effects. When applied to the skin, clotrimazole can cause stinging, erythema, edema, urticaria, pruritus, and peeling. However, the incidence of these reactions is low. Intravaginal administration is occasionally associated with burn-

Table 83–3. Topical Drugs for Vaginal Candidiasis

Generic Name	Trade Name	Formulation	Dosage
Nystatin	generic	100,000 U vaginal tablet	1 tablet at HS × 14 days
	Mycostatin	100,000 U vaginal tablet	1 tablet at HS × 14 days
	Nilstat	100,000 U vaginal tablet	1 tablet at HS × 14 days
	O-V Statin	100,000 U vaginal tablet	1 tablet at HS × 14 days
Butoconazole	Femstat	2% vaginal cream	5 gm at HS × 6 days (pregnant)
			5 gm at HS × 3 days (nonpregnant)
Clotrimazole	Gyne-Lotrimin	100-mg vaginal tablet	1 tablet at HS × 7 days *or*
			2 tablets at HS × 3 days
		500-mg vaginal tablet	1 tablet at HS once
		1% vaginal cream	5 gm at HS × 7–14 days
	Mycelex-G	100-mg vaginal tablet	1 tablet at HS × 7 days *or*
			2 tablets at HS × 3 days
		500-mg vaginal tablet	1 tablet at HS once
		1% vaginal cream	5 gm at HS × 7–14 days
Miconazole	Monistat 3	200-mg vaginal suppository	1 suppository at HS × 3 days
	Monistat 7	100-mg vaginal suppository	1 suppository at HS × 7 days
	Monistat 7	2% vaginal cream	5 gm at HS × 7 days
Terconazole	Terazol 3	80-mg vaginal suppository	1 suppository at HS × 3 days
		0.8% vaginal cream	5 gm at HS × 3 days
	Terazol 7	0.4% vaginal cream	5 gm at HS × 7 days
Tioconazole	Vagistat	6.5% vaginal ointment	4.6 gm at HS once

ing sensations and lower abdominal cramps. The oral formulation can cause gastrointestinal distress.

Preparations, Dosage, and Administration. Clotrimazole is available as an oral troche, a cream or tablet for intravaginal use, and in three formulations (cream, lotion, solution) for application to the skin. For fungal infections of the skin, the drug is applied twice daily for 1 week or longer. Several dosing schedules have been employed for vaginal candidiasis, including (1) intravaginal insertion of 1 tablet nightly for 7 days, and (2) application of 5 gm of cream once a day for 1 to 2 weeks. Trade names for clotrimazole include Lotrimin, Gyne-Lotrimin, and Mycelex.

Ketoconazole

Ketoconazole [Nizoral] is the only azole antifungal drug approved for both oral and topical therapy of superficial mycoses. Oral ketoconazole provides effective treatment of dermatophytic infections and candidiasis of the skin, mouth, and vagina. However, because of the toxicity associated with oral use, this route should be reserved for infections that have failed to respond to topical agents (e.g., clotrimazole, miconazole). Ketoconazole is available in cream and shampoo formulations for topical therapy of dermatophytic infections and for candidiasis of the skin. The basic pharmacology of ketoconazole is discussed in the section on systemic mycoses.

Miconazole

Therapeutic Uses. Miconazole is an azole antifungal drug available for topical and systemic administration. Topical miconazole is a drug of choice for dermatophytic infections as well as for cutaneous and vaginal candidiasis. Systemic uses of miconazole are discussed above.

Adverse Effects. Untoward effects of topical miconazole are generally mild. Intravaginal administration causes burning, itching, and irritation in about 7% of patients. When applied to the skin, miconazole occasionally causes irritation, burning, and maceration. Topical application is not associated with systemic toxicity.

Preparations, Dosage, and Administration. Miconazole is available in cream, liquid, and powder formulations for application to the skin, and in cream and suppository formulations for intravaginal application. Cutaneous mycoses are treated with twice daily applications for 2 to 4 weeks. For vaginal candidiasis, miconazole cream or a 100-mg suppository is administered nightly for 1 week. Alternatively, a 200-mg suppository can be administered nightly for 3 days. Trade names for topical miconazole are Micatin, Monistat-Derm, Monistat 3, and Monistat 7.

Newer Azole Drugs

Econazole. Econazole [Spectazole] is available for topical application only. The drug is indicated for tinea infections and superficial candidiasis. Local adverse effects (burning, erythema, stinging, itching) occur in about 3% of patients. Less than 1% of topical econazole is absorbed, and systemic toxicity has not been reported. Econazole, dispensed as a 1% cream, is applied twice daily for 2 to 4 weeks.

Oxiconazole and Sulconazole. Oxiconazole [Oxistat] and sulconazole [Exelderm] are broad-spectrum antifungal drugs. Both are approved for topical treatment of tinea infections. Local adverse effects (itching, burning, irritation, erythema) occur in less than 3% of those treated. Neither drug is absorbed to a significant degree, and systemic toxicity has not been reported. Oxiconazole is dispensed as a cream, and sulconazole is dispensed as a cream and in solution. Both drugs are applied once daily for 2 to 4 weeks.

Butoconazole, Terconazole, and Tioconazole. These azole drugs are approved only for topical treatment of vaginal candidiasis. All three are fungicidal. Local adverse effects (burning, itching) occur in 2% to 6% of those treated. Absorption following intravaginal administration is low, and systemic reactions are rare (except for headache from terconazole). Because of a small risk of fetal injury, these drugs are not recommended for use during the first trimester of pregnancy. Trade names, formulations, and dosages are presented in Table 83–3.

GRISEOFULVIN

Griseofulvin is administered orally for treatment of superficial mycoses. The drug is inactive against organisms that cause systemic fungal infections.

Mechanism of Action. Following absorption, griseofulvin is deposited in the keratin precursor cells of skin, hair, and nails. Because of the presence of griseofulvin, newly formed keratin is resistant to fungal invasion. Hence, as infected keratin is shed, it is replaced by fungus-free tissue.

Griseofulvin produces its fungicidal effects by inhibiting fungal mitosis. The drug inhibits mitosis by binding to components of microtubules, the structures that form the mitotic spindle. Because griseofulvin acts by disrupting mitosis, the drug only affects fungi that are actively growing.

Pharmacokinetics. Griseofulvin is administered orally. Absorption can be enhanced by taking the drug with a fatty meal. As noted, griseofulvin is deposited in the keratin precursor cells of skin, hair, and nails. Elimination is by hepatic metabolism and renal excretion.

Therapeutic Uses. Griseofulvin is employed orally to treat dermatophytic infections of the skin, hair, and nails. The drug is not active against *Candida* species, nor is it useful for treating systemic mycoses. Dermatophytic infections of the skin respond relatively quickly (in 3 to 8 weeks). However, infections of the palms may require 2 to 3 months of treatment, and a year or more may be needed to eliminate infections of the toenails.

Adverse Effects. Most untoward effects are not serious. Transient headache is common, occurring in about 15% of patients. Other mild reactions include rash, insomnia, tiredness, and gastrointestinal effects (nausea, vomiting, diarrhea). Griseofulvin may cause hepatotoxicity and photosensitivity in patients with porphyria. The drug is contraindicated for individuals with a history of porphyria or hepatocellular disease.

Drug Interactions. Griseofulvin induces hepatic drug-metabolizing enzymes and can thereby decrease the effects of *warfarin*. When this combination is used, the dosage of warfarin may need to be increased.

Preparations, Dosage, and Administration. Griseofulvin is prepared in two particle sizes: microsized and ultramicrosized. The microcrystalline form [Fulvicin-U/F, Grifulvin V, Grisactin] is dispensed in tablets (250 and 500 mg), capsules (125 and 250 mg), and in suspension (125 mg/ml). The ultramicrocrystalline form [Fulvicin P/G, Grisactin Ultra, Gris-PEG] is dispensed in tablets, ranging in size from 125 to 330 mg.

Dosage depends to some degree upon which formulation (microsized or ultramicrosized) is being used. With the *microsized* formulations, the usual *adult* dosage is 500 mg to 1 gm per day; the usual dosage for *children* is 11 mg/kg/day. The ultramicro-

sized particles are better absorbed than the microsized particles. As a result, doses of *ultramicrocrystalline* griseofulvin are about 30% lower than doses of the microcrystalline form.

POLYENE ANTIBIOTICS

Amphotericin B

Amphotericin B [Fungizone] is a broad-spectrum antifungal drug available for intravenous and topical use. As discussed above, intravenous amphotericin B is the drug of choice for most systemic mycoses. In contrast, topical amphotericin is limited to treatment of candidiasis of the skin. The drug is not employed to treat vaginal candidiasis, and is ineffective against dermatophytic infections. Adverse effects (burning, itching, erythema) from topical application occur occasionally. Absorption following topical application is minimal, and does not result in systemic toxicity. Topical amphotericin B is dispensed in cream, lotion, and ointment formulations. The drug is applied two to four times each day. Duration of treatment is 1 to 4 weeks.

Nystatin

Actions, Uses, and Adverse Effects. Nystatin is a polyene antibiotic. Use is limited to treatment of candidiasis. This agent is the drug of choice for chemotherapy of intestinal candidiasis, and is also employed to treat candidal infections of the skin, mouth, esophagus, and vagina. Nystatin can be administered orally, intravaginally, and topically. There is no significant absorption associated with any of these routes. Oral nystatin occasionally causes gastrointestinal disturbance (nausea, vomiting, diarrhea). Topical application may produce local irritation.

Preparations, Dosage, and Administration. For oral administration, nystatin is dispensed as a suspension and in tablets and lozenges; dosages range from 100,000 units to 1,000,000 units three to four times a day. Vaginal tablets are employed for vaginal candidiasis; the usual dosage is 100,000 units once a day for 2 weeks. Nystatin is dispensed as a cream, ointment, and powder to treat candidiasis of the skin. The cream and ointment formulations are applied twice daily; the powder is applied three times daily. Trade names for nystatin include Mycostatin, Nilstat, and O-V Statin.

OTHER DRUGS FOR SUPERFICIAL MYCOSES

Tolnaftate

Tolnaftate is employed topically to treat a variety of superficial mycoses. The drug is active against dermatophytes, but not against *Candida* species. The mechanism of antifungal action is unknown. Adverse effects (sensitization, irritation) are extremely rare. Tolnaftate is available in several formulations. Creams, gels, and solutions are most effective; powders are used adjunctively. The drug is applied twice daily for 2 to 3 weeks. Trade names include Aftate, Tinactin, and Zeasorb-AF.

Haloprogin

Haloprogin [Halotex] is a topical antifungal agent that is active against dermatophytes and *Candida* species. The primary indication for this drug is tinea pedis (athlete's foot). Principal side effects are irritation, burning sensations, and peeling of skin. The drug is dispensed as a cream and in solution. Treatment consists of twice daily application for 2 to 3 weeks.

Undecylenic Acid

Undecylenic acid [Desenex, Cruex, others] is a topical agent used to treat superficial mycoses. The drug is active against dermatophytes but not *Candida* species. The major indication for this agent is tinea pedis (athlete's foot). However, other drugs (tolnaftate, haloprogin, the imidazoles) are more effective.

Ciclopirox Olamine

Ciclopirox olamine [Loprox], a broad-spectrum antifungal drug, is active against dermatophytes and *Candida* species. This agent is applied topically to treat superficial candidiasis and tinea pedis, tinea cruris, tinea corporis, and tinea versico-

lor. The drug penetrates the epidermis to the dermis, but absorption is minimal and no significant systemic accumulation occurs. There is no toxicity from local application. Ciclopirox olamine is dispensed in cream and lotion formulations. Treatment consists of twice daily application for 2 to 4 weeks.

Naftifine

Naftifine [Naftin] is the first representative of a new class of antifungal drugs, the allylamines. Although approved only for topical treatment of dermatophytic infections, naftifine is active against a broad spectrum of pathogenic fungi. The drug acts by inhibiting the biosynthesis of ergosterol, but by a mechanism different from that of the azole antifungal drugs. The most common adverse effects are burning and stinging. Absorption following topical administration is low (about 6%), and systemic effects have not been reported. Naftifine is dispensed in two formulations: 1% cream and 1% gel. The cream is applied once daily; the gel is applied twice daily. The usual duration of treatment is 4 weeks.

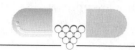 # Summary of Major Nursing Implications

The implications summarized below pertain only to use of antifungal drugs in the treatment of *systemic* mycoses.

AMPHOTERICIN B

 ✓ **Preadministration Assessment**

Therapeutic Goal

Treatment of progressive and potentially fatal systemic fungal infections. Flucytosine may be employed concurrently to enhance therapeutic effects.

Identifying High-Risk Patients

When amphotericin B is used as it should be (i.e., for treatment of life-threatening infections), there are no contraindications to its use.

✓ **Implementation: Administration**

Routes

Intravenous, intrathecal.

Intravenous Administration

Use aseptic technique when preparing infusion solutions. Infuse slowly (over 2 to 4 hours). Check the solution periodically for a precipitate; if a precipitate is seen, discontinue the infusion immediately. Therapy lasts for several months; rotate the infusion site to insure availability of a usable vein. Dosages must be individualized. Alternate-day dosing may be ordered to reduce adverse effects. Heparin may be combined with amphotericin B to reduce phlebitis.

 ✓ **Ongoing Evaluation and Interventions**

Minimizing Adverse Effects

General Considerations. Amphotericin can produce serious adverse effects. The patient should be under close supervision, preferably in a hospital.

Effects Associated with Intravenous Infusion. Infusion of amphotericin can cause chills, nausea, and headache. Mild reactions can be reduced by pretreatment with *aspirin* or *acetaminophen*; more intense reactions may require *meperidine* or *hydrocortisone*. Amphotericin infusion can cause thrombophlebitis; infusion of *heparin* can reduce this reaction.

Nephrotoxicity. Almost all patients experience renal impairment. Monitor and record intake and output. Kidney function should be tested weekly; if plasma creatinine content rises above 3.5 mg/dl, amphotericin dosage should be reduced. The risk of renal damage can be decreased by maintaining adequate hydration and by avoiding other nephrotoxic drugs (e.g., aminoglycosides, cyclosporine).

Renal injury may cause hypokalemia; serum potassium content should be measured frequently. Hypokalemia can be corrected with potassium supplements.

Hematologic Effects. Normocytic, normochromic anemia has occurred secondary to amphotericin-induced depression of bone marrow. Hematocrit determinations should be performed to monitor for this anemia.

Minimizing Adverse Interactions

Unless clearly required, amphotericin should not be combined with other nephrotoxic drugs, such as the *aminoglycosides* and *cyclosporine*.

FLUCYTOSINE

 Preadministration Assessment

Therapeutic Use

Treatment of serious infections caused by *Candida* species and *Cryptococcus neoformans*. Flucytosine is usually combined with amphotericin B.

Baseline Data

Obtain baseline tests of *renal function, hematologic status,* and *serum electrolytes.*

Identifying High-Risk Patients

Use with *extreme caution* in patients with *kidney disease* or *bone marrow depression.*

 Implementation: Administration

Route

Oral.

Dosage and Administration

Treatment may require administration of 20 or more capsules four times per day; advise patients to take capsules a few at a time over a 15-minute interval to minimize nausea and vomiting. Dosage must be reduced in patients with renal impairment.

 Ongoing Evaluation and Interventions

Monitoring Summary

Obtain weekly tests of liver function (serum transaminase and alkaline phosphatase levels) and hematologic status (leukocyte counts). In patients receiving amphotericin B concurrently, and in those with pre-existing renal impairment, monitor kidney function and flucytosine levels.

Minimizing Adverse Effects

Hematologic Effects. Flucytosine-induced bone marrow depression can cause neutropenia, thrombocytopenia, and fatal agranulocytosis. The risk of these effects can be minimized by adjusting the dosage to keep plasma flucytosine levels below 100 µg/ml. Obtain weekly leukocyte counts to monitor hematologic effects.

Hepatotoxicity. Mild and reversible liver dysfunction occurs frequently; severe hepatic damage is rare. Obtain weekly determinations of serum transaminase and alkaline phosphatase levels to evaluate liver function.

Minimizing Adverse Interactions

Amphotericin B. Kidney damage from amphotericin B may decrease flucytosine excretion, thereby promoting toxicity secondary to flucytosine accumulation. When these drugs are combined, renal function and flucytosine levels must be monitored.

KETOCONAZOLE

 Preadministration Assessment

Therapeutic Use

Treatment of systemic and superficial mycoses. Because of its slow onset, ketoconazole is best suited for long-term therapy of chronic fungal infections.

Baseline Data

Obtain baseline tests of liver function.

Identifying High-Risk Patients

Ketoconazole is *contraindicated* for patients taking *terfenadine* or *astemizole*. Use with *caution* in patients with *liver disease*.

 Implementation: Administration

Route

Oral.

Administration

Advise patients to take ketoconazole with food to minimize nausea and vomiting.

An acidic environment is needed for absorption: instruct patients with achlorhydria to dissolve ketoconazole tablets in 4 ml of 0.2 N HCl and to sip this solution through a glass or plastic straw (to protect the teeth), and to follow drug administration with a glass of water.

Minimizing Adverse Effects

 Ongoing Evaluation and Interventions

Hepatotoxicity. Hepatotoxicity is rare but potentially serious; fatal hepatic necrosis has occurred. Tests of liver function should be obtained prior to treatment and at intervals of 1 month or less thereafter. At the first indication of liver injury, ketoconazole should be withdrawn. Inform patients about symptoms of liver dysfunction (e.g., unusual fatigue, anorexia, nausea, vomiting, jaundice, dark urine, pale stools), and advise them to notify the physician if these occur.

Minimizing Adverse Interactions

Drugs That Raise Gastric pH. Antacids, H_2 antagonists, omeprazole, and *anticholinergic drugs* can reduce ketoconazole absorption. These drugs should be administered no sooner than 2 hours after ingestion of ketoconazole.

Rifampin. This drug reduces plasma levels of ketoconazole. Ketoconazole dosage should be increased if these agents are used concurrently.

Terfenadine and Astemizole. Concurrent use of terfenadine or astemizole with ketoconazole is contraindicated because of the risk of severe cardiac dysrhythmias.

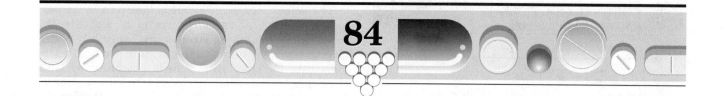

84

Antiviral Agents

SYSTEMIC ANTIVIRAL AGENTS
Acyclovir
Zidovudine (Azidothymidine, AZT)
Didanosine
Zalcitabine
Ganciclovir
Foscarnet
Ribavirin
Vidarabine
Amantadine
Rimantadine
Interferon Alfa

OPHTHALMIC ANTIVIRAL AGENTS
Trifluridine
Vidarabine
Idoxuridine

O ur ability to treat viral infections is quite limited. In contrast to the dramatic advances made in antibacterial therapy over the past 45 years, efforts to develop safe and effective antiviral drugs have been largely unsuccessful. A major reason for this lack of success resides in the process of viral replication: viruses are obligate intracellular parasites that must use the biochemical machinery of host cells for reproduction. Because the viral growth cycle employs host-cell enzymes and substrates, it is extremely difficult to suppress viral replication without also doing significant harm to the host. The few useful antiviral drugs that have been developed act by affecting biochemical processes unique to viral reproduction. As our knowledge of viral molecular biology advances, it is likely that additional virus-specific processes will be discovered, thereby giving us new targets against which to direct our drugs.

At this time, only 14 antiviral agents are approved for use in the United States. These drugs are active against a narrow spectrum of viruses, and their clinical applications are limited to just a few types of viral infections. Eleven of these drugs are employed to treat systemic infections. Three are employed locally for infections of the eye. Drugs of first choice for systemic infections are summarized in Table 84–1.

SYSTEMIC ANTIVIRAL AGENTS

ACYCLOVIR

Acyclovir [Zovirax] is the agent of first choice for infections caused by herpes simplex viruses and

1041

Table 84–1. Drugs of Choice for Viral Infections

Virus and Infection	Drug of Choice
Herpes Simplex Virus	
Genital herpes	
First episode	Acyclovir
Recurrence	Acyclovir
Frequent recurrences	Acyclovir
Encephalitis	Acyclovir
Mucocutaneous disease in the immunocompromised host	Acyclovir
Neonatal	Acyclovir
Acyclovir-resistant	Foscarnet
Keratoconjunctivitis	Trifluridine
Varicella-Zoster Virus	
Varicella (chickenpox)	Acyclovir
Herpes zoster (shingles)	Acyclovir
Varicella or zoster in the immunocompromised host	Acyclovir
Acyclovir-resistant	Foscarnet
Human Immunodeficiency Virus	
Symptomatic, AIDS or advanced AIDS-related complex	Zidovudine *or* didanosine
Asymptomatic, CD4 <500/mm³	Zidovudine
Influenza A Virus	
Respiratory tract infection	Amantadine
Respiratory Syncytial Virus	
Bronchiolitis, pneumonia	Ribavirin
Cytomegalovirus	
Retinitis	Ganciclovir *or* foscarnet
Hepatitis Viruses B and C	
Chronic hepatitis	Interferon alfa-2b

varicella-zoster virus. The drug can be administered topically, orally, and intravenously. Serious side effects are uncommon.

Antiviral Spectrum

Acyclovir is active only against members of the herpesvirus family, a group that includes *herpes simplex viruses* (HSV), *varicella-zoster virus* (VZV), and *cytomegalovirus* (CMV). Of these viruses, HSV are most sensitive; VZV is moderately sensitive; and most strains of CMV are resistant.

Mechanism of Action

Acyclovir inhibits viral replication by suppressing synthesis of viral DNA. To exert its antiviral effects, acyclovir must first be activated. The critical step in activation is conversion of acyclovir to acyclo-GMP by *thymidine kinase*. Once formed, acyclo-GMP is converted to acyclo-GTP, the compound directly responsible for inhibiting DNA synthesis. Acyclo-GTP suppresses DNA synthesis by (1) inhibiting viral DNA polymerase, and (2) becoming incorporated into the growing strand of viral DNA, where it then acts to block further strand growth.

The selectivity of acyclovir is based in large part on the ability of certain viruses to activate the drug. Herpes simplex viruses are especially sensitive to acyclovir because the drug is a much better substrate for thymidine kinase produced by HSV than it is for mammalian thymidine kinase. Hence, formation of acyclo-GMP, the limiting step in the activation of acyclovir, occurs almost exclusively in cells infected with HSV. Cytomegalovirus is inherently resistant to the drug because acyclovir is a poor substrate for the form of thymidine kinase produced by this virus.

Resistance

Herpesviruses develop resistance to acyclovir by three mechanisms: decreased production of thymidine kinase, alteration of thymidine kinase such that it no longer converts acyclovir to acyclo-GMP, and alteration of viral DNA polymerase such that it is less sensitive to inhibition. Of these mechanisms, thymidine kinase deficiency is by far the most common. Resistance is rare in immunocompetent patients, but many cases have been reported in transplant patients and patients with AIDS. Lesions caused by resistant HSV can be extensive and severe, progressing despite continued acyclovir therapy. Acyclovir-resistant HSV and VZV usually respond to intravenous *foscarnet*, a new antiviral drug.

Therapeutic Uses

Herpes Simplex Genitalis. Genital herpes infections are caused by *type 2 HSV* (HSV-2). For patients with *initial* infection, *topical* acyclovir reduces the duration of viral shedding, but does not accelerate healing. Topical acyclovir is not effective for *recurrent* genital infections. *Oral* acyclovir is superior to topical therapy for initial genital infections and recurrent infections. For patients with initial infection, oral therapy decreases formation of additional lesions and decreases the duration and severity of the initial episode. For patients with recurrent herpes genitalis, continuous oral therapy reduces the frequency at which lesions appear. When initial genital infection is especially severe, *intravenous* acyclovir may be indicated. Patients with primary or recurrent herpes genitalis should be informed that although acyclovir can decrease symptoms, the drug does not eliminate the virus and does not produce cure. Also, patients should be advised to avoid sexual contact when lesions are present.

Mucocutaneous Herpes Simplex Infections. Herpes infections of the face and oropharynx are usually caused by HSV-2. For immunocompetent patients, *oral* acyclovir can be used to treat primary infections of the gums and mouth. Oral acyclovir can also be taken *prophylactically* to prevent episodes of *recurrent* herpes labialis (fever blisters). However, there is no effective treatment for *active* herpes labialis. Mucocutaneous herpes infections can be especially severe in immunocompromised patients. For these people, *intravenous* acyclovir is the treatment of choice.

Varicella-Zoster Infections. High-dose *oral* acyclovir is effective therapy for herpes zoster (shingles) in older adults. Oral therapy is also effective for varicella (chickenpox) in children, adolescents, and adults, provided that dosing is begun early (within 24 hours of rash onset). *Intravenous* acyclovir is the treatment of choice for varicella-zoster infection in the immunocompromised host.

Pharmacokinetics

Acyclovir is administered topically, orally, and intravenously. Oral bioavailability is low (about 20%). No significant absorption occurs with topical use. Once in the blood, acyclovir is distributed widely to body fluids and tissues. Levels achieved in cerebrospinal fluid are 50% of those in plasma. Elimination is renal, primarily as the unchanged drug. In patients with normal kidney function, acyclovir has a half-life of 2.5 hours. The half-life is prolonged by renal impairment, reaching 20 hours in anuric patients. Accordingly, dosages should be reduced in patients with kidney disease.

Adverse Effects

Intravenous Therapy. Intravenous acyclovir is generally well tolerated. The most common reactions are *phlebitis* and *inflammation* at the site of infusion. Reversible *nephrotoxicity*, manifested as elevations in creatinine and blood urea nitrogen (BUN), occurs in some patients. The cause of nephrotoxicity is deposition of acyclovir in renal tubules. The risk of renal injury is increased by dehydration and use of other nephrotoxic drugs. Kidney damage can be minimized by infusing acyclovir slowly (over 1 hour) and by insuring adequate hydration during the infusion and for 2 hours after.

Oral and Topical Therapy. Oral acyclovir is devoid of serious adverse effects. Renal impairment has not been reported. The most common reactions to oral therapy are *nausea, vomiting, diarrhea, headache,* and *vertigo.* Topical acyclovir frequently causes transient *burning or stinging sensations*; systemic reactions do not occur.

Preparations, Dosage, and Administration

Topical. Acyclovir [Zovirax] is dispensed as a 5% ointment for topical use. This formulation is indicated for initial episodes of herpes genitalis and for mild mucocutaneous herpes simplex infections in the immunocompromised host. The drug is applied six times a day at 3-hour intervals. Patients should be advised to apply the drug with a finger cot or rubber glove to avoid viral transfer to other body sites or other people.

Oral. Oral acyclovir [Zovirax] is available in 200-mg capsules, 800-mg tablets, and a suspension (200 mg/5 ml). Dosages for patients with normal kidney function are given below. Dosages must be reduced for patients with renal impairment.

For *initial episodes of herpes genitalis*, the usual dosage is 200 mg five times a day (at 4-hour intervals) for 10 days.

For *long-term suppressive therapy of recurrent genital infections*, the usual dosage is 400 mg twice daily for up to 12 months. Alternative dosages range from 200 mg three times a day to 200 mg five times a day.

For acute therapy of *herpes zoster*, the dosage is 800 mg five times a day (at 4-hour intervals) for 7 to 10 days.

For *varicella* (chickenpox) the dosage is 20 mg/kg (but no more than 800 mg) four times a day for 5 days. Treatment should begin at the earliest sign of rash.

Intravenous. Acyclovir [Zovirax] is dispensed as a powder (500 mg per 10-ml vial) to be reconstituted for IV administration. *The drug is administered by slow IV infusion* (over 1 hour or more). It must not be given as an IV bolus or by IM or SC injection. To minimize the risk of renal damage, hydrate the patient during the infusion and for 2 hours after. Dosages for patients with normal kidney function are given below. Dosages should be reduced for patients with renal impairment.

For *mucocutaneous herpes simplex infection in the immunocompromised host*, the *adult* dosage is 5 mg/kg infused every 8 hours for 7 days. The dosage for *children under 12 years* is 250 mg/m^2 infused every 8 hours for 7 days.

For *varicella-zoster infection in the immunocompromised host*, the *adult* dosage is 10 mg/kg infused every 8 hours for 7 days. The dosage for *children under 12 years* is 500 mg/m^2 infused every 8 hours for 7 days.

For *severe initial episodes of herpes genitalis in the immunocompetent host*, the *adult* dosage is 5 mg/kg infused every 8 hours for 5 days. The dosage for *children under 12 years* is 250 mg/m^2 infused every 8 hours for 5 days.

ZIDOVUDINE (AZIDOTHYMIDINE, AZT)

Zidovudine [Retrovir], formerly called azidothymidine (AZT), is the current drug of choice for initial therapy of patients infected with the *human immunodeficiency virus* (HIV), the causative agent of acquired immunodeficiency syndrome (AIDS). The drug's principal dose-limiting toxicities are *severe anemia* and *granulocytopenia*.

Mechanism of Antiviral Action

Zidovudine inhibits HIV replication by suppressing synthesis of viral DNA. To do this, the drug must first undergo intracellular conversion to its active form, zidovudine triphosphate (ZTP). ZTP then blocks viral DNA synthesis by (1) inhibiting reverse transcriptase, the enzyme employed by HIV to make DNA, and (2) becoming incorporated into the growing strand of viral DNA where it then blocks further strand growth. There is speculation that certain adverse effects of zidovudine may result from inhibiting the type of DNA polymerase found in mitochondria of host cells.

Therapeutic Use: HIV Infection

Zidovudine is the drug of first choice for initial therapy of patients with symptomatic or asymptomatic HIV infection. The drug can delay onset of symptoms, reduce the severity of symptoms, and significantly prolong life. In asymptomatic patients, low-dose therapy delays symptom onset. In symptomatic patients with advanced infection (AIDS or AIDS-related complex [ARC]), zidovudine can improve clinical, immunologic, and virologic status. Treatment can increase CD4 lymphocyte counts, reduce the incidence of opportunistic infections, and reduce titers of p24 antigen (a marker for HIV). In addition, zidovudine promotes weight gain and may temporarily improve neurologic status. Reductions in mortality have been dramatic: in one study, the mortality rate after 9 months of zidovudine was only 6% as compared with 39% in the control group. It should be noted, however, that despite these important benefits, zidovudine is not a cure for AIDS: the drug suppresses HIV replication but does not produce outright kill. Accordingly, patients should be told that treatment will not prevent transmission of HIV by sexual contact. Also, patients should be informed that they may still acquire serious opportunistic infections and, hence, must remain under close medical supervision. Although zidovudine-resistant strains of HIV have been isolated from patients taking the drug, this resistance has not been directly associated with a decline in clinical status. The characteristics of AIDS are discussed further in Chapter 80 (Drugs for Sexually Transmitted Diseases). Drugs of choice for AIDS-associated infections are summarized in Table 80–2 and discussed throughout the chapters on antimicrobials.

Pharmacokinetics

Zidovudine is readily absorbed following oral administration. After entering the blood, some of the drug is taken up by cells and converted to the active form. The remainder undergoes rapid hepatic conversion to an inactive metabolite. Both zidovudine and its inactive metabolite are eliminated by renal excretion. The plasma half-life of the drug is approximately 1 hour.

Adverse Effects

Anemia and Granulocytopenia. Severe anemia and granulocytopenia are zidovudine's principal toxic effects. Multiple transfusions may be required. The risk of hematologic toxicity is increased by high-dose therapy, advanced HIV infection (indicated by low CD4 lymphocyte counts), deficiencies in vitamin B_{12} and folic acid, and concurrent use of drugs that are myelosuppressive, nephrotoxic, or directly toxic to circulating blood cells (see below). Anemia and granulocytopenia generally resolve following zidovudine withdrawal.

Hematologic status (hemoglobin concentration and granulocyte counts) should be determined before treatment and at least every 4 weeks thereafter. Hemoglobin levels may fall significantly within 2 to 4 weeks; granulocyte counts may not fall until after week 6. For patients who develop severe anemia (hemoglobin <7.5 gm/dl or down 25% from the pretreatment baseline) or severe neutropenia (granulocyte count <750/mm^3 or down 50% from the pretreatment baseline), zido-

vudine should be interrupted until there is evidence of bone marrow recovery. If neutropenia and anemia are less severe, a reduction in dosage may be sufficient. Transfusions may permit some patients to continue drug use.

Recently, *granulocyte colony-stimulating factors* have been given to reverse zidovudine-induced neutropenia. Also, if erythropoietin levels are not already elevated, *epoetin* (recombinant erythropoietin) can be given to reduce transfusion requirements in patients with anemia. Granulocyte colony-stimulating factors and epoetin are discussed in Chapter 48.

Other Adverse Effects. *Gastrointestinal effects* (anorexia, nausea, vomiting, diarrhea, abdominal pain, stomach upset) occur on occasion. Possible *CNS reactions* include *headache, confusion, anxiety, insomnia, nervousness,* and *seizures. Rash, muscle pain,* and *changes in nail pigmentation* may also occur.

Drug Interactions

Drugs that are myelosuppressive, nephrotoxic, or directly toxic to circulating blood cells can increase the risk of hematologic toxicity from zidovudine. Notable among these drugs is *ganciclovir,* a new antiviral agent used to treat cytomegalovirus retinitis, a common infection in patients with AIDS. Other drugs of concern include *dapsone, pentamidine, pyrimethamine, trimethoprim-sulfamethoxazole, amphotericin B, flucytosine, vincristine, vinblastine,* and *doxorubicin.*

Preparations, Dosage, and Administration

Preparations. Zidovudine [Retrovir] is available in capsules (100 mg) and a syrup (10 mg/ml) for oral therapy and in solution (10 mg/ml) for IV use.

Oral Therapy. For *adults* with *symptomatic* HIV infection (AIDS or advanced ARC), the recommended dosage is 200 mg every 4 hours around the clock for 1 month, after which the dosage can be reduced to 100 mg every 4 hours. For *adults* with *asymptomatic* HIV infection, the recommended dosage is 100 mg every 4 hours while awake (500 mg/day). For *children* (3 months to 12 years) with HIV infection, the dosage is 180 mg/ $\cdot$m^2 every 6 hours (720 mg/m^2/day), but it should not exceed 200 mg every 6 hours.

Hematologic monitoring should be done every 2 weeks. If severe anemia or severe granulocytopenia develops, treatment should be interrupted until there is evidence of bone marrow recovery. If anemia or granulocytopenia is mild, a reduction in dosage may be sufficient.

Intravenous Therapy. Intravenous zidovudine is indicated for adults with AIDS or advanced ARC who have a history of cytologically confirmed *Pneumocystis carinii* pneumonia or a CD4 lymphocyte count of less than 200/mm^3 in peripheral blood. The IV dosage is 1 to 2 mg/kg (infused over 1 hour) every 4 hours around the clock. Rapid infusion and bolus injection must be avoided. Intravenous therapy should be stopped as soon as oral therapy is appropriate.

Intravenous solutions are prepared by withdrawing the calculated dose from the stock vial and diluting it to 4 mg/ml or less in 5% dextrose for injection. The solution should not be mixed with biologic or colloidal fluids (e.g., blood products, protein solutions) and should be administered within 8 hours (if held at room temperature) or within 24 hours (if held under refrigeration).

DIDANOSINE

Actions and Uses. Didanosine [Videx], also known as dideoxyinosine or ddI, is approved for patients with advanced HIV infection who cannot tolerate zidovudine or have experienced significant deterioration despite zidovudine therapy. The drug is also indicated for patients with HIV infection who have received zidovudine for more than 4 months. Didanosine is taken up by host cells where it undergoes conversion to its active form, dideoxyadenosine triphosphate (ddATP). The active drug blocks synthesis of viral DNA by (1) inhibiting HIV reverse transcriptase, the enzyme that makes viral DNA, and (2) undergoing incorporation into the growing DNA strand, thereby causing premature chain termination. In clinical trials, didanosine has increased CD4 cell counts, decreased viremia, and reduced symptoms in patients with AIDS and severe AIDS-related complex.

Pharmacokinetics. Didanosine is administered orally and bioavailability is low (about 35%). Absorption is greatly reduced by gastric acidity and food. The drug crosses the blood-brain barrier poorly; levels in cerebrospinal fluid are only 20% of those in plasma. Much of the drug (35% to 60%) is excreted unchanged in the urine. There are no data on metabolism of didanosine in humans. The drug's half-life in patients with normal renal function is 1.6 hours. The half-life is three times longer in patients with uremia.

Adverse Effects. *Pancreatitis*, which can be fatal, is the major dose-limiting toxicity. The incidence is 3% to 17%. Patients should be monitored for indications of developing pancreatitis (increased serum amylase in association with increased serum triglycerides, decreased serum calcium, and nausea, vomiting, or abdominal pain). If evolving pancreatitis is diagnosed, didanosine should be withdrawn. The risk of pancreatitis is increased by a history of pancreatitis or alcoholism and by use of IV pentamidine. Caution should be exercised with these patients. Additional adverse effects include *diarrhea* (28%), *peripheral neuropathy* (20%), *leukopenia* (16%), *chills or fever* (12%), and *rash or pruritus* (9%). Less common effects include *headache*, *insomnia*, and *hyperuricemia*. In contrast to zidovudine, didanosine causes minimal bone marrow suppression.

Preparations, Dosage, and Administration. Didanosine [Videx] is available in three formulations: *chewable buffered tablets* (25, 50, 100, and 150 mg), *buffered powder for oral solution* (100, 167, 250, and 375 mg in single-dose packets), and *pediatric powder for oral solution* (in 2-gm and 4-gm bottles). Bioavailability with the tablets is about 20% greater than with the oral solution. Since absorption is greatly reduced by food, administration should be done 1 hour before meals or 2 hours after. Instruct patients using the tablets to either (1) chew them thoroughly, or (2) manually crush or disperse them in at least 1 ounce of water. Instruct patients using powdered didanosine to (1) pour the contents of one packet into 4 ounces of water (not fruit juice or any other acid-containing beverage), (2) stir the mixture until the drug dissolves (about 2 to 3 minutes), and (3) drink the solution immediately.

Dosage is based on body weight. For adults over 60 kg, the dosage is 200 mg twice daily. For adults under 60 kg, the dosage is 125 mg twice daily. Dosages should be reduced in patients with renal impairment. To insure adequate buffering of gastric acid, patients using didanosine tablets must take *two* tablets (of appropriate size) for each dose.

ZALCITABINE

Actions and Uses. Zalcitabine [Hivid], also known as dideoxycytidine or ddC, is approved for combined use with zidovudine to treat patients with advanced HIV infection (CD4 count <300/mm³) who have shown significant clinical or immunologic deterioration. As of this writing, there have been no controlled clinical studies demonstrating the efficacy of the combination. Zalcitabine is a prodrug that undergoes conversion to its active form (ddC triphosphate) within host cells. The active form inhibits viral DNA synthesis by (1) inhibiting HIV

reverse transcriptase, and (2) causing premature termination of the growing DNA chain. Toxicity of zalcitabine results in part from inhibiting mitochondrial DNA polymerase in host cells.

Pharmacokinetics. Zalcitabine is administered orally and bioavailability is 80%. Food delays absorption and reduces the amount absorbed by 14%. The drug crosses the blood-brain barrier poorly; levels in cerebrospinal fluid are only 20% of those in blood. Elimination is primarily by renal excretion. Hepatic metabolism is minimal. The elimination half-life is approximately 2 hours.

Adverse Effects. The major toxicities are *peripheral neuropathy* and, less commonly, *pancreatitis*. The neuropathy, which develops in 10% to 30% of patients, manifests initially as numbness and burning sensations in the extremities. These symptoms may progress to sharp shooting pain and severe continuous burning if the drug is not withdrawn. Pain of severe neuropathy requires opioid (narcotic) analgesics for control. Patients should be informed about the early symptoms of neuropathy and instructed to report them immediately. Neuropathy reverses slowly if zalcitabine is withdrawn early, but may become irreversible if the drug is continued.

Zalcitabine-induced *pancreatitis* is uncommon (<1% incidence), but can be fatal. Patients should be monitored for indications of impending pancreatitis (rising serum amylase in association with rising serum triglycerides, decreasing serum calcium, and nausea, vomiting, or abdominal pain). If evolving pancreatitis is diagnosed, zalcitabine should be withdrawn. Caution is required in patients with a history of pancreatitis or alcoholism and in those receiving IV pentamidine.

Preparations, Dosage, and Administration. Zalcitabine [Hivid] is available in tablets (0.375 and 0.75 mg) for oral administration. The recommended dosage is 0.75 mg zalcitabine plus 200 mg zidovudine every 8 hours.

GANCICLOVIR

Ganciclovir [Cytovene] is a synthetic antiviral agent with activity against herpesviruses, including *cytomegalovirus* (CMV). Because the drug can cause serious adverse effects, especially *granulocytopenia* and *thrombocytopenia*, use should be restricted to prevention and treatment of CMV infection in the immunocompromised patient.

Mechanism of Action. Ganciclovir is a prodrug that undergoes conversion to its active form (ganciclovir triphosphate) within host cells. Ganciclovir triphosphate then inhibits replication of viral DNA by (1) competing with deoxyguanosine triphosphate for binding to viral DNA polymerase, and (2) becoming incorporated into the growing DNA chain, thereby causing premature chain termination.

Pharmacokinetics. Ganciclovir is absorbed very poorly from the gastrointestinal tract. Hence, administration is parenteral (IV). Following IV infusion, the drug is widely distributed to body fluids and tissues. Ganciclovir is excreted unchanged in the urine. In patients with normal renal function, the drug's half-life is about 3 hours. The half-life is prolonged in patients with renal impairment.

Therapeutic Use. Ganciclovir has two approved indications: (1) treatment of CMV retinitis in immunocompromised patients, including those with AIDS, and (2) prevention of CMV infection in transplant patients. In patients with AIDS, CMV retinitis has an incidence of up to 30%. Although most AIDS patients respond initially, the relapse rate is high, even with continued maintenance therapy. To reduce the risk of relapse, patients with AIDS must continue maintenance therapy with ganciclovir for life. Ganciclovir has been used investigationally to treat other CMV infections, including pneumonitis, gastroenteritis, radiculitis, and hepatitis. Since viral resistance can develop during treatment, this possibility should be considered if the patient responds poorly.

Adverse Effects. *Granulocytopenia and Thrombocytopenia.* The adverse effect of greatest concern is *bone marrow suppression*, which can result in *granulocytopenia* (40%) and *thrombocytopenia* (20%). These hematologic responses can be exacerbated by concurrent therapy with zidovudine. Conversely, granulocytopenia can be reduced with granulocyte colony-stimulating factors (see Chapter 48). Because of the risk of hematologic effects, blood cell counts must be monitored. Treatment should be interrupted if the absolute neutrophil count falls below 500/mm^3 or if the platelet counts falls below 25,000/mm^3. Cell counts usually begin to recover within 3 to 5 days. Ganciclovir should be used with caution in patients with pre-existing cytopenias and in those with a history of cytopenic reactions to other drugs.

Reproductive Toxicity. Ganciclovir is *teratogenic* and *embryotoxic* in laboratory animals and probably in humans. Women should be advised to avoid pregnancy during therapy and for 90 days after ceasing treatment. At doses equivalent to those used therapeutically, ganciclovir *inhibits spermatogenesis* in mice; sterility is reversible with low doses and irreversible with high doses. *Female infertility* may also occur. Patients should be forewarned of these effects.

Other Adverse Effects. Incidental effects include *nausea, fever, rash, anemia, liver dysfunction,* and *confusion and other CNS symptoms.*

Preparations, Dosage, and Administration. Ganciclovir [Cytovene] is available as a powder to be reconstituted for IV infusion. Solutions are alkaline and must be infused into a freely flowing vein to avoid local injury. For treatment of CMV retinitis, the *initial dosage* for *adults* with normal renal function is 5 mg/kg (infused over 1 hour) every 12 hours for 14 to 21 days. Two *maintenance dosages* can be used: (1) 5 mg/kg infused over 1 hour once every day, or (2) 6 mg/kg infused over 1 hour once a day, 5 days each week. Dosages must be reduced for patients with renal impairment. Since patients with AIDS must continue maintenance therapy for life, they need a permanent IV line and equipment for home infusion. Adequate hydration must be maintained in all patients to insure the drug's renal excretion.

FOSCARNET

Actions and Use. Foscarnet [Foscavir] is an intravenous antiviral drug indicated only for *cytomegalovirus (CMV) retinitis in patients with AIDS.* This infection, which carries a high risk of blindness, affects up to 30% of AIDS patients. Foscarnet is active against strains of CMV that are resistant to ganciclovir, the other drug used to treat CMV retinitis. Compared with ganciclovir, foscarnet is more difficult to administer, less well tolerated, and much more expensive (the cost to the *pharmacy* is about $20,000 a year). For patients with AIDS, treatment of CMV retinitis must continue for life. Although use of foscarnet is limited to CMV retinitis, the drug is active against all herpesviruses as well as HIV. Antiviral effects result from inhibiting viral DNA polymerase.

Pharmacokinetics. Foscarnet has low oral bioavailability and must be administered intravenously. The drug is poorly soluble in water and does not penetrate cells easily. Accordingly, it must be given in large doses and large volumes of fluid. Between 10% and 28% of each dose is deposited in bone; the remainder is excreted unchanged in the urine. Because foscarnet is eliminated by the kidneys, dosages must be reduced in patients with renal impairment. The drug's plasma half-life is 3 to 5 hours.

Adverse Effects and Interactions. Foscarnet is generally less well tolerated than ganciclovir. However, unlike ganciclovir, foscarnet does *not* cause granulocytopenia or thrombocytopenia.

Nephrotoxicity. Renal injury, as evidenced by a rise in serum creatinine concentration, is the most common dose-limiting toxicity. Renal impairment develops most often during the second week of therapy. The risk of nephrotoxicity is increased by concurrent use of other nephrotoxic drugs, including *amphotericin B, aminoglycosides* (e.g., gentamicin), and *pentamidine.* Prehydration with intravenous saline may reduce the risk of renal injury. Renal function (creatinine clearance) should be

monitored closely. The dosage should be reduced if renal impairment develops.

Electrolyte and Mineral Imbalances. Foscarnet frequently causes *hypocalcemia, hypokalemia, hypomagnesemia,* and *hypo- or hyperphosphatemia. Ionized* serum calcium may be reduced despite normal levels of *total* serum calcium. Patients should be informed about symptoms of low ionized calcium (e.g., paresthesias, numbness in the extremities, perioral tingling) and instructed to report these. Severe hypocalcemia can result in dysrhythmias, tetany, and seizures. Serum levels of calcium, magnesium, potassium, and phosphorus should be measured frequently. Special caution is required in patients with pre-existing electrolyte, cardiac, or neurologic abnormalities. The risk of hypocalcemia is increased by concurrent use of *pentamidine.*

Other Adverse Effects. Common reactions include fever (65%), nausea (47%), anemia (33%), diarrhea (30%), vomiting (26%), and headache (26%). In addition, foscarnet can cause fatigue, tremor, irritability, genital ulceration, abnormal liver function tests, neutropenia, anemia, and seizures.

Preparations, Dosage, and Administration. Foscarnet [Foscavir] is dispensed in solution (24 mg/ml) for IV infusion. An infusion pump is essential to reduce the risk of accidental overdosage. Infusions may be administered through a central venous line or a peripheral vein. When a central venous line is used, a concentrated (24 mg/ml) solution may be given. When a peripheral vein is used, the solution should be diluted to 12 mg/ml. For patients with normal kidney function, the *initial* dosage is 60 mg/kg (infused over 1 hour) every 8 hours for 2 to 3 weeks. The *maintenance* dosage is 90 to 120 mg/kg (infused over 2 hours) once daily for life. Dosages must be reduced for patients with renal impairment.

RIBAVIRIN

Antiviral Actions. Ribavirin [Virazole] is virustatic. The drug is active against *respiratory syncytial virus* (RSV), *influenza virus* (types A and B), and *herpes simplex virus.* Although several biochemical actions of the drug have been described, it is not known which (if any) of these are responsible for antiviral effects.

Therapeutic Uses. Ribavirin is labeled only for *severe viral pneumonia caused by RSV in carefully selected, hospitalized infants and young children.* The drug may be of special value for premature infants and for pediatric patients who have cardiopulmonary disease or other conditions that can increase the severity of RSV pneumonia. Ribavirin should not be used for mild RSV infections.

Ribavirin has been employed investigationally to treat influenza A and B. Administration should be initiated within 24 hours of the onset of symptoms. Additional unlabeled uses include measles, herpes genitalis, acute and chronic hepatitis, Lassa fever, and Korean hemorrhagic fever.

Pharmacokinetics. Ribavirin is administered by oral inhalation. The drug is absorbed from the lungs and achieves high concentrations in respiratory tract secretions and erythrocytes. Concentrations in plasma remain low. The drug is metabolized to active and inactive products. Excretion is via the urine (30% to 55%) and feces (15%). Ribavirin that is sequestered in erythrocytes remains in the body for weeks.

Adverse Effects. Inhalation of ribavirin produces little or no systemic toxicity. However, although generally safe, inhaled ribavirin does pose a hazard to infants undergoing mechanical assistance of ventilation: the drug can precipitate in the respiratory apparatus, thereby interfering with safe and effective respiratory support. Consequently, ribavirin should not be administered to infants who need respiratory assistance. In some infants and in adults who have asthma or chronic obstructive lung disease, ribavirin has caused deterioration of pulmonary function. Accordingly, respiratory function should be carefully monitored. If deterioration occurs, ribavirin should be discontinued. When administered systemically (orally or IV), ribavirin frequently causes anemia. This effect has not been reported with inhalational therapy.

Use in Pregnancy. Ribavirin is contraindicated for use during pregnancy. Although studies in primates indicate no effect on the developing fetus, ribavirin has proved either teratogenic or embryolethal in nearly all other species tested. No studies in humans have been performed. Ribavirin is classified under FDA Pregnancy Category X: the risk of use during pregnancy clearly outweighs any potential benefits. Because of the risk of significant drug exposure, pregnant women should not directly care for patients undergoing ribavirin aerosol therapy.

Preparations, Dosage, and Administration. Ribavirin [Virazole] is dispensed as a powder (6 gm/100-ml vial) to be reconstituted for aerosol administration. According to the manufacturer, only one device—the Viratek Small Particle Aerosol Generator (SPAG) Model SPAG-2—should be employed for ribavirin administration. The SPAG-2 is used to deliver ribavirin to an infant oxygen hood. Treatment is given 12 to 18 hours a day for no less than 3 days and no more than 1 week. The drug should not be administered to patients who require ventilatory assistance. To reconstitute powdered ribavirin, dissolve 6 gm of the drug in sterile water for injection or inhalation, transfer this concentrated solution to the SPAG-2 reservoir, and dilute to a final volume of 300 ml using sterile water for injection or inhalation. The final concentration of ribavirin is 20 mg/ml. This solution is aerosolized and inhaled by the patient.

VIDARABINE

Mechanism of Antiviral Action. Vidarabine [Vira-A] is active against several DNA viruses but not RNA viruses. To be effective, the drug must undergo intracellular conversion to its active form, vidarabine triphosphate. Vidarabine triphosphate then blocks synthesis of viral DNA by (1) inhibiting viral DNA polymerase, and (2) becoming incorporated into the growing DNA chain, where it causes premature chain termination.

Therapeutic Use. Intravenous. Intravenous vidarabine is labeled only for *herpes simplex encephalitis*. When therapy is begun early, the drug can decrease mortality and morbidity. However when administered to patients who are already comatose, vidarabine may decrease mortality, but is not likely to decrease morbidity or prevent serious neurologic sequelae. It should be noted that vidarabine is not the treatment of choice for herpes simplex encephalitis; IV acyclovir is more effective and is preferred.

Topical. Vidarabine is available in an ophthalmic ointment for treating keratitis and keratoconjunctivitis caused by HSV. These ophthalmic uses are discussed later in the chapter. Although topical vidarabine is effective against herpes infections of the eye, the preparation is of no benefit to patients with recurrent herpes simplex infections of the lips or genitalia.

Pharmacokinetics. Because vidarabine is poorly soluble in water, it must be diluted in a large volume of fluid for intravenous use. Once in the body, the drug is rapidly metabolized to arabinosyl hypoxanthine (Ara-Hx). Both the parent drug and Ara-Hx are widely distributed. Concentrations in cerebrospinal fluid are about one half those in plasma. Elimination is primarily renal.

Adverse Effects. At usual therapeutic doses, IV vidarabine is well tolerated by most patients. *Gastrointestinal effects* (nausea, vomiting, diarrhea) and *thrombophlebitis* occur on occasion. *Neurotoxicity* develops at high doses and is rare; symptoms include tremor, weakness, ataxia, confusion, hallucinations, and seizures. Animal studies indicate that vidarabine is *mutagenic*, *teratogenic*, and *carcinogenic*.

Preparations, Dosage, and Administration. Vidarabine [Vira-A] is dispensed in a concentrated suspension (200 mg/ml) and must be diluted for IV administration. Solubilization requires 2.22 ml of IV fluid for each mg of vidarabine. Administration is done slowly (over 12 to 24 hours). For herpes simplex encephalitis, the usual dosage is 15 mg/kg/day for 15 days. For herpes zoster, the usual dosage is 10 mg/kg/day for 5 days.

AMANTADINE

Amantadine [Symmetrel, Symadine] is an antiviral drug employed for prophylaxis and treatment of infections caused by type A influenza virus. As discussed in Chapter 21, the drug is also used to treat Parkinson's disease.

Mechanism of Antiviral Action. Just how amantadine suppresses viral growth is not completely understood. The drug can prevent penetration of influenza A virus into host cells and can inhibit viral uncoating. Replication of viral components may also be suppressed.

Therapeutic Use. Antiviral applications of amantadine are limited to prophylaxis and treatment of respiratory tract infections caused by *type A influenza virus* strains. The drug is not active against type B influenza. Prophylaxis should be instituted only in the presence of a documented influenza A epidemic. Candidates for prophylaxis include (1) individuals at high risk of developing complications from influenza (e.g., elderly patients and those with cardiopulmonary disease), and (2) health care workers and family members who make extensive contact with patients at risk. Prophylaxis is continued until the epidemic abates (usually in 5 to 6 weeks). It should be noted that immunization against influenza A is preferred to prophylaxis with amantadine. Since amantadine does not impede the immune response to influenza A vaccine, individuals at risk can be vaccinated while receiving amantadine for prophylaxis. Amantadine can be discontinued 2 weeks after vaccination. For treatment of active influenza A infection, amantadine is most effective when therapy is instituted early (within 48 hours of the onset of symptoms).

Pharmacokinetics. Amantadine is well absorbed following oral administration and is distributed widely to body fluids and tissues. The drug crosses the blood-brain barrier and the placenta. It also appears in saliva, nasal secretions, and breast milk. Amantadine is not metabolized. Excretion of unaltered drug is via the kidneys. In patients with renal impairment, amantadine will accumulate to high levels if the dosage is not reduced.

Adverse Effects. Amantadine is generally well tolerated when given in the doses employed for prophylaxis and treatment of influenza.

Central Nervous System Effects. CNS effects occur in 10% to 30% of patients. Reactions include dizziness, nervousness, insomnia, and difficulty in concentrating. Individuals involved in hazardous activities should exercise appropriate caution. More serious CNS effects (depression, hallucinations, seizures) have occurred. Accordingly, care should be exercised in patients with a history of epilepsy or psychosis.

Cardiovascular Effects. Rarely, amantadine has caused *congestive heart failure* (CHF). The drug should be used with caution in patients with CHF or peripheral edema. Patients should be instructed to contact their physician if they experience shortness of breath or swelling of the extremities.

Orthostatic hypotension has occurred. Patients should be advised to move slowly when assuming an upright position. Also, they should be advised to sit or lie down if dizziness or light-headedness occurs.

Use in Pregnancy and Lactation. Amantadine is teratogenic and embryotoxic in rats. Adequate studies during human pregnancy have not been performed. The drug crosses the placenta and is classified in FDA Pregnancy Category C. It should be avoided by pregnant women unless the benefits of treatment are deemed to outweigh the potential risks to the fetus. Amantadine is secreted in breast milk and should not be used by nursing mothers.

Drug Interactions. Amantadine can intensify the peripheral and CNS effects of *anticholinergic drugs*. When amantadine has been combined with anticholinergic drugs, psychotic reactions resembling those associated with atropine poisoning have occurred. Such responses can be reduced by lowering the dosage of amantadine or the anticholinergic agent.

Preparations, Dosage, and Administration. Amantadine [Symmetrel, Symadine] is dispensed in 100-mg capsules and a syrup (10 mg/ml) for oral use. For treatment or prophylaxis of influenza A, the dosage for patients older than 9 years is 100 mg twice daily. For children aged 1 to 9 years, the dosage is 4.4

to 8.8 mg/kg/day in two or three divided doses. The dosage must be reduced in patients with kidney dysfunction. Prophylactic administration should commence prior to anticipated viral exposure and should continue for as long as the influenza A epidemic lasts. For treatment of active influenza A infection, therapy should begin within 48 hours of the onset of symptoms and should continue for 4 to 5 days.

RIMANTADINE

Rimantadine [Flumadine], an investigational drug, is very similar to amantadine in structure, actions, and uses. Like amantadine, rimantadine is indicated only for prophylaxis and treatment of *influenza A virus infections*. Administration is oral and bioavailability appears to be greater than 90%. In contrast to amantadine, which is not metabolized, rimantadine undergoes extensive metabolism prior to excretion in the urine. Primary adverse effects are nervousness, lightheadedness, difficulty in concentration, sleep disturbances, and fatigue. However, these CNS effects occur much less frequently than with amantadine (3% versus up to 30%). Suggested dosages are 200 mg twice daily for adults, and 5 to 7 mg/kg/day for children. The duration of therapy is 5 days for treatment of active infections, and up to 6 weeks for prophylaxis.

INTERFERON ALFA

Human interferons are naturally occurring compounds with complex antiviral, immunomodulatory, and antineoplastic actions. The interferon family has three major classes, designated alfa, beta, and gamma. Currently, all interferons employed clinically belong to the alfa class. Three forms of interferon alfa are available: alfa-2a [Roferon-A], alfa-2b [Intron A], and alfa-n3 [Alferon N]. In the discussion below, these compounds are referred to collectively as interferon alfa. Commercial production is by recombinant DNA technology. Interferons are used to treat a variety of viral infections (see below) and neoplastic diseases (Chapter 91).

Mechanism of Antiviral Action. Interferon alfa has multiple effects on the viral replication cycle. After binding to receptors on host cell membranes, the drug blocks (1) viral entry into cells, (2) synthesis of viral messenger RNA and viral proteins, and (3) viral assembly and release.

Pharmacokinetics. Interferon alfa is not absorbed orally. Hence administration is parenteral (IM and SC). Plasma drug levels peak in 4 to 8 hours. Inactivation occurs rapidly in body fluids and tissues. No intact drug appears in the urine.

Antiviral Uses and Dosages. Principal systemic antiviral applications are *chronic hepatitis B* and *chronic hepatitis C*. In patients with *chronic hepatitis B*, parenteral interferon alfa-2b (5 million IU/day for 4 months) has produced biochemical and histologic improvement in about 40% of recipients. Remissions have been prolonged. In patients with *chronic hepatitis C*, interferon alfa-2b (2 or 3 million IU 3 times a week for 6 months) has caused biochemical and histologic improvement in about 50% of recipients. Unfortunately, approximately half of these responders relapsed when treatment stopped. There is some indication that giving interferon alfa during acute hepatitis C decreases the risk of progression to chronic disease. Additional antiviral applications include *cytomegalovirus, herpes simplex, varicella-zoster, herpes keratoconjunctivitis*, and *condylomata acuminata* (genital warts).

Adverse Effects. Interferon alfa causes multiple adverse effects. The most common is a *flulike syndrome* characterized by fever (74%–98%), fatigue (89%–98%), myalgia (69%–73%), headache (66%–71%), and chills (41%–64%). Symptoms tend to diminish with continued therapy. Some symptoms (fever, headache, myalgia) can be reduced with acetaminophen. Other common effects include *anorexia, weight loss, diarrhea, abdominal pain, dizziness*, and *cough*. Prolonged or high-dose therapy can cause *bone marrow suppression; neurotoxicity*, including profound fatigue and depression; *hair loss; thyroid dysfunction*; and, possibly, *cardiotoxicity*.

OPHTHALMIC ANTIVIRAL AGENTS

TRIFLURIDINE

Trifluridine [Viroptic] is indicated only for topical treatment of ocular infections caused by HSV types 1 and 2. The drug is given to treat *acute keratoconjunctivitis* and *recurrent epithelial keratitis*. Antiviral actions result from inhibiting DNA synthesis. The most common side effects are localized burning and stinging. Edema of the eyelid occurs in about 3% of patients. Systemic absorption is minimal following topical administration. Hence, the drug is devoid of systemic toxicity. Trifluridine is dispensed in a 1% ophthalmic solution. Treatment consists of placing 1 drop on the cornea every 2 hours (while the patient is awake) for a maximum of 9 drops/day. Once re-epithelialization of the cornea has occurred, the dosage is reduced to 5 drops/day administered one at a time every 4 hours. Treatment continues for 7 days.

VIDARABINE

Like trifluridine, topical vidarabine [Vira-A] is indicated for *acute keratoconjunctivitis* and *recurrent epithelial keratitis* caused by HSV types 1 and 2. Antiviral effects result from inhibition of viral DNA polymerase and from premature termination of the growing viral DNA chain. The most frequent side effects are burning sensations, photophobia, and lacrimation. Absorption of topical vidarabine is insignificant, and systemic toxicity has not been reported. Vidarabine is available in a 3% ointment for application to the eye. About one-half inch of ointment is administered into the lower conjunctival sac five times a day at 3-hour intervals. As a rule, treatment lasts for no more than 3 weeks. Use of vidarabine for *systemic* viral infections is discussed above.

IDOXURIDINE

Idoxuridine [Herplex Liquifilm, Stoxil] was the first effective antiviral drug for use in humans. Antiviral effects result from incorporation of a metabolite of idoxuridine into viral DNA. Idoxuridine is indicated only for *keratitis caused by type 1 HSV*. The drug is inactive against type 2 HSV. Because vidarabine and trifluridine are more effective and less toxic than idoxuridine, these newer agents have largely replaced idoxuridine for treating herpes simplex keratitis. Side effects of idoxuridine include inflammation, itching, photophobia, edema of the eyelid, lacrimal duct occlusion, and punctate defects in the corneal epithelium. Topical application has not been associated with systemic toxicity. Idoxuridine is dispensed in a 0.5% ointment and a 0.1% solution.

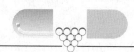

Summary of Major Nursing Implications

ACYCLOVIR

Preadministration Assessment

Therapeutic Goal

Treatment of infections caused by herpes simplex viruses and varicella-zoster virus.

Identifying High-Risk Patients

Use with *caution* in patients who are *dehydrated, have renal impairment,* or are *receiving other nephrotoxic drugs.*

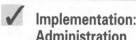
Implementation: Administration

Routes

Topical, oral, IV.

Dosage

Oral and IV dosages must be reduced in patients with renal impairment.

Administration

Topical. Advise patients to apply the drug with a finger cot or rubber glove to avoid viral transfer to other body sites and other people.

Oral. Note that dosages vary widely for different indications.

Intravenous. Give by slow IV infusion (over 1 hour or more). Never administer by IV bolus.

Implementation: Measures to Enhance Therapeutic Effects

Inform patients with *herpes simplex genitalis* that acyclovir only decreases symptoms; the drug does not eliminate the virus and does not produce cure. Advise patients to cleanse the affected area with soap and water three to four times a day, drying thoroughly after each wash. Advise patients to avoid sexual contact while lesions are present.

Ongoing Evaluation and Interventions

Evaluating Therapeutic Effects

Observe for decreased clinical manifestations of herpes simplex and varicella-zoster infection. Virologic testing may also be performed.

Minimizing Adverse Effects

Nephrotoxicity. *Intravenous* acyclovir can precipitate in renal tubules, causing reversible kidney damage. To minimize the risk of injury, infuse acyclovir slowly and insure adequate hydration during the infusion and for 2 hours after. Exercise caution in patients with pre-existing renal impairment and in those who are dehydrated or taking other nephrotoxic drugs.

ZIDOVUDINE (AZIDOTHYMIDINE, AZT)

Preadministration Assessment

Therapeutic Goal

Zidovudine is given to delay the progression of HIV infection in patients with early HIV disease and to improve the clinical, immunologic, and virologic status of patients with advanced HIV disease.

Baseline Data

Assess the patient's clinical status and obtain baseline laboratory values for hemoglobin, granulocyte counts, and CD4 lymphocyte counts.

Identifying High-Risk Patients

The risk of hematologic toxicity is increased by *low granulocyte counts, low hemoglobin levels, low CD4 lymphocyte counts, low levels of vitamin B_{12} or folic acid*, and *concurrent use of drugs that are myelosuppressive, nephrotoxic, or toxic to circulating blood cells*.

Implementation: Administration

Routes

Oral, intravenous.

Administration

Oral. Instruct patients with *symptomatic* HIV infection (AIDS or advanced ARC) to take 6 doses a day at 4-hour intervals around the clock, even if sleep must be interrupted. Instruct patients with *asymptomatic* HIV infection to take 5 doses a day at 4-hour intervals.

If hematologic monitoring indicates severe anemia or severe granulocytopenia, treatment should be interrupted until there is evidence of bone marrow recovery. If anemia and granulocytopenia are mild, a reduction in dosage may be sufficient.

Intravenous. Administer IV doses every 4 hours around the clock. Infuse each dose slowly (over 1 hour). Avoid rapid infusion and bolus injection. Switch to oral therapy as soon as appropriate.

Prepare the IV solution by withdrawing the calculated dose from the stock vial and diluting it to 4 mg/ml or less in 5% dextrose for injection. Do not mix the solution with biologic or colloidal fluids (e.g., blood products, protein solutions). Administer within 8 hours (if stored at room temperature) or within 24 hours (if stored under refrigeration).

Implementation: Measures to Enhance Therapeutic Effects

Inform patients that although zidovudine can reduce symptoms of HIV infection and prolong life, the drug is not a cure for AIDS and does not eliminate the risk of transmitting HIV through sexual contact. Warn patients that they may still acquire serious opportunistic infections, and, hence, must remain under close medical supervision.

Ongoing Evaluation and Interventions

Evaluating Therapeutic Effects

In asymptomatic patients, success is indicated by continued absence of symptoms. In symptomatic patients, success is indicated by improvements in clinical, immunologic, and virologic status.

Minimizing Adverse Effects

Hematologic Effects. Zidovudine can cause *severe anemia* and *granulocytopenia*. Hematologic status should be determined before treatment and at least every 4 weeks thereafter. In the event of severe anemia (hemoglobin <7.5 gm/dl or down 25% from the pretreatment baseline) or severe neutropenia (granulocyte count <750/mm³ or down 50% from the pretreatment baseline), interrupt treatment until there is evidence of bone marrow recovery. If neutropenia and anemia are less severe, a reduction in dosage may be sufficient. Some patients may require multiple transfusions. Granulocyte colony-stimulating factors can be used to reverse neutropenia. Epoetin (recombinant erythropoietin) can be given to reduce transfusion requirements in patients with anemia, provided endogenous erythropoietin levels are not already elevated.

Minimizing Adverse Interactions

Drugs that are *myelosuppressive, nephrotoxic,* or *directly toxic to circulating blood cells* can increase the risk of hematologic toxicity from zidovudine. Drugs of concern include *ganciclovir, dapsone, pentamidine, pyrimethamine, trimethoprim-sulfamethoxazole, amphotericin B, flucytosine, vincristine, vinblastine,* and *doxorubicin.*

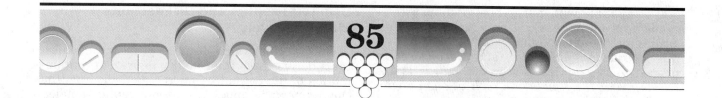

Antiseptics and Disinfectants

Antiseptics and disinfectants are locally acting drugs that are toxic to microorganisms. These agents are used to reduce acquisition and transmission of infection. Drugs suitable for antisepsis and disinfection cannot be used internally because of toxicity.

GENERAL CONSIDERATIONS

Terminology

The terms *antiseptic* and *disinfectant* are not synonymous. In common usage, the term *antiseptic* is reserved for agents *applied to living tissue*. *Disinfectants* are preparations *applied to inanimate objects*. As a rule, agents used as disinfectants are too harsh for application to living tissue. Disinfectants are employed most frequently to decontaminate surgical instruments and to cleanse hospitals and other medical facilities. Most uses of antiseptics are prophylactic. For example, antiseptics are used to cleanse the hands of medical personnel; they are applied to the skin prior to invasive procedures (surgery, insertion of needles); and they are used to bathe neonates. Rarely, antiseptics are employed to treat an existing local infection. However, in most cases, established infections are best treated with a systemic antimicrobial drug.

Several related terms may need clarification. *Sterilization* indicates complete destruction of all microorganisms. In contrast, *sanitization* implies only that contamination has been reduced to a level compatible with public health standards. A *germicide* is a drug that *kills* microorganisms. Germicides may be divided into subcategories: *bactericides, virucides, fungicides,* and *amebicides.* In contrast to a germicide, a *germistatic drug* is one that *decreases the growth and replication* of microorganisms but does not produce kill.

Properties of an Ideal Antiseptic

The ideal antiseptic, like any other ideal drug, should be safe, effective, and selective. The preparation should be germicidal (rather than germistatic) and should have a broad spectrum of antimicrobial activity: the drug should kill bacteria and their spores, as well as viruses, protozoa, yeasts, and fungi. Drug actions should be rapid and sustained. Development of microbial resistance to the drug should be low. The drug should have no harmful effects on humans: it should not produce local damage, impair healing, or produce systemic toxicity following topical application. Lastly, the drug should not cause stains, and should be devoid of offensive odor. No antiseptic has all these characteristics.

Time Course of Action

Toxicity to microorganisms is determined in part by duration of exposure to an antiseptic or disinfectant. Some agents act much more quickly than others. For example, ethanol (70% solution) reduces the cutaneous bacterial count by 50% in just 36 seconds. In contrast, benzalkonium chloride (at a dilution of 1:1000) requires 7 minutes to produce an equivalent effect. Because such differences in time course exist, effective use of antiseptics and disinfectants requires that health personnel acquaint themselves with the exposure requirements of these agents.

Use of Antiseptics to Treat Established Local Infection

In the past, topical agents were used routinely to treat established local infection. Today, *systemic* anti-infective drugs are the treatment of choice. Systemic agents are preferred for two reasons: systemic agents are more effective than topical drugs, and they are less damaging to inflamed or abraded tissue. Experience has shown that antiseptics do little to reduce infection in wounds, cuts, and abrasions. This lack of efficacy is attributed to poor penetration into the site of infection, and to diminished activity in the presence of wound exudates. Although of limited value for *established* local infection, antiseptics are quite useful as *prophylaxis*: when applied properly, antiseptics can help cleanse wounds and decrease microbial contamination.

Using Antiseptics and Disinfectants Most Effectively

The principal value of antiseptics and disinfectants derives from their ability to prevent contamination of the patient by microorganisms from the *environment*; it appears that antiseptics applied directly to the *patient* contribute relatively little to prophylaxis against infection. A number of clinical studies support this conclusion. In one study, over 5000 preoperative patients were bathed with hexachlorophene. Although this treatment greatly reduced the concentration of surface bacteria, it had no effect on the incidence of postoperative infection. Similarly, in a study of patients who had undergone cardiothoracic surgery, it was found that most postoperative infections were caused by organisms not present at the site of the incision. From these studies and others, we can conclude that infections are caused primarily by environmental microorganisms rather than by organisms living on the skin of the patient. Consequently, use of antiseptics by nurses, physicians, and others who contact the patient is of much greater importance than application of antiseptics to the patient. Patients also benefit greatly by the rigorous use of disinfectants to decontaminate surgical supplies and medical buildings.

PROPERTIES OF INDIVIDUAL ANTISEPTICS AND DISINFECTANTS

Antiseptics and disinfectants belong to a variety of chemical families, ranging from alcohols to iodine compounds to phenols. The various antiseptics and disinfectants differ from one another with respect to mechanism of action, time course of effects, and antimicrobial spectra. In almost all cases, the drugs employed as disinfectants are not used for antisepsis and vice versa. The more commonly employed antiseptics and disinfectants are listed in Table 85–1. For each drug, the table indicates chemical family and clinical application (antisepsis, disinfection, or both). The pharmacology of individual antiseptics and disinfectants is discussed below.

ALCOHOLS

Ethanol

Ethanol (ethyl alcohol) is an effective virucide and also kills most common pathogenic bacteria. The drug is inactive against bacterial spores, and its activity against fungi is erratic. Bactericidal effects result from precipitation of bacterial protein and from dissolution of membranes. Ethanol

		Application	
Chemical Category	**Drug**	*Antisepsis*	*Disinfection*
Alcohols	Ethanol	✓	
	Isopropanol	✓	
Aldehydes	Glutaraldehyde		✓
	Formaldehyde		✓
Iodine Compounds	Iodine tincture	✓	
	Iodine solution	✓	
	Povidone iodine	✓	✓
Chlorine Compounds	Oxychlorosene	✓	
	Sodium hypochlorite	✓	✓
Phenolic Compounds	Hexachlorophene	✓	
	Parachlorometaxylenol	✓	
	Hexylresorcinol	✓	
Miscellaneous Agents	Chlorhexidine	✓	
	Thimerosal	✓	
	Hydrogen peroxide		✓
	Benzalkonium chloride	✓	✓

Table 85–1. Antiseptics and Disinfectants: Chemical Category and Application

can enhance the effects of several other antimicrobial preparations (e.g., chlorhexidine, hexachlorophene, benzalkonium chloride).

Ethanol is employed almost exclusively for antisepsis. The most frequent use is cleansing of the skin prior to needle insertion and minor surgery. Because of its limited activity against bacterial spores and fungi, ethanol is poorly suited for use as a disinfectant.

Optimal bacterial kill requires that ethanol be present in the proper concentration and for a sufficient length of time. The drug is most effective at a concentration of 70%. Higher concentrations are *less* active. To produce 90% kill of surface bacteria, the skin must be kept moist with ethanol for 2 minutes. This extended exposure can be accomplished by use of ethanol foam. Exposure is prolonged because evaporation from this formulation is slower than from ethanol solution.

Ethanol should not be applied to open wounds. The drug can increase tissue damage and, by causing coagulation of proteins, can form a mass under which bacteria can multiply.

Isopropanol

Isopropanol (isopropyl alcohol) is employed primarily as an antiseptic. When applied in concentrations greater than 70%, isopropanol is somewhat more germicidal than ethanol. Like ethanol, isopropanol can increase the effects of other antiseptics. Isopropanol promotes local vasodilation and can thereby

increase bleeding from needle punctures and incisions. Isopropanol is available in concentrations ranging from 70% to 100%.

ALDEHYDES

Glutaraldehyde

Glutaraldehyde [Cidex] is lethal to all microorganisms; the drug kills bacteria, bacterial spores, viruses, and fungi. Antimicrobial effects result from cross-linking and precipitation of proteins. Glutaraldehyde is used to disinfect and sterilize surgical instruments and other medical supplies, such as respiratory and anesthetic equipment, catheters, and thermometers. The drug is too harsh for use as an antiseptic. To completely eliminate bacterial spores, instruments and equipment must be immersed in glutaraldehyde for 10 hours or more. Glutaraldehyde is most active at alkaline pH. However, under alkaline conditions, glutaraldehyde eventually becomes inactive because of gradual polymerization. Consequently, alkaline solutions of glutaraldehyde are active for only 2 to 4 weeks. Glutaraldehyde should be used with adequate ventilation, since fumes can irritate the respiratory tract.

Formaldehyde

Formaldehyde kills bacteria, bacterial spores, viruses, and fungi. Like glutaraldehyde, formaldehyde is too harsh for application to the skin. Accordingly, use is limited to disinfection and sterilization of equipment and instruments. For two reasons, formaldehyde is less desirable than glutaraldehyde. First, formaldehyde acts slowly: destruction of bacterial spores may take 2 to 4 days. Second, because of its greater volatility, formaldehyde tends to cause more respiratory irritation than glutaraldehyde.

IODINE COMPOUNDS

Iodine Solution and Iodine Tincture

Iodine was first employed as an antiseptic more than 150 years ago. Despite the introduction of numerous other drugs, iodine remains one of our most widely used germicidal agents. The drug is extremely effective, having the ability to kill all known bacteria, fungi, protozoa, viruses, and yeasts. Additional assets are low cost and relative lack of toxicity.

The composition of iodine solution and iodine tincture is very similar. Iodine *solution* consists of 2% elemental iodine and 2.4% sodium iodide in water. Iodine *tincture* contains the same amounts of elemental iodine and sodium iodide and also contains 47% ethanol. The ethanol enhances the antimicrobial activity of iodine tincture.

The germicidal activity of iodine tincture and iodine solution is due only to *free* (dissolved) *elemental* iodine. In both the tincture and the solution, the concentration of free elemental iodine is only about 0.15%. This low figure reflects the poor solubility of iodine. Since only free iodine is active, most of the elemental iodine and all of the sodium iodide present in iodine tincture and iodine solution do not contribute *directly* to microbicidal activity. However, these components do contribute *indirectly* by serving as reservoirs from which free elemental iodine can be released.

Iodine tincture and iodine solution are employed primarily for antisepsis of the skin, a use for which these drugs are the most effective agents available. When the skin is *intact*, iodine *tincture* is preferred. This preparation is commonly employed to cleanse the skin prior to intravenous injection and withdrawal of blood for microbial culture. For treatment of *wounds* and *abrasions*, iodine *solution* should be employed. (Because of the irritant properties of alcohol, iodine tincture is less appropriate for application to broken skin.)

Povidone-Iodine

Povidone-iodine is a complex of elemental iodine with povidone (an organic polymer). Povidone-iodine has no antimicrobial activity of its own, but rather serves as a reservoir from which elemental iodine can be released. Free elemental iodine is the active germicide. The concentration of free iodine achieved through application of povidone-iodine is lower than that produced with iodine tincture or iodine solution. Hence, povidone-iodine is less effective than these other iodine preparations. Povidone-iodine is employed primarily for prophylaxis against postoperative infection. Additional uses include hand washing, surgical scrubbing, and preparation of the skin prior to invasive procedures (e.g., surgery, aspiration, injection). In addition, povidone-iodine is employed to sterilize equipment. However, superior disinfectants are available. The drug is dispensed in a variety of formulations (ointments, solutions, aerosols, gels). It is also available impregnated in swabs, sponges, and wipes. Trade names include ACU-dyne, Betadine, and Operand.

CHLORINE COMPOUNDS

Chlorine is lethal to a wide variety of microbes. Chlorine is active both as elemental chlorine and as hypochlorous acid, the acid formed by reaction of chlorine with water. Chlorine is used extensively to sanitize water supplies and swimming pools. However, because of physical properties that make working with chlorine difficult, chlorine itself is rarely used clinically. Instead, chlorine-containing compounds with the ability to release hypochlorous acid are employed.

Oxychlorosene Sodium

Oxychlorosene sodium [Clorpactin] is a complex mixture of hypochlorous acid with alkylphenyl sulfonates. Antimicrobial effects derive from release of hypochlorous acid. Oxychlorosene is lethal to bacteria, yeast, fungi, viruses, molds, and spores. This agent is employed as a topical antiseptic and can be especially useful for treating localized infection caused by drug-resistant microbes. Oxychlorosene is also employed to irrigate and cleanse fistulas, sinus tracts, wounds, and empyemas (pus-filled cavities).

Sodium Hypochlorite

Sodium hypochlorite kills bacteria, spores, fungi, protozoa, and viruses. Undiluted (5%) solutions are employed commonly as household bleach. These concentrated solutions are too irritating for application to human tissue. For antiseptic use, dilute solutions (0.5%) are employed. These dilute preparations can be used to irrigate wounds and to cleanse and deodorize necrotic tissue. To minimize local irritation, solutions of sodium hypochlorite should be rinsed off promptly. A 1% solution can be used to sterilize equipment. Solutions of sodium hypochlorite are unstable and must be prepared fresh for each use.

PHENOLS

The family of phenolic compounds consists of phenol itself together with several phenol derivatives. Following its introduction in 1867, phenol rapidly became both the antiseptic and disinfectant of choice. Today, use of phenol for antiseptic purposes is rare. However, the drug is still employed in some hospitals as a disinfectant. Three phenol derivatives are discussed below.

Hexachlorophene

Actions. Hexachlorophene is *bacteriostatic*, not bactericidal. The drug is quite active against gram-positive bacteria—the bacteria found most frequently on the skin. However, hexachlorophene has little or no effect on gram-negative bacteria. In fact, when used on a regular basis, hexachlorophene encourages overgrowth with gram-negative organisms. (By killing off gram-positive bacteria, hexachlorophene makes conditions more conducive for gram-negative growth.)

Uses. Hexachlorophene is employed most commonly as a hand-washing preparation for health personnel. Although the effects of a single wash are minimal, with repeated use hexachlorophene can produce significant reductions in the population of cutaneous gram-positive bacteria. This cumulative effect results from residual hexachlorophene retained on the skin. Hexachlorophene has been employed to prepare the skin prior to surgery. However, availability of superior antiseptics (e.g., chlorhexidine) makes this use inappropriate.

Adverse Effects. Hexachlorophene can be absorbed through intact skin and mucous membranes. Absorption through denuded areas can be especially great. If absorbed in sufficient amounts, hexachlorophene causes central nervous system stimulation. Responses range from confusion to twitching to seizures. Death has occurred. To minimize systemic toxicity, hexachlorophene should not be applied extensively to burns, wounds, cuts, or mucous membranes. Total body bathing, especially of infants, should be avoided. For bathing infants, chlorhexidine is safer and more effective.

Preparations. Hexachlorophene is available only by prescription. The drug is dispensed as a solution and a foam. Trade names are pHisoHex, Septisol, and Septi-Soft.

Other Phenol Derivatives

Parachlorometaxylenol (PCMX). PCMX, also known as chloroxylenol, is a phenol derivative with a spectrum of antibacterial action broader than that of hexachlorophene. When combined with hexachlorophene, PCMX helps prevent overgrowth with gram-negative organisms. PCMX is employed as a hand-washing preparation for health personnel. In addition, the drug is present in dermatologic preparations used to treat acne, eczema, seborrheic dermatitis, and superficial burns.

Hexylresorcinol. This drug is less toxic than phenol and exerts greater antibacterial action. Hexylresorcinol is employed as an antiseptic mouthwash and to cleanse wounds. Application to broken skin can be irritating.

MISCELLANEOUS AGENTS

Chlorhexidine

Actions. Chlorhexidine is an important surgical antiseptic. The drug is fast-acting and lethal to most gram-positive and gram-negative bacteria. Virucidal activity is lacking. Antibacterial effects are reduced somewhat in the presence of soap, blood, and pus. Chlorhexidine that remains on the skin after rinsing is sufficient to exert continuing germicidal effects.

Uses. Chlorhexidine is used for preoperative preparation of the skin and as a surgical scrub, hand-wash preparation, and wound cleanser.

Adverse Effects. Chlorhexidine is very safe. Routine preoperative use only rarely causes local adverse effects. Inadvertent IV injection has been reported twice: in one patient, hemolysis occurred; in the other, no ill effects were observed.

Preparations. Chlorhexidine gluconate (0.5%, 2%, 4%) is dispensed in combination with isopropanol (4% or 70%). Trade names include Exidine Scrub, Dyna-Hex Skin Cleanser, Hibistat Germicidal Hand Rinse, and Hibiclens.

Hydrogen Peroxide

Hydrogen peroxide is an excellent disinfectant and sterilizing agent, but is useless as an antiseptic. The entity in hydrogen peroxide solution responsible for antimicrobial effects is the hydroxyl free radical. These free radicals are destroyed when hydrogen peroxide is acted upon by catalase, an enzyme found in all tissues. Hence, contact with tissue terminates hydrogen peroxide's germicidal actions. The only benefit resulting from application of hydrogen peroxide to wounds derives from liberation of oxygen (by the reaction with catalase). This oxygen causes frothing that is sufficient to loosen debris and thereby facilitate cleansing. The principal use of hydrogen peroxide is disinfection and sterilization of instruments. A 3% to 6% solution is employed.

Thimerosal

Thimerosal is an organic compound that contains 49% mercury, the active antimicrobial factor. Thimerosal has only weak bacteriostatic and fungistatic properties; it does not kill bacteria or fungi. Antimicrobial actions are reduced in the presence of blood and tissue proteins. Thimerosal is less effective than ethanol. Use on large areas of denuded skin may yield systemic toxicity from absorption of mercury. Poisoning from thimerosal ingestion can be treated with dimercaprol (see Chapter 93). Thimerosal has been employed as a wound irrigant and to prepare the skin prior to surgery. It has also been employed as an antiseptic for the eyes, nose, throat, and genitourinary tract. Trade names are Mersol and AeroAid.

Benzalkonium Chloride

Actions. Benzalkonium chloride (BAC) is an organic quaternary ammonium compound that has antimicrobial and detergent properties. BAC is active against many gram-positive and gram-negative bacteria as well as some fungi, protozoa, and viruses. The drug is relatively inactive against *Mycobacterium tuberculosis*, *Clostridium*, and other spore-forming bacteria. Germicidal effects result from disruption of membranes, and are enhanced in the presence of ethanol. BAC is inactivated by soaps and organic material. The actions of BAC are slow compared with those of iodine.

Antiseptic Uses. BAC is employed for preoperative preparation of the skin and mucous membranes; as a surgical scrub; as an antiseptic for abrasions and minor wounds; as a vaginal douche; and for irrigation of the eyes, body cavities, and genitourinary tract. Since BAC is inactivated by soap, all soap must be removed by rinsing with water and 70% alcohol prior to BAC application. *Concentrated* solutions of BAC can cause severe local damage. Hence, care must be taken to use solutions of appropriate dilution. For several reasons (limited antimicrobial spectrum, lack of rapid action, potential for toxicity, availability of superior agents), there seems to be little to recommend BAC for antiseptic use.

Disinfectant Use. Immersion in BAC solution is employed for sterile storage of instruments and supplies. Adsorption of BAC onto porous material can significantly reduce the concentration of BAC in solutions. To insure continuing efficacy, solutions should be changed or replenished with BAC on a regular basis.

Preparations and Dosage. BAC is dispensed in concentrated (17%) and diluted (1:750) solution. Trade names are Benza and Zephiran. Recommended dilutions are 1:750 (for application to intact skin and to minor wounds and abrasions); 1:2000 to 1:5000 (for application to mucous membranes and diseased or seriously damaged skin); and 1:750 to 1:5000 (for storage of instruments and supplies).

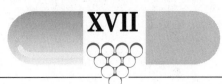

Chemotherapy of Parasitic Diseases

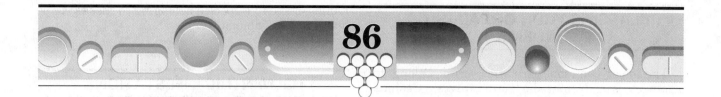

Anthelmintics

CLASSIFICATION OF PARASITIC WORMS

HELMINTHIC INFESTATIONS

DRUGS OF CHOICE FOR HELMINTHIASIS
  Mebendazole
  Thiabendazole
  Pyrantel Pamoate
  Niclosamide
  Praziquantel
  Diethylcarbamazine

H elminths are parasitic worms; *anthelmintics* are the drugs used against them. Helminthiasis (worm infestation) is the most common affliction of humans, affecting more than 2 billion people worldwide. The intestine is a frequent site of infestation. Other sites include the liver, lymphatic system, and blood vessels. Infestation is frequently asymptomatic. However, infection with some parasites can cause severe complications. Helminthiasis is most prevalent where sanitation is poor. Cleanliness greatly reduces the risk of infestation.

Treatment of helminthiasis is not always indicated. Most parasitic worms do not reproduce within the human body. Hence, in the absence of reinfestation, many infections subside on their own as adult worms die. Since many infestations abate spontaneously, treatment may be optional. In countries where physicians and medication are readily available, drug therapy is definitely indicated. However, in less fortunate locales, several factors—cost of medication, limited medical facilities, high probability of reinfestation—may render individual treatment impractical. In these places, preventative measures, such as improved hygiene and elimination of carriers, may be the most valuable means of controlling infestation.

In approaching the anthelmintic drugs, we will begin by reviewing classification of the parasitic worms. Next we will briefly discuss the characteristics of the more common helminthic infestations. After this, we will discuss the drugs of choice for helminthiasis.

CLASSIFICATION OF PARASITIC WORMS

The most common parasitic worms belong to three classes: Nematoda (roundworms), Cestoda (tapeworms), and Trematoda (flukes). Nematodes belong to the phylum Nemathelminthes. Cestodes and trematodes belong to the phylum Platyhelminthes (flat worms).

Nematodes. Parasitic nematodes can be subdivided into two groups: (1) those that infest the intestinal lumen, and (2) those that inhabit tissues. There are five major species of intestinal nematodes. Common names for these organisms are giant roundworm, pinworm, hookworm, whipworm, and threadworm. Official names of these parasites are listed in Table 86–1. Two types of nematodes invade tissues: (1) pork roundworms (responsible for trichinosis), and (2) filariae. The three species of filariae encountered most commonly are listed in Table 86–1.

Cestodes. Three species of cestodes infest humans. Common names for these parasites are beef tapeworm, pork tapeworm, and fish tapeworm. Official names of these organisms appear in Table 86–1.

Trematodes. Five species of trematodes infest humans. These organisms fall into four groups having the following common names: blood fluke, liver fluke, intestinal fluke, and lung fluke. Official names of the five species belonging to these groups are given in Table 86–1.

HELMINTHIC INFESTATIONS

This section describes the major characteristics of infestation by specific helminths. These infestations can differ with respect to anatomic site and danger to the host. Infestations also differ with respect to the drugs employed for treatment (see Table 86–1 for a summary).

The name applied to an infestation is based on the official name of the invading organism. For example, infestation with the giant roundworm, whose official name is *Ascaris lumbricoides*, is referred to as ascariasis.

In the discussion below, the helminthic infestations are grouped in four categories: (1) nematode infestations of the intestine, (2) nematode infestations at extraintestinal sites, (3) cestode infestations, and (4) trematode infestations.

Nematode Infestations (Intestinal)

Ascariasis (Giant Roundworm Infestation). Ascariasis is the most prevalent helminthic infestation. Worldwide, one of every three people is affected. Adult worms inhabit the small intestine. Ascariasis is usually asymptomatic. However, serious complications can result if worms migrate into the pancreatic duct, bile duct, gallbladder, or liver. In addition, if infestation is extremely heavy, intestinal blockage may occur. Because of these potential hazards, ascariasis should always be treated. Drugs of choice are *mebendazole* and *pyrantel*.

Table 86–1. Drugs of Choice for Parasitic Worms

| Worm Class | Parasitic Organism | | Drugs of Choice |
	Common Name	Official Name	
Nematodes (roundworms): Intestinal	Giant roundworm Pinworm Hookworm	*Ascaris lumbricoides* *Enterobius vermicularis* *Ancylostoma duodenale* *Necator americanus*	Mebendazole or pyrantel pamoate
	Whipworm	*Trichuris trichiura*	Mebendazole
	Threadworm	*Strongyloides stercoralis*	Thiabendazole
Nematodes: Tissue invading	Pork roundworm	*Trichinella spiralis*	Thiabendazole
	Filariae	*Wuchereria bancrofti* *Brugia malayi* *Loa loa*	Diethylcarbamazine
Cestodes (tapeworms)	Beef tapeworm Pork tapeworm Fish tapeworm	*Taenia saginata* *Taenia solium* *Diphyllobothrium latum*	Niclosamide or praziquantel
Trematodes (flukes)	Blood fluke Liver fluke Intestinal fluke Lung fluke	*Schistosoma* species *Fasciola hepatica* *Clonorchis sinensis* *Fasciolopsis buski* *Paragonimus westermani*	Praziquantel

Enterobiasis (Pinworm Infestation). Enterobiasis is the most common helminthic infestation in the United States. Adult pinworms inhabit the ileum and large intestine. Their life span is approximately 2 months. Although usually asymptomatic, enterobiasis may cause intense perineal itching in some patients. Serious complications are rare. Drugs of choice are *mebendazole* and *pyrantel*. Because enterobiasis is readily transmitted, all family members of an infected individual should be treated simultaneously.

Ancylostomiasis and Necatoriasis (Hookworm Infestation). Hookworm infestation is most common in rural areas where hygiene is poor and people go barefoot. Adult hookworms attach to the wall of the small intestine and suck blood. As a result, infestation is associated with chronic blood loss and progressive anemia. Symptomatic anemia is most likely in menstruating women and people who are undernourished. Nausea, vomiting, and abdominal pain may accompany the infestation. *Mebendazole* and *pyrantel* are the treatments of choice.

Trichuriasis (Whipworm Infestation). Trichuriasis is extremely common, affecting about 1 billion people worldwide. Larvae and adult worms inhabit the large intestine. Mature worms may live for 10 or more years. The disease is usually devoid of symptoms. However, when the worm burden is very large, rectal prolapse may occur. Patients with severe infestation require therapy. *Mebendazole* is the treatment of choice.

Strongyloidiasis (Threadworm Infestation). Strongyloidiasis is common in the southern United States. Larval and adult threadworms inhabit the small intestine. The disease can be very dangerous, although symptoms are usually absent. Mild infestation may cause abdominal pain and occasional diarrhea. Severe infestation can cause vomiting, massive diarrhea, dehydration, electrolyte imbalance, and secondary bacteremia. Death has occurred. Affected individuals should always be treated. *Thiabendazole* is the agent of choice.

Nematode Infestations (Extraintestinal)

Trichinosis (Pork Roundworm Infestation). Trichinosis is acquired by eating undercooked pork that is infested with encysted larvae of *Trichinella spiralis*. Adult worms reside in the intestine, whereas larvae migrate to skeletal muscle and become encysted. Some encysted larvae live for years. Others die and calcify within months. Symptoms of trichinosis include gastrointestinal upset, fever, muscle pain, and sore throat. Potentially lethal complications (congestive heart failure, meningitis, neuritis) arise in some patients. *Thiabendazole* is the drug of choice for killing adult worms and migrating larvae. However, this agent is not active against those larvae that have become encysted. *Glucocorticoids* are given to reduce inflammation during larval migration.

Wuchereriasis and Brugiasis (Lymphatic Filarial Infestation). *Wuchereria bancrofti* and *Brugia malayi* are filarial nematodes that invade the lymphatic system. Infestation with either organism can cause severe complications. When infestation is heavy, lymphatic obstruction occurs, resulting in elephantiasis (usually of the scrotum or legs). In addition, "filarial fever" may develop. Symptoms include chills, fever, headache, nausea, vomiting, constipation, and lymphadenitis. The drug of choice for use against both filarial species is *diethylcarbamazine*.

Cestode Infestations

Taeniasis (Beef and Pork Tapeworm Infestation). Taeniasis is acquired by eating undercooked beef or pork that contains tapeworm larvae. Adult tapeworms live attached to the wall of the small intestine. Infestation is usually asymptomatic. Taeniasis can be treated with *niclosamide* and *praziquantel*.

Diphyllobothriasis (Fish Tapeworm Infestation). Diphyllobothriasis is acquired by ingestion of undercooked fish that is infested with tapeworm larvae. Adult worms inhabit the ileum. Infestation is usually devoid of symptoms. Worms can be killed with *niclosamide* or *praziquantel*.

Trematode Infestations

Schistosomiasis (Blood Fluke Infestations). The term *schistosomiasis* refers to infestation with blood flukes of any species (e.g., *Schistosoma mansoni, S. japonicum*). Specific snails serve as intermediate hosts for these flukes. Schistosomiasis cannot be acquired in the continental United States because of an absence of the appropriate snails.

Schistosomiasis has an acute and a chronic phase. The acute phase subsides in 3 to 4 months. Symptoms that accompany this phase include lymphadenopathy, fever, anorexia, malaise, muscle pain, and rash. During the chronic phase, schistosomes take up residence in the vascular system, primarily in the veins of the intestines and liver. This late infestation can produce intestinal polyposis, hepatosplenomegaly, and portal hypertension. For either the acute or the chronic stage, *praziquantel* is the treatment of choice.

Fascioliasis (Liver Fluke Infestation). Fascioliasis is the only fluke infestation indigenous to the United States. Parasites inhabit the biliary tract. Symptoms (anorexia, mild fever, fatigue, aching in the region of the liver) are delayed for 1 to 3 months. *Praziquantel* is the treatment of choice.

Fasciolopsiasis (Intestinal Fluke Infestation). Fasciolopsiasis is most common in Southeast Asia. Adult worms inhabit the small intestine. The disease is usually asymptomatic. In some people, ulcer-like pain is experienced. Disruption of bowel function (constipation or diarrhea) may occur. In the presence of massive infestation, bowel obstruction may develop; clearance may require surgery. *Praziquantel* is the treatment of choice.

DRUGS OF CHOICE FOR HELMINTHIASIS

The six most commonly employed anthelmintic drugs are considered below. These agents differ from one another in antiparasitic spectra: some agents are active against several worms, whereas others are more selective. Because of these differences, it is important to identify the invading organism so that the most appropriate therapeutic agent can be chosen. Table 86–2 lists the major anthelmintic drugs and indicates the parasites against which each is most effective. Although the discussion that follows is limited to drugs of choice, be aware that additional anthelmintics are available.

MEBENDAZOLE

Target Organisms. Mebendazole is a drug of choice for most *intestinal roundworms*. This agent clears infestation with *pinworms, hookworms, whipworms,* and *giant roundworms*. Because of its relatively broad spectrum of action, mebendazole is especially useful for treatment of mixed infestations.

Mechanism of Action. Mebendazole prevents uptake of glucose by susceptible intestinal worms. Lack of glucose results in immobilization followed by death. Worms die slowly. Hence, up to 3 days may elapse between initiation of treatment and complete clearance of parasites. Mebendazole does not influence glucose uptake or utilization by humans.

Pharmacokinetics. Only a small fraction (5% to 10%) of orally administered mebendazole is absorbed. The fraction absorbed undergoes rapid metabolism. Consequently, plasma levels of mebendazole remain low.

		Table 86–2. First Choice Anthelmintic Drugs: Target Organisms and Dosages		
Generic Name [Trade Name]	**Target Organism**	**Adult Dosge**	**Pediatric Dosage**	
Mebendazole [Vermox]	Giant roundworm Whipworm Hookworm	100 mg bid for 3 days	Same as adult	
	Pinworm	100 mg; repeat in 2 weeks	Same as adult	
Thiabenzadole [Mintezol]	Threadworm	25 mg/kg bid for 2 days	Same as adult	
	Pork roundworm	25 mg/kg bid for 5 days	Same as adult	
Pyrantel pamoate [Antiminth]	Giant roundworm	11 mg/kg; (once)	Same as adult	
	Hookworm	11 mg/kg for 3 days	Same as adult	
	Pinworm	11 mg/kg; repeat in 2 weeks	Same as adult	
Niclosamide [Niclocide]	Beef tapeworm Pork tapeworm Fish tapeworm	4 tablets (2 gm) taken at one time and chewed thoroughly	11–34 kg: 2 tablets Over 34 kg: 3 tablets	
Praziquantel [Biltricide]	Beef tapeworm Pork tapeworm Fish tapeworm	10–20 mg/kg (once)	Same as adult	
	Blood flukes	20 mg/kg tid for 1 day	Same as adult	
	Liver fluke Intestinal fluke Lung fluke	25 mg/kg tid for 1 or 2 days	Same as adult	
Diethylcarbamazine [Hetrazan]	Filariae	Day 1: 50 mg Day 2: 50 mg tid Day 3: 100 mg tid Days 4 to 21: 2 mg/kg tid	Day 1: 1 mg/kg Day 2: 1 mg/kg tid Day 3: 1–2 mg/kg tid Days 4 to 21: 2 mg/kg tid	

Adverse Effects. Systemic effects are rare at usual doses, perhaps because the drug is so poorly absorbed. In patients with massive parasitic infestations, transient abdominal pain and diarrhea may occur.

Relatively low doses of mebendazole are embryotoxic and teratogenic in rats. However, these effects have not been observed in dogs, sheep, or horses. Limited experience with mebendazole in pregnant women has shown no increase in spontaneous abortion or fetal malformation. Nonetheless, it is recommended that pregnant women avoid this drug, especially during the first trimester.

Preparations, Dosage, and Administration. Mebendazole [Vermox] is available in 100-mg tablets for oral administration. Tablets may be chewed, crushed, or swallowed whole. The usual dosage for adults and children is 100 mg taken mornings and evenings for 3 days.

THIABENDAZOLE

Target Organisms. Thiabendazole is the drug of choice for *threadworms*. This agent is also the treatment of choice for *trichinosis*. In trichinosis, thiabendazole is active against adult worms and migrating larvae, but not against larvae that are encysted.

Mechanism of Action. Thiabendazole can inhibit helminth-specific fumarate reductase, but the contribution of this action to therapeutic effects is not known. Symptomatic improvement in patients with trichinosis may result in part from the analgesic, antipyretic, and anti-inflammatory actions of thiabendazole.

Pharmacokinetics. Thiabendazole undergoes rapid absorption and metabolism. Most of each dose is excreted in the urine as metabolites within 24 hours.

Adverse Effects. The incidence of adverse reactions is high: as many as one third of those treated become incapacitated for several hours. The most common effects are gastrointestinal (anorexia, nausea, vomiting) and neurologic (dizziness, drowsiness). Because of the potential for reduced alertness, patients should avoid hazardous activities (e.g., driving). Hepatotoxicity with jaundice has been reported. Accordingly, thiabendazole should be avoided in patients with liver dysfunction.

Preparations, Dosage, and Administration. Thiabendazole [Mintezol] is available in 500-mg chewable tablets and an oral suspension (100 mg/ml). Patients should be instructed to chew the tablets thoroughly. Gastrointestinal discomfort can be reduced by administering thiabendazole with food. Dosages for threadworm infestation and trichinosis are presented in Table 86–2.

PYRANTEL PAMOATE

Target Organisms. Pyrantel is active against *intestinal nematodes*. The drug is an alternative to mebendazole for infestations with *hookworms, pinworms,* and *giant roundworms*.

Mechanism of Action. Pyrantel is a depolarizing neuromuscular blocking agent that causes spastic paralysis of intestinal parasites. The paralyzed worms are cleared in the feces.

Pharmacokinetics. Pyrantel is poorly absorbed, and plasma levels remain low. Most of an administered dose is excreted unchanged in the feces.

Adverse Effects. Serious reactions are rare. The most common effects are gastrointestinal (nausea, vomiting, diarrhea, stomach pain, cramps). Possible central nervous system (CNS) effects include dizziness, drowsiness, headache, and insomnia.

Preparations, Dosage, and Administration. Pyrantel pamoate [Antiminth, Reese's Pinworm] is dispensed in liquid formulations (50 mg/ml) for oral use. The entire prescribed dose should be taken at one time. Dosages for intestinal nematodes are given in Table 86–2.

NICLOSAMIDE

Target Organisms. Niclosamide is a drug of choice for *cestode* infestations. The drug is active against pork, beef, and fish tapeworms.

Mechanism of Action. Niclosamide inhibits mitochondrial oxidative phosphorylation in tapeworms. This results in cessation of ATP production, followed by death.

Adverse Effects. Niclosamide is devoid of serious adverse effects. Absorption is poor. Hence, systemic effects are minimal. The most common reactions are gastrointestinal (nausea, vomiting, anorexia).

Preparations, Dosage, and Administration. Niclosamide [Niclocide] is available in 500-mg tablets. Tablets should be chewed thoroughly and swallowed with a small volume of water. Administration with food reduces gastrointestinal upset. Dosages are presented in Table 86–2.

PRAZIQUANTEL

Target Organisms. Praziquantel is very active against nematodes (flukes) and cestodes (tapeworms). This agent is a drug of choice for *schistosomiasis* and other *fluke infestations*. Also, praziquantel is an alternative to niclosamide for removal of *tapeworms*.

Mechanism of Action. Praziquantel is readily absorbed by helminths. At low therapeutic concentrations, the drug produces spastic paralysis, causing detachment of worms from body tissues. At high therapeutic concentrations, praziquantel disrupts the integument of the worms, rendering the parasites vulnerable to lethal attack by host defenses.

Pharmacokinetics. Praziquantel is rapidly absorbed from the GI tract. The drug undergoes extensive hepatic metabolism. Metabolites are excreted in the urine.

Adverse Effects. Praziquantel is relatively free of toxicity. Transient headache and abdominal discomfort are the most frequent reactions. Drowsiness may occur, and patients should avoid driving and other hazardous activities.

Preparations, Dosage, and Administration. Praziquantel [Biltricide] is available in 600-mg tablets for oral administration. Tablets should be swallowed intact. Dosages for tapeworm and fluke infestations are presented in Table 86–2.

DIETHYLCARBAMAZINE

Target Organisms. Diethylcarbamazine is the drug of choice for filarial infestations. The drug destroys microfilariae of *Wuchereria bancrofti, Brugia malayi,* and *Loa loa.* Adult females of these species are also killed.

Mechanism of Action. Diethylcarbamazine has two antifilarial actions. First, the drug reduces muscular activity, thereby causing parasites to be dislodged from their site of attachment. Second, by altering the surface properties of the parasites, the drug renders the organisms more vulnerable to attack by host defenses.

Pharmacokinetics. Diethylcarbamazine is readily absorbed and undergoes rapid and extensive metabolism. Metabolites are excreted in the urine.

Adverse Effects. Reactions caused directly by diethylcarbamazine are minor (headache, weakness, dizziness, nausea, vomiting). Indirect effects, occurring secondary to death of the parasites, can be more serious. These effects include rashes, intense itching, encephalitis, fever, tachycardia, lymphadenitis, leukocytosis, and proteinuria. These reactions are transient, however, lasting only a few days. Pretreatment with glucocorticoids can minimize these responses.

Preparations, Dosage, and Administration. Diethylcarbamazine citrate [Hetrazan] is dispensed in 50-mg tablets for oral use. The drug is available without charge from Lederle Laboratories. Dosages for treatment of filarial infestations are presented in Table 86–2.

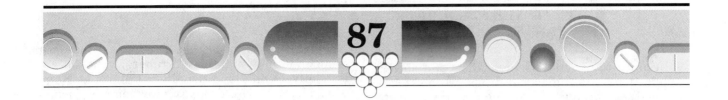

Antiprotozoal Drugs I: Antimalarial Agents

Malaria is a parasitic disease caused by protozoa of the genus *Plasmodium*. Worldwide, malaria is responsible for more death and suffering than any other infectious disease. Malaria afflicts over 800 million people, killing more than 2 million each year.

Large-scale attempts to eradicate the disease have achieved only partial success. Eradication programs have been directed at the malarial parasite as well as the *Anopheles* mosquito, the insect that transmits malaria to humans. Failure to produce complete control has resulted largely from development of drug resistance by both the parasite and the mosquito. The incidence of malaria is now rising in some regions where it had once been suppressed. There remains a great need for safe, effective, and affordable agents capable of killing the malaria parasite and its mosquito carrier.

In approaching the antimalarial drugs, we will begin by reviewing the life cycle of the malaria parasite. After that we will discuss the two major subtypes of malaria: falciparum malaria and vivax malaria. Next we will consider basic principles of treatment, focusing on therapeutic objectives and drug selection. Having established this background, we will discuss the pharmacology of the major antimalarial drugs.

LIFE CYCLE OF THE MALARIA PARASITE

In order to understand the actions and specific applications of antimalarial drugs, we must first understand the life cycle of the malaria parasite. As indicated in Figure 87–1, this cycle takes place in two hosts: humans and the female *Anopheles* mosquito. In the human host, the parasite undergoes asexual reproduction. Sexual reproduction occurs in the mosquito.

The human phase of the life cycle begins when sporozoites are injected into the bloodstream by a feeding *Anopheles* mosquito. These sporozoites invade parenchymal cells of the liver, where they multiply and transform into merozoites. This process, which takes from 12 to 26 days (depending upon the species of parasite), is referred to as the pre-erythrocytic or exoerythrocytic phase of the life cycle. Upon release from the liver, merozoites infect erythrocytes. Within the erythrocyte, each parasite differentiates and divides, becoming first a trophozoite and then a multinucleated schizont. The schizont then evolves into new merozoites. This process of asexual reproduction takes 2 to 3 days. At the end of this time, red blood cells burst and release the new merozoites into the blood. These new merozoites then infect fresh erythrocytes, thereby establishing an escalating cycle of red cell invasion and lysis. Each time the erythrocytes rupture, they release pyrogenic agents. These substances induce the repeating episodes of fever that characterize malaria. After several cycles of asexual reproduction, a few parasites differentiate into male and female gametocytes.

Sexual reproduction occurs following ingestion of gametocyte-containing blood by a female *Anopheles* mosquito. Within the mosquito, the gametocytes differentiate into mature forms, after which fertilization takes place. The resulting zygote then produces sporozoites, thus completing sexual reproduction.

TYPES OF MALARIA

Malaria is caused by four different species of *Plasmodium*. We will limit discussion to the two species encountered most frequently: *Plasmodium vivax* and *Plasmodium falciparum*. Malaria caused by either species is characterized by high fever, chills, and profuse sweating. However, despite similarity of symptoms, these two forms of malaria are very different. They differ most with regard to severity of symptoms, occurrence of relapse, and drug resistance. These and other differences are summarized in Table 87–1.

VIVAX MALARIA

Vivax malaria, caused by *P. vivax*, is the most common form of malaria. Fortunately, the disease is relatively mild and usually self-limiting. Since drug resistance by *P. vivax* is uncommon, symptoms can be readily suppressed with medication.

Infection begins when the host is inoculated with *P. vivax* sporozoites. After 26 days, merozoites emerge from the liver and begin their attack on erythrocytes. Symptoms of malaria (chills, fever, sweating) commence as infected erythrocytes rupture, releasing pyrogens and other substances into the blood. Symptoms peak, decline, and peak again every 48 hours in response to cyclic reinfection and lysis of red cells. This cycle continues until terminated by drugs or by acquired immunity. Unfortunately, relapse is likely following termination of the acute attack. Relapse is possible because dormant forms of *P. vivax* remain in the liver. These dormant forms periodically evolve into merozoites, emerge from the liver, and start the erythrocyte cycle anew. Relapse becomes less frequent with the passage of time, and, after 2 or more years, ceases entirely. Relapse can be stopped with drugs capable of killing the dormant hepatic parasites.

FALCIPARUM MALARIA

Malaria caused by *P. falciparum* is less common than malaria caused by *P. vivax*, but is also more severe. In the absence of treatment, the disease is lethal to about 10% of its victims. This infection is made even more dangerous by the emergence of drug-resistant strains of *P. falciparum*. Unlike the symptoms of vivax malaria, which peak every 48 hours, the symptoms of falciparum malaria occur at irregular intervals. The erythrocyte cycle of *P. falciparum* can destroy up to 60% of circulating red blood cells, resulting in profound anemia and weakness. The hemoglobin released from these cells causes the urine to darken, giving rise to the term *blackwater fever*. Falciparum malaria can produce serious complications, including pulmonary edema, hypoglycemia, and toxic encephalopathy, characterized by confusion, coma, and convulsions. When treated early, falciparum malaria usually responds well. However, if treatment is delayed, the disease may progress rapidly to irreversible shock and death. In contrast to infection with *P. vivax*, infection with *P. falciparum* does not relapse. This is because there are no dormant forms of *P. falciparum* in the liver. Hence, once the erythrocytic forms have been eliminated, the patient is free of the infection.

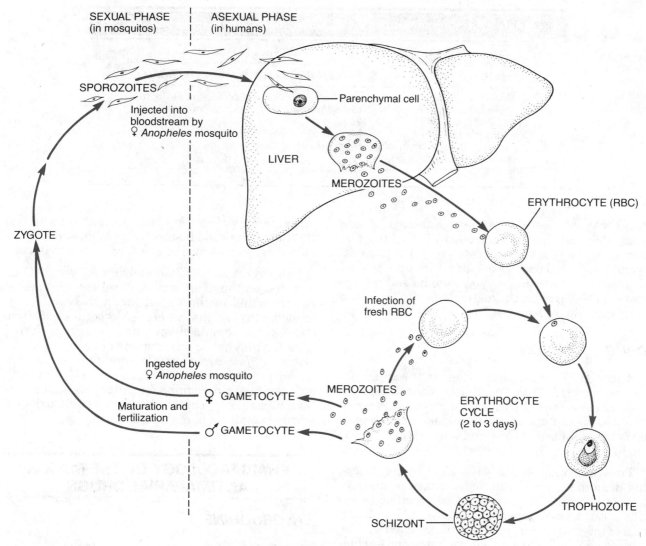

Figure 87–1. Life cycle of the malaria parasite.

PRINCIPLES OF ANTIMALARIAL THERAPY

THERAPEUTIC OBJECTIVES

Drug responsiveness of the malaria parasite changes as the parasite goes through its life cycle. The *erythrocytic* stages are killed most easily, whereas the *exoerythrocytic* (hepatic) stages are more difficult to kill. *Sporozoites* do not respond to drugs at all. Because of these differences in drug sensitivity, antimalarial therapy has three separate objectives: (1) treatment of an acute attack (clinical cure), (2) prevention of relapse (radical cure), and (3) prophylaxis (suppressive therapy). Because sporozoites are insensitive to drugs, therapy cannot prevent primary infection of the liver.

Treatment of Acute Attack. Clinical cure is accomplished with drugs that are active against erythrocytic forms of the malaria parasite. By eliminating parasites from red blood cells, the erythrocytic cycle is stopped and symptoms cease. For patients with vivax malaria, clinical cure will not prevent relapse, since dormant parasites remain in the liver. However, for patients with falciparum malaria, successful treatment of the acute attack will prevent further episodes (unless the patient is reinoculated by another infected mosquito).

Prevention of Relapse. People infected with *P. vivax* harbor dormant parasites in the liver. In order to prevent relapse, a drug capable of killing these hepatic forms must be taken. The use of drugs to eradicate hepatic *P. vivax* is referred to as radical cure. Since reinfection by a mosquito bite is a virtual certainty as long as one remains in a region where malaria is endemic, radical cure is usually postponed until departure from the region.

Prophylaxis. Persons anticipating travel to an area where malaria is endemic should take antimalarial medication for prophylaxis. Although

Table 87–1. Comparison of Vivax Malaria and Falciparum Malaria

| Characteristics | Type of Malaria | |
	Vivax Malaria	Falciparum Malaria
Causative organism	*Plasmodium vivax*	*Plasmodium falciparum*
Frequency of infection	More common	Less common
Latency of symptoms	26 days	12 days
Intensity of symptoms	Mild	Severe
Timing of febrile paroxysms	Every 2 days	Irregular
Probability of relapse	High	None
Drug resistance	Uncommon	Common

drugs cannot prevent primary infection of the liver, they *can* prevent infection of erythrocytes. Hence, although the parasite may be present, symptoms of malaria are avoided. Since prophylactic treatment prevents only symptoms and not invasion of the liver, such treatment is often referred to as *suppressive therapy*.

DRUG SELECTION

Selection of antimalarial drugs is based largely on two factors: (1) the goal of treatment, and (2) drug resistance of the causative strain of *Plasmodium*. Drugs of choice for treatment and prophylaxis are discussed below and summarized in Table 87–2.

Treatment of Acute Attacks. Chloroquine is the drug of choice for an acute attack of malaria caused by either *P. vivax* or by chloroquine-sensitive strains of *P. falciparum*. As a rule, a 3-day course of treatment produces clinical cure. For strains of *P. falciparum* that are resistant to chloroquine, a combination of three drugs is employed: quinine plus pyrimethamine plus a sulfonamide (e.g., sulfadoxine).

Prevention of Relapse. The drug of choice for preventing relapse of vivax malaria is primaquine, a drug that is highly active against the hepatic

stages *of P. vivax*. For falciparum malaria, no treatment is needed, since relapse does not occur following clinical cure of this form of the malaria.

Prophylaxis. Selection of drugs for prophylaxis is based on the drug sensitivity of the plasmodial species found in the region to which travel is intended. In regions where chloroquine-sensitive strains are found, chloroquine is the preferred drug for prophylaxis. In regions of chloroquine-resistant *P. falciparum*, mefloquine is now the preferred prophylactic agent. Alternatively, the traveler can take chloroquine for prophylaxis and then take Fansidar (pyrimethamine plus sulfadoxine) if febrile symptoms of malaria develop.

PHARMACOLOGY OF THE MAJOR ANTIMALARIAL DRUGS

CHLOROQUINE

Actions and Use. Chloroquine [Aralen] is the most generally useful of the antimalarial drugs. This agent is highly active against *erythrocytic* forms of the malaria parasite. Consequently, chloroquine is the drug of choice for treating acute attacks caused by *P. vivax* and by chloroquine-sensitive strains of *P. falciparum*. Chloroquine is also

Table 87–2. Drugs of Choice for Treatment and Prevention of Malaria

| Plasmodial Strain | Drugs of Choice | | |
	Treatment of Acute Attack	Prevention of Relapse	Prophylaxis
P. vivax	Chloroquine	Primaquine*	Chloroquine
P. falciparum: chloroquine sensitive	Chloroquine	NA†	Chloroquine
P. falciparum: chloroquine resistant	Quinine *plus* pyrimethamine/sulfadoxine	NA†	Mefloquine

*Primaquine is given following control of the acute attack.
†Not applicable. Malaria caused by *P. falciparum* does not relapse following successful treatment of the acute attack.

the drug of first choice for prophylaxis (suppressive therapy).

Chloroquine is not active against *exoerythrocytic* forms of the malaria parasite. Hence, the drug is unable to prevent primary infection by *P. vivax* or *P. falciparum*. Nor is it able to prevent relapse of vivax malaria, which is caused by emergence of dormant hepatic parasites.

Lethal effects on erythrocytic stages of the malaria parasite are thought to result from binding of chloroquine to DNA, an action that inhibits replication of DNA and synthesis of RNA. Chloroquine concentrates in parasitized erythrocytes. This phenomenon may explain the selective actions against erythrocytic forms of *Plasmodium*.

Pharmacokinetics. Chloroquine is rapidly and completely absorbed from the gastrointestinal tract. A substantial fraction of absorbed drug is deposited in certain tissues (e.g., lung, spleen, liver, kidney). Slow release from these sites helps maintain therapeutic plasma levels of the drug. Hence, when used for prophylaxis, chloroquine need be administered only once weekly. Excretion is primarily by nonrenal routes.

Adverse Effects. Since the doses required for prophylaxis are low, and since the higher doses required for treatment are taken only briefly, chloroquine rarely causes serious adverse effects. When employed to treat an acute malarial attack, chloroquine may cause visual disturbances, pruritus, headache, and gastrointestinal effects (abdominal discomfort, nausea, diarrhea). These effects can be minimized by taking the drug with meals. Because chloroquine concentrates in the liver, it should be used with caution in patients with hepatic disease.

Routes of Administration. Chloroquine may be administered orally and IM. The oral route is preferred. Intramuscular administration is employed only when emesis precludes oral treatment or when infection is especially severe.

Preparations and Dosage. Chloroquine phosphate [Aralen] is dispensed in tablets (250 and 500 mg) for oral administration. Chloroquine hydrochloride (50 mg/ml in 5-ml ampuls) is employed for IM injection.

For *prophylaxis* of malaria, the adult dosage is 500 mg of chloroquine phosphate once a week. The pediatric dosage is 8.3 mg/kg once a week. Treatment should commence 1 week before expected exposure to malaria and should continue for 4 weeks after leaving the endemic region.

To *treat an acute attack*, the adult dosage is 1 gm of chloroquine phosphate (PO) initially followed in 6 hours by a dose of 500 mg. Additional 500-mg doses are given on days 2 and 3.

PRIMAQUINE

Actions and Use. Primaquine is highly active against *hepatic* forms of *P. vivax*. Effects against *erythrocytic* forms are less profound. The drug is used to eradicate *P. vivax* from the liver, thereby preventing relapse. Primaquine is similar to chloroquine in structure, and may act by the same mechanism (inhibition of DNA and RNA synthesis following binding of the drug to DNA).

Pharmacokinetics. Primaquine is well absorbed following oral administration. Absorbed drug is rapidly metabolized to products of low antimalarial activity. Metabolites are excreted in the urine.

Adverse Effects. The most serious and frequent response to primaquine is *hemolysis*. This reaction develops in patients whose red blood cells are deficient in an enzyme named glucose-6-phosphate dehydrogenase (G-6-PD). Deficiency of G-6-PD is an inherited trait, occurring most commonly in black populations and in darker-skinned whites (e.g., Sardinians, Greeks, Iranians, Sephardic Jews). When possible, patients suspected of G-6-PD deficiency should be screened for this trait before treatment. During primaquine therapy, periodic blood counts should be performed. Also, the urine should be monitored (darkening indicates the presence of hemoglobin). If severe hemolysis develops, primaquine should be discontinued.

Preparations, Dosage, and Administration. Primaquine phosphate is dispensed in tablets that contain 26.3 mg of the drug. Administration is oral. For radical cure (prevention of relapse) of vivax malaria, the usual adult dosage is 26.3 mg/day for 2 weeks. The pediatric dosage is 0.53 mg/kg/day for 2 weeks.

MEFLOQUINE

Actions and Uses. Mefloquine [Lariam] kills erythrocytic forms of *P. vivax* and *P. falciparum*. The mechanism of action is unknown. Currently, mefloquine is the drug of choice for prophylactic therapy of *P. falciparum* infections. It can also be used to treat an acute attack. Unfortunately, resistance to mefloquine may emerge rapidly. The mechanism of resistance is not known.

Pharmacokinetics. Mefloquine is well absorbed following oral administration. The drug undergoes hepatic metabolism and is excreted in the bile and feces. Mefloquine has a prolonged half-life, ranging from 1 to 4 weeks. This allows the dosing interval to be long.

Adverse Effects. Adverse effects are dose related. At the low doses employed for prophylaxis, reactions are generally mild (nausea, dizziness, syncope). At the higher doses used for treatment of acute attacks, more intense reactions may occur, including gastrointestinal disturbances, nightmares, altered vision, and headache. Some of these effects may be indistinguishable from symptoms of malaria.

Toxicity to the central nervous system is a concern. Therapeutic doses have caused vertigo, confusion, psychosis, and convulsions. Mefloquine should not be given to people with epilepsy or psychiatric disorders.

Drug Interactions. Mefloquine, like quinine, can slow cardiac conduction. Accordingly, the drug should not be combined with other cardiosuppressants, including beta blockers and calcium-channel blockers. Also, mefloquine should not be combined with quinine or quinidine. Furthermore, caution is needed if quinine or quinidine is used to treat an active infection in a patient who had taken mefloquine for prophylaxis.

Preparations, Dosage, and Administration. Mefloquine [Lariam] is available in 250-mg tablets for oral administration.

For *prophylaxis,* the adult dosage is 250 mg once a week. Treatment should begin 1 week prior to travel to an endemic region and should continue for 4 weeks after leaving.

The adult dose for *acute treatment* of *P. falciparum* malaria is 1250 mg (5 tablets) taken all at once with at least 8 ounces of water.

QUININE

At one time, quinine was the only drug available to treat malaria. Today, quinine has been largely replaced by more effective and less toxic agents (e.g., chloroquine). However, quinine still has an important role: treatment of chloroquine-resistant falciparum malaria. Quinine occurs naturally in the bark of the cinchona tree. Commercial preparations are derived from this source.

Actions and Use. Quinine is active against erythrocytic forms of *Plasmodium* but has little effect on sporozoites and hepatic forms. The drug concentrates in parasitized red blood cells and may be selective against erythrocytic parasites for this reason. Like chloroquine, quinine can bind to DNA, causing inhibition of RNA synthesis and DNA replication. However, it is not known if this is the mechanism by which quinine kills the malaria parasite.

The principal application of quinine is malaria caused by chloroquine-resistant *P. falciparum.* Because quinine is not highly active, it must be combined with pyrimethamine plus a sulfonamide (e.g., sulfadoxine). Although quinine can produce effective prophylaxis against falciparum malaria, the drug is not used for this purpose: toxicity and poor compliance make quinine less desirable than chloroquine for prophylaxis.

Pharmacokinetics. Quinine is well absorbed from the gastrointestinal tract, even in the presence of diarrhea. The drug is metabolized by the liver, and metabolites are excreted in the urine. Plasma levels of quinine fall rapidly upon discontinuation of drug use.

Adverse Effects. At usual therapeutic doses, quinine frequently causes mild *cinchonism,* a syndrome characterized by tinnitus (ringing in the ears), headache, visual disturbances, nausea, and diarrhea. The physician should be notified if these symptoms develop. Because of its adverse effects on vision and hearing, quinine is contraindicated for patients with optic neuritis or tinnitus.

Quinine has *quinidine-like effects on the heart* and must be used cautiously in patients with atrial fibrillation: by increasing A-V conduction, quinine can promote passage of atrial impulses to the ventricles, thereby causing a dangerous increase in ventricular rate.

Like primaquine, quinine can cause *hemolysis* in patients whose red blood cells are deficient in G-6-PD. Patients using the drug should be monitored for hemolytic anemia. Quinine is contraindicated in the presence of G-6-PD deficiency.

Intravenous administration may cause *hypotension* and *acute circulatory failure.* To minimize these responses, IV quinine should be diluted and injected slowly. Patients should be transferred to oral medication as soon as possible.

Quinine is classified in FDA Pregnancy Category X: the risks of use during pregnancy clearly outweigh any possible benefits. The drug has caused fetal abnormalities, the most common being deafness from damage to the auditory nerve. Quinine can stimulate the uterus, and might thereby induce premature labor. *The drug must not be taken by pregnant women.*

Preparations, Dosage, and Administration. Quinine is available as two salts. *Quinine sulfate* is used for *oral* administration. *Quinine hydrochloride* is used for *intravenous* administration. The oral route is preferred. Intravenous administration is employed primarily when vomiting precludes absorption of oral drugs.

For chloroquine-resistant falciparum malaria, the adult dosage (PO or IV) is 650 mg every 8 hours for 3 days. The pediatric dosage is 8 mg/kg every 8 hours for 3 days. When used to treat chloroquine-resistant falciparum malaria, quinine should be combined with pyrimethamine and a sulfonamide.

PYRIMETHAMINE

Therapeutic Use. Pyrimethamine is used against chloroquine-resistant *P. falciparum.* It is a drug of choice for acute attacks and an alternative to mefloquine for prophylaxis. When taken for *prophylaxis,* pyrimethamine is combined with a sulfonamide (e.g., sulfadoxine). When used for *treatment,* pyrimethamine is combined with quinine as well as a sulfonamide.

In addition to its antimalarial use, pyrimethamine is the drug of first choice for toxoplasmosis (see Chapter 88).

Mechanism of Action. Pyrimethamine inhibits dihydrofolate reductase, an enzyme that converts folic acid into its active form. Without active folic acid, cells are unable to synthesize DNA, RNA, and proteins. Pyrimethamine rarely disrupts host biochemistry because the concentration of pyrimethamine required to inhibit human dihydrofolate reductase is about 1000 times greater than the concentration needed to inhibit plasmodial dihydrofolate reductase.

The effects of pyrimethamine are potentiated by concurrent use of a sulfonamide. Unlike humans, the malaria parasite is unable to take up pre-formed folic acid from its environment. Consequently, the parasite must synthesize folic acid of its own. Sulfonamides inhibit this synthesis. Hence, the combination of a sulfonamide with pyrimethamine produces a *sequential block* in a critical biochemical pathway. In step one, sulfonamides inhibit folic acid synthesis, thereby reducing folic acid levels. In step two, pyrimethamine prevents conversion of the reduced pool of folic acid into an active form. This sequential block has devastating effects on the parasite.

Pharmacokinetics. Pyrimethamine is well absorbed following oral administration. The drug is highly bound to plasma proteins, and its elimination is therefore slow. The plasma half-life of the drug is approximately 4 days. Pyrimethamine undergoes limited hepatic metabolism. Metabolites and parent drug are excreted in the urine.

Adverse Effects. At the doses employed for treatment or prophylaxis of malaria, pyrimethamine produces few adverse effects. However, at high doses, such as those used to treat toxoplasmosis, pyrimethamine can produce symptoms of *folic acid deficiency*. Symptoms result from effects on the bone marrow and the gastrointestinal mucosa, tissues that have a high percentage of cells undergoing division. Effects on the bone marrow manifest as leukopenia, thrombocytopenia, and anemia. Effects on the gastrointestinal mucosa manifest as ulcerative stomatitis, atrophic glossitis, pharyngitis, and diarrhea. These responses reverse upon discontinuation of treatment, and can be prevented by giving folic or folinic acid.

Preparations. Pyrimethamine is dispensed alone and in combination with sulfadoxine. The combination preparation, known as *Fansidar*, contains 25 mg of pyrimethamine and 500 mg of sulfadoxine. Tablets containing pyrimethamine alone (25 mg) are marketed under the trade name *Daraprim*.

Dosage and Administration. Administration is oral. When used to treat malaria, pyrimethamine is almost always taken in combination with a sulfonamide. The doses presented here refer to the combination of pyrimethamine with sulfadoxine [Fansidar]. To treat an acute attack of chloroquine-resistant falciparum malaria, Fansidar is administered as a single dose in the following amounts: for adults, 2 to 3 tablets; for children aged 9 to 14 years, 2 tablets; for children aged 4 to 8 years, 1 tablet; and for children under 4 years, one-half tablet.

The dosage for toxoplasmosis is given in Chapter 88.

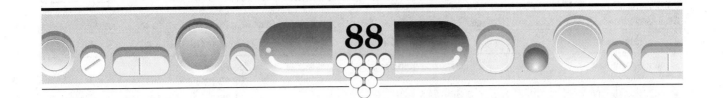

Antiprotozoal Drugs II: Miscellaneous Agents

PROTOZOAL INFECTIONS

DRUGS OF CHOICE FOR PROTOZOAL
INFECTIONS
Iodoquinol
Metronidazole
Pentamidine
Quinacrine
Other Drugs of Choice

Because of increasing world travel by Americans, and because of increased immigration by individuals from regions where infectious protozoa are endemic (South America, Asia, Africa), the incidence of protozoal infection in the United States is rising. The organisms encountered most frequently are *Entamoeba histolytica*, *Trichomonas vaginalis*, and *Giardia lamblia*. Infections with most other protozoa (e.g., *Leishmania* species, trypanosomes) are rare in North America. In approaching the antiprotozoal drugs, we will begin by discussing the diseases that protozoa produce. After that we will discuss the drugs used for treatment.

PROTOZOAL INFECTIONS

Our goal in this section is to describe the major protozoal infections (except for malaria, which is the subject of Chapter 87). Discussion focuses on causative organisms, sites of infection, symptoms of disease, and preferred drug therapy. Causative organisms and drugs of choice are summarized in Table 88–1.

1075

Table 88–1. Drugs of Choice for Protozoal Infection

Disease	Causative Protozoan	Drugs of Choice
Amebiasis	*Entamoeba histolytica*	Iodoquinol* Metronidazole*
Giardiasis	*Giardia lamblia*	Quinacrine Metronidazole†
Leishmaniasis	*Leishmania* species	Sodium stibogluconate
Pneumocystis carinii pneumonia	*Pneumocystis carinii*	Trimethoprim plus sulfamethoxazole; pentamidine‡
Toxoplasmosis	*Toxoplasma gondii*	Pyrimethamine plus a sulfonamide
Trichomoniasis	*Trichomonas vaginalis*	Metronidazole
Trypanosomiasis, African (sleeping sickness)	*Trypanosoma brucei gambiense* *Trypanosoma brucei rhodesiense*	Suramin§ Melarsoprol§
Trypanosomiasis, American (Chagas' disease)	*Trypanosoma cruzi*	Nifurtimox

*For asymptomatic disease, use iodoquinol by itself; for symptomatic disease, use metronidazole followed by iodoquinol.
†Metronidazole is an alternative drug of choice for moderate giardiasis.
‡Pentamidine is an alternative to trimethoprim plus sulfamethoxazole for severely immunocompromised patients.
§Suramin is useful only during the early phase of the disease; melarsoprol is required once CNS involvement has developed.

Amebiasis

Amebiasis is an infestation with *Entamoeba histolytica*. In the United States, the disease affects between 2% and 4% of the population. The principal site of infestation is the intestine. However, amebas may migrate to other tissues, most commonly to the liver, where abscesses may form. Amebiasis is usually asymptomatic. When symptoms are present, the most characteristic are diarrhea and abdominal pain.

Drugs of choice for amebiasis are *iodoquinol* and *metronidazole*. Iodoquinol is active only against amebas residing in the intestine. Metronidazole is active against amebas that inhabit the intestine, liver, and all other sites. For individuals who are asymptomatic, therapy with iodoquinol alone is sufficient. When symptoms are present, metronidazole is given initially, followed by iodoquinol.

Giardiasis

Giardiasis is an infection with *Giardia lamblia*. In the United States, giardiasis has an incidence of 2% to 10%. Infestation usually occurs by contact with contaminated objects or by drinking contaminated water. The primary habitat of *Giardia lamblia* is the upper small intestine. Occasionally, organisms migrate to the bile ducts and gallbladder. As many as 50% of affected individuals remain free of symptoms. However, symptoms that are both unpleasant and uncomfortable can develop. These include profound malaise; heartburn; vomiting; colicky pain after eating; and malodorous belching, flatulence, and diarrhea. The pain associated with giardiasis may mimic that of gallstones, appendicitis, peptic ulcers, or hiatal hernia. The drug of choice for treatment is *quinacrine*. For individuals who cannot tolerate quinacrine and whose disease is relatively mild, *metronidazole* is an alternative treatment of choice.

Leishmaniasis

The term *leishmaniasis* refers to infestation by certain protozoal species belonging to the genus *Leishmania*. Worldwide, the incidence of leishmaniasis is estimated at 100 million. The disease is acquired through the bite of sand flies indigenous to tropical and subtropical regions. In the human host, the parasites take up residence inside cells of the reticuloendothelial system.

Leishmaniasis has three different forms: cutaneous, mucocutaneous, and visceral. The particular form acquired is determined by the species of *Leishmania* involved. These forms vary greatly in severity, ranging from mild (cutaneous leishmaniasis) to potentially fatal (visceral leishmaniasis). In *cutaneous* leishmaniasis, a nodule forms at the site of inoculation; later, this nodule may evolve into an ulcer that is very slow to heal. *Mucocutaneous* leishmaniasis is characterized by ulceration in the mucosa of the mouth, nose, and pharynx. Symptoms of *visceral* leishmaniasis include fever, hepatosplenomegaly, liver dysfunction, hypoalbuminemia, pancytopenia, lymphadenopathy, and hemorrhage. The disease is frequently fatal when left untreated. For all forms of leishmaniasis, *sodium stibogluconate* is the treatment of choice.

Pneumocystis carinii Pneumonia

Pneumocystis pneumonia is caused by *Pneumocystis carinii*, an organism of uncertain classification. (It has been classified as both a protozoan and a fungus.) Infection occurs primarily in the immunocompromised host. The incidence of *Pneumocystis carinii* pneumonia (PCP) is extremely high (80%) in patients with AIDS. Those at highest risk have a CD4 lymphocyte count below 200 cells/mm³. Following control of an initial infection, the rate of recurrence is 60% within the first year. Because of the high risk of PCP in people with AIDS, prophylactic therapy is recommended for all patients who have had PCP before or whose CD4 lymphocyte count is low.

Clinical manifestations of PCP are generally nonspecific. Early symptoms include cough, dyspnea, chest discomfort, pallor, and cyanosis. In advanced infection, lung morphology is altered. Left untreated, the disease has a mortality rate of 90%.

The treatment of choice for PCP is *trimethoprim plus sulfamethoxazole*. For patients who are severely immunocompromised, *pentamidine* may be preferred. Alternative regimens include *trimethoprim plus dapsone*, *primaquine plus clindamycin*, and *trimetrexate plus folinic acid*. For prophylaxis of PCP, *trimethoprim plus sulfamethoxazole* is the treatment of choice. Alternative prophylactic drugs are *dapsone* and *aerosolized pentamidine*.

Toxoplasmosis

Toxoplasmosis is caused by infection with *Toxoplasma gondii*, a protozoan of the class Sporozoa. The parasite is harbored by many animals as well as by humans. Infection is acquired most commonly by eating undercooked meat. Toxoplasmosis may also be congenital. Congenital infection can damage the brain, eyes, liver, and other organs. Extensive disease is usually fatal. In adults, infection is frequently asymptomatic. However, in some individuals the disease progresses to encephalitis and death. The treatment of choice is *pyrimethamine* combined with a *sulfonamide*.

Trichomoniasis

Trichomoniasis is caused by *Trichomonas vaginalis*, a flagellated protozoan. Trichomoniasis is a common disease, affecting about 200 million people worldwide. The usual site of infestation is the genitourinary tract. Parasites may also inhabit the rectum. In females, infection results in vaginitis. Urethritis occurs in males. The disease is usually transmitted sexually but can also be acquired by contact with contaminated objects (e.g., toilet seats). Oral *metronidazole* is the treatment of choice.

Trypanosomiasis

There are two major forms of trypanosomiasis: African trypanosomiasis and American trypanosomiasis. Both forms are caused by protozoal species belonging to the genus *Trypanosoma*.

African Trypanosomiasis (Sleeping Sickness). African trypanosomiasis, transmitted by the bite of the tsetse fly, is caused by two subspecies of *Trypanosoma brucei: T. brucei rhodesiense* and *T. brucei gambiense*. Trypanosomiasis caused by either subspecies has similar symptoms. Early symptoms include fever, lymphadenopathy, hepatosplenomegaly, dyspnea, and tachycardia. Late symptoms, which result from involvement of the central nervous system (CNS), include mental dullness, incoordination, and apathy. As CNS involvement advances, sleep becomes constant and death may eventually follow. During the early phase of African trypanosomiasis, *suramin* is the treatment of choice. *Melarsoprol* is the preferred agent for the late (CNS) stage. Both suramin and melarsoprol can produce serious side effects, and both agents require prolonged use. Treatment is difficult and frequently unsuccessful.

American Trypanosomiasis (Chagas' Disease). Chagas' disease is caused by infection with *Trypanosoma cruzi*, a protozoan of the class Sporozoa. The disease is prevalent in South America and the Caribbean, where it affects some 10 million people. The parasites are harbored in the digestive tract of certain blood-sucking bugs, and are transmitted as follows: the bug bites a sleeping person (usually on the face) and also defecates; the parasites, which are contained in the bug's feces, are then forced into the bite wound by rubbing or scratching. An early sign of the disease is swelling and severe inflammation at the site of inoculation. Over time, parasites invade cardiac cells and neurons of the myenteric plexus. Destruction of these cells can cause cardiomyopathy, megaesophagus, and megacolon. Death has occurred, usually as a result of injury to the heart. In its early phase, Chagas' disease can be treated with *nifurtimox*. Unfortunately, neither this drug nor any other is very effective against chronic infection.

DRUGS OF CHOICE FOR PROTOZOAL INFECTIONS

The major antiprotozoal drugs are discussed below. Most of these agents are active against only one organism. The principal exception to this rule is metronidazole. Although consideration here is limited to drugs of choice, be aware that additional antiprotozoal drugs are available.

IODOQUINOL

Actions and Use. Iodoquinol [Yodoxin] is the drug of choice for asymptomatic intestinal amebiasis. In addition, the drug is employed in conjunction with metronidazole to treat symptomatic intestinal infection and systemic amebiasis. In these last two cases, iodoquinol is administered after treatment with metronidazole to eliminate any surviving intestinal parasites. The mechanism of amebicidal action is not known.

Pharmacokinetics. Only a small fraction (5% to 8%) of oral iodoquinol is absorbed. The fraction absorbed is excreted as metabolites in the urine.

Adverse Effects. Mild reactions occur occasionally. These include rash, acne, slight thyroid enlargement, and gastrointestinal (GI) effects (nausea, vomiting, diarrhea, cramps, pruritus ani). Rarely, prolonged therapy at very high doses has caused optic atrophy with permanent loss of vision.

Preparations, Dosage, and Administration. Iodoquinol [Yodoxin] is available in tablets (210 and 650 mg) and as a powder for oral administration. The usual adult dosage is 650 mg three times a day for 20 days. The dosage for children is 10 to 13 mg/kg three times a day for 20 days.

METRONIDAZOLE

Therapeutic Uses. Metronidazole [Flagyl, others] is the drug of choice for symptomatic intestinal amebiasis and systemic amebiasis. Because most of an administered dose is absorbed in the small intestine, concentrations in the colon remain low. Consequently, for treatment of amebiasis, metronidazole is followed by iodoquinol, an amebicidal drug that achieves high colonic levels. As a result, iodoquinol kills those intestinal parasites that may have survived therapy with metronidazole.

Metronidazole is the agent of choice for infection with *Trichomonas vaginalis*. The drug is effective against trichomoniasis in males as well as in females.

Metronidazole is an alternative to quinacrine for moderate giardiasis. The drug is almost as active as quinacrine and produces fewer severe side effects.

Many pathogenic bacteria are sensitive to metronidazole. Antibacterial applications are discussed in Chapter 82.

Mechanism of Action. To be effective, metronidazole must first be converted to a more chemically reactive form. This reactive form interacts with DNA, causing strand breakage and loss of helical structure. The resulting impairment of DNA function is thought responsible for the antimicrobial and mutagenic actions of the drug.

Pharmacokinetics. Metronidazole is readily absorbed from the GI tract. The drug undergoes extensive hepatic metabolism. Metabolites and unchanged drug are excreted in the urine.

Adverse Effects. Metronidazole produces a variety of untoward effects, but these rarely preclude continued treatment. The most common side effects are nausea, headache, dry mouth, and an unpleasant metallic taste. Other common responses include stomatitis, vomiting, diarrhea, insomnia, vertigo, and weakness. Harmless darkening of the urine may occur; patients should be forewarned of this effect. Certain neurologic effects (numbness in the extremities, ataxia, convulsions) occur rarely;

metronidazole should be withdrawn if these develop. Metronidazole should not be used by patients with active disease of the CNS. Carcinogenic effects have been observed in rodents; however, there is no evidence for increased incidence of cancer in humans.

Use in Pregnancy. Metronidazole readily crosses the placenta, and is mutagenic in bacteria. However, experience to date has shown no effect on the developing fetus following treatment of pregnant women. Nonetheless, it is recommended that metronidazole be avoided during the first trimester, and employed with caution throughout the rest of pregnancy.

Drug Interactions. Metronidazole has disulfiram-like effects and can therefore produce unpleasant or dangerous reactions if taken in conjunction with alcohol. Accordingly, patients must be warned against consuming alcohol.

Metronidazole inhibits metabolic inactivation of oral anticoagulants (e.g., warfarin). Dosages of these agents must be lowered.

Preparations, Dosage, and Administration. Metronidazole [Flagyl, others] is available in tablets (250 and 500 mg), as a powder (to be reconstituted for injection), and as a ready-to-use injection. For treatment of protozoal infections, the oral tablets are used. Antibacterial therapy usually requires IV administration. Dosages for antiprotozoal therapy are given below. Antibacterial dosages are presented in Chapter 82.

Amebiasis. The usual adult dosage is 750 mg three times daily for 10 days. The pediatric dosage is 12 to 17 mg/kg three times daily for 10 days. Following treatment with metronidazole, iodoquinol is given for 20 days.

Trichomoniasis. Treatment for adults consists of either (1) a single 2-gm dose or (2) doses of 250 mg three times a day for 7 days. The pediatric dosage is 5 mg/kg three times daily for 7 days.

Giardiasis. The adult dosage is 250 mg three times daily for 5 days. The pediatric dosage is 5 mg/kg three times daily for 5 days.

PENTAMIDINE

Actions. Pentamidine [Pentam 300, NebuPent] is active against *Pneumocystis carinii*. The drug disrupts synthesis of DNA, RNA, phospholipids, and proteins. We do not know if these actions underlie antiprotozoal effects.

Uses. Pentamidine is given by injection (IM or IV) and by inhalation. Pentamidine *injection* is used to treat active *Pneumocystis carinii* pneumonia (PCP). *Inhaled* pentamidine is used to *prevent* PCP in high-risk, HIV-positive patients. High-risk patients are those with (1) a history of one or more episodes of PCP, or (2) peripheral CD4 lymphocyte counts less than 200 cells/mm^3. In addition to its use against PCP, pentamidine has been used on an investigational basis against leishmaniasis and trypanosomiasis.

Pharmacokinetics. For treatment of active PCP, pentamidine is administered IM or IV. Equivalent blood levels are achieved with both routes. The drug is extensively bound in tissues. Penetration to the brain and cerebrospinal fluid is poor. Between 50% and 65% of an administered dose is excreted rapidly in the urine. The remaining drug is excreted slowly, over 1 month or more.

Adverse Effects Associated with Parenteral Administration. Pentamidine can produce serious side effects when given IM or IV. Caution must be exercised.

Sudden and severe *hypotension* occurs in about 1% of those treated. The fall in blood pressure may cause tachycardia, dizziness, and fainting. To minimize hypotensive responses, patients should receive the drug while lying down. Blood pressure should be monitored closely.

Hypoglycemia (0.4%) and *hyperglycemia* have occurred. Hypoglycemia has been associated with necrosis of pancreatic islet cells and excessive levels of insulin. The cause of hyperglycemia is not known. Because of possible fluctuations in blood glucose levels, blood glucose should be monitored daily.

Intramuscular administration is painful. Necrosis at the injection site followed by formation of a sterile abscess is common.

Some adverse effects can be life-threatening when severe. The incidence of their occurrence is as follows: leukopenia (2.8%), thrombocytopenia (1.7%), acute renal failure (0.5%), hypocalcemia (0.2%), and dysrhythmias (0.2%).

Adverse Effects Associated with Aerosolized Pentamidine. Inhaled pentamidine does not cause the severe adverse effects associated with injected pentamidine. The most common reactions are cough (38%) and bronchospasm (15%). These are more pronounced in patients with asthma and in those with a history of smoking. Both reactions can be controlled with an inhaled bronchodilator, and rarely necessitate pentamidine withdrawal.

Preparations, Dosage, and Administration. Pentamidine isethionate *for injection* [Pentam 300] is dispensed in 300-mg single-dose vials. Administration is IM or IV. For treatment of active PCP, the dosage for adults and children is 4 mg/kg daily for 2 weeks. Intravenous administration must be done slowly (over 60 minutes).

Pentamidine isethionate *aerosol* [NebuPent] is used for prophylaxis of PCP in patients with AIDS. The dosage is 300 mg once every 4 weeks. Administration is performed with a Respirgard II nebulizer by Marquest. Solutions should be freshly prepared.

QUINACRINE

Actions and Use. Quinacrine [Atabrine HCl] is a drug of choice for giardiasis. In the past, the drug was used to treat tapeworm infestation and malaria; these applications are now obsolete. Antiparasitic actions are thought to result from interaction with DNA.

Pharmacokinetics. Quinacrine is well absorbed from the GI tract and becomes distributed throughout the body. Extensive binding to tissues results in drug accumulation. Excretion is primarily renal. Because of slow release from sites of tissue binding, quinacrine can be detected in urine for more than 2 months after therapy has ceased.

Adverse Effects. When used to treat giardiasis, quinacrine rarely causes serious adverse effects. The most common reactions are dizziness, headache, diarrhea, and vomiting. Deposition of quinacrine in the skin may cause yellow staining. This pigmentation should not be confused with jaundice. Toxic psychosis may occur but is rare at the doses employed in giardiasis. Quinacrine should be avoided by patients with a history of psychosis. Quinacrine can seriously exacerbate psoriasis, sometimes causing exfoliative lesions; caution should be exercised in patients with psoriasis. Quinacrine crosses the placenta and may pose a hazard to the fetus; since giardiasis is seldom a threat to life, treatment should be postponed until parturition.

Preparations, Dosage, and Administration. Quinacrine hydrochloride [Atabrine HCl] is dispensed in 100-mg tablets for oral administration. For giardiasis, the adult dosage is 100 mg three times daily (after meals) for 7 days. The pediatric dosage is 2 mg/kg three times daily (after meals) for 5 days.

OTHER DRUGS OF CHOICE

Melarsoprol

Therapeutic Use. Melarsoprol is a drug of choice for African trypanosomiasis (sleeping sickness). The drug is employed during the late stage of the disease (i.e., after CNS involvement has developed). For earlier stages of the disease, suramin, which is less toxic than melarsoprol, is the treatment of choice.

Mechanism of Action. Melarsoprol is an organic arsenical compound that reacts with sulfhydryl groups of proteins. Antiparasitic effects result from inactivation of enzymes. This same action appears to underlie the serious toxicity of the drug. Melarsoprol is more toxic to parasites than to humans because it penetrates parasitic membranes more easily than human cells.

Adverse Effects. Melarsoprol is quite toxic, and adverse reactions are common. Frequent responses include hypertension, albuminuria, peripheral neuropathy, myocardial damage, and Herxheimer-type reactions. Reactive encephalopathy may develop during the first course of treatment. Although fatalities have occurred, they are much less common than in the past.

Preparations, Dosage, and Administration. Melarsoprol [Arsobal] is administered by slow IV injection. The drug is highly irritating to tissues, and care must be taken to avoid extravasation. Because of its toxicity, melarsoprol should be administered in a hospital setting. Treatment for adults begins with 2 to 3.6 mg/kg IV daily for 3 days. Seven days later a second course (3.6 mg/kg IV daily for 3 days) is given. This is repeated once more after 10 to 21 days. Melarsoprol can be obtained through the Centers for Disease Control and Prevention. The drug is not available commercially.

Nifurtimox

Therapeutic Use. Nifurtimox is the drug of choice for American trypanosomiasis (Chagas' disease). The drug is most effective in the acute stage of the disease, curing about 80% of patients. Chronic disease is less responsive.

Pharmacokinetics. Nifurtimox is well absorbed from the GI tract and undergoes rapid and extensive metabolism. Metabolites are excreted in the urine.

Adverse Effects. Therapy is prolonged, and significant untoward effects occur frequently. Gastrointestinal effects (anorexia, nausea, vomiting, abdominal pain) and peripheral neuropathy are especially common. Weight loss resulting from GI effects may require discontinuation of treatment. Additional common reactions include rashes and CNS effects (memory loss, insomnia, vertigo, headache).

Preparations, Dosage, and Administration. Nifurtimox [Bayer 2502, Lampit] is dispensed in 100-mg tablets. In the United States, the drug is available only from the Centers for Disease Control and Prevention. The adult dosage is 2 to 2.5 mg/kg four times daily for 120 days. For young children (ages 1 through 10 years), the usual dosage is 4 to 5 mg/kg four times daily for 90 days. For older children (ages 11 to 16 years), the usual dosage is 3 to 4 mg/kg four times daily for 90 days.

Pyrimethamine

Pyrimethamine [Daraprim] is the drug of choice for toxoplasmosis. This drug is also important for treating malaria. For toxoplasmosis, the adult dosage is 25 to 100 mg daily for 3 to 4 weeks. The dosage for children is 2 mg/kg/day for 3 days followed by 1 mg/kg/day for 4 weeks. The pharmacology of pyrimethamine is discussed in Chapter 87.

Sodium Stibogluconate

Sodium stibogluconate [Pentostam] is the drug of choice for leishmaniasis. The mechanism of action is not known. The drug is poorly absorbed from the GI tract and, hence, must be administered parenterally (IM or IV). Stibogluconate undergoes little metabolism and is excreted rapidly in the urine. Although severe side effects can occur, the drug is generally well tolerated. The most frequent untoward reactions are muscle pain, joint stiffness, and bradycardia. Changes in the EKG are common and occasionally precede serious dysrhythmias. Liver and renal dysfunction, shock, and sudden death occur rarely. Sodium stibogluconate is dispensed in aqueous solution for IM and IV injection. For leishmaniasis, the usual dosage (adult and pediatric) is 20 mg/kg/day (IM or IV) for 20 to 28 days. In the United States, the drug is available only from the Centers for Disease Control and Prevention.

Suramin

Actions and Uses. Suramin sodium is the drug of choice for treating the early phase of African trypanosomiasis (sleeping sickness); for the late phase of the disease (i.e., the stage of CNS involvement), melarsoprol is the preferred treatment. Suramin is known to inhibit many trypanosomal enzymes; however, its primary mechanism of action has not been established.

Pharmacokinetics. The drug is poorly absorbed from the GI tract, and therefore must be administered parenterally (IV). Suramin binds tightly to plasma proteins and remains in the bloodstream for months. Penetration into cells is low. Excretion is renal.

Adverse Effects. Side effects can be severe, and treatment should take place in a hospital. Frequent reactions include vomiting, itching, rash, paresthesias, photophobia, and hyperesthesia of the palms and soles. Suramin concentrates in the kidney and can cause local damage, resulting in the appearance of protein, blood cells, and casts in the urine. If urinary casts are observed, treatment should cease. Rarely, a shock-like syndrome develops after IV administration. To minimize the risk of this reaction, a small test dose (200 mg) is administered; in the absence of a severe reaction, full doses may follow.

Preparations, Dosage, and Administration. Suramin sodium [Germanin] is available from the Centers for Disease Control and Prevention. The drug is dispensed in 1-gm ampuls. Administration is by slow IV infusion. Suramin is unstable, and fresh solutions must be made daily. The adult dosage is 1 gm IV on days 1, 3, 7, 14, and 21. The pediatric dosage is 20 mg/kg IV administered by the same schedule employed for adults.

Trimethoprim plus Sulfamethoxazole

The combination of trimethoprim plus sulfamethoxazole is the treatment of choice for *Pneumocystis carinii* pneumonia

(PCP). This drug combination is also important for bacterial infections. The pharmacology of the combination is discussed in Chapter 78. For therapy of PCP, the *total daily* dose for adults and children is 15 to 20 mg/kg of trimethoprim and 75 to 100 mg/kg of sulfamethoxazole. The total daily dose is given in three or four divided doses. Treatment lasts for 2 to 3 weeks. Administration may be oral or intravenous.

Ectoparasiticides

E ctoparasites are parasites that live on the surface of the host. Most ectoparasites that infest humans live on the skin and hair. Some live on clothing and bedding, moving to the host only to feed. The principal ectoparasites that infest humans are mites and lice. Infestation with mites is known as *scabies*. Infestation with lice is known as *pediculosis*. Both conditions are characterized by intense pruritus (itching). Infestations with mites and with lice can be eradicated with topical drugs.

ECTOPARASITIC INFESTATIONS

SCABIES

Scabies is caused by infestation with *Sarcoptes scabiei*, an organism known commonly as the itch mite. Irritation occurs as a result of the female mite burrowing beneath the skin to lay eggs. Burrows may be visible as small ridges or dotted lines. In adults, the most common sites of infestation are the wrists, elbows, nipples, navel, genital region, and webs of the fingers. In children, infestation is most likely on the head, neck, and buttocks.

The primary symptom of scabies is pruritus. Itching is most intense just after going to bed. Scratching may result in abrasion and secondary infection.

Transmission of scabies is usually by direct contact. This contact may be sexual or of a less intimate nature. Scabies may also be transmitted through contact with infested linen, towels, or clothing.

Scabies is best treated using a pesticide-containing lotion or cream. To eradicate mites, the entire body surface must be treated (excluding the face and scalp in adults). To prevent reinfestation, bedding and intimate clothing should be machine washed and dried.

Several drugs can kill mites. Permethrin (5% cream formulation) is the drug of choice. This preparation is effective in just one application. Crotamiton and lindane are alternatives.

PEDICULOSIS

Pediculosis is a general term referring to infestation with any of several kinds of lice. The types of lice encountered most frequently are *Pediculus humanus capitis* (head louse), *Pediculus humanus corporis* (body louse), and *Phthirus pubis* (pubic or crab louse). Infestation with any of these insects causes pruritus. Infestations with head, pubic, and body lice differ with regard to method of treatment and mode of acquisition.

Pubic Lice

Pubic lice, commonly known as crabs, usually reside on the skin and hair of the pubic region. However, pubic lice may also be found on the eyelashes and other parts of the body. As a rule, infestation is transmitted through sexual contact. Consequently, crabs are most common among people who have multiple sexual partners. Two preparations—*lindane* and *malathion* (0.5% lotion)—are drugs of choice for eliminating crabs. Infestation of the eyelashes is treated with *petrolatum ophthalmic ointment*. Clothing and linen should be disinfected by washing in very hot water, followed by machine drying at high temperature.

Head Lice

Head lice reside on the scalp and lay their nits (eggs) on the hair. Adult lice may be difficult to observe. Nits, however, are usually visible. Infestation may be associated with hives, boils, impetigo, and other skin disorders. The head louse is more democratic than the pubic or body louse and can be found infesting people from all socioeconomic groups. Head lice may be transmitted by close personal contact and by contact with infested clothing, hairbrushes, furniture, and other objects. Treatments of choice are *permethrin* and *malathion*. Both drugs kill adult lice as well as nits. Eradication of head lice does not require shaving or cutting the hair.

Body Lice

Despite their name, body lice reside not on the body but on clothing. These lice move to the body only to feed. Consequently, body lice are rarely seen on the skin. Rather, these insects can be found in bed linens and in the seams of garments. Transmission of body lice is by contact with infested clothing or bedding. Body lice are relatively uncommon in the United States, where regular laundering precludes infestation. Infestation is most likely among vagrants and other people whose clothes may not be frequently washed. The majority of body lice can be removed from the host simply by removal of clothing. Those lice that remain on the body can be killed by application of a pesticide (lindane or pyrethrins fortified with piperonyl butoxide). Clothing and bedding should be disinfected by washing and drying at high temperature.

PHARMACOLOGY OF ECTOPARASITICIDES

Ectoparasitic infestations are treated with topical drugs. These agents are dispensed in the form of creams, gels, lotions, and shampoos. The pharmacology of scabicides and pediculicides is discussed below. Properties of the five major ectoparasiticides are summarized in Table 89–1.

LINDANE

Actions and Uses

Lindane is absorbed through the chitin shell of adult mites and lice and causes death by inducing convulsions. The drug is also lethal to the eggs. Until the recent introduction of the 5% formulation of permethrin, lindane had been the drug of choice for scabies. Lindane is also active against lice.

Adverse Effects

Irritation. Lindane is irritating to the eyes and mucous membranes. Application to the face should be avoided. If contact occurs, the affected area should be flushed with water.

Convulsions. Lindane can penetrate the intact skin and, if absorbed in sufficient amounts, can cause convulsions. Seizures can also occur following lindane ingestion. Fortunately, convulsions are rare, resulting most often from drug ingestion or inappropriate administration. Premature infants are particularly vulnerable to lindane-induced seizures. This is because the drug can penetrate the skin of these infants with relative ease, and because limited liver function prevents the premature infant from detoxifying absorbed drug. Accordingly, lindane should be applied with caution to the premature infant. Caution should also be exercised when treating individuals with pre-exist-

		Indications			
Generic Name	**Trade Names**	*Scabies (Mites)*	*Pediculosis (Lice)*	**Dosage Forms**	**Adverse Effects**
Lindane	Kwell G-well Scabene	√	√	Cream: 1% Lotion: 1% Shampoo: 1%	Occasional: rash, conjunctivitis Rare: convulsions, aplastic anemia
Crotamiton	Eurax	√		Cream: 10% Lotion: 10%	Occasional: rash, conjunctivitis
Permethrin	Nix Elimite	√	√	Liquid: 1% Cream: 5%	Occasional: burning, stinging, itching, numbness, pain, rash, erythema, edema
Pyrethrins plus piperonyl butoxide	A-200 R&C Others		√	Gel Liquid Shampoo	Occasional: irritation to eyes and mucous membranes following inadvertent contact
Malathion	Ovide		√	Lotion: 0.5%	Occasional: local irritation

Table 89–1. Ectoparasiticides: Trade Names, Indications, Dosage Forms, and Adverse Effects

ing seizure disorders. If a seizure develops, it can be controlled with an IV barbiturate (e.g., phenobarbital) or IV diazepam.

Preparations and Administration

Preparations. Lindane [Kwell, Scabene, G-well] is dispensed as a lotion, cream, and shampoo. The concentration of lindane in all formulations is 1%.

Administration. *Scabies.* To treat scabies, a thin layer of cream or lotion is applied to the entire body below the head. No more than 30 gm (1 oz) should be used. The drug is removed by washing 8 to 12 hours later. As a rule, only one application is required. Pruritus may persist because of residual insect products. This itching does not indicate a need for additional treatment.

Head Lice. To kill head lice and their nits, lindane shampoo (30 to 60 gm) should be worked into *dry* hair and left in place for 4 minutes. After this, the shampoo should be rinsed off with warm water. Dead nits can be removed with a comb or tweezers. Lindane *cream* can be employed to treat head lice, but this formulation is less convenient than the shampoo.

Pubic Lice. The affected region should receive the same treatment employed for the removal of head lice. Shampoo is preferred to lotion. Although one treatment is usually sufficient, a second application in 7 days may be required. Sexual partners should be treated simultaneously. Lindane should not be used to treat infestation of the eyelashes by the pubic louse. For this condition, petrolatum ophthalmic ointment is employed.

Body Lice. Body lice can be killed by applying a thin layer of lindane ointment or cream to the affected areas. The drug should be washed off 8 to 12 hours after application.

PERMETHRIN

Basic Pharmacology

Actions and Uses. Permethrin is toxic to mites, lice, and their ova. The drug kills adult insects by disrupting nerve traffic, thereby causing paralysis. In addition to killing mites and lice, permethrin is active against fleas and ticks. The 1% formulation is a drug of choice for head lice. The new 5% for-

mulation has replaced lindane as the drug of choice for scabies. As a rule, only one application is required.

Pharmacokinetics. Very little (about 2%) of topically applied permethrin is absorbed. The fraction absorbed is rapidly inactivated and excreted in the urine.

Adverse Effects. Topical permethrin is devoid of serious adverse effects. The drug may cause some exacerbation of the itching, erythema, and edema normally associated with pediculosis. Other reactions include temporary sensations of burning, stinging, and numbness.

Preparations and Administration

Preparations. Permethrin is dispensed in two concentrations: (1) a 1% liquid [Nix] used for lice, and (2) a 5% cream [Elimite] used for scabies.

Administration. *Head Lice.* Before applying permethrin (1% liquid) to remove head lice, the hair should be washed, rinsed, and towel dried. Permethrin is then applied in an amount sufficient to saturate the hair and scalp. After 10 minutes, permethrin should be removed with a warm-water rinse. If needed, retreatment can be performed in 7 days. However, reapplication is required in less than 1% of cases.

Scabies. The 5% cream [Elimite] is massaged into the skin, from the head to the soles of the feet. After 8 to 14 hours, the cream is removed by washing. Thirty grams is sufficient for the average adult. Only one application is needed.

MALATHION

Actions and Uses. Malathion is an organophosphate cholinesterase inhibitor (see Chapter 16). The drug kills lice and their ova. Humans and other mammals are not harmed because an enzyme in their blood converts malathion to nontoxic metabolites. The drug is approved for treatment of head lice. It is also used widely as an insecticide.

Adverse Effects and Interactions. The preparation used topically for head lice is devoid of significant adverse effects. Scalp irritation occurs occasionally. No systemic toxicity has been reported. Likewise, no drug interactions have been reported.

Preparations and Administration. Malathion [Ovide] is dispensed in a 5% lotion. The preparation is applied to dry hair, gently massaged until the scalp is moist, and allowed to dry naturally. (The lotion is flammable because of its 78% alcohol content. Hence, hair dryers and other sources of heat should be avoided until the alcohol has dried.) Eight to 12 hours after application, malathion is washed off with shampoo. Dead lice and ova can then be removed with a fine-tooth comb. Treatment may be repeated in 7 to 9 days if needed.

OTHER ECTOPARASITICIDES

Crotamiton

Crotamiton [Eurax] is used to treat scabies. The drug is not indicated for pediculosis. This agent has scabicidal actions and may also relieve itching by an independent mechanism. Mild adverse reactions (dermatitis, conjunctivitis) occur occasionally. Crotamiton is dispensed in cream and lotion formulations.

To treat scabies, crotamiton is massaged into the skin of the entire body, starting with the chin and working down. The head and face are treated only if needed. Special attention should be given to skin folds and creases. Contact with the eyes, mucous membranes, and any regions of inflammation should be avoided. A second application is made 24 hours after the first. A cleansing bath should be taken 48 hours after the second application. If needed, treatment can be repeated in 7 days.

Pyrethrins plus Piperonyl Butoxide

The combination of pyrethrins with piperonyl butoxide is used to remove pubic or head lice. Pyrethrins are the components of this preparation that are toxic to lice. The piperonyl butoxide enhances pyrethrins' action by decreasing the ability of insects to metabolize pyrethrins to inactive products. Pyrethrins undergo little transcutaneous absorption and are one of the safest insecticides available. Principal adverse effects are irritation to the eyes and mucous membranes. Accordingly, contact with these areas should be avoided. Pharmaceutical preparations vary in their content of pyrethrins (0.17% to 0.33%) as well as in their content of piperonyl butoxide (2% to 4%). Treatment consists of applying the preparation (gel, liquid, shampoo) to the infested region, followed later by a warm-water rinse. The procedure should be repeated in a week. Nits are removed by combing.

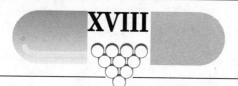

Cancer Chemotherapy

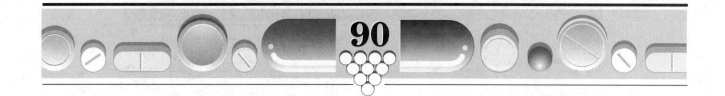
Basic Principles of Cancer Chemotherapy

As mortality from infectious diseases has declined, thanks to the development of antimicrobial drugs, cancer has emerged as a leading cause of death. In the United States the number of deaths from cancer is about 500,000 a year—second only to deaths from heart disease. Among women aged 30 to 74, neoplastic diseases lead all other causes of mortality. Among children aged 1 to 14 years, cancer is the leading nonaccidental cause of death. As shown in Table 90–1, the three most common cancers in women are breast, lung, and colorectal cancers. In men, the most common are prostate, lung, and colorectal cancers.

We have three major modalities for treating cancer: *surgery*, *radiotherapy*, and *chemotherapy* (drug therapy). Surgery and/or irradiation are preferred for most *solid* cancers. Drug therapy is the treatment of choice for *disseminated* cancers (leukemias, disseminated lymphomas, widespread metastases) and a few localized cancers (e.g., choriocarcinoma, testicular carcinoma). Drug therapy also has an important role as an adjunct to surgery and irradiation: by killing malignant cells that surgery and irradiation leave behind, adjuvant chemotherapy can significantly prolong life.

The modern era of cancer chemotherapy dates from 1942, the year in which "nitrogen mustards" were first used to treat cancer. Since the introduction of nitrogen mustards, chemotherapy has made significant advances. Patients with some neoplas-

	Females		Males	
Table 90–1. Cancer Incidence and Deaths in Females and Males				
Type of Cancer	*Incidence*	*Deaths*	*Incidence*	*Deaths*
Breast	32%	18%	–	–
Prostate	–	–	22%	12%
Colorectal	14%	13%	14%	11%
Lung	11%	21%	19%	34%
Uterus	8%	4%	–	–
Leukemias/lymphomas	6%	7%	7%	8%
Urinary tract	4%	3%	10%	5%
Ovary	4%	5%	–	–
Pancreas	3%	5%	3%	4%
Stomach	–	–	3%	3%
Melanoma of skin	3%	2%	3%	2%
Oral	2%	1%	4%	2%
All others	13%	22%	15%	19%

tic diseases now have a good chance of being cured (Table 90–2). Cancers with a high cure rate include Hodgkin's disease, Ewing's sarcoma, and acute lymphocytic leukemia. For many patients whose cancer is not yet curable, chemotherapy can still be of value, offering realistic hopes of palliation and prolongation of useful life. However, although progress in chemotherapy has been encouraging, the ability to cure most cancers with drugs remains elusive. At this time, the major impediment to successful chemotherapy is toxicity of anticancer drugs to normal tissues.

Our principal objectives in this chapter are to examine the major obstacles confronting success in chemotherapy, the strategies being employed to overcome those obstacles, and the major toxicities of the anticancer drugs, along with the steps that can be taken to minimize their harm and discomfort. As preparation for discussing these issues, we will begin the chapter by considering the nature of cancer itself, and the tissue growth fraction and its relationship to cancer chemotherapy.

WHAT IS CANCER?

In the discussion below, we will consider properties shared by neoplastic cells as a group. Although we will be addressing cancers in general, be aware that the term *cancer* refers to a group of disorders and not to a single disease entity. The various forms of cancer differ both in phenotype and aggressiveness. Cancers also differ in responsiveness to drugs.

Characteristics of Neoplastic Cells

Persistent Proliferation. Unlike normal cells, whose proliferation is carefully controlled, cancer cells undergo unrestrained growth and division. This capacity for persistent proliferation is the most distinguishing property of malignant cells. In the absence of intervention, cancerous tissues will continue to grow until they cause death.

It was once believed that cancer cells divided more rapidly than normal cells and that this excessive rate of division was responsible for the abnormal growth patterns of cancerous tissues. We now know that this concept is not correct. Division of neoplastic cells is not necessarily rapid: although some cancers are composed of cells that divide rapidly, others are composed of cells that divide slowly. The correct explanation for the relentless growth of tumors is that *malignant cells are unresponsive to the feedback mechanisms that regulate cellular proliferation in healthy tissue.* Hence, cancer cells are able to continue multiplying under conditions that would suppress further growth and division of normal cells.

Invasive Growth. In the absence of malignancy, the various types of cells that compose a tissue remain segregated from one another; cells of one type do not invade territory that belongs to cells of a different type. In contrast, malignant cells are free of the constraints that inhibit invasive growth. As a result, cells of a solid tumor can penetrate adjacent tissues, thereby allowing the cancer to spread.

Formation of Metastases. Metastases are secondary tumors that appear at sites distant from the primary tumor. Metastases result from the unique ability of malignant cells to break away from their site of origin, migrate to other parts of the body (via the lymphatic and circulatory systems), and then reimplant to form a new tumor.

Etiology of Cancer

The abnormal behavior of cancer cells results from alterations in their DNA. These genetic alterations are caused by chemical carcinogens, viruses, and radiation (x-rays, ultraviolet light, radioiso-

Table 90–2. Some Cancers for Which Drugs May Be Curative	
Type of Cancer	**Drug Therapy**
Hodgkin's disease	Mechlorethamine + vincristine + procarbazine + prednisone
Burkitt's lymphoma	Cyclophosphamide + vincristine + methotrexate + doxorubicin + prednisone
Choriocarcinoma	Methotrexate ± leucovorin
Small cell cancer of lung	Etoposide + cisplatin
Testicular cancer	Cisplatin + etoposide + bleomycin
Wilms' tumor*	Dactinomycin + vincristine
Ewing's sarcoma*	Cyclophosphamide + doxorubicin + vincristine
Acute lymphocytic leukemia	Vincristine + prednisone, followed by methotrexate + 6-mercaptopurine

*Chemotherapy is combined with surgery and/or radiotherapy in these cancers.

topes). Malignant transformation occurs in three major stages, called *initiation, promotion,* and *progression.* These stages suggest that DNA in cancer cells undergoes sequential modification. Evidence gathered in recent years indicates that *oncogenes* (cancer-causing genes) have an important role in malignant transformation. Oncogenes are formed by mutation of proto-oncogenes, which are present in all cells and serve to regulate their function.

THE GROWTH FRACTION AND ITS RELATIONSHIP TO CHEMOTHERAPY

The growth fraction of a tissue is a major determinant of its responsiveness to chemotherapy. Consequently, before we discuss the anticancer drugs, we need to understand the growth fraction. In order to define the growth fraction, we need to review the cell cycle.

The Cell Cycle

The cell cycle is the sequence of events that a cell goes through from one mitotic division to the next. As shown in Figure 90–1, the cell cycle consists of four major phases, named G_1, S, G_2, and M. (The length of the curved arrows in the figure is proportional to the time spent in each phase.) For purposes of discussion, we can imagine the cycle as beginning with G_1, the phase in which the cell prepares to make DNA. Following G_1, the cell enters S phase, the phase in which DNA synthesis actually takes place. Once synthesis of DNA is complete, the cell enters G_2 and prepares for mitosis. Mitosis (cell division) occurs next during M phase. Upon completion of mitosis, the resulting daughter cells have two options: they can enter G_1 and repeat the cycle, or they can enter the phase known as G_0. Cells that enter G_0 become mitotically dormant; these cells do not replicate and are

not considered to be participating in the cell cycle. Cells may remain in G_0 for days, weeks, or even years. Under appropriate conditions, resting cells may leave G_0 and resume active participation in the cycle.

The Growth Fraction

If we were to examine any tissue, we would observe that some cells are going through the cell cycle, whereas others are "resting" in G_0. The ratio of proliferating cells to G_0 cells is called the *growth fraction.* A tissue with a large percentage of proliferating cells and few cells in G_0 would have a *high*

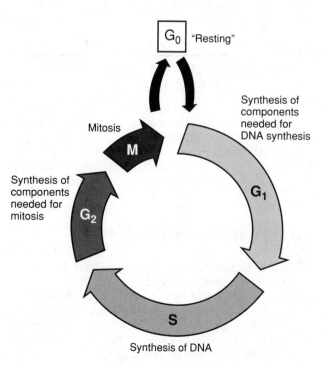

Figure 90–1. The cell cycle.

growth fraction. Conversely, a tissue composed mostly of G_0 cells would have a *low* growth fraction.

Impact of Tissue Growth Fraction on Responsiveness to Anticancer Drugs

As a general rule, *anticancer drugs are much more toxic to tissues that have a high growth fraction than to tissues that have a low growth fraction.* This is because most anticancer agents are more active against proliferating cells than they are against cells in G_0. Proliferating cells are especially sensitive to chemotherapy because anticancer drugs usually act by disrupting DNA synthesis or mitosis—activities that only proliferating cells carry out. Unfortunately, toxicity of anticancer drugs is not restricted to *cancers* that have a high growth fraction: these drugs are also toxic to *normal tissues* whose growth fraction is high (e.g., bone marrow, gastrointestinal epithelium, hair follicles, sperm-forming cells).

Having established the relationship between growth fraction and drug sensitivity, we can apply this knowledge to predict how specific cancers will respond to chemotherapy. As a rule, *solid tumors* have a *low* growth fraction and, therefore, tend to respond *poorly*. In contrast, *disseminated cancers* have a *high* growth fraction and generally respond *well*. In practical terms, this means that the leukemias and lymphomas, which are disseminated forms of cancer, represent the majority of cancers that can be successfully treated with drugs. Conversely, and unfortunately, the most common cancers—solid tumors of the breast, lung, prostate, colon, and rectum—are much less responsive to drugs.

OBSTACLES TO SUCCESSFUL CHEMOTHERAPY

Our objective in this section is to examine the major factors that make success in cancer chemotherapy difficult. Foremost among these factors is the serious and unavoidable toxicity to normal cells caused by currently available anticancer drugs.

TOXICITY TO NORMAL CELLS

Toxicity to normal cells is the biggest barrier to success in chemotherapy. Injury to normal cells occurs primarily in tissues whose growth fraction is high (bone marrow, gastrointestinal epithelium, hair follicles, germinal epithelium of the testes). Drug-induced injury to each of these tissues is discussed in detail later in the chapter. For now we will consider injury to normal cells as a group.

Toxicity to normal cells is dose limiting. That is, drug dosage cannot exceed an amount that produces the maximally tolerated degree of injury to normal cells. Hence, although very large doses of anticancer agents might be able to produce 100% kill of malignant cells, such doses cannot be given because of the very real risk of killing the patient.

Why is it that anticancer drugs are so harmful to normal tissues? These drugs injure normal tissue because they lack *selective toxicity*, a property that can be defined as *the ability to kill one kind of cell* (target cell) *without killing other cells with which the target cell is in intimate contact.* We first encountered this concept in Chapter 73 (Basic Considerations in the Chemotherapy of Infectious Diseases). In that chapter we noted that the great success that has been achieved in antimicrobial therapy has been possible because antimicrobial drugs are highly selective in their toxicity. Penicillin, for example, can readily kill infectious bacteria while being virtually harmless to cells of the host. This high degree of selective toxicity stands in sharp contrast to the lack of selectivity displayed by most anticancer drugs.

Why have we been unable to develop drugs that are selectively toxic to neoplastic cells? Achieving selective toxicity has been elusive because normal cells and malignant cells are very much alike. Production of a selectively toxic drug requires that the target cell have some biochemical feature that normal cells lack. By way of illustration, let's consider how penicillin achieves its selectively toxic effects. Penicillin kills bacteria by disrupting the bacterial cell wall. Since our cells have no cell wall, penicillin can't hurt us. Our current understanding of cancer cells offers no such basis for creating selectively toxic anticancer drugs: we have yet to identify a unique biochemical characteristic of cancer cells that would render them vulnerable to selective attack with chemotherapeutic agents. Thus, until means of selective attack are discovered, we will be unable to kill or injure malignant cells without causing harm to many noncancer cells as well.

CURE REQUIRES 100% CELL KILL

To cure a patient of cancer we must eliminate virtually every malignant cell from the body; just one remaining cell can proliferate and cause relapse. For most patients, 100% cell kill cannot be achieved. Factors that make it difficult to produce complete cell kill include (1) the kinetics of drug-induced cell kill, (2) minimal participation of the immune system in eliminating malignant cells, and (3) disappearance of symptoms before all cancer cells are gone.

Kinetics of Drug-Induced Cell Kill. Killing of cancer cells follows *first-order kinetics*. That is, at any given dose, a drug will kill a *constant percent-*

age of malignant cells, *regardless of how many cells are actually present.* This means that the dose required to shrink a cancer from 10^3 cells down to 10 cells will be just as big, for example, as the dose required to reduce that cancer from 10^9 cells down to 10^7 cells. Hence, with each successive round of chemotherapy, drug dosage must remain the same, even though the cancer is getting progressively smaller. This means that if treatment is to continue, the patient must be able to tolerate the same degree of toxicity late in therapy as he or she could when therapy began. For many patients, this is not possible.

Nonparticipation of Host Defenses in Cell Kill. In contrast to the antimicrobial drugs, anticancer agents receive very little help from host defenses. Accordingly, anticancer agents must produce cell kill almost entirely on their own. There are two reasons why host defenses contribute so little. First, because of their immunosuppressant actions, anticancer drugs seriously compromise immune function. Second, because malignant cells are so much like normal cells, the immune system generally fails to identify cancer cells as appropriate for attack.

When Should Treatment Stop? We have no way of knowing when 100% cell kill has been achieved. As a result, there is no definitive method for deciding just when chemotherapy should stop. As indicated in Figure 90–2, symptoms disappear long before the last malignant cell has been eliminated. Once a cancer has been reduced to less than 1 million cells, it becomes virtually undetectable; all signs of disease are absent, and the patient is considered to be in complete remission. It is obvious, however, that a patient harboring a million malignant cells is by no means cured. It is also obvious that further chemotherapy is indicated. However, what is not so obvious is just how long therapy should last: since the patient is already asymptomatic, we have no objective means of determining when to discontinue drug use. The clinical dilemma is this: if therapy is continued too long, the patient will be needlessly exposed to serious toxicity; conversely, if drugs are withdrawn prematurely, relapse will take place.

FAILURE OF EARLY DETECTION

Early detection of cancer is rare. At this time, cancer of the cervix, which can be diagnosed with a Pap smear, is the only neoplastic disease capable of truly early detection. All other forms of cancer are significantly advanced by the time they have grown large enough for discovery. The smallest detectable cancers are about 1 cm in diameter, have a mass of 1 gm, and consist of about one billion cells (see Fig. 90–2). Detection at this stage cannot be considered early.

Late detection has three important consequences. First, by the time the primary tumor is discovered, metastases may have formed. Second, the tumor will be less responsive to drugs than it would have been at an earlier stage (see below). Third, since cancer has been present for a long time, the patient may be debilitated by the disease, and therefore less able to tolerate treatment.

SOLID TUMORS RESPOND POORLY

As noted earlier, solid tumors have a low growth fraction (high percentage of G_0 cells) and are generally unresponsive to chemotherapy. There are two reasons for this low responsiveness. First, G_0 cells do not perform the activities that most anticancer drugs are designed to disrupt. Second, because G_0 cells are not active participants in the cell cycle, they have time to repair drug-induced damage before that damage can do them serious harm.

Not all solid tumors are equally unresponsive: as a rule, *large tumors are even less responsive than small tumors.* This difference occurs because as solid tumors increase in size, many of their cells leave the cell cycle and enter G_0, causing the growth fraction to decline. Tumor growth slows, in large part, because blood flow in the tumor core is low, depriving cells of nutrients and oxygen. The decrease in growth fraction in older tumors is a major reason that therapeutic success is more likely when cancers are detected early. Because the rate of growth declines as a tumor gets larger, the tumor growth curve is said to follow *Gompertzian kinetics* (see Fig. 90–2).

The drug sensitivity of a solid tumor can be enhanced by *debulking*. When a solid tumor is reduced in size by surgery or irradiation, many of the remaining cells leave G_0 and re-enter the cell cycle, thereby increasing their sensitivity to chemotherapy. This phenomenon is known as *recruitment*. It is because of recruitment that chemotherapy can be very useful as an adjunct to surgery or irradiation even though drugs may have been largely ineffective before debulking was done.

DRUG RESISTANCE

During the course of chemotherapy, cancer cells can develop resistance to the drugs used against them. Drug resistance can be a significant cause of therapeutic failure. Mechanisms of resistance include reduced drug uptake, increased drug efflux, reduced drug activation, reduced target molecule sensitivity to a drug, and increased repair of drug-induced damage to DNA.

Cellular production of a drug transport molecule, known as *P-glycoprotein*, can confer *multiple drug resistance* upon cells. P-glycoprotein is a large molecule that spans the cytoplasmic membrane

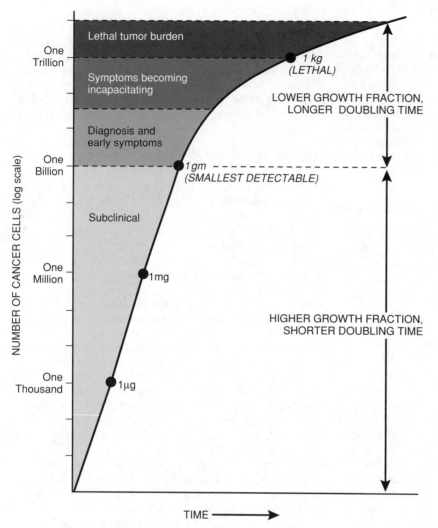

Figure 90–2. Gompertzian tumor growth curve showing the relationship between tumor size and clinical status.

and serves to pump drugs out of the cell. Induction of P-glycoprotein synthesis following exposure to a single anticancer drug produces cross-resistance to many structurally unrelated agents. Several drugs, including calcium channel blockers, have been used investigationally to inhibit the P-glycoprotein pump and reverse multiple drug resistance.

Drug resistance usually results from a change in DNA. Mutation to a drug-resistant form is a spontaneous event and is not caused by the anticancer drugs themselves. However, although drugs do not *cause* the mutations that render cells resistant, drugs do *create selection pressure* favoring the drug-resistant mutants. That is, by killing drug-sensitive cells, anticancer agents create a competition-free environment in which drug-resistant mutants can flourish.

Since the presence of anticancer agents favors the growth of drug-resistant cells, as therapy proceeds, the number of resistant cells will increase. Because resistant cells cannot be killed with drugs, the risk of therapeutic failure becomes greater with each course of therapy. Since patients are usually exposed to drugs over an extended time, therapeutic failure owing to drug resistance is a significant problem.

HETEROGENEITY OF TUMOR CELLS

Tumors do not consist of a single population of identical cells. Rather, because of ongoing mutation, tumors are composed of subpopulations of dissimilar cells. These subpopulations can differ in morphology, growth rate, and metastatic ability. More importantly from our perspective, they can differ in responsiveness to drugs (primarily because of increased resistance). As a tumor ages, cellular heterogeneity increases.

LIMITED DRUG ACCESS TO TUMOR CELLS

Because of a tumor's location or blood supply, drugs may have limited access to its cells. Large solid tumors have poor vascularization, especially toward the core. Hence, cells within these tumors are difficult to reach with drugs. Similarly, tumors of the central nervous system (CNS) are difficult to reach because most anticancer drugs have difficulty crossing the blood-brain barrier.

STRATEGIES FOR ACHIEVING MAXIMUM BENEFITS FROM CHEMOTHERAPY

INTERMITTENT CHEMOTHERAPY

The goal of chemotherapy is to produce 100% kill of neoplastic cells while causing limited injury to normal tissues (especially the bone marrow and gastrointestinal epithelium). Intermittent therapy is the primary technique for achieving this goal. When anticancer drugs are administered on an intermittent schedule, normal cells are given the opportunity to repopulate between rounds of therapy. However, for this approach to succeed, one obvious requirement must be met: *normal cells must repopulate faster than the malignant cells*. If the malignant cells grow back faster than normal cells, there can be no reduction in tumor burden between rounds of treatment. The successful use of intermittent therapy is depicted in Figure 90–3.

COMBINATION CHEMOTHERAPY

Chemotherapy employing a combination of drugs is generally much more effective than therapy with just one drug. Accordingly, most patients are now treated with two or more agents.

Benefits of Drug Combinations

Combination chemotherapy offers three major advantages: (1) suppression of drug resistance, (2) increased cancer cell kill, and (3) reduced injury to normal cells (at any given level of anticancer effect).

Suppression of Drug Resistance. Drug resistance occurs less frequently with multiple-drug therapy than with single-drug therapy. To understand why, we need to recall that resistance is acquired through random mutational events. The probability of a cell undergoing two or more mutations, and therefore developing resistance to a combination of drugs, is smaller than the probability of a cell undergoing the single mutation needed to develop resistance to one drug. Because drug resistance is reduced with combination chemotherapy, the chances of therapeutic success are increased.

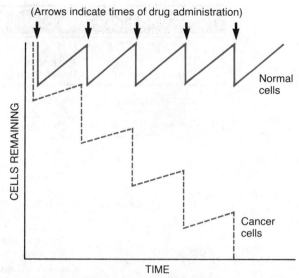

(Arrows indicate times of drug administration)

Figure 90–3. Recovery of critical normal cells during intermittent chemotherapy. Cancer cells and normal cells (e.g., cells of the bone marrow) are killed with each drug administration. In the intervals between doses, both types of cells proliferate. Since, in this example, normal cells repopulate faster than cancer cells, normal cells are able to recover entirely between doses, whereas regrowth of the cancer cells is only partial. Hence, with each succeeding round of treatment, the total number of cancer cells becomes smaller, whereas the number of normal cells remains within a tolerable range. Note that differential loss of malignant cells is possible only if these cells repopulate more slowly than normal cells. If cancer cells grow back as fast as normal cells, intermittent chemotherapy will fail.

Increased Cancer Cell Kill. If we administer several anticancer drugs, each with a different mechanism of action, we will kill more malignant cells than if we use only one drug. Therapeutic effects are enhanced because the combination attacks the cancer in several ways instead of just one. Greater cell kill is especially likely if a drug-resistant subpopulation of cells is present. The superiority of drug combinations over single-drug therapy is illustrated by the data in Table 90–3.

Reduced Injury to Normal Cells. By using a combination of drugs *that do not have overlapping toxicities*, we can achieve a greater anticancer effect than we could *safely* achieve using any of the agents alone. Why this is so is illustrated by the data in Table 90–4. This table summarizes responses to two drugs—vincristine and cyclophosphamide—when given individually and in combination. Both drugs kill malignant cells, but they act by different mechanisms: cyclophosphamide damages DNA, whereas vincristine blocks mitosis. Furthermore, these drugs have different toxicities: cyclophosphamide causes *neutropenia*, whereas vincristine is *neurotoxic*. In the table, the intensity of effects is indicated by plus (+) symbols; the more plusses, the more intense the response. With either drug, 2+ represents the maximum degree of toxicity that can be tolerated. When adminis-

Table 90–3. Single-Drug Treatment versus Combination Chemotherapy

Type of Cancer	Method of Treatment and Drugs Employed	Percent of Patients with Complete Remission
Acute lymphocytic leukemia of childhood	**Single-Drug Therapy**	
	Daunorubicin	38
	Prednisone	63
	Vincristine	57
	Combination Chemotherapy	
	Prednisone + vincristine	90
	Prednisone + vincristine + daunorubicin	97
Hodgkin's disease	**Single-Drug Therapy**	
	Vincristine	<10
	Prednisone	<5
	Procarbazine	<10
	Mechlorethamine	20
	Combination Chemotherapy	
	Vincristine + prednisone + mechlorethamine + procarbazine	81

Data from DeVita, V. T., Young, R. C., and Canellos, G. P. Combination versus single agent chemotherapy: A review of the basis for selection of drug treatment of cancer. Cancer 35:98, 1975.

tered alone in doses that produce 2+ toxicity, each drug produces an anticancer effect of 2+ intensity; this is the greatest therapeutic effect that we can safely achieve with either drug by itself. Now let's consider the effect of combining these drugs, giving each in its maximally tolerated dose. The total anticancer effect of the combination is 4+, twice the effect that could be achieved safely with either agent alone. Since the toxicities of these agents do not overlap, overall toxicity of the combination remains at a tolerable level—although the patient is now exposed to two kinds of toxicity rather than one.

Guidelines for Drug Selection

From the preceding discussion, we can extract three guidelines for selecting drugs for use in combination: (1) each drug should be effective by itself, (2) each drug should have a different mechanism of action, and (3) the drugs should have minimally overlapping toxicities.

OPTIMIZATION OF DOSING SCHEDULES

The schedule by which an anticancer drug is administered is an important determinant of the outcome of treatment. The experiment summarized in Table 90–5 provides a dramatic illustration of this point. In the experiment, two groups of mice were inoculated with cancer cells and then treated with cytarabine. Mice in group I received *a single large dose* of cytarabine on days 2, 6, 10, and 14 after being inoculated with cancer cells. The group II mice were treated on the same days as the group I mice but, rather than receiving one large dose of cytarabine, they were given *8 small doses*, one every 3 hours. By the end of the study, all of the group II mice were cured. In stark contrast, all of the group I mice were dead. Since the two groups had the same disease and were given the same drug, we must conclude that the life and death difference in outcome was due to the dosing schedules employed.

Table 90–4. Responses to Cyclophosphamide and Vincristine Alone and in Combination

Therapeutic Regimen	Anticancer Effect	Toxicity	
		Neutropenia	*Neurotoxicity*
Cyclophosphamide	+ +	+ +	"0"
Vincristine	+ +	"0"	+ +
Cyclophosphamide + vincristine	+ + + +	+ +	+ +

Table 90–5. Effect of Dosing Schedule on Therapeutic Response			
Experimental Group	Dosage Size	Dosing Schedule	Mice Surviving
I	240 mg/kg	1 dose/day*	None
II	15 mg/kg	8 doses/day*	100%

*Cytarabine was administered on days 2, 6, 10, and 14 after mice were inoculated with leukemia cells. See text for further details.

To understand these results, we need to know two properties of cytarabine: (1) the drug kills cells by disrupting DNA synthesis, and (2) it undergoes rapid inactivation. Since cytarabine acts by disrupting DNA synthesis, it can only affect cells while they are in the S phase of the cell cycle. Since the drug is rapidly inactivated, and since many cells will not be in S phase during the short time before inactivation occurs, many cells will escape injury following each dose. The group I mice died because administration of just one large dose every 4 days did not maintain active drug in the body for a time sufficient to catch all of the cancer cells as they cycled through S phase. Since the group II mice received multiple doses over a 24-hour period on each of 4 days, the presence of active drug was sustained. Hence, the chance of cancer cells being in S phase while active drug was present was greatly increased, thereby leading to enhanced cell kill with resultant cure.

The message from this experiment is that selection of the right drugs for cancer therapy is only one of the requirements for success; those drugs must also be administered according to schedules that will maximize their effects. Dosing schedules are especially critical for drugs that, like cytarabine, act during a specific phase of the cell cycle.

REGIONAL DRUG DELIVERY

By using special techniques for drug delivery, we can increase drug access to tumors, thereby increasing cell kill and reducing systemic toxicity.

Intra-arterial Delivery. Local intra-arterial infusion can be used to treat solid tumors. This technique has the advantage of establishing a high concentration of drug in the vicinity of the tumor while minimizing toxicity to the rest of the body. Specific routes include carotid artery delivery (for brain tumors) and hepatic artery delivery (for liver metastases). Clearly, intra-arterial therapy is suitable only for localized cancers.

Intrathecal Delivery. As noted previously, many anticancer agents are unable to cross the blood-brain barrier and, therefore, cannot reach malignant cells within the CNS. To enhance ther-

apy of CNS cancers, drugs can be administered intrathecally (by injection directly into the subarachnoid space). This technique bypasses the blood-brain barrier, thereby giving drugs better access to cells within the CNS.

Other Specialized Routes. Anticancer agents can be administered via the portal vein to treat liver metastases, and directly into the bladder to treat bladder cancer. Neoplasms located in the pleural and peritoneal cavities can be treated by direct intracavitary drug administration.

MAJOR TOXICITIES OF ANTICANCER DRUGS AND THEIR MANAGEMENT

As a group, the anticancer drugs are our most toxic medicines. Serious injury occurs most to tissues that have a high growth fraction (bone marrow, gastrointestinal epithelium, hair follicles, and sperm-forming cells). In the discussion below, we will consider the more common toxicities of the anticancer drugs along with steps that can be taken to minimize harm and discomfort.

BONE MARROW SUPPRESSION

Anticancer drugs are highly toxic to the bone marrow, a tissue with a high proportion of proliferating cells. Myelosuppression reduces the number of circulating neutrophils, thrombocytes, and erythrocytes. Loss of these cells has three major consequences: (1) infection (from loss neutrophils), (2) bleeding (from loss of thrombocytes), and (3) anemia (from loss of erythrocytes).

Neutropenia

Neutrophils (neutrophilic granulocytes) are white blood cells that play an essential role in fighting infection. In patients with neutropenia (a reduction in circulating neutrophils), both the incidence and severity of infection are increased. Infections that are normally benign (e.g., candidiasis) can become life-threatening. There is no question that infection secondary to neutropenia is the most serious complication of cancer chemotherapy. The grim reality of this problem cannot be stressed too much.

With most anticancer drugs, onset of neutropenia is *rapid* and recovery develops relatively *quickly*. Neutropenia begins to develop a few days after drug administration, and the lowest neutrophil count, called the *nadir*, occurs between days 10 and 14. Neutrophil counts then recover in 3 to 4 weeks. Patients are at highest risk during the nadir, and special care should be taken to avoid contagion during this time.

With some anticancer drugs, neutropenia is *delayed*. Neutrophil counts begin to fall in 1 to 2 weeks, and reach their nadir between weeks 3 and 4. Full recovery may not occur until after week 7.

Monitoring of neutrophil counts is essential. Normal counts range from 2500 to 7000/mm³. If neutropenia is substantial (absolute neutrophil count below 500/mm³), the next round of chemotherapy should be delayed until neutrophil counts return toward normal.

Lack of neutrophils confounds the diagnosis of infection. This is because the usual signs of infection (e.g., pus, abscesses, infiltrates on the chest x-ray) depend on having neutrophils present. In the absence of neutrophils, *fever* is the principal early sign of infection.

Patients must be their own first line of defense against infection. They should be made aware of the serious risk they face and should be taught how to minimize contagion. They should be informed that fever may be the only indication of infection and instructed to notify the physician immediately if fever develops. Since infection is commonly acquired through contact with other people, hospitalized patients should be instructed to refuse direct contact with anyone who has not washed his or her hands in the patient's presence. This rule applies not only to visiting friends and relatives but also to nurses, physicians, and all other hospital staff. The normal flora of the body are a major source of infection; the risk of acquiring an infection with these microbes can be reduced by daily examination and cleansing of the skin and oral cavity.

Hospitalization of the infection-free neutropenic patient is controversial. Some physicians feel that hospitalization will *increase* the risk of acquiring a serious infection. This is because hospitals harbor drug-resistant microbes, which can make hospital-acquired (nosocomial) infections especially difficult to treat. Accordingly, these physicians recommend that neutropenic patients stay at home as long as they remain infection-free.

If neutropenic patients *are* hospitalized, every precaution must be taken to prevent them from acquiring a nosocomial infection. They should be given an isolation room and monitored frequently for fever. Certain foods (e.g., salads) abound in pathogenic bacteria and must be avoided.

When a neutropenic patient develops an infection, immediate and vigorous intervention is required. Specimens for culture should be taken to identify the infecting organism and determine its drug sensitivity. While awaiting reports on the cultures, empiric therapy with intravenous antibiotics should be instituted. The drugs selected should cover all likely pathogens.

In recent years, *colony-stimulating factors* have been employed to minimize neutropenia. Two preparations are available: *granulocyte colony-stimulating factor* (G-CSF, filgrastim) and *granulocyte-monocyte colony-stimulating factor* (GM-CSF, sargramostim). Both drugs act on the bone marrow to enhance granulocyte (neutrophil) production. Colony-stimulating factors can decrease the incidence, magnitude, and duration of neutropenia. As a result, they can decrease the incidence and severity of infection as well as the need for IV antibiotics and hospitalization. The basic pharmacology of G-CSF and GM-CSF is discussed in Chapter 48 (Hematopoietic Growth Factors).

Thrombocytopenia

Bone marrow suppression can cause thrombocytopenia (a reduction in circulating platelets), thereby increasing the risk of serious bleeding. Bleeding from the nose and gums is relatively common. Bleeding from the gums can be reduced by avoiding vigorous tooth brushing. Drugs that promote bleeding (e.g., aspirin, anticoagulants) should not be used. When a mild analgesic is required, acetaminophen, which does not promote bleeding, is preferred to aspirin. For patients with severe thrombocytopenia, platelet infusion is the mainstay of treatment.

Caution should be exercised when performing procedures that might promote bleeding. Intravenous needles should be inserted with special care. Intramuscular injections should be avoided if possible. Blood pressure cuffs should be applied cautiously, since overinflation may cause bruising or bleeding.

Anemia

Anemia is defined as a reduction in the number of circulating erythrocytes (red blood cells). Although anticancer drugs can suppress erythrocyte production, anemia is much less common than neutropenia or thrombocytopenia. This is because circulating erythrocytes have a long life span (120 days), which usually allows erythrocyte production to recover before levels of existing erythrocytes decline.

DIGESTIVE TRACT INJURY

The epithelial lining of the gastrointestinal tract has a very high growth fraction, and, therefore, is exquisitely sensitive to cytotoxic drugs. Stomatitis and diarrhea are common. Severe gastrointestinal injury can be life-threatening.

Stomatitis. Stomatitis (inflammation of the oral mucosa) often develops a few days after the onset of chemotherapy and may persist for 2 or more weeks after treatment has ceased. Inflammation can progress to denudation and ulceration. Pain can be severe, inhibiting eating, speaking, and swallowing. Management measures include good oral hygiene and a bland diet. A combination of topical anesthetics and systemic analgesics may be required to relieve pain. Topical antifungal drugs may be needed to control infection with *Candida albicans*. Severe stomatitis may necessitate interrupting chemotherapy.

Diarrhea. By injuring the epithelial lining of the intestine, anticancer drugs can impair absorption of fluids and other nutrients, thereby causing diarrhea. Diarrhea can be reduced with a diet high in fiber (which gives the stool a more firm consistency) and by consumption of constipating foods (e.g., cheeses).

NAUSEA AND VOMITING

Nausea and vomiting are common sequelae of cancer chemotherapy. These responses, which result in part from stimulation of the chemoreceptor trigger zone, can be both immediate and dramatic, and may persist for hours. In some cases, discomfort is so great as to prompt refusal of further treatment.

It is important to appreciate that the nausea and vomiting associated with anticancer drugs are typically much more severe than with most other medicines. Hence, whereas these reactions are generally unremarkable with most drugs, they must be considered major and characteristic side effects of cancer chemotherapy.

Nausea and vomiting can be reduced by premedication with antiemetics. These drugs offer three benefits: (1) reduction of anticipatory nausea and vomiting, (2) prevention of dehydration and malnutrition secondary to frequent nausea and vomiting, and (3) promotion of compliance with anticancer therapy by reducing discomfort. Of the antiemetics in use, *ondansetron* [Zofran] is unusually effective. Other antiemetics employed during chemotherapy include *metoclopramide* [Reglan], *prochlorperazine*, *methylprednisolone*, *dexamethasone*, and *lorazepam* [Ativan]. In addition, two cannabinoids (marijuana-like drugs) are available: *dronabinol* [Marinol] and *nabilone* [Cesamet]. Combinations of antiemetics may be more effective than single-drug therapy. The basic pharmacology of the antiemetics is discussed in Chapter 68.

OTHER IMPORTANT TOXICITIES

Alopecia. Alopecia (hair loss) results from injury to hair follicles. Reversible alopecia can occur with nearly all anticancer drugs. While alopecia is not dangerous, it is nonetheless very upsetting. If treatment is expected to cause hair loss, the patient should be forewarned. For patients who wish to wear a wig, it is recommended that the wig be selected before hair loss occurs.

Reproductive Toxicity. The developing fetus and the germinal epithelium of the testes have high growth fractions. As a result, both are highly susceptible to injury by anticancer drugs. These drugs can interfere with embryogenesis, causing death of the early embryo. They may also cause fetal malformation. Accordingly, women undergoing chemotherapy should be warned against becoming pregnant. If pregnancy occurs, the possibility of terminating the pregnancy should be discussed. Drug effects on the ovaries may result in amenorrhea, menopausal symptoms, and atrophy of the vaginal epithelium. Anticancer drugs can cause irreversible sterility in males. Men should be forewarned of this effect and counseled about sperm banking.

Hyperuricemia. Hyperuricemia is defined as an excessive level of uric acid in the blood. Uric acid, a compound with low solubility, is formed by the breakdown of DNA following cell death. Hyperuricemia is especially common following treatment for leukemias and lymphomas, since therapy results in massive cell kill. The major concern with hyperuricemia is injury to the kidneys secondary to deposition of uric acid crystals in renal tubules. The risk of crystal formation can be reduced by increasing fluid intake. If necessary, uric acid levels can be lowered with *allopurinol*, a drug that suppresses uric acid formation. The basic pharmacology of allopurinol is discussed in Chapter 63.

Local Injury from Extravasation of Vesicants. Certain anticancer drugs, known as *vesicants*, are highly chemically reactive. These drugs can cause severe local injury if they make direct contact with tissues. Vesicants are administered intravenously, since dilution in venous blood decreases the risk of injury. Administration is usually by injection (IV push) through a sidearm in a freely flowing IV line. Sites of previous irradiation should be avoided. Extreme care must be exercised to prevent extravasation, since leakage can produce high local concentrations, resulting in prolonged pain, infection, and loss of mobility. Severe injury can lead to necrosis and sloughing, requiring surgical debridement and skin grafting. If extravasation occurs, the infusion should be stopped immediately. Vesicants should be administered only by clinicians specially trained in their safe handling and use.

Unique Toxicities. In addition to the toxicities discussed above, most of which apply to the anticancer drugs as a group, some agents produce unique toxicities. Daunorubicin, for example, can cause serious harm to the heart, whereas vincristine can injure peripheral nerves. Special toxicities of individual drugs are considered in Chapter 91.

Carcinogenesis. Along with their other adverse actions, anticancer drugs have one final and ironic toxicity: these drugs, which are used to *treat* cancer, have *caused* cancer in some patients. Cancer results from drug-induced damage to DNA. Cancers caused by anticancer drugs may take many years to appear.

MAKING THE DECISION TO TREAT

From the preceding discussion of toxicities, it is clear that anticancer drugs can cause great harm. Given the known dangers of these drugs, we must ask ourselves why such toxic substances are administered to sick people at all. The answer to this question lies with the primary dictum of therapeutics, which states that the benefits of therapy must outweigh the risks. For most patients undergoing chemotherapy, the conditions of this rule are met. That is, although the toxicities of the anticancer drugs can be very bad, the potential benefits (cure, prolonged life, palliation) justify the risks. However, the desirability of treating cancer with drugs is not always obvious. There are patients whose chances of being helped by chemotherapy may be very remote, while their chances of experiencing serious injury remain ever present. Since the potential benefits for some patients are small and the risks are large, the decision to institute chemotherapy must be made with careful deliberation.

Before the decision to treat can be made, the patient must be given some idea of the probable benefits that the proposed therapy has to offer. There are three basic benefits that chemotherapy can provide: cure, palliation, and prolongation of useful life. For treatment to be justified, there should be reason to believe that at least one of these benefits will be forthcoming. If a patient cannot be offered some reasonable hope of cure, palliation, or prolongation of useful life, it would be difficult to justify treatment.

The most important factors for predicting the outcome of chemotherapy are (1) the general health status of the patient, and (2) the responsiveness of the particular cancer the patient has. General health status can be assessed with the Karnofsky Performance Scale (Table 90–6). A Karnofsky rating of less than 40 indicates that the patient is very debilitated and not likely to tolerate the additional stress of chemotherapy. Patients with a low Karnofsky rating should receive anticancer drugs only if the type of cancer they have is known to be especially responsive.

The responsiveness of some common cancers is indicated in Table 90–7. Patients with highly responsive types of cancer should almost always be treated, regardless of their Karnofsky rating. In contrast, patients with minimally responsive types of cancer should be treated only after careful consideration. It may well be that such patients are better off limiting their problems to the cancer itself, without adding the dangers and discomforts of a course of treatment that has little to offer.

An important requirement for deciding in favor of chemotherapy is that the impact of treatment be measurable. That is, there must be some objective

Table 90–6. Karnofsky Performance Scale		
Definition	**Percentage**	**Criteria**
Able to carry on normal activity and work; no special care needed	100	Normal; no complaints; no evidence of disease
	90	Able to carry on normal activity; minor signs or symptoms of disease
	80	Normal activity with effort; some signs or symptoms of disease
Unable to work; able to live at home and care for most personal needs; a varying amount of assistance needed	70	Cares for self; unable to carry on normal activity or do active work
	60	Requires occasional assistance; able to care for most needs
	50	Requires considerable assistance and frequent medical care
Unable to care for self; requires equivalent of institutional or hospital care; disease may be progressing rapidly	40	Disabled; requires special care and assistance
	30	Severely disabled; hospitalization is indicated although death not imminent
	20	Very sick, hospitalization necessary; active supportive treatment necessary
	10	Moribund; fatal processes progressing rapidly
	0	Dead

Table 90–7. Responsiveness of Some Cancers to Chemotherapy		
Responsiveness to Chemotherapy	Type of Cancer	Probable Benefits of Chemotherapy
High	Hodgkin's disease Burkitt's lymphoma Acute lymphocytic leukemia Choriocarcinoma Wilms' tumor Ewing's sarcoma	Cure or substantial prolongation of life
Moderate	Breast cancer Cervical carcinoma Chronic lymphocytic leukemia Bladder cancer Multiple myeloma Prostate carcinoma	Prolongation of life; palliation
Minimal	Colorectal cancer Hepatocellular carcinoma Melanoma Pancreatic cancer Renal cancer Osteogenic sarcoma	Palliation; minimal prolongation of life

means of determining the cancer's response to therapy. For solid tumors, we should be able to measure a decrease in tumor size. For hematologic cancers, we should be able to measure a decrease in the number of circulating neoplastic cells. If we have no way to measure the response of a cancer, then we have no way of knowing if treatment has done any good. If we cannot determine that drugs are doing something beneficial, there is little justification for giving them.

Clearly, not all patients are candidates for chemotherapy. The decision to institute treatment must be made on an individual basis. Patients should be informed as accurately as possible about the potential risks and benefits of the therapy under consideration. When the decision to treat is made, it should be the result of collaboration between the patient, family, and physician, and should reflect a conviction on the part of the patient that within his or her set of values the potential benefits outweigh the inherent risks.

LOOKING AHEAD

Does the future offer hope of developing chemotherapeutic cures for all forms of cancer? This question can be cautiously answered in the affirmative. There is no theoretical reason to believe that cancers are inherently incapable of cure. On the contrary, there is good reason to believe that cancers are in fact curable diseases. We have discussed the issue of selective toxicity and concluded that the absence of selectively toxic anticancer drugs constitutes the primary obstacle to truly curative therapy. We currently lack selectively toxic drugs because we have yet to identify biochemical characteristics of cancer cells that would render them vulnerable to selective attack. However, although we have yet to discover a chink in cancer's biochemical armor, it is not unreasonable to think that one nonetheless exists. Cancer cells are, after all, different from normal cells. This difference, manifested as unrestrained growth, must have a biochemical basis. That biochemical basis, when it is finally understood, may well provide the basis for making chemotherapeutic agents that are truly selective in their toxicity—drugs that are as selective for cancer cells as, for example, penicillin G is for gram-positive bacteria. Drugs with this degree of selectivity will offer a cure for neoplastic diseases. It is not completely naive to believe that such drugs will be developed.

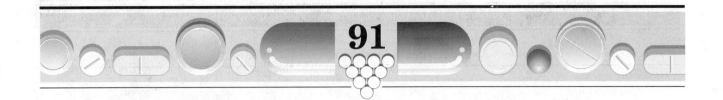

91

Representative Anticancer Drugs

The family of anticancer drugs is large and diverse. We will not attempt to consider all of these agents in detail. Rather, discussion will focus primarily on selected representative drugs. Basic principles of cancer chemotherapy are considered in Chapter 90.

INTRODUCTION TO THE ANTICANCER DRUGS

DRUG CLASSIFICATION

The anticancer drugs fall into three major classes: (1) cytotoxic agents, (2) hormones and hormone antagonists, and (3) biologic response modifiers. The cytotoxic agents, which constitute the largest group of anticancer drugs, can be subclassified as follows: (1) alkylating agents, (2) antimetabolites, (3) antitumor antibiotics, (4) mitotic inhibitors, and (5) miscellaneous cytotoxic drugs. Individual cytotoxic agents are listed in Table 91–1.

MECHANISMS OF CYTOTOXIC ACTION

Table 91–2 summarizes the principal mechanisms by which the cytotoxic anticancer drugs act. As the table shows, most cytotoxic agents disrupt

Table 91–1. Anticancer Drugs: Cytotoxic Agents

Generic Name	Trade Name	Cell-Cycle Phase Specificity	Route	Dose-Limiting Toxicity
Alkylating Agents				
Nitrogen Mustards				
Cyclophosphamide	Cytoxan, Neosar	Phase nonspecific	PO, IV	Bone marrow depression
Chlorambucil	Leukeran	Phase nonspecific	PO	Bone marrow depression
Ifosfamide	Ifex	Phase nonspecific	IV	Bone marrow depression
Melphalan	Alkeran	Phase nonspecific	PO, IV	Bone marrow depression
Mechlorethamine	Mustargen	Phase nonspecific, but M and G_1 most sensitive	IV, IC, T	Bone marrow depression
Nitrosoureas				
Carmustine	BiCNU	Phase nonspecific	IV, T	Bone marrow depression
Lomustine	CeeNU	Phase nonspecific	PO	Bone marrow depression
Streptozocin	Zanosar	Phase nonspecific	IV	Nephrotoxicity
Others				
Busulfan	Myleran	Phase nonspecific	PO	Bone marrow depression
Carboplatin	Paraplatin	Phase nonspecific	IV	Bone marrow depression
Cisplatin	Platinol	Phase nonspecific	IV	Nephrotoxicity
Antimetabolites				
Folic Acid Analogue				
Methotrexate	Folex	S-phase specific	IV, IM, PO, IT	Bone marrow depression, oral and GI ulceration
Pyrimidine Analogues				
Cytarabine	Cytosar-U	S-phase specific	IV, SC, IT	Bone marrow depression
Fluorouracil	Adrucil	Phase nonspecific, but cell must be cycling	IV	Bone marrow depression, oral and GI ulceration
Floxuridine	FUDR	Phase nonspecific, but cell must be cycling	IA	Bone marrow depression, oral and GI ulceration
Purine Analogues				
Mercaptopurine	Purinethol	S-phase specific	PO	Bone marrow depression
Thioguanine	generic only	S-phase specific	PO, IV	Bone marrow depression
Fludarabine	Fludara	S-phase specific	IV	Bone marrow depression
Pentostatin	Nipent	S-phase specific	IV	Bone marrow depression, CNS depression
Antitumor Antibiotics				
Bleomycin	Blenoxane	G_2-phase specific	IV, IM, SC	Pneumonitis and pulmonary fibrosis
Dactinomycin	Cosmegen	Phase nonspecific	IV	Bone marrow depression, oral ulceration
Daunorubicin	Cerubidine	Phase nonspecific	IV	Bone marrow depression, cardiotoxicity
Doxorubicin	Adriamycin, Rubex	Phase nonspecific	IV	Bone marrow depression, cardiotoxicity
Idarubicin	Idamycin	Phase nonspecific, but S phase most sensitive	IV	Bone marrow depression
Mitomycin	Mutamycin	Phase nonspecific	IV	Bone marrow depression
Mitoxantrone	Novantrone	Phase nonspecific	IV	Bone marrow depression
Plicamycin	Mithracin	Phase nonspecific	IV	Bone marrow depression, bleeding disorders
Mitotic Inhibitors				
Vinblastine	Oncovin, Vincasar	M-phase specific	IV	Bone marrow depression
Vincristine	Velban, others	M-phase specific	IV	Peripheral neuropathy
Miscellaneous				
Altretamine	Hexalen	Mechanism unknown	PO	Bone marrow depression
Asparaginase	Elspar	G_1-phase specific	IV, IM	None
Dacarbazine	DTIC-Dome	Phase nonspecific	IV	Bone marrow depression
Etoposide	VePesid	G_2-phase specific	PO, IV	Bone marrow depression
Hydroxyurea	Hydrea	S-phase specific	PO	Bone marrow depression
Procarbazine	Matulane	Phase nonspecific	PO	Bone marrow depression
Mitotane	Lysodren	Phase nonspecific	PO	CNS depression
Teniposide	Vumon	G_2-phase specific	IV	Bone marrow depression
Paclitaxel	Taxol	G_2-phase specific	IV	Bone marrow depression, peripheral neuropathy

Key to routes: IA = intra-arterial, IC = intracavitary, IM = intramuscular, IT = intrathecal, IV = intravenous, PO = oral, SC = subcutaneous, T = topical.

Table 91–2. Actions of Representative Cytotoxic Anticancer Drugs		
Drug	**Drug Action**	**Cellular Process Disrupted**
Cyclophosphamide, cisplatin	Alkylates DNA, causing cross-links and strand breakage	DNA and RNA synthesis
Methotrexate	Inhibits one-carbon transfer reactions	Synthesis of DNA precursors (purines, dTMP)
Hydroxyurea	Inhibits ribonucleotide reductase	Synthesis of DNA precursors (blocks conversion of ribonucleotides into deoxyribonucleotides)
Thioguanine, mercaptopurine	Inhibits purine ring synthesis and nucleotide interconversion	Synthesis of DNA precursors (purines, pyrimidines, ribonucleotides, and deoxyribonucleotides)
Fluorouracil	Inhibits thymidylate synthetase	Synthesis of dTMP, a DNA precursor
Cytarabine	Inhibits DNA polymerase	DNA synthesis
Bleomycin	Breaks DNA strands and prevents their repair	DNA synthesis
Plicamycin	Binds to DNA	DNA and RNA synthesis
Dactinomycin, daunorubicin, doxorubicin	Intercalates between base pairs of DNA	DNA and RNA synthesis
Vinblastine, vincristine	Blocks microtubule assembly	Mitosis
Asparaginase	Deaminates asparagine, depriving cells of this amino acid	Protein synthesis

processes related to synthesis of DNA or its precursors. In addition, some agents (e.g., vinblastine, vincristine) act specifically to block mitosis, and one drug—asparaginase—disrupts synthesis of proteins. Note that with the exception of asparaginase, all of these drugs disrupt processes carried out exclusively by cells that are undergoing proliferation. This explains why anticancer drugs are most toxic to tissues that have a high growth fraction (i.e., a high proportion of proliferating cells).

CELL-CYCLE PHASE SPECIFICITY

As we discussed in Chapter 90, the cell cycle is the sequence of events that a cell goes through from one mitotic division to the next. Some anticancer agents, known as *cell-cycle phase specific drugs,* are effective only during a specific phase of the cell cycle. Other anticancer agents, known as *cell-cycle phase nonspecific drugs,* can affect cells during any phase of the cell cycle. All of the hormones, hormone antagonists, and biologic response modifiers are phase nonspecific. In contrast, about half of the cytotoxic anticancer drugs are phase nonspecific, whereas the other half are phase specific. The phase specificity of individual cytotoxic agents is summarized in Table 91–1.

Cell-Cycle Phase Specific Drugs. Phase-specific agents are toxic only to cells that are passing through a particular phase of the cell cycle. Vincristine, for example, acts by causing mitotic arrest; hence, the drug is effective only during M phase. Other agents act by disrupting DNA syn-

thesis; hence, they are effective only during S phase. Because of their phase specificity, these drugs are toxic only to cells that are active participants in the cell cycle; cells that are "resting" in G_0 will not be harmed. Obviously, if these drugs are to be effective, they must be present as neoplastic cells cycle through the specific phase in which they act. This means that these drugs must be present for an extended time. To accomplish this, phase-specific drugs are often administered by prolonged infusion. Alternatively, they can be given in multiple small doses at short intervals over an extended time. Because the dosing schedule is so critical to therapeutic response, phase-specific drugs are also known as *schedule-dependent drugs.*

Cell-Cycle Phase Nonspecific Drugs. The phase-nonspecific drugs can act during any phase of the cell cycle, including G_0. Among the phase-nonspecific drugs are the alkylating agents and most antitumor antibiotics. Since phase-nonspecific drugs can injure G_0 cells, whereas phase-specific drugs cannot, phase-nonspecific drugs can increase cell kill when used together with phase-specific drugs.

Although the phase-nonspecific drugs can inflict biochemical lesions at any time during the cell cycle, *as a rule these drugs are more toxic to proliferating cells than to cells in G_0.* There are two reasons for the greater sensitivity of proliferating cells. First, cells in G_0 often have time to repair drug-induced damage before it can result in significant harm. In contrast, proliferating cells lack time for repair. Second, toxicity may not become manifested until the cell attempts to proliferate. For example, many alkylating agents act by producing cross-links between DNA strands. Although these biochemical lesions can be made at any time, they are largely without effect until cells attempt to replicate DNA. This is much like inflicting a flat tire on an automobile: the tire can be deflated at any time; however, loss of air is consequential only if the car is moving. Carrying the analogy further, if the flat occurs while the car is stopped, and is repaired before travel is attempted, the flat will have no functional impact at all.

TOXICITY

As discussed in Chapter 90, many anticancer drugs are toxic to normal tissues—especially tissues that have a high percentage of proliferating cells (bone marrow, hair follicles, gastrointestinal epithelium, and germinal epithelium). The common major toxicities of the anticancer drugs, together with management procedures, are discussed at length in Chapter 90. Accordingly, as we consider individual anticancer agents in this chapter, discussion of most toxicities will be brief.

DOSAGE, HANDLING, AND ADMINISTRATION

Dosage and Administration. Cancer chemotherapy is a highly specialized field. Accordingly, in a general text such as this, presentation of detailed information on dosage and administration of specific agents would be inappropriate. Be aware that dosages for anticancer agents must be individualized and that timing of administration may vary with the particular protocol being followed. Because of the complex and hazardous nature of cancer chemotherapy, anticancer drugs should be administered under the direct supervision of a physician experienced in their use.

Handling of Cytotoxic Drugs. Antineoplastic drugs are often mutagenic, teratogenic, and carcinogenic. In addition, direct contact with the skin, eyes, and mucous membranes can result in local injury. Accordingly, it is imperative that health care personnel involved in the preparation and administration of these drugs follow safe handling procedures. Risks of injury from contact with parenteral chemotherapeutic drugs can be minimized by use of containment equipment and approved technique.

Administration of Vesicants. As discussed in Chapter 90, extravasation of vesicants can cause severe local injury, sometimes requiring surgical debridement and skin grafting. Drugs with strong vesicant properties include carmustine, dacarbazine, dactinomycin, daunorubicin, doxorubicin, mechlorethamine, mitomycin, plicamycin, strepto-

zocin, vinblastine, and vincristine. To minimize the risk of injury, IV administration should be performed only into veins with good flow. Sites of previous irradiation should be avoided. If extravasation occurs, administration should be discontinued immediately.

ALKYLATING AGENTS

The family of alkylating agents consists of nitrogen mustards, nitrosoureas, and other compounds. Before considering the properties of individual alkylating agents, we will discuss the characteristics of the group as a whole. The alkylating agents are listed in Table 91–1.

SHARED PROPERTIES

Mechanism of Action. The alkylating agents are highly reactive compounds that have the ability to transfer an alkyl group to a variety of cell constituents. Cell kill results primarily from alkylation of DNA. As a rule, alkylating agents interact with DNA by forming a covalent bond with a specific nitrogen atom in guanine (Fig. 91–1). Those alkylating agents that have *two* reactive sites (*bifunctional* agents) are able to bind DNA in two places to form *cross-links*. These bridges may be formed within a single strand of DNA or between parallel DNA strands. Figure 91–1 illustrates the production of interstrand cross-links by nitrogen mustard. *Monofunctional* alkylating agents (agents with only one reactive group) lack the ability to form cross-links, but are still able to bind to a single guanine in DNA. The consequences of guanine alkylation are miscoding, scission of DNA strands, and, if cross-links have been formed, inhibition of DNA replication. Since cross-linking of DNA is especially injurious, cell death is more likely with bifunctional agents than with monofunctional agents.

Because alkylation reactions can take place at any time during the cell cycle, alkylating agents are considered *cell-cycle phase nonspecific*. However, *most of these drugs are more toxic to proliferating cells than to cells in G_0*. This is because (1) alkylation of DNA produces its most detrimental effects when cells attempt to replicate DNA, and because (2) resting cells are often able to repair damage to DNA before that damage can affect cell function. Because alkylating agents are phase nonspecific, they needn't be present over an extended time. Accordingly, they can be administered in a single bolus dose.

Resistance. Development of resistance to alkylating agents is common. A major cause of resistance is increased production of enzymes that per-

A

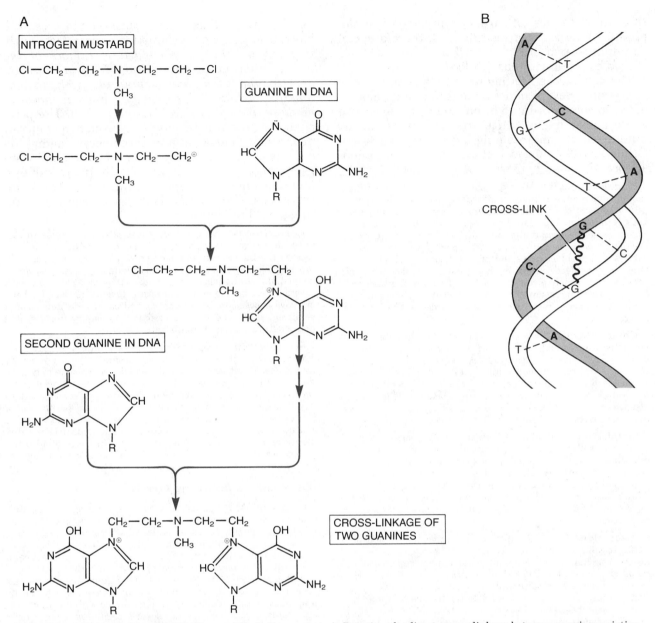

Figure 91–1. Cross-linking of DNA by an alkylating agent. *A,* Reactions leading to cross-linkage between guanine moieties in DNA. *B,* Schematic representation of interstrand cross-linking within the DNA double helix. (A = adenine, C = cytosine, G = guanine, T = thymine)

form DNA repair. Resistance may also result from decreased uptake of alkylating agents and from increased production of nucleophiles (compounds that act as substitute targets for alkylation).

Toxicities. Alkylating agents are toxic to tissues that have a high growth fraction. Hence, these drugs may injure cells of the bone marrow, hair follicles, gastrointestinal mucosa, and germinal epithelium. Blood dyscrasias (neutropenia, thrombocytopenia, anemia) caused by bone marrow depression are of greatest concern. Nausea and vomiting occur with all alkylating agents, and can be especially severe with cisplatin. Practically all of these drugs are vesicants and, therefore, must be administered intravenously.

PROPERTIES OF INDIVIDUAL ALKYLATING AGENTS

Nitrogen Mustards

Cyclophosphamide. Cyclophosphamide [Cytoxan, Neosar] is a bifunctional agent active against a *broad spectrum* of neoplastic diseases. Indications include *Hodgkin's disease, non-Hodgkin's lymphomas, multiple myeloma,* and *solid tumors of the head, neck, ovary, and breast.* Of all the alkylating agents, cyclophosphamide is the most widely employed.

Cyclophosphamide is a prodrug that undergoes conversion to its active form in the liver. Because activation is required, onset of effects is delayed.

In contrast to most other alkylating agents, cyclophosphamide is not a vesicant and, therefore, can be administered orally as well as IV. Oral doses should be administered with food.

The major dose-limiting toxicity is bone marrow depression. Severe nausea, vomiting, and alopecia are also common. In addition, the drug can cause acute hemorrhagic cystitis; renal damage can be minimized by maintaining adequate hydration. Other adverse effects include sterility, immunosuppression, and hypersensitivity reactions.

Mechlorethamine. Mechlorethamine [Mustargen], a bifunctional compound, was the first alkylating agent employed clinically. Applications include *Hodgkin's disease* and *non-Hodgkin's lymphomas*. Mechlorethamine is a powerful vesicant and can cause severe local injury. Accordingly, for systemic therapy, the drug must be administered intravenously. Caution must be exercised to avoid extravasation or direct contact with the skin. Once in the bloodstream, mechlorethamine undergoes rapid conversion to inactive compounds. The dose-limiting toxicity is bone marrow depression. Other major toxicities include nausea, vomiting, alopecia, diarrhea, stomatitis, amenorrhea, and sterility.

Chlorambucil. Chlorambucil [Leukeran] is the safest nitrogen mustard available. Bone marrow depression is the major dose-limiting toxicity. Other adverse effects include hepatotoxicity, sterility, pulmonary infiltrates, and pulmonary fibrosis. Nausea and vomiting are usually mild. Chlorambucil is a drug of choice for *chronic lymphocytic leukemia*. The drug is also used to treat *Hodgkin's disease, non-Hodgkin's lymphomas*, and *ovarian cancers*. Administration is oral.

Melphalan. Melphalan [Alkeran], a bifunctional agent, is generally well tolerated. Bone marrow depression is major dose-limiting toxicity. The drug has caused leukemia and may also be mutagenic. Melphalan is not a vesicant. Severe nausea and vomiting are rare. Administration is oral and IV. Melphalan is a drug of choice for palliative therapy of *multiple myeloma*. The drug is also active against *carcinoma of the ovary and breast*.

Ifosfamide. Ifosfamide [Ifex], a derivative of cyclophosphamide, is approved only for refractory *germ-cell cancer of the testes*. Dose-limiting toxicities are bone marrow depression and hemorrhagic cystitis. The risk of cystitis is minimized by concurrent therapy with *mesna* [Mesnex] and by extensive hydration (at least 2 L of oral or IV fluid daily). Because of the risk of cystitis, urinalysis should be performed before each dose. If the analysis reveals microscopic hematuria, dosing should be postponed until the hematuria resolves. Additional adverse effects include nausea, vomiting, metabolic acidosis, and central nervous system (CNS) toxicity (confusion, hallucinations, blurred vision, coma). Administration is intravenous.

Nitrosoureas

The nitrosoureas are bifunctional agents that are active against a broad spectrum of neoplastic diseases. Cell kill results from cross-linking of DNA. Unlike most anticancer drugs, the nitrosoureas are highly lipophilic and, therefore, can readily penetrate the blood-brain barrier. As a result, these drugs are especially useful against *cancers of the CNS*. The major dose-limiting toxicity is *delayed bone marrow depression*.

Carmustine (BCNU). Carmustine [BiCNU] was the first nitrosourea to undergo extensive clinical testing, and can be considered the prototype for the group. Because of its ability to cross the blood-brain barrier, carmustine is used frequently to treat *primary and metastatic tumors of the brain*. Other indications include *Hodgkin's disease, non-Hodgkin's lymphomas, multiple myeloma, malignant melanoma, hepatoma*, and *adenocarcinoma of the stomach, colon, and rectum*. The principal dose-limiting toxicity is delayed bone marrow depression; leukocyte and thrombocyte nadirs occur 4 to 6 weeks after treatment. Nausea and vomiting can be severe. Injury to the liver, kidneys, and lungs has been reported. Administration is intravenous. Carmustine is not a vesicant but can cause local phlebitis.

Lomustine (CCNU). Lomustine [CeeNU] is similar to carmustine in actions and uses. Like carmustine, lomustine crosses the blood-brain barrier and can be used to treat *CNS cancers*. The drug also has activity against *lymphomas, melanomas*, and *carcinomas of the breast, lung, and colon*. As with carmustine, the major dose-limiting toxicity is delayed bone marrow depression. Additional toxicities include nausea and vomiting, renal and hepatic toxicity, pulmonary fibrosis, and neurologic reactions. Administration is oral.

Streptozocin. Streptozocin [Zanosar] differs significantly from the other nitrosoureas. The drug contains a glucose moiety that causes selective drug uptake by islet cells of the pancreas. This selective uptake underlies the drug's principal use: *metastatic islet-cell tumors*. The major dose-limiting toxicity is kidney damage. Accordingly, renal function should be monitored in all patients. As with other nitrosoureas, nausea and vomiting can be severe. Additional toxicities include hypoglycemia, hyperglycemia, diarrhea, chills, and fever. In contrast to other nitrosoureas, streptozocin causes minimal bone marrow depression. Administration is intravenous.

Miscellaneous Alkylating Agents

Cisplatin. Although not a true alkylating agent, cisplatin [Platinol] is discussed in this section because, like the true alkylating agents, the drug kills cells primarily by forming cross-links between and within strands of DNA. Cisplatin's principal indications are *testicular carcinoma* (primary and metastatic) and *metastatic breast carcinoma*. Other indications include *carcinomas of the bladder, head, and neck*. The major dose-limiting toxicity is damage to the kidney, which can be minimized with extensive hydration coupled with diuretic therapy. Nausea and vomiting are severe, beginning about 1 hour after administration and persisting for 1 to 2 days. Other adverse effects include neurotoxicity, bone marrow depression, and toxicity to the ear (manifested as tinnitus and high-frequency hearing loss). Administration is by IV infusion.

Carboplatin. Carboplatin [Paraplatin] is an analogue of cisplatin. Cell kill appears to result from cross-linking of DNA. The drug's only approved indications are initial and palliative therapy of *ovarian cancer*. Unlabeled uses include *small cell cancer of the lung, squamous cell cancer of the head and neck*, and *endometrial cancer*. The major dose-limiting toxicity is bone marrow depression. Nausea and vomiting occur, but are less severe than with cisplatin. Similarly, nephrotoxicity, neurotoxicity, and hearing loss are less frequent than with cisplatin. Carboplatin is administered by intravenous infusion. Anaphylactic reactions have occurred minutes after administration; symptoms can be managed with epinephrine, glucocorticoids, and antihistamines.

Busulfan. Busulfan [Myleran] is a bifunctional agent whose cytotoxic effects are limited almost exclusively to the bone marrow. Because it causes selective attack on the bone marrow, busulfan is a drug of choice for *chronic myelogenous leukemia*. The remission rate is 90% with one course of therapy. Dose-limiting toxicities are bone marrow depression, pulmonary infiltrates, and pulmonary fibrosis. Other toxicities include nausea, vomiting, alopecia, gynecomastia, male and female sterility, skin hyperpigmentation, cataracts, and hepatitis. Administration is oral.

ANTIMETABOLITES

Antimetabolites are structural analogues of important natural metabolites. This structural similarity allows these drugs to disrupt critical metabolic processes. Some antimetabolites inhibit enzymes that synthesize essential cellular constituents. Others undergo incorporation into DNA, thereby disrupting DNA replication and function.

Antimetabolites are effective only against cells that are active participants in the cell cycle. Several antimetabolites are S-phase specific. Others can act during any phase of the cycle, except G_0. To be effective, agents that are S-phase specific must be present for a prolonged time.

There are three classes of antimetabolites: (1) folic acid analogues, (2) purine analogues, and (3) pyrimidine analogues. Members of each class are listed in Table 91–1.

FOLIC ACID ANALOGUES

Folic acid, in its active form, is needed for several essential biochemical reactions. The folic acid analogues act by preventing the conversion of folic acid to its active form. Methotrexate is the only folate analogue employed in cancer chemotherapy. Other folate analogues are used to treat bacterial infections (trimethoprim) and malaria (pyrimethamine).

Methotrexate

Mechanism of Action. As shown in Figure 91–2, methotrexate [Folex] *inhibits dihydrofolate reductase*, the enzyme that converts dihydrofolic acid (FH_2) into tetrahydrofolic acid (FH_4). Since production of FH_4 is a necessary step in the activation of folic acid, and since activated folic acid is required for biosynthesis of essential cellular constituents (DNA, RNA, proteins), inhibition of FH_4 production has multiple effects on the cell. Of all the processes that are suppressed by methotrexate, biosynthesis of thymidylate appears most critical. Suppression of thymidylate synthesis is critical because, in the absence of thymidylate, cells are unable to make DNA. Because cell kill results primarily from disruption of DNA synthesis, methotrexate is considered S-phase specific.

An investigational technique known as *leucovorin rescue* has been employed to enhance the effects of methotrexate. Some neoplastic cells are unresponsive to methotrexate because they lack the transport system required for active uptake of the drug. By giving massive doses of methotrexate, the drug can be forced into these cells by passive diffusion. However, since this process also exposes normal cells to extremely high concentrations of methotrexate, these cells are also at risk. To save normal cells, leucovorin (citrovorum factor, folinic acid) is given. As shown in Figure 91–2, leucovorin bypasses the metabolic block caused by methotrexate, thereby permitting normal cells to synthesize thymidylate and other compounds. Malignant cells are not saved because leucovorin uptake requires the same transport system employed for methotrexate uptake, a transport system that these cells lack. It should be noted that leucovorin rescue is potentially hazardous: *failure to administer leucovorin in the right dose at the right time can be fatal.*

Resistance. Acquired resistance to methotrexate can result from three mechanisms: (1) decreased uptake of methotrexate, (2) increased synthesis of dihydrofolate reductase (the target enzyme for methotrexate), and (3) synthesis of a modified form of dihydrofolate reductase that has a reduced affinity for methotrexate.

Pharmacokinetics. Methotrexate can be administered orally, IM, IV, and intrathecally. For most cancers of the CNS, intrathecal administration is employed. Metabolism of methotrexate is minimal. Most of each dose is excreted intact in the urine. Because elimination is renal, methotrexate can accumulate to dangerous levels in patients with kidney dysfunction; hence, the dosage must be reduced.

Therapeutic Uses. Neoplastic Diseases. Methotrexate is curative for women with *choriocarcinoma*. The drug is also active against *non-Hodgkin's lymphomas* and *acute lymphocytic leukemia of childhood*. Very large doses coupled with leucovorin rescue have been employed to treat *head and neck sarcomas* and *osteogenic sarcoma*.

Other Indications. Low doses are used to control *severe psoriasis* (see Chapter 70). Higher doses are used to treat *severe rheumatoid arthritis* (see Chapter 63).

Toxicity. The usual dose-limiting toxicities are bone marrow depression, pulmonary infiltrates and fibrosis, and oral and gastrointestinal ulceration. Death may result from intestinal perforation and hemorrhagic enteritis. Nausea and vomiting may occur shortly after administration. High doses can cause direct injury to the kidneys. To promote drug excretion, and thereby minimize renal damage, the urine should be alkalinized and adequate hydration should be maintained. Methotrexate has been associated with fetal malformation and death. Accordingly, pregnancy should be avoided until at least 6 months after completing treatment.

PYRIMIDINE ANALOGUES

Pyrimidines (cytosine, thymine, uracil) are bases employed in the biosynthesis of nucleic acids (DNA and RNA). The pyrimidine analogues, because of their structural similarity to naturally occurring pyrimidines, can act in several ways: (1) they can

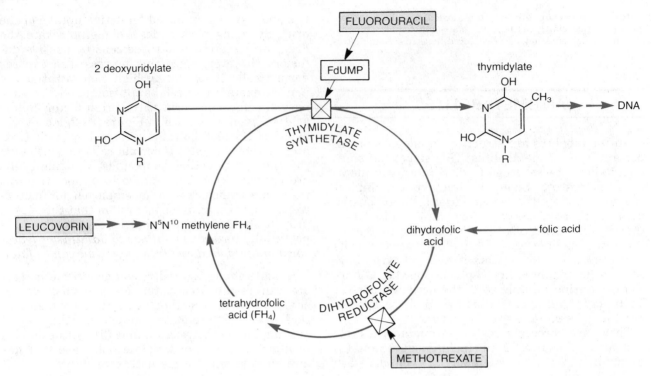

Figure 91–2. Actions of methotrexate, leucovorin, and fluorouracil. (FdUMP = 5-flouro-2'-deoxyuridine-5'-monophosphate, ⊠ = blockade of reaction)

inhibit biosynthesis of pyrimidines, (2) they can inhibit biosynthesis of nucleic acids, and (3) they can undergo incorporation into DNA and RNA, thereby disrupting nucleic acid function. All of the pyrimidine analogues are prodrugs that must be converted to their active forms within the body.

Cytarabine

Cytarabine [Cytosar-U], also known as *cytosine arabinoside* and *Ara C*, is an analogue of deoxycytidine. The drug has an established role in treating acute myelogenous leukemia.

Mechanism of Action. Cytarabine is converted to its active form—Ara-CTP—within the body. As Ara-CTP, the drug becomes incorporated into DNA. By a mechanism that is not fully understood, this incorporation suppresses further DNA synthesis. Ara-CTP may also impede DNA synthesis by a second mechanism: inhibition of DNA polymerase. Cytarabine is highly S-phase specific.

Resistance. Decreased conversion of cytarabine to Ara-CTP is a major cause of resistance. Other mechanisms include decreased uptake of cytarabine, increased conversion of cytarabine to an inactive product, and increased production of dCTP (the natural metabolite with which Ara-CTP competes for incorporation into DNA).

Pharmacokinetics. Administration may be IV, SC, or intrathecal. Cytarabine is not active orally. Drug that is not taken up by cells undergoes rapid deamination in the liver. Metabolites are excreted in the urine.

Therapeutic Uses. The principal indication for cytarabine is *acute myelogenous leukemia*. The drug has been combined with thioguanine and daunorubicin or doxorubicin to treat this disease. Other applications include *acute lymphocytic leukemia, chronic myelogenous leukemia*, and *non-Hodgkin's lymphomas*.

Toxicity. Bone marrow suppression (neutropenia, thrombocytopenia) is the usual dose-limiting toxicity. Nausea, vomiting, and fever may develop, especially after bolus IV injection. Other toxicities include stomatitis, liver injury, and conjunctivitis. High doses may cause pulmonary edema and central and peripheral neurotoxicity.

Fluorouracil

Fluorouracil [Adrucil] is a fluorinated derivative of uracil. The drug is employed extensively to treat solid tumors.

Mechanism of Action. In order to exert cytotoxic effects, fluorouracil must be converted to its active form, 5-fluoro-2'-deoxy-5'-monophosphate (FdUMP). As shown in Figure 91–2, FdUMP inhibits thymidylate synthetase, thereby depriving cells of thymidylate needed to make DNA. Fluorouracil is active only against cells that are going through the cell cycle. However, the drug lacks phase specificity.

Resistance. Potential mechanisms for resistance are (1) decreased activation of fluorouracil, and (2) production of altered thymidylate synthetase that has a low affinity for FdUMP. The clinical significance of these mechanisms has not been established.

Therapeutic Uses. Chemotherapeutic use of fluorouracil is limited to solid tumors. The drug is employed for palliative therapy of *carcinomas of the colon, rectum, breast, stomach, and pancreas*. In addition to therapy of cancer, fluorouracil is employed topically to treat *premalignant keratoses* (see Chapter 70).

Pharmacokinetics. Administration is intravenous. Continuous infusion is more effective and less toxic than bolus administration. Fluorouracil is distributed widely and enters the CNS with ease. Elimination is by rapid hepatic metabolism.

Toxicity. The usual dose-limiting toxicities are bone marrow depression (neutropenia) and oral and gastrointestinal (GI) ulceration. To minimize GI injury (e.g., ulceration of the oropharynx or bowel), fluorouracil should be discontinued as soon as mild reactions (stomatitis, diarrhea) occur. Other adverse effects include alopecia, hyperpigmentation, and neurologic deficits.

Floxuridine

Floxuridine [FUDR], like fluorouracil, is converted to FdUMP within the body. Hence, the pharmacologic effects of floxuridine and fluorouracil are nearly identical. Floxuridine has been used for palliation of *primary gastrointestinal carcinomas and their metastases to the liver*. Beneficial effects are no greater than with IV fluorouracil. Floxuridine is administered only by intra-arterial infusion.

PURINE ANALOGUES

Like the pyrimidines, the purines (adenine, guanine, hypoxanthine) are bases employed for biosynthesis of nucleic acids. The three drugs discussed below—thioguanine, mercaptopurine, and fludarabine—are analogues of guanine, hypoxanthine, and adenine, respectively. All three agents are prodrugs that become activated in the body.

Mercaptopurine

Mechanisms of Action and Resistance. Mercaptopurine [Purinethol] is a prodrug that undergoes conversion to its active form within cells. Following activation, the drug can disrupt multiple biochemical processes, including purine biosynthesis, nucleotide interconversion, and biosynthesis of nucleic acids. All of these actions probably contribute to cytotoxic effects. Mercaptopurine is S-phase specific. Mechanisms of resistance include reduced activation of the drug and accelerated deactivation.

Pharmacokinetics. Mercaptopurine is administered orally and undergoes erratic absorption. Absorbed drug is distributed widely, but not to the CNS. Extensive metabolism occurs in the liver; an important reaction is catalyzed by xanthine oxidase. Accordingly, for patients receiving allopurinol (an inhibitor of xanthine oxidase), mercaptopurine dosage should be reduced.

Therapeutic Uses. The principal indication for mercaptopurine is *acute lymphocytic leukemia* in children and adults. The drug may also be of some

benefit in *acute and chronic myelogenous leukemia* in adults.

Toxicity. Bone marrow depression (neutropenia, thrombocytopenia, anemia) is the principal dose-limiting toxicity. Hepatic dysfunction, which usually manifests as cholestatic jaundice, occurs in about 30% of patients. Other adverse effects include, nausea, vomiting, and oral and intestinal ulceration. Concurrent use of allopurinol increases the overall risk of toxicity. Mercaptopurine is mutagenic; hence, women should be warned against becoming pregnant.

Thioguanine

Actions and Uses. Thioguanine acts much like mercaptopurine. Following conversion to its active form, thioguanine inhibits purine synthesis and the interconversion of nucleotides. DNA synthesis is also inhibited. Like mercaptopurine, thioguanine is S-phase specific. The drug is used primarily for *acute lymphocytic and myelogenous leukemias*.

Pharmacokinetics. Administration is oral; absorption is erratic and incomplete. Thioguanine does not distribute to the CNS. Inactivation is by hepatic metabolism. In contrast to mercaptopurine, thioguanine is not degraded by xanthine oxidase. Thus, the drug can be employed concurrently with allopurinol without a reduction in dosage.

Toxicity. The usual dose-limiting toxicity is bone marrow depression. Gastrointestinal reactions (nausea, vomiting, diarrhea) may develop, but these are less severe than with mercaptopurine. Liver injury, manifesting as cholestatic jaundice, may occur.

Fludarabine

Fludarabine [Fludara] is an analogue of adenosine. The drug is approved only for *chronic lymphocytic leukemia*. Following IV infusion, fludarabine undergoes rapid conversion to its active form, 2-fluoro-ara-ATP. Cell kill appears to result from inhibition of DNA replication. Hence, the drug is probably S-phase specific. The major dose-limiting toxicity is bone marrow depression (neutropenia, thrombocytopenia, anemia). Other common toxicities include nausea, vomiting, and chills. When given in especially high doses during clinical trials, fludarabine caused severe neurologic effects, including blindness, coma, and death. However, neurologic effects are rare (0.2%) at maximal recommended therapeutic doses.

Pentostatin

Pentostatin [Nipent] is an analogue of adenosine. The drug inhibits adenosine deaminase and thereby suppresses synthesis of DNA. The only approved indication for pentostatin is *hairy cell leukemia* that has not responded to interferon alfa. The major dose-limiting toxicities are bone marrow depression and CNS depression. Other toxicities include nausea, vomiting, rash, and fever. Administration is by IV bolus or IV infusion. Pentostatin is expensive; the cost to the pharmacist for a single course of therapy is approximately $1400.

ANTITUMOR ANTIBIOTICS AND RELATED AGENTS

The antitumor antibiotics are cytotoxic drugs that were originally isolated from cultures of *Streptomyces*. In this section we will consider six antitumor antibiotics along with three of their derivatives. The antitumor antibiotics and their derivatives are used only to treat cancer; they are not used to treat infections. All of these drugs injure cells through direct interaction with DNA. Because of poor gastrointestinal absorption, they are all administered parenterally (almost always IV).

Dactinomycin (Actinomycin D)

Mechanism of Action. Dactinomycin [Cosmegen] is a planar molecule that kills cells through *intercalation* with DNA. We can understand intercalation by envisioning the stacked base pairs of DNA as having a structure like that of a stack of coins. Having a coin-like shape itself, dactinomycin is able to slip between base pairs of DNA, after which the drug becomes bound to DNA. This process (intercalation) distorts DNA structure. Because of this distortion, RNA polymerase is unable to use DNA as a template. Hence, synthesis of RNA is inhibited. Unlike RNA polymerase, DNA polymerase is relatively insensitive to the change in DNA. Consequently, DNA synthesis is not suppressed. Dactinomycin is phase *nonspecific*.

Pharmacokinetics. Administration is by intravenous infusion. Because of tissue uptake and binding to DNA, dactinomycin is rapidly cleared from the blood. The drug does not cross the blood-brain barrier. Elimination occurs slowly by biliary and renal excretion.

Therapeutic Uses. Major indications for dactinomycin are *Wilms' tumor* and *rhabdomyosarcoma*. Other indications include *choriocarcinoma*, *Ewing's sarcoma*, *Kaposi's sarcoma*, and *testicular cancer*.

Toxicity. Dose-limiting toxicities are bone marrow depression and oral and gastrointestinal mucositis. Other toxicities include nausea, vomiting, diarrhea, alopecia, folliculitis, and, in previously irradiated areas, dermatitis. Dactinomycin is extremely corrosive to soft tissue. Hence, extravasation will cause severe local injury.

Doxorubicin

Doxorubicin [Adriamycin, Rubex] is active against a broad spectrum of neoplastic diseases. Unfortunately, cardiotoxicity limits the drug's utility.

Mechanism of Action. Like dactinomycin, doxorubicin intercalates with DNA, causing distortion of DNA structure. As a result, DNA is unable to function as a template for synthesis of DNA and RNA. Doxorubicin also acts on DNA to cause strand scission.

Pharmacokinetics. Doxorubicin is administered by intravenous infusion, and undergoes rapid uptake by tissues. The drug does not cross the blood-brain barrier. Much of each dose is metabolized in the liver. Hence, dosages must be reduced for patients with hepatic impairment. Doxorubicin and its metabolites are eliminated primarily by biliary excretion.

Therapeutic Uses. Doxorubicin is active against many neoplastic diseases. The drug is employed to treat solid tumors and disseminated cancers. Specific indications include *Hodgkin's and non-Hodgkin's lymphomas, acute lymphoblastic and myeloblastic leukemias, sarcomas of soft tissue and bone, and various carcinomas, including carcinoma of the lung, stomach, breast, ovary, testes, and thyroid.*

Toxicity. The usual dose-limiting toxicity is bone marrow depression. Neutropenia develops in about 70% of patients. Thrombocytopenia and anemia may occur also. Additional delayed toxicities include alopecia, stomatitis, anorexia, conjunctivitis, and pigmentation in the extremities.

Acute toxicity usually manifests as nausea and vomiting. Because of its vesicant properties, doxorubicin can cause severe local injury if extravasation occurs. In addition, the drug imparts a harmless red coloration to urine and sweat; patients should be forewarned.

Doxorubicin can cause *acute and delayed injury to the heart*. Acute effects (dysrhythmias, EKG changes) can develop within minutes of administration. These reactions are usually transient, lasting for no more than 2 weeks. Delayed cardiotoxicity manifests as congestive heart failure secondary to diffuse cardiomyopathy (myofibril degeneration). This reaction is often unresponsive to treatment. Delayed cardiac injury is directly related to the total cumulative dose: the risk of heart failure increases significantly as the cumulative lifetime dose rises above 550 mg/m^2. Accordingly, the total dose should not exceed this amount. A drug named *dexrazoxane* has been used on an investigational basis to prevent delayed cardiotoxicity. This drug is effective, but may interfere with the antitumor activity of doxorubicin.

Daunorubicin

Daunorubicin [Cerubidine] is nearly identical in structure to doxorubicin, and shares many of that drug's properties. Like doxorubicin, daunorubicin intercalates with DNA and thereby inhibits DNA and RNA synthesis. The drug can act during all phases of the cell cycle, but cytotoxicity is greatest during S phase. The only indications for daunorubicin are *acute lymphocytic leukemia* and *acute myelogenous leukemia*. In contrast to doxorubicin, daunorubicin is not used to treat solid tumors. As with doxorubicin, the major dose-limiting toxicities are bone marrow depression and congestive heart failure. In addition, daunorubicin may cause nausea, vomiting, stomatitis, and alopecia. Like doxorubicin, daunorubicin imparts a harmless red coloration to urine and tears; patients should be forewarned. Daunorubicin is administered intravenously and can cause severe local injury upon extravasation. Part of each dose is metabolized in the liver. Metabolites and parent drug are excreted in the urine and bile.

Idarubicin

Idarubicin [Idamycin] is a structural analogue of daunorubicin and doxorubicin. The drug's only indication is *acute myelogenous leukemia*. Cell kill results from intercalation with DNA and subsequent inhibition of nucleic acid synthesis. Idarubicin is most effective during S phase, but is not considered to be phase specific. Following IV infusion, the drug undergoes rapid and widespread distribution. Elimination is by hepatic metabolism followed by biliary excretion. The principal dose-limiting toxicity is bone marrow depression. Like daunorubicin and doxorubicin, idarubicin is cardiotoxic, but the maximal cumulative dose has not been determined. Additional toxicities include nausea, vomiting, alopecia, and stomatitis. Idarubicin is a vesicant and can cause severe local injury upon extravasation.

Mitoxantrone

Mitoxantrone [Novantrone] is a structural analogue of doxorubicin and daunorubicin, but is less toxic than those drugs. Mitoxantrone appears to act by two mechanisms: (1) intercalation of DNA, and (2) promotion of DNA strand breakage secondary to activation of topoisomerase II. The drug is cell-cycle phase *nonspecific*. Principal applications are *acute nonlymphocytic leukemias, lymphomas,* and *breast cancer.* Mitoxantrone is administered intravenously and undergoes rapid and widespread distribution. Elimination occurs slowly, primarily by hepatic metabolism and biliary excretion. The major dose-limiting toxicity is bone marrow depression. Other important toxicities—nausea, vomiting, alopecia, mucositis, and cardiotoxicity—are less severe than with doxorubicin. Mitoxantrone imparts a harmless blue-green tint to the urine, skin, and sclera; patients should be forewarned.

Bleomycin

The preparation of bleomycin [Blenoxane] used clinically contains a mixture of glycopeptides. The major components of the mixture are bleomycin A_2 and bleomycin B_2. Bleomycin is unusual among the anticancer drugs in that it causes very little bone marrow suppression. However, it *can* cause severe injury to the lungs. Because myelosuppression is minimal, bleomycin is especially useful in combination chemotherapy. Bleomycin binds to DNA, causing chain scission and fragmentation. The drug is most effective during G_2.

Bleomycin is indicated for *testicular carcinoma* and *squamous cell carcinomas of the head, neck, larynx, cervix, penis, vulva, and skin.* The drug is also used for *Hodgkin's and non-Hodgkin's lymphomas.*

Administration is parenteral (IM, IV, and SC). High concentrations are achieved in the skin and lungs. The drug does not enter the CNS. Most tissues contain large amounts of bleomycin hydrolase, an enzyme that renders the drug inactive; cells of the skin and lungs, which are sites of toxicity, lack this enzyme. Most of each dose is excreted unchanged in the urine.

The major dose-limiting toxicity is injury to the lungs, which occurs in about 10% of patients. Injury manifests initially as pneumonitis. In about 1% of patients, pneumonitis progresses to severe pulmonary fibrosis and death. Pulmonary function should be monitored, and drug use should cease at the first sign of adverse changes.

Additional toxicities include stomatitis, alopecia, and skin reactions (hyperpigmentation, hyperkeratosis, pruritus erythema, ulceration, vesiculation). Nausea and vomiting are usually mild. Unlike most other anticancer agents, bleomycin exerts minimal toxicity to bone marrow. About 1% of patients with lymphomas experience a unique hypersensitivity reaction, characterized by fever, chills, confusion, hypotension, and wheezing.

Mitomycin

Mitomycin [Mutamycin] is a prodrug that is converted to its active form within cells. Following activation, the drug functions as a bifunctional or trifunctional alkylating agent. Cell death is caused by cross-linking of DNA with resultant blockade of DNA synthesis. Mitomycin may also induce strand scission. The drug is active during all phases of the cell cycle, but toxicity is greatest during late G_1 and early S phase.

Mitomycin is labeled for *adenocarcinoma of the stomach and pancreas.* Unlabeled uses include *carcinomas of the colon, rectum, esophagus, lung, breast, cervix, and bladder.*

Mitomycin is administered by intravenous infusion and is distributed widely, but not to the CNS. The drug is rapidly metabolized by the liver. Metabolites are excreted in the urine.

The major dose-limiting toxicity is delayed bone marrow depression; nadirs for neutropenia and thrombocytopenia usually occur 3 to 4 weeks after treatment. Other toxicities include nausea, vomiting, stomatitis, alopecia, renal toxicity, and pulmonary toxicity. Mitomycin is a vesicant and can cause severe local injury upon extravasation.

Plicamycin (Mithramycin)

Plicamycin [Mithracin] is a highly toxic drug whose use in cancer chemotherapy is restricted to *testicular carcinoma.* Cell kill results from binding to DNA with subsequent inhibition of DNA and RNA synthesis. The drug is cell-cycle phase *nonspecific.* Dose-related bleeding is the most serious toxicity. Bleeding results from thrombocytopenia and deficiencies of several clotting factors. Because of the risk of hemorrhage, plicamycin should be used only in a hospital setting. Patients with coagulation disorders and pre-existing thrombocytopenia should not receive the drug. Additional toxicities include nausea, vomiting, stomatitis, renal injury, and disruption of calcium metabolism. Plicamycin is administered intravenously and little is known about its fate. Elimination is renal. In addition to management of testicular cancer, plicamycin is used to manage hypercalcemia of malignancy. This application is considered in Chapter 52 (Drugs Affecting Calcium Levels and Utilization).

MITOTIC INHIBITORS

Mitotic inhibitors are drugs that act during M phase to prevent cell division. The principal mitotic inhibitors are *vincristine* and *vinblastine.* Both drugs are derived from *Vinca rosea* (the periwinkle plant) and, therefore, are known as *vinca alkaloids.* Vincristine and vinblastine have nearly identical structures and share the same mechanism of action. However, these drugs have quite different toxicities. Vincristine is toxic to peripheral nerves, but does little damage to bone marrow. Conversely, vinblastine can cause significant bone marrow depression, but is relatively harmless to nerves. The basis for these differences in toxicity is not understood. Vincristine and vinblastine do not share the same indications.

Vincristine

Mechanism of Action. Vincristine [Oncovin, Vincasar] blocks mitosis during metaphase. The drug does this by preventing the assembly of microtubules (the filaments that move chromosomes during cell division). In the absence of microtubules, distribution of chromosomes to daughter cells becomes random. This failure to correctly allocate chromosomes is the presumed cause of cell death. Vincristine disrupts microtubule assembly by binding to *tubulin*, the major protein of which microtubules are composed. The drug is M-phase specific.

Pharmacokinetics. Because of low and erratic oral absorption, vincristine must be given intravenously. The drug leaves the blood rapidly and enters tissues, where it becomes tightly but reversibly bound. Penetration to the CNS is poor. Most of each dose undergoes hepatic metabolism followed by biliary excretion. Only 12% of the drug is eliminated in the urine.

Therapeutic Uses. Vincristine is bone marrow–sparing. Accordingly, the drug is ideal for combination chemotherapy. Indications include *Hodgkin's and non-Hodgkin's lymphomas, acute lymphocytic leukemia, Wilms' tumor, rhabdomyosarcoma, Kaposi's sarcoma, breast cancer,* and *bladder cancer.*

Toxicity. Peripheral neuropathy is the major dose-limiting toxicity. Vincristine injures neurons by disrupting neurotubules, structures that are required for axonal transport of enzymes and organelles. Injury to neurotubules results from binding to tubulin, the same protein found in microtubules. Nearly all patients experience symptoms of sensory or motor nerve injury (e.g., decreased reflexes, weakness, paresthesias, sensory loss). Symptoms of injury to autonomic nerves (e.g., constipation, urinary hesitancy) are less common, occurring in 30% to 50% of those treated. Since vincristine does not readily enter the CNS, injury to the brain is minimal.

In contrast to most anticancer drugs, vincristine causes little toxicity to bone marrow. As a result, the drug is especially desirable for combined therapy with other anticancer drugs.

Vincristine is a powerful irritant and can cause severe local injury if extravasation occurs. Alopecia develops in about 20% of patients. Nausea and vomiting are rare.

Vinblastine

Vinblastine [Velban, Velsar, Alkaban] is a structural analogue of vincristine. The two drugs share the same mechanism of action: production of metaphase arrest through blockade of microtubule assembly. Like vincristine, vinblastine is administered intravenously, does not cross the blood-brain barrier, and is eliminated by biliary and urinary excretion. Indications for vinblastine include *Kaposi's sarcoma, Hodgkin's and non-Hodgkin's lymphomas,* and *carcinoma of the breast and testes.* The major dose-limiting toxicity is bone marrow depression. (Note that vinblastine differs markedly from vincristine in this action.) Neurotoxicity can occur but is much less severe than with vincristine. Additional adverse effects include nausea, vomiting, alopecia, stomatitis, and severe local injury if extravasation should occur.

MISCELLANEOUS CYTOTOXIC AGENTS

Paclitaxel

Sources. Paclitaxel [Taxol] is a natural product currently prepared by extraction from the bark of the Western yew (*Taxus brevifolia*), a tree native to the Pacific Northwest. A full course of treatment for a single patient requires the bark of 3 to 4 trees, which die as a result of harvesting the bark. A drug very similar to paclitaxel, known as *taxotere*, is prepared from *needles* of the European yew tree, allowing the tree to be spared. Recently, a paclitaxel-producing fungus (*Taxomyces andreanae*) that grows naturally on the Pacific yew was shown to continue producing paclitaxel when grown in culture, thereby representing a potentially limitless source of the drug.

Actions and Uses. Paclitaxel acts during late G_2 to cause formation of stable microtubule bundles, thereby inhibiting cell replication. The drug is approved only for *metastatic ovarian cancer* that has not responded to other drugs. However, early clinical studies indicate that paclitaxel is also active against *metastatic breast cancer, advanced non-small cell lung cancer, malignant melanoma,* and *head and neck cancer.*

Treatment is expensive. Patients require a series of 3 to 6 infusions, each costing over $1000 for the drug and another $1000 or more for hospitalization and physician's fees.

Pharmacokinetics. Paclitaxel is administered by 24-hour infusion. The drug undergoes wide distribution, but not to the CNS. Very little is known about how paclitaxel is eliminated; small amounts appear in the urine and bile, but the fate of the remainder is not understood.

Toxicity. Severe hypersensitivity reactions (hypotension, dyspnea, angioedema, urticaria) have occurred during the infusion, probably in response to the vehicle (castor oil) rather than to paclitaxel itself. The risk of severe hypersensitivity reactions can be minimized by performing the infusion slowly and by pretreatment with a glucocorticoid (dexamethasone), a histamine$_1$-receptor antagonist (diphenhydramine), and a histamine$_2$-receptor antagonist (cimetidine).

The major dose-limiting toxicity is bone marrow depression (neutropenia). Peripheral neuropathy develops with repeated infusions and may also be dose limiting. Paclitaxel can affect the heart, causing bradycardia, second- and third-degree heart block, and even fatal myocardial infarction. Muscle pain and joint pain have occurred. Practically all patients experience sudden but reversible alopecia, which frequently involves the entire body as well as the scalp. Gastrointestinal reactions (nausea, vomiting, diarrhea, mucositis) are generally mild.

Asparaginase

Mechanism of Action. Asparaginase [Elspar] is an enzyme that converts the amino acid asparagine into aspartic acid. By doing so, the drug deprives cells of asparagine needed to synthesize proteins. Since most normal cells contain asparagine synthetase, an enzyme that enables them to produce their own asparagine, normal cells are largely insensitive to the drug. Obviously, only those neoplastic cells that lack asparagine synthetase will be hurt by asparaginase. Asparaginase appears to act selectively during G_1.

Pharmacokinetics. Administration is parenteral (IM and IV). Distribution is restricted to the vascular system. The drug does not cross the blood-brain barrier. Asparaginase is inactivated by serum proteases.

Therapeutic Use. The only indication for asparaginase is *acute lymphocytic leukemia.* The drug is most effective when combined with other agents (e.g., prednisone and vincristine).

Toxicity. Asparaginase can cause severe adverse effects. However, the spectrum of toxicities differs from that of other anticancer drugs. By inhibiting protein synthesis, the drug can cause coagulation deficiencies and injury to the liver, pancreas, and kidneys. Symptoms of CNS depression, ranging from confusion to coma, develop in about 30% of those treated. Nausea and vomiting can be intense and may limit the dose that can be tolerated. Since asparaginase is a foreign protein, hypersensitivity reactions are common; fatal anaphylaxis can occur, and facilities for resuscitation should be immediately available. In contrast to most other anticancer drugs, asparaginase does not depress the bone marrow nor does it cause alopecia, oral ulceration, or intestinal ulceration.

Hydroxyurea

Mechanism of Action. Hydroxyurea [Hydrea] inhibits DNA replication by suppressing synthesis of DNA precursors. Specifically, the drug inhibits ribonucleoside diphosphate reductase, the enzyme that converts ribonucleotides into their corresponding deoxyribonucleotides. In the absence of deoxyribonucleotides, DNA cannot be made. Hydroxyurea is S-phase specific.

Pharmacokinetics. Hydroxyurea is rapidly absorbed following oral administration. Unlike most anticancer agents, hydroxyurea crosses the blood-brain barrier with ease. Part of each dose is metabolized in the liver. Parent drug and metabolites are eliminated primarily in the urine.

Therapeutic Uses. The principal indication for hydroxyurea is *chronic myelocytic leukemia*. The drug is also used for recurrent, metastatic, or inoperable *carcinoma of the ovary*.

Toxicity. The principal dose-limiting toxicity is bone marrow depression. The drug also causes nausea, vomiting, and dysuria. Neurologic deficits and stomatitis may occur, but these are rare. Hydroxyurea is teratogenic in experimental animals. Hence, like most other anticancer agents, the drug should be avoided during pregnancy.

Mitotane

Chemistry, Actions, and Uses. Mitotane [Lysodren] is a structural analogue of two insecticides: DDD and DDT. For reasons that are not understood, the drug is selectively toxic to cells of the adrenal cortex; normal cells and neoplastic cells are both injured. The only indication for mitotane is palliative therapy of *inoperable adrenocortical carcinoma*.

Pharmacokinetics. Mitotane is administered orally, and about 40% of each dose is absorbed. The drug is distributed widely, but not to the CNS. Because of storage in tissues (primarily fat), active drug remains in the body for weeks after administration has ceased. Elimination is by hepatic metabolism and renal excretion.

Toxicity. The principal dose-limiting toxicities are CNS depression, nausea, and vomiting. Because mitotane injures the adrenal cortex, adrenal insufficiency is likely. Accordingly, patients will require supplemental glucocorticoids, especially at times of stress. Dermatitis is common. Other adverse effects include visual disturbances; orthostatic hypotension; and renal damage, manifested as hematuria, hemorrhagic cystitis, and albuminuria. Mitotane does not cause the toxicities associated with most other anticancer drugs (bone marrow depression, alopecia, oral and gastrointestinal ulceration).

Procarbazine

Mechanism of Action. Procarbazine [Matulane] is a prodrug that is converted to active metabolites in the liver. The metabolites cause chromosomal damage and suppress synthesis of DNA, RNA, and proteins. The precise cause of cell death is not known. Procarbazine is cell-cycle phase *non*specific.

Pharmacokinetics. Procarbazine is readily absorbed following oral administration, but undergoes rapid and extensive hepatic metabolism. Active metabolites are highly lipid soluble and cross the blood-brain barrier with ease. Procarbazine and its metabolites are excreted primarily in the urine.

Therapeutic Uses. The major indication for procarbazine is advanced *Hodgkin's disease*. Other uses include *non-Hodgkin's lymphomas* and *brain tumors*. For treating Hodgkin's disease, procarbazine is combined with mechlorethamine, vincristine [Oncovin], and prednisone, in the so-called MOPP regimen.

Toxicity. The usual dose-limiting toxicity is bone marrow depression. Nausea and vomiting may also be dose limiting. Other adverse effects include peripheral neuropathy, CNS depression, secondary leukemias, and sterility, especially in males.

Procarbazine can interact with other drugs. Because of its CNS effects, procarbazine should not be combined with CNS depressants (e.g., barbiturates, phenothiazines, opioids). Ingestion of alcohol can induce a disulfiram-like response. Because procarbazine inhibits monoamine oxidase, there is a risk of severe hypertension in response to sympathomimetic drugs, tricyclic antidepressants, and tyramine-rich foods.

Dacarbazine

Actions and Uses. Dacarbazine [DTIC-Dome] is a prodrug that is activated by the liver. Although the precise mechanism of cell kill is not known, there is evidence for alkylation of DNA, inhibition of DNA and RNA synthesis, and interaction with sulfhydryl groups on proteins. Dacarbazine is considered cell-cycle phase *non*specific. The principal indication for the drug is

metastatic malignant melanoma, but the response rate is low (about 20%).

Pharmacokinetics. Since gastrointestinal absorption is erratic, procarbazine is administered IV. Penetration to the CNS is poor. Elimination is by hepatic metabolism and renal excretion.

Toxicity. Bone marrow depression is the usual dose-limiting toxicity. Nausea and vomiting occur in most patients, occasionally requiring cessation of treatment. Other toxicities include a flulike syndrome, hepatic necrosis, photosensitivity, and burning pain along the injection site.

Etoposide

Etoposide [VePesid] is derived from podophyllotoxin, a naturally occurring plant alkaloid. The drug inhibits DNA topoisomerase II, and thereby prevents resealing of DNA strand breaks. The resultant damage to DNA arrests the cell cycle in G_2 phase. Etoposide is approved only for *refractory testicular cancer* and *small cell cancer of the lung*.

Administration is oral and intravenous. Penetration to the CNS is low. Most of the drug is eliminated intact in the urine. Hence, dosages must be reduced in patients with renal impairment.

The major dose-limiting toxicity is bone marrow depression. Other toxicities include alopecia, peripheral neuropathy, and mucositis. Early adverse effects include nausea, vomiting, diarrhea, and fever. Hypotension can occur with rapid IV administration.

Teniposide

Teniposide [Vumon] is an analogue of etoposide and shares that drug's mechanism of action: inhibition of DNA topoisomerase II with resultant DNA strand scission and G_2 arrest. The only indication for teniposide is *refractory acute lymphoblastic leukemia of childhood*.

Administration is by slow IV infusion. Most of each dose becomes bound to plasma proteins. Penetration to the CNS is poor. Elimination is by hepatic metabolism and renal excretion.

The major dose-limiting toxicity is bone marrow depression (neutropenia, thrombocytopenia, anemia). Severe hypersensitivity reactions (urticaria, angioedema, bronchospasm, hypotension) occur in about 5% of patients; symptoms can be suppressed with epinephrine. Secondary leukemias have developed within 8 years of initial drug exposure. Other toxicities include nausea, vomiting, diarrhea, and alopecia.

Altretamine (Hexamethylmelamine)

Altretamine [Hexalen], formerly known as hexamethylmelamine, is indicated for palliative therapy of persistent or recurrent ovarian cancer. Altretamine is a prodrug that is converted to active metabolites in the body. The mechanism by which the metabolites act is not known. Altretamine is well absorbed following oral administration, but undergoes rapid and extensive hepatic metabolism. The metabolites are excreted in the urine. The principal dose-limiting toxicity is bone marrow depression. Nausea and vomiting can also be dose limiting. Peripheral sensory neuropathy is common. Central neurotoxicity (tremors, ataxia, vertigo, hallucinations, seizures, depression) is less common. Because of peripheral and central neurotoxicity, patients should receive regular neurologic evaluations.

HORMONES AND HORMONE ANTAGONISTS

The hormones and hormone antagonists are the least toxic of all anticancer drugs. Because these agents act through specific hormone receptors on target tissues, their effects are relatively selective. As a result, these drugs are generally devoid of the severe systemic toxicities that characterize most anticancer agents. The hormonal anticancer drugs fall into five basic categories: (1) androgens and antiandrogens, (2) estrogens and antiestrogens, (3) progestins, (4) gonadotropin-releasing hormone analogues, and (5) glucocorticoids. The principal indications for these drugs are cancers of the breast, endometrium, and prostate. In addition, the glucocorticoids are used against lymphomas and certain leukemias. Trade names, routes of administration, and indications are summarized in Table 91–3.

ANDROGENS AND ANTIANDROGENS

Androgens

The basic pharmacology of the androgens is discussed in in Chapter 54. Consideration here is limited to therapy of cancer.

Therapeutic Use. Androgens are employed for palliative therapy in women with *advanced or metastatic carcinoma of the breast.* It should be noted, however, that tamoxifen is the preferred drug for this indication. Androgen therapy should be instituted only if surgery and irradiation are deemed inappropriate. After a delay of several weeks, objective responses are obtained in 50% to 60% of those treated. Beneficial effects persist for 12 to 14 months. The androgens employed most frequently are *fluoxymesterone* [Halotestin] and *testosterone.*

Adverse Effects. The doses used for breast cancer are high, making virilization is a common side effect. Symptoms include clitoral enlargement, proliferation of facial and body hair, deepening of the voice, increased libido, and male-pattern baldness.

The effects of androgens coupled with the effects of osteolytic metastases can result in severe hypercalcemia. Principal dangers are ectopic calcification (especially in the urinary tract) and disruption of calcium-dependent physiologic processes. If hypercalcemia develops, androgen therapy should be temporarily interrupted and large volumes of fluids should be administered. Androgen therapy may resume once calcium levels have normalized.

Flutamide

Flutamide [Eulexin] is an *antiandrogen.* The drug is indicated only for *metastatic prostate cancer*, and then only in combination with a gonadotropin-releasing hormone agonist, such as leuprolide or goserelin. Flutamide acts by blocking receptors for androgens. Since prostate cells require stimulation of androgen receptors to flourish,

receptor blockade suppresses their growth. In one clinical study, patients receiving flutamide plus leuprolide had a mean survival time of nearly 3 years, compared with 2.3 years for those receiving leuprolide alone.

Flutamide is administered orally and undergoes rapid and complete absorption. Most of each dose is converted to an active metabolite on the first pass through the liver. Parent drug and metabolites are excreted in the urine.

The most common adverse effect is gynecomastia. Nausea, vomiting, and diarrhea are less frequent. Toxic hepatitis has occurred, killing some patients. Hence, liver function should be monitored.

ESTROGENS AND ANTIESTROGENS

Estrogens

Estrogens are used to treat two forms of cancer: *prostate cancer* and *advanced carcinoma of the breast in postmenopausal women.* For patients with either disease, estrogens can offer palliation, and may also induce tumor regression. The estrogen preparations employed most frequently are *diethylstilbestrol diphosphate* [Stilphostrol] and *ethinyl estradiol* [Estinyl]. Adverse effects include nausea, fluid retention, hypercalcemia, depression, and thromboembolic disorders. Gynecomastia may develop in males. Treatment of prostate and breast cancer with estrogens is discussed further in Chapter 55 (Estrogens and Progestins).

Estramustine

Estramustine [Emcyt] is a hybrid molecule composed of estradiol (an estrogen) coupled to nornitrogen mustard (an alkylating agent). The only indication for the drug is palliative therapy of *advanced prostate cancer.* Following oral administration, estramustine becomes concentrated in prostate cells, apparently through the actions of a unique "estramustine binding protein." Cell injury appears to result from two mechanisms. First, estramustine acts as a weak alkylating agent. Second, hydrolysis of estramustine releases free estradiol, which suppresses gonadotropin release, thereby depriving prostate cells of hormonal support.

Adverse effects are caused primarily by free estradiol. Gynecomastia is common. The most serious effect is increased risk of thrombosis, with resultant myocardial infarction and stroke. Other adverse effects include fluid retention, nausea, vomiting, diarrhea, and hypercalcemia.

Tamoxifen

Tamoxifen [Nolvadex] is an *antiestrogen.* The drug binds to estrogen receptors and thereby pre-

Generic Name	Trade Name	Route	Indications
Androgens			
Fluoxymesterone	Halotestin	PO	Breast cancer
Testosterone	generic only	PO	Breast cancer
Antiandrogen			
Flutamide	Eulexin	PO	Metastatic prostate cancer
Estrogens			
Diethylstilbestrol diphosphate	Stilphostrol	PO, IV	Prostate and breast cancer
Ethinyl estradiol	Estinyl	PO	Prostate and breast cancer
Estrogen Mustard			
Estramustine	Emcyt	PO	Prostate cancer
Antiestrogen			
Tamoxifen	Nolvadex	PO	Breast cancer
Progestins			
Medroxyprogesterone acetate	Depo-Provera	PO, IM	Endometrial cancer
Megestrol	Megace	PO	Breast and endometrial cancer
Gn-RH Analogues*			
Leuprolide	Lupron	IM, SC	Prostate cancer
Goserelin	Zoladex	SC	Prostate cancer
Glucocorticoid			
Prednisone	Deltasone, others	PO	Acute and chronic lymphocytic leukemias, Hodgkin's and non-Hodgkin's lymphomas

*Gonadotropin-releasing hormone analogues.

vents their activation by estradiol, the major naturally occurring estrogen. If tamoxifen is to be of benefit, target cells must be estrogen-receptor (ER) positive. That is, they must possess receptors for estrogens. In pre- and postmenopausal women with *advanced ER-positive carcinoma of the breast*, tamoxifen is the current treatment of choice. The most common adverse effects are nausea, vomiting, hot flushes, and menstrual irregularities. In bone, tamoxifen acts like a weak estrogen. Hence, the drug does not promote osteoporosis. Administration is oral.

PROGESTINS

Two progestins are employed to treat cancers: *medroxyprogesterone acetate* [Depo-Provera] and *megestrol* [Megace]. Both drugs are indicated for *advanced endometrial carcinoma*. Megestrol is also indicated for *advanced breast cancer*. In women with metastatic endometrial cancer, progestins can cause palliation and tumor regression. About 30% of patients have objective responses. Among those who respond, survival time is increased to about 2 years. This compares with survival times of 6 months among nonresponders. Patients with

tumors that test positive for progesterone receptors are most likely to respond. However, the exact mechanism by which progestins suppress tumor growth is not known. The principal adverse effects of progestins are fluid retention and nonfluid weight gain. Hypercalcemia may occur if bone metastases are present. Progestins are teratogens and should be avoided during the first 4 months of pregnancy. The basic pharmacology of the progestins is discussed in Chapter 55 (Estrogens and Progestins).

GONADOTROPIN-RELEASING HORMONE ANALOGUES

Leuprolide

Therapeutic Use. Leuprolide [Lupron] is a synthetic analogue of *gonadotropin-releasing hormone* (GnRH), which is also known as *luteinizing hormone releasing hormone* (LH-RH). Leuprolide is indicated for *advanced carcinoma of the prostate*. Although the drug does not alter the course of this disease, it does offer palliation. For patients with prostate cancer, leuprolide is an alternative to orchiectomy (castration) and estrogen therapy. Since the drug does not produce the emotional trauma of orchiectomy or the thromboembolic disorders associated with estrogens, leuprolide is often preferred to these other treatments. Leuprolide may be administered daily (by SC injection) or monthly (by IM injection using a depot formulation).

Mechanism of Action. Cells of the prostate, both normal and neoplastic, are testosterone dependent. Leuprolide provides palliation by suppressing testosterone production. During the initial phase of treatment, leuprolide *mimics* the actions of GnRH. That is, the drug acts on the pituitary to *stimulate* release of interstitial cell-stimulating hormone (ICSH), which acts on the testes to *increase* production of testosterone. However, with continuous exposure to leuprolide, pituitary GnRH receptors become desensitized. As a result, release of ICSH *declines*, causing testosterone production to decline as well. After several weeks of treatment, testosterone levels are equivalent to those seen after castration.

Adverse Effects. Leuprolide is generally well tolerated. Hot flushes are the most common adverse effect, but these usually attenuate as treatment progresses. Impotence and loss of libido may occur. During the initial weeks of treatment, *elevation* of testosterone levels may aggravate symptoms (bone pain, urinary obstruction) of prostate cancer. As a result, patients with vertebral metastases or pre-existing obstruction of the urinary tract may find treatment intolerable.

Goserelin

Goserelin [Zoladex], like leuprolide, is a GnRH analogue used for *advanced prostate cancer*. Both drugs share the same mechanism of action and adverse effects. Administration of goserelin is unique. The drug is formulated as a pellet that is dispensed in a syringe with a 16-gauge needle. The pellet is implanted by SC injection in the upper abdominal wall. Local anesthesia may be used prior to the injection.

GLUCOCORTICOIDS

The basic pharmacology of the glucocorticoids is discussed in Chapter 62 (Glucocorticoids in Nonendocrine Diseases). Discussion here is limited to the use of glucocorticoids in cancer.

Glucocorticoids (e.g., *prednisone*) are used in combination with other agents to treat cancers arising from lymphoid tissue. Specific indications are *acute and chronic lymphocytic leukemias, Hodgkin's disease,* and *non-Hodgkin's lymphomas.* Glucocorticoids are beneficial in these cancers because of their direct toxicity to lymphoid tissues: high-dose therapy causes suppression of mitosis, dissolution of lymphocytes, regression of lymphatic tissue, and cell death. When used acutely, glucocorticoids are devoid of significant adverse effects. However, with prolonged treatment, these drugs can cause a broad spectrum of serious toxicities,

including adrenal insufficiency, increased susceptibility to infection, peptic ulcers, fluid and electrolyte disturbances, osteoporosis, myopathy, growth retardation, and cutaneous atrophy.

In addition to their use against lymphoid-derived cancers, glucocorticoids are used to manage complications of cancer and cancer therapy. Specific benefits include suppression of chemotherapy-induced nausea and vomiting, reduction of cerebral edema secondary to irradiation of the cranium, reduction of pain secondary to nerve compression or edema, and suppression of hypercalcemia in steroid-responsive tumors. In addition, glucocorticoids can improve appetite, promote weight gain, and impart a generalized sense of well-being.

BIOLOGIC RESPONSE MODIFIERS

Biologic response modifiers are drugs that alter host responses to cancer. Many of these drugs are immunostimulants that enhance host defenses against cancer. Some render cancer cells nonmalignant by causing them to differentiate into nonproliferative forms. Some (hematopoietic growth factors) enable the host to better tolerate the myelosuppressive actions of anticancer drugs (see Chapter 48). All of the biologic response modifiers discussed in this chapter are immunostimulants. Their trade names, indications, and routes of administration are summarized in Table 91–4.

Interferon Alfa-2a and Interferon Alfa-2b

Interferons are naturally occurring proteins with complex antiviral, anticancer, and immunomodulatory actions. Release of endogenous interferons is triggered by viral infections and other stimuli. Interferons are active against a variety of solid tumors and hematologic malignancies. They are also active against several viruses (see Chapter 84).

Description. Interferon alfa-2a [Roferon-A] and interferon alfa-2b [Intron A] are glycoproteins that contain 165 amino acids. These two drugs, referred to collectively as interferon alfa-2, are identical except for 1 amino acid. Commercial production is by recombinant DNA technology.

Mechanism of Action. Anticancer effects are thought to result from two basic processes: (1) enhancement of host immune responses, and (2) direct antiproliferative effects on cancer cells. Both processes are mediated by binding of interferons to cell-surface receptors, with resultant increased expression of certain genes and reduced expression of other genes. Interferons can cause G_0 cells to remain dormant, thereby preventing their prolif-

Table 91–4. Anticancer Drugs: Biologic Response Modifiers

Generic Name	Trade Name	Route	Indications
Interferon Alfa-2a	Roferon-A	IM, IV , SC	Hairy cell leukemia, AIDS-related Kaposi's sarcoma*
Interferon Alfa-2b	Intron A		
Aldesleukin (Interleukin-2)	Proleukin	IV	Metastatic renal cell cancer
Levamisole	Ergamisol	PO	Stage II colon cancer (combination therapy with fluorouracil)
BCG Live	TheraCys	Intravesical	In situ bladder cancer
BCG Vaccine	TICE BCG		

*In addition to these approved indications, interferons have been used to treat many other cancers, including acute leukemias, chronic myelogenous leukemia, and cancers of the bladder, ovary, and kidney.

eration. In addition, interferons can cause proliferating cells to differentiate into nonproliferative mature forms.

Antineoplastic Uses. Interferons alfa-2a and alfa-2b are approved only for *hairy cell leukemia* and *AIDS-related Kaposi's sarcoma*. However, these drugs are active against many other cancers, including *acute leukemias, chronic myelogenous leukemia,* and *cancers of the bladder, ovary, and kidney.* Response rates are generally higher with hematologic cancers than with solid tumors.

Pharmacokinetics. Interferon alfa-2 is administered by IM or SC injection. Plasma drug levels peak in 4 to 8 hours. Inactivation occurs rapidly in body fluids and tissues. No intact drug appears in the urine.

Adverse Effects. Interferon alfa-2 causes multiple adverse effects. The most common is a flulike syndrome characterized by fever, fatigue, myalgia, headache, and chills. Symptoms tend to diminish with continued therapy. Some symptoms (fever, headache, myalgia) can be reduced with acetaminophen. Other common effects include anorexia, weight loss, diarrhea, abdominal pain, dizziness, and cough. Prolonged or high-dose therapy can cause bone marrow depression, thyroid dysfunction, alopecia, cardiotoxicity, and neurotoxicity, including profound fatigue and depression.

Aldesleukin (Interleukin-2)

Aldesleukin [Proleukin], also known as interleukin-2, is an immunostimulant used for advanced renal carcinoma. Because severe adverse effects are very common, the drug must be administered in a hospital that has an intensive care facility; a specialist in cardiopulmonary or intensive care medicine must be available.

Description and Actions. Aldesleukin is a large glycoprotein nearly identical in structure and actions to human interleukin-2. The drug is produced by recombinant DNA technology. Like interleukin-2, aldesleukin stimulates immune function. Specific responses include increased production and cytotoxicity of lymphocytes; increased production of interleukin-1, interferon gamma, and tumor necrosis factor; and induction of lymphokine-activated killer (LAK) cell activity. The exact mechanism of antitumor action is not known.

Therapeutic Use. Aldesleukin is approved only for *metastatic renal cell cancer in adults.* Objective responses occur in about 15% of patients (4% respond completely and 11% partially). The median duration of responses (complete and partial) is approximately 2 years. Investigational uses include *Kaposi's sarcoma, melanoma,* and *colorectal cancer.*

Pharmacokinetics. Aldesleukin is administered by intravenous infusion and distributes throughout the extracellular space. About 70% of each dose undergoes preferential uptake by the liver, kidneys, and lungs. Renal enzymes convert the drug into inactive metabolites, which are then excreted in the urine. Aldesleukin has an elimination half-life of just 85 minutes.

Adverse Effects. Practically all patients experience significant toxicity, and the fatality rate is high (4%). Effects seen most frequently are fever and chills (89%), nausea and vomiting (87%), hypotension (85%), anemia (77%), diarrhea (76%), altered mental status (76%), sinus tachycardia (70%), impaired renal function (61%), impaired liver function (56%), pulmonary congestion (54%), dyspnea (52%), and pruritus (48%).

Capillary leak syndrome (CLS) is of particular concern. This potentially fatal reaction is characterized by hypotension and reduced organ perfusion secondary to loss of vascular tone and extravasation of plasma proteins and fluid. Symptoms begin to develop immediately after treatment. CLS may be associated with angina pectoris, cardiac dysrhythmias, myocardial infarction, pronounced respiratory insufficiency, renal insufficiency, GI bleeding, and altered mental status. Because of the risk of CLS, aldesleukin must not be given to patients with cardiac, pulmonary, renal, hepatic, or CNS impairment. Careful monitoring is essential.

Levamisole

Actions. Levamisole [Ergamisol] is an immunostimulant. The drug can help restore immune responses that are depressed, but does not enhance responses that are normal. Specific effects include increased antibody formation, increased proliferation and activity of T-cells, and increased function of neutrophils, monocytes, and macrophages. The precise mechanism underlying these effects is not known.

Therapeutic Use. Levamisole, in combination with fluorouracil, is approved only for adjuvant therapy following surgical resection of *stage III colon cancer.* Although levamisole or fluorouracil *alone* has little effect, the *combination* produces a 41% decrease in the risk of cancer recurrence and a 33% decrease in mortality (as compared with surgical controls who received no adjuvant therapy).

Pharmacokinetics. Levamisole is administered orally and is rapidly absorbed. The drug undergoes extensive hepatic metabolism followed by urinary excretion. Fluorouracil, which is used together with levamisole, is administered IV.

Adverse Effects. Reactions to levamisole alone are infrequent and mild. In contrast, reactions to levamisole plus fluorouracil can be severe, but these are due primarily to the fluorouracil. The principal dose-limiting toxicity of the combination is bone marrow suppression. The most common responses to the combination are nausea, vomiting, and diarrhea. Other reactions include alopecia, oral and GI ulceration, flulike symptoms, metallic taste, dizziness, and arthralgia.

BCG Live and BCG Vaccine

Description and Therapeutic Use. BCG live [TheraCys] and BCG vaccine [TICE BCG] are freeze-dried preparations of attenuated strains of *Mycobacterium bovis* (bacillus of Calmette and Guerin). Both preparations are approved for primary and relapsed *carcinoma in situ of the bladder*, both in the presence and absence of associated papillary tumors. However, neither preparation should be used for papillary tumors alone. To treat bladder cancers, BCG is administered intravesically (i.e., directly into the bladder through a urethral catheter).

Mechanism of Action. BCG is a nonspecific immunostimulant. Instillation in the bladder produces a local inflammatory response that, by an unknown mechanism, promotes regression of tumor lesions in the urothelial lining.

Adverse Effects. The most common adverse effects, which result from bladder irritation, are dysuria, urinary frequency, urinary urgency, and hematuria. Urinary status should be monitored closely. The most common systemic reactions are malaise, fatigue, fever, and chills.

Since BCG live and BCG vaccine consist of live *Mycobacterium bovis*, therapy carries a risk of systemic infection, including fatal septic shock. Accordingly, these BCG preparations are contraindicated for (1) immunocompromised patients (e.g., those taking immunosuppressant drugs, those with symptomatic or asymptomatic HIV infection), (2) patients with fever of unknown origin (since it may signify infection), and (3) patients with urinary tract infections (since there is an increased risk of systemic absorption of BCG).

Since BCG preparations are infectious, they must be handled using aseptic technique. All materials employed during administration should be disposed of in plastic bags labeled "Infectious Waste." Urine voided within 6 hours of BCG instillation should be disinfected with an equal volume of 5% hypochlorite before flushing.

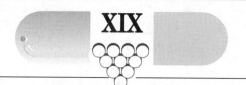

Immunosuppressive Drugs

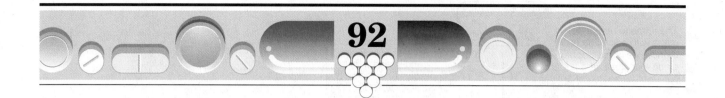

92

Immunosuppressive Drugs

THE IMMUNE RESPONSE AND SITES OF
DRUG ACTION

PHARMACOLOGY OF THE
IMMUNOSUPPRESSIVE DRUGS
  Cyclosporine
  Glucocorticoids
  Cytotoxic Drugs
  Antibodies

Immunosuppressive drugs inhibit immune responses. These agents have two principal applications: (1) prevention of organ rejection in transplant patients, and (2) treatment of autoimmune disorders (e.g., rheumatoid arthritis, systemic lupus erythematosus). At the doses required to suppress allograft rejection, all of these drugs are toxic. Two toxicities are of particular concern: (1) increased risk of infection, and (2) increased risk of neoplasms.

THE IMMUNE RESPONSE AND SITES OF DRUG ACTION

Four major cell types participate in the immune response. These are (1) macrophages and monocytes, (2) helper T lymphocytes, (3) cytotoxic T lymphocytes, and (4) B lymphocytes (Fig. 92–1). The roles of these cells and the effects of immunosuppressive drugs on them are discussed below.

Macrophages and Monocytes. The immune response begins with macrophages and monocytes. These cells phagocytize antigen, process it, and then present it to helper T cells. At the same time, these macrophages and monocytes elaborate interleukin-1 and other small proteins. As indicated in Figure 92–1, we can block these initial steps with *glucocorticoids* (e.g., prednisone).

Helper T Lymphocytes. T lymphocytes are derived from the thymus. Activation of helper T cells by macrophages and monocytes requires stimula-

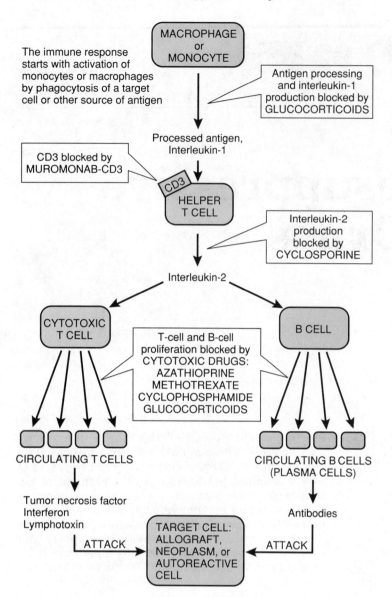

The immune response starts with activation of monocytes or macrophages by phagocytosis of a target cell or other source of antigen

MACROPHAGE or MONOCYTE

Antigen processing and interleukin-1 production blocked by GLUCOCORTICOIDS

Processed antigen, Interleukin-1

CD3 blocked by MUROMONAB-CD3

CD3

HELPER T CELL

Interleukin-2 production blocked by CYCLOSPORINE

Interleukin-2

CYTOTOXIC T CELL

B CELL

T-cell and B-cell proliferation blocked by CYTOTOXIC DRUGS: AZATHIOPRINE METHOTREXATE CYCLOPHOSPHAMIDE GLUCOCORTICOIDS

CIRCULATING T CELLS

CIRCULATING B CELLS (PLASMA CELLS)

Tumor necrosis factor Interferon Lymphotoxin

ATTACK

Antibodies

TARGET CELL: ALLOGRAFT, NEOPLASM, or AUTOREACTIVE CELL

ATTACK

Figure 92–1. Sites of action of immunosuppressive drugs. The figure depicts the cells of the immune system and the points at which immunosuppressive drugs act to inhibit immune responses. See text for details.

tion of a surface receptor, part of which is designated *cell differentiation complex 3* (CD3). We can prevent this activation by blocking CD3 with a drug called *muromonab-CD3*, a monoclonal antibody that selectively binds to CD3.

Once the helper T cell is activated, it acts on cytotoxic T lymphocytes and B lymphocytes to stimulate their proliferation. This stimulation is accomplished in part through production of interleukin-2. We can block production of interleukin-2 and subsequent activation of B cells and cytotoxic T cells with *cyclosporine* (see Fig. 92–1).

Cytotoxic T Lymphocytes. Cytotoxic or "killer" T cells are responsible for cellular immunity. These cells do not make antibodies. Rather, they act directly to kill target cells. Cytotoxic T lymphocytes destroy their targets by direct cell-to-

cell contact and by secretion of toxic compounds (lymphotoxin, interferon, tumor necrosis factor).

Following activation, the cytotoxic T cell undergoes rapid proliferation to produce the cells that are actually responsible for killing target cells. We can block this proliferative stage with *cytotoxic drugs* (azathioprine, methotrexate, cyclophosphamide) and *glucocorticoids* (see Fig. 92–1).

B Lymphocytes. B cells, which are derived from bone marrow, are responsible for humoral immunity. It is the B lymphocytes that make antibodies. Following activation by helper T cells, B cells undergo proliferation to produce plasma cells, the cells ultimately responsible for antibody production. Like the proliferation of T cells, the proliferation of B cells can be blocked with *cytotoxic drugs* and *glucocorticoids*.

PHARMACOLOGY OF THE IMMUNOSUPPRESSIVE DRUGS

CYCLOSPORINE

Cyclosporine [Sandimmune] is the most effective immunosuppressant available, and is the drug of choice for preventing organ rejection following allogenic transplants. Major adverse effects are nephrotoxicity and increased risk of infection.

Mechanism of Action

Cyclosporine acts on helper T cells to suppress production of interleukin-2 and other lymphokines. The drug's primary molecular target on helper T cells appears to be a group of proteins known as *cyclophilins*. In contrast to cytotoxic immunosuppressants (e.g., methotrexate), cyclosporine does not depress the bone marrow.

Therapeutic Uses

Cyclosporine is our most effective immunosuppressant. The drug is used primarily to prevent rejection of allogenic kidney, liver, and heart transplants. A glucocorticoid (prednisone) is usually given concurrently. In addition to its use in transplant patients, cyclosporine has been employed on an investigational basis to treat autoimmune diseases, including rheumatoid arthritis, psoriasis, myasthenia gravis, and early stages of insulin-dependent diabetes.

Pharmacokinetics

Oral administration is preferred; intravenous administration is reserved for patients who cannot take the drug orally. Absorption from the gastrointestinal (GI) tract is incomplete (about 30%) and variable. Accordingly, to avoid toxicity (from high drug levels) and organ rejection (from low drug levels), blood levels of cyclosporine should be measured periodically during long-term use.

Most cyclosporine in the body is bound. In the blood the drug is bound to red cells (60% to 70%), leukocytes (10% to 20%), and plasma lipoproteins. Outside the vascular system the drug is bound to tissues.

Cyclosporine undergoes extensive metabolism by hepatic microsomal enzymes. Hence, drugs that increase or decrease the activity of microsomal enzymes can have a significant impact on cyclosporine levels. Excretion of cyclosporine and its metabolites is via the bile. Practically none of the drug appears in the urine.

Adverse Effects

The most common adverse effects are nephrotoxicity, infection, hypertension, tremor, and hirsu-tism. Of these, nephrotoxicity and infection are the most serious.

Nephrotoxicity. Renal damage occurs in 25% to 38% of patients. Injury manifests as reduced renal blood flow and reduced glomerular filtration rate. These effects are dose dependent and usually reverse following a decrease in cyclosporine dosage.

Nephrotoxicity is evaluated by monitoring for elevated blood urea nitrogen (BUN) and serum creatinine. However, be aware that a rise in these values could also indicate rejection of a kidney transplant. Patients should be informed about the possibility of kidney damage and the importance of periodic tests for BUN and creatinine.

Infection. Cyclosporine increases the risk of infection, although less so than the cytotoxic immunosuppressants. Infectious complications occur in 74% of those treated. Except for glucocorticoids, other immunosuppressants (e.g., cyclophosphamide, azathioprine) should not be combined with cyclosporine. Patients should be warned about early signs of infection (fever, sore throat) and instructed to report these immediately.

Hepatotoxicity. Liver damage occurs in 4% to 7% of patients. Injury is evaluated by monitoring for serum bilirubin and liver transaminases. Signs of liver injury reverse rapidly with a reduction in dosage. Inform the patient about the need for periodic tests of liver function.

Lymphomas. Cyclosporine and other immunosuppressants can cause lymphoproliferative diseases. The incidence with cyclosporine alone is low. However, when cyclosporine is combined with other immunosuppressants, the risk of malignant lymphomas increases.

Other Common Adverse Effects. *Hypertension*, indicated by a 10% to 15% increase in blood pressure, develops in 13% to 53% of patients. *Tremor* (21% to 55%) and *hirsutism* (21% to 45%) are also common. Less frequently, patients experience *leukopenia* (6%), *gingival hyperplasia* (4%), *gynecomastia* (4%), *sinusitis* (3% to 7%), and *hyperkalemia*.

Use in Pregnancy and Lactation. At doses 2 to 5 times those used clinically, cyclosporine is embryotoxic and fetotoxic to rats and rabbits. However, experience to date shows minimal fetal risk in humans. Nonetheless, prudence dictates that the drug be avoided during pregnancy if possible. Patients taking cyclosporine should be advised to use a mechanical form of contraception (condom, diaphragm); oral contraceptives should not be used. Cyclosporine is classified in FDA Pregnancy Category C. The drug is excreted in breast milk and nursing should be avoided.

Anaphylactic Reactions. These reactions are rare, occurring in 1 patient per 1000 treated. Signs of anaphylaxis are flushing, respiratory distress, hypotension, and tachycardia. Anaphylaxis occurs only with IV therapy—not with oral cyclosporine. Patients should be monitored for 30 minutes after the onset of IV treatment. If anaphylaxis develops, discontinue the infusion and treat with epinephrine and oxygen.

Drug Interactions

Many interactions with other drugs have been reported. However, only a few appear to be of clinical significance. Important interactions are considered below.

Drugs That Can Decrease Cyclosporine Levels. Drugs that induce hepatic microsomal enzymes can accelerate metabolism of cyclosporine, causing cyclosporine levels to fall. This can result in organ rejection. Drugs known to lower cyclosporine levels include *phenytoin*, *phenobarbital*, *rifampin*, and *trimethoprim-sulfamethoxazole*. Cyclosporine levels should be monitored and the dosage adjusted in patients taking these drugs.

Drugs That Can Increase Cyclosporine Levels. *Ketoconazole* and *erythromycin* can elevate cyclosporine levels (by inhibiting hepatic microsomal enzymes). When either of these drugs is combined with cyclosporine, the dosage of cyclosporine must be reduced to prevent accumulation to toxic levels.

Some physicians administer ketoconazole concurrently with cyclosporine for the express purpose of permitting a reduction in cyclosporine dosage. By slowing metabolism of cyclosporine, ketoconazole permits cyclosporine dosage to be reduced by up to 88%, while continuing to maintain cyclosporine levels within the therapeutic range. The lowered dosage greatly reduces the cost of treatment—from between $5000 and $8000 per year to about $1000 per year.

Nephrotoxic Drugs. Renal damage may be intensified by concurrent use of other nephrotoxic drugs. These include *amphotericin B*, *aminoglycosides*, and *nonsteroidal anti-inflammatory drugs*.

Preparations, Dosage, and Administration

Preparations and Storage. Cyclosporine [Sandimmune] is available in capsules (25 and 100 mg) and solution (100 mg/ml) for oral use, and in a 50 mg/ml solution for IV use. The drug should be stored at room temperature.

Oral Therapy. To improve palatability, the oral solution can be mixed with milk, chocolate milk, or orange juice just before administration. The initial dose is 15 mg/kg given 4 to 24 hours prior to surgery. This dose is continued once daily for 1 to 2 weeks. Dosage is then gradually reduced to a maintenance level of 3 to 10 mg/kg/day.

Intravenous Therapy. One ml of concentrate is diluted in 20 to 100 ml of 0.9% sodium chloride or 5% dextrose. The initial dose is 5 to 6 mg/kg (one-third the oral dose) administered over 2 to 6 hours. The solution should be protected from light. Because of the risk of anaphylaxis, epinephrine and oxygen must be immediately available. The patient should be switched to oral therapy as soon as possible.

Monitoring. Dosage is adjusted on the basis of nephrotoxicity and cyclosporine levels. Blood for drug levels is drawn just prior to the next dose. Target levels are generally 50 to 100 ng/ml in *plasma* or 250 to 800 ng/ml in *whole blood*.

GLUCOCORTICOIDS

Glucocorticoids are used widely to suppress immune responses. Immunosuppressant applications range from suppression of transplant rejection to treatment of asthma to treatment of autoimmune disorders, such as rheumatoid arthritis and systemic lupus erythematosus.

Glucocorticoids have multiple effects on elements of the immune system. They cause lysis of antigen-activated lymphocytes, suppression of lymphocyte proliferation, and sequestration of lymphocytes at extravascular locations. In addition, they reduce production of interleukin-2 by monocytes and lymphocytes, and they reduce the responsiveness of T lymphocytes to interleukin-1.

Immunosuppressive doses are large. For example, to prevent organ rejection, an initial dose of 0.5 to 2 mg/kg of prednisone is employed. To treat episodes of acute organ rejection, 500 to 1500 mg of IV methylprednisolone is given.

Because large doses are employed, the full range of glucocorticoid adverse effects can be expected. These include increased risk of infection, thinning of the skin, bone dissolution with resultant fractures, impaired growth in children, and suppression of the hypothalamic-pituitary-adrenal axis.

The pharmacology of glucocorticoids is discussed at length in Chapter 62 (Glucocorticoids in Nonendocrine Diseases).

CYTOTOXIC DRUGS

Cytotoxic drugs suppress immune responses by killing T and B lymphocytes that are undergoing proliferation. Unfortunately, these drugs, like the anticancer drugs, are also toxic to all other proliferating cells. As a result, they can cause bone marrow depression, gastrointestinal disturbances, reduced fertility, and alopecia. Neutropenia and thrombocytopenia from bone marrow suppression are of particular concern. Because of their serious adverse effects, the cytotoxic drugs are usually reserved for patients who do not respond to safer immunosuppressants (cyclosporine and glucocorticoids).

Azathioprine

Mechanism of Action. Azathioprine suppresses cell-mediated and humoral immune responses by inhibiting the proliferation of T and B lymphocytes. Azathioprine is a prodrug and must be converted to its active form—mercaptopurine—in the body. Mercaptopurine suppresses cell proliferation by inhibiting DNA synthesis. Hence, the drug acts selectively during the S phase of the cell cycle. As discussed in Chapter 91, mercaptopurine itself is used to treat cancer.

Therapeutic Uses. Prior to the advent of cyclosporine, azathioprine (combined with prednisone) was the principal drug employed to suppress rejection of renal transplants. The drug still has this indication. In addition, azathioprine is approved for severe refractory rheumatoid arthritis in nonpregnant adults (see Chapter 63). Azathioprine has been used on an investigational basis to treat various autoimmune diseases, including myasthenia gravis, systemic lupus erythematosus, Crohn's disease, and insulin-dependent diabetes.

Adverse Effects and Interactions. Although uncommon at usual therapeutic doses, neutropenia and thrombocytopenia from bone marrow suppression can be serious concerns. Accordingly, patients should receive complete blood counts at regular intervals. Azathioprine is mutagenic and teratogenic in animals, and should be avoided during pregnancy. Long-term therapy is associated with an increased incidence of neoplasms.

Allopurinol delays conversion of mercaptopurine to inactive products, increasing the risk of toxicity. If allopurinol and azathioprine are used concurrently, the dose of azathioprine must be reduced by about 70%.

Preparations, Dosage, and Administration. Azathioprine [Imuran] is available in 50-mg tablets for oral administration, and as a powder to be reconstituted with sterile water for IV administration. Immunosuppressive therapy is initiated with a single daily dose of 3 to 5 mg/kg, usually beginning on the day of renal transplantation. Daily maintenance doses range from 1 to 3 mg/kg. Oral administration is preferred to intravenous.

Cyclophosphamide

Cyclophosphamide, an anticancer drug, is discussed at length in Chapter 91. Discussion here is limited to its immunosuppressant actions. Cyclophosphamide is a prodrug that is converted to its active form by the liver. The active form is an alkylating agent that cross-links DNA, leading to cell injury and death. Immunosuppressant effects result from a decrease in the number and activity of B and T lymphocytes. Toxicity to other cells produces adverse effects. These include neutropenia (from bone marrow suppression), hemorrhagic cystitis, and sterility in males and females. Cyclophosphamide has been used for its immunosuppressant actions to treat rheumatoid arthritis, systemic lupus erythematosus, and multiple sclerosis. The drug is as effective as azathioprine for suppressing rejection of renal transplants.

Methotrexate

Methotrexate is an anticancer drug (see Chapter 91) that is also employed for immunosuppression. As an immunosuppressant, the drug is approved for severe, refractory rheumatoid arthritis (see Chapter 63) and psoriasis. Methotrexate has also been used to suppress graft-versus-host disease in bone marrow recipients. These beneficial effects result from suppression of B and T lymphocytes secondary to interference with folate metabolism. The doses employed for immunosuppression are lower than those employed to treat cancers. As a result, toxicities differ with the two applications: in cancer therapy, bone marrow suppression, ulcerative stomatitis, and renal damage are primary concerns, whereas in immunosuppressive therapy, hepatic fibrosis and cirrhosis are primary concerns.

ANTIBODIES

Antibodies directed against components of the immune system can suppress immune responses. Three preparations are considered here. Two of these—muromonab-CD3 and antithymocyte globulin—are used to manage allograft rejection in renal transplant recipients. The third—Rh$_o$(D) immune globulin—is used to prevent reactions to Rh-positive blood in Rh-negative women.

Muromonab-CD3

Actions and Uses. Muromonab-CD3 is a monoclonal antibody developed in mice and directed against the CD3 site on human T lymphocytes. Upon binding to the CD3 site, the antibody blocks all T cell functions. All T cells—both those in the circulation and those in tissues—are affected. Muromonab-CD3 is approved for treatment of acute allograft rejection of renal transplants. In addition,

the drug has been used with success on an investigational basis to prevent rejection of heart and liver transplants.

Adverse Effects. Relatively mild reactions are common. These include fever (73%), chills (59%), dyspnea (21%), chest pain (14%), and nausea and vomiting (12%). These effects are most intense on the first day of treatment and then rapidly subside. In addition to these moderate reactions, severe pulmonary edema can occur. This reaction, although relatively rare (2%), can be fatal. Accordingly, patients should be monitored closely.

Preparations, Dosage, and Administration. Muromonab-CD3 [Orthoclone OKT3] is dispensed in solution (5 mg/5 ml) for IV administration. The usual dosage is 5 mg/day for 10 to 14 days. Administration is by IV bolus. The preparation should be drawn through a filter before injection. Treatment is begun following diagnosis of acute transplant rejection. To minimize first-dose adverse reactions, the patient should be pretreated with IV glucocorticoids.

Lymphocyte Immune Globulin, Antithymocyte Globulin (Equine)

Basic Pharmacology. Lymphocyte immune globulin is used to suppress rejection of renal transplants. The drug is prepared by immunizing horses with human T lymphocytes. Beneficial effects of the drug derive from a decrease in the number and activity of thymus-derived lymphocytes. Lymphocyte immune globulin is usually employed together with glucocorticoids and azathioprine. Because these other immunosuppressants are present, immune reactions to this horse-derived drug are generally mild (chills, fever, leukopenia, skin reactions). However, anaphylactic reactions can occur. Accordingly, epinephrine and facilities for respiratory support should be immediately available.

Preparations, Dosage, and Administration. Lymphocyte immune globulin [Atgam] is dispensed in solution (50 mg/ml) for IV administration. The concentrate should be diluted in saline according to the manufacturer's instructions, and the infusion apparatus should have an in-line filter. The usual adult dosage is 10 to 30 mg/kg/day administered over 4 hours or more. To minimize phlebitis, a high-flow vein should be employed. The patient must be monitored for anaphylaxis.

Rh$_o$(D) Immune Globulin

Actions and Uses. Rh$_o$(D) immune globulin (RhIG) is a concentrated preparation of immune globulin containing antibodies to Rh$_o$(D). RhIG is given to prevent development of antibodies to Rh$_o$(D) in Rh$_o$(D)-negative women following exposure to Rh$_o$(D)-positive blood. Such exposure can occur in association with an Rh$_o$(D)-positive pregnancy (as a result of the pregnancy itself, full-term delivery, spontaneous or induced abortion, or amniocentesis). RhIG acts by suppressing the immune response of Rh-negative women to Rh-positive blood cells. In many medical centers, RhIG is administered routinely at 28 weeks of gestation to all Rh$_o$(D)-negative women.

Adverse Effects, Precautions, Contraindications. Undesired reactions are uncommon and mild. Temperature may rise slightly. RhIG is contraindicated for Rh-positive women and must not be administered to newborns.

Preparations, Dosage, and Administration. Rh$_o$(D) immune globulin [Gamulin, RhoGAM, others] is dispensed in vials and prefilled syringes. Administration is intramuscular—never intravenous. Prevention of anti-Rh$_o$(D) antibody formation is most successful if the drug is administered twice: at 28 weeks of gestation and again within 72 hours after delivery.

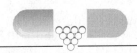

Summary of Major Nursing Implications

CYCLOSPORINE

 Preadministration Assessment

Therapeutic Goal

Prevention of allograft rejection.

Baseline Data

Obtain baseline data on kidney function (serum creatinine, BUN), liver function (AST, ALT, serum amylase, bilirubin, alkaline phosphatase), and serum potassium levels.

Identifying High-Risk Patients

Cyclosporine is *contraindicated* in the presence of *hypersensitivity to cyclosporine or to its intravenous vehicle (polyoxyethylated castor oil), pregnancy, recent inoculation with live-virus vaccines,* and *recent contact with or active infection with chickenpox or herpes zoster.*

The drug should be used with *caution* in patients using *potassium-sparing diuretics* and in those with *intestinal malabsorption, hypertension, hyperkalemia, active infection,* and *renal or hepatic dysfunction.*

 Implementation: Administration

Routes

Oral, intravenous.

Patient Education for Oral Administration

Dispense the oral liquid into a glass container using the specially calibrated pipette. Mix well and drink immediately. Rinse the container with diluent and drink to insure ingestion of the complete dose. Dry the outside of the pipette and return to its cover for storage.

To improve palatability, mix the concentrated drug solution with milk, chocolate milk, or orange juice just before administration.

Intravenous Dosage and Administration

Dilute 1 ml of concentrate in 20 to 100 ml of 0.9% sodium chloride or 5% dextrose. Protect from light. Administer the initial dose (5 to 6 mg/kg) slowly—over 2 to 6 hours. Because of the risk of anaphylactic reactions, monitor the patient closely for 30 minutes after beginning administration; have epinephrine and oxygen available. Switch to oral therapy as soon as possible.

Dosage Adjustment

Adjust dosage on the basis of nephrotoxicity and cyclosporine levels. Draw blood for drug levels just prior to the next dose. Target levels are 50 to 100 ng/ml in *plasma* or 250 to 800 ng/ml in *whole blood.*

Storage

Store at room temperature — do not refrigerate or freeze.

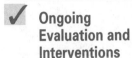

Ongoing Evaluation and Interventions

Evaluating Therapeutic Effects

Graft tenderness or fever may indicate rejection. In renal transplant patients, elevated BUN and elevated serum creatinine in conjunction with low cyclosporine may indicate rejection. Therapeutic failure can be confirmed with ultrasound, a biopsy, or renal flow scan.

Minimizing Adverse Effects

Nephrotoxicity. Cyclosporine can cause a dose-dependent reduction in kidney function. Monitor for elevation of serum creatinine and BUN. Inform outpatients about the importance of receiving periodic tests of kidney function.

Infection. Cyclosporine increases the risk of infection. Inform patients about early signs of infection (fever, sore throat), and instruct them to report these immediately.

Hepatotoxicity. Cyclosporine causes reversible liver damage. Monitor for elevation of serum bilirubin and liver transaminases. Inform patients about the need for periodic tests of liver function.

Hirsutism. Cyclosporine promotes hair growth. Assure the patient that this effect is reversible.

Use in Pregnancy and Lactation. Cyclosporine is embryotoxic. Advise women of child-bearing age to use a mechanical form of contraception (diaphragm, condom) and avoid oral contraceptives. Cyclosporine is excreted in breast milk; warn the patient against breast-feeding.

Anaphylactic Reactions. See *Intravenous Dosage and Administration.*

Minimizing Adverse Interactions

Drugs That Can Decrease Cyclosporine Levels. Phenytoin, phenobarbital, rifampin, and *trimethoprim-sulfamethoxazole* can reduce cyclosporine levels, leading to organ rejection. Monitor cyclosporine levels and increase the dosage as needed.

Drugs That Can Increase Cyclosporine Levels. Ketoconazole and *erythromycin* can elevate cyclosporine levels, increasing the risk of toxicity. Monitor cyclosporine levels and reduce the dosage as needed.

Nephrotoxic Drugs. Amphotericin B, aminoglycosides, and *nonsteroidal anti-inflammatory drugs* increase the risk of cyclosporine-induced kidney damage. Monitor renal function.

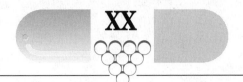

Toxicology

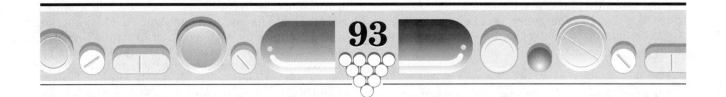

93

Management of Poisoning

P oisoning is defined as a pathologic state caused by a toxic agent. Sources of poisoning include medications, plants, environmental pollutants, and drugs of abuse. These toxicants may enter the body orally, by inhalation, and by absorption through the skin. Poisoning may be accidental or intentional. Symptoms of poisoning often mimic those of disease. Hence, the possibility of poisoning should be considered whenever a diagnosis is made.

Poisonings occur at an estimated rate of 5 million per year, and about 5000 deaths result. Approximately 60% of these fatalities are due to ingestion of drugs, either prescription medicines or over-the-counter (OTC) preparations. The remaining deaths are caused by other chemicals. The *incidence* of poisoning is highest in young children; however, the *mortality* rate in this group is low. Most poisoning-related hospital admissions result from suicide attempts by adults.

POISON CONTROL CENTERS

In the United States there are more than 500 local poison control centers and over 40 certified regional centers. All of these centers are accessible by telephone, and can provide immediate instruction on the management of acute poisoning. In the majority of cases, the information supplied will permit successful treatment at home. By facilitating rapid treatment, poison control centers can decrease morbidity and mortality and can help reduce the cost of emergency care. Phone numbers for regional poison control centers are given in Appendix E.

FUNDAMENTALS OF TREATMENT

Poisoning is a medical emergency and requires rapid treatment. Management has five basic elements: (1) supportive care, (2) identification of the poison, (3) prevention of further absorption, (4) promotion of poison removal, and (5) use of specific antidotes. These essentials are discussed below.

Supportive Care

Supportive care is the most important element in the management of acute poisoning. Support is based on the clinical status of the patient and requires no knowledge specific to the poison involved. Maintenance of respiration and circulation are the primary concerns. Measures for support of breathing include insertion of an airway, administration of humidified oxygen, and mechanical ventilation. Volume depletion (resulting from vomiting, diarrhea, or sweating) can compromise circulation. Volume should be restored by administering normal saline or Ringer's solution. Severe hypoglycemia may occur, resulting in coma. Levels of blood glucose should be monitored. For coma of unknown etiology, IV dextrose should be given immediately—even if information on blood glucose is lacking. Acid-base disturbances may occur; determination of arterial blood gases will facilitate diagnosis and management. If convulsions develop, IV diazepam is the treatment of choice.

Poison Identification

Treatment of poisoning is facilitated by knowledge of the identity and amount of the ingested toxicant. Efforts to obtain this information should proceed concurrently with medical management.

A history is one means by which a toxic agent may be identified. However, experience has shown that histories taken at times of poisoning are frequently inaccurate. That is, statements about the nature or quantity of poison may be incorrect.

Positive identification can be made using analytical techniques. The gas chromatograph/mass spectrometer can provide qualitative and quantitative information. Analyses can be performed on specimens of blood, urine, or gastric contents. To determine whether poison levels are rising or falling, analyses should be performed on sequential blood samples taken about 2 hours apart.

Prevention of Further Absorption

By reducing the absorption of a poison, we can minimize its blood levels and thereby significantly

decrease morbidity and mortality. Five procedures are available for reducing absorption: (1) induction of emesis (usually with syrup of ipecac), (2) gastric lavage, (3) administration of activated charcoal, (4) purgation (with a saline cathartic), and (5) surface decontamination when exposure is topical. Details of these procedures are discussed in the next section.

Promotion of Poison Removal

Measures that help eliminate poison from the body shorten the duration of exposure and, if implemented before plasma levels have peaked, can reduce the maximal level of poison achieved. By shortening exposure and reducing maximal poison levels, these measures can decrease the severity of symptoms.

Removal of poison can be promoted with drugs and nonpharmacologic techniques. The drugs used to promote poison removal act by increasing renal excretion of toxic agents. Nonpharmacologic methods of poison removal include peritoneal dialysis, hemodialysis, and exchange transfusion. Details on methods of poison removal are presented later in the chapter.

Use of Specific Antidotes

An antidote is an agent administered to counteract the effects of a poison. Examples include naloxone (used to reverse poisoning by heroin and other opioids) and physostigmine (used to treat poisoning by atropine and other anticholinergic drugs). Several specific antidotes are discussed later in this chapter. Unfortunately, although antidotes can be extremely valuable, these agents are rare: for most poisons, we have no specific antidote. Hence, for most patients, treatment is limited to the general measures described above.

DRUGS AND PROCEDURES USED TO MINIMIZE ABSORPTION OF POISONS

SYRUP OF IPECAC

Actions and Uses. Syrup of ipecac is the drug of choice for induction of emesis. Ipecac is indicated following ingestion of practically all poisons. Emesis is caused by stimulation of the chemoreceptor trigger zone of the medulla and by an irritant action exerted in the stomach. Vomiting usually occurs 20 to 30 minutes after drug administration. After vomiting has finished, activated charcoal can be administered to remove residual poison from the stomach and intestine. (Charcoal should not be administered prior to emesis since it can adsorb the ipecac and may thereby reduce ipecac's effects.) If ipecac fails to provoke vomiting, gastric lavage can be used to empty the stomach of poison (see below). The most common side effects of ipecac are sedation and diarrhea.

Contraindications. Although generally indicated in cases of poison ingestion, induction of vomiting can be hazardous in some situations. Ipecac is contraindicated following ingestion of strong acids or bases. Under these circumstances, regurgitation increases the risk of gastric perforation and esophageal necrosis. Ipecac is also contraindicated for patients who are comatose, delirious, or experiencing convulsions. Under these conditions, induction of vomiting may result in aspiration of gastric contents.

Preparations, Dosage, and Administration. Ipecac syrup is dispensed in 15- and 30-ml containers. The drug is available without prescription and should be kept in all households that have children over the age of 1 year. The presence of fluid in the stomach increases the effects of ipecac. Hence, administration should be accompanied by an appropriate volume of water. The dose of ipecac syrup for children under 1 year of age is 5 to 10 ml followed by one-half to 1 glass of water. The dose for older children and adults is 15 ml followed by 1 to 2 glasses of water. If vomiting does not occur within 20 minutes dosing should be repeated.

ACTIVATED CHARCOAL

Activated charcoal is an inert substance that adsorbs drugs and other chemicals. Binding of toxicants to charcoal is essentially irreversible. Since the charcoal particles cannot be absorbed into the blood, adsorption of poisons onto charcoal prevents toxicity. The charcoal-poison complex is eliminated in the stool. Patients should be advised that charcoal will turn the feces black. When ipecac is being used, charcoal should be administered only after vomiting has taken place. Charcoal is nontoxic and there are no contraindications to its use.

Activated charcoal has the consistency of a fine powder and is mixed with water for oral administration. The adult dose is 50 to 100 gm. Pediatric doses range from 25 to 50 gm. For toxicants that are slowly absorbed, and for ones that undergo enterohepatic recirculation or secretion from the blood into the stomach, sequential doses can be beneficial. Since charcoal is devoid of toxicity, there is no upper limit to the amount that may be given.

SALINE CATHARTICS

Cathartics hasten passage of toxicants through the intestine, and thereby minimize absorption. Saline cathartics (e.g., sodium sulfate, magnesium sulfate) are the agents of choice. These preparations act rapidly and have little toxicity. For patients on a low sodium regimen (e.g., patients with hypertension or congestive heart failure), magnesium sulfate (Epsom salt) is preferred to sodium sulfate. Cathartics do not reduce adsorption onto charcoal, and will accelerate charcoal elimination. When a cathartic is administered simultaneously with charcoal, the interval between administration and the appearance of black stool provides an index of intestinal transit time.

GASTRIC LAVAGE

Gastric lavage (irrigation of the stomach) is indicated in cases of significant poisoning when induction of emesis cannot be performed. Since emesis is more effective than lavage, ipecac is preferred to lavage except when emesis is contraindicated. Although early use of lavage or ipecac is desirable, these procedures can still be beneficial many hours after poison has been ingested.

Lavage is accomplished using a large-bore orogastric tube (36 to 42 French for adults, 26 to 28 French for children). Smaller tubes should be avoided since they may not permit removal of solids (food, pills, capsules, tablets) and because their small diameter will impede flow of the lavage fluid. If the patient is comatose, an endotracheal tube with an inflatable cuff should be installed to protect the airway. Because of the anatomy of the stomach, the patient should be placed on the left side with the head down. Prior to initiation of lavage, stomach contents should be aspirated and sent for toxicologic analysis. Lavage may be performed employing tap water or saline solution. Multiple washes are instilled using 100 to 300 ml of fluid per wash. Larger volumes should be avoided since they may push stomach contents into the small intestine. Washes should be repeated until the fluid retrieved from the stomach is clear. About 10 to 12 washes are required. The total volume of fluid employed should be about 2 L for children and 5 L for adults.

SURFACE DECONTAMINATION

Topical exposure to toxicants can cause local and systemic injury. To prevent both local damage and systemic effects, contaminated clothing should be removed, and the poison should be washed from the victim. The recommended procedure is to alternate soap and water washes with alcohol washes. Health personnel performing these washes should take precautions to avoid becoming contaminated themselves. If the eyes have been exposed, they should be flushed with water for at least 15 minutes. Shampoo should be employed to remove toxic agents from the hair and scalp.

DRUGS AND PROCEDURES USED FOR POISON REMOVAL

DRUGS THAT ENHANCE RENAL EXCRETION

Drugs that alter the pH of urine can accelerate the excretion of organic acids and bases. Agents that *elevate* urinary pH (i.e., make the urine more alkaline) will promote the excretion of *acids*. Drugs that *lower* urinary pH will promote the excretion of *bases*. The mechanism underlying these effects is called ion trapping. This mechanism is discussed in Chapter 5.

The drugs employed most frequently to alter urinary pH are *sodium bicarbonate* and *ammonium chloride*. Both agents are administered IV. Sodium bicarbonate renders the urine more alkaline, an effect that decreases the passive reabsorption of acids (e.g., aspirin, phenobarbital), and thereby enhances their excretion. Ammonium chloride acidifies the urine, and thereby increases the excretion of bases (e.g., amphetamines, phencyclidine). Because of the buffer systems present in blood, sodium bicarbonate and ammonium chloride have a relatively small effect on the pH of blood.

NONDRUG METHODS OF POISON REMOVAL

Several nondrug procedures—peritoneal dialysis, hemodialysis, hemoperfusion, exchange transfusion—can be employed to remove toxicants from the body. Although these procedures are usually of limited value, they can be lifesaving in some situations. Nondrug procedures are most effective (1) when binding of toxicants to plasma proteins is low, and (2) when blood levels of toxicants are high (i.e., when distribution of the toxic agent is restricted to the blood and extracellular fluid).

Each of the nondrug methods of poison removal has its benefits and drawbacks. *Peritoneal dialysis* has two advantages: the procedure is relatively simple to perform, and it occupies a minimum of staff time. *Hemodialysis*, although more difficult than peritoneal dialysis, is considerably more effective. As a result, use of hemodialysis in the management of acute poisoning is increasing. *Hemoperfusion* is a process in which blood is passed over a column of charcoal or absorbent resin. If the affinity of the resin for a particular poison is sufficiently high, this procedure can strip a toxicant from binding sites on plasma proteins. The principal disadvantage of hemoperfusion is loss of plate-

lets. When binding of a poison to plasma proteins is particularly avid, *exchange transfusion* can be an effective method of removal.

SPECIFIC ANTIDOTES

HEAVY-METAL ANTAGONISTS

The heavy metals most frequently responsible for poisoning are lead, iron, mercury, arsenic, gold, and copper. These metals produce their toxic effects by forming complexes with enzymes and other physiologically important molecules, thereby impairing their function. Poisoning may result from environmental exposure, intentional overdosage, or therapeutic use of heavy metals.

The drugs given to treat heavy-metal poisoning are called *chelating agents* or *chelators*. These agents interact with metals to form *chelates*. A chelate is a ring structure in which there are two or more points of attachment between the metal and the chelating agent. The chelate formed by the interaction of mercury with dimercaprol illustrates this concept (Fig. 93–1).

Useful chelating agents have a high affinity for heavy metals and can therefore compete successfully with endogenous molecules for metal binding. By preventing initial binding of metals to endogenous molecules, and by stripping metals that have already become bound, chelators can prevent toxicity from heavy metals and can enhance their excretion.

The selectivity of a heavy-metal antagonist is determined by its affinity for specific metals. Some antagonists are selective for only one metal, whereas others can form chelates with several heavy metals. Deferoxamine, for example, binds selectively to iron. In contrast, dimercaprol is relatively nonselective, binding tightly with arsenic, mercury salts, and gold.

Properties desirable in a heavy-metal antagonist include (1) affinity for a toxic metal that is higher than the affinity of endogenous molecules for that metal, (2) low affinity for essential endogenous metals (e.g., magnesium, zinc), (3) an ability to reach sites of metal storage, (4) high activity at the pH of body fluids, (5) formation of chelates that are less toxic than the free metal, and (6) formation of chelates that are easily excreted.

Deferoxamine

Actions and Uses. Deferoxamine has a high affinity for ferric iron. The drug will chelate free iron and will also strip iron

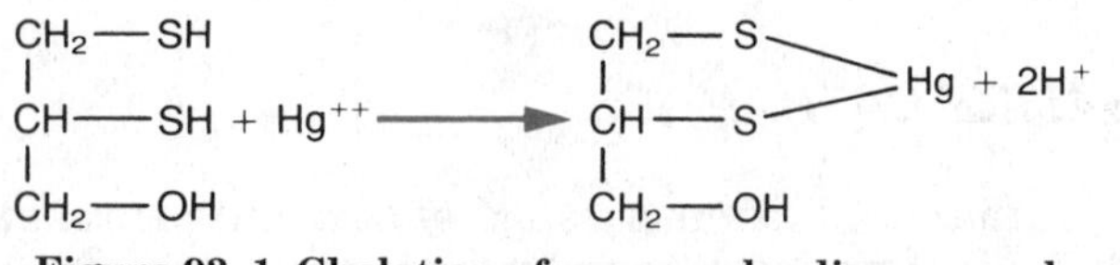

Figure 93–1. Chelation of mercury by dimercaprol.

from ferritin and hemosiderin. In contrast, iron present in hemoglobin and cytochromes is not affected. Deferoxamine is employed to treat acute and chronic iron toxicity.

Pharmacokinetics. Deferoxamine is poorly absorbed from the gastrointestinal tract. Hence, administration is parenteral. The chelate formed between deferoxamine and iron is excreted primarily in the urine.

Adverse Effects. Deferoxamine is generally well tolerated. Pain may occur at the site of injection. Rapid IV infusion may cause hypotension, tachycardia, erythema, and urticaria. Prolonged therapy may be associated with allergic reactions, abdominal discomfort, leg cramps, fever, and dysuria.

Contraindications. Because deferoxamine is excreted by the kidneys, the drug should not be given to patients with renal insufficiency. Deferoxamine has caused fetal malformation in experimental animals and is not recommended for use during pregnancy.

Preparations, Dosage, and Administration. Deferoxamine mesylate [Desferal Mesylate] is dispensed as a powder to be reconstituted for injection. The drug can be administered by IM injection or by IV or SC infusion. Intramuscular injection is preferred for most patients. Intravenous infusion is usually reserved for patients in shock. The dosage for IM or IV administration is the same. The initial dose for adults and children is 1 gm. This is followed 4 and 8 hours later with 0.5-gm doses. For IV administration, the maximum rate of infusion is 15 mg/kg/hr.

Dimercaprol

Actions and Uses. Dimercaprol binds to arsenic, gold, and mercury. The resulting chelates are excreted in the urine. The drug is used as the sole chelator to rid the body of arsenic, mercury, or gold. In addition, dimercaprol can be combined with edetate calcium disodium to treat poisoning with lead. Since dimercaprol is more effective at *preventing* binding of metals to endogenous molecules than it is at reversing binding that has already taken place, benefits are greatest when the drug is administered early (within 1 to 2 hours after metal ingestion).

Pharmacokinetics. Administration is by deep IM injection. Dimercaprol cannot be used orally. The drug has a short plasma half-life; complete elimination occurs in approximately 4 hours.

Adverse Effects. At recommended doses, dimercaprol is generally well tolerated. Tachycardia and elevation of blood pressure occur frequently; blood pressure returns to normal values within hours. Pain and sterile abscesses may occur at sites of injection. Fever is common in children. High doses produce a broad spectrum of untoward effects.

Chelates formed with dimercaprol are unstable at acidic pH. Hence, if the urine is acidic, heavy metals may dissociate from dimercaprol, resulting in renal toxicity. To protect the kidneys, the urine should be kept alkaline.

Preparations, Dosage, and Administration. Dimercaprol [BAL In Oil] is dispensed in ampuls containing 300 mg of the drug in 3 ml of peanut oil. The preparation is administered by deep IM injection. For *mild poisoning with gold or arsenic*, doses of 2.5 mg/kg are administered according to the following schedule: 4 times daily on days 1 and 2, twice daily on day 3, and once daily on days 4 through 13. For *acute poisoning with mercury*, the initial dose is 5 mg/kg. Subsequent doses of 2.5 mg/kg are administered 1 or 2 times daily for 10 days.

Edetate Calcium Disodium (Calcium EDTA)

Actions and Uses. Calcium EDTA is used primarily for lead poisoning. The drug combines with lead to form a stable chelate that is excreted in the urine.

Pharmacokinetics. Calcium EDTA may be administered IV or IM. The drug is poorly absorbed from the GI tract and is not administered orally. Elimination is by glomerular filtration. Because calcium EDTA is excreted by the kidneys, the drug

should employed only if urine flow is adequate. If urine flow is insufficient, it should be restored with IV fluids prior to administration of the chelator. If anuria develops during the course of treatment, administration of calcium EDTA should cease.

Adverse Effects. The principal toxicity of calcium EDTA is renal tubular necrosis. Signs of renal damage include hematuria and proteinuria. Daily urinalysis should be performed to monitor for these effects. If renal toxicity develops, the drug should be discontinued immediately.

Preparations, Dosage, and Administration. Calcium EDTA [Calcium Disodium Versenate] is dispensed in 5-ml ampuls containing 1000 mg of the drug. Administration may be IV or IM. The IV route is preferred for adults, whereas IM injection is preferred for children.

For IV use, the contents of 1 ampul are diluted in 250 to 500 ml of 5% dextrose solution or normal saline. Infusion should be done slowly (over 1 hour or more). The adult dosage is 1 gm twice daily for 5 days. After a 2-day hiatus, a second course can be given if needed.

The IM dosage for children is 35 mg/kg (or less) administered twice daily for 3 to 5 days. After a pause of 4 days or more, a second course is given.

Penicillamine

Actions. Penicillamine is a breakdown product of penicillin. Commercial preparations are made synthetically. Penicillamine forms water-soluble chelates with copper, iron, lead, arsenic, gold, and mercury. These complexes are excreted in the urine.

Therapeutic Uses. The principal indication for penicillamine is Wilson's disease, a disorder of copper metabolism. Individuals with this disease are deficient in ceruloplasmin, a plasma protein that serves as a carrier for copper. Symptoms result from deposition of copper in the liver, brain, kidneys, eyes, and other organs. Penicillamine relieves symptoms by promoting copper excretion. Therapeutic effects may take several months to develop. Additional uses for the drug are *rheumatoid arthritis* and *cystinuria*. Beneficial effects in these disorders are not related to chelation of heavy metals.

Pharmacokinetics. Penicillamine is well absorbed following oral administration. Food greatly reduces the extent of absorption. Once absorbed, penicillamine is rapidly excreted in the urine.

Adverse Effects. With prolonged use, penicillamine can cause varied and serious toxicity. Death has occurred. The drug should be employed only with close medical supervision. Possible cutaneous reactions include urticaria, maculopapular and morbilliform rashes, pemphigoid lesions, and pruritus. Bone marrow suppression can result in leukopenia, agranulocytosis, and aplastic anemia—reactions that can be fatal. Autoimmune and immune complex disorders have been associated with penicillamine; these include dermatomyositis, polymyositis, lupus erythematosus, alveolitis, and myasthenia gravis. Renal toxicity may occur.

Contraindications. Penicillamine is contraindicated for patients who have experienced agranulocytosis or aplastic anemia when receiving penicillamine in the past. The drug is also contraindicated for patients with rheumatoid arthritis who are pregnant or have renal insufficiency.

Preparations, Dosage, and Administration. Penicillamine [Cuprimine, Depen] is dispensed in 125-mg capsules and 250-mg tablets for oral administration. For Wilson's disease, the usual dosage is 250 mg 4 times a day. Doses should be administered 1 hour before meals and at bedtime. Dosage is adjusted on the basis of untoward effects and urinary copper content. Treatment is long term.

Succimer

Actions and Uses. Succimer is a new heavy-metal chelating agent. The drug binds avidly with lead, mercury, and arsenic. Binding is less avid with copper and zinc. Binding to iron, calcium, and magnesium is minimal; hence, succimer presents no risk of depleting these essential minerals.

Succimer is approved for treatment of lead poisoning in children. The drug may also be useful against poisoning with arsenic and mercury.

Pharmacokinetics. Succimer is rapidly but variably absorbed following oral administration. The drug undergoes extensive metabolism. Metabolites and parent drug are eliminated slowly in the urine.

Adverse Effects. Adverse effects appear to be mild. About 10% of patients experience gastrointestinal reactions (nausea, diarrhea, cramps). Other moderate reactions include nasal congestion, muscle pain, and rash. Succimer has caused temporary elevations in serum transaminases, indicating possible liver injury. Accordingly, serum transaminases should be monitored before treatment and weekly thereafter. Caution should be exercised in patients with liver disease. In mice, the drug is teratogenic and fetotoxic. Since succimer is a relatively new drug, it may be able to cause as-yet unreported adverse effects. Be alert for this possibility.

Preparations, Dosage, and Administration. Succimer [Chemet] is dispensed in 100-mg capsules for oral use. For children over 1 year of age, a course of treatment consists of 10 mg/kg or 350 mg/m^2 every 8 hours for 5 days, followed by the same dose every 12 hours for 14 more days. If needed, the course can be repeated after a minimum hiatus of 2 weeks.

OTHER IMPORTANT ANTIDOTES

Throughout this text we have considered the toxic effects of various drugs. Where appropriate, we have discussed specific antidotes used to treat these toxicities. For example, when discussing the adverse effects of opioids, we also discussed treatment of opioid overdosage with naloxone. Similarly, when discussing heparin toxicity, we discussed the use of protamine sulfate as treatment. The major specific antidotes presented in previous chapters are listed in Table 93–1. This table indicates generic and trade names, the substances whose toxicity these antidotes are used to treat, and the chapters in which these antidotes are discussed.

Table 93–1. Specific Antidotes Discussed in Previous Chapters

Antidote			
Generic Name	*Trade Name*	*Toxic/Overdosed Substance*	*Chapter*
Atropine		Muscarinic agonists, cholinesterase inhibitors	13
Physostigmine salicylate	Antilirium	Anticholinergic drugs	16
Neostigmine	Prostigmin	Nondepolarizing neuromuscular blocking agents	16
Pralidoxime	Protopam	Organophosphate cholinesterase inhibitors	16
Naloxone	Narcan	Opioids	28
Ethanol		Methanol	33
Vitamin K		Oral anticoagulants	46
Protamine sulfate		Heparin	46
Glucagon		Insulin	49
Acetylcysteine	Mucomyst	Acetaminophen	61
Leucovorin calcium	Wellcovorin	Folic acid antagonists	91

Weights and Measures

Volume Equivalents

1 milliliter	= 0.034	fluid ounce
	= 0.271	fluid dram
	= 16.2	minims
1 liter	= 1000	milliliters
	= 33.8	fluid ounces
	= 2.11	pints
	= 1.06	quarts
	= 0.26	gallon
1 cubic centimeter	= 1	milliliter
1 minim	= 0.062	milliliter
1 fluid dram	= 3.70	milliliters
	= 60	minims
1 fluid ounce	= 29.6	milliliters
	= 2	tablespoons
	= 8	fluid drams
1 teaspoon	= 5	milliliters
1 tablespoon	= 15	milliliters
	= 3	teaspoons
1 cup	= 237	milliliters
	= 8	fluid ounces
	= 16	tablespoons
1 pint	= 473	milliliters
	= 16	fluid ounces
	= 2	cups
1 quart	= 946	milliliters
	= 32	fluid ounces
	= 2	pints
1 gallon	= 3785	milliliters
	= 128	fluid ounces
	= 4	quarts

Mass Equivalents

1 milligram	= 0.0154	grain (apothecaries')
	= 1000	micrograms
1 gram	= 15.4	grains (apothecaries')
	= 0.0322	ounce (apothecaries')
	= 0.0353	ounce (avoirdupois)
	= 0.257	dram (apothecaries')
1 grain (apothecaries')	= 64.8	milligrams
	= 0.0021	ounce (apothecaries')
	= 0.0023	ounce (avoirdupois)
	= 0.0167	dram (apothecaries')
1 dram (apothecaries')	= 3.89	grams
1 ounce (apothecaries')	= 31.1	grams
1 ounce (avoirdupois)	= 28.4	grams
1 pound (avoirdupois)	= 454	grams
	= 0.454	kilogram
	= 16	ounces (avoirdupois)
1 kilogram	= 2.20	pounds (avoirdupois)

Temperature Conversion

Celsius degrees $\times$ 9/5 + 32 = Fahrenheit degrees

(Fahrenheit degrees $-$ 32) $\times$ 5/9 = Celsius degrees

Normal Laboratory Values

Part I. Hematology

Measurement	Normal Laboratory Values*	
	Traditional Units	*SI Units*†
Cell Counts		
Erythrocytes		
Adult female	4.2–5.4 million/mm³	4.2–5.4 × 10¹²/L
Adult male	4.2–6.2 million/mm³	4.2–6.2 × 10¹²/L
Newborn	4.8–7.2 million/mm³	4.8–7.2 × 10¹²/L
Child	3.8–5.5 million/mm³	3.8–5.5 × 10¹²/L
Leukocytes		
Total		
Adult	5000–10,000/mm³	5–10 × 10⁹/L
Newborn	9000–30,000/mm³	9–30 × 10⁹/L
Differential (% total leukocytes)		
Neutrophils	50%–70%	0.50–0.70
Segments	50%–65%	0.50–0.65
Bands	0%–5%	0.0–0.05
Eosinophils	0%–3%	0.0–0.03
Basophils	1%–3%	0.01–0.03
Lymphocytes	25%–35%	0.25–0.35
Monocytes	2%–6%	0.02–0.06
Platelets		
Adult	150,000–400,000/mm³	150–400 × 10⁹/L
Newborn	150,000–300,000/mm³	150–300 × 10⁹/L
Infant	200,000–475,000/mm³	200–475 × 10⁹/L
Reticulocytes		
Adult	10,000–75,000/mm³ (0.1%–2.4% of all RBCs)	10–75 × 10⁹/L
Newborn	2.5%–6.5% of all RBCs	2.5%–6.5% of all RBCs
Infant	0.5%–3.5% of all RBCs	0.5%–3.5% of all RBCs
Coagulation-Related Tests		
Bleeding time	3–9.5 min	180–570 sec
Activated partial thromboplastin time (APTT)	25–35 sec	25–35 sec
Prothrombin time	<2 sec from control	<2 sec from control
Corpuscular Values of Erythrocytes		
Mean corpuscular volume (MCV)		
Adult	80–96 μm³	80–96 fl
Newborn	96–108 μm³	96–108 fl
Child	82–92 μm³	82–92 fl
Mean corpuscular hemoglobin (MCH)		
Adult	27–31 pg/RBC	27–31 pg/RBC
Newborn	32–34 pg/RBC	32–34 pg/RBC
Child	27–31 pg/RBC	27–31 pg/RBC
Mean corpuscular hemoglobin concentration (MCHC)	32–36 gm/dl	320–360 gm/L
Erythrocyte Sedimentation Rate		
Wintrobe method		
Adult female	0–15 mm/hr	0–15 mm/hr
Adult male	0–7 mm/hr	0–7 mm/hr
Newborn	0–2 mm/hr	0–2 mm/hr
Westergren method		
Female	0–20 mm/hr	0–20 mm/hr
Male	0–15 mm/hr	0–15 mm/hr

Part I. Hematology Continued

Measurement	Normal Laboratory Values*	
	Traditional Units	*SI Units†*
Hematocrit		
Adult female	36%–48%	0.36–0.48
Adult male	42%–53%	0.42–0.53
Newborn	42%–54%	0.42–0.54
Child (1–3 yr)	29%–40%	0.29–0.40
Child (4–10 yr)	36%–48%	0.36–0.48
Hemoglobin Concentration		
Adult female	12–16 gm/dl	120–160 gm/L
Adult male	13–18 gm/dl	130–180 gm/L
Newborn	14–24 gm/dl	140–240 gm/L

Part II. Blood Chemistry

Measurement	Normal Laboratory Values*	
	Traditional Units	*SI Units†*
Adrenocorticotropic hormone (ACTH)		
6 AM	10–80 pg/ml	2–16 pmol/ml
6 PM	<50 pg/ml	<10 pmol/ml
Aldosterone		
Normal sodium diet	8.1–15.5 ng/dl	220–430 pmol/L
Restricted sodium diet	20.8–44.4 ng/dl	580–1240 pmol/L
Ammonia	10–80 μg/dl	5–50 μmol/L
Amylase	0–125 U/L	0–2.17 μkat/L
Bicarbonate	22–26 mEq/L	22–26 mEq/L
Bilirubin		
Adult		
Direct	0.1–0.4 mg/dl	1.7–6.8 μmol/L
Indirect	0.2–0.7 mg/dl	3.4–12.0 μmol/L
Total	0.3–1.1 mg/dl	5.1–18.8 μmol/L
Newborn (total)	1–12 mg/dl	17–205 μmol/L
Child (total)	0.2–0.8 mg/dl	3.4–13.7 μmol/L
Calcitonin		
Female	0–28 pg/ml	0–8.2 pmol/L
Male	0–14 pg/ml	0–4.1 pmol/L
Calcium	8.8–10.3 mg/dl	2.2–2.6 mmol/L
Carbon dioxide content		
Adult	24–40 mEq/L	24–40 mmol/L
Infant	20–28 mEq/L	20–28 mmol/L
Chloride	96–106 mEq/L	96–106 mmol/L
Cholesterol	See Table 45–2	
Cholinesterase, plasma	620–1370 U/L	10.3–22.8 μkat/L
Copper, total		
Adult female	70–140 μg/dl	11–22 μmol/L
Adult male	85–155 μg/dl	13–24 μmol/L
Newborn	20–70 μg/dl	3–11 μmol/L
Child	30–150 μg/dl	5–24 μmol/L
Cortisol		
Adult		
8 AM	4–19 μg/dl	110–520 nmol/L
4 PM	2–15 μg/dl	50–410 nmol/L
10 PM	<50% of AM value	<50% of AM value
Child		
8 AM	10–25 μg/dl	280–700 nmol/L
4 PM	5–10 μg/dl	140–280 nmol/L
Creatine phosphokinase (CK, CPK)		
Female	10–55 U/L (30°)	10–55 U/L (30°)
	30–135 U/L (37°)	30–135 U/L (37°)
Male	12–80 U/L (30°)	12–80 U/L (30°)
	55–170 U/L (37°)	55–170 U/L (37°)
Creatinine	0.6–1.2 mg/dl	50–110 μmol/L
Ferritin (serum)		
Iron deficiency	0–12 ng/ml	0–4.8 nmol/L
Borderline	13–20 ng/ml	5.2–8 nmol/L
Iron excess	>400 ng/ml	>160 nmol/L

Table continued on following page

Part II. Blood Chemistry Continued

Measurement	Normal Laboratory Values*	
	Traditional Units	*SI Units†*
Fibrinogen	200–400 mg/dl	2.0–4.0 gm/L
Folic acid	2–10 ng/ml	4–22 nmol/L
Follicle-stimulating hormone (FSH)		
Female	2–15 IU/L	2–15 IU/L
Peak production	20–50 IU/L	20–50 IU/L
Male	1–10 IU/L	1–10 IU/L
Free fatty acids	8–20 mg/dl	80–200 mg/L
Gases		
pCO_2	33–44 mm Hg	4.4–5.9 kPa
pO_2	75–105 mm Hg	10–14 kPa
Glucose, fasting		
Adult	60–115 mg/dl	3.4–6.6 mmol/L
Newborn	30–80 mg/dl	1.7–4.6 mmol/L
Child	60–100 mg/dl	3.4–5.7 mmol/L
Glucose-6-phosphate dehydrogenase (G-6-PD)	5–15 U/gm hemoglobin	5–15 U/gm hemoglobin
Insulin (fasting)	5–20 mU/L	35–145 pmol/L
Iron		
Adult female	60–160 μg/dl	11–29 μmol/L
Adult male	80–180 μg/dl	14–32 μmol/L
Newborn	100–200 μg/dl	18–36 μmol/L
Child (6 months–2 years)	40–100 μg/dl	7–18 μmol/L
Iron-binding capacity		
Adult	250–450 μg/dl	45–80 μmol/L
Newborn	60–175 μg/dl	11–31 μmol/L
Child (6 months–2 years)	100–300 μg/dl	17–53 μmol/L
Lactate dehydrogenase (LDH)	50–150 U/L	0.82–2.66 μkat/L
Lipoprotein cholesterol		
LDL cholesterol	See Table 45–2	
HDL cholesterol	See Table 45–2	
Magnesium	1.6–2.4 mEq/L	0.8–1.2 mmol/L
Osmolality, plasma	280–300 mOsm/kg of serum water	280–300 mmol/kg
pH	7.35–7.45	7.35–7.45
Phosphatase		
Acid	0–5.5 U/L	0–90 nkat/L
Alkaline	30–120 U/L	0.5–2.0 μkat/L
Potassium		
Adult	3.5–5.0 mEq/L	3.5–5.0 mmol/L
Infant	3.6–5.8 mEq/L	3.6–5.8 mmol/L
Child	3.5–5.5 mEq/L	3.5–5.5 mmol/L
Progesterone		
Follicular phase	<2 ng/ml	<6 nmol/L
Luteal phase	2–20 ng/ml	6–64 nmol/L
Prolactin	2–15 ng/ml	80–600 pmol/L
Protein		
Total	6.0–8.0 gm/dl	60–80 gm/L
Albumin	3.5–5.5 gm/dl	35–55 gm/L
Globulin		
Alpha₁	0.2–0.4 gm/dl	2–4 gm/L
Alpha₂	0.5–0.9 gm/dl	5–9 gm/L
Beta	0.6–1.1 gm/dl	6–11 gm/L
Gamma	0.7–1.7 gm/dl	7–17 gm/L
Renin activity		
Normal sodium diet	1.1–4.1 ng/ml/hr	0.3–1.1 ng/(L-s)
Restricted sodium diet	6.2–12.4 ng/ml/hr	1.7–3.4 ng(L-s)
Sodium	135–145 mEq/L	135–145 mmol/L
Testosterone		
Female	0.6 ng/ml	2 nmol/L
Male	4.6–8 ng/ml	14–28 nmol/L
Thyroid function tests		
Thyroid-stimulating hormone	2–11 μU/ml	2–11 mU/L
Thyroxine (T₄)		
Adult	4.4–9.9 μg/dl	57–127 nmol/L
Newborn	11–23 μg/dl	142–296 nmol/L
1–4 months	7.5–16.5 μg/dl	97–212 nmol/L
4–12 months	5.5–14.5 μg/dl	71–187 nmol/L
1–6 years	5.5–13.5 μg/dl	71–174 nmol/L
6–10 years	5–12.5 μg/dl	64–161 nmol/L

Part II. Blood Chemistry Continued

Measurement	Normal Laboratory Values*	
	Traditional Units	*SI Units†*
Thyroid function tests *Continued*		
Thyroxine binding globulin	12–28 μg/dl	150–360 nmol/L
Triiodothyronine (T₃)	75–220 μg/dl	1.2–3.4 nmol/L
T₃ resin uptake	25%–38%	0.25–0.35
Transaminases		
AST (aspartate aminotransferase)		
Adult	8–20 U/L (30°)	0.13–0.33 μkat/L (30°)
	7–40 U/L (37°)	0.12–0.67 μkat/L (37°)
Newborn	4 times adult value	4 times adult value
ALT (alanine aminotransferase)	8–20 U/L (30°)	0.13–0.33 μkat/L (30°)
	5–37 U/L (37°)	0.08–0.62 μkat/L (37°)
Triglycerides	See Table 45–2	
Urea nitrogen, blood (BUN)		
Adult female	8–20 mg/dl	2.9–7.1 mmol/L
Adult male	10–25 mg/dl	3.6–8.9 mmol/L
Infant	5–15 mg/dl	1.8–5.4 mmol/L
Child	5–20 mg/dl	1.8–7.1 mmol/L
Uric acid	2–7 mg/dl	120–420 μmol/L
Vitamin B₁₂	205–876 pg/ml	150–674 pmol/L

Part III. Urine Chemistry

Measurement	Normal Laboratory Values*	
	Traditional Units	*SI Units†*
Aldosterone	3–20 μg/24 hr	8.3–55.5 nmol/day
Calcium	<250 mg/24 hr	<6.2 mmol/day
Catecholamines		
Epinephrine	<20 μg/24 hr	<109 nmol/day
Norepinephrine	<100 μg/24 hr	<590 nmol/day
Cortisol	10–100 μg/24 hr	30–300 nmol/day
Creatine		
Female	0–80 mg/24 hr	0–600 μmol/day
Male	0–40 mg/24 hr	0–3000 μmol/day
Creatinine	15–25 mg/kg/24 hr	0.13–0.22 nmol/kg/day
Creatinine clearance		
Female	105–132 ml/min	1.2–2.2 ml/sec
Male	110–150 ml/min	1.8–2.5 ml/sec
17-Hydroxycorticosteroids		
Female	2–8 mg/24 hr	2–25 μmol/day
Male	3–10 mg/24 hr	10–30 μmol/day
17-Ketosteroids		
Female		
10 yr	1–4 mg/24 hr	3.5–14 μmol/day
20 yr	4–16 mg/24 hr	14–56 μmol/day
30 yr	4–14 mg/24 hr	14–49 μmol/day
50 yr	3–9 mg/24 hr	10–32 μmol/day
70 yr	1–7 mg/24 hr	3.5–25 μmol/day
Male		
10 yr	1–4 mg/24 hr	3.5–14 μmol/day
20 yr	6–21 mg/24 hr	21–74 μmol/day
30 yr	8–26 mg/24 hr	28–91 μmol/day
50 yr	5–18 mg/24 hr	18–63 μmol/day
70 yr	2–10 mg/24 hr	7–35 μmol/day
Potassium	25–100 mEq/24 hr	25–100 mmol/day
Sodium	(diet dependent)	(diet dependent)

*The values presented are intended as guidelines only. Laboratory values may vary with the method employed and among different laboratories using the same method. When a laboratory issues a report, the report will include normal values for that laboratory.
†Système International d'Unités (International System of Units)

APPENDIX C

Commonly Used Abbreviations

ac	before meals	FDA	Food and Drug Administration
ACh	acetylcholine	g (gm)	gram
ad lib	freely as desired	G-6-PD	glucose-6-phosphate dehydrogenase
ADP	adenosine diphosphate	GABA	gamma-aminobutyric acid
AED	antiepileptic drug	GFR	glomerular filtration rate
AIDS	acquired immunodeficiency syndrome	GI	gastrointestinal
ALT	alanine aminotransferase	gm (g)	gram
	(also known as SGPT)	GMP	guanosine monophosphate
AMP	adenosine monophosphate	gr	grain
ANA	antinuclear antibodies	GTP	guanosine triphosphate
ARC	AIDS-related complex	GU	genitourinary
AST	aspartate aminotransferase	HBGM	home blood glucose monitoring
	(also known as SGOT)	HDL	high-density lipoprotein
ATP	adenosine triphosphate	HIV	human immunodeficiency virus
A-V	atrioventricular	hr	hour
bid	two times a day	H$_2$RA	histamine$_2$-receptor antagonist
bin	two times a night	hs	at bedtime (hora somni)
bol	bolus	HSV	herpes simplex virus
BP	blood pressure	IBD	inflammatory bowel disease
BUN	blood urea nitrogen	IDDM	insulin-dependent diabetes mellitus
C	Celsius (centigrade)	IM	intramuscular, intramuscularly
cAMP	cyclic adenosine 3′,5′ monophosphate	IOP	intraocular pressure
CAT	computerized axial tomography	ISA	intrinsic sympathomimetic activity
cc	cubic centimeter (milliliter)	IU	international units
CDC	Centers for Disease Control and	IUD	intrauterine device
	Prevention	IV	intravenous, intravenously
CHF	congestive heart failure	kg	kilogram
CNS	central nervous system	KVO	keep vein open
COMT	catechol-o-methyltransferase	L	liter
COPD	chronic obstructive pulmonary	LDL	low-density lipoprotein
	disease	LGV	lymphogranuloma venereum
CPK	creatine phosphokinase	LSD	d-lysergic acid diethylamide
CSF	cerebrospinal fluid	m	minim
CTZ	chemoreceptor trigger zone	MAC	minimum alveolar concentration
CVA	cerebrovascular accident	MAO	monoamine oxidase
DBP	diastolic blood pressure	MAOI	monoamine oxidase inhibitor
DC	direct current	MBC	minimum bactericidal concentration
DKA	diabetic ketoacidosis	mcg (μg)	microgram
dl	deciliter (100 ml)	MDI	metered-dose inhaler
DMARD	disease-modifying anti-rheumatic	MEC	minimum effective concentration
	drug	mEq	milliequivalent
DNA	deoxyribonucleic acid	μg	microgram
DPI	dry-powder inhaler	(mcg)	
ECG	electrocardiogram	mg	milligram
(EKG)		MI	myocardial infarction
ECT	electroconvulsive therapy	MIC	minimum inhibitory concentration
EEG	electroencephalogram	ml	milliliter
EKG	electrocardiogram	mM	millimole
(ECG)		mOsm	milliosmole
F	Fahrenheit	MRI	magnetic resonance imaging

1142

ng	nanogram
NGU	nongonococcal urethritis
NIDDM	noninsulin-dependent diabetes mellitus
NPO	nothing by mouth
NSAID	nonsteroidal anti-inflammatory drug
OD	right eye
OS	left eye
OTC	over-the-counter
OU	both eyes
PABA	para-aminobenzoic acid
pc	after meals (post cibum)
PCP	*Pneumocystis carinii* pneumonia
PET	positron emission tomography
pg	picogram
PG	prostaglandin
PID	pelvic inflammatory disease
PO	by mouth (per os)
PR	by the rectum
PRN	as needed (pro re nata)
PT	prothrombin time
PTT	partial thromboplastin time
PVC	premature ventricular complex
qd	every day
qh	every hour
qid	four times a day

qod	every other day
RBC	red blood cell (erythrocyte)
RDA	recommended dietary allowance
REM	rapid eye movement
RNA	ribonucleic acid
S-A	sinoauricular
SAARD	slow-acting anti-rheumatic drug
SBP	systolic blood pressure
SC	subcutaneous, subcutaneously
SGOT	serum glutamic-oxaloacetic transaminase (also known as AST)
SGPT	serum glutamic-pyruvic transaminase (also known as ALT)
SLE	systemic lupus erythematosus
SPF	sun protection factor
SR	sarcoplasmic reticulum
SSRA	selective serotonin reuptake antagonist
stat	immediately
STD	sexually transmitted disease
SVT	supraventricular tachycardia
tid	three times a day
UTI	urinary tract infection
VLDL	very-low-density lipoprotein
VSM	vascular smooth muscle
WBC	white blood cell (leukocyte)

Techniques of Drug Administration

Linda Moore, M.S.N., Ed.D., R.N.

Type of Administration	Technique to Be Used

Oral

Liquids

General Considerations
1. Perform any required dilution using appropriate liquid. Avoid liquids that can reduce drug absorption (e.g., milk will decrease absorption of tetracyclines).
2. Measure using medicine cup or device supplied with medication.
3. Pour medication away from label/directions.
4. Read amount at bottom of meniscus (see diagram).

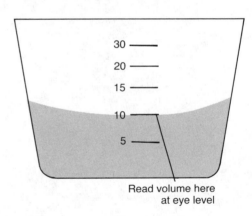

Read volume here
at eye level

5. Do not leave patient before medication is taken.

Infants
Do not mix medication with formula or juice in bottle (you cannot be sure of amount taken if all of the liquid is not swallowed).

Nasogastric Tube Administration
1. Insure correct location of the tube.
2. Follow directions for diluting (e.g., Metamucil becomes thick rapidly and should be mixed at time of administration, not before).
3. Follow with sufficient liquid to clear the tube (stay within fluid restrictions).

Tablets, Capsules

1. If possible, have the patient in a sitting position to facilitate swallowing.
2. Check requirement for administration with food or liquids (e.g., medications that irritate often need to be given with food; some medications may have decreased absorption with food).

Type of Administration	Technique to Be Used
	3. Provide proper liquid for swallowing (stay within fluid restrictions, or, if patient needs increased fluids, this is a good time to provide extra fluid).
Chewable Tablets	Be sure tablet is completely chewed before it is swallowed.

Sublingual and Buccal

Sublingual	1. Place tablet under tongue, and instruct patient to hold it there until dissolved.
	2. Swallowing of residual should then occur.
Buccal	1. Instruct patient to hold medication between teeth and cheek until it is dissolved.
	2. Residual can then be swallowed.

Rectal (Suppository)

1. Patient is to lie in left lateral Sims' position.
2. Nurse to wear gloves during procedure.
3. Lubricate suppository and glove fingertip with water-soluble lubricant.
4. Insert suppository when rectal sphincter is relaxed (see diagram).

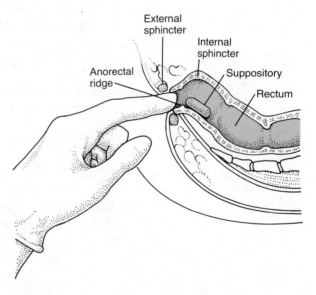

5. Instruct patient as to length of time to retain medication (about 20 to 30 minutes for defecation stimulation and about 60 minutes for systemic absorption).

Vaginal

1. Wear gloves during procedure.
2. Insert foam or suppository into vagina.
3. Instruct patient as to length of time to remain lying down.

Type of Administration	**Technique to Be Used**

Topical

    1. Wear gloves when applying *any* topical ointment.
    2. Apply with applicator, gauze, or gloved hand.
    3. Apply a thin layer by patting, not rubbing.
    4. Take care to protect the patient's clothing.
    5. Certain medications require plastic wrap to increase absorption (e.g., nitroglycerin ointment).

Otic

    1. Medication should be at body temperature.
    2. Patient should lie on side with appropriate ear up.
    3. Instill drops toward auditory canal wall, not on eardrum. Procedure varies for adults and children. *Adults:* The auricle is pulled back and posteriorly. *Infants:* The auricle is pulled down and posteriorly (see diagram).

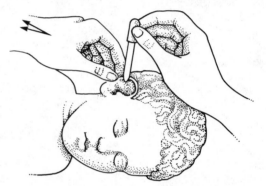

    4. Rest hand administering drops lightly against the patient's head to prevent injury from dropper should the patient suddenly move.
    5. Patient should remain in this position for about 15 minutes.

Optic

    1. Have patient lying on back with eyes facing up.
    2. Do not touch tip of dropper to patient or to any object.

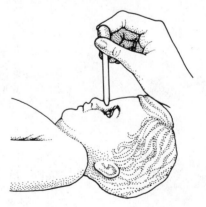

    3. Have tissues available to blot any overflow from eyes (use separate tissue for each eye).

Type of Administration	**Technique to Be Used**

4. Rest hand instilling drops on patient's forehead to stabilize dropper and to prevent injury due to sudden patient movement.
5. Instill drops into conjunctival pouch while patient looks upward (see diagram).
6. To decrease systemic absorption, light pressure may be applied to lacrimal sac for about a minute.
7. *Ointment* is applied as a thin "ribbon" along inner aspect of lower lid. Do not touch tube to eye or other surface.

Intradermal

1. Select an appropriate site. (Usual sites for *skin testing* are shown in the diagram.)

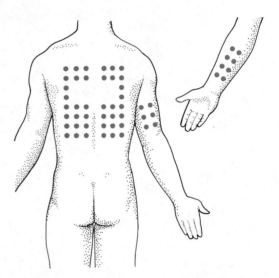

2. Use a short-bevel (26-gauge, ⅜-in) needle.
3. Amount of medication is limited to 1 ml or less.
4. If skin testing is being done, have emergency medication (epinephrine) available.
5. With bevel of needle pointed up, inject medication into layers of the skin (see diagram).

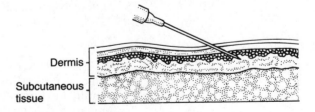

6. Use dry wipe to wipe area following injection.

| **Type of Administration** | **Technique to Be Used** |

Subcutaneous

1. Select a needle size (usually 25- to 27-gauge, ½- to ⅝-in).
2. Select a site that has adequate subcutaneous tissue and that is away from bony prominences, major nerves, and blood vessels (see diagram).

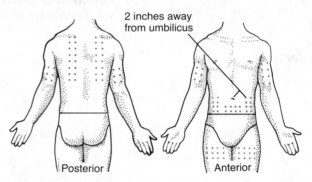

3. Angle of needle insertion depends on size of the individual. Obese people will require needle inserted at 90° angle, whereas very thin people will require pinching of the skin, with insertion at a 90° angle to the pocket pinched. Individuals who are neither fat nor very thin require a 45° angle for needle insertion (see diagram).

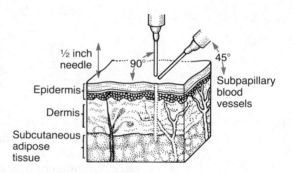

4. Aspiration for blood depends on substance being injected. Follow protocol.
5. Do not rub most SC injection sites.

Intramuscular

1. Select a needle length appropriate to size of patient. The needle should be long enough to reach to the middle of the muscle. Measure the circumference of the arm and select appropriate needle length. The average person requires a 1½- to 2-inch needle. Muscular males require 2- to 3-inch needles or as long as 3- to 5-inches in some cases.
2. Select technique of injection.
   a. *Standard*—insert needle at 90° angle to the muscle after area is cleaned.
   b. *Z-track method*—pull tissue to one side, insert needle, inject medication, and allow tissue to return to original position as needle is removed. (Used for medications that damage tissue and as method to decrease pain of injection.)

Type of Administration	**Technique to Be Used**

3. Select site of injection:
   a. *Dorsogluteal*—to locate, draw a diagonal line between the superior iliac spine and the greater trochanter of the femur (see diagram). Patient should be prone with toes turned inward. *Do not use this site for children less than 2 years of age or for children who are emaciated.*
   b. *Ventrogluteal*—to locate, place palm of hand over the greater trochanter of the femur with thumb pointing to patient's abdomen, index finger placed over the anterior iliac spine, and middle finger spread back toward the iliac crest. The V-shaped area between the fingers is the ventrogluteal site. Direct needle toward largest muscle mass (see diagram).

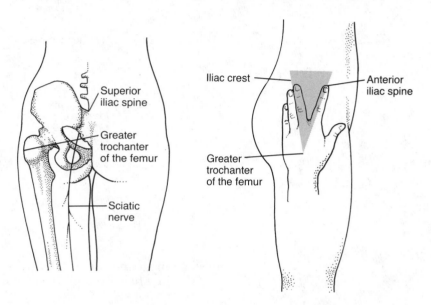

   c. *Anteriolateral thigh*—to locate, area is one third the distance from the greater trochanter and the knee and is between the midline of the anterior and lateral thighs (see diagram). *This is a good site for infants and children.*

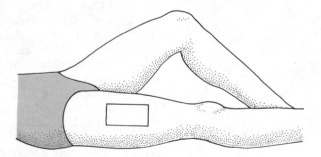

Type of Administration	**Technique to Be Used**

d. *Deltoid*—to locate, bordered above by 2 fingerbreadths below the acromion process and below by 2 fingerbreadths above the insertion of the deltoid (see diagram). Injection site must be in lateral aspect of the arm.

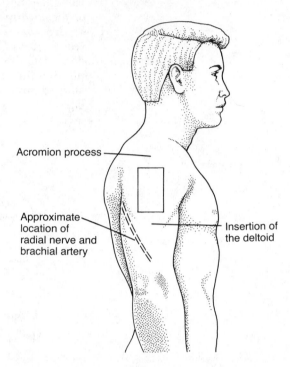

Acromion process

Approximate location of radial nerve and brachial artery

Insertion of the deltoid

4. Insert needle at 90° angle. Aspirate to be sure the needle is not in a blood vessel. Inject slowly. Withdraw needle, and apply pressure to site.

Intravenous

1. Only clinicians with specific training should inject medication intravenously.
2. Medications can be administered into a continuous IV or a heparin lock designed for intermittent administration. Be sure medication is compatible with solution being infused. Check for infiltration prior to administering medication.
3. Do not administer medications that have precipitates or discoloration.
4. Dilute according to directions. Certain medications are not to be diluted. Be sure to check specifics.
5. If "piggybacking" medication, set drip rate for proper infusion time. Note drop rate on IV tubing package.
6. Tape IV securely but with some flexibility in the tubing.
7. Check IV frequently for correct infusion rate. Discontinue when complete dose has been delivered.
8. Record the name of the medication and volume of fluid administered.

Certified Regional Poison Control Centers

Regional poison centers certified by the American Association of Poison Control Centers are accessible 24 hours a day; have a specially trained, full-time staff (usually nurses, pharmacists, or both); are directed by a board-certified physician-toxicologist; and are associated with a medical center that has laboratory facilities and personnel needed for the diagnosis and management of poisoning. In addition, certified poison centers participate in the toxic exposure surveillance system, and offer poison-prevention education to the public and poison-treatment education to health professionals.

Alabama

Regional Poison Control Center
The Children's Hospital of Alabama
1600 7th Avenue South
Birmingham, AL 35233-1711
(205) 939-9201
(800) 292-6678 (AL only)
(205) 933-4050

Arizona

Arizona Poison and Drug Information Center
Arizona Health Sciences Center, Rm #3204-K
1501 N. Campbell Avenue
Tucson, AZ 85724
(800) 362-0101 (AZ only)
(602) 626-6016

Samaritan Regional Poison Center
Good Samaritan Regional Medical Center
1130 E. McDowell, Suite A-5
Phoenix, AZ 85006
(602) 253-3334

California

Fresno Regional Poison Control Center
Fresno Community Hospital and Medical Center
2823 Fresno Street
Fresno, CA 93721
(800) 346-5922
(209) 445-1222

San Diego Regional Poison Center
UCSD Medical Center
225 Dickinson Street
San Diego, CA 92103-8925
(619) 543-6000
(800) 876-4766 (in 619 area code only)

San Francisco Bay Area Regional Poison Control Center
San Francisco General Hospital
1001 Potrero Avenue
Building 80, Room 230
San Francisco, CA 94122
(415) 476-6600

Santa Clara Valley Medical Center Regional Poison Center
751 South Bascom Avenue
San Jose, CA 95128
(408) 299-5112
(800) 662-9886 (CA only)

University of California, Davis, Medical Center Regional Poison Control Center
2315 Stockton Boulevard
Sacramento, CA 95817
(916) 734-3692
(800) 342-9293 (Northern California only)

Colorado

Rocky Mountain Poison and Drug Center
645 Bannock Street
Denver, CO 80204
(303) 629-1123

District of Columbia

National Capital Poison Center
Georgetown University Hospital
3800 Reservoir Road, NW
Washington, DC 20007
(202) 625-3333
(202) 784-4660 (TTY)

Florida

The Florida Poison Information Center at Tampa General Hospital
P.O. Box 1289
Tampa, FL 33601
(813) 253-4444 (Tampa)
(800) 282-3171 (Florida)

Georgia

Georgia Poison Center
Grady Memorial Hospital
80 Butler Street, SE
P.O. Box 26066
Atlanta, GA 30335-3801
(800) 282-5846 (GA only)
(404) 589-4400

Indiana

Indiana Poison Center
Methodist Hospital of Indiana
1701 N. Senate Boulevard
P.O. Box 1367
Indianapolis, IN 46206-1367
(800) 382-9097 (IN only)
(317) 929-2323

Maryland

Maryland Poison Center
20 N. Pine Street
Baltimore, MD 21201
(410) 528-7701
(800) 492-2414 (MD only)

***National Capital Poison Center
(DC suburbs only)***
Georgetown University Hospital
3800 Reservoir Road, NW
Washington, DC 20007
(202) 625-3333
(202) 784-4660 (TTY)

Massachusetts

Massachusetts Poison Control System
300 Longwood Avenue
Boston, MA 02115
(617) 232-2120
(800) 682-9211

Michigan

Blodgett Regional Poison Center
1840 Wealthy, SE
Grand Rapids, MI 49506-2968
(800) 632-2727 (Michigan only)
(800) 356-3232 (TTY)

Poison Control Center
Children's Hospital of Michigan
3901 Beaubien Boulevard
Detroit, MI 48201
(313) 745-5711

Minnesota

Hennepin Regional Poison Center
Hennepin County Medical Center
701 Park Avenue
Minneapolis, MN 55415
(612) 347-3141
(612) 337-7387 (Petline)
(612) 337-7474 (TTD)

Minnesota Regional Poison Center
St. Paul–Ramsey Medical Center
640 Jackson Street
St. Paul, MN 55101
(612) 221-2113

Missouri

***Cardinal Glennon Children's Hospital
Regional Poison Center***
1465 S. Grand Boulevard
St. Louis, MO 63104
(314) 772-5200
(800) 366-8888

Montana

Rocky Mountain Poison and Drug Center
645 Bannock Street
Denver, CO 80204
(303) 629-1123

Nebraska

The Poison Center
8301 Dodge Street
Omaha, NE 68114
(402) 390-5555 (Omaha)
(800) 955-9119 (NE)

New Jersey

***New Jersey Poison Information and
Education System***
201 Lyons Avenue
Newark, NJ 07112
(800) 962-1253

New Mexico

***New Mexico Poison and Drug Information
Center***
University of New Mexico
Albuquerque, NM 87131-1076
(505) 843-2551
(800) 432-6866 (NM only)

New York

Hudson Valley Poison Center
Nyack Hospital
160 N. Midland Avenue
Nyack, NY 10960
(800) 336-6997
(914) 353-1000

Long Island Regional Poison Control Center
Winthrop University Hospital
259 First Street
Mineola, NY 11501
(516) 542-2323, 2324, 2325, 3813

New York City Poison Control Center
NYC Department of Health
455 First Avenue, Room 123
New York, NY 10016
(212) 340-4494
(212) P-O-I-S-O-N-S
(212) 689-9014 (TTD)

Ohio

Central Ohio Poison Center
700 Children's Drive
Columbus, OH 43205-2696
(614) 228-1323
(800) 682-7625
(614) 228-2272 (TTY)
(614) 461-2012

*Cincinnati Drug & Poison Information
Center and Regional Poison Control System*
231 Bethesda Avenue, ML 144
Cincinnati, OH 45267-0144
(513) 558-5111
(800) 872-5111 (OH only)

Oregon

Oregon Poison Center
Oregon Health Sciences University
3181 S.W. Sam Jackson Park Road
Portland, OR 97201
(503) 494-8968
(800) 452-7165 (OR only)

Pennsylvania

Central Pennsylvania Poison Center
University Hospital
Milton S. Hershey Medical Center
Hershey, PA 17033
(800) 521-6110

*The Poison Control Center serving the
greater Philadelphia metropolitan area*
One Children's Center
Philadelphia, PA 19104-4303
(215) 386-2100

Pittsburgh Poison Center
3705 Fifth Avenue at DeSoto Street
Pittsburgh, PA 15213
(412) 681-6669

Rhode Island

Rhode Island Poison Center
593 Eddy Street
Providence, RI 02903
(401) 277-5727

Texas

North Texas Poison Center
5201 Harry Hines Boulevard
P.O. Box 35926
Dallas, TX 75235
(214) 590-5000
(800) 441-0040 (Texas Watts)

Texas State Poison Center
The University of Texas Medical Branch
Galveston, TX 77550-2780
(409) 765-1420 (Galveston)
(713) 654-1702 (Houston)

Utah

*Intermountain Regional Poison Control
Center*
50 North Medical Drive
Salt Lake City, UT 84132
(801) 581-2151
(800) 456-7707 (UT only)

Virginia

Blue Ridge Poison Center
Box 67
Blue Ridge Hospital
Charlottesville, VA 22901
(804) 924-5543
(800) 451-1428

*National Capital Poison Center
(Northern VA only)*
Georgetown University Hospital
3800 Reservoir Road, NW
Washington, DC 20007
(202) 625-3333
(202) 784-4660 (TTY)

West Virginia

West Virginia Poison Center
3110 MacCorkle Avenue, SE
Charleston, WV 25304
(800) 642-3625 (WV only)
(304) 348-4211

Wyoming

The Poison Center
8301 Dodge Street
Omaha, NE 68114
(402) 390-5555 (Omaha)
(800) 955-9119 (NE)

Canadian Drug Information

Alfred J. Rémillard, Pharm.D.

INTERNATIONAL SYSTEM OF UNITS

In an attempt to standardize the large number of different units used worldwide and thus improve communication, the *Système International d'Unités* (International System of Units, SI) was recommended in 1954. In 1971, the mole (mol) was adopted as the standard for designating the amount of substance present, and the liter (L) was adopted as the standard for designating volume. The World Health Organization recommended the adoption of SI units in 1977. However, Canada had already implemented an equivalent system in 1971.

In therapeutics, the major change caused by adopting the SI was to express drug concentrations present in body fluids in molar units (e.g., μmol/L) rather than in mass units (e.g., mg/L). This allows us to better compare the pharmacologic and pharmacodynamic effects of different drugs, since these effects are now related to the number of molecules (e.g., μmol) of drug present rather than to the number of mass units (e.g., mg).

DRUG SERUM CONCENTRATIONS

Many drugs have known therapeutic or toxic levels that are monitored in patients to insure safety and efficacy. In Canada, clinical laboratories report these levels in SI units. Levels traditionally reported as μg/ml can be converted to μmol/L once the conversion factor (CF) is calculated:

$$CF = \frac{1000}{\text{molecular weight of the drug}}$$

To convert from μg/ml to SI units:

$$\mu g/ml \times CF = \mu mol/L$$

To convert from SI units to μg/ml:

$$\frac{\mu mol/L}{CF} = \mu g/ml$$

Table F–1 lists some important drugs for which therapeutic or toxic levels have been established. For most of these drugs, the levels presented are *trough* (minimum) values, which are measured in blood samples drawn just prior to the next dose. For the aminoglycosides and vancomycin, two levels are listed: a *trough* level and a *peak* (maximum) level. Levels must remain between the peak and trough to maintain efficacy of these drugs and to minimize toxicity.

References

1. SI Manual in Health Care, 2nd ed. Subcommittee of Metric Commission Canada, Sector 9.10, Health and Welfare, Ottawa, Canada, June 1, 1982.
2. McLeod DC: SI units in drug therapeutics. Drug Intell Clin Pharm 22:990–993, 1988.
3. Evans WE, Schentag JJ, Jusko WJ (eds): Applied Pharmacokinetics: Principles of Therapeutic Drug Monitoring. Applied Therapeutics, Inc., Spokane, WA, 1992.

CANADIAN DRUG LEGISLATION

In Canada, two acts form the basis of drug laws. The Food and Drug Act, which was amended in 1953, controls the manufacture, distribution, and sale of all drugs except narcotics. The Narcotic Control Act (1961) controls the manufacture, distribution, and sale of narcotic drugs. The responsibility for administering these Acts rests with the Health Protection Branch, Department of National Health and Welfare. Both acts contain general statements relating to the safety and efficacy of drugs. Detailed requirements are outlined in the Regulations.

	Table F–1. Therapeutic Serum Drug Concentrations				
Drugs	**SI Reference Interval**	**SI Unit**	**Conversion Factor**	**Traditional Reference Interval**	**Traditional Reference Unit**
Acetaminophen	13–40	μmol/L	66.16	0.2–0.6	mg/dl
Acetylsalicylic acid	7.2–21.7	μmol/L	0.0724	100–300	mg/dl
Amikacin*	—	—	—	15–25†; <8‡	μg/ml
Amitriptyline	430–900§	nmol/L	3.605	120–250§	ng/ml
Carbamazepine	17–42	μmol/L	4.233	4–10	μg/ml
Desipramine	430–750	nmol/L	3.754	115–200	ng/ml
Digoxin	0.6–2.8	nmol/L	1.282	0.5–2.2	ng/ml
Disopyramide	6–18	μmol/L	2.946	2–6	μg/ml
Gentamicin*	—	—	—	6–10†; <2‡	μg/ml
Imipramine	640–1070§	nmol/L	3.566	180–300§	ng/ml
Lidocaine	4.5–21.5	μmol/L	4.267	1–5	μg/ml
Lithium	0.4–1.2	mmol/L	1.0	0.4–1.2	mEq/L
Netilmicin*	—	—	—	6–10†; <2‡	μg/ml
Nortriptyline	190–570	nmol/L	3.797	50–150	ng/ml
Phenobarbital	65–170	μmol/L	4.306	15–40	μg/ml
Phenytoin	40–80	μmol/L	3.964	10–20	μg/ml
Primidone	25–46	μmol/L	4.582	6–10	μg/ml
Procainamide	17–34§	μmol/L	4.249	4–8§	μg/ml
Qunidine	4.6–9.2	μmol/L	3.082	1.5–3	μg/ml
Theophylline	55–110	μmol/L	5.55	10–20	μg/ml
Tobramycin*	—	—	—	6–10†; <2‡	μg/ml
Valproic acid	300–700	μmol/L	6.934	50–100	μg/ml
Vancomycin*	—	—	—	25–40†; <10‡	μg/ml

*Aminoglycosides (amikacin, gentamicin, netilmicin, tobramycin) and vancomycin are not reported in SI units because of the variability of their molecular weights.
†Peak drug level.
‡Trough drug level.
§Drug level reported as the total of the parent drug and its active metabolite.

PRESCRIPTION DRUGS (SCHEDULE F)

The Food and Drug Regulations separate drugs sold in Canada into several categories, referred to as Schedules. Schedule F lists all prescription drugs, and includes a wide diversity of classes, such as antihypertensives, hormonal preparations, and psychotropic medications. These drugs are available to the general public only with a prescription from a medical practitioner. Prescriptions for Schedule F medications may be written or verbal (i.e., telephone order to the pharmacist) and can be refilled as often as indicated by the physician. More than 350 drugs are listed in Schedule F, which is subject to frequent changes. The symbol Pr must appear on all manufacturing labels. Although some drugs may be classified *federally* as nonprescription, the *provinces* may nonetheless require a prescription, as occurs with digoxin, for example.

CONTROLLED DRUGS (SCHEDULE G)

Controlled drugs, listed in Schedule G of the Food and Drug Act, have a moderate potential for abuse. Accordingly, these agents require greater control than Schedule F drugs (prescription drugs), which have essentially no potential for abuse.

Schedule G contains about 14 drugs, including potent analgesics (nalbuphine, butorphanol), amphetamine and its congeners, and the barbiturates (phenobarbital, amobarbital, secobarbital). The distribution of controlled substances is more restricted than the distribution of Schedule F drugs. Schedule G drugs can be obtained by a written or verbal prescription, but refills are only allowed on a written order. The symbol ◈ must appear on the labels of these drugs. Schedule G is similar to Schedule III of the Controlled Substances Act in the United States.

RESTRICTED DRUGS (SCHEDULE H)

These agents are hallucinogenic, potentially dangerous, and have no recognized medicinal use. Examples include LSD, peyote, and mescaline. These chemicals are available legally only to medical institutions involved in specialized research. This category is similar to Schedule I of the Controlled Substances Act in the United States.

NARCOTIC DRUGS

Narcotic drugs are controlled by the Narcotic Control Act and Regulations. Examples include coca leaves (cocaine), opium, codeine, morphine, phencyclidine, and Cannabis (marijuana). The major clinical use for these drugs is strong analgesia. However, they all have potent psychotropic effects and addictive potential. As a result, their availability must be strictly controlled. Narcotic agents can be dispensed only with a written prescription. No refills are allowed. The letter **N** must appear on all labels and professional advertisements.

An exception to the narcotic drug regulations is low-dose codeine (8-mg tablets and 20 mg/30 ml liquid), which can be purchased without a prescription. The codeine must be in a preparation that contains at least two additional medicinal ingredients (acetylsalicylic acid and caffeine) and can be sold only by a pharmacist.

NONPRESCRIPTION DRUGS

Nonprescription drugs, also known as over-the-counter (OTC) medications, can be purchased without a prescription. These drugs represent an interesting class of compounds, as several prescription drugs shown to have a proven safety record are, in low-dose formulations, gradually being transferred to the OTC category. Examples include ibuprofen [Motrin] in 200-mg tablets and hydrocortisone in 0.5% topical preparations.

Although the Food and Drug Act and Regulations place no restrictions on how OTC drugs are sold, most provinces have drug schedules—administered by their respective Pharmacy Acts—to determine the conditions and place of sale. As a result, there are three categories of nonprescription medications in Canada. These are described below.

The first category represents general proprietary (GP) medicines and can be purchased at any retail outlet. These products are intended for the symptomatic treatment of self-limiting minor illness, injury, or discomfort. Proprietary medications have adequate information on the packages so that they can be administered without the assistance of a health professional. Examples include medicated shampoos, minor analgesics, and cough drops.

Agents in the second category are generally available only in pharmacies. Although these drugs are intended for treating minor self-limiting conditions, it is recommended that the advice of a health professional be obtained concerning their proper use. Examples of this category include laxatives, cough and cold preparations, disinfectants, and many vitamins.

The third category consists of medicines that should be taken only on the recommendation of a physician. These drugs, which are available in pharmacies, include insulin, nitroglycerin, muscle relaxants, and antispasmodics. Also in this category are medications that are not accessible to the public but may be purchased after consultation with the pharmacist. These include ibuprofen, hydrocortisone, and low-dose preparations of codeine.

SCHEDULE HARMONIZATION

The Health Protection Branch (HPB) has expressed concern about the proliferation of differing provincial schedules that regulate the sale of nonprescription drugs. In an attempt to address the problems of the current regulatory system at both the federal and provincial levels, the HBP has proposed to harmonize drug schedules throughout the country, using a three-Schedule system. Schedule I would include all prescription drugs (Schedules F and G, and Narcotics); Schedule II would consist of pharmacist-monitored nonprescription drugs; and Schedule III would consist of nonprescription drugs that are not appropriate for inclusion in Schedule I or II. For Schedule III drugs, there would be no restrictions on the place of sale.

The first step toward harmonization is to develop scientific criteria to determine the degree of professional involvement required for the sale and judicious use of drug products. Criteria for determining which drugs will be assigned to Schedule II will be the greatest challenge. Creation of Schedule II represents a very progressive step in drug regulation, as it is anticipated that many prescription drugs with a proven safety profile, such as cimetidine, may be transferred to this Schedule. The HPB is currently reviewing comments received and is expected to publish its proposals soon in the form of draft regulations.

References

1. Health Protection and Drug Laws. Health and Welfare Canada, Canadian Publishing Center, Ottawa, Canada, 1988.
2. Johnson GE, Hannah KJ, Zerr SR: Pharmacology and the Nursing Process. 3rd ed. WB Saunders, Philadelphia, 1992.
3. Health Protection Branch, Information Newsletter. Issue No. 798, September 9, 1991.

NEW DRUG DEVELOPMENT IN CANADA

The process for approving a new drug in Canada is very similar, if not identical, to the process in the United States. The same drug data that are required for approval by the Food and Drug Administration in the United States are required by the Health Protection Branch (HPB) in Canada. The principal difference between Canada and the U.S. is one of nomenclature: once preclinical testing is completed, the manufacturer in Canada applies for a *Preclinical New Drug Submission*, versus an Investigational New Drug in the United States; at the end of clinical testing, the manufacturer in Canada seeks a *New Drug Submission* (NDS), versus a New Drug Application in the United States.

After all the information on a new drug has been submitted—including results of preclinical and clinical testing, method of manufacturing, packaging, labeling, and results of stability testing—the pharmaceutical company receives a *Notice of Compliance* (NOC) from the HPB, and the drug enters the market.

Although data collection for a new drug is thorough, there is no guarantee that all adverse reactions are known, especially when the drug is used concurrently with other drugs. Also, long-term effects are not fully appreciated. For these reasons, postmarketing surveillance plays a major role in monitoring these drugs. The manufacturer must immediately report any new clinical findings, unexpected adverse effects, or therapeutic failures to the HPB.

PATENT LAWS

In 1969, changes were made to the Patent Act, and Compulsory Licensing was introduced. The license allowed generic drug companies to manufacture and distribute patented drugs in Canada, provided that a minimal 4% royalty fee was paid to the patent holder. This system was introduced to help control drug prices. Unfortunately, the system caused a decline in revenue to "innovative" pharmaceutical companies, with a resultant decline in research on new drug development. After much debate, and retroactive to June 1987, the Patent Act was amended to allow market exclusivity for either (1) 7 to 10 years, or (2) until the 17-year patent (from date of filing) expires, whichever comes first. A Price Review Board was created to monitor the prices of new drugs and those under Compulsory Licensing.

ANTICIPATED PATENT LAW CHANGES

Further changes in the Patent Act are expected. As a result of extensive lobbying from representatives of the pharmaceutical industry, provisions were included in the North American Free Trade Agreement (1992) and the General Agreement on Tariffs and Trade (1991) that require Canada to repeal its patent laws and bring them into agreement with international rules on the protection of intellectual property. At the time of this writing, the Canadian Parliament approved Bill C-91, which will extend patent protection by 3 years, thereby providing 20 years of exclusivity for companies that develop new drugs. This would be consistent with patent laws in the United States and other industrialized nations.

References

1. Health Protection and Drug Laws. Health and Welfare Canada, Canadian Publishing Center, Ottawa, Canada, 1988.
2. Mailhot R: The Canadian drug regulatory process. J Clin Pharmacol 26:232–239, 1986.
3. Sullivan P: CMA to support increased patent protection for drugs but will attach strong qualifications. Can Med Assoc J 147:1669–1701, 1992.

SOME IMPORTANT CANADIAN TRADE NAMES

The list below contains common trade names that are employed in Canada but not in the United States. Trade names that are employed in *both* countries appear in the index, but are not included here.

In the list, trade names are presented in SMALL CAPITAL LETTERS and generic names are presented in standard type. Canadian trade names that are formed simply by affixing a manufacturer's prefix to a generic name are not included in the list; examples of such names are APO-FLURAZEPAM (flurazepam), NOVODIGOXIN (digoxin), PMS-ISONIAZID (isoniazid), and SYN-DILTIAZEM (diltiazem).

An asterisk (*) indicates drugs that are available in Canada but not in the United States. These drugs are not discussed in the text.

Acebutolol, MONITAN, SECTRAL, RHOTRAL
Acetaminophen, ATASOL, PANADOL
ACETAZOLAM, Acetazolamide
Acetazolamide, ACETAZOLAM
Acetohexamide, DIMELOR
ACETOXYL, Benzoyl peroxide
Acetylcysteine, AIRBRON, PARVOLEX
Acetylsalicylic acid, ENTROPHEN, ECOTRIN
ACHROMYCIN, Tetracycline
ACILAC, Lactulose
ACTIFED, Tripolidine
ACTIPROFEN, Ibuprofen
ACULAR, Ketorolac
AEROSPORIN, Polymyxin B
AIRBRON, Acetylcysteine
AKARPINE, Pilocarpine
AK-CON, Naphazoline
AK-DEX, Dexamethasone
AK-DILATE, Phenylephrine
AKINETON, Biperiden
AK-PENTOLATE, Cyclopentolate
AK-SULF, Sulfacetamide
ALBERT TIAFEN, Tiaprofenic acid*
Albuterol, See Salbutamol
Alfacalcidol, ONE-ALPHA
ALLERDRYL, Diphenhydramine
ALLOPRIN, Allopurinol
Allopurinol, ALLOPRIN, PURINOL
ALOMIDE, Lodoxamide* (antiallergy eye drops)
ALOPHEN, Phenolphthalein
Alpha$_1$ proteinase inhibitor, PROLASTIN

Alprazolam, NOVO-ALPRAZOL
AMATINE, Midodrine* (vasopressor)
Ambenonium, MYTELASE
AMERSOL, Ibuprofen
Aminoglutethimide, CYTADREN
Aminophylline, PHYLLOCONTIN
5-Aminosalicylic Acid, ASACOL, SALOFALK, MESASAL, PENTASA
Amitriptyline, LEVATE
Amoxicillin, APO-AMOXI, NOVAMOXIN, NU-AMOXI
Amoxicillin/clavulanate, CLAVULIN
Ampicillin, AMPICIN, APO-AMPI, NU-AMPI, PENBRITIN
AMPICIN, Ampicillin
ANAFRANIL, Clomipramine* (antidepressant)
ANANDRON, Nilutamide* (antiandrogen)
ANAPOLON 50, Oxymetholone
ANCOTIL, Flucytosine
Ancrod* (anticoagulant), ARVIN
ANDRIOL, Testosterone
ANDROCUR, Cyproterone* (antiandrogen)
ANEXATE, Flumazenil
Anileridine* (narcotic), LERITINE
ANTHRANOL, Dithranol
ANTIVERT, Meclizine
ANTURAN, Sulfinpyrazone
APARKANE, Trihexyphenidyl
APO-ALPRAZ, Alprazolam
APO-AMOXI, Amoxicillin
APO-AMPI, Ampicillin
APO-CAPTO, Captopril
APO-CHLORAX, Clidinium
APO-CLOXI, Cloxacillin
APO-DICLO, Diclofenac
APO-DILTIAZ, Diltiazem
APO-DOXY, Doxycycline
APO-ERYTHRO, Erythromycin
APO-HYDRO, Hydrochlorthiazide
APO-ISDN, Isosorbide
APO-KETO, Ketoprofen
APO-METOCLOP, Metoclopramide
APO-NADOL, Nadolol
APO-NIFED, Nifedipine
APO-PEN-VK, Penicillin V
APO-PRAZO, Prazosin
APO-SALVENT, Salbutamol (Albuterol in U.S.)
APO-SULIN, Sulindac
APO-TAMOX, Tamoxifen
APO-TETRA, Tetracycline
APO-TRIAZIDE, Triamterene
APO-TRIAZO, Triazolam
APO-TRIHEX, Trihexyphenidyl
APO-TRIMIP, Trimipramine
APO-VERAP, Verapamil
Apraclonidine* (alpha-adrenergic, ophthal.), IOPIDINE
APRESOLINE, Hydralazine
ARLIDIN, Nylidrin
ARVIN, Ancrod* (anticoagulant)
ASACOL, 5-Aminosalicylic Acid
Asparaginase, KIDROLASE
ATASOL, Acetaminophen
Atovaquone* (*Pneumocystis carinii* therapy), MEPRON
Atropine, ATROPISOL
ATROPISOL, Atropine
ATROVENT, Ipratropium* (asthma inhaler)
AUREOMYCIN, Chlortetracycline
AVLOSULFON, Dapsone
AXSAIN, Capsaicin
Azatadine, OPTIMINE
Bacampicillin, PENGLOBE
BACIGUENT, Bacitracin
BACITIN, Bacitracin
Bacitracin, BACIGUENT, BACITIN
BACTROBAN, Mupirocin* (antibiotic)
BANLIN, Propantheline
BCG, IMMUCYST
BECLOFORTE, Beclomethasone

Beclomethasone, BECLOFORTE
BENOXYL, Benzoyl peroxide
Benserazide* (antiparkinson), PROLOPA
BENTYLOL, Dicyclomine
BENYLIN, Dextromethorphan
Benzoyl peroxide, ACETOXYL, BENOXYL
BEROTEC, Fenoterol* (asthma inhaler)
BETAGAN, Levobunolol
BETALOC, Metoprolol
Betamethasone, CELESTONE, DIPROSONE
BICILLIN, Penicillin G
Biperiden, AKINETON
BIQUIN, Quinidine
BONAMINE, Meclizine
BONEFOS, Clodronate* (for hypercalcemia)
BRETYLATE, Bretylium
Bretylium, BRETYLATE
BRICANYL, Terbutaline
BRIETAL, Methohexital
Bromazepam* (benzodiazepine), LECTOPAM
Brompheniramine, DIMETANE
BRONKAID, Epinephrine
Budesonide* (steroid inhaler), PULMICORT, RHINOCORT
Bufexamac* (NSAID, topical), NORFEMAC
BUSCOPAN, Scopolamine
Buserelin* (LH-RH analogue), SUPREFACT
CANESTEN, Clotrimazole
CANTHACUR, Cantharidin
Cantharidin, CANTHACUR, CANTHARONE
CANTHARONE, Cantharidin
Capsaicin, AXSAIN, ZOSTRIX
Captopril, APO-CAPTO, NU-CAPTO
Carbamazepine, NOVO-CARBAMAZ
CARBOCAINE, Mepivacaine
CARBOLITH, Lithium carbonate
CATARASE, Chymotrypsin
CEDOCARD, Isosorbide
CEDOCARD-SR, Isosorbide dinitrate
CEFOMONIL, Cefsulodin
Cefsulodin, CEFOMONIL
Ceftazidime, FORTAZ
CELESTONE, Betamethasone
CELONTIN, Methsuximide
Cephalexin, NOVO-LEXIN
CEPHULAC, Lactulose
CEREVON, Ferrous succinate
Cetirizine* (antihistamine), REACTINE
Chloramphenicol, SOPAMYCETIN
Chlordiazepoxide, SOLIUM
Chlorothiazide, SUPRES
Chlorphenesin, MYCIL
Chlorpheniramine, CHLOR-TRIPOLON
Chlorpromazine, LARGACTIL
Chlorpropamide, NOVO-PROPAMIDE
Chlortetracycline, AUREOMYCIN
CHLOR-TRIPOLON, Chlorpheniramine
Cholecalciferol, OS-CAL D
CHOLEDYL, Oxtriphylline
Choline magnesium salicylate, TRILISATE
CHOLOXIN, Dextrothyroxine
CHOPHYLLIN, Oxtriphylline
CHRONULAC, Lactulose
CHYMODIACTIN, Chymopapain
Chymopapain, CHYMODIACTIN
Chymotrypsin, CATARASE, ZONULYN
CIDOMYCIN, Gentamicin
Cilazapril* (ACE inhibitor), INHIBACE
Cimetidine, PEPTOL, NU-CIMET
CITANEST, Prilocaine
Cladribine* (cancer chemotherapy), LEUSTATIN
CLARITIN, Loratadine* (antihistamine)
CLAVULIN, Amoxicillin/clavulanate
Clidinium, APO-CHLORAX, CORIUM, LIBRAX
Clindamycin, DALACIN C
Clobazam* (benzodiazepine, anticonvulsant), FRISIUM

Clodronate* (for hypercalcemia), BONEFOS
Clofibrate, NOVO-FIBRATE
Clomipramine* (antidepressant), ANAFRANIL
Clonazepam, RIVOTRIL
Clonidine, DIXARIT
Clorazepate, NOVO-CLOPATE
CLOTRIMADERM, Clotrimazole
Clotrimazole, CANESTEN, CLOTRIMADERM, MYCLO, NEO-ZOL
Cloxacillin, APO-CLOXI, ORBENIN, NOVO-CLOXIN, NU-CLOXI
COMBANTRIN, Pyrantel
CORADUR, Isosorbide dinitrate
CORAMINE, Nikethamide
CORIUM, Clidinium
CORONEX, Isosorbide dinitrate
CORTATE, Hydrocortisone
CORTEF, Hydrocortisone
Cortisone, CORTONE
CORTONE, Cortisone
CORTROSYN, Cosyntropin
Cosyntropin, CORTROSYN, SYNACTHEN DEPOT
Cyanocobalamin, RUBION, RUBRAMIN
Cyclizine, MARZINE
CYCLOGYL, Cyclopentolate
CYCLOMEN, Danazol
Cyclopentolate, AK-PENTOLATE, CYCLOGYL
Cyclophosphamide, PROCYTOX
CYKLOKAPRON, Tranexamic acid* (hemostatic)
Cyproheptadine, PERIACTIN
Cyproterone* (antiandrogen), ANDROCUR
CYTADREN, Aminoglutethimide
CYTOTEC, Misoprostol
DALACIN C, Clindamycin
Danazol, CYCLOMEN
Dapsone, AVLOSULFON
DARBID, Isopropamide
Deferoxamine, DESFERAL
DELALUTIN, Hydroxyprogesterone
DELATESTRYL, Testosterone
DELSYM, Dextromethorphan
DELTASONE, Prednisone
DESFERAL, Deferoxamine
Desipramine, NORPRAMIN
Dexamethasone, AK-DEX, DEXASONE, HEXADROL, ORADEXON, SPERSADEX
DEXASONE, Dexamethasone
Dexbrompheniramine* (antihistamine), DRIXORAL, DRIXTAB
Dexchlorpheniramine, POLARAMINE
Dextromethorphan, BENYLIN, DELSYM, ROBIDEX
Dextrothyroxine, CHOLOXIN
DIABETA, Glyburide
DIAZEMULS, Diazepam
Diazepam, DIAZEMULS, VIVOL
DICLECTIN, Doxylamine
Diclofenac, NOVO-DIFENAC
Dicyclomine, BENTYLOL, FORMULEX
DIDRONEL, Etidronate
Dienestrol, ORTHO DIENESTROL
Diethylcarbamazine, HETRAZAN
Diethylpropion, TENUATE
Diethylstilbestrol, HONVOL
DIGITALINE, Digitoxin
Digitoxin, DIGITALINE
Dihydroergotoxine, see Ergoloid mesylates
DILOSYN, Methdilazine
Diltiazem, APO-DILTIAZ, NU-DILTIAZ
DIMELOR, Acetohexamide
Dimenhydrinate, GRAVOL, NAUSEATOL, TRAVEL AID
DIMETANE, Brompheniramine
Dinoprostone, PREPIDIL, PROSTIN
Diphenhydramine, ALLERDRYL
DIPROSONE, Betamethasone
Dipyridamole, NOVO-DIPIRADOL
DISIPAL, Orphenadrine
Disopyramide, RYTHMODAN

Dithranol, ANTHRANOL
DIXARIT, Clonidine
DOPAMET, Methyldopa
Dopamine, REVIMINE
Doxepin, TRIADAPIN
DOXIDAN, Phenolphthalein
Doxycycline, APO-DOXY
Doxylamine, DICLECTIN
DRISDOL, Ergocalciferol
DRIXORAL, Dexbrompheniramine* (antihistamine)
DRIXTAB, Dexbrompheniramine* (antihistamine)
DURALITH, Lithium carbonate
DURETIC, Methyclothiazide
Echothiophate, PHOSPHOLINE IODIDE
Econazole, ECOSTATIN
ECOSTATIN, Econazole
ECOTRIN, Acetylsalicylic acid
Edoxudine* (antiviral), VIROSTAT
Edrophonium, ENLON
ELDISINE, Vindesine
ELTOR, Pseudoephedrine
ELTROXIN, Levothyroxine
ENLON, Edrophonium
Enoxaparin, LOVENOX
ENTROPHEN, Acetylsalicylic acid
Epinephrine, BRONKAID, SUS-PHRINE
EQUANIL, Meprobamate
ERGAMISOL, Levamisole
Ergocalciferol, DRISDOL, OSTOFORTE
Ergoloid mesylates, HYDERGINE
ERGOMAR, Ergotamine
Ergotamine, ERGOMAR, GYNERGEN
ERYC, Erythromycin
ERYTHROMID, Erythromycin
Erythromycin, ERYTHROMID, APO-ERYTHRO, ERYC
ESTINYL, Ethinyl estradiol
Estrone, FEMOGEN
Estropipate, OGEN
Ethambutol, ETIBI
Ethinyl estradiol, ESTINYL
Ethopropazine, PARSITAN
ETIBI, Ethambutol
Etidronate, DIDRONEL
EUFLEX, Flutamide
EUGLUCON, Glyburide
FACTREL, Gonadorelin
FASTIN, Phentermine
Felodipine, PLENDIL
FEMOGEN, Estrone
Fenfluramine, PONDERAL, PONDIMIN
Fenoterol* (asthma inhaler), BEROTEC
Ferrous fumarate, PALAFER
Ferrous succinate, CEREVON
FIBREPUR, Psyllium
FLAMAZINE, Silver sulfadiazine
Flavoxate* (antispasmodic), URISPAS
Floctafenine* (NSAID), IDARAC
FLUANXOL, Flupenthixol* (antipsychotic)
FLUCLOX, Flucloxacillin* (antibiotic)
Flucloxacillin* (antibiotic), FLUCLOX
Flucytosine, ANCOTIL
Flumazenil, ANEXATE
Flunisolide, RHINALAR
Fluorescein, FLUORESCITE, FLUOR-I-STRIP
FLUORESCITE, Fluorescein
FLUOR-I-STRIP, Fluorescein
Flupenthixol* (antipsychotic), FLUANXOL
Fluphenazine, MODECATE, MODITEN
Flurazepam, NOVO-FLUPAM, SOMNOL
Flurbiprofen, FROBEN
Fluspirilene* (antipsychotic), IMAP
Flutamide, EUFLEX
Fluvoxamine, LUVOX
Folic acid, NOVO-FOLACID

FORANE, Isoflurane
FORMULEX, Dicyclomine
FORTAZ, Ceftazidime
FRISIUM, Clobazam* (benzodiazepine, anticonvulsant)
FROBEN, Flurbiprofen* (NSAID)
Furosemide, URITOL
GEN-GLYBE, Glyburide
GENTACIDIN, Gentamicin
GENTAK, Gentamicin
Gentamicin, CIDOMYCIN, GENTACIDIN, GENTAK, GENTRASUL
GENTRASUL, Gentamicin
GESTEROL, Progesterone
GLUCOPHAGE, Metformin* (hypoglycemic)
Glyburide, DIABETA, EUGLUCON, GEN-GLYBE
Gonadorelin, FACTREL
GRAVOL, Dimenhydrinate
Griseofulvin, GRISOVIN-FP
GRISOVIN-FP, Griseofulvin
GYNERGEN, Ergotamine
GYNO-TROSYD, Tioconazole
Haloperidol, NOVO-PERIDOL
HEPALEAN, Heparin
Heparin, HEPALEAN
HERPLEX, Idoxuridine
HETRAZAN, Diethylcarbamazine
HEXADROL, Dexamethasone
HEXIT, Lindane
HISTANTIL, Promethazine
HONVOL, Diethylstilbestrol
HYCODAN, Hydrocodone
HYCORT, Hydrocortisone
HYDERGINE, Ergoloid mesylates (formerly Dihydroergotoxine)
Hydralazine, APRESOLINE, NOVO-HYLAZIN, NU-HYDRAL
Hydrochlorothiazide, APO-HYDRO
Hydrocodone, HYCODAN, ROBIDONE
Hydrocortisone, CORTATE, CORTEF, HYCORT
Hydroxyprogesterone, DELALUTIN
Hydroxyzine, MULTIPAX
HYGROTON, Chlorthalidone
HYPRHO-D, Rho(D) immune globulin
Ibuprofen, ACTIPROFEN, AMERSOL, MEDIPREN, NOVO-PROFEN
IDARAC, Floctafenine* (NSAID)
Idoxuridine, HERPLEX, STOXIL
IMAP, Fluspirilene* (antipsychotic)
IMFERON, Iron dextran
Imipenem, PRIMAXIN
IMMUCYST, BCG
IMOVANE, Zopiclone* (hypnotic)
Indapamide, LOZIDE
INDOCID, Indomethacin
Indomethacin, INDOCID, NOVO-METHACIN, NU-INDO
INFLAMASE, Prednisolone
INHIBACE, Cilazapril* (ACE inhibitor)
Interferon alfa-n1, WELLFERON
IONAMIN, Phentermine
IOPIDINE, Apraclonidine* (alpha-adrenergic, ophthal.)
Iron dextran, IMFERON
Iron sorbitex, JECTOFER
Isoflurane, FORANE
Isoniazid, ISOTAMINE
Isoproterenol, MEDIHALER-ISO
Isosorbide, APO-ISDN, CEDOCARD
Isosorbide dinitrate, CEDOCARD-SR, CORADUR, CORONEX
ISOTAMINE, Isoniazid
Isoxsuprine, VASODILAN
JECTOFER, Iron sorbitex
KEMADRIN, Procyclidine
Ketazolam* (benzodiazepine), LOFTRAN
Ketoprofen, APO-KETO, ORUVAIL, RHODIS
Ketorolac, ACULAR
Ketotifen* (anti-allergy), ZADITEN
KIDROLASE, Asparaginase
KONAKION, Phytomenadione
KWELLADA, Lindane

Lactulose, ACILAC, CEPHULAC, CHRONULAC, RHODIALOSE
LANVIS, Thioguanine
LARGACTIL, Chlorpromazine
LECTOPAM, Bromazepam* (benzodiazepine)
LERITINE, Anileridine* (narcotic)
LEUSTATIN, Cladribine* (cancer chemotherapy)
Levamisole, ERGAMISOL
Levarterenol, See Norepinephrine
LEVATE, Amitriptyline
Levobunolol, BETAGAN
Levocabastine* (antihistamine), LIVOSTIN
Levodopa/benserazide* (antiparkinson), PROLOPA
LEVOPHED, Norepinephrine
Levothyroxine, ELTROXIN
LIBRAX, Clidinium
Lidocaine, XYLOCARD
Lindane, HEXIT, KWELLADA
Lisinopril, PRINIVIL
Lithium carbonate, CARBOLITH, DURALITH, LITHIZINE
LITHIZINE, Lithium carbonate
LIVOSTIN, Levocabastine* (antihistamine)
Lodoxamide* (antiallergy eye drops), ALOMIDE
LOFTRAN, Ketazolam* (benzodiazepine)
LONITEN, Minoxidil
Loratadine* (antihistamine), CLARITIN
Lorazepam, NOVO-LORAZEM, NU-LORAZ
Lovastatin, MEVACOR
LOVENOX, Enoxaparin
LOXAPAC, Loxapine
Loxapine, LOXAPAC
LOZIDE, Indapamide
LUVOX, Fluvoxamine
MAJEPTIL, Thioproperazine* (antipsychotic)
MANERIX, Moclobemide* (MAOI)
MARZINE, Cyclizine
MAXERAN, Metoclopramide
MEBARAL, Mephobarbital
Meclizine, ANTIVERT, BONAMINE
MEDIHALER-ISO, Isoproterenol
MEDIPREN, Ibuprofen
MEDROL, Methylprednisolone
Mefenamic acid, PONSTAN
MEGACILLIN, Penicillin G
Menadiol, SYNKAVITE
Mephenytoin, MESANTOIN
Mephobarbital, MEBARAL
Mepivacaine, CARBOCAINE
Meprobamate, EQUANIL
MEPRON, Atovaquone* (*Pneumocystis carinii* therapy)
MESANTOIN, Mephenytoin
MESASAL, 5-Aminosalicylic acid
Mesna, UROMITEXAN
MESTINON, Pyridostigmine
METANDREN, Methyltestosterone
Metformin* (hypoglycemic), GLUCOPHAGE
Methazolamide, NEPTAZANE
Methdilazine, DILOSYN
Methocarbamol, ROBAXIN
Methohexital, BRIETAL
Methotrimeprazine, NOZINAN
Methoxamine* (vasopressor), VASOXYL
Methsuximide, CELONTIN
Methyclothiazide, DURETIC
Methyldopa, DOPAMET, NOVO-MEDOPA, NU-MEDOPA
Methylprednisolone, MEDROL
Methyltestosterone, METANDREN
Metoclopramide, APO-METOCLOP, MAXERAN
Metolazone, ZAROXOLYN
Metoprolol, BETALOC, NOVO-METOPROL
Metronidazole, NOVO-NIDAZOL, TRIKACIDE
MEVACOR, Lovastatin
MICRONOR, Norethindrone
Midodrine* (vasopressor), AMATINE
Minoxidil, LONITEN

MIOCARPINE, Pilocarpine
Misoprostol, CYTOTEC
MOBENOL, Tolbutamide
MOBIFLEX, Tenoxicam* (NSAID)
Moclobemide* (MAOI), MANERIX
MODECATE, Fluphenazine
MODITEN, Fluphenazine
MOGADON, Nitrazepam
MONITAN, Acebutolol
MULTIPAX, Hydroxyzine
Mupirocin* (antibiotic), BACTROBAN
MYCIFRADIN, Neomycin
MYCIGUENT, Neomycin
MYCIL, Chlorphenesin
MYCLO, Clotrimazole
MYSOLINE, Primidone
MYTELASE, Ambenonium
Nadolol, APO-NADOL
NADOSTINE, Nystatin
Nafarelin, SYNAREL
NAFRINE, Oxymetazoline
Naphazoline, AK-CON, PRIVINE, RHINO-MEX-N, VASOCON
Naproxen, NAXEN, NEOPROX, NOVO-NAPROX, NU-NAPROX
NATULAN, Procarbazine
NAUSEATOL, Dimenhydrinate
NAXEN, Naproxen
NEBCIN, Tobramycin
NEO-PAUSE, Testosterone/estradiol
NEO-PROX, Naproxen
NEO-ZOL, Clotrimazole
Neomycin, MYCIFRADIN, MYCIGUENT
NEPTAZANE, Methazolamide
NEULEPTIL, Pericyazine* (antipsychotic)
Nicotinyl alcohol tartrate, RONIACOL
Nifedipine, APO-NIFED, NOVO-NIFEDIN, NU-NIFED
Nikethamide, CORAMINE
Nilutamide* (antiandrogen), ANANDRON
Nitrazepam, MOGADON
Nitrofurantoin, NOVO-FURAN
Nitroglycerin (intravenous), NITROSTAT
NITROSTAT, Nitroglycerin (intravenous)
NOLVADEX, Tamoxifen
Norepinephrine, LEVOPHED
Norethindrone, MICRONOR, NORLUTATE
NORFEMAC, Bufexamac* (NSAID, topical)
NORFLEX, Orphenadrine
NORLUTATE, Norethindrone
NORPRAMIN, Desipramine
NOVAMOXIN, Amoxicillin
NOVA-RECTAL, Pentobarbital
NOVO-ALPRAZOL, Alprazolam
NOVO-AZT, Zidovudine
NOVO-BUTAMIDE, Tolbutamide
NOVO-BUTAZONE, Phenylbutazone
NOVO-CARBAMAZ, Carbamazepine
NOVO-CLOPATE, Clorazepate
NOVO-CLOXIN, Cloxacillin
NOVO-DIFENAC, Diclofenac
NOVO-DIPIRADOL, Dipyridamole
NOVO-FIBRATE, Clofibrate
NOVO-FLUPAM, Flurazepam
NOVO-FOLACID, Folic acid
NOVO-FURAN, Nitrofurantoin
NOVO-HYLAZIN, Hydralazine
NOVO-LEXIN, Cephalexin
NOVO-LORAZEM, Lorazepam
NOVO-MEDOPA, Methyldopa
NOVO-METHACIN, Indomethacin
NOVO-METOPROL, Metoprolol
NOVO-MUCILAX, Psyllium
NOVO-NAPROX, Naproxen
NOVO-NIDAZOL, Metronidazole
NOVO-NIFEDIN, Nifedipine
NOVO-PENTOBARB, Pentobarbital

NOVO-PEN-VK, Penicillin V
NOVO-PERIDOL, Haloperidol
NOVO-PIROCAM, Piroxicam
NOVO-PRANOL, Propranolol
NOVO-PRAZIN, Prazosin
NOVO-PRED, Prednisolone
NOVO-PROFEN, Ibuprofen
NOVO-PROPAMIDE, Chlorpropamide
NOVO-PYRAZONE, Sulfinpyrazone
NOVO-SALMOL, Salbutamol (Albuterol in U.S.)
NOVO-SECOBARB, Secobarbital
NOVO-SPIROTON, Spironolactone
NOVO-SUNDAC, Sulindac
NOVO-TETRA, Tetracycline
NOVO-TRIOLAM, Triazolam
NOVO-TRIPRAMINE, Trimipramine
NOVO-VERAMIL, Verapamil
NOZINAN, Methotrimeprazine or Levomepromazine
NU-ALPRAZ, Alprazolam
NU-AMOXI, Amoxicillin
NU-AMPI, Ampicillin
NU-CAPTO, Captopril
NU-CIMET, Cimetidine
NU-CLOXI, Cloxacillin
NU-DICLO, Diclofenac
NU-DILTIAZ, Diltiazem
NU-HYDRAL, Hydralazine
NU-INDO, Indomethacin
NU-LORAZ, Lorazepam
NU-MEDOPA, Methyldopa
NU-NAPROX, Naproxen
NU-NIFED, Nifedipine
NU-PEN-VK, Penicillin V
NU-PINDOL, Pindolol
NU-PIROX, Piroxicam
NU-PRAZO, Prazosin
NU-RANIT, Ranitidine
NU-TETRA, Tetracycline
NU-TRIAZO, Triazolam
NU-VERAP, Verapamil
NYADERM, Nystatin
Nylidrin, ARLIDIN
Nystatin, NADOSTINE, NYADERM
OCUCLEAR, Oxymetazoline
OGEN, Estropipate
ONE-ALPHA, Alfacalcidol
OPHTHO-SULF, Sulfacetamide
OPTICROM, Cromolyn
OPTIMINE, Azatadine
ORADEXON, Dexamethasone
ORBENIN, Cloxacillin
Orciprenaline, see Metaproterenol
ORNADE, Phenylpropanolamine
Orphenadrine, DISIPAL, NORFLEX
ORTHO DIENESTROL, Dienestrol
ORUVAIL, Ketoprofen
OS-CAL-D, Cholecalciferol
OSTOFORTE, Ergocalciferol
OTRIVIN, Xylometazoline
OVOL, Simethicone
Oxprenolol, TRASICOR
Oxtriphylline, CHOLEDYL, CHOPHYLLIN
OXYBUTAZONE, Oxyphenbutazone
Oxycodone, PERCOCET
Oxymetazoline, NAFRINE, OCUCLEAR
Oxymetholone, ANAPOLON 50
Oxyphenbutazone, OXYBUTAZONE, TANDERIL
PALAFER, Ferrous fumarate
PANADOL, Acetaminophen
PANECTYL, Trimeprazine
PARSITAN, Ethopropazine
PARVOLEX, Acetylcysteine
PENBRITIN, Ampicillin
PENGLOBE, Bacampicillin

Penicillin G, BICILLIN, MEGACILLIN
Penicillin V, APO-PEN-VK, NOVO-PEN-VK, NU-PEN-VK, PEN-VEE, PVF
PENTACARINAT, Pentamidine
Pentaerythritol tetranitrate, PERITRATE
Pentamidine, PENTACARINATE, PNEUMOPENT
PENTASA, 5-Aminosalicylic acid
Pentobarbital, NOVO-PENTOBARB, NOVA-RECTAL
Pentoxifylline, TRENTAL
PEN-VEE, Penicillin V
PEPTOL, Cimetidine
PERCOCET, Oxycodone
Pergolide, PERMAX
PERIACTIN, Cyproheptadine
Pericyazine* (antipsychotic), NEULEPTIL
PERITRATE, Pentaerythritol tetranitrate
PERMAX, Pergolide
Perphenazine, PHENAZINE
PHENAZINE, Perphenazine
PHENAZO, Phenazopyridine* (urinary analgesic)
Phenazopyridine* (urinary analgesic), PHENAZO, PYRIDIUM
Phenolphthalein, ALOPHEN, DOXIDAN
Phentermine, FASTIN, IONAMIN
Phentolamine, ROGITINE
Phenylbutazone, NOVO-BUTAZONE
Phenylephrine, AK-DILATE
Phenylpropanolamine, ORNADE, SINE-OFF
PHOSPHOLINE IODIDE, Echothiophate
PHYLLOCONTIN, Aminophylline
Phytomenadione, KONAKION
Pilocarpine, AKARPINE, MIOCARPINE, SPERSACARPINE
Pindolol, VISKEN, NU-PINDOL
PIPORTIL L4, Pipotiazine* (antipsychotic)
Pipotiazine* (antipsychotic), PIPORTIL- L4
Piroxicam, NOVO-PIROCAM, NU-PIROX
Pivampicillin* (antibacterial), PONDOCILLIN
Pizotyline* (antimigraine), SANDOMIGRAN
PLENDIL, Felodipine
PNEUMOPENT, Pentamidine
PODOFILM, Podophyllum resin
Podophyllum resin, PODOFILM
POLARAMINE, Dexchlorpheniramine
Polymyxin B, AEROSPORIN
PONDERAL, Fenfluramine
PONDIMIN, Fenfluramine
PONDOCILLIN, Pivampicillin* (antibacterial)
PONSTAN, Mefenamic acid
Pramoxine, TRONOTHANE
Prazosin, APO-PRAZO, NOVO-PRAZIN, NU-PRAZO
PRED, Prednisolone
Prednisolone, INFLAMASE, NOVO-PRED, PRED
Prednisone, DELTASONE, WINPRED
PREPIDIL, Dinoprostone
PRESSYN, Vasopressin
Prilocaine, CITANEST
PRIMAXIN, Imipenem
Primidone, MYSOLINE, SERTAN
PRINIVIL, Lisinopril
PRIVINE, Naphazoline
Procainamide, PROCAN SR
PROCAN SR, Procainamide
Procarbazine, NATULAN
Prochlorperazine, STEMETIL
PROCYCLID, Procyclidine
Procyclidine, KEMADRIN, PROCYCLID
PROCYTOX, Cyclophosphamide
PRODIEM, Psyllium
Progesterone, GESTEROL
PROLASTIN, Alpha₁ proteinase inhibitor
PROLOPA, Levodopa/benserazide* (antiparkinson)
Promethazine, HISTANTIL
Propantheline, BANLIN
Propranolol, NOVO-PRANOL
PROPYL-THYRACIL, Propylthiouracil
Propylthiouracil, PROPYL-THYRACIL

PROSTIN, Dinoprostone
Protriptyline, TRIPTIL
Pseudoephedrine, ELTOR
Psyllium, FIBREPUR, NOVO-MUCILAX, PRODIEM
PULMICORT, Budesonide* (steroid inhaler)
PULMOPHYLLINE, Theophylline
PURINOL, Allopurinol
PVF, Penicillin V
Pyrantel, COMBANTRIN
Pyrazinamide, TEBRAZID
PYRIBENZAMINE, Tripelennamine
PYRIDIUM, Phenazopyridine* (urinary analgesic)
Pyridostigmine, MESTINON, REGONOL
Pyrvinium pamoate, VANQUIN
Quinidine, BIQUIN
Ranitidine, NU-RANIT
REACTINE, Cetirizine* (antihistamine)
RECTOVALONE, Tixocotrol* (mineralocorticoid)
REGONOL, Pyridostigmine
REVIMINE, Dopamine
RHINALAR, Flunisolide
RHINOCORT, Budesonide* (steroid inhaler)
RHINO-MEX-N, Naphazoline
Rho(D) immune globulin, HYPRHO-D, WINRHO
RHODIALOSE, Lactulose
RHODIS, Ketoprofen
RHOTRAL, Acebutolol
RHOTRIMINE, Trimipramine
Rifampin, ROFACT
RIOPAN, Simethicone
RISPERDAL, Risperidone
Risperdone, RISPERDAL
RIVOTRIL, Clonazepam
ROBAXIN, Methocarbamol
ROBIDEX, Dextromethorphan
ROBIDONE, Hydrocodone
ROFACT, Rifampin
ROGITINE, Phentolamine
RONIACOL, Nicotinyl alcohol tartrate
ROVAMYCINE, Spiramycin* (antibiotic)
RUBION, Cyanocobalamin
RUBRAMIN, Cyanocobalamin
RYNACROM, Cromolyn
RYTHMODAN, Disopyramide
SALAZOPYRIN, Sulfasalazine
Salbutamol (Albuterol in U.S.), APO-SALVENT, NOVO-SALMOL, VENTOLIN
SALOFALK, 5-Aminosalicylic acid
SANDOMIGRAN, Pizotyline* (antimigraine)
SANDOSTATIN, Octreotide
Scopolamine, BUSCOPAN, TRANSDERM-V
Secobarbital, NOVO-SECOBARB
SECTRAL, Acebutolol
SERTAN, Primidone
Silver sulfadiazine, FLAMAZINE
Simethicone, OVOL, RIOPAN
SINE-OFF, Phenylpropanolamine
SLOW-FE, Ferrous sulfate
SOLIUM, Chlordiazepoxide
SOMNOL, Flurazepam
SOMOPHYLLIN, Theophylline
SOPAMYCETIN, Chloramphenicol
SOTACOR, Sotalol
Sotalol, SOTACOR
Spectinomycin* (antibiotic), TROBICIN
SPERSACARPINE, Pilocarpine
SPERSADEX, Dexamethasone
Spiramycin* (antibiotic), ROVAMYCINE
Spironolactone, NOVO-SPIROTON
Stanozolol, WINSTROL
STEMETIL, Prochlorperazine
STIEVAA, Tretinoin
STOXIL, Idoxuridine
Streptozocin, ZANOSAR

SULCRATE, Sucralfate
Sulfacetamide, AK-SULF, OPHTHO-SULF, SULFEX
Sulfasalazine, SALAZOPYRIN
SULFEX, Sulfacetamide
Sulfinpyrazone, ANTURAN, NOVO-PYRAZONE
Sulindac, APO-SULIN, NOVO-SUNDAC
SUPREFACT, Buserelin* (LH-RH analogue)
SUPRES, Chlorothiazide
SURGAM, Tiaprofenic acid* (NSAID)
SUS-PHRINE, Epinephrine
SYNACTHEN DEPOT, Cosyntropin
SYNAREL, Nafarelin
SYNKAVITE, Menadiol
TAMOFEN, Tamoxifen
TAMONE, Tamoxifen
Tamoxifen, APO-TAMOX, NOLVADEX, TAMOFEN, TAMONE
TANDERIL, Oxyphenbutazone
TEBRAZID, Pyrazinamide
Tenoxicam* (NSAID), MOBIFLEX
TENUATE, Diethylpropion
TERAZOL, Terconazole
Terbutaline, BRICANYL
Terconazole, TERAZOL
Testosterone, ANDRIOL, DELATESTRYL
Testosterone/estradiol, NEO-PAUSE
Tetracycline, ACHROMYCIN, APO-TETRA, NOVO-TETRA, NU-TETRA, TETRACYN
TETRACYN, Tetracycline
THEOLAIR, Theophylline
Theophylline, PULMOPHYLLINE, SOMOPHYLLIN, THEOLAIR
Thiethylperazine, TORECAN
Thioguanine, LANVIS
Thioproperazine* (antipsychotic), MAJEPTIL
Tiaprofenic acid* (NSAID), ALBERT TIAFEN, SURGAM
Tioconazole, GYNO-TROSYD, TROSYD
Tixocotrol* (mineralocorticoid), RECTOVALONE
Tobramycin, NEBCIN
Tolbutamide, MOBENOL, NOVO-BUTAMIDE
TORECAN, Thiethylperazine
Tranexamic acid* (hemostatic), CYKLOKAPRON
TRANSDERM-V, Scopolamine
TRASICOR, Oxprenolol
TRAVEL AID, Dimenhydrinate
TRENTAL, Pentoxifylline
Tretinoin, STIEVAA, VITAMIN A ACID
TRIADAPIN, Doxepin
Triamterene, APO-TRIAZIDE
Triazolam, APO-TRIAZO, NOVO-TRIOLAM, NU-TRIAZO
Trihexyphenidyl, APARKANE, APO-TRIHEX
TRIKACIDE, Metronidazole

TRILISATE, Choline magnesium salicylate
Trimeprazine, PANECTYL
Trimipramine, APO-TRIMIP, NOVO-TRIPRAMINE, RHOTRIMINE
Tripelennamine, PYRIBENZAMINE
Tripolidine, ACTIFED
TRIPTIL, Protriptyline
TROBICIN, Spectinomycin* (antibiotic)
TRONOTHANE, Pramoxine
TROPICACYL, Tropicamide
Tropicamide, TROPICACYL
TROSYD, Tioconazole
TUBARINE, Tubocurarine
Tubocurarine, TUBARINE
URISPAS, Flavoxate* (antispasmodic)
URITOL, Furosemide
UROMITEXAN, Mesna
Ursodiol, URSOFALK
URSOFALK, Ursodiol
VANQUIN, Pyrvinium pamoate
VASOCON, Naphazoline
VASODILAN, Isoxsuprine
Vasopressin, PRESSYN
VASOXYL, Methoxamine* (vasopressor)
VELBE, Vinblastine
VENTOLIN, Salbutamol (Albuterol in U.S.)
Verapamil, APO-VERAP, NOVOVERAMIL, NU-VERAP
Vinblastine, VELBE
Vindesine, ELDISINE
VIROSTAT, Edoxudine* (antiviral)
VISKEN, Pindolol
VITAMIN A ACID, Tretinoin
VIVOL, Diazepam
Warfarin, WARFILONE
WARFILONE, Warfarin
WELLFERON, Interferon alfa-n1
WINPRED, Prednisone
WINRHO, Rho(D) immune globulin
WINSTROL, Stanozolol
XYLOCARD, Lidocaine
Xylometazoline, OTRIVIN
YOCON, Yohimbine
Yohimbine, YOCON
ZADITEN, Ketotifen* (anti-allergy)
ZANOSAR, Metolazone
ZESTRIL, Lisinopril
Zidovudine, NOVO-AZT
ZONULYN, Chymotrypsin
Zopiclone* (hypnotic), IMOVANE
ZOSTRIX, Capsaicin
ZYLOPRIM, Allopurinol

DRUGS THAT ARE MENTIONED IN THE TEXT BUT ARE NOT AVAILABLE IN CANADA

Adenosine
Aldesleukin
Altretamine
Amyl nitrate
Anisindione
Azithromycin
Azlocillin
Aztreonam
Benazepril
Benzphetamine
Benzquinamide
Benzthiazide
Bishydroxycoumarin
Bisoprolol
Bitolterol
Bumetanide
Buprenorphine
Capreomycin
Carbinoxamine
Carboprosts tromethamine
Carteolol
Cefmetazole
Cefpodoxime
Cefprozil
Clofazimine
Cycloserine
Cyclothiazide
Demecarium
Dezocine
Dichlorphenamide
Difenoxin plus atropine

Dromostanolone
Enoxacin
Epoetin
Epoprostenol
Ethaverine
Ethionamide
Ethotoin
Etidocaine
Etodolac
Floxuridine
Foscarnet
Gitalin
Glipizide
Glutethimide
Guanabenz
Hexocyclium
Hydroflumethiazide
Interferon alfa-n3
Isoetharine
Isoflurophate
Isradipine
Itraconazole
Kanamycin
Lithium citrate
Lomefloxacin
Loracarbef
Lypressin
Mecamylamine
Melarsoprol
Mepenzolate

Methacycline
Methamphetamine
Methantheline
Methicillin
Methoxyflurane
Methscopolamine
Metipranolol
Mezlocillin
Milrinone
Mivacurium
Molindone
Monooctanoin
Moricizine
Nabumetone
Naftifine
Niclosamide
Osalazine
Oxacillin
Oxandrolone
Oxaprozin
Oxyphenonium
Oxytetracycline
Paramethasone
Paromomycin
Penbutolol
Pentostatin
Phenacemide
Phendimetrazine
Phenindione
Phenmetrazine

Phenoxybenzamine
Phenprocoumon
Physostigmine
Pipecuronium
Polyestradiol
Polythiazide
Praziquantel
Progestin implants
Propylhexedrine
Pyrilamine
Quazepam
Ramipril
Remoxipride
Rimantadine
Sargramostim
Siccimer
Sulfacytine
Sulfamethizole
Suramin
Testolactone
Tetrahydrozoline
Thyroid USP
Tolazamide
Trichlormethiazide
Tridihexethyl
Triflupromazine
Trilostane
Trimethadione
Trimethobenzamide
Zolpidem

Index

Note: **Boldface** page numbers indicate prototypes, other important drugs, and main topics. *Italic* page numbers refer to illustrations. Page numbers followed by t refer to tables. Trade names appear in SMALL CAPITAL LETTERS followed by generic name in parentheses; check for further information under the generic name.

MAJOR DRUG CLASSES AND THEIR PROTOTYPES

ENDOCRINE DRUGS (continued)

Drugs That Affect Uterine Motility
  Uterine Stimulants
    Oxytocin
    Ergonovine
  Uterine Relaxants
    Ritodrine

DRUGS FOR INFLAMMATION AND ALLERGIES

Antihistamines (H₁ Antagonists)
  Traditional H₁ Antagonists
    Diphenhydramine
  Nonsedative H₁ Antagonists
    Terfenadine
Aspirin-Like Drugs
  Nonsteroidal Anti-inflammatory Drugs
    Aspirin
    Ibuprofen
  Drugs That Lack Anti-inflammatory Actions
    Acetaminophen
Glucocorticoids
    Hydrocortisone
Drugs for Rheumatoid Arthritis
  Nonsteroidal Anti-inflammatory Drugs
    Aspirin (a salicylate)
    Naproxen (a nonsalicylate)
  Disease-Modifying Antirheumatic Drugs
    Hydroxychloroquine
    Gold salts
  Glucocorticoids
    Prednisone

RESPIRATORY TRACT DRUGS

Drugs for Asthma
  Beta₂-Adrenergic Agonists
    Terbutaline
  Methylxanthines
    Theophylline
  Glucocorticoids
    Beclomethasone (inhaled)
    Prednisone (oral)
  Muscarinic Antagonist
    Ipratropium
  Other
    Cromolyn sodium

GASTROINTESTINAL DRUGS

Drugs for Peptic Ulcer Disease
  H₂ Antagonists
    Cimetidine
  Proton Pump Inhibitors
    Omeprazole

  Muscarinic Antagonists
    Pirenzepine
  Mucosal Protectants
    Sucralfate
  Antacids
    Aluminum hydroxide/magnesium hydroxide
  Drug for NSAID-Induced Ulcers
    Misoprostol
  Antibiotics (for Helicobacter pylori)
    Triple therapy: metronidazole plus
      tetracycline plus amoxicillin
Laxatives
  Bulk-Forming Agents
    Methylcellulose
  Surfactants
    Docusate sodium
  Contact Laxatives
    Bisacodyl
  Saline Laxatives
    Magnesium hydroxide
Antiemetics
  Antidopaminergics
    Prochlorperazine
    Metoclopramide
  Cannabinoids
    Dronabinol
  Antiserotonergics
    Ondansetron
  Glucocorticoids
    Dexamethasone
  Benzodiazepines
    Diazepam

DRUGS FOR INFECTIOUS DISEASES

Penicillins, Cephalosporins, and Other Drugs
That Weaken the Bacterial Cell Wall
  Penicillins
    Penicillin G
  Cephalosporins
    Cephalothin
  Others
    Imipenem
    Vancomycin
Bacteriostatic Inhibitors of Protein Synthesis
  Tetracyclines
    Tetracycline
  Macrolides
    Erythromycin
  Others
    Clindamycin
Aminoglycosides (Bactericidal Inhibitors of
Protein Synthesis)
    Gentamicin
Fluoroquinolones
    Ciprofloxacin